GOUT AND OTHER CRYSTAL ARTHROPATHIES

GOUT AND OTHER CRYSTAL ARTHROPATHIES

Robert Terkeltaub, MD
Chief, Rheumatology Section
San Diego Veterans Affairs Medical Center;
Professor of Medicine, Interim Chief
Division of Rheumatology, Allergy and Immunology
University of California San Diego School of Medicine
La Jolla, California, USA

ELSEVIER
SAUNDERS

ELSEVIER
SAUNDERS

1600 John F. Kennedy Blvd.
Ste 1800
Philadelphia, PA 19103-2899

GOUT AND OTHER CRYSTAL ARTHROPATHIES, First edition ISBN: 978-1-4377-2864-4
Copyright © 2012 by Saunders, an imprint of Elsevier Inc.

Notice

Knowledge and best practice in this field are constantly changing. As new research and experience broaden our knowledge, changes in practice, treatment and drug therapy may become necessary or appropriate. Readers are advised to check the most current information provided (i) on procedures featured or (ii) by the manufacturer of each product to be administered, to verify the recommended dose or formula, the method and duration of administration, and contraindications. It is the responsibility of the practitioner, relying on their own experience and knowledge of the patient, to make diagnoses, to determine dosages and the best treatment for each individual patient, and to take all appropriate safety precautions. To the fullest extent of the law, neither the Publisher nor the Editors assumes any liability for any injury and/or damage to persons or property arising out of or related to any use of the material contained in this book.

The Publisher

Library of Congress Cataloging-in-Publication Data

Gout and other crystal arthropathies / [edited by] Robert Terkeltaub.
  p. ; cm.
 Includes bibliographical references and index.
 ISBN 978-1-4377-2864-4 (hardcover : alk. paper)
 1. Gout. 2. Chondrocalcinosis. I. Terkeltaub, Robert.
 [DNLM: 1. Gout. 2. Calcium Compounds--metabolism. 3.
Chondrocalcinosis. 4. Hyperuricemia. WE 350]
 RC629.G683 2012
 616.3′999--dc23

2011032013

Acquisitions Editor: Pamela Hetherington
Developmental Editor: Roxanne Halpine Ward
Publishing Services Manager: Peggy Fagen
Project Manager: Siva Raman Krishnamoorthy
Design Direction: Steven Stave

Printed in the United States of America

Last digit is the print number: 9 8 7 6 5 4 3 2 1

I dedicate this book to my patients, mentors, colleagues in the field, and students and research trainees, who have inspired me and taught me so much about these disorders. I also dedicate the work to my wife Barbara, whose support was integral to the success of this endeavor.

Acknowledgments

I am grateful to acknowledge Robyn Austin and Wendy Geolina, who provided administrative support and editing assistance, as well as Pamela Hetherington for her strong vision and support, Roxanne Ward for manuscript preparation, and Peggy Fagen and the production staff at Elsevier for their hard work in bringing this book to print.

Contributors

Naohiko Anzai, MD, PhD
Professor and Chairman
Department of Pharmacology and Toxicology
Dokkyo Medical University School of Medicine
Tochigi, Japan

Joana Atxotegi Saenz de Buruaga, MD
Assistant Physician
Rheumatology Division
Hospital de Cruces
Vizcaya, Spain

Hyon K. Choi, MD, DrPH
Professor of Medicine
Section of Rheumatology and the Clinical
Epidemiology Unit
Boston University school of Medicine
Boston, Massachusetts, USA

Nicola Dalbeth, MBChB, MD, FRACP
Associate Professor and Rheumatologist
Department of Medicine, Faculty of Medical and
Health Sciences
University of Auckland
Auckland, New Zealand

Hitoshi Endou, MD, PhD
Professor Emeritus
Department of Pharmacology and Toxicology
Kyorin University School of Medicine
Tokyo, Japan

Angelo L. Gaffo, MD, MSPH
Assistant Professor of Medicine
Division of Rheumatology
University of Alabama at Birmingham
Staff Rheumatologist
Birmingham VA Medical Center
Birmingham, Alabama, USA

Amilcare Gentili, MD
Professor of Clinical Radiology
Department of Radiology
University of California San Diego
Chief, Radiology Service
San Diego VA Health Care System
San Diego, California, USA

**Rebecca Grainger, BMedSci, PhD,
MBChB, FRACP**
Senior Lecturer
Department of Medicine
University of Otago Wellington
Consultant Rheumatologist
Wellington Regional Rheumatology Unit
Hutt Valley District Health Board
Wellington, New Zeland

Pierre-André Guerne, MD
Professor of Internal Medicine
and Rheumatology
Associate Medical Officer
Division of Rheumatology
University Hospitals of Geneva
Geneva, Switzerland

Ana Maria Herrero-Beites, MD
Senior Assistant
Rehabilitation Division
Hospital de Górliz
Vizcaya, Spain

Tudor H. Hughes, MD, FRCR
Professor of Clinical Radiology
Radiology Resident Program Director
Vice Chair of Education
Department of Radiology
University of California at San Diego
San Diego, California, USA

Dinesh Khanna, MD, MSc
Associate Professor of Medicine
Marvin and Betty Danto Research Professor
Director
University of Michigan Scleroderma Program
Division of Rheumatology
Department of Internal Medicine
University of Michigan School of Medicine
Ann Arbor, Michigan, USA

Puja Khanna, MD, MPH
Assistant Professor
Division of Rheumatology
Department of Internal Medicine
University of Michigan School of Medicine
Ann Arbor, Michigan, USA

Eswar Krishnan, MD, MPhil
Assistant Professor of Medicine
Stanford University
Stanford, California, USA

Diego F. Lemos, MD
Assistant Professor of Radiology
Section Head Musculoskeletal Imaging
Department of Radiology
Fletcher Allen Health Care and the University of
Vermont
Burlington, Vermont, USA

Frédéric Lioté, MD, PhD
Professor of Rheumatology
Paris Diderot University
President, Sorbonne Paris Cité
Deputy Head
Centre Viggo Petersen, Service de Rhumatologie
(Pôle Appareil Locomoteur)
Hôpital Lariboisière (Assistance Publique-
Hôpitaux de Paris)
Paris, France

Ru Liu-Bryan, PhD
Associate Professor of Medicine
University of California San Diego
San Diego, California, USA

**Paul MacMullan, BComm, BSc
(Physio), MBChB, BAO**
Research Fellow
Department of Molecular and Cellular
Therapeutics
Royal College of Surgeons in Ireland
Rheumatology Department
Mater Misericordiae University Hospital
Dublin, Ireland

Elisabeth Matson, DO
Rheumatology Fellow
Division of Rheumatology
The Warren Alpert Medical School at Brown
University
Providence, Rhode Island, USA

Geraldine M. McCarthy, MD
Consultant Rheumatologist
Department of Medicine
Mater Misericordiae University Hospital
Clinical Professor of Medicine
UCD School of Medicine
and Medical Science
University of College Dublin
Honorary Associate Professor
Molecular and Cellular Therapeutics
Royal College of Surgeons in Ireland
Dublin, Ireland

Gillian McMahon, BSc, PhD, MRSC, CChem, FICI
Analytical Chemistry Lecturer
School of Chemical Sciences
Dublin City University
Dublin, Ireland

Tuhina Neogi, MD, PhD, FRCPC
Associate Professor of Medicine
Sections of Clinical Epidemiology Research
and Training Unit and Rheumatology
Department of Medicine
Boston University School of Medicine
Associate Professor of Epidemiology
Department of Epidemiology
Boston University School of Public Health
Boston, Massachusetts, USA

George Nuki, MB, FRCP
Emeritus Professor of Rheumatology
Rheumatic Diseases Unit
Western General Hospital
Emeritus Professor of Rheumatology
Osteoarticular Research Group
Institute of Genetics and Molecular Medicine
University of Edinburgh
Edinburgh, Scotland, UK

Eliseo Pascual, MD, PhD
Professor of Medicine
Universidad Miguel Hernández
Head, Rheumatology Section
Hospital General Universitario de Alicante
Alicante, Spain

Fernando Perez-Ruiz, MD, PhD
Specialist Faculty
Rheumatology Division
Hospital de Cruces
Vizcaya, Spain

Kenneth P.H. Pritzker, MD, FRCPC
Professor, Laboratory Medicine
and Pathobiology; Surgery
University of Toronto
Pathologist
Mount Sinai Hospital
Toronto, Ontario, Canada

Juan Garcia Puig, MD, PhD
Associate Professor
Division of Internal Medicine
Metabolic and Vascular Unit
Hospital Universitario La Paz, IdiPAZ
Universidad Autónoma
Madrid, Spain

Supriya G. Reddy, MPH
Program Administrator
Clinical Immunology and Rheumatology
University of Alabama
at Birmingham
Birmingham, Alabama, USA
Doctoral Student (PhD candidate)
Department of Health Science
The University of Alabama
Tuscaloosa, Alabama, USA

Anthony M. Reginato, PhD, MD
Director, Rheumatology Research
and Musculoskeletal Ultrasound
Division of Rheumatology
University of Medicine Foundation
Rhode Island Hospital
The Warren Alpert School of Medicine
at Brown University
Staff Physician
Medical Service/Rheumatology
Providence VA Medical Center
Providence, Rhode Island, USA

Philip L. Riches, BSc, MRCP
Consultant Rheumatologist
Rheumatic Diseases Unit
Western General Hospital
Honorary Senior Lecturer
Institute of Genetics and Molecular Medicine
University of Edinburgh
Edinburgh, Scotland, UK

Naomi Schlesinger, MD
Professor of Medicine
Chief, Division of Rheumatology
Department of Medicine
Robert Wood Johnson Medical School
University of Medicine and Dentistry
of New Jersey
New Brunswick, New Jersey, USA

Jasvinder A. Singh, MBBS, MPH
Staff Physician
Medicine Service and Center for Surgical
Medical Acute Care Research
and Transitions
Birmingham VA Medical Center;
Associate Professor of Medicine
and Epidemiology
Department of Medicine
Division of Rheumatology
University of Alabama at Birmingham
Birmingham, Alabama, USA
Research Collaborator
Department of Orthopedic Surgery
Mayo Clinic Collage of Medicine
Rochester, Minnesota, USA

Francisca Sivera, MD
Consultant in Rheumatology
Rheumatology Unit
Hospital del Vinalopó
Clinical Assistant Professor
Department of Internal Medicine
(Rheumatology)
Universidad Miguel Hernandez
Alicante, Spain

Lisa K. Stamp, MBChB, FRACP, PhD
Associate Professor
Department of Medicine
University of Otago Christchurch
Rheumatologist
Department of Rheumatology, Immunology
and Allergy
Christchurch Hospital
Christchurch, New Zealand

William J. Taylor, PhD, MBChB, FRACP, FAFRM
Associate Professor and Head of Unit
Rehabilitation Teaching and Research Unit
Department of Medicine
University of Otago Wellington
Rheumatologist and Rehabilitation Physician
Wellington Regional Rheumatology Unit
Hutt Valley District Health Board
Wellington, New Zealand

Robert Terkeltaub, MD
Chief, Rheumatology Section
San Diego Veterans Affairs Medical Center
Professor of Medicine, Interim Chief
Division of Rheumatology, Allergy,
and Immunology
University of California San Diego School
of Medicine
La Jolla, California, USA

Ralf G. Thiele, MD, FACR
Assistant Professor of Medicine
Department of Medicine
Allergy/Immunology & Rheumatology Division
University of Rochester School of Medicine
and Dentistry
Rochester, New York, USA

Rosa J. Torres, MD, PhD
Biomedical Researcher
Biochemistry Laboratory, Metabolic Vascular
Unit, Idipaz
La Paz University Hospital
Madrid, Spain

Foreword

Gouty arthritis was among the earliest of diseases to be recognized as a clinical entity; there is a description of gout in ancient Egypt in the second millennium BC attributable to Imhotep (the "Father of Medicine"). However, the role of crystals of monosodium urate (MSU) in the pathogenesis of gout and recognition of other crystal-associated deposition arthropathies emerged much later. Drawings of crystals taken from a tophus from a patient with gout were made by the pioneer Dutch microscopist Antoni Van Leeuwenhoek in 1769, although he was unaware that they were crystals and ignorant of their chemical composition. A century later, the English chemist Wollaston was able to show that a gouty tophus from his own ear was composed of sodium urate, following chemical identification of uric acid in urinary calculi by the Swedish apothecary Scheele in 1776. Elevated levels of uric acid in the serum of patients with gout were first demonstrated by Sir Alfred Baring Garrod in 1848 using a semiquantitative "thread test"—an early milestone in the development of the discipline of clinical chemistry.

In a set of remarkably prescient propositions published in 1859 in his book *A Treatise on Gout and Rheumatic Gout*, A. B. Garrod was the first to show a clear understanding of the importance of hyperuricemia and the pivotal role of urate crystals in the pathogenesis of gout. At the turn of the nineteenth century, Freudweiler demonstrated that intra-articular injections of crystals of sodium urate could mimic acute attacks of gout and showed that subcutaneous injections of microcrystals were followed by the development of tophus-like lesions. The historical importance of these experiments only came to light, however, in the early 1960s after rediscovery of the capacity of microcrystals of sodium urate to induce inflammation in joints, skin, and subcutaneous tissues by Faires and McCarty and by Seegmiller and his colleagues. These experiments followed publication of McCarty and Hollander's seminal paper demonstrating the diagnostic value of detecting negatively birefringent crystals of MSU, by polarizing light microscopy, within synovial fluid leukocytes during acute attacks of gouty arthritis, and a series of landmark publications demonstrating the presence of positively birefringent microcrystals, which were confirmed by x-ray diffraction to be calcium pyrophosphate dihydrate (CPPD) in patients with acute synovitis and "pseudogout."

Although experiments demonstrating that acute synovitis could also be induced by injections of microcrystals of CPPD into normal canine and human joints appeared to confirm a pathogenic role for CPPD crystals in patients with pseudogout, the extent to which deposition of CPPD crystals are the cause, or the consequence, of other pathology in the wide range of clinical settings subsequently described and classified by McCarty as manifestations of CPPD deposition disease remains much less certain. Cadaver studies undertaken more than 80 years ago had shown that meniscus calcification in the knee was a frequent age-related finding, and recent community-based epidemiologic studies have demonstrated an age-related radiographic prevalence of chondrocalcinosis of approximately 10% in persons in the seventh decade of life. CPPD deposition in the form of chondrocalcinosis is positively associated with osteoarthritis (OA) but is also seen in the absence of OA and variably influences progression of articular cartilage loss in patients with knee OA. Basic calcium phosphate (BCP) crystals are also frequently associated with OA as well as with age-related calcific periarthritis and a destructive form of age-related, apatite-associated arthritis.

Fifty years ago, gout became a paradigm for understanding, treating, and preventing a chronic rheumatic disease after the development of allopurinol as an effective uricostatic drug. A decade later, Seegmiller's discovery that primary purine overproduction and severe premature gout in boys with Lesch-Nyhan syndrome resulted from an inherited deficiency of the purine salvage enzyme hypoxanthine guanine phosphoribosyltransferase led to an explosion of knowledge and scientific literature about the regulation of purine metabolism that was characterized as the "purine revolution." Much of this was included in a comprehensive monograph, *Gout and Hyperuricemia*, by Wyngaarden and Kelley published in 1976, and evolving knowledge of calcium crystal deposition and disease, which was slower to develop, was included in a shorter monograph, *Crystals and Joint Disease,* by Dieppe and Calvert published in 1986.

Following the introduction and use of allopurinol 40 years ago, a widespread perception developed that gout was no longer a clinical problem. For many years, gout has been largely managed in general practice and has ceased to be at the forefront of interest for rheumatologists and clinical investigators. Recent studies have, however, shown that this potentially curable condition is being inadequately treated and that the incidence and prevalence of gout have doubled over the past 30 years. Gout is now the most common inflammatory joint disease in men and an increasingly frequent cause of inflammatory joint disease in postmenopausal women. The changing epidemiology of gout is largely attributable to rising levels of serum urate, associated with the changing age structure of the population, as well as with the worldwide epidemic of obesity and a dramatic increase in the prevalence of the metabolic syndrome. Additional risk factors include the use of diuretics, consumption of alcoholic beverages (especially beer), diets containing increased quantities of red meat or shellfish purines, and heavy consumption of fructose-sweetened soft drinks. Complicated gout associated with comorbidities such as hypertension and cardiovascular and renal disease is also an increasing problem. Overt tophi are now seen in 30% of untreated patients within 5 years of the first acute attack. Developments in imaging with ultrasound, computed tomography, and magnetic resonance imaging are also revealing more widespread evidence of crystal deposition in patients with gout much earlier in the course of the disease.

Other developments have recently stimulated renewed interest in gout and crystal deposition diseases. In the past few years, there have been important new insights into the genes responsible for urate transport in the kidney and into the mechanisms involved in the induction of inflammation by microcrystals. The latter have included new data on the generation of cytokines following activation of complement and intracellular signaling molecules, such as the MAP kinases and NF-κB, and the role of innate immunity, via induction of interleukin-1β following activation of the NLRP3 inflammasome by urate crystals, with or without the need for additional innate immune signals such as free fatty acids. This has led to studies and therapeutic trials of interleukin-1 blockade with the interleukin-1 receptor antagonist anakinra, the interleukin-1 soluble receptor antagonist fusion protein rilonacept, and an anti-interleukin-1β antibody canakinumab.

The development of new urate-lowering drugs for the first time in 40 years has also stimulated a great deal of clinical interest and new clinical research. The nonpurine xanthine oxidase inhibitor febuxostat is now being widely used, and the pegylated uricase, pegloticase, has recently received US Food and Drug Administration approval for the treatment of patients with severe and previously treatment-resistant gout.

Novel uricosurics are on the horizon, and oral combination therapy with xanthine oxidase inhibition and uricosuric agents has been "re-discovered" after being largely abandoned since the late 1970s as a therapeutic strategy for tophaceous gout.

Progress in research in the calcium crystal arthropathies has been less dramatic. However, recent genetic and physico-chemical studies suggest that we have a better understanding of how extracellular inorganic pyrophosphate (PPi) is generated and degraded and the mechanisms whereby it promotes CPPD deposition and inhibits the formation of apatite crystals. Hopefully, this will lead to new therapeutic approaches for controlling CPPD and BCP crystal deposition.

This book covers all these advances and presents a timely and authoritative set of updates and reviews of many aspects of gout and other crystal deposition diseases. It is written by an international panel of authors, each of whom is an expert in his or her area. It will be a useful source of information for all physicians who have to deal with these common conditions, as well as for investigators in this field.

George Nuki
Edinburgh, UK
January 2011

Contents

Introduction and Overview

"….Gout will seize you and plague you both…"

Benjamin Franklin

Gout and other crystal deposition arthropathies, the subject of this book, are significant medical disorders and health problems that plague the population and have seized the imagination of biomedical researchers. Crystal deposition is produced by supersaturation of different solutes in tissue extracellular fluids. A substantial variety of crystals (or stones, alternatively termed "calculi") can be formed, and at different locations, such as pathologic deposition of crystalline salts in the biliary tract and urinary tract. Pathologic calcification with hydroxyapatite in the extracellular matrix in arteries in atherosclerosis, diabetes mellitus, chronic kidney disease, and aging, and calcification at sites of tissue degeneration of necrosis is a very common form of crystal deposition.

Gout is the oldest recognized example of a systemic crystal-deposition disorder that causes arthritis, and gout is the major intensively covered topic in this book. In gout, serum (and tissue) concentrations of the monosodium salt of uric acid increases beyond its solubility threshold (which has been defined as greater than 6.8-7.0 mg/dL (~408-420 micromolar) in vitro), termed "hyperuricemia." This situation consequently promotes deposition of monosodium urate (MSU) monohydrate crystals that aggregate into tophi. The connective tissues of the joint are primary sites of urate crystal deposition, and gout is principally a rheumatic disease. However, gout also affects the kidney via interstitial urate crystal deposition or tubular formation of uric acid urolithiasis and promotion of oxalate urolithiasis. Furthermore, there is a large and growing body of evidence, reviewed here, that renal and vascular effects of soluble urate in hyperuricemic individuals promote hypertension, renal dysfunction, and cardiovascular disease complications that are linked to elevated risk of mortality.

Gout has been recognized since antiquity and had previously been affectionately stereotyped as the "disease of kings, and king of diseases." Progress in gout had been hampered by the outdated caricature of the average patient as a wealthy, powerful middle-aged man and the mistaken impression that gout was simply a self-limiting problem and relatively easy to control via temperance in diet, alcohol, and other pleasures of life. However, the last three decades have seen gout markedly increased in not only prevalence but also clinical complexity in the USA and other countries.

A new epidemiology and clinical landscape in gout is being carved by a perfect storm of dietary megatrends, increased longevity, increasingly prevalent co-morbidities (such as hypertension, obesity, metabolic syndrome, and chronic kidney disease), and iatrogenic factors including prescription diuretic use. Also, as reviewed in this book, the gout algorithm is being redefined by evolving diagnostic criteria and imaging tools, such as high-resolution articular ultrasound and dual energy computed tomography (DECT). Treatment-refractory gouty arthritis and hyperuricemia are now large challenges. Fortunately, this situation is prompting tremendous advances in understanding of therapeutic outcomes benchmarks and quality measures in gout that are reviewed here. Furthermore, new treatments have been approved (febuxostat, pegloticase) and are emerging (eg, IL-1 antagonism, novel uricosurics) and available for difficult gouty arthritis and hyperuricemia.

Recent advances in diagnosis and treatment of gout and hyperuricemia make it an exciting era to see gout in the clinic. The same is becoming the case for the other crystal deposition arthropathies reviewed here (calcium pyrophosphate dihydrate [CPPD], basic calcium phosphate, and oxalate crystal deposition disease). In particular, new understanding of the molecular genetics and pathogenesis of CPPD crystal deposition disease has the potential to lead to targeted new therapies to suppress crystal deposition. Some of the anti-inflammatory therapies being developed for gout may well be useful in other crystal deposition arthropathies, with IL-1 antagonism a prime example. Furthermore, high resolution ultrasound has emerged as a highly useful tool for rapid diagnosis of CPPD deposition disease, with DECT useful for specific diagnosis of pathologic calcification.

I, and the distinguished international group of clinicians and scholars that have written this book, welcome you to enjoy the cohesive reviews herein of critical areas in the field of crystal deposition arthropathies. The reviews encompass genetic, epidemiologic, pathologic, mechanistic, clinical, diagnostic, therapeutic, and outcomes issues in these diseases. Some of the "hot" research areas addressed include molecular and genetic epidemiologic aspects of renal urate anion transporters (Chapters 4 and 7, respectively), innate immunity in crystal-induced arthritis pathogenesis and the role of the NLRP3 inflammasome and IL-1b axis (Chapter 5), and ANKH and PP_i metabolism in CPPD crystal deposition disease (Chapter 20).

Practical subjects covered include synovial fluid crystal analysis (Chapter 2), diagnostic criteria for gout (Chapter 8), and plain radiography and CT and MRI as diagnostic imaging tools (Chapters 24 and 25). High resolution ultrasound is given individual attention in Chapter 26. Different pharmacologic and diet and lifestyle approaches to gouty arthritis and hyperuricmia treatment are covered in Chapters 10 to 15, with a comprehensive overview of gout therapy provided in Chapter 16, and crystal arthropathies in advanced renal disease reviewed in Chapter 23. Quality of life and quality of care issues are reviewed (Chapters 17 and 18, respectively). The highly topical subject of linkages between hyperuricemia and renal, vascular, and metabolic disorders is discussed in Chapter 18. The complex relationship between basic calcium phosphate (BCP) crystal deposition and osteoarthritis is reviewed in Chapter 22. The book concludes with a forward-looking, integrative and translational view of the discussions presented.

Taken together, this textbook endeavors to convey the excitement and promise of the work in a dynamic field of medicine. We hope this book serves and inspires in your pursuits of better diagnosis, research, understanding, and treatment of these fascinating disorders.

Robert Terkeltaub

GOUT AND OTHER CRYSTAL ARTHROPATHIES

Section I

Basic Concepts

Articular Pathology of Gout, Calcium Pyrophosphate Dihydrate and Basic Calcium Phosphate Crystal Deposition Arthropathies

Kenneth P.H. Pritzker

KEY POINTS

- Each crystal type associated with arthritis forms in specific joint tissues dependent on the distinct metabolic environment.
- Crystals require additional factors beyond tissue deposition to incite inflammation.
- Crystals within cartilage can lead to degenerative changes resulting from both metabolic and physical effects.
- Monosodium urate monohydrate (MSU) crystals have the potential to precipitate in loose connective tissues of joints and bursae.
- Calcium pyrophosphate dihydrate crystal deposition is restricted to hyaline cartilage, fibrocartilage, and fibrous tissue environments. Acute arthritis is believed to be triggered by crystal shedding from cartilage into the joint space.
- Basic calcium phosphate crystals within synovial fluid may be derived from bone and calcified cartilage fragments exposed to the articular surface, or from periarticular or bursal basic calcium phosphate deposition.

General Pathology of Crystal-Associated Joint Disease

It is fascinating to consider that almost all the advances recorded in this chapter stem from the pioneering studies half a century ago of Zitnan and colleagues[1-3] on chondrocalcinosis and of McCarty and colleagues[4-8] on the detection and separation of calcium pyrophosphate dihydrate (CPPD) crystals from monosodium urate (MSU) crystals in synovial fluid (SF).

Common to the pathogenesis of crystal-associated arthropathy is a local tissue metabolic environment that is supersaturated with ions of at least one of the crystal components[9] and an event or series of events that facilitates crystal precipitation from a supersaturated state[10] (Fig. 1-1). Regardless of systemic metabolic abnormalities or systemic ion saturation, the supersaturated metabolic environment must be local to the tissues in which the crystals deposit: elevated tissue urate concentration (urate) in gout, elevated tissue inorganic pyrophosphate ion concentration (PP_i) associated with CPPD crystal deposition, and increased inorganic phosphate ion concentration (P_i) associated with basic calcium phosphate (BCP) crystal formation.

Under normal conditions, ions can remain in a supersaturated state until an environmental event occurs that renders the ions less soluble and promotes crystal nucleation. This event may be the increased kinetic energy of sudden mechanical force or increased free ion concentration associated with tissue dehydration, pH change, decreased temperature, enzymatic activity, concentration change in secondary ions, or absorption of ions on solid particles. This results in initial formation of molecular clusters (nuclei).[10] From molecular clusters, depending on relative molecular solubilities between larger particles and smaller ones, as well as molecular diffusion rate, crystals rapidly grow to sizes specific to each crystal phase (Ostwald ripening factor).[11] Under some conditions, new crystals grow on preexisting crystals (epitaxial growth). Crystals elongate on the face with the highest energy. Adhesion of proteins and other substances has crystal face specificity that can be disrupted by local ionic conditions.[12,13] With crystal formation, there is local tissue depletion of the contributing ions as they are incorporated into the crystals. In gout, this shift in equilibrium brings in more urate from systemic interstitial fluid, stabilizing and amplifying the crystal deposition; in CPPD deposition disease, the local cartilage or tendon tissue matrix may remain depleted of PP_i.

The biologic reactions that follow depend not only on crystal size and charge but also on the tissue environment in which crystals are deposited. In synovial or bursal spaces including the synovial spaces associated with tendons, acute inflammation can occur. In cartilage or fibrous tissue environments such as tendon insertions or intervertebral disc, slower, more chronic reactions to the crystals and/or the crystal-associated inflammation lead to impaired functionality of the tissue (degeneration) (see Fig. 1-1).

Crystal formation does not necessarily lead to immediate tissue reaction. When crystals form in connective tissues, the crystal surfaces rapidly become covered with matrix material, usually hyaluronate proteoglycan, present in the tissue space.[14,15] Proteoglycan has at least two functions related to crystal reactions. First, intact proteoglycan increases hydration in the local environment via coordination of water with its negative charge groups; second, proteoglycan provides a barrier to cells by physical gelation. To incite inflammation in synovial spaces, it has been suggested that crystals must first become coated (opsonized) with proteins that promote cell adhesion or inflammatory response,[16] such as IgG, or that urate crystals must shed surface proteins that inhibit cell interaction such as low-density lipoprotein apolipoprotein B (see Chapter 5). This occurs when there is increased vascular permeability to proteins adjacent to the space where crystals precipitate. This may be related to low-grade inflammation from other causes or from rapid crystal precipitation, which by itself may induce increased vascular permeability, perhaps via pH change. However, if crystals form slowly or if the SF is particularly viscous, the crystals could become coated with sufficient proteoglycan to act as a barrier to both acute reactant proteins and inflammatory cells.

CRYSTAL-ASSOCIATED ARTHRITIS

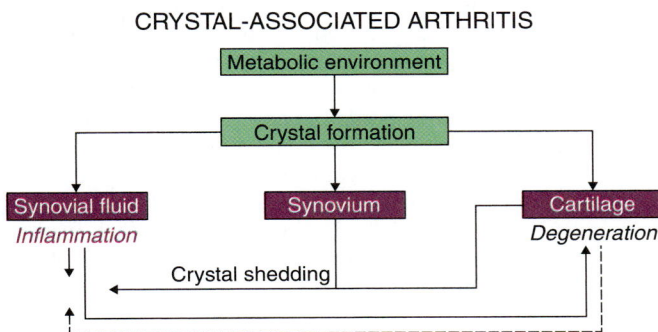

Figure 1-1 The metabolic environment favorable for crystal formation in joints is specific to the crystal type. Monosodium urate crystals form initially in synovial fluid; calcium pyrophosphate dihydrate (CPPD) crystals form in hyaline cartilage, fibrocartilage, and synovium with chondroid metaplasia. Basic calcium phosphate (BCP) crystals form in cartilage. CPPD crystals are shed from cartilage into synovial fluid. BCP crystals can be shed from exposed bone, calcified cartilage, or periarticular soft tissue.

Therefore, without inducing acute inflammation, crystals can be present in the synovial space, in gout, even producing a thick layer on the cartilage surface (Fig. 1-2),[14] which is also detectable by high-resolution ultrasound in gout. Similarly, quiescence of crystal-induced inflammation (see Chapter 5) may well involve large proteoglycans that separate crystals from cells.

Although the amount of inflammation varies with crystal type, crystal aggregation,[17] the volume and rapidity of crystal precipitation or shedding, and innate immune inflammatory mechanisms are common to both urate and CPPD crystals, with BCP crystals having multiple distinctions, resulting in a less inflammatory picture in the joint space (see Chapters 6, 21, and 23). The acute inflammatory mechanisms in crystal-associated arthritis have been documented extensively using morphologic, biochemical, cell biology, and molecular biologic techniques.[18-35] This is of great interest for understanding inflammation biology and its control by drugs. In fact, as pathologic agents to study inflammation mechanisms, crystals are ideal because their composition and surfaces are known in precise atomic detail. Further, for CPPD in particular[36] but also for other pathologic crystals, the crystal size, shape, and surface can be modified experimentally to help understand the effect of each parameter of the inflammatory stimulus.

Briefly, under the appropriate conditions described earlier, crystals precipitate or, in the crystal "autoinjection" model, free non-aggregated crystals are shed into loci in the joint where synovial lining cells and resident phagocytes are able to interact with the crystals, With changes in vascular permeability, the crystal surfaces become coated with blood-derived proteins.[22,37-39] As reviewed in Chapter 5, for gout, products of resident cells, such as mast cells, synovial lining cells, macrophages, and complement activation are major factors in attracting blood monocytes and neutrophils with phagocytosis capability to the joint. The phagocytes bind to the crystal surface and, recognizing the crystal as a foreign substance, phagocytose or, with larger crystals such as urate or CPPD, attempt to phagocytose the crystals. Amplification of inflammation ensues, with monocyte and neutrophil recruitment, phagocyte activation,[22,40] with elaboration of increased lysosomes within the cell, focal cell membranolysis facilitated by crystal physical properties,[41] incorporation of the crystal within the phagosome, merging of the lysososome with the phagosome,[42] as well as, in macrophage lineage cells, activation of the NLRP3 inflammasome.[43-46]

From a pathology perspective, because the crystals are relatively insoluble, this process is often not successful, resulting

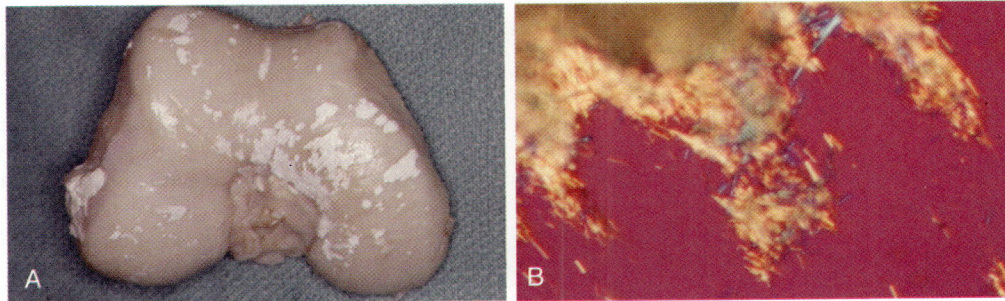

Figure 1-2 Femoral condyle from intercritical gout. **A,** Monosodium urate (MSU) crystals form a white paste on the cartilage surface. Note absence of cartilage fibrillation or erosion. These changes occur at a later stage when the crystals cover the surface entirely. **B,** MSU crystals from the cartilage surface are arranged in parallel sheaves similar to MSU deposits in tophi. Note the absence of inflammatory cells. Compensated polarized light microscopy, original magnification ×100. (*A* from Pritzker KPH. Patogenesis de la Gota y la pseudogota. In Seminarios de Reumatologia. Fundación Instituto de Reumatología e Inmunología. Bogotá, Colombia: Ediciones Lerner; 1980:83-93.)

in increased cell membrane permeability, with consequent cell death and fragmentation. The released lysosomal enzymes bind to extracellular crystals and, along with hydrogen peroxide, facilitate crystal dissolution.[13,47] The cell debris and released intracellular enzymes act to attract more phagocytes and increase vascular congestion and permeability, further resulting in acute inflammation characterized clinically by the familiar characteristics of joint pain, swelling, redness, warmth, and loss of function. After the neutrophils and monocytes are recruited into the space containing the crystals and monocytes differentiate to mature macrophages, over time, usually a few days, the extracellular enzymes and reactive oxygen species break down the inflammatory proteins[48]; the crystals are cleared by phagocytosis followed by crystal dissolution within the cell phagolysosomes, by crystal dissolution in the extracellullar space facilitated by increased solute (synovial effusion), pH change, and, for CPPD at least, extracellular enzymes.[13] Under appropriate conditions, crystals become sequestered from the inflammatory cells by hyaluronate and proteoglycans,[49] newly secreted from synovial cells.

In the usual circumstance, crystal-associated inflammation resolves completely with substantial clearance of crystals from the joint space (although not typically complete in patients with gout as a prime example), and without residual chronic, clinical inflammation or synovial effusion. Eliseo Pascual and colleagues have observed that SF leukocyte counts can remain mildly elevated relative to normal joints in patients with gout.[15] Nevertheless, the synovial tissue structure is usually restored to its state before the acute inflammation. This means that the synovial cell proliferation and fibrosis in crystal arthropathy are associated with persistence of crystals or have been caused by other, indirectly crystal-related pathology.

When crystals form in dense connective tissue rich in proteoglycans and collagen, it has been thought that the crystals are inaccessible to proinflammatory proteins, neutrophils, and macrophages. However, the work of Nicola Dalbeth and colleagues, reviewed in Chapter 5, indicates that tophi are more dynamic structures than previously suspected, even in those in which typical acute inflammatory reactions do not occur. However, crystals are involved in degenerative reactions, which, over time, disrupt and alter the composition of extracellular matrix, producing irregular matrix heterogeneity resulting in decreased mechanical functionality. These reactions may be caused by crystal presence within cartilage or tendon insertion matrix or by chronic inflammation associated with crystals sequestrated in adjacent loose connective tissue spaces. This is described later in the sections on specific pathology of urate and CPPD crystals.

Gout (Monosodium Urate Crystal Deposition)

Since the discoveries of Garrod,[50,51] it has been recognized that gout results from systemic disorders of uric acid metabolism, which manifest as hyperuricemia. However, it has also been recognized since the 19th century that patients may have hyperuricemia without gout, that acute gout can occur without hyperuricemia,[52-55] that gout and osteoarthritis can coexist,[56] and that urate crystals can be present on cartilage surfaces in the absence of episodes of acute gout.[57,58] This indicates that local tissue urate supersaturation[59] and other local factors must be present to enable urate crystal deposition.[60] Crystals in

acute gout and tophi have been definitively identified by x-ray diffraction analysis as monosodium urate monohydrate.[61]

Acute Gouty Arthritis

In acute gout, MSU crystals appear in the synovial fluid, a local tissue space that becomes supersaturated in urate[62] usually related to a systemic increase in urate in interstitial fluid and blood.[59] MSU crystals seen in acute gout typically have a needle-shaped habit and are about 5 to 15 μm in length.[63] In contrast to tophaceous gout, urate crystals in acute gout are distributed individually in random orientation.

The predilection of acute gouty arthritis for certain joints such as the big toe (podagra) and time of onset (night) illustrates the pathogenesis of acute urate crystal deposition. During the day, it is likely that small effusion develops in the first metatarsalphalangeal joint or adjacent bursa. At night, with elevation of the foot, the fluid drains. As urate diffuses through synovial tissues at less than 50% the rate of water, the urate concentration rises substantially. Another contributing factor may be decreased temperature, which lowers urate solubility. In the presence of supersaturation, minor trauma or a solid tissue component, such as collagen fragments, could serve to initiate crystal nucleation.[64]

Acute gouty arthritis appears to be mediated by both the presence of crystals with elevated inflammatory potential in the synovial space, with additional triggers, such as elevated free fatty acids, helping to mediate induction of interleukin (IL)-1β secretion.[34,35] Experimentally, the acute inflammatory reaction of model gout enters the cellular phase usually within a few hours of initial crystal injection.[20,65,66] Single urate crystals are phagocytosed or partially phagocytosed principally by neutrophils.[67] Later, smaller crystals are observed intracellularly and extracellularly. Unsuccessful phagocytic activity leads to inflammatory cell destruction with release of cell debris, lysosomal enzymes, and partially dissolved crystals, which further amplifies the inflammatory response and, later, crystal clearance.[21,25,29,68,69] During the acute inflammation, the blood vessels in the synovium itself become dilated and congested. A neutrophil and fibrinous exudate can be observed within the synovium and in the SF.[70,71] The SF can have cell counts well above 10,000 and can even simulate acute septic arthritis. While reported, coincident acute gout or pseudogout and septic arthritis is uncommon.[72,73] Further, released lysosomal enzymes break down existing SF proteoglycan, decreasing urate crystal solubility and promoting additional crystal precipitation.[74]

The acute inflammation is resolved by mechansms that include clearance of crystals via either dissolution or sequestration. As inflammation resolves, hyaluronate proteoglycan secretion from the synovium increases hydration and urate solubility.[75] With crystal clearance, the synovial space and synovium are usually restored to its original state. With crystal sequestration that is present in recurrent acute gout, crystals tend to accumulate in the synovial recesses at the cartilage–synovium junction. Crystal persistence in this location can give rise later to tophaceous urate deposits and their cellular reaction, and be manifest by imaging.[76,77]

Intercritical Gout

Intercritical gout refers to the quiescent period between attacks of acute gouty arthritis. It is now known that urate crystals can remain on the surface of articular cartilage during the intercritical period[14,78-80] (see Fig. 1-2). However, these crystals are present as aggregates. Release of these crystals into the synovial space is thought to produce only low-grade inflammation,[81] because the crystals remain aggregated and coated with proteoglycan. Accordingly, one school of thought is that recurrent acute gouty arthritis with presence of individual urate crystals in random arrangement may reflect recurrent precipitation of urate in the synovial space. The other, and dominant, school of thought, reviewed in Chapter 5, is that various triggers, including crystal "autoinjection" via crystal shedding (from synovial microscopic tophi and possibly cartilage surface deposits) and tophus remodeling by serum urate lowering and trauma, or proinflammatory triggers, are the primary stimuli of acute gouty inflammation. The latter model fits better with the fact that so many gout flares are triggered by drops rather than acute increases in serum urate. Moreover, many joint fluids in acute gout do not have large amounts of urate crystals on microscopic exam. As such, physical increases in the inflammatory potential of urate crystals in the synovium, and other inciting factors such as local or systemic inflammatory mediator generation, are held to be major drivers of acute gout attacks.

Chronic Tophaceous Gout

With the advent of effective urate-lowering drugs over the past 50 years, end-stage tophaceous gout, fortunately, is now often preventable.[82-84] However, tophaceous gout remains a common presentation of the disease. Tophaceous gout can occur without previous history of acute gout,[85] and urate crystal deposits with similar characteristics to tophi can be seen on articular cartilage surfaces of untreated patients with intercritical gout[14] and even in some subjects with asymptomatic hyperuricemia. Excellent descriptions of tophaceous gout pathology and the effects of urate and urate crystal injections into articular tissues extend back in the scientific literature over 100 years.[86-92]

In tophaceous gout, urate crystals precipitate in a matrix usually containing proteoglycans (Figs. 1-3 to 1-7). Where

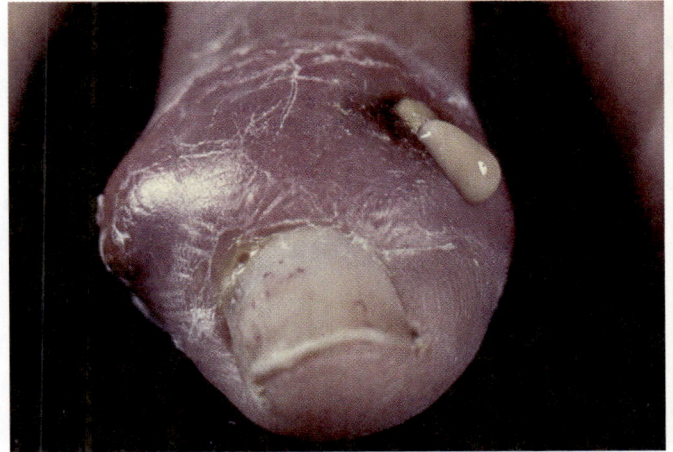

Figure 1-3 Tophaceous gout. Note that the digit appears enlarged with a nodular mass. The white paste oozing from the ulcer consists entirely of monosodium urate crystals.

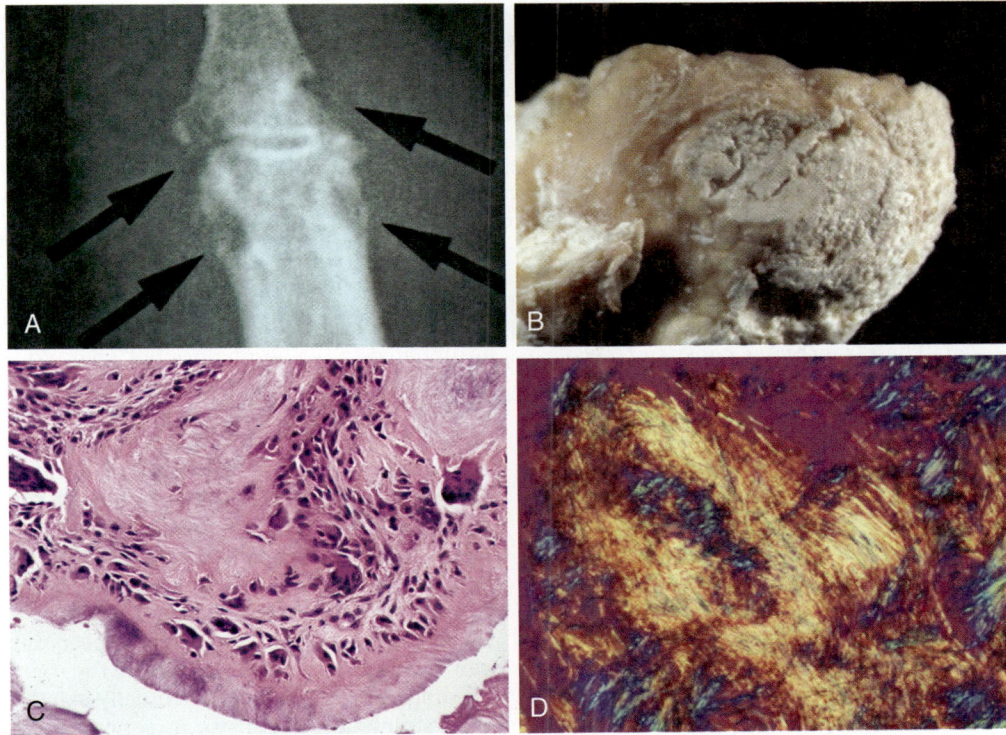

Figure 1-4 Tophaceous gout. **A,** Radiograph of digit demonstrates mass and erosions. The erosions are subjacent to the articular margin and originate in the synovial recesses. **B,** Tophaceous gout. Note the circumscribed white mass of monosodium urate (MSU) crystals. Macroscopic photograph. **C** and **D,** The tophus consists of masses of needle-shaped MSU crystals arranged in parallel sheaves. Macrophages and occasional giant cells surround the tophus. **C,** Light microscopy, hematoxylin and eosin stain. **D,** Compensated polarized light microscopy, unstained, coverslipped. **C** and **D,** Alcohol-fixed tissue, original magnification ×10.

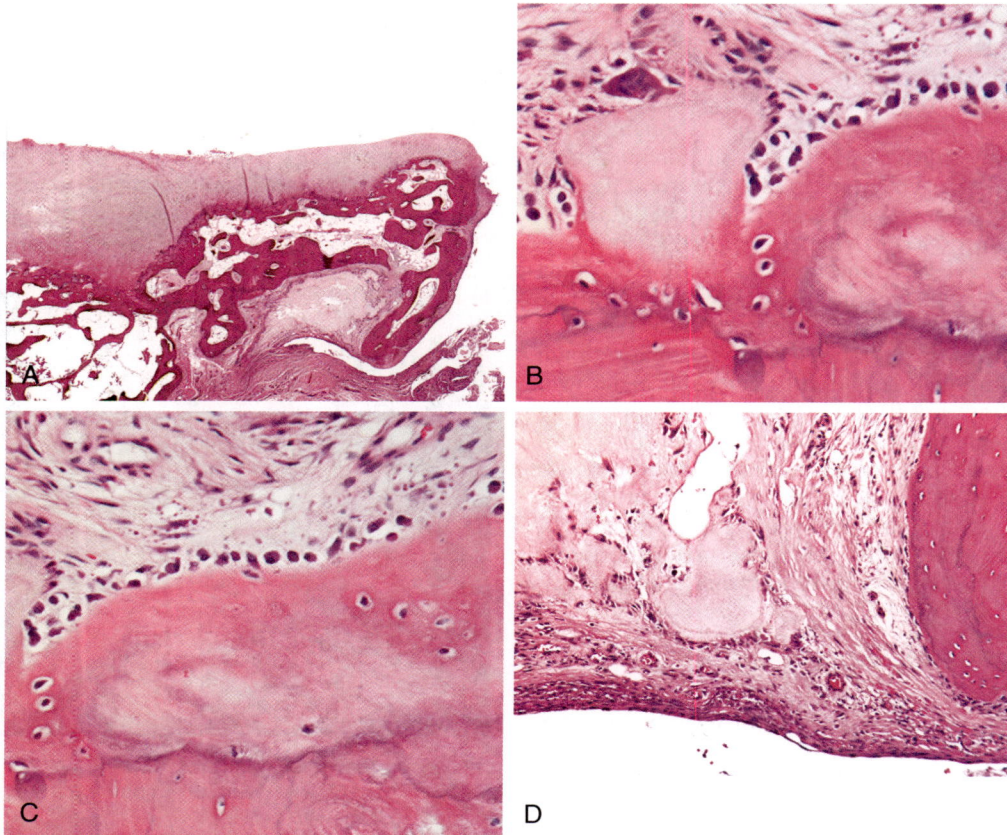

Figure 1-5 Tophaceous gout with subarticular erosion, knee joint. **A,** Articular cartilage and bone with tophaceous monosodium urate (MSU) deposits. The erosion is located adjacent to the synovial recess. The tissue overlying the tophus is fibrocartilage and bone of a chondroosteophyte. No inflammation is seen in the synovial space. Original magnification ×1. **B,** Tophaceous tissue. The matrix where the MSU crystals have dissolved out has pale amphophilic staining. Ghosts of crystal clusters can be observed. A portion of the tophus is surrounded by a mild chronic inflammatory infiltrate consisting of macrophages and occasional giant cells. The macrophages are elongate; the giant cell, derived from macrophages, resembles a foreign body giant cell and osteoclast. Adjacent to this, a portion of the tophus is being incorporated within new reparative bone. Original magnification ×40. **C,** Tophaceous matrix is being incorporated into new bone. The new bone is lined by osteoblasts. Original magnification ×40. **D,** Tophaceous tissue adjacent to synovium and bone. Note that the synovial lining is thin and that the synovium demonstrates fibrosis. The bone, which is located on the inner edge of the osteophyte, shows active new bone formation. The changes in both the synovium and bone are reparative. This indicates that the tophus has ceased to expand and that the MSU crystals have been sequestered from the synovial space. Original magnification ×10. **A–D,** Decalcified sections, light microscopy, hematoxylin and eosin stain.

crystals are uncovered, epitaxial precipitation of urate crystal aggregates is observed. These aggregates consist of needle-shaped crystals up to 20 μm × 1 μm × 1 μm aligned in parallel arrays (see Fig. 1-4). As the aggregates grow, groups of crystals become oriented to the characteristics of the tissue space. In the loose soft tissues such as bursa or synovium, the crystals may form spherical aggregates of crystal sheaves. On articular cartilage, the aggregates contain crystals aligned parallel to the joint surface. In both situations, urate crystals appear to bind extracellular proteoglycan as they are deposited.[14]

The reactions to tophaceous urate deposits are very different depending on whether the crystals deposit in avascular or vascular tissue spaces. In avascular spaces such as articular cartilage surfaces, the crystal aggregates form first without any reaction of the underlying cartilage. With the accumulation of more urate crystals, necrosis of adjacent chondrocytes is seen (see Figs. 1-6 and 1-7). This pathophysiologic sequence is confirmed by old experimental evidence that urates do not deposit in necrotic tissues.[86]

On morphologic observation, chondrocyte death subjacent to urate crystal deposits does not relate to mechanical pressure, osmotic effects of dissolved urate, or direct urate toxicity itself but likely results from interference with cell nutrition (nutrients must diffuse past the crystal aggregate barrier into the cartilage matrix). Regardless of the mode, chondrocyte necrosis results in failure to maintain the adjacent extracellular matrix. The matrix becomes physically weaker and has less capacity to retain water. At these sites, with time, these matrix features permit the crystal aggregates to enlarge and extend deeper into the cartilage, eventually reaching subchondral bone (see Fig. 1-7). At the most advanced stage, urate deposits can extend into the bone, replacing the trabecular spaces and eroding the cortical bone, eventually expanding to a nodular mass simulating tumor[92] or osteomyelitis,[93] and can advance across the joint space resulting in bony ankylosis.[94] Rarely, fractures can occur through tophaceous bony deposits.[95]

In contrast, where tophi form in connective tissue spaces that have a vascular supply, chronic inflammation characterized by C68+ macrophage, giant cell, and lymphocyte reaction

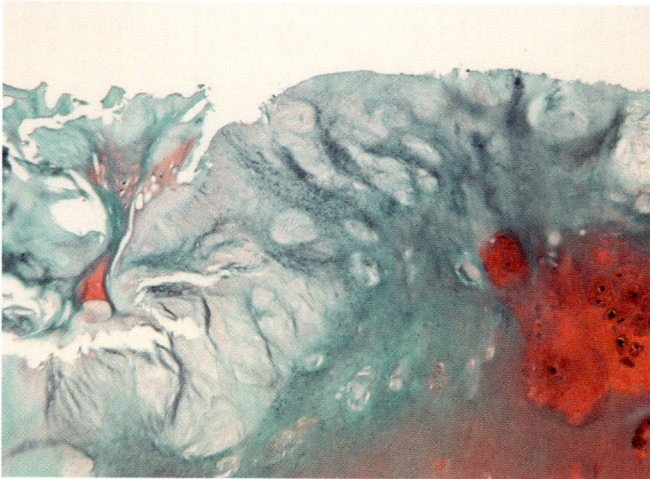

Figure 1-6 Chronic gout, articular cartilage surface. The pale staining matrix with "ghosts" of needlelike crystal is the site of monosodium urate (MSU) crystal deposition. The MSU crystals are deposited first on the articular surface. The subjacent chondrocytes are necrotic and the matrix adjacent to the crystal deposits becomes depleted of Safranin O–positive sulfated proteoglycans. This permits the MSU crystal deposits to enlarge and erode the cartilage matrix. Note the absence of inflammation. Decalcified formalin-fixed block. Safranin O, light green stain. Original magnification ×20.

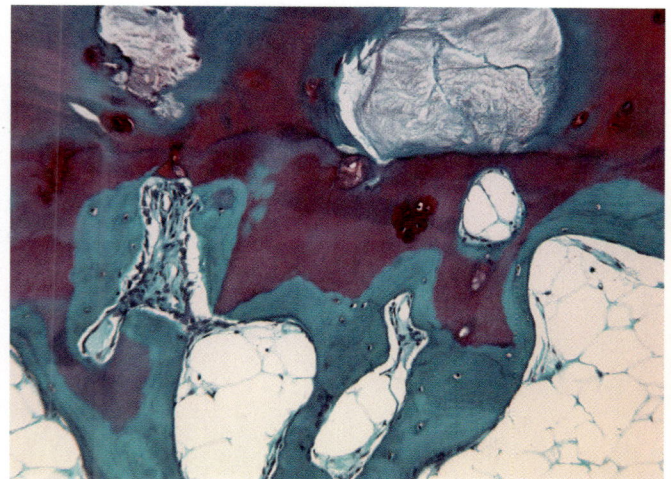

Figure 1-7 Chronic gout, deep articular cartilage and subchondral bone plate. The monosodium urate (MSU) crystal deposits have eroded the cartilage down to the calcified cartilage tidemark. Active bone remodeling characterized by osteoclasts and osteoblasts in process of focally resorbing subchondral bone is observed. Decalcified formalin-fixed block. Safranin O, light green stain. Original magnification ×20.

is seen on the border (corona)[71,83,96-98] of the tophaceous deposit (also discussed in Chapter 5). Without dissolution, chronic inflammation persists at the tophus–tissue interface (see Fig. 1-5). Successive generations of macrophages, unable to digest the crystal aggregates, die. Lipid from the residual cell membranes coalesces and precipitates to form cholesterol crystals, which in turn have surfaces that elicit macrophage and giant cell reactions as well as BCP calcification on the cholesterol crystal surfaces.[99,100] Similar reactions to cholesterol crystals occur with atheroma.[101] In advanced cases, clinical imaging can demonstrate the calcification surrounding the tophaceous deposits.[77] On ultrasound, tophi are hyperechoic but may have a hypoechoic border,[102] perhaps related to cholesterol crystal deposition.

Where urates become sequestered in the synovial recesses at the joint margins, a synovial lining grows over the tophus, further isolating the crystals from the joint surface. However, the macrophage giant cell reaction persists and through cytokine production, particularly IL-1β, enables bone resorption and remodeling in the bone at the edge of the joint.[103] This can result in joint erosions that superficially imitate those of rheumatoid arthritis (see Fig. 1-5). The erosions of tophaceous gout can be distinguished on imaging from those of rheumatoid arthritis by adjacent structural features.[76] Unlike rheumatoid arthritis, there is no synovial hyperplasia or preferential erosion of articular cartilage at the joint margin; osteoporosis is not usually seen. With the treatment of gout, the erosions persist but contain loose fibrous connective tissue rather than crystals. The adjacent bone may demonstrate sclerosis.

Gouty tophi can form in any connective tissue but does have predilection, perhaps because of lower temperature and decreased vascular circulation, for certain sites such as the helix of the external ear, the olecranon bursa, and extensor surface of the elbows. Clinical diagnostic confusion with

rheumatoid arthritis is exacerbated by the frequent presence of rheumatoid factor in patients with tophaceous gout.[104]

As noted earlier, gouty tophi can result in persistent chronic inflammation but can also result in an immune response. Immunoglobulin can adhere, through simple electrostatic interaction, to the highly negatively charged surface of urate crystals.[39] Whether immune response to the immunoglobulin on the urate crystal surface, or other adjuvant effects of urate crystals on adaptive immunity, give rise to the presence of rheumatoid factor in patients with gout is not clear.[37,38]

Some specific clinicopathologic presentations of tophaceous gout are noteworthy. Tophaceous gout can occur at acral sites, specifically the finger pads, with or without previous history of gouty arthritis.[105,106] As well, tophaceous material can erode through skin, simulating pus from a sinus tract or an open wound.[107] Not widely recognized, tophaceous gout can occur in the spinal intervertebral discs. Expansion of the tophus can lead to radiculopathy and cord compression.[108]

Gout and osteoarthritis are common forms of arthritis and can coexist, but their pathologic features are entirely different. Nonetheless, the relative contribution of each disease to a patient's arthritis can be a diagnostic challenge, particularly in patients with nodal osteoarthritis[108,109]—tophaceous deposits can occur in or around Bouchard or Heberden nodes, as just one example.

Calcium Pyrophosphate Dihydrate Crystal Deposition Disease and Pseudogout

CPPD crystal deposition disease shares with gout the acute inflammatory reaction to the presence of crystals in the synovial space—hence, the clinical term pseudogout for the acute monoarticular arthritis presentation of the disease. The mechanisms of acute inflammation and resolution are also similar to those for urate crystals.

However, CPPD crystal deposition disease differs greatly from gout not only in the type of crystal formed but also

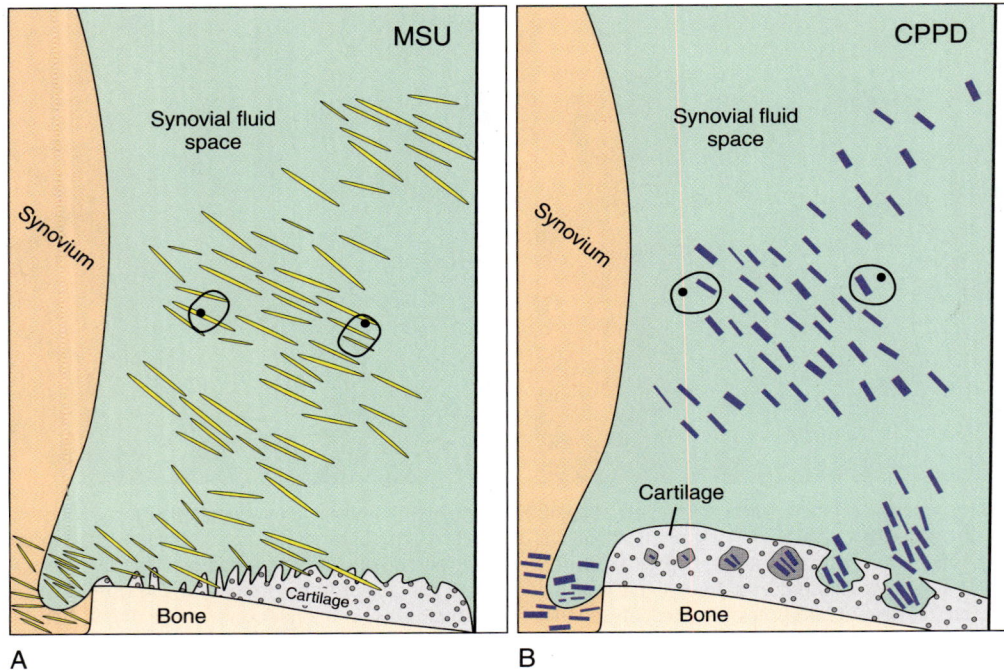

Figure 1-8 Comparison of monosodium urate (MSU) and calcium pyrophosphate dihydrate (CPPD) crystal formation in synovial joints. **A,** MSU crystals form in synovial fluid. MSU crystals usually dissolve during acute gouty inflammation. However, MSU crystal precipitation may cause minimal inflammation. In these cases, MSU crystals may remain on the articular cartilage sequestrated by proteoglycan. Accumulation of MSU crystals leads to chondrocyte necrosis and cartilage erosion forming MSU tophaceous deposits within cartilage. In addition, MSU crystals collect in the synovial recess where the crystals become walled off by chronic inflammation and fibrosis. These tophaceous deposits result in subarticular erosions. **B,** In contrast, CPPD crystals form within the matrix of hyaline cartilage and fibrocartilage. Subsequently, CPPD crystals are shed into the synovial space, resulting in acute inflammation. Also, CPPD crystals can collect in the synovial recess and later may be incorporated into the synovium. With chondroid metaplasia of synovial fibroblasts, the tissue conditions can also favor de novo CPPD crystal deposition within the synovium.

in the tissue sites and mechanisms of crystal formation, the resulting clinical manifestations,[110] and the associations with other diseases[110-112] (Fig. 1-8). This is reviewed in more detail in Chapters 20 and 21.

CPPD crystal formation is restricted to only a few connective tissues: hyaline cartilage, fibrocartilage (meniscus, symphyses, entheses), intervertebral disc annulus, and, occasionally, fibrotic synovium with cartilaginous metaplasia[113] (Figs. 1-9 to 1-11). These tissues are avascular, with the cells receiving nutrition via diffusion. However, related to the high negative charge associated with the proteoglycan component, diffusion is limited to small molecules.

In blood, and in most connective tissues of the body, phosphatases, particularly alkaline phosphatases, are present. In these tissues, pyrophosphate (PP_i) secreted by cells or formed extracellularly on the cell surface, rapidly hydrolyzes to an equilibrium concentration, $PP_i < 10 \ \mu mol/L$. This concentration is far below the value of $PP_i > 200 \mu mol/L$ necessary for CPPD crystal deposition.

Alkaline phosphatases formed on chondrocytes are bound to the outer cell membrane by phosphoinositol linkages. These high-molecular-weight molecules, when released from their phosphoinositol linkages to the cell membrane by phospholipases, diffuse slowly, and only for limited distances, through the matrix in the affected tissues.[114] Smaller molecules such as PP_i can diffuse faster than the phosphatases, thereby escaping local hydrolysis by enzymes. PP_i that has diffused beyond pyrophosphatase can become sequestered in the matrix and increase to supersaturation

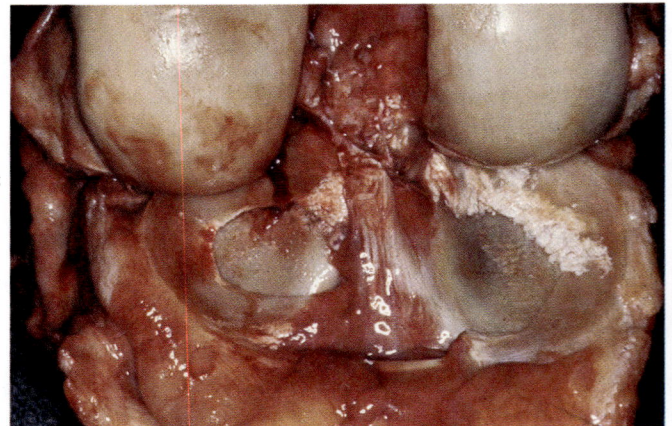

Figure 1-9 Calcium pyrophosphate dihydrate (CPPD) crystal arthropathy, knee joint. White CPPD crystal deposits are seen within meniscus, hyaline cartilage, and synovium. Note that the normal synovium, uninvolved with crystal deposits, is translucent, indicating the absence of chronic inflammation and fibrosis. *(From Pritzker KPH. Patogenesis de la gota y la pseudogota. In Seminarios de Reumatología. Fundación Instituto de Reumatología e Inmunología. Bogotá, Colombia: Ediciones Lerner; 1980:83-93, Figure 2.)*

concentration by coordinating to calcium bound to the matrix proteoglycans.

Crystal deposition is then initiated by local events such as increased impact force, delivering increased energy, local dehydration, local changes in concentrations of secondary ion

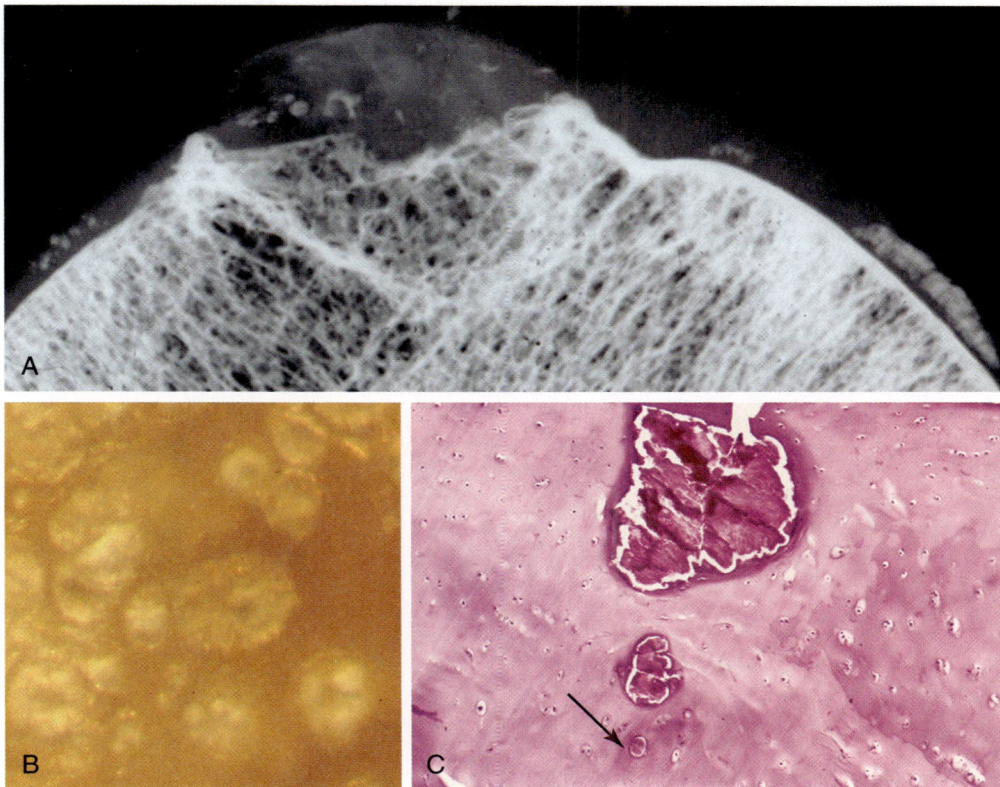

Figure 1-10 Calcium pyrophosphate dihydrate (CPPD) crystal arthropathy, femoral head. **A,** Chondrocalcinosis. Punctuate CPPD crystal deposits are seen as chondrocalcinosis in the articular cartilage mid-zone. As the deposits enlarge, there is coalescence to larger deposits and the crystal deposits appear closer to the articular surface. Note that fibrocartilage adjacent to central osteophyte and fibrous tissue at the base of ligamentum teres also shows chondrocalcinosis deposits. The articular cartilage has retained its normal thickness and the articular surface is intact. Specimen radiograph, 5-mm block. **B,** Articular cartilage surface, CPPD crystal shedding. CPPD crystal deposits are observed in "geodes" within the cartilage. Above the geodes, matrix translucency is observed. Focally, matrix holes are observed above the geodes at sites where the CPPD crystals are eroding through to the surface. Dissecting microscopy, original magnification ×10. **C,** Articular cartilage. CPPD crystal deposits are seen in mid-zone with extension toward cartilage surface. The cartilage surface is intact, indicating that erosion follows rather than precedes crystal deposition. The chondrocytes appear to be of normal size, although some chondrons are enlarged. The smallest CPPD deposit observed occupies a single chondron (*arrow*). Undecalcified section, hematoxylin and eosin stain, original magnification ×40. (**A** *from Pritzker KPH, Cheng PT, Renlund RC. Calcium pyrophosphate crystal deposition in hyaline cartilage: ultrastructural analysis and implications for pathogenesis. J Rheumatol 1988;15:828-35.*)

(ions in the tissue environment not directly incorporated into the crystals), or local increase in PP_i making the supersaturated state less stable.[115]

As tissue Ca^{2+} remains constant within narrow limits, local changes in extracellular secondary ions appear extremely important to CPPD crystal formation. Increased keratan sulfate–to–chondroitin sulfate ratio, commonly seen in aged cartilage, favors CPPD crystal formation,[116,117] as does decreased Mg^{2+}.[118] Increased P_i > 3 mmol/L strongly inhibits CPPD formation with the consequence that the formation conditions for CPPD and BCP crystals are mutually exclusive,[119] a finding recently confirmed in matrix vesicle studies.[120,121] Decreased P_i as seen in hyperparathyroidism favors CPPD crystal formation.[122] Secondary ions determine the kinetics of crystal formation and the exquisite crystal phase sensitivity of calcium pyrophosphate crystal formation. Of the more than 30 calcium pyrophosphate crystal phases, only two, calcium pyrophosphate dihydrate, monoclinic CPPD(M), and calcium pyrophosphate dihydrate, triclinic CPPD(T), form in biologic tissues.[123] The increased association of CPPD crystal deposition disease with hypomagnesemia,[122,124-126] hyperparathyroidism,[122] and hypothyroidism[127] may relate largely to secondary ion imbalances. The association of CPPD with hemochromatosis is more complicated[128] and may relate to secondary hyperparathyroidism rather than direct effects of Fe^{2+} ions.[129]

As extracellular Ca^{2+} is constant, CPPD crystal formation is dependent on increased extracellular pyrophosphate concentration ePP_i. In turn, this relates to increased ePP_i production by cell secretion or production on outer cell membrane as well as persistence of ePP_i in the extracellular fluid. As reviewed in Chapter 20, there are two sources for generation of extracellular PP_i in the vicinity of the chondrocyte: PP_i secretion from the chondrocyte via the phosphate pyrophosphate cell membrane transporter containing the ANKH protein and increased PP_i generation at the cell membrane facilitated by the enzyme ectonucleotide pyrophosphatase/phosphodiesterase 1 (ENPP1). Both mechanisms are enhanced by upregulated ATP production.[130,131]

Alkaline phosphatase is the key chondrocyte extracellular enzyme that promotes both PP_i destruction and CPPD crystal dissolution, as it has PP_i phosphatase activity at normal tissue pH.[114,132,133] Alkaline phosphatase directly dissolves CPPD crystals by hydrolyzing PP_i at the crystal surface

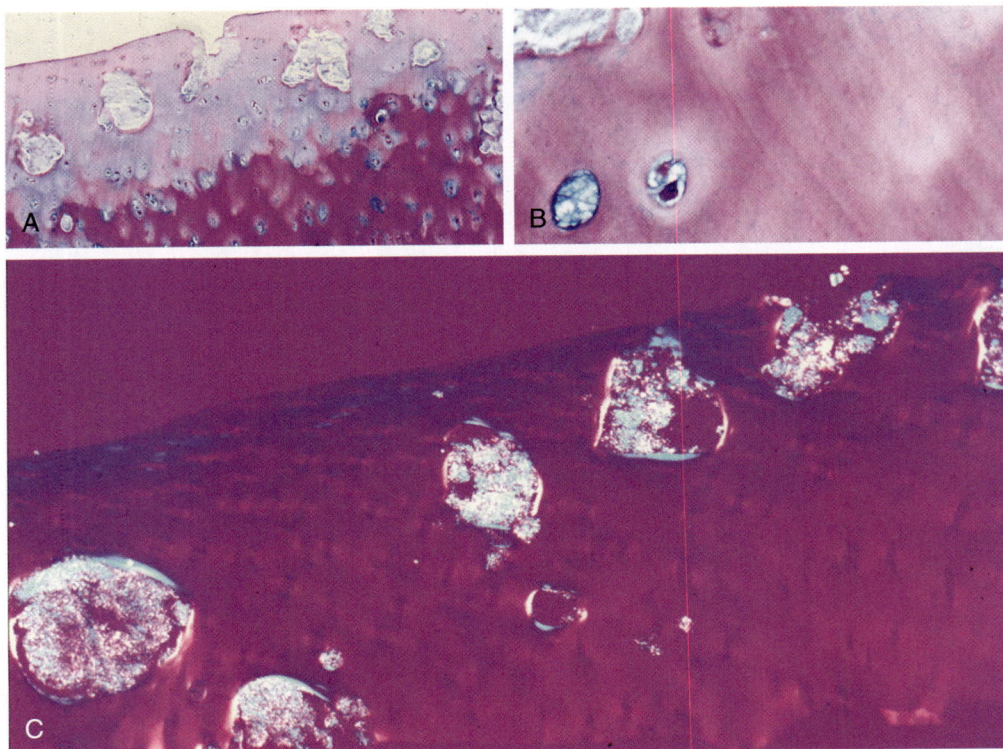

Figure 1-11 Calcium pyrophosphate dihydrate (CPPD) crystal arthropathy, femoral head. **A,** The matrix in which the crystals deposit as well as the adjacent matrix stains blue, indicating the presence of acid proteoglycans. The more distant non–crystal-bearing matrix is pale staining, indicating proteoglycan depletion. The deeper mid-zone cartilage shows normal purple red staining. Original magnification ×5. **B,** The matrix where CPPD crystals deposit stains blue, as does the pericellular matrix of adjacent chondrocytes, indicating a high concentration of acid proteoglycans. Original magnification ×40. **A, B,** Alcian blue/periodic acid-Schiff stain. **C,** CPPD crystal deposits within hyaline articular cartilage. The CPPD crystals are deposited randomly as agglomerates within geodes in the mid-zone. Enlarged crystal deposits erode through the articular surface. The smallest crystal deposit occupies the volume of a chondron, which suggests that the fibrous capsule of the chondron limits the volume of initial CPPD crystal deposition. Even the smallest CPPD crystals are much larger (in the micron range) than basic calcium phosphate crystals (in the nanometer range). As discussed in Chapter 20 regarding the pathogenesis of CPPD crystal deposition, this is consistent with different mechanisms of crystal formation. CPPD crystals appear far too large to form inside matrix vesicles. Undecalcified, unstained 5-μm section. Compensated polarized light microscopy.

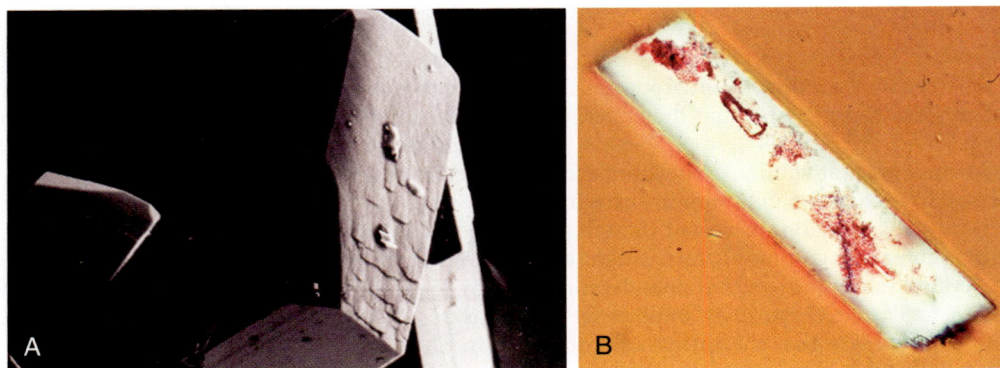

Figure 1-12 Alkaline phosphatase dissolution effects on calcium pyrophosphate dihydrate (CPPD)(M) crystal. **A,** Alkaline phosphatase (red stain) is seen on the crystal surface at sites of etch pit dissolution. Interference contrast, compensated polarized light microscopy, original magnification ×500. **B,** Step dislocations indicative of crystal dissolution are observed preferentially on the short face of the crystal. This crystal face at the site of crystal growth is the face with the highest energy potential. This demonstrates the face stereospecificity of CPPD crystal deposition by alkaline phosphatase. Scanning electron microscopy, original magnification ×2000. (**B** from Shinozaki T, Xu Y, Cruz TF, et al. Calcium pyrophosphate dihydrate [CPPD] crystal dissolution by alkaline phosphatase: interaction of alkaline phosphatase on CPPD crystals. J Rheumatol 1995;22:117-23.)

(Fig. 1-12). To have this effect, alkaline phosphatase must be in very close proximity or actually on the surface of CPPD crystals.[13] Therefore, decreased alkaline phosphatase in the presence of increased ePP_i are the prerequisite conditions for CPPD crystal formation in cartilage. At sites of CPPD crystal formation, alkaline phosphatase may be decreased because of insufficient enzyme synthesis or by enzyme inhibition from endogenous substances or by ePP_i diffusion into the matrix beyond the reach of the enzyme. Similarly, without the presence of alkaline phosphatase in the immediate

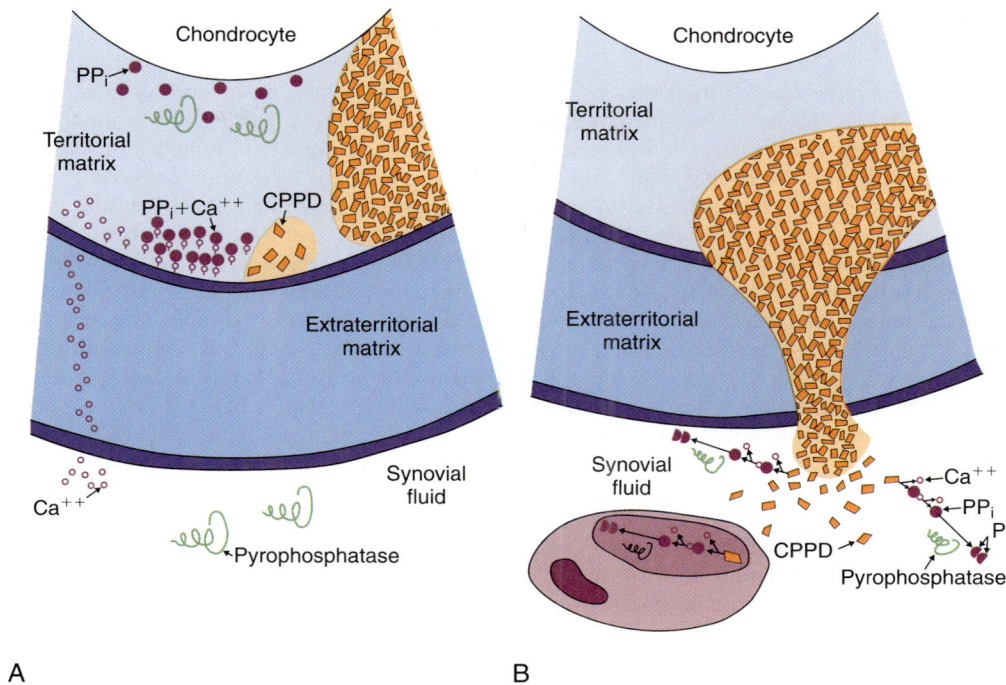

A   B

Figure 1-13 **A,** Calcium pyrophosphate dihydrate (CPPD) crystal formation within articular cartilage. The key conditions favoring CPPD crystal formation are low availability of alkaline phosphase and the increased availability of pyrophosphate PP_i within the matrix. Alkaline phosphatase activity may be decreased because alkaline phosphatase synthesis and export to chondrocyte cell membrane are decreased or inhibitors of the enzyme are present or diffusion of the enzyme beyond the immediate vicinity of the cell is restricted. Decreased availability of alkaline phosphates in the presence of normal or increased PP_i generation will result in increased PP_i sufficient to form CPPD crystals. Once CPPD crystals are formed, the crystal agglomerates expand toward the cartilage surface, where the crystals are shed into the synovial fluid. **B,** CPPD crystal dissolution within the synovial fluid space. CPPD crystals incite acute inflammation as described in the text. CPPD crystals incorporated into neutrophil and macrophage phagolysosomes dissolve by the action of intracellular phosphatases. CPPD crystals free in synovial fluid are dissolved by the action of phosphatases derived from blood and interstitial fluid as well as phosphatases released from inflammatory cells.

vicinity, CPPD crystal dissolution does not occur within cartilage matrix.

Selective inhibition of alkaline phosphatase activity by endogenous substances such as cysteine[134] or mercaptopyruvate[135] favors both increased extracellular PP_i and inhibition of CPPD crystal dissolution. There is some early evidence that this mechanism can apply in vivo as tissue cysteine and mercaptopyruvate may be generated under hypoxic conditions as a response to free radical formation.[136] As well, transforming growth factor (TGF)-β1 upregulation in chondrocytes by ionic ePi leads to increased ePP_i and decreased alkaline phosphatase expression, two preconditions for CPPD crystal formation and inhibition of CPPD crystal dissolution[137-139] Normal adult[114] and aged mid-zone chondrocytes do not express alkaline phosphatase activity.[133] Cartilage extracellular ionic Pi can become decreased in aging and various disease states, further setting up the local environment for CPPD crystal deposition (Fig. 1-13).

In contrast to osteoarthritis, the chondrocytes in aged and CPPD crystal bearing cartilage do not appear to have as much hypertrophic differentiation or to be expressing significant alkaline phosphatase, which is a marker of chondrocyte hypertrophy.[140-142] Some authors did consider CPPD-associated chondrocytes to be hypertrophic.[143,144] However, this observation was relative to smaller superficial zone chondrocytes. Chondrocytes adjacent to crystals measured greater than 15 μm in diameter, which is within the upper normal range of human articular cartilage chondrocytes.[145] Hence,

chondrocyte hypertrophy linkage to CPPD crystal deposition is not fully established through differentiation analyses. Chondrocytes in the vicinity of CPPD crystals have been shown to be associated with increased lipid but the biologic significance in CPPD crystal deposition is as yet unknown.[146]

Typically, in both hereditary and the more common sporadic disease, CPPD crystals first form extracellularly in the cartilage mid zone[142,147-153] (see Figs. 1-10 and 1-11). This is the tissue domain where the matrix is at the greatest distance from phosphatase activity in overlying SF or underlying bone. CPPD crystal deposition in both sporadic and hereditary disease is associated with matrix rich in keratan sulfate proteoglycan,[153-156] a finding that is in accord with experimental studies.[116] CPPD crystals precipitate as agglomerates of randomly oriented needle-shaped or rhomboidal crystals approximately 10 to 12 μm in longest dimension. While there is some experimental evidence suggesting that CPPD crystals may form in association with matrix vesicles (see Chapter 20),[157-160] CPPD crystals in adult human articular cartilage form free in the extracellular space unassociated with cells, collagen, or matrix vesicles. Similar agglomerates can be formed in cell-free gels with high PP_i concentrations simply through the differential diffusion of Ca^{2+} ions.[161-164] The smallest crystal agglomerate fills the space of a chondron, obliterating the chondrocyte. As the disease progresses, the agglomerates enlarge via epitaxial growth on existing crystals.

CPPD crystals are extremely insoluble in aqueous solution[165] but can readily be dissolved by extracellular phosphatases including chondrocyte alkaline phosphatase.[13,36,114,132,166-168] Polyamines, molecules found in cell nuclei, enhance CPPD crystal dissolution.[169]

When the CPPD agglomerates reach sufficient size and proximity to the cartilage surface, the crystals are shed into the synovial space.[170] Softening of cartilage matrix with increased hydration as may be seen in hypothyroidism[127] will facilitate CPPD crystal shedding. CPPD crystals in the SF may be present without symptoms. However, CPPD crystals can induce low-grade cellular inflammation[15] or incite an episode of acute inflammation, presenting clinically as acute pseudogout.

Similar CPPD crystal formation conditions are seen in meniscus, symphysis, or enthesis. However, CPPD crystals can also be observed in fibrocartilage overlying hyaline cartilage and in areas of chondrometaplasia in the meniscus,[171] tendon insertions,[172,173] flexor retinaculum and triangular cartilage of the wrist,[174] annulus fibrosus,[156,175-177] cartilage endplate[156] and ligamentum flavum of the intervertebral disc, and occasionally synovium.[113] Where the tissue environment is constrained by densely aligned collagen fibers such as tendon and fibrous synovium, CPPD crystals will tend to deposit in similar alignment. In more proteoglycan-rich environments such as cartilage, the crystals will precipitate in random agglomerates.[142,149,171] Chondrometaplasia[113] at these sites is associated with compressive forces and degeneration of tissues with fraying of collagen fibers and generation of matrix rich in proteoglycan.

CPPD crystal formation is to some extent species limited. CPPD crystals have been definitively identified in humans, monkeys,[178-182] and dogs.[183,184] Rabbits,[185] rats, and mice form BCP crystals at the same sites. In part, these differences could be ascribed to the thickness of the crystal-bearing tissues, which have an increased distance from interstitial fluid phosphatase, and in part to differences in PP_i metabolism between species.

Acute Pseudogout

In contrast to urate crystals that form in the SF, CPPD crystals are extruded into the synovial space from the adjacent hyaline articular cartilage or meniscal fibrocartilage. CPPD crystals incite acute inflammation via similar mechanisms to MSU crystals.[31,186] In some cases, the synovial neutrophil count can exceed 50,000 cells/mm³ and the arthritis can simulate septic arthritis.[187] Phosphatases liberated from exudated neutrophils and phosphatase diffusing into the SF from permeable blood vessels likely act to dissolve CPPD crystals and help resolve the inflammation. As the inflammation progresses, the crystals become smaller and more difficult to recognize with light microscopy techniques.[188]

Whatever the anatomic location, at each crystal deposition site, shedding of CPPD crystals into adjacent synovial or bursal[189] space can incite acute inflammation. As well, CPPD crystals, like urate crystals, can be sequestered in synovial recesses and covered with fibrous tissue. Unlike urates, under most circumstances, the CPPD "pseudotophus" does not subsequently enlarge.

Chronic CPPD Crystal Deposition Disease

Unlike osteoarthritis (OA), which is a disorder with onset in middle age,[190] CPPD crystal deposition disease commonly has onset after age 55. It also increases with aging, affecting more than 20% of the population older than 70 years, regardless of the joints affected,[177,191-201] as reviewed in Chapter 21. Pathologic CPPD crystal deposition disease is more common than that detected by radiologic chondrocalcinosis, since approximately 50% of the tissue density must be affected to observe chondrocalcinosis in a conventional radiograph.[147,202-204] Chondrocalcinosis in radiologic OA is more closely associated with aging than with OA progression.[205,206]

Considerable controversy exists about the overlap between the common diseases osteoarthritis and CPPD.[207] CPPD crystals are observed occasionally in OA SF.[208] In a longitudinal study, 25% of patients with knee joint OA developed CPPD.[209] This approximates the prevalence of CPPD in elderly populations. CPPD crystal deposition in hyaline articular cartilage appears to be a distinct disease. Most surgically removed femoral heads that have been observed with CPPD crystal deposits have been removed for osteoporotic fracture. These femoral heads show intact cartilage thickness and articular surfaces rather than OA.[142,194]

Two general patterns of CPPD crystal deposition are seen in knee joints removed for "degenerative" arthritis—a younger group with crystal deposition affecting predominantly meniscal fibrocartilage, coexistent with histologic OA, and an older group lacking cartilage radiologic and histologic features for OA[210] but demonstrating CPPD arthropathy affecting fibrocartilage, hyaline cartilage, and synovium.[211] With advanced arthritis, these patients typically present with CPPD crystals within the cartilage and extensive areas of sclerotic, eburnated bone articular surface.[202,203,212] It remains to be determined whether or how much CPPD crystal deposits in cartilage stimulate cartilage matrix degradation via chondrocyte upregulation, "microcrystal-induced stress."[207] CPPD crystal deposits have very much different compliance from adjacent tissues and therefore can contribute to matrix degradation through physical wear.

Our observations are that some elderly patients with OA do have CPPD in knee meniscal fibrocartilage but only rarely is CPPD observed in hyaline cartilage affected by OA. As well, CPPD meniscal deposition is seen patients with OA associated with joint hypermobility.[213] This distinction is important as typically CPPD diseased cartilage lacks the features of chondrocyte proliferation and increased chondrocyte alkaline phosphatase expression, characteristic changes seen in OA cartilage.[214] As well, OA cartilage binds increased calcium, phosphorus, and magnesium compared to normal subjects,[215] an ionic environment that inhibits CPPD calcification. From experimental evidence, episodes of pseudogout in OA patients may aggravate OA synovitis.[216]

A second controversy relates to the simultaneous presence of CPPD and BCP crystals in OA SF.[217,218] BCP crystals can be observed adjacent to CPPD crystal agglomerates, but this is very unusual as the formation conditions for these crystals are mutually exclusive. When this is seen, it implies that the crystals formed at different times. CPPD and BCP can be seen together in SF in advanced arthritis where a portion of the articular surface consists of exposed bone. Under these circumstances, BCP from the bone surfaces and CPPD from within cartilage can reach the SF.

While rheumatoid arthritis patients may have CPPD crystal deposition,[219,220] CPPD also can present as pseudo–rheumatoid arthritis (Chapter 21). As in chronic gout, patients may be seropositive for the rheumatoid factor. Pseudo–rheumatioid arthritis is characterized by extensive synovial deposition of CPPD crystals, accompanied by radiographic erosions similar to those in tophaceous gout.[221] However, synovial inflammation is highly attenuated, and pannus formation is not observed.

CPPD crystal deposition is observed in the intervertebral discs and other soft tissue structures of the aged spine and can be a source of back or neck pain.[125,156,175-177,193,222-228] CPPD crystal deposition at the cranial cervical junction such as in the transverse ligament of C1 and the periodontoid tissues can cause pain, myelopathy, and radiculopathy.[125,226-228] Recently recognized radiologically, these patients can present with "crowned dens syndrome."[125,227,228] Of particular interest are linear and nodular CPPD deposits in the ligamentum flavum, which may account for the majority of cases of ligamentum flavum calcification commonly seen in Japan.[229-231] As with CPPD deposition in other spinal tissues, large deposits with crystal shedding can lead to spinal cord compression and radiculopathy.[230] The pathogenic relationship, if any, to the hierarchial culture of bowing remains to be understood. CPPD crystal deposits within tendons, like urate tophi, can lead to tendon rupture.[232]

From clinical reports of CPPD following surgery for osteochondritis dissecans,[233] meniscectomy,[234] or intervertebral disc extrusion,[235,236] CPPD crystals may form preferentially at sites of previous injury and fibrous repair.

CPPD has also been associated with rapidly destructive arthritis affecting the femoral head[237] and other joints, predominantly in elderly woman.[238-240] It is likely that this is a sequela of insufficiency fracture through the osteoporotic articular plate.[241]

Familial CPPD crystal deposition disease is rare but has been much studied[219,242] and is reviewed in Chapters 20-21.

From a pathology perspective, it is useful to classify familial CPPD into those families with CPPD and cartilage dysplasia, those with premature chondrocalcinosis younger than 30 years old, and those with familial occurrence as adults. Hypophosphatasia,[112,243,244] where there is relative deficiency of alkaline phosphatase, is in the latter group and reinforces the role of decreased extracellular alkaline phosphatase activity in the pathogenesis of CPPD arthropathy.[167]

CPPD arthropathy can present rarely as a "tumor" involving a single joint, raising the clinical and radiologic suspicion of neoplasia.[222,245-247] As with the initially recognized case,[222] more than 50% of known cases involve the temporomandibular joint.[246-249] The pathogenesis of this condition is unknown but typically the connective tissue cells in the vicinity of the crystal deposits exhibit chondroid metaplasia.

Basic Calcium Phosphate (Calcium Apatite) Crystal Deposition

An extensive discussion of BCP-associated arthropathy (see Chapter 23) degradation effects on articular tissues is beyond the scope of this chapter. BCP is the mineral deposited in bone formation. Under these circumstances, BCP crystals deposit in a highly ordered fashion with very well defined and limited crystal size and structure. BCP can be present in SF, as a result of breakdown product of bone fragments produced in advanced arthritis, of adjacent BCP deposits in periarticular connective tissues, or of pathologic[250,251] BCP deposits in hyaline or fibrocartilage[252-259] (Fig. 1-14). BCP crystals from bone can be recognized by their orderly array and alignment,

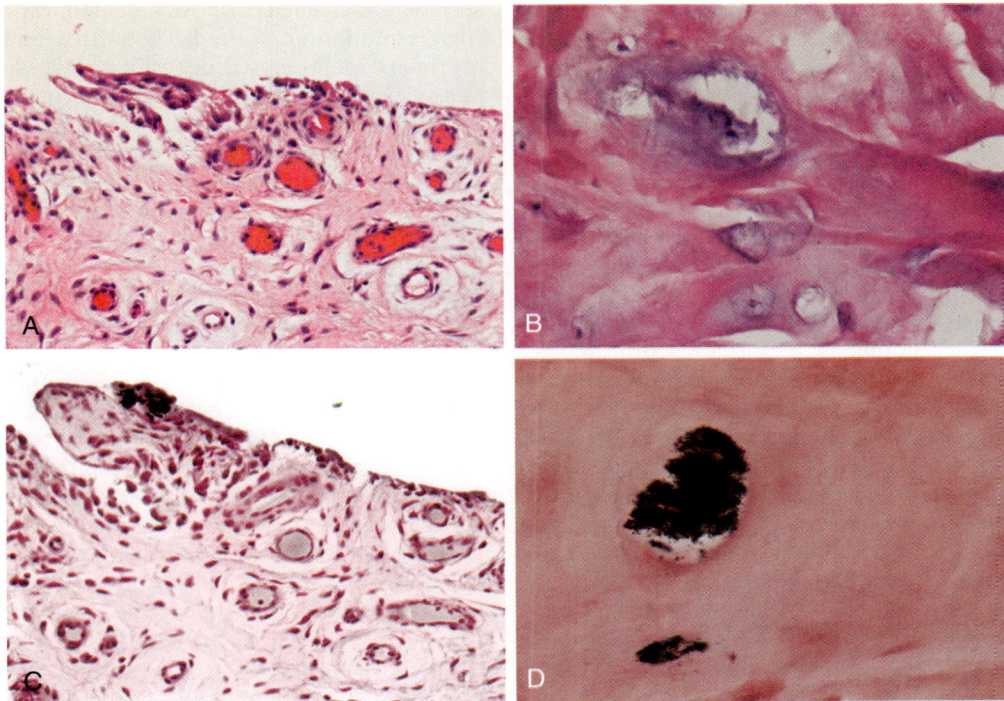

Figure 1-14 Basic calcium phosphate (BCP) arthropathy. **A** and **C**, Synovium. The synovium shows an increase in size of synovial lining cells with vascular dilation and slight fibrosis. The BCP crystal deposition has dissolved out of the section. **C**, BCP crystal aggregates are seen as black staining material adjacent to the synovial cells. **B** and **D**, Cartilage. **B**, BCP deposits are observed adjacent to chondrocytes within and adjacent to the chondron. **D**, BCP crystal aggregates are seen as black staining material. **A** and **B**, Hematoxylin and eosin stain. **C** and **D**, Von Kossa stain. **A–D**, original magnification ×100.

the consistent size of single crystals of 10 to 40 nm × 10 nm, and the irregular size of the bone fragments. In contrast, BCP crystals forming de novo, depending on circumstances, may be associated with cell membranes or, especially in growing tissues, matrix vesicles. BCP crystals in pathologic circumstances may vary in size and crystal orientation and occasionally may demonstrate spherulitic forms.

The relationships of BCP crystal deposition to gout, CPPD, and OA continue to be controversial,[207,217,260,261] in part because of the technical difficulties of finding BCP crystals in SF in these conditions.[262] As noted earlier, similar to other chronic inflammation including atheroma, BCP can precipitate on the cholesterol crystals that are associated with the granulomatous inflammation of gouty tophi. BCP can form in hyaline cartilage and fibrocartilage where there is cell death, extensive matrix dehydration, or fibrosis. These conditions are present in OA cartilage with advanced disease.[259] Extensive corticosteroid administration can facilitate BCP deposition in articular cartilage tissues. BCP crystals in experimental systems can induce microcrystal-induced stress in chondrocytes.[207] In both advanced CPPD and OA, bone is exposed to the articular surface and microfractures are common. Under these circumstances, bone fragments are resorbed by synovium. During either microfracture or resorption of bone fragments in the synovium, aggregations of BCP crystals can be released to the SF. BCP crystals can induce upregulation of synovial macrophages, producing chronic inflammation and fibrosis.[263] Like urate and CPPD crystals, these fragments can incite acute inflammation and can be sequestered in synovial recesses. Unlike urate and CPPD, BCP crystals are readily dissolved in the acidic environment of joint inflammation. Exposure of chondrocytes to BCP crystals in vitro can upregulate cell reactivity.[264]

Considerations for Detection of MSU, CPPD, and BCP Crystals in Tissues

Tophi (MSU Crystals)

If a tophaceous nodule undergoes a biopsy, crystal deposition can be inferred by the white, firm appearance on the fresh cut surface. In these circumstances, a definitive diagnosis can be made by scraping the whitish material on the cut surface onto a slide and examining the material with the use of polarized light microscopy. If the nodule is to be examined histologically, it should be fixed in alcohol, not formalin, as formalin has been demonstrated to dissolve urate crystals.[56,265] Similarly, the whitish paste seen on the cartilage surfaces in gout can be mistaken by the uninitiated for pus and can be diagnosed by examining the fresh material scraped onto a slide with the use of polarized light microscopy.

Frequently, the white material in a tophaceous nodule is not recognized on gross examination, particularly if the tissue is submitted as a rheumatoid nodule and the tissue is not bisected. In these cases, if the nodule has not been fixed in formalin for long or if the formalin is insufficient, crystals may survive processing. Residual urate crystals may be identifiable in these circumstances if an unstained deparaffinized 5-μm section is examined with a polarized microscope. Using an unstained slide is essential, as staining involves washing the section in water, thereby dislodging the crystals.

Even if crystals have been dissolved out, a tophaceous nodule can be distinguished from a palisading granuloma of rheumatoid nodule by the presence of needle-shaped crystal ghosts and the relative absence of fibrinoid and cell debris[96] in the matrix.

Calcium Crystals (CPPD, BCP)

Decalcification procedures remove CPPD and BCP crystals from tissues. To examine tissues for calcium crystals, undecalcified blocks must be prepared. Optimal detection for CPPD is facilitated by preparing a 5-μm unstained, deparaffinized slide, which is subsequently coverslipped and examined with compensated polarized light microscopy.[266] BCP crystals fail to polarize, whereas urate crystals are yellow and CPPD crystals are blue when the crystal long axes are aligned to the axis of the compensating plate. For BCP crystals, a 5-μm slide treated with Alizarin red or Von Kossa stain will demonstrate the calcifications. When the nature of the crystal is in doubt, x-ray or electron diffraction can be performed on the crystal deposits within the section (see Chapter 22).[266,267]

Editor's Note

A major issue in the pathology of gout, discussed in this chapter, also highly relevant to the discussion of molecular pathogenesis of gouty inflammation in Chapter 5, is the net role, in triggering gouty inflammation, of urate crystal deposition developing directly in joint fluid. Importantly, Chapter 26 highlights the diagnostic value of the settling and/or deposition and embedding of urate crystals at the cartilage surface, seen as the characteristic "double contour" sign of gout on high resolution ultrasound. The cartilage surface may not be a primary site of crystal deposition; indeed, seed urate crystals formed primarily in synovial fluid could "settle" and then substantially grow on the cartilage surface as proposed by Dr. Pritzker from analyses of fine structure of urate crystals. In addition, major questions remain on whether new urate crystals formed in joint fluid or those "loosened" from cartilage surface deposits, or both, help to ignite gouty attacks by interacting with synovial fluid phagocytes and synovial lining cells, as well as complement. Alternatively, does gouty joint inflammation principally result from synovium-driven inflammation triggered by "remodeling" or breakdown of microscopic tophi, particularly in response to changes in ambient urate levels? This scenario is exemplified by gout attacks precipitated by a large drop in serum urate with initiation of pharmacologic urate-lowering drugs. In reality, quite often the amounts of urate crystals in the joint fluid actually seen by rheumatologists and other clinicians in acute gout are not large. Conversely, clinicians can see urate crystals in asymptomatic joint fluids, and sometimes in massive amounts in "joint milk" that is aspirated from joints that are not inflamed. In addition, high resolution ultrasound detects clinically silent urate crystal deposits at the cartilage surface even in many patients with asymptomatic hyperuricemia. The Editor's opinion is that it is not clear that primary urate crystal deposition in the synovial fluid is the triggering force in most cases of either acute or chronic gouty arthritis, and many questions remain to be resolved.

Response by Author

Urate crystal formation in tissues follows the general principles of crystal formation beautifully. When individual urate crystals are seen in synovial fluid in random orientation, these crystals have precipitated in the fluid recently. Some crystals may then adhere to the cartilage surface where there is further precipitation of crystals aligned parallel to the first crystals, a process called epitaxy.

It is possible that some crystals on the cartilage surface are derived from the crystals initially precipitated in the synovial fluid but relatively few, as there is no evidence of cellular debris in the cartilage surface crystals that are epitaxially aligned. This means that most urate crystals on the cartilage surface are forming from nidal sites on previously deposited crystals and are growing from precipitation of soluble urate. Release of these crystals from the cartilage surface into the synovial space shows clusters of aligned crystals similar to tophi.

As these two patterns of crystals are seen in synovial fluid aspirates, at least in some cases of acute gout, it is likely there is no prior crystal deposition on the cartilage surface. That is the crux of uncertainty and disagreement among investigators. By the time ultrasound or other imaging findings of urate deposition on cartilage surfaces are seen, the patient essentially has gout with a measurable crystal burden. Some patients with acute gout, with no prior history, will show synovial fluid inflammation with randomly oriented crystals. Others, also with no history, may show aligned crystals indicative of previous asymptomatic urate crystal deposition on the cartilage surface. Whether acute gout in both situations is initiated by the same mechanisms, and the mechanisms themselves, remain as open questions.

References

1. Valsik J, Zitnan D, Sit'Aj S. Chondrocalcinosis articularis. Section II. Genetic study. Ann Rheum Dis 1963;22:153–7.
2. Zitnan D, Sit'Aj S. Chondrocalcinosis articularis. Section I. Clinical and radiological study. Ann Rheum Dis 1963;22:142–52.
3. Zitnan D, Sit'Aj S, Huttl S, et al. Chondrocalcinosis articularis. Section III. Physiopathological study. Ann Rheum Dis 1963;22:158–64.
4. McCarty Jr DJ, Kohn NN, Faires JS. The significance of calcium phosphate crystals in the synovial fluid of arthritic patients: the "pseudogout syndrome." I. Clinical aspects. Ann Intern Med 1962;56:711–37.
5. Kohn NN, Hughes RE, McCarty Jr DJ, et al. The significance of calcium phosphate crystals in the synovial fluid of arthritic patients: the "pseudogout syndrome." II. Identification of crystals. Ann Intern Med 1962;56:738–45.
6. McCarty Jr DJ, Gatter RA, Hughes RE. Pseudogout syndrome, IV. Early (perilacunar) and "mature" cartilaginous deposits of monoclinic and triclinic crystals of calcium pyrophosphate dihydrate; Koch's postulates and possible pathogenesis. Ann Rheum Dis 1963;6:287.
7. McCarty Jr DJ, Haskin ME. The roentgenographic aspects of pseudogout (articular chondrocalcinosis). An analysis of 20 cases. Am J Roentgenol Radium Ther Nucl Med 1963;90:1248–57.
8. McCarty Jr DJ. Crystal-induced inflammation; syndromes of gout and pseudogout. Geriatrics 1963;18:467–78.
9. Robertson WG. The solubility concept. In: Nancollas GH editor. Biological Mineralization and Demineralization. Berlin, Germany: Springer-Verlag; 1982:17.
10. Garside J. Nucleation. In: Nancollas GH, editor. Biomineralization and Demineralization. Berlin, Germany: Springer-Verlag; 1982:13.
11. Finsy R. On the critical radius of Ostwald ripening. Langmuir 2004;20:22.
12. Perl-Treves D, Addadi L. A structural approach to pathological crystallizations. Gout: the possible role of albumin in sodium urate crystallization. Proc R Soc Lond 1988;B235:145–59.
13. Shinozaki T, Xu Y, Cruz TF, et al. Calcium pyrophosphate dihydrate (CPPD) crystal dissolution by alkaline phosphatase: interaction of alkaline phosphatase on CPPD crystals. J Rheumatol 1995;22:117–23.
14. Pritzker KPH, Zahn CE, Nyburg SC, et al. The ultrastructure of urate crystals in gout. J Rheumatol 1978;5:7–18.
15. Martinez Sanchis A, Pascual E. Intracellular and extracellular CPPD crystals are a regular feature in synovial fluid from uninflamed joints of patients with CPPD related arthropathy. Ann Rheum Dis 2005;64:1769–72.
16. Kozin F, McCarty DJ. Protein binding to monosodium urate monohydrate, calcium pyrophosphate dihydrate, and silicon dioxide crystals. I. Physical characteristics. J Lab Clin Med 1977;89:1314–25.
17. Fam AG, Schumacher Jr HR, Clayburne G, et al. A comparison of five preparations of synthetic monosodium urate monohydrate crystals. J Rheumatol 1992;19:780–7.
18. McCarty DJ, Kozin F. An overview of cellular and molecular mechanisms in crystal-induced inflammation. Arthritis Rheum 1975;18:757–64.
19. McCarty Jr DJ. The inflammatory reaction to microcrystalline sodium urate. Arthritis Rheum 1965;8:726–35.
20. McCarty Jr DJ. Mechanisms of the crystal deposition diseases: gout and pseudogout. Ann Intern Med 1973;78:767–70.
21. Buchanan WW, Klinenberg JR, Seegmiller JE. The inflammatory response to injected microcrystalline monosodium urate in normal, hyperuricemic, gouty, and uremic subjects. Arthritis Rheum 1965;8:361–7.
22. Burt HM, Jackson JK, Rowell J. Calcium pyrophosphate and monosodium urate crystal interactions with neutrophils: effect of crystal size and lipoprotein binding crystals. J Rheumatol 1989;16:809–17.
23. Beck C, Morbach H, Richl P, et al. How can calcium pyrophosphate crystals induce inflammation in hypophosphatasia or chronic inflammatory joint diseases? Rheumatol Int 2009;29:229–38.
24. McCarty DJ. Calcium pyrophosphate dihydrate crystal deposition disease: 1975. Arthritis Rheum 1976;19:275–85.
25. Liote F, Ea HK. Recent developments in crystal-induced inflammation pathogenesis and management. Curr Rheumatol Rep 2007;9:243–50.
26. Akahoshi T, Murakami Y, Kitasato H. Recent advances in crystal-induced acute inflammation. Curr Opin Rheumatol 2007;19:146–50.
27. Martin WJ, Harper JL. Innate inflammation and resolution in acute gout. Immunol Cell Biol 2010;88:15–9.
28. VanItallie TB. Gout: epitome of painful arthritis. Metabolism 2010;59(Suppl. 1):S32–6.
29. Busso N, So A. Mechanisms of inflammation in gout. Arthritis Res Ther 2010;12:206.
30. Liu-Bryan R, Liote F. Monosodium urate and calcium pyrophosphate dihydrate (CPPD) crystals, inflammation, and cellular signaling. Joint Bone Spine J 2005;72:295–302.
31. Liu-Bryan R, Pritzker K, Firestein GS, et al. TLR2 signaling in chondrocytes drives calcium pyrophosphate dihydrate and monosodium urate crystal-induced nitric oxide generation. J Immunol 2005;174:5016–23.
32. Cherian PV, Schumacher Jr HR. Immunochemical and ultrastructural characterization of serum proteins associated with monosodium urate crystals (MSU) in synovial fluid cells from patients with gout. Ultrastruct Pathol 1986;10:209–19.
33. Spilberg I. Current concepts of the mechanism of acute inflammation in gouty arthritis. Arthritis Rheum 1975;18:129–34.
34. Dinarello CA. How interleukin-1beta induces gouty arthritis. Arthritis Rheum 2010;62:3140–4.
35. Joosten LA, Netea MG, Mylona E, et al. Engagement of fatty acids with Toll-like receptor 2 drives interleukin-1beta production via the ASC/caspase 1 pathway in monosodium urate monohydrate crystal-induced gouty arthritis. Arthritis Rheum 2010;62:3237–48.
36. Pritzker KPH, Amjad Z. Calcium Pyrophosphate Crystal Formation and Dissolution. Boston, MA: Kluwer Academic Publishers; 1998:277–301.
37. Hasselbacher P. C3 activation by monosodium urate monohydrate and other crystalline material. Arthritis Rheum 1979;22:571–8.
38. Hasselbacher P. Binding of IgG and complement protein by monosodium urate monohydrate and other crystals. J Lab Clin Med 1979;94:532–41.
39. Hasselbacher P, Schumacher HR. Immunoglobulin in tophi and on the surface of monosodium urate crystals. Arthritis Rheum 1978;21:353–61.
40. Popa-Nita O, Naccache PH. Crystal-induced neutrophil activation. Immunol Cell Biol 2010;88:32–40.
41. Burt HM, Kalkman PH, Mauldin D. Membranolytic effects of crystalline monosodium urate monohydrate. J Rheumatol 1983;10:440–8.
42. Andrews R, Phelps P. Release of lysosomal enzymes from polymorphonuclear leukocytes (PMN) after phagocytosis of monosodium urate (MSU) and calcium pyrophosphate dihydrate (CPPD) crystals: effect of colchicine and indomethacin. Arthritis Rheum 1971;14:368.

43. Shi Y, Mucsi AD, Ng G. Monosodium urate crystals in inflammation and immunity. Immunol Rev 2010;233:203–17.
44. Ng G, Chau EM, Shi Y. Recent developments in immune activation by uric acid crystals. Arch Immunol Ther Exp (Warsz) 2010;58:273–7.
45. Latz E. The inflammasomes: mechanisms of activation and function. Curr Opin Immunol 2010;22:28–33.
46. Liu-Bryan R. Intracellular innate immunity in gouty arthritis: role of NALP3 inflammasome. Immunol Cell Biol 2010;88:20–3.
47. Ginsberg MH, Kozin F, Chow D, et al. Adsorption of polymorphonuclear leukocyte lysosomal enzymes to monosodium urate crystals. Arthritis Rheum 1977;20:1538–42.
48. Ortiz-Bravo E, Sieck MS, Schumacher Jr HR. Changes in the proteins coating monosodium urate crystals during active and subsiding inflammation. Immunogold studies of synovial fluid from patients with gout and of fluid obtained using the rat subcutaneous air pouch model. Arthritis Rheum 1993;36:1274–85.
49. Brandt K. Modification of chemotaxis by synovial fluid hyaluronate. Arthritis Rheum 1970;13:2.
50. Garrod AB. Observations on certain pathological conditions of the blood and urine, in gout, rheumatism, and Bright's disease. Med Chir Trans 1848;31:83–97.
51. Garrod AB. On gout and rheumatism. the differential diagnosis, and the nature of the so-called rheumatic gout. Med Chir Trans 1854;37:181–220.
52. Luff AP. The Goulstonian Lectures on the Chemistry and Pathology of Gout: delivered before the Royal College of Physicians, March, 1897. Br Med J 1897;1:904–7.
53. Luff AP. The Goulstonian Lectures in the Chemistry and Pathology of Gout: delivered before the Royal College of Physicians, March, 1897. Br Med J 1897;1:838–42.
54. Luff AP. The Goulstonian Lectures on the Chemistry and Pathology of Gout: delivered before the Royal College of Physicians, March, 1897. Br Med J 1897;1:769–72.
55. Meldon A. Pathology and treatment of gout. Br Med J 1881;1:466–7.
56. Nowatzky J, Howard R, Pillinger MH, et al. The role of uric acid and other crystals in osteoarthritis. Curr Rheumatol Rep 2010;12:142–8.
57. Barwell RA. Treatise on Diseases of the Joints. New York, NY: William Wood & Co; 1881:252–73.
58. Pritzker KP. Gout and the gullible. J Rheumatol 1994;21:2175–6.
59. Perez-Ruiz F. Treating to target: a strategy to cure gout. Rheumatology (Oxf) 2009;48(Suppl. 2):ii9–14.
60. Wilcox WR, Khalaf AA. Nucleation of monosodium urate crystals. Ann Rheum Dis 1975;34:332–9.
61. Howell RR, Eanes ED, Seegmiller JE. X-ray diffraction studies of the tophaceous deposits in gout. Arthritis Rheum 1963;6:97–103.
62. Simkin PA. Local concentration of urate in the pathogenesis of gout. Lancet 1973;2:1295–8.
63. McCarty Jr DJ, Gatter RA, Brill JM, et al. Crystal deposition diseases: sodium urate (gout) and calcium pyrophosphate (chondrocalcinosis, pseudogout). JAMA 1965;193:129–32.
64. Simkin PA. The pathogenesis of podagra. Ann Intern Med 1977;86:230–3.
65. Seegmiller JE. The acute attack of gouty arthritis. Arthritis Rheum 1965;8:714–25.
66. Malawista SE. Gouty inflammation. Arthritis Rheum 1977;20:9.
67. Riddle JM, Bluhm GB, Barnhart MI. Ultrastructural study of leucocytes and urates in gouty arthritis. Ann Rheum Dis 1967;26:389–401.
68. Shirahama T, Cohen AS. Ultrastructural evidence for leakage of lysosomal contents after phagocytosis of monosodium urate crystals. A mechanism of gouty inflammation. Am J Pathol 1974;76:501–20.
69. Rajan KT. Observations on phagocytosis of urate crystals by polymorphonuclear leucocytes. Ann Rheum Dis 1975;34:54–61.
70. Agudelo CA, Schumacher HR. The synovitis of acute gouty arthritis. A light and electron microscopic study. Hum Pathol 1973;4:265–79.
71. Schumacher HR. Pathology of the synovial membrane in gout. Light and electron microscopic studies. Interpretation of crystals in electron micrographs. Arthritis Rheum 1975;18:771–82.
72. Lurie DP, Musil G. Staphylococcal septic arthritis presenting as acute flare of pseudogout: clinical, pathological and arthroscopic findings with a review of the literature. J Rheumatol 1983;10:503–6.
73. Weng CT, Liu MF, Lin LH, et al. Rare coexistence of gouty and septic arthritis: a report of 14 cases. Clin Exp Rheumatol 2009;27:902–6.
74. Brandt KD. The effect of synovial hyaluronate on the ingestion of monosodium urate crystals by leukocytes. Clin Chim Acta 1974;55:307–15.
75. Katz WA. Deposition of urate crystals in gout. Altered connective tissue metabolism. Arthritis Rheum 1975;18:751–6.
76. Barthelemy CR, Nakayama DA, Carrera GF, et al. Gouty arthritis: a prospective radiographic evaluation of sixty patients. Skeletal Radiol 1984;11:1–8.
77. Perez-Ruiz F, Dalbeth N, Urresola A, et al. Imaging of gout: findings and utility. Arthritis Res Ther 2009;11:232.
78. Weinberger A, Schumacher HR. Urate crystals in asymptomatic metatarsophalangeal joints. Ann Intern Med 1979;91(1):56–7.
79. Rouault T, Caldwell DS, Holmes EW. Aspiration of the asymptomatic metatarsophalangeal joint in gout patients and hyperuricemic controls. Arthritis Rheum 1982;25(2):209–12.
80. Gordon TP, Bertouch JV, Walsh BR, et al. Monosodium urate crystals in asymptomatic knee joints. J Rheumatol 1982;9:967–9.
81. Pascual E. Persistence of monosodium urate crystals and low-grade inflammation in the synovial fluid of patients with untreated gout. Arthritis Rheum 1991;34:141–5.
82. Lichtenstein L, Scott HW, Levin MH. Pathologic changes in gout. Am J Pathol 1956;XXXII:871–95.
83. Sokoloff L. The pathology of gout. Metabolism 1957;6:230–43.
84. Sokoloff L. Pathology of gout. Arthritis Rheum 1965;8:707–13.
85. Hollingworth P, Scott JT, Burry HC. Nonarticular gout: hyperuricemia and tophus formation without gouty arthritis. Arthritis Rheum 1983;26:98–101.
86. Ebstein W. Der Natur und Behandlung der Gicht Dtsch med Wochenschr 1882;8:683–683 Georg Thieme Verlag.
87. Hiss W. Schicksal und Wirkungen des Sauren Harnsauren Natrons in Bauch-und Gelenkhohale des Kaminchens. Deutches Arch Klin Med 1900;67.
88. Freudweiler M. Studies on the nature of gouty tophi. Deutsches Arch Klin Med 1899;63.
89. Freudweiler M. Experimentelle Inersuchungen uber die Entstehung der Gichtknoten. Deutches Arch Klin Med 1901;69.
90. Brill JM, McCarty DJ. "Studies on the nature of Gouty Tophi" by Max Freudweiler. Ann Intern Med 1964;60:19.
91. Brill JM, McCarty DJ. "Experimental Investigations into the origin of gouty tophi" by Max Freudweiler. Arthritis Rheum 1965;8:18.
92. Kawenoki-Minc E, Maldyk E, Polowiec Z. Consecutive stages of arthropathy progression in patients with gout. Z Rheumatol 1977;36:106–11.
93. Kunkel G. Tophaceous gout mimicking osteomyelitis: the value of musculoskeletal ultrasound in establishing the diagnosis. J Clin Rheumatol 2010;16:295–7.
94. Cortet B, Duquesnoy B, Amoura I, et al. Ankylosing gout. Apropos of 2 cases. Rev Rhum Ed Fr 1994;61:49–52.
95. Nguyen C, Ea HK, Palazzo E, et al. Tophaceous gout: an unusual cause of multiple fractures. Scand J Rheumatol 2010;39:93–6.
96. Palmer DG, Highton J, Hessian PA. Development of the gout tophus. An hypothesis. Am J Clin Pathol 1989;91:190–5.
97. Dalbeth N, Pool B, Gamble GD, et al. Cellular characterization of the gouty tophus: a quantitative analysis. Arthritis Rheum 2010;62:1549–56.
98. Diaz-Flores LL, Alonso J, Camara J, et al. Gout tophi histogenesis based on its light and electron microscopy. Morfol Normal Patolog 1977;1:16.
99. Rajamaki K, Lappalainen J, Oorni K, et al. Cholesterol crystals activate the NLRP3 inflammasome in human macrophages: a novel link between cholesterol metabolism and inflammation. PLoS One 2010;5:e11765.
100. Pritzker KP, Fam AG, Omar SA, et al. Experimental cholesterol crystal arthropathy. J Rheumatol 1981;8:281–90.
101. Abela GS. Cholesterol crystals piercing the arterial plaque and intima trigger local and systemic inflammation. J Clin Lipidol 2010;4:156–64.
102. de Avila Fernandes E, Kubota ES, Sandim GB, et al. Ultrasound features of tophi in chronic tophaceous gout. Skeletal Radiol 2010;40:309–15.
103. Schlesinger N, Thiele RG. The pathogenesis of bone erosions in gouty arthritis. Ann Rheum Dis 2010;69:1907–12.
104. Talbott JH, Altman RD, Yu TF. Gouty arthritis masquerading as rheumatoid arthritis or vice versa. Semin Arthritis Rheum 1978;8:77–114.
105. Holland NW, Jost D, Beutler A, et al. Finger pad tophi in gout. J Rheumatol 1996;23:690–2.
106. Shmerling RH, Stern SH, Gravallese EM, et al. Tophaceous deposition in the finger pads without gouty arthritis. Arch Intern Med 1988;148:1830–2.
107. Patel GK, Davies WL, Price PP, et al. Ulcerated tophaceous gout. Int Wound J 2010;7:423–7.
108. Saketkoo LA, Robertson HJ, Dyer HR, et al. Axial gouty arthropathy. Am J Med Sci 2009;338:140–6.
109. Fam AG, Stein J, Rubenstein J. Gouty arthritis in nodal osteoarthritis. J Rheumatol 1996;23:684–9.
110. Pritzker KP. Calcium pyrophosphate dihydrate crystal deposition and other crystal deposition diseases. Curr Opin Rheumatol 1994;6:442–7.
111. Jones AC, Chuck AJ, Arie EA, et al. Diseases associated with calcium pyrophosphate deposition disease. Semin Arthritis Rheum 1992;22:188–202.
112. Abhishek A, Doherty M. Pathophysiology of articular chondrocalcinosis: role of ANKH. Nat Rev Rheumatol 2010;7(2):96–104.

113. Beutler A, Rothfuss S, Clayburne G, et al. Calcium pyrophosphate dihydrate crystal deposition in synovium. Relationship to collagen fibers and chondrometaplasia. Arthritis Rheum 1993;36:704–15.

114. Xu Y, Pritzker KP, Cruz TF. Characterization of chondrocyte alkaline phosphatase as a potential mediator in the dissolution of calcium pyrophosphate dihydrate crystals. J Rheumatol 1994;21:912–9.

115. Boskey AL. Pathogenesis of cartilage calcification: mechanisms of crystal deposition in cartilage. Curr Rheumatol Rep 2002;4:245–51.

116. Hunter GK, Grynpas MD, Cheng PT, et al. Effect of glycosaminoglycans on calcium pyrophosphate crystal formation in collagen gels. Calcif Tissue Int 1987;41:164–70.

117. Cheng PT, Pritzker KPH. Inhibition of calcium pyrophosphate dihydrate crystal formation: effects of carboxylate ions. Calcif Tiss Int 1988;42:46–52.

118. Cheng PT, Pritzker KPH. The effect of calcium and magnesium ions on calcium pyrophosphate crystal formation in aqueous solutions. J Rheumatol 1981;8:772–82.

119. Cheng PT, Pritzker KP. Pyrophosphate, phosphate ion interaction: effects on calcium pyrophosphate and calcium hydroxyapatite crystal formation in aqueous solutions. J Rheumatol 1983;10:769–77.

120. Garimella R, Bi X, Anderson HC. Nature of phosphate substrate as a major determinant of mineral type formed in matrix vesicle-mediated in vitro mineralization: an FTIR imaging study. Bone 2006;38:811–7.

121. Thouverey C, Bechkoff G, Pikula S, et al. Inorganic pyrophosphate as a regulator of hydroxyapatite or calcium pyrophosphate dihydrate mineral deposition by matrix vesicles. Osteoarthrit Cartil 2009;17:64–72.

122. Grahame R, Sutor DJ, Mitchener MB. Crystal deposition in hyperparathyroidism. Ann Rheum Dis 1971;30:597–604.

123. Cheng PT, Pritzker KP, Adams ME, et al. Calcium pyrophosphate crystal formation in aqueous solutions. J Rheumatol 1980;7:609–16.

124. Milazzo SC, Ahern MJ, Cleland LG, et al. Calcium pyrophosphate dihydrate deposition disease and familial hypomagnesemia. J Rheumatol 1981;8: 767–71.

125. Gutierrez M, Silveri F, Bertolazzi C, et al. Gitelman syndrome, calcium pyrophosphate dihydrate deposition disease and crowned dens syndrome. A new association? Rheumatology (Oxf) 2010;49:610–3.

126. Terkeltaub R. Pseudogout, hypomagnesemia, and liver transplantation. Curr Rheumatol Rep 2002;4:243–4.

127. Dorwart BB, Schumacher HR. Joint effusions, chondrocalcinosis and other rheumatic manifestations in hypothyroidism. A clinicopathologic study. Am J Med 1975;59:780–90.

128. Atkins CJ, McIvor J, Smith PM, et al. Chondrocalcinosis and arthropathy: studies in haemochromatosis and in idiopathic chondrocalcinosis. Q J Med 1970;39:71–82.

129. Cheng PT, Pritzker KPH. Ferrous Fe++ but not ferric Fe+++ ions inhibit de novo formation of calcium pyrophosphate dihydrate crystals: possible relationships to chondrocalcinosis and hemochromatosis. J Rheumatol 1988;15:321–4.

130. Costello JC, Rosenthal AK, Kurup IV, et al. Parallel regulation of extracellular ATP and inorganic pyrophosphate: roles of growth factors, transduction modulators, and ANK. Connect Tiss Res 2011;52(2):139–461.

131. Rosenthal AK, Hempel D, Kurup IV, et al. Purine receptors modulate chondrocyte extracellular inorganic pyrophosphate production. Osteoarthrit Cartil 2010;18:1496–501.

132. Xu Y, Cruz TF, Pritzker KP. Alkaline phosphatase dissolves calcium pyrophosphate dihydrate crystals. J Rheumatol 1991;18:1606–10.

133. Caswell A, Guilland-Cumming DF, Hearn PR, et al. Pathogenesis of chondrocalcinosis and pseudogout. Metabolism of inorganic pyrophosphate and production of calcium pyrophosphate dihydrate crystals. Ann Rheum Dis 1983;42(Suppl. 1):27–37.

134. So PP, Tsui FW, Vieth R, et al. Inhibition of alkaline phosphatase by cysteine: implications for calcium pyrophosphate dihydrate crystal deposition disease. J Rheumatol 2007;34:1313–22.

135. Kannampuzha JV, Tupy JH, Pritzker KP. Mercaptopyruvate inhibits tissue-nonspecific alkaline phosphatase and calcium pyrophosphate dihydrate crystal dissolution. J Rheumatol 2009;36:2758–65.

136. Nagahara N, Sawada N. The mercaptopyruvate pathway in cysteine catabolism: a physiologic role and related disease of the multifunctional 3-mercaptopyruvate sulfurtransferase. Curr Med Chem 2006;13:1219–30.

137. Cailotto F, Bianchi A, Sebillaud S, et al. Inorganic pyrophosphate generation by transforming growth factor-beta-1 is mainly dependent on ANK induction by Ras/Raf-1/extracellular signal-regulated kinase pathways in chondrocytes. Arthritis Res Ther 2007;9:R122.

138. Hamade T, Bianchi A, Sebillaud S, et al. Inorganic phosphate (Pi) modulates the expression of key regulatory proteins of the inorganic pyrophosphate (PPi) metabolism in TGF-beta1-stimulated chondrocytes. Biomed Mater Eng 2010;20:209–15.

139. Cailotto F, Sebillaud S, Netter P, et al. The inorganic pyrophosphate transporter ANK preserves the differentiated phenotype of articular chondrocyte. J Biol Chem 2010;285:10572–82.

140. Stockwell R. Biology of Cartilage Cells. Cambridge: UK. Cambridge University Press; 1979:25.

141. Keen CE, Crocker PR, Brady K, et al. Calcium pyrophosphate dihydrate deposition disease: morphological and microanalytical features. Histopathology 1991;19:529–36.

142. Pritzker KPH, Cheng PT, Renlund RC. Calcium pyrophosphate crystal deposition in hyaline cartilage: ultrastructural analysis and implications for pathogenesis. J Rheumatol 1988;15:828–35.

143. Ishikawa K, Masuda I, Ohira T, et al. A histological study of calcium pyrophosphate dihydrate crystal-deposition disease. J Bone Joint Surg Am 1989;71:875–86.

144. Masuda I, Koichiro I, Usuku G. A histologic and immunohistochemical study of calcium pyrophosphate dihydrate crystal deposition disease. Clin Orthop Rel Res 1991;263:272–87.

145. Stockwell RA. Biology of Cartilage Cells. Cambridge, UK: Cambridge University Press; 1979: 256.

146. Ohira T, Ishikawa K, Masuda I, et al. Histologic localization of lipid in the articular tissues in calcium pyrophosphate dihydrate crystal deposition disease. Arthritis Rheum 1988;31:1057–62.

147. Bundens Jr WD, Brighton CT, Weitzman G. Primary articular-cartilage calcification with arthritis (pseudogout syndrome). J Bone Joint Surg Am 1965;47:111–22.

148. Pritzker KP. Calcium pyrophosphate crystal arthropathy: a biomineralization disorder. Hum Pathol 1986;17:543–5.

149. Lagier R. L'approche anatomo-pathologique du concept de chondrocalcinose articulaire. Rhumatologie 1981;33:18.

150. Schumacher HR. Ultrastructural findings in chondrocalcinosis and pseudogout. Arthritis Rheum 1976;19(Suppl. 3):413–25.

151. Bjelle AO. Morphological study of articular cartilage in pyrophosphate arthropathy. (Chondrocalcinosis articularis or calcium pyrophosphate dihydrate crystal deposition diseases). Ann Rheum Dis 1972;31:449–56.

152. Bjelle AO, Sundstrom KG. An ultrastructural study of the articular cartilage in calcium pyrophosphate dihydrate (CPPD) crystal deposition disease (chondrocalcinosis articularis). Calcif Tiss Res 1975;19:63–71.

153. Bjelle A. Cartilage matrix in hereditary pyrophosphate arthropathy. J Rheumatol 1981;8:959–64.

154. Bjelle AO. The glycosaminoglycans of articular cartilage in calcium pyrophosphate dihydrate (CPPD) crystal deposition disease (chondrocalcinosis articularis or pyrophosphate arthropathy. Calcif Tiss Int 1973;12: 37–46.

155. Mitrovic DR. Pathology of articular deposition of calcium salts and their relationship to osteoarthrosis. Ann Rheum Dis 1983;42(Suppl. 1):19–26.

156. Pritzker KPH. Aging and degeneration in the lumbar intervertebral disc. Orthop Clin North Am 1977;8:66–77.

157. Howell DS. Articular cartilage calcification and matrix vesicles. Curr Rheumatol Rep 2002;4:265–9.

158. Anderson HC. Matrix vesicles and calcification. Curr Rheumatol Rep 2003;5:222–6.

159. Anderson HC, Harmey D, Camacho NP, et al. Sustained osteomalacia of long bones despite major improvement in other hypophosphatasia-related mineral deficits in tissue nonspecific alkaline phosphatase/nucleotide pyrophosphatase phosphodiesterase 1 double-deficient mice. Am J Pathol 2005;166:1711–20.

160. Anderson HC, Mulhall D, Garimella R. Role of extracellular membrane vesicles in the pathogenesis of various diseases, including cancer, renal diseases, atherosclerosis, and arthritis. Lab Invest 2010;90:1549–57.

161. Pritzker KP, Cheng PT, Adams ME, et al. Calcium pyrophosphate dihydrate crystal formation in model hydrogels. J Rheumatol 1978;5:469–73.

162. Omar SA, Cheng PT, Nyburg SC, et al. Application of scanning and transmission electron microscopy, x-ray energy spectroscopy, and x-ray diffraction to calcium pyrophosphate crystal formation in vitro. Scand Electron Microsc 1979:745–9.

163. Pritzker KP, Cheng PT, Omar SA, et al. Calcium pyrophosphate crystal formation in model hydrogels. II. Hyaline articular cartilage as a gel. J Rheumatol 1981;8:451–5.

164. Pritzker KPH, Cheng PT, Hunter GK, et al. In Vitro and In Vivo Models of Calcium Pyrophosphate Crystal Formation. Birmingham, UK. Ebsco Media; 1985:381-4.

165. Grynpas MD, Cheng PT, Pritzker KPH. Dissolution of calcium pyrophosphate crystals by free radicals generated by neutron irradiation. J Rheumatol 1987;14:1073–4.

166. Xu Y, Cruz T, Cheng PT, et al. Effects of pyrophosphatase on dissolution of calcium pyrophosphate dihydrate crystals. J Rheumatol 1991;18:66–71.

167. Shinozaki T, Pritzker KP. Regulation of alkaline phosphatase: implications for calcium pyrophosphate dihydrate crystal dissolution and other alkaline phosphatase functions. J Rheumatol 1996;23:677–83.

168. Holmyard DP, Shinozaki T, Pritzker KPH. FE-SEM examination of calcium pyrophosphate dihydrate crystal dissolution. Proc Microsc Soc Can 1997;24:86–7.

169. Shinozaki T, Pritzker KP. Polyamines enhance calcium pyrophosphate dihydrate crystal dissolution. J Rheumatol 1995;22:1907–12.

170. Bennett RM, Lehr JR, McCarty DJ. Crystal shedding and acute pseudogout. An hypothesis based on a therapeutic failure. Arthritis Rheum 1976;19: 93–7.

171. Boivin G, Lagier R. An ultrastructural study of articular chondrocalcinosis in cases of knee osteoarthritis. Virchows Arch A Pathol Anat Histopathol 1983;400:13–29.

172. Gerster JC, Baud CA, Lagier R, et al. Tendon calcifications in chondrocalcinosis. A clinical, radiologic, histologic, and crystallographic study. Arthritis Rheum 1977;20:717–22.

173. Gerster JC, Lagier R, Boivin G. Achilles tendinitis associated with chondrocalcinosis. J Rheumatol 1980;7:82–8.

174. Gerster JC, Lagier R, Boivin G, et al. Carpal tunnel syndrome in chondrocalcinosis of the wrist. Clinical and histologic study. Arthritis Rheum 1980;23:926–31.

175. Lagier R, Wildi E. Incidence of chondrocalcinosis in a series of 1,000 surgically excised intervertebral disks. Rev Rhum Mal Osteoartic 1979;46: 303–7.

176. Lagier R, MacGee W. Erosive intervertebral osteochondrosis in association with generalized osteoarthritis and chondrocalcinosis; anatomico-radiological study of a case. Z Rheumatol 1979;38:405–14.

177. Mohr W, Oehler K, Hersener J, et al. Chondrocalcinose der Zwischenwirbelscheiben. Z Rheumatol 1979;38:16.

178. Kandel RA, Renlund RC, Cheng PT, et al. Calcium pyrophosphate dihydrate crystal deposition disease with concurrent vertebral hypertosis in a barbary ape. Arthritis Rheum 1983;26:682–7.

179. Renlund RC, Pritzker KP, Cheng PT, et al. Rhesus monkeys (Macaca mulatta) as a model for calcium pyrophosphate dihydrate crystal deposition disease. J Lab Invest 1985;52:155.

180. Renlund RC, Pritzker KPH, Kessler MJ. Rhesus monkey (Macaca mulatta) as a model for calcium pyrophosphate dihydrate crystal deposition disease. J Med Primatol 1986;15:11–6.

181. Roberts ED, Baskin GB, Watson E, et al. Calcium pyrophosphate deposition disease (CPPD) in nonhuman primates. Am J Pathol 1984;116:359–61.

182. Roberts ED, Baskin GB, Watson E, et al. Calcium pyrophosphate deposition in non-human primates. Vet Pathol 1984;21:592–6.

183. Gibson JP, Roenigk WJ. Pseudogout in a dog. J Am Vet Med Assoc 1972;161:912–5.

184. de Haan JJ, Andreasen CB. Calcium crystal-associated arthropathy (pseudogout) in a dog. J Am Vet Med Assoc 1992;200:943–6.

185. Yosipovitch ZH, Glimcher MJ. Articular chondrocalcinosis, hydroxyapatite deposition disease, in adult mature rabbits. J Bone Joint Surg Am 1972;54:841–53.

186. Liu R, O'Connell M, Johnson K, et al. Extracellular signal-regulated kinase 1/extracellular signal-regulated kinase 2 mitogen-activated protein kinase signaling and activation of activator protein 1 and nuclear factor kappaB transcription factors play central roles in interleukin-8 expression stimulated by monosodium urate monohydrate and calcium pyrophosphate crystals in monocytic cells. Arthritis Rheum 2000;43:1145–55.

187. Frischnecht J, Steigerwald JC. High synovial fluid white blood cell counts in pseudogout; Possible confusion with septic arthritis. Arch Intern Med 1975;135:298–9.

188. Bjelle A, Crocker P, Willoughby D. Ultra-microcrystals in pyrophosphate arthropathy. Crystal identification and case report. Acta Med Scand 1980;207:89–92.

189. Gerster JC, Lagier R, Boivin G. Olecranon bursitis related to calcium pyrophosphate dihydrate crystal deposition disease. Arthritis Rheum 1982;25:989–96.

190. Hogan DB, Pritzker KP. Synovial fluid analysis: another look at the mucin clot test. J Rheumatol 1985;12:242–4.

191. Pritzker KP. Crystal-associated arthropathies: what's new in old joints. J Am Geriatr Soc 1980;28:439–45.

192. Renlund RC, Pritzker KPH, Kessler MJ. Calcium pyrophosphate dihydrate crystal deposition disease: a common disease of aging human and non-human primates. Lab Investig 1989;60:78A.

193. Pritzker KPH, Nyburg SC, et al. Intervertebral disc calcifications in the elderly: calcium pyrophosphate dihydrate arthropathy. Lab Investig 1977; 36:1.

194. Pritzker KPH, Renlund RC, Cheng P-T, et al. Calcium pyrophosphate crystal arthropathy in femoral heads. Lab Investig 1980;42:1.

195. Mohr WH, Wilke W, Weinland G, et al. Pseudogicht (Chondrokalzinose). Z Rheumatol 1974;33:23.

196. Wilkins E, Dieppe P, Maddison P, et al. Osteoarthritis and articular chondrocalcinosis in the elderly. Ann Rheum Dis 1983;42:280–4.

197. Dieppe PA, Alexander GJ, Jones HE, et al. Pyrophosphate arthropathy: a clinical and radiological study of 105 cases. Ann Rheum Dis 1982;41: 371–6.

198. Doherty M, Dieppe P, Watt I. Pyrophosphate arthropathy: a prospective study. Br J Rheumatol 1993;32:189–96.

199. Ellman MH, Levin B. Chondrocalcinosis in elderly persons. Arthritis Rheum 1975;18:43–7.

200. Memin Y, Monville C, Ryckewaert A. Articular chondrocalcinosis after 80 years of age. Rev Rhum Mal Osteoartic 1978;45:77–82.

201. Mitrovic DR, Stankovic A, Iriarte-Borda O, et al. The prevalence of chondrocalcinosis in the human knee joint. An autopsy survey. J Rheumatol 1988;15:633–41.

202. Steinbach LS, Resnick D. Calcium pyrophosphate dihydrate crystal deposition disease revisited. Radiology 1996;200:1–9.

203. Genant HK. Roentgenographic aspects of calcium pyrophosphate dihydrate crystal deposition disease (pseudogout). Arthritis Rheum 1976;19(Suppl. 3):307–28.

204. Gutierrez M, Di Geso L, Filippucci E, et al. Calcium pyrophosphate crystals detected by ultrasound in patients without radiographic evidence of cartilage calcifications. J Rheumatol 2010;37:2602–3.

205. Mitsuyama H, Healey RM, Terkeltaub RA, et al. Calcification of human articular knee cartilage is primarily an effect of aging rather than osteoarthritis. Osteoarthr Cartil 2007;15:559–65.

206. Neogi T, Nevitt M, Niu J, et al. Lack of association between chondrocalcinosis and increased risk of cartilage loss in knees with osteoarthritis: results of two prospective longitudinal magnetic resonance imaging studies. Arthritis Rheum 2006;54:1822–8.

207. Ea HK, Nguyen C, Bazin D, et al. Articular cartilage calcification in osteoarthritis: insights into crystal-induced stress. Arthritis Rheum 2011;63: 10–8.

208. Schlesinger N, Hassett AL, Neustadter L, et al. Does acute synovitis (pseudogout) occur in patients with chronic pyrophosphate arthropathy (pseudo-osteoarthritis)? Clin Exp Rheumatol 2009;27:940–4.

209. Reuge L, Van Linthoudt D, Gerster JC. Local deposition of calcium pyrophosphate crystals in evolution of knee osteoarthritis. Clin Rheumatol 2001;20:428–31.

210. Halverson PB, McCarty DJ. Patterns of radiographic abnormalities associated with basic calcium phosphate and calcium pyrophosphate dihydrate crystal deposition in the knee. Ann Rheum Dis 1986;45:603–5.

211. Pritzker KP, et al. Osteoarthritis and calcium pyrophosphate dihydrate crystal arthropathy. Osteoarthr Cartil 2004;12:1.

212. Resnick D, Niwayama G, Goergen TG, et al. Clinical, radiographic and pathologic abnormalities in calcium pyrophosphate dihydrate deposition disease (CPPD): pseudogout. Radiology 1977;122:1–15.

213. Bird HA, Tribe CR, Bacon PA. Joint hypermobility leading to osteoarthrosis and chondrocalcinosis. Ann Rheum Dis 1978;37:203–11.

214. Pritzker KP, Gay S, Jimenez SA, et al. Osteoarthritis cartilage histopathology: grading and staging. Osteoarthr Cartil 2006;14:13–29.

215. Pritzker KPH, Chateauvert JMD, Grynpas MD. Osteoarthritic cartilage contains increased calcium, magnesium and phosphorus. J Rheumatol 1987;14:806–10.

216. Fam AG, Morava-Protzner I, Purcell C, et al. Acceleration of experimental lapine osteoarthritis by calcium pyrophosphate microcrystalline synovitis. Arthritis Rheum 1995;38:201–10.

217. Dieppe P, Campion G, Doherty M. Mixed crystal deposition. Rheum Dis Clin North Am 1988;14:415–26.

218. Rosenthal AK. Crystals, inflammation, and osteoarthritis. Curr Opin Rheumatol 2011;23(2):140–3.

219. Gerster JC, Varisco PA, Kern J, et al. CPPD crystal deposition disease in patients with rheumatoid arthritis. Clin Rheumatol 2006;25:468–9.

220. Su KY, Lee HT, Tsai CY. Recurrent calcium pyrophosphate dihydrate crystal deposition disease in a patient with rheumatoid arthritis–associated osteoporosis. Eur J Intern Med 2008;19:555–6.

221. Resnick D, Williams G, Weisman MH, et al. Rheumatoid arthritis and pseudo-rheumatoid arthritis in calcium pyrophosphate dihydrate crystal deposition disease. Radiology 1981;140:615–21.

222. Pritzker KPH, Phillips H, Luk SC, et al. Pseudotumor of temporomandibular joint: destructive calcium pyrophosphate dihydrate arthropathy. J Rheumatol 1976;3:70–81.

223. Ferrer-Roca O, Brancos MA, Franco M, et al. Massive articular chondro-calcinosis. Its occurrence with calcium pyrophosphate crystal deposits in nucleus pulposus. Arch Pathol Lab Med 1982;106:352–4.

224. Resnick D, Pineda C. Vertebral involvement in calcium pyrophosphate dihydrate crystal deposition disease. Radiographic-pathological correlation. Radiology 1984;153:55–60.

225. Sekijima Y, Yoshida T, Ikeda S. CPPD crystal deposition disease of the cervical spine: a common cause of acute neck pain encountered in the neurology department. J Neurol Sci 2010;296:79–82.

226. Fenoy AJ, Menezes AH, Donovan KA, et al. Calcium pyrophosphate dihydrate crystal deposition in the craniovertebral junction. J Neurosurg Spine 2008;8:22–9.

227. Salaffi F, Carotti M, Guglielmi G, et al. The crowned dens syndrome as a cause of neck pain: clinical and computed tomography study in patients with calcium pyrophosphate dihydrate deposition disease. Clin Exp Rheumatol 2008;26:1040–6.

228. Viana SL, Fernandes JL, De Araujo Coimbra PP, et al. The "crowned dens" revisited: imaging findings in calcium crystal deposition diseases around the odontoid. J Neuroimaging 2010;20:311–23.

229. Kawano N, Matsuno T, Miyazawa S, et al. Calcium pyrophosphate dihydrate crystal deposition disease in the cervical ligamentum flavum. J Neurosurg 1988;68:613–20.

230. Nagashima C, Takahama M, Shibata T, et al. Calcium pyrophosphate dihydrate deposits in the cervical ligamenta flava causing myeloradiculopathy. J Neurosurg 1984;60:69–80.

231. Mwaka ES, Yayama T, Uchida K, et al. Calcium pyrophosphate dihydrate crystal deposition in the ligamentum flavum of the cervical spine: histopathological and immunohistochemical findings. Clin Exp Rheumatol 2009;27:430–8.

232. Ariyoshi D, Imai K, Yamamoto S, et al. Subcutaneous tendon rupture of extensor tendons on bilateral wrists associated with calcium pyrophosphate crystal deposition disease. Mod Rheumatol 2007;17:348–51.

233. Linden B, Telhag H. Morphology and crystal composition of chondrocalcinosis after osteochondritis dissecans. Clin Orthop Relat Res 1977:243–7.

234. Doherty M, Watt I, Dieppe PA. Localised chondrocalcinosis in post-meniscectomy knees. Lancet 1982;1:1207–10.

235. Andres TL, Trainer TD. Intervertebral chondrocalcinosis: a coincidental finding possibly related to previous surgery. Arch Pathol Lab Med 1980;104:269–71.

236. Ellman MH, Vazques LT, Brown NL, et al. Calcium pyrophosphate dihydrate deposition in lumbar disc fibrocartilage. J Rheumatol 1981;8:955–8.

237. Doherty M, Watt I, Dieppe PA. Chondrocalcinosis and rapid destruction of the hip. J Rheumatol 1986;13:669–71.

238. Menkes C-JS, Chouraki M, Ecoffet M, et al. Les arthropies destructrices de la chondrocalcinose. Rev Rheumat 1973;40:9.

239. Gaucher A, Faure G, Netter P, et al. Identification of the crystals observed in the destructive arthropathies of chondrocalcinosis. Rev Rhum Mal Osteoartic 1977;44:407–14.

240. Villiaumey JG, Amourtoux J, Larget-Piet B, et al. Arthropathies Lytiques et Chondrocalcinose Articulare. Semin Hop Paris 1974;50:16.

241. Yamamoto T, Bullough PG. The role of subchondral insufficiency fracture in rapid destruction of the hip joint: a preliminary report. Arthritis Rheum 2000;43:2423–7.

242. Couto AR, Brown MA. Genetic factors in the pathogenesis of CPPD crystal deposition disease. Curr Rheumatol Rep 2007;9:231–6.

243. Eade AW, Swannell AJ, Williamson N. Pyrophosphate arthropathy in hypophosphatasia. Ann Rheum Dis 1981;40:164–170.

244. O'Duffy JD. Hypophosphatasia associated with calcium pyrophosphate dihydrate deposits in cartilage. Report of a case. Arthritis Rheum 1970;13:381–8.

245. Lambert RG, Becker EJ, Pritzker KP. Case report 597: Calcium pyrophosphate deposition disorder (CPPD) of the right temporomandibular joint. Skeletal Radiol 1990;19:139–141.

246. Sissons HA, Steiner GC, Bonar F, et al. Calcium pyrophosphate deposition disease. Skeletal Radiol 1989;18:79–87.

247. Yamakawa K, Iwasaki H, Ohjimi Y, et al. Tumoral calcium pyrophosphate dihydrate crystal deposition disease. A clinicopathologic analysis of five cases. Pathol Res Pract 2001;197:499–506.

248. Dijkgraaf LC, Liem RSB, De Bont LGM, et al. Calcium pyrophosphate dihydrate crystal deposition disease: a review of the literature and a light and electron microscopic study of a case of the temporomandibular joint with numerous intracellular crystals in the chondrocytes. Osteoarthr Cartil 1995;3:35–45.

249. Athanasou NA, Caughey M, Burge P, et al. Deposition of calcium pyrophosphate dihydrate crystals in a soft tissue chondroma. Ann Rheum Dis 1991;50:950–952.

250. Schumacher HR, Miller JL, Ludivico C, et al. Erosive arthritis associated with apatite crystal deposition. Arthritis Rheum 1981;24:31–37.

251. Schumacher HR, Somlyo AP, Tse RL, et al. Arthritis associated with apatite crystals. Ann Intern Med 1977;87:411–6.

252. Fam AG, Pritzker KPH, Stein JL, et al. Apatite-associated arthropathy: a clinical study of 14 cases and of 2 patients with calcific bursitis. J Rheumatol 1979;6:461–471.

253. Fam AG, Rubenstein J. Hydroxyapatite pseudopodagra. A syndrome of young women. Arthritis Rheum 1989;32:741–747.

254. Kandel RA, Cheng PT, Pritzker KPH. Localized apatite synovitis of the wrist. J Rheumatol 1986;13:667–9.

255. McCarty DJ, Halverson PB, Carrera GF, et al. "Milwaukee shoulder": association of microspheroids containing hydroxyapatite crystals, active collagenase, and neutral protease with rotator cuff defects. Arthritis Rheum 1981;24:464–473.

256. Molloy ES, McCarthy GM. Hydroxyapatite deposition disease of the joint. Curr Rheumatol Rep 2003;5:215–21.

257. Ohira T, Ishikawa K. Hydroxyapatite deposition in articular cartilage by intra-articular injections of methylprednisolone. A histological, ultrastructural, and x-ray microprobe analysis in rabbits. J Bone Joint Surg Am 1986;68:509–20.

258. Pritzker KPH, Luk SC. Apatite associated arthropathies: preliminary ultrastructural studies. Scan Electron Microsc 1976:493–500.

259. Fuerst M, Bertrand J, Lammers L, et al. Calcification of articular cartilage in human osteoarthritis. Arthritis Rheum 2009;60:2694–703.

260. Pritzker KP. Counterpoint: Hydroxyapatite crystal deposition is not intimately involved in the pathogenesis and progression of human osteoarthritis. Curr Rheumatol Rep 2009; 11:148–53.

261. McCarthy GM, Cheung HS. Point: Hydroxyapatite crystal deposition is intimately involved in the pathogenesis and progression of human osteoarthritis. Curr Rheumatol Rep 2009;11:141–147.

262. Yavorskyy A, Hernandez-Santana A, McCarthy G, et al. Detection of calcium phosphate crystals in the joint fluid of patients with osteoarthritis: analytical approaches and challenges. Analyst 2008;133:302–18.

263. Bondeson J, Blom AB, Wainwright S, et al. The role of synovial macrophages and macrophage-produced mediators in driving inflammatory and destructive responses in osteoarthritis. Arthritis Rheum 2010;62:647–57.

264. Liu YZ, Jackson AP, Cosgrove SD. Contribution of calcium-containing crystals to cartilage degradation and synovial inflammation in osteoarthritis. Osteoarthr Cartil 2009;17:1333–1340.

265. Simkin PA, Bassett JE, Lee QP. Not water, but formalin, dissolves urate crystals in tophaceous tissue samples. J Rheumatol 1994;21:2320–1.

266. Markel SF, Hart WR. Arthropathy in calcium pyrophosphate dihydrate crystal deposition disease. Pathologic study of 12 cases. Arch Pathol Lab Med 1982;106:529–33.

267. Bjelle A, Sundstrom B. Micro x-ray diffraction of cartilage biopsy specimens in articular chondrocalcinosis. Acta Pathol Microbiol Scand 1969;76:497–500.

Chapter 2

Synovial Fluid Crystal Analysis

Eliseo Pascual and Francisca Sivera

KEY POINTS

- The identification of monosodium urate (MSU) and calcium pyrophosphate dihydrate (CPPD) crystals in synovial fluid or tissue biopsy samples is central to the definitive diagnosis of gout and CPPD deposition disease.
- Basic calcium phosphate crystals are too small to be viewed with an optical microscope other than as crystal aggregates that appear as amorphous clumps.
- Synovial fluid crystal analysis performed with a compensated polarized light microscopy is the gold standard for identifying MSU and CPPD crystals and for distinguishing these pathologic crystals from a variety of other particles present in the synovial fluid. However, this simple and rapid diagnostic approach is markedly underused in clinical practice.
- The strong negative birefringence of MSU crystals and the weak positive birefringence of CPPD crystals, as well as differences in crystal shape under many, but not all, circumstances, helps distinguish MSU from CPPD crystals.
- A rotating microscope stage is helpful to distinguish MSU and CPPD crystals from birefringent debris in the joint fluid. MSU and CPPD crystals have characteristic angles of extinction of birefringence that can be seen when rotated between angles parallel and perpendicular to the axis of slow vibration of light of the first-order red plate compensator.

Introduction

The identification of monosodium urate (MSU) and calcium pyrophosphate dihydrate (CPPD) crystals is clinically relevant when performing a synovial fluid (SF) analysis for crystals. The search for apatite and other basic calcium phosphate (BCP) crystals remains of less certain clinical relevance at this point, but this issue is addressed in Chapter 22. BCP crystals are too small to be seen with an optical microscope as anything more, at the most, as crystal aggregates in amorphous clumps. The occasional finding of other, rarer crystals plays only an anecdotal role. Hence, this review focuses on the search for MSU and CPPD crystals.

SF analysis for crystals has received little critical attention since its initial description, and the technique remains essentially unchanged. Crystal identification in SF is included in the core curricula in rheumatology, by both the American College of Rheumatology[1] and the European Board of Rheumatology, UEMS Section of Rheumatology.[2] SF analysis is a simple procedure requiring only a microscope fitted with polarized filters and a first-order red compensator; the identification of MSU and CPPD crystals provides an unequivocal diagnosis of gout and CPPD crystal arthritis. Using an adequately equipped microscope in the clinic allows an immediate and definitive diagnosis of crystal arthritis. There is no other immediate procedure that allows such an unequivocal etiologic diagnosis in any other arthritic disease.

Despite its immediacy and elegance, SF analysis is inconsistently implanted among rheumatologists,[3] who as a community appear to have many that consider it dispensable. The reasons for this (other than the general low profile, in the past, of crystal arthritis) remain unclear, but as early as 1974 this lack of interest was noted.[4] The authors have participated in the organization and tutoring of a good number of introductory workshops on crystal identification, including those held at the European League Against Rheumatism (EULAR) international congress meetings since 2002; key difficulties encountered among the attendants include (1) lack of familiarity with the use of the microscope, (2) the widespread concept that SF analysis is impossible without the fully equipped compensated polarized microscope, which is unavailable in many units, and (3) (for younger trainees) the lack of interest of their senior colleagues. In this chapter, we will review the current state of MSU and CPPD crystal identification—with a short review of other, rarer crystals—and specifically focus on practical aspects. We will also address some of the difficulties likely to be encountered by trainees and other less-experienced users. Currently at EULAR workshops, the possibility of detecting both crystal types—and even quite reasonably of distinguishing MSU from CPPD—by means of an ordinary microscope is being highlighted, as well as the availability of simple polarized microscopy at most pathology departments. By providing motivated trainees with such simple starting tools, we hope that they will feel motivated to start by themselves and, if successful, will be encouraged to perfect their technique and then to acquire the microscope necessary to comply with the standards.

MSU crystals were first seen in the 17th century by the inventor of the modern microscope (Leeuwenhoek), and their inflammatory potential in animal models had been noted by the end of the 19th century. MSU crystals were first identified in SF samples from gouty patients with acute arthritis with the use of a compensated polarized microscope by Daniel McCarty, Jr.,[5] after being noted with the use of an ordinary microscope by his mentor, Joseph Hollander.[6] CPPD crystals were detected by McCarty while studying SF samples from patients with acute arthritis and presumed gout.[6-8] The nature of both the MSU and CPPD crystals was confirmed by their x-ray diffraction pattern and by the capability of uricase to dissolve MSU crystals.[9,10] However, their differing appearance and type of birefringence under the compensated polarized microscope allowed an easy and accurate distinction, and this microscope became the standard for crystal identification in SF.

MSU crystals in joint fluids have not been described outside of gout or some cases of asymptomatic hyperuricemia. Small numbers of CPPD crystals have been noted in the SF of patients with osteoarthritic joints[11] and in other conditions such as the "Milwaukee shoulder syndrome"[12] or in patients years after surgical knee meniscectomy[13]; the meaning of these findings remains undefined, and the identification of occasional CPPD crystals in a noninflammatory SF sample remains difficult to interpret. The presence of intracellular MSU and CPPD crystals in SF had been considered indicative of active joint inflammation of gout and pseudogout, but in SF drawn from asymptomatic joints, intracellular MSU and CPPD crystals are common in patients with gout and CPPD deposition disease.[14,15] Of interest, the presence of either type of crystal in asymptomatic joints is associated with mild subclinical inflammation, as shown by a raised cellularity.[15,16] Of particular clinical interest, when a joint containing either MSU or CPPD crystals is the seat of an infectious arthritis, the crystals will nevertheless be apparent in the SF analysis; if cultures are not obtained, the infection may easily be missed.

Crystal Identification, Validation Studies, and Quality Control

Real-life quality audits of SF analysis have been performed in Finland,[17,18] Sydney (Australia),[19] and different areas of the United States.[20,21] SF samples were sent to laboratories considered to routinely perform SF analysis; the results were then compared to a gold standard, obtained from an experienced analyst. Both false-negative and false-positive results are common in all studies, and the rate of correct MSU crystal identification can be as low as 50% in some laboratories. These studies show the status of crystal analysis in real life and the results are worrisome. The studies were performed a few decades ago, but there is little to indicate that circumstances have changed. Different issues—methodological and otherwise—could partly account for these poor results. Observers were not identified; therefore, training and experience could not be evaluated, and in some laboratories, as many as 12 people participated in the analysis of a single SF sample. The microscopes that were used were not evaluated, and in numerous cases the technique might not have been as recommended, with no first-order red compensator available[20] or with ordinary or simple polarized light inspection being omitted.[19] So, even though the study results are poor, we are left wondering what would happen if current standards were applied and observers were appropriately trained. These surveys highlight the need to implement quality control programs in SF analysis rather than evaluate the reliability of the technique itself.

At least two other studies have been undertaken to evaluate the reliability of crystal detection. In the largest study to date, six observers with different experiences evaluated 143 unstained slides with MSU crystals, CPPD crystals, or no crystals.[22] Results were unsatisfactory, with a low sensitivity for MSU detection and a moderate to low sensitivity and specificity for CPPD identification.[23] Crystals were synthetically fabricated and then added to samples of SF obtained from patients. Data must be interpreted with caution as synthetic crystals can be larger and more irregular in shape and the larger crystals remain outside the cells and are not phagocytosed. A curious finding was that the rheumatologist with many years of experience in SF analysis had the lowest false-positive ratio but was most likely to miss crystals at low concentrations, suggesting a greater reluctance to report occasional particles or equivocal findings. In a recent study, we have shown that for trained observers, the detection and identification of natural crystals in fresh SF samples can be a consistent procedure.[24] The training of the observers—four clinical analysis residents who were familiar with the ordinary microscope—consisted of a short course in crystal identification followed by a 3-month period of sample analysis. Then the participants examined 64 fresh SF samples containing MSU, CPPD, or no crystals. Sensitivities and specificities for both MSU and CPPD crystal identification were greater than 90%, although CPPD remained the more difficult crystal to identify.

Technical Considerations

The Microscope

Four microscope settings are useful in crystal analysis and in the training process: ordinary microscopy, simple polarized microscopy, compensated polarized microscopy (Fig. 2-1, *A* and *B*), and phase microscopy. These four settings are usually achieved with the same microscope and different filters, except phase microscopy, which requires specific lenses and condenser. The basic laboratory microscope of most brands can adapt polarized filters for simple polarized microscopy, and many can also incorporate a first-order compensator (also known as retardation plate or lambda [λ] plate) to allow for compensated light microscopy. Many microscopes can also be fitted with phase lenses and condenser; phase microscopy is good to have, especially at the learning stage, but it is not necessary for crystal analysis.

Before starting training on crystal analysis, it is necessary to become acquainted with the use of the ordinary light microscope. The initial tool for crystal analysis was the geological polarized microscope, fitted with a rotating stage. It allows measurement of the angle of extinction of the birefringence (see later) and allows orientation of the crystals in relation to the axis of the compensator through rotation of the stage. These measurements are especially useful when there is a need to distinguish among a number of different crystal types, as a geologist may need to do, but in the joint we are essentially concerned with MSU or CPPD crystals, from which artifacts or the sporadic previously injected corticosteroid crystals are readily distinguished. In this context, corticosteroid crystals such as those of triamcinolone often have bright positive birefringence rather than the weak positive birefringence of CPPD. We believe that an ordinary microscope fitted with the appropriate lenses and filters is an adequate tool for crystal analysis.

To better understand our observations, the basic tool is described—the ordinary brightfield microscope—and then built-in complexity.

1. *Brightfield microscopy:* This is the illumination of conventional microscopes. Because SF preparations are fresh and unstained, detection of crystals with this illumination is based solely on shape.[5,6,8] Cells and crystals are essentially transparent, so the height of the microscope condenser and aperture of the diaphragm must be regulated to obtain the best detail and contrast of the SF elements. Crystals are seen as regular structures with sharp edges, which can be found both inside and outside cells.

MSU crystals are always seen as thin needles of different sizes, intracellular or extracellular, and occasionally forming groups (with spherulites of MSU an infrequent finding). MSU crystals observed in SF from inflamed or uninflamed joints are smaller than those obtained by needling a tophus, which can be very large in comparison (Fig. 2-2).

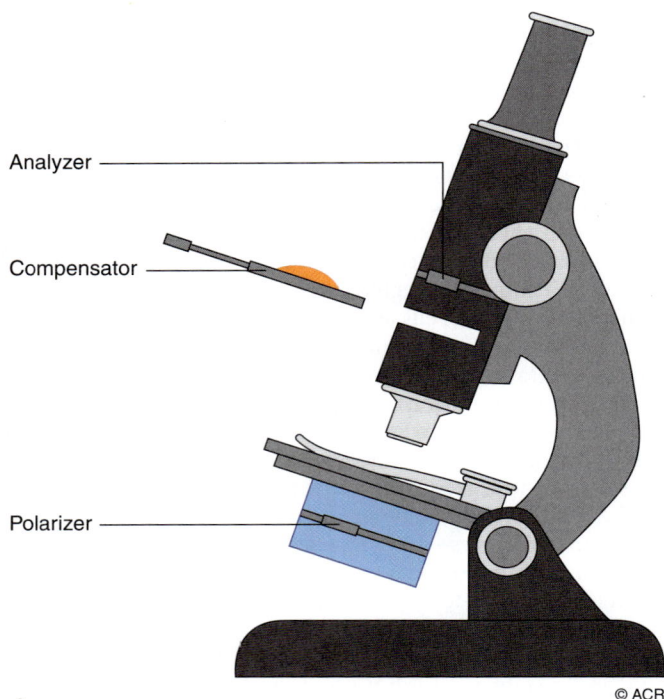

A

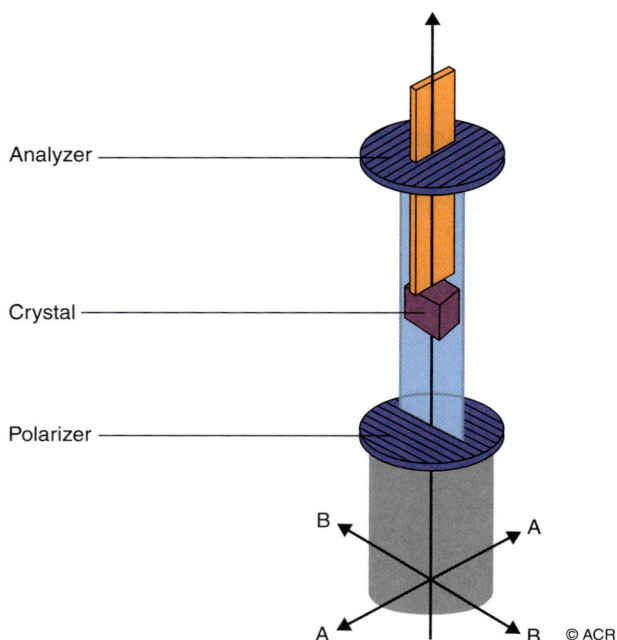

B

Figure 2-1 **A,** Compensated polarized light microscope, set up in the standard manner, with two crossed polarized light filters (termed the "polarizer" and the "analyzer") and a first-order red plate compensator filter. **B,** Compensated polarized light microscopy used to detect and identify synovial fluid crystals. The crystals, interposed in a darkfield of crossed polarizing filters, bend light into slow and fast components. The figure illustrates that the slow vibration of light by the crystal allows the crystal to be detected in the darkfield, and this phenomenon is termed "birefringence." Comparison with the axis of slow vibration of polarized light by a compensator filter (see **A**), typically using a first-order red plate compensator, allows definition of whether the crystal is negatively or positively birefringent. *(Redrawn from American College of Rheumatology Image Bank © 2009. A, Available at http://images .rheumatology.org/viewphoto.php?imageId=2861705. B, Available at http://images.rh eumatology.org/viewphoto.php?imageId=2861704.)*

Figure 2-2 Monosodium urate (MSU) crystals. **A–C,** From synovial fluid. Brightfield microscopy, ×400. **D,** From synovial fluid. Brightfield microscopy, ×600. **E,** From an aspirate of a tophus. Brightfield microscopy, ×400. **F–H,** From synovial fluid. Same microscope fields as **A–C,** simple polarized microscopy, ×400. **I,** From synovial fluid. Same microscope fields as **D,** simple polarized microscopy, ×600. **J,** From an aspirate of a tophus. Same microscope field as **E,** simple polarized microscopy, ×400. **K,** From an aspirate of a tophus. Simple polarized microscopy, ×400. MSU crystals from tophus aspirates can be very large. **L,** From synovial fluid. Same microscope field as **D** and **I.** Compensated polarized microscopy, ×400. **M,** From synovial fluid. Compensated polarized microscopy, ×400. **N, O,** From an aspirate of a tophus. Same microscope fields as **E, J,** and **K.** Compensated polarized microscopy, ×400. **P,** From synovial fluid. Compensated phase microscopy ×1000. These figures show that brightfield allows very close detection and identification of MSU crystals by shape and that simple polarized microscopy shows them well by their bright shine. Compensated polarized microscopy remains the standard for crystal identification. Compensated phase microscopy shows well the acicular MSU crystals but do not add to detection or identification.

On Photographing Crystals in Synovial Fluid
The depth of field (depth of the area in focus) of the microscope lenses is very thin. When observing through the microscope, we compensate for that fine-focusing with the micrometric knob (fine focusing), so only a very thin layer of synovial fluid in the preparation is in focus; many crystals and cells in the photographs are out of focus. When photographing with simple polarized microscopy, if the polarized filters are fully crossed, the background is too dark and the photographic image has excess contrast. Thus, a proper contrast to show some background detail can be obtained by slightly uncrossing the polarized filters until one obtains the proper contrast. This may result in the photograph losing some brilliancy of birefringent crystals in relation to the original. When photographing through the compensated polarized microscope, if the polarized filters are fully crossed, the color saturation in the photograph can be too high. Some uncrossing of the polarized filters—or rotation of the compensator if possible—helps to obtain images that represent better the original. In the photographs, the polarized filters are not fully crossed, to allow some background detail. Fully crossing the polarized filters, and with intense light, allows faint birefringence to be better appreciated, but it is always fainter than the birefringence of MSU crystals.

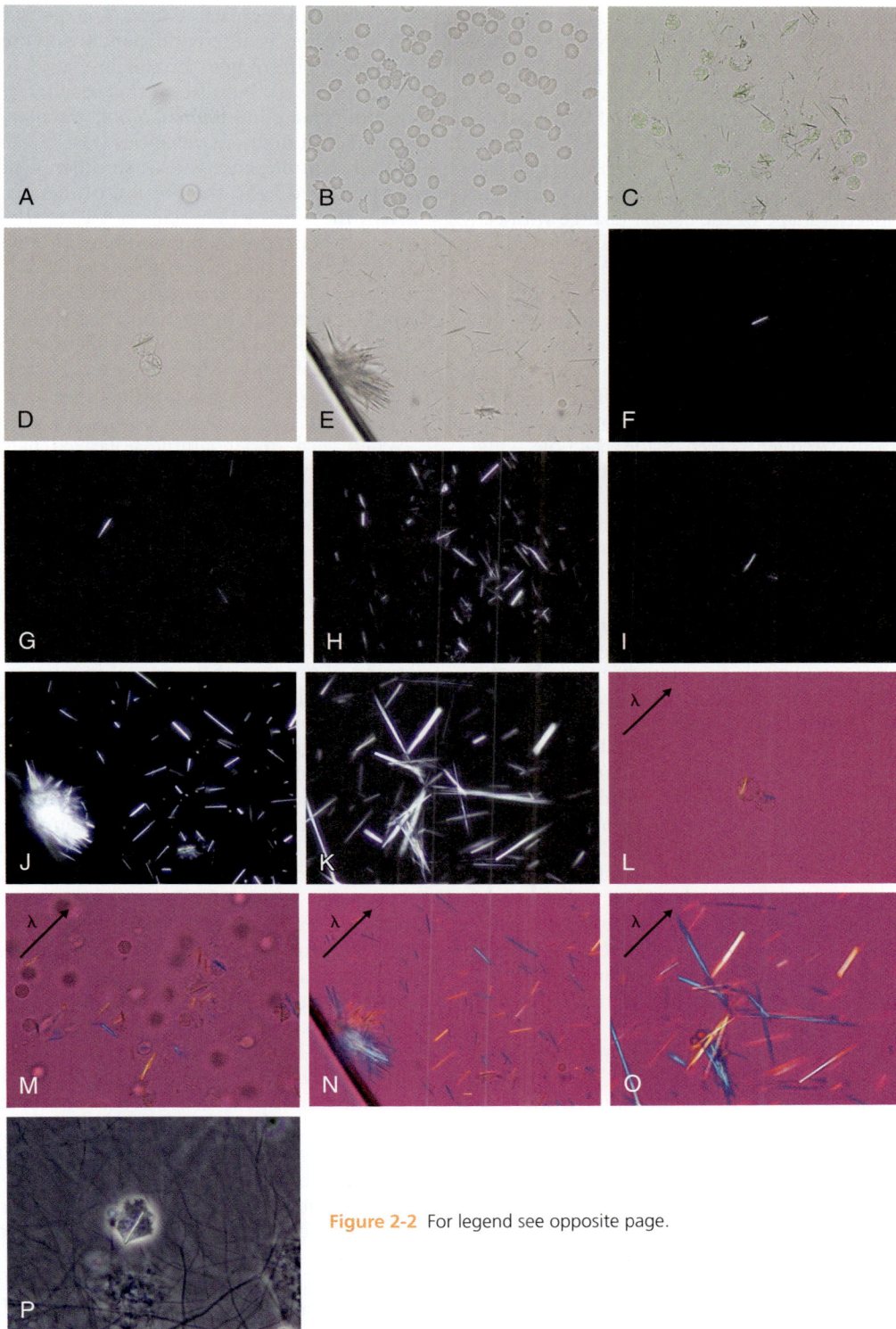

Figure 2-2 For legend see opposite page.

The polymorphic CPPD crystals may pose more difficulties. Observed under brightfield microscopy, typical crystals are rhombi or parallelepipeds. Some very thin and long parallelepipeds can look like rods or even needles; these are the only CPPD crystals that can be mistaken for MSU crystals. Often, CPPD crystals show a less regular shape, likely because of their position (it is a learning experience to observe typical crystals in a fresh preparation while the cells are still moving and watch the apparent shape of the crystal change with cell movement). In addition, some crystals may have broken off of larger crystals and therefore have a more irregular shape. Very small intracellular CPPD crystals are common and are seen as distinct inclusions that may have one or more linear borders or angles; tiny needles are also common. These smaller crystals are much better seen under a higher magnification with the ×1000 oil lens. The ×600 or ×630 lens (a good magnification level for crystal analysis) also shows them well. CPPD crystals are quite frequently seen inside a vacuole, while this appears not to be the case with MSU crystals (Figs. 2-3, 2-4, A–C, 2-5, A, and 2-6, A). The particularly inflammatory osmotic and membranolytic effects of MSU crystals discussed in Chapter 5 may account for this phenomenon.

The morphologic identification under ordinary light of CPPD crystals should be done only when enough typical crystals are seen; the finding of very small or less "typical"-looking crystals should prompt the observer to keep searching until he or she can identify an unquestionable crystal. In a small trial, both types of crystals were reasonably well distinguished with brightfield microscopy by their shape—63 SF samples (13 from patients with gout; 14, CPPD arthopathy; 1, both MSU and CPPD crystals; 35, different noncrystalline inflammatory arthritides) were blindly examined with brightfield microscopy by two different observers. The observers detected the presence of crystals in 100% (observer 1) and 97% (observer 2, who was a resident) of the samples; the crystals were properly identified with the brightfield microscope (in relation with the compensated polarized microscope) as MSU or CPPD in 92% (observer 1) and 87% (observer 2) of the occasions. In the sample containing MSU and CPPD crystals, both observers perceived the presence of both crystals.[25]

2. *Simple polarized light microscopy:* Simple polarized light can identify crystals due to the intensity of their birefringence; it is often used to identify foreign material in pathologic specimens. Simple polarized microscopy is obtained when two polarized filters are added to the brightfield microscope. One of the filters is placed between the light source and the microscope slide (polarizer), while the second is placed above the lens (analyzer). A polarized filter is one that allows only the light vibrating in a plane parallel to its axis to pass through. In essence, you can imagine a polarized filter as a comb whose teeth are very closely packed and only the light vibrating parallel to its teeth is allowed to pass through. When the axes of the two polarized filters are placed perpendicular to each other, the light that passed through the polarizer is retained by the analyzer and the observer sees a dark microscope field (also known as crossed polarization). When the axes of the two filters are parallel to each other, observations can be made as with ordinary light. In an optic microscope, one of the filters is movable, allowing a change between brightfield

and simple polarized light. The mechanism for crossing the filters is different depending on the microscope.

When a birefringent crystal is placed on the stage, the already polarized light beam that reaches it is split into two perpendicular components, none parallel to the incident ray, and with different velocities (fast ray and slow ray) and therefore out of phase with each other. The result is elliptically polarized light; the portion of this light vibrating parallel to the axis of the analyzer passes through it as plane polarized light, producing an image of a white crystal on a darkfield.[4,26] In short, birefringent crystals seem to shine on a dark background because the microscope light can be seen through the crystal. By partially uncrossing one of the filters, less polarization is obtained; this allows the viewer to simultaneously distinguish the SF elements and the birefringence of crystals, which can occasionally be useful, especially for photography.

When seen under simple polarized light, MSU crystals shine brightly over the dark background. Brilliance, however, also depends on the intensity of the light source of the microscope—showing higher luminosity with the microscopes fitted with a stronger light source such as halogen lighting—and the height of the microscope condenser, which should be graduated to obtain the best image. Occasional MSU crystals may show no birefringence; this depends on crystal mass (very small crystals may be anisotropic) but also on the position of the axes of the crystal in relation with the axis of either the polarizer or the analyzer filters. When the crystal axis is positioned parallel to the axes of crossed polarized filters, birefringence disappears and the crystal is said to be in a position of extinction.[27] On occasion, a crystal moving in the microscope field can fall in and out of the position of extinction and therefore show oscillating birefringence. Spherical aggregates of MSU crystals, all radiating from a center, have been reported,[28] and incomplete radiating appearances are occasionally seen (an irregular radiating structure seen in a tophus is shown in Fig. 2-6 D–F). After the viewer gains some experience, the bright MSU crystals are usually well detected at a magnification of ×200 with simple polarized microscopy. A better image is obtained at ×400; when searching for MSU crystals, there is rarely a need to use higher magnifications (see Fig. 2-2, F–K).

In the early descriptions of CPPD crystals, it was noted that under the simple polarized microscope they show only a weak birefringence, which is often absent.[7,19,29] In a more recent trial, 10 SF samples from patients with CPPD crystal–proved acute arthritis were examined separately by two observers. First, a brightfield microscope was used; then, the same area was examined with a simple polarized microscope. Crystals showing any birefringence were annotated. Both observers found that less that 20% of CPPD crystals showed any birefringence. Ten SF samples from patients with crystal-proved gouty attacks were also examined; examination under simple polarized microscopy showed more crystals than observation by brightfield, indicating that some MSU crystals had passed unseen under the brightlight.[30] Therefore, for CPPD, careful observation under brightfield appears to be the best method for detecting the crystals; when MSU is the suspected crystal, observation under simple polarized light is clearly better. It follows that before deciding that an SF sample has no crystals, it should be examined under both brightfield and simple polarized microscopy (see Figs. 2-4, D–F, 2-5, B, and 2-6, C).

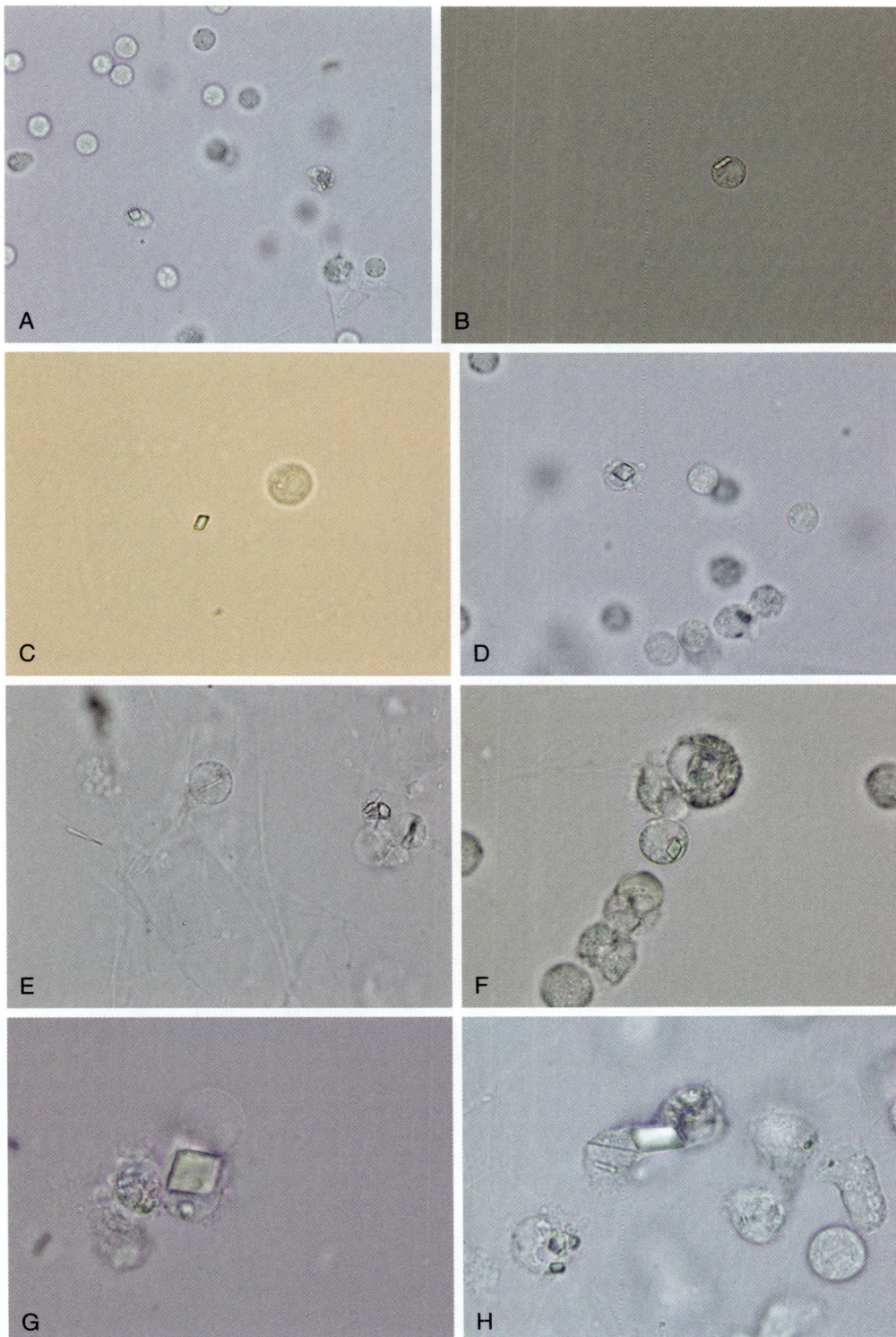

Figure 2-3 Calcium pyrophosphate dihydrate (CPPD) identification by shape with a brightfield microscope. **A–D,** CPPD crystals intracellularly and extracellularly, ×400. **E,** Two needle-shaped CPPD crystals (intracellular and extracellular) (*left*); the shape of the crystals (*right*) is important clue for identification; absence of birefringence or faint one, another. Compensated polarized microscopy helps to determine the coincidence of MSU and CPPD crystals, ×600. **F,** Rhomboidal crystal at ×600. **G, H,** CPPD at ×1000. Smaller crystals are also seen. These figures show that brightfield allows very close detection and identification of CPPD crystals by shape: ×400 allows good distinction of the crystals, especially the large ones, but ×600 and ×1000 in particular show much better detail and are important means of observation, allowing beginners to become closely acquainted with the different shapes and sizes of CPPD crystals.

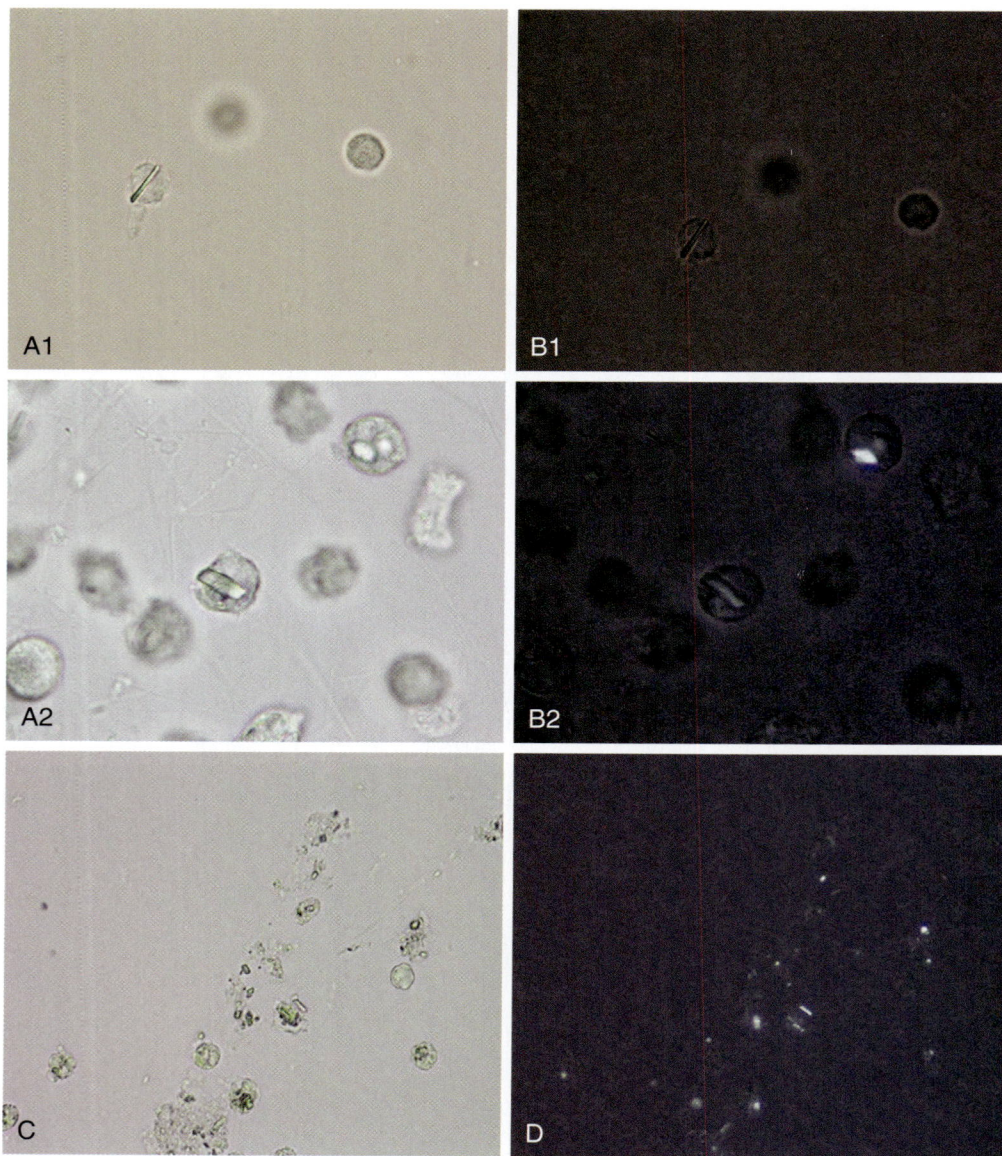

Figure 2-4 Calcium pyrophosphate dihydrate (CPPD) by brightfield and simple polarized microscopy. **A1** and **A2,** CPPD crystals seen by brightfield microscopy (A1, ×400; A2, ×600). **B1** and **B2,** Same microscope fields by simple polarized microscopy: the crystals do not show birefringence—an out-of-focus crystal on **E,** top right, does. **C,** Abundant CPPD crystals brightfield ×400. **D,** Same microscope field seen by simple polarized microscopy—and showing that only a minority of crystals show any birefringence. These figures illustrate that CPPD crystals often do not show birefringence under simple polarized light. For beginners it is convenient to carefully observe the lesser to very faint to absent birefringence of CPPD crystals and become acquainted with it.

3. *Compensated polarized microscopy:* This method remains the current standard for crystal identification; it adds to the previously discussed system a first-order red compensator (λ or retardation plate), which helps to determine the amount of retardation in the wavelength of the compound ray emerging from the long dimension of the birefringent crystal. When this ray has a raised wavelength, it is viewed as yellow when parallel to the compensator axis (usually marked by a λ and an arrow) and as blue if perpendicular and the crystal is said to have negative birefringence or elongation. When the vibration of the slow ray is parallel to the long dimension of the crystal, it has a positive birefringence or

elongation. Compensated polarized microscopy helps in the distinction between MSU and CPPD crystals, because the crystals have different birefringence: in MSU, it is negative (and bright) birefringence (see Fig. 2-2, *L* and *M*), while in CPPD, it is positive (and weak) birefringence (see Figs. 2-5, *C–E,* and 2-6, *D* and *F*).[4,27,31,26,32] The axis of the compensator can also be determined by keeping reference MSU crystals (a dried imprint of material needled from a tophi provides abundant MSU crystals for reference). Although it remains the standard tool for definitive crystal distinction, the crystal nature is already evident in most occasions based on the shape and intensity of birefringence under simple polarized

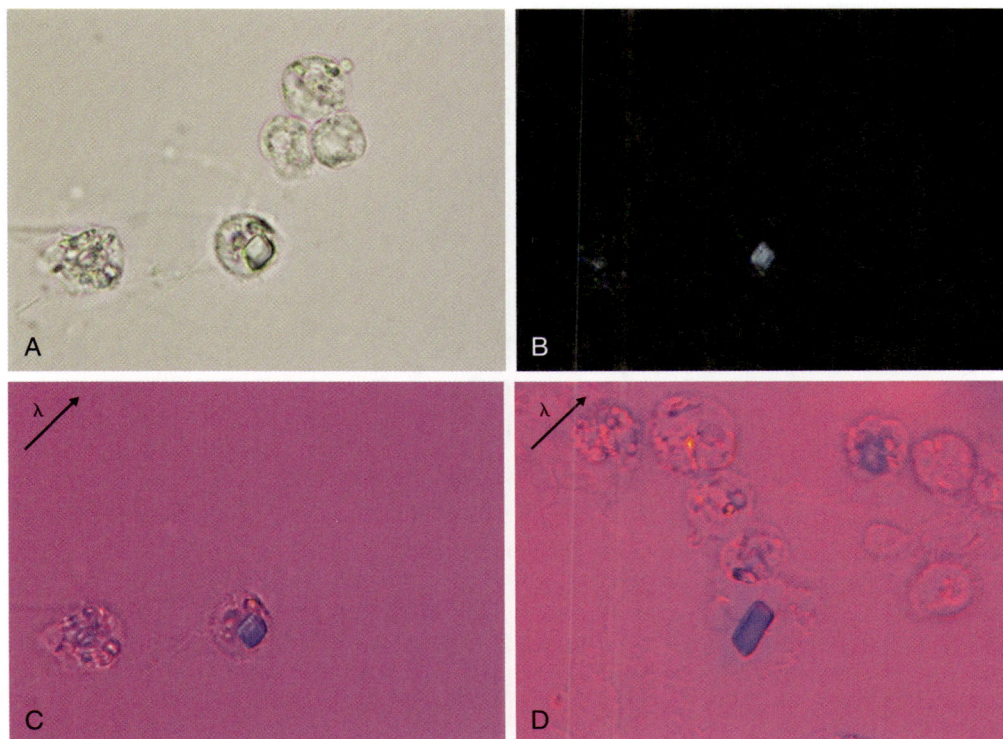

Figure 2-5 Calcium pyrophosphate dihydrate (CPPD) compensated polarized microscope. **A,** Rhomboidal CPPD crystal seen by brightfield microscopy, ×1000. **B,** Same as **A** by simple polarized microscopy (×1000) showing faint birefringence (taken in reference to the birefringence shown by monosodium urate crystals). **C,** Same as **A** by compensated polarized microscopy, ×1000. The shape of the crystal does not allow determination of its orientation in relation to the compensator axis (λ marked by an *arrow*). **D,** Parallelepipedic CPPD crystal by compensated polarized microscopy, ×1000. The long axis of the crystal lies parallel to the axis of the compensator (λ marked by an *arrow*); the blue color shown by the crystal indicates positive elongation (also referred as birefringence) characteristic of CPPD crystals. These figures show the positive birefringence shown by CPPD crystals. Only parallelepipedic and rod-shaped crystals can be oriented in relation to the compensator axis.

light. Compensated polarized microscopy is most useful in the identification of very occasional needlelike artefacts or when MSU and CPPD crystals coincide in the same SF; this occurrence appears sporadic and no report on its clinical consequences has been published. A recent report examining SF from a patient with gout after cytocentrifugation also found a few CPPD crystals in patients with associated moderate to severe osteoarthritis, and possibly related to the osteoarthritis.[33]

4. *Phase contrast microscopy:* This is a contrast-enhancing technique that produces high-contrast images of transparent specimens using ordinary light. When light waves that passed through the phase condenser pass through the preparation, some of its elements diffract and retard the phase (i.e., retard the wavelength). These retarded emerging waves are invisible to the naked eye but are transformed by the phase plate in the lens into amplitude differences observable at the oculars.[34,35] Objects that modify the light phase—as do crystals—are seen lighter (see Fig. 2-6, *A2, B2, E,* and *G–K*). Phase microscopy was recommended by McCarty[27] and shows the crystal's shape particularly well; if available, phase microscopy and observation at ×1000 can be very good teaching instruments to familiarize a beginner with the different crystal shapes, particularly with CPPD crystals, including the very small intracellular ones. On occasion, it can also be useful for the expert analyst.

An ordinary microscope can be polarized by fitting it with polarized filters (obtainable online from commercial vendors) and cellophane tape can be used as a makeshift compensator.[36-38] These are improvised polarized and compensated polarized microscopes, although the image quality may be inferior. Polarized filters can be cut by opticians from a large photographic polarized filter and adapted to the filter lodges of the microscope. Two filters are necessary—one under the stage, in the usual filter lodge of the microscope, and the other over it (most microscopes have a filter lodge in the inside of the piece that holds the lenses).

Additional Practical Tips

Initial Approach

It is practical to approach crystal analysis in two separate steps: (1) *crystal detection* (if crystals are present in SF, they will be detected, so crystal arthritis will not be missed) and (2) *crystal identification* (the detected crystals will be properly identified as MSU or CPPD).[39,40] It must be noted that reviews and book chapters tend to show figures of MSU and CPPD crystals in their most typical form. For MSU crystals, book descriptions fit quite well, with the great majority of the crystals—all acicular and strongly birefringent under simple polarized light—but as described earlier, CPPD crystals vary in size, shape, and characteristics of birefringence.

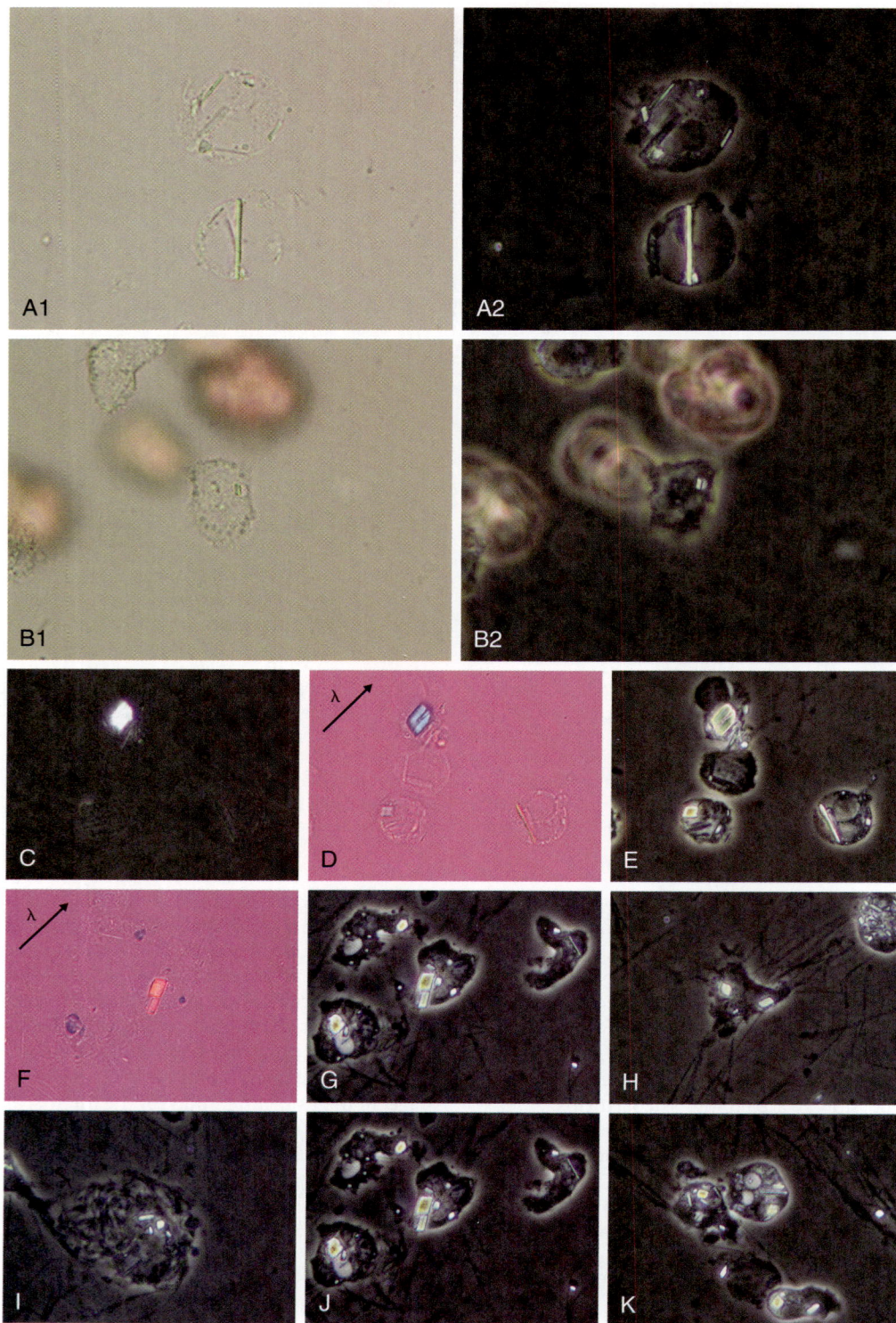

Figure 2-6 Calcium pyrophosphate dihydrate (CPPD) as seen with phase contrast microscopy. **A1,** Brightfield microscopy, ×1000. Several rod-shaped CPPD crystals. **A2,** Phase contrast microscopy, ×1000. Same microscope field. **B1,** Brightfield microscopy, ×1000. A single small intracellular CPPD crystal in a vacuole. **B2,** Phase contrast microscopy, ×1000. Same microscope field. The crystal and vacuole are now more clearly distinguished. **C,** Simple polarized microscopy, ×1000. Only one parallelepipedic CPPD crystal shows clear birefringence. **D,** Compensated polarized microscopy, ×1000. Same field as **C**. Only two crystals (showing + elongation or birefringence—yellow when perpendicular to the compensator axis [λ] and blue if parallel) can be identified as CPPD crystals. **E,** Phase contrast microscopy. Same field as **C** and **D**. A larger number of crystals are now clearly seen. **F,** Compensated polarized microscopy, ×1000. Only two crystals can be identified as CPPD by their birefringence (+ elongation; yellow when parallel to the compensator axis [λ]). **G,** Phase contrast microscopy, ×1000. Same microscope field as **F**. More crystals are now distinguished. **H–K,** Phase contrast microscopy, ×1000. Several images showing the capability of phase contrast microscopy to distinguish CPPD crystals by shape, even if small. All these figures show the clear vision obtained by phase contrast microscopy, ×1000. It may help to identify small crystals, but its advantages for routine synovial fluid analysis remain unproved. Our practice is to look for CPPD crystals by brightfield microscopy, and for long rod-shaped crystals, to check (absence or faint birefringence) under simple polarized microscopy. Compensated polarized microscopy remains useful for occasional doubtful crystals.

Samples

Crystal identification is usually made with SF samples from inflamed joints, but both MSU and CPPD crystals are also found in asymptomatic joints. In gout, their presence is regular in joints previously inflamed but currently asymptomatic in patients untreated with serum urate–lowering agents, allowing gout diagnosis during intercritical periods.[16,41] Such a finding is not surprising because ultrasound studies[42,43] and arthroscopic observations[44] show that MSU crystals deposit at the surface of the joint cartilage, directly bathed by SF, and in an area of pressure and friction during joint movements.

CPPD crystals are also found regularly in the SF of inflamed joints; these crystals usually lie deeper in joint cartilage than do MSU crystals, but after an episode of joint inflammation has occurred, the crystals are also regularly found in the SF of asymptomatic joints.[15] Very thin (25- to 29-gauge) needles allow arthrocentesis of asymptomatic first metatarsophalangeal (MTP) joints with only modest discomfort,[45,46] and arthrocentesis of asymptomatic knees is also reasonably simple.[46] Needling of a tophus (with a 21- or 23-gauge needle) most often yields abundant MSU crystals (often seen inside the needle as a white material; Fig. 2-7). High resolution ultrasonography (Chapter 26) can show deeper crystal deposits, which can easily be sampled, allowing definitive MSU crystal identification. Finally, MSU and CPPD crystals can also be seen in biopsy specimens processed in the pathology department. But MSU crystals are dissolved by formalin[47] and, if they are contemplated, the sample should be cut by freezing or by fixation with alcohol (which does not dissolve urate crystals) (Fig. 2-8).

SF is ideally examined in fresh state with no centrifugation, fixation, or staining required, but after its extraction, SF decays steadily, and preparations should ideally be examined promptly—preferably within the day—because crystals are often intracellular and the integrity of cells is important (especially for CPPD crystal identification). Nevertheless, both CPPD and MSU crystals have been readily identified after 24 hours in refrigerated or frozen SF samples or on Gram stain samples.[48] A small drop of SF must be placed on a clean glass slide and covered by a coverslip; this can be done directly from the syringe.

Dirty slides often have birefringent artefacts. Smaller drops of SF result in thinner preparations and this allows less superimposition of SF elements and better detail. Sealing the periphery of the cover slide with nail polish is not usually done, but helps to delay drying and can be useful occasionally. Even the smallest amount of SF may be examined, and if crystals are suspected, it should never be discarded. After an apparent dry tap, the fluid inside the needle can often be recovered and analyzed after flushing air through it onto a glass slide. Typical elements of SF include leukocytes, and erythrocytes may be present, especially because CPPD deposition disease can present with hemarthrosis. Crystals can also be seen in cytocentrifuged preparations or in stained slides,[33] but these modes of observation have not been properly evaluated against the standard fresh SF observation.

Magnification

When white SF is obtained from a joint or white speckles are seen floating in an SF sample, most likely these are composed of MSU crystals (although it must be confirmed with the

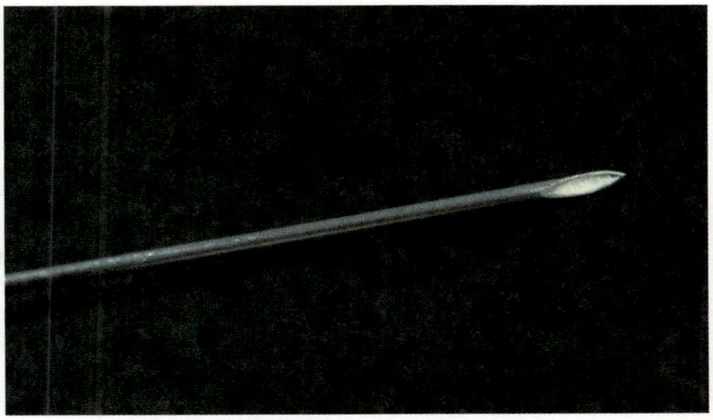

Figure 2-7 After needling a tophus, the microscopic analysis of the white material recovered inside this 21-gauge showed packed monosodium urate crystals (same as the material obtained from a draining tophus).

microscope). White specks are also occasionally seen by the naked eye in a preparation ready for microscopic observation.

Changing to a higher-power lens to better view a doubtful crystal is a useful practice; ×1000 oil lenses show excellent detail but oil is messy and it is difficult after oil observation to return to dry lenses. Observation at ×400 is adequate and often the standard, showing CPPD crystals well under bright-light and MSU crystals under uncompensated, polarized light, although strongly birefringent crystals of MSU are also clearly visible at ×200. Observation under ordinary light at ×1000 assists in the assessment of polymorphic (rhomboidal, parallelepipedic, and needle-shaped) CPPD crystals; a ×600 to ×630 dry lens is a useful option (and used by the authors). At ×1000, phase contrast microscopy shows the crystals in their best detail and, if available, is an excellent tool to become acquainted with CPPD crystals, but it remains uncertain whether it is advantageous for routine use.

Effort Needed to Detect Crystals

The effort needed to detect the presence of crystals—when scarce—or to decide their absence has received little critical attention. In case crystals are not identified in the first SF sample and clinical suspicion remains high, examination of SF samples obtained from different time points has been recommended. In a report in which SF samples were obtained from the joints of 77 asymptomatic patients with crystal-proved gout, the crystals were found in the first microscope field examined in 61% of the samples and in the first five microscope fields in 90%[41]; these data cannot be extrapolated to SF from inflamed joints, but crystals are often easily found there, too. It may help standardization to consider the number of ×400 microscope fields examined rather than the minutes dedicated to an SF examination before deciding the sample does not contain crystals. Thirty such fields have been applied,[16] but this number may be conservative.

When crystals are scarce, they are often found in clumps of cells or small tissue pieces brought along with the SF. Perhaps a more definitive proof of the absence of MSU crystals can be obtained by centrifuging an SF sample and looking under simple polarized light at the pellet, where crystals concentrate, although this has not been critically evaluated.

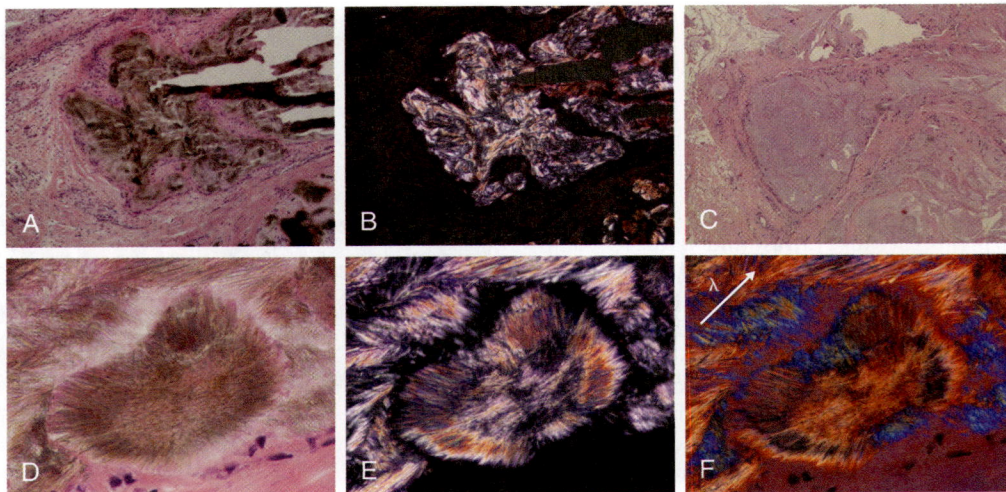

Figure 2-8 Tophus. **A,** Frozen section, hematoxylin and eosin (HE). Brightfield microscopy. Crystals are seen as dark purplish areas in the center of the figure ×200. **B,** Simple polarized (incompletely crossed polarized filters to allow detail in the tissue) monosodium urate (MSU) crystals in the deposit show bright birefringence ×200. **C,** A different fragment of the same tissue sample, formalin fixed. HE. Brightfield microscopy. Crystals have now dissolved, and a homogeneous acellular central area marks the site of their previous place, ×100. These figures show that formalin fixation results in dissolution of MSU crystals (**C**), which are well seen by simple polarized microscopy in a stained frozen section. Tophus (same tissue sample as **A–C**) detail, frozen section, HE, ×400. **D,** Brightfield microscopy, ×400. **E,** Simple polarized microscopy, ×400. **F,** Compensated polarized microscopy, ×400. The λ indicates the axis of the compensator. These three images show a radiating arrangement of MSU crystals inside a tophus, which may be similar to the spherical MSU crystal arrangement described as spherulites.[28] The large size of the crystals seen explains the larger size of MSU crystals obtained by needling a tophus in comparison with those generally seen in synovial fluid samples.

Training in Crystal Analysis

The training process in SF examination for crystals has received little attention. In a recent study,[24] we have shown that analyst training results in very acceptable consistency in the identification of both MSU and CPPD crystals, but the previous expertise in microscopy of the trainees (laboratory residents) undoubtedly influenced the favorable results. It would appear that the problems reported with crystal identification may be more related to the training—or lack of training—than to the technique itself.

Other Crystals and Particles in Synovial Fluid

There are other crystals and particles to be identified in SF (Fig. 2-9).

BCP Crystals

BCP crystals—which include apatite—can commonly be found in osteoarthritic joints or with rapidly destructive arthritis. Their small size makes them undetectable with light microscopy, although amorphous aggregates of the crystals are well seen by brightfield microscopy. Staining with Alizarin red, which stains calcium salts, might be useful to detect apatite crystal aggregates (see Chapter 22, but Alizarin red also weakly stains the calcium in CPPD crystals.

Corticosteroid Crystals

Intraarticular injection of corticosteroid crystals is a frequent procedure; it can occasionally result in an acute arthritis that can simulate infection.[49,50] The crystals can persist in the joint for an undefined period of time[51] after their injection. Steroid crystals can be seen under light microscopy and usually appear strongly birefringent and predominantly positively birefringent; however, this varies from one preparation to another.[52] It is wise to become familiar with corticosteroid preparations most commonly used in your area and to specifically ask the patient regarding previous injections when an unexpected crystal is seen in the SF analysis.

Cholesterol

Cholesterol crystals can be found in chronic effusions of any long-standing arthopathy,[53,54] most commonly rheumatoid arthritis.[55,56] They might be more common in the shoulders[57] and periarticular bursae.[58] They appear as large rhomboidal plates with a notched corner and are variably birefringent.[59] Their pathogenic potential appears small, although some studies in animals have shown that cholesterol crystals can produce an acute synovitis and a chronic proliferative synovitis with granulomas and fibrosis.[60] Recently, cholesterol crystals were suggested to be implicated in the pathogenesis of murine atherosclerosis.[60a]

Calcium Oxalate

Calcium oxalate crystals were identified in joints of patients undergoing hemodialysis decades ago[61] (see Chapter 23 for more details). However, a modification of the filtering system has permitted adequate clearance of oxalate; oxalate arthopathy therefore has been largely eliminated. Sporadic cases have also been described in patients undergoing peritoneal dialysis[62] or in patients with primary hyperoxaluria.[63,64] Only a few crystals show their characteristic bipyramidal shape, which permits morphologic identification, while many are irregular

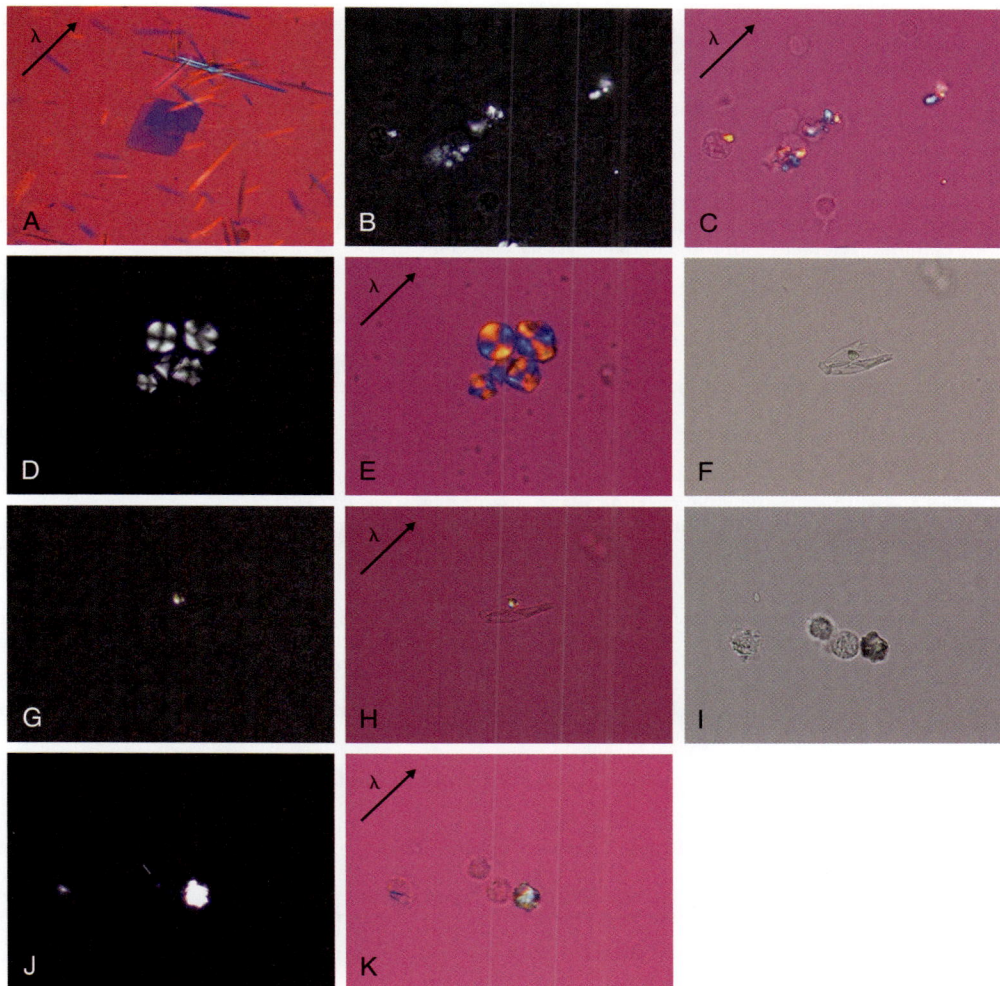

Figure 2-9 Other crystals and artefacts. **A,** Monosodium urate (MSU) crystals obtaining by needling a tophus. A platelike notched corner cholesterol crystal is seen in the center. Compensated polarized microscopy ×400. **B, C,** Triamcinolone acetonide crystals, ×400. **B,** Simple polarized microscopy, **C,** Compensated polarized microscopy. **D, E,** Starch from latex gloves, ×400. **D,** Simple polarized microscopy, **E,** Compensated polarized microscopy. These particles are easily distinguished from liquid lipid crystals because the lipid crystals are round and starch is irregular. **F–H,** Dust particle. ×400. **F,** Brightfield microscopy, **G,** Simple polarized microscopy, **H,** Compensated polarized microscopy. **I–K,** Dust particle, ×400. **I,** Brightfield microscopy, **J,** Simple polarized microscopy, **K,** Compensated polarized microscopy. Note urate crystals well seen by simple polarized microscopy and by compensated polarized microscopy—two blue crystals inside the left cell.

Table 2-1

	Brightfield Microscope	**Simple Polarized**	**Compensated Polarized**	**Phase Contrast**
MSU	All needles Easy to miss if few crystals	Very bright birefringence Best for detection; sufficient for identification	Current standard for identification Negative elongation Screening samples	Does not add much
CPPD	Parallelepipeds, rods, or needles; very well seen Best for detection; sufficient for identification	Only about one fifth show any birefringence. Easy to miss if few crystals	Current standard for identification Positive elongation Nonbirefringent crystals under simple polarized light may show color	Very clear distinction of crystals Good tool to become familiar with CPPD crystals

CPPD, Calcium pyrophosphate dihydrate; *MSU,* monosodium urate.

Table 2-2 Checklist for Crystal Detection in Synovial Fluid

1. Before starting
   - Become acquainted with your microscope and the role of its different parts.
   - Become familiar with the elements of synovial fluid in fresh preparations and with different magnifications (mostly white blood cells of different shapes and red blood cells).
2. The fresh slide
   - Clean the glass slide and coverslip (or use precleaned ones); dust particles are seen as birefringent and are distracting.
   - Synovial fluid for examination is ideally fresh (i.e., optimally obtained within 1 day); delay results in cell decay that can hamper (but not totally eliminate) detection of intracellular crystals, especially CPPD.
3. When CPPD crystals are suspected
   - Examine the preparation under brightfield at ×400.
   - Crystals are very often intracellular (and in a fresh sample, any intracellular inclusion is not an artefact).
   - Large (sometimes larger than the diameter of a white blood cell) clearly distinct rhomboidal or parallelepipedic crystals are typical CPPD crystals.
   - Very small crystals are seen as rhombi or tiny rods or needles (if difficult to distinguish, it could be worthwhile looking with a ×1000 oil lens).
   - Observation at ×1000 with a phase contrast microscope offers the best vision and is very useful to become initially acquainted with the crystals.
   - Needle- or rod-shaped CPPD can be confused with MSU under brightfield microscopy. Several things help in the distinction:
     o If these crystals are accompanied by typical clinical and imaging features of CPPD
     o Most CPPD crystals show no or a faint birefringence under simple polarized light
     o Under compensated polarized light, the long crystals have positive elongation (blue when parallel to the axis of slow rotation of light of the compensator, yellow when perpendicular to it)
4. When MSU crystals are suspected
   - Initial detection is easier with simple polarized light, although MSU crystals can also be seen with brightfield microscopy.
   - All MSU crystals are needle shaped, and all are strongly birefringent (with occasional exceptions described in the text).
   - MSU crystals are well detected at ×200 (especially useful if crystals are scarce) and at ×400.
   - Higher magnifications or phase microscopy do not add in the detection or identification of these MSU crystals.
   - A compensated polarized microscope shows a negative elongation (yellow if the crystal lies parallel to the compensator axis of slow rotation of light and blue if perpendicular).
5. Other points to consider
   - If you detect a crystal that is not clearly identifiable (because of shape or birefringence), continue searching until you see a characteristic crystal.
   - A microscope with a rotating stage is ideal, since it allows for detection of characteristic birefringence extinction angles of MSU and CPPD crystals, whereas other birefringent particles do not similarly extinguish birefringence upon rotation of the microscope stage.
   - It is a good practice never to diagnose a crystal arthritis based on one crystal.

CPPD, Calcium pyrophosphate dihydrate; *MSU,* monosodium urate.

or rod-shaped. Chondrocalcinosis can sometimes be seen with oxalate deposition.[65]

Other Crystals

Most of the information on other crystal types is anecdotal. Hematoidin crystals are seen as golden brown crystals with positive birefringence and can sometimes be seen in joints with bloody effusions.[66] Charcot-Leyden crystals are sometimes found in eosinophilic synovitis.[67-69] Cryoglobulin crystals—nonbirefringent or with weak positive birefringence rhomboid crystals—have been sporadically reported in patients with type I cryoglobulinemia.[70,71] Lipid crystals—also known as "Maltese cross" crystals because of their appearance under polarized light—have been found in patients with acute monoarthritis[72] or intraarticular fractures.[73] One of the most common artefacts—starch from gloves used in the handling of the SF sample—also exhibit a Maltese cross appearance under simple polarized light.[74,75] However, they seem to be more spherical and larger than lipid crystals.[76,77] Silicon dioxide crystals have been identified in some osteoarthritic SF samples. Under polarized light, they appear as irregular, polymorphic crystals.[78] They cannot be identified by their shape or polarization characteristics alone, so other, more sophisticated identification techniques are required. Their identification, however, is currently irrelevant for clinical practice.

References

1. American College of Rheumatology. Core Curriculum Outline for Rheumatology Fellowship Programs: a Competency-Based Guide to Curriculum Development. http://www.rheumatology.org/educ/training/cco.doc
2. European Board of Rheumatology, UEMS Section of Rheumatology. Core curriculum for specialist training. http://www.uems-rheumatology.net/
3. Amer H, Swan A, Dieppe P. The utilization of synovial fluid analysis in the UK. Rheumatology (Oxford) 2001;40:1060–3.
4. Gatter RA. The compensated light microscope in clinical rheumatology. Arthritis Rheum 1974;17:253–5.
5. McCarty DJ, Hollander JL. Identification of urate crystals in gouty synovial fluid. Ann Intern Med 1961;54:452–60.
6. McCarty D. Crystals, joints, and consternation. Ann Rheum Dis 1983;42:243–53.
7. McCarty DJ, Kohn NN, Faires JS. The significance of calcium phosphate crystals in the synovial fluid of arthritis patients: the "pseudogout syndrome." I. Clinical aspects. Ann Intern Med 1962;56:711–37.
8. Kohn N, Hughes R, McCarty DJ. The significance of calcium phosphate crystals in the synovial fluid of arthritic patients: the "pseudogout syndrome." II. Identification of crystals. Ann Intern Med 1962;56:738–45.
9. Gatter RA, McCarty Jr DJ. Pathological tissue calcifications in man. Arch Pathol 1967;84:346–53.
10. McCarty Jr DJ, Gatter RA. Pseudogout syndrome (articular chondrocalcinosis). Bull Rheum Dis 1964;14:331–4.
11. Nalbant S, Martinez JA, Kitumnuaypong T, et al. Synovial fluid features and their relations to osteoarthritis severity: new findings from sequential studies. Osteoarthritis Cartilage 2003;11:50–4.
12. Halverson PB, Carrera GF, McCarty DJ. Milwaukee shoulder syndrome. Fifteen additional cases and a description of contributing factors. Arch Intern Med 1990;150:677–82.
13. Doherty M, Watt I, Dieppe PA. Localised chondrocalcinosis in postmeniscectomy knees. Lancet 1982;29:1207–10.

14. Pascual E, Jovaní V. A quantitative study of the phagocytosis of urate crystals in the synovial fluid of asymptomatic joints of patients with gout. Br J Rheumatol 1995;34:724–6.

15. Martinez-Sanchis A, Pascual E. Intracellular and extracellular CPPD crystals are a regular feature in synovial fluid from uninflamed joints of patients with CPPD related arthropathy. Ann Rheum Dis 2005;64:1769–72.

16. Pascual E. Persistence of monosodium urate crystals, and low grade inflammation, in the synovial fluid of untreated gout. Arthritis Rheum 1991;34:141–5.

17. Von Essen R, Holtta AMH. Quality control of the laboratory diagnosis of gout by synovial fluid microscopy. Scand J Rheumatol 1990;19:232–4.

18. Von Essen R, Holtta AMH, Pikkarainen R. Quality control of synovial fluid crystal identification. Ann Rheum Dis 1998;57:107–9.

19. McGill NW, York HF. Reproducibility of synovial fluid examination for crystals. Aust N Z J Med 1991;21:10–3.

20. Hasselbacher P. Variation in synovial fluid analysis by hospital laboratories. Arthritis Rheum 1987;30:637–42.

21. Schumacher HR, Sieck MS, Rothfuss C, et al. Reproducibility of synovial fluid analyses; a study among our laboratories. Arthritis Rheum 1986;29:770–4.

22. Gordon C, Swan A, Dieppe P. Detection of crystals in synovial fluids by light microscopy: sensitivity and reliability. Ann Rheum Dis 1989;48:737–42.

23. Segal JB, Albert D. Diagnosis of crystal-induced arthritis by synovial fluid examination for crystals: lessons from an imperfect test. Arthritis Care Res 1999;12:376–80.

24. Lumbreras B, Pascual E, Frasquet J, et al. Analysis for crystals in synovial fluid: training of the analysts results in high consistency. Ann Rheum Dis 2005;64:612–5.

25. Pascual E, Tovar J, Ruiz MT. The ordinary light microscope: an appropriate tool for the detection and identification of crystals in synovial fluid. Ann Rheum Dis 1989;48:983–5.

26. Olympus Microscopy Resource Center. Polarized microscopy. http://www.olympusmicro.com/primer/techniques/polarized/polarizedhome.html

27. McCarty DJ. Synovial fluid. In: Arthritis and Allied Conditions. 9th ed. Philadelphia, PA: Lea & Febiger; 1979:51–69

28. Fiechtner JJ, Simkin PA. Urate spherulites in gouty synovia. JAMA 1981;245:1533–6.

29. Schumacher HR, Reginato A. Calcium phosphate dihydrate crystals. In: Schumacher HR, Reginato A, editors. Atlas of Synovial Fluid Analysis and Crystal Identification. Philadelphia, PA: Lea & Febiger; 1991.

30. Ivorra J, Rosas E, Pascual E. Most calcium pyrophosphate crystals appear as non-birefringent. Ann Rheum Dis 1999;58:582–4.

31. Phelps P, Steele AD, McCarty Jr DJ. Compensated polarized light microscopy. Identification of crystals in synovial fluids from gout and pseudogout. JAMA 1968;203:508–12.

32. Nikon Microscopy U. Polarized light microscopy. http://www.microscopyu.com/articles/polarized/index.html

33. Robier C, Neubauer M, Quehenberger F, et al. Coincidence of calcium pyrophosphate and monosodium urate crystals in the synovial fluid of patients with gout determined by the cytocentrifugation technique. Ann Rheum Dis 2010 Oct 21:[Epub ahead of print].

34. Nikon Microscopy U. Introduction to phase contrast microscopy. http://www.microscopyu.com/articles/phasecontrast/phasemicroscopy.html

35. Olympus Microscopy Resource Center. Contrast in optical microscopy. http://www.olympusmicro.com/primer/techniques/contrast.html

36. Owen DS. A cheap and useful compensated polarizing microscope. N Engl J Med 1971;285:1152.

37. Owen Jr DS. Proceedings: new and simple polarized microscope. Arthritis Rheum 1974;17:323–4.

38. Fagan TJ, Lidsky MD. Compensated polarized light microscopy using cellophane adhesive tape. Arthritis Rheum 1974;17:256–62.

39. Pascual E, Jovaní V. Synovial fluid analysis. Best Pract Res Clin Rheumatol 2005;19:371–86.

40. Courtney P, Doherty M. Joint aspiration and injection and synovial fluid analysis. Best Pract Res Clin Rheumatol 2009;23:161–92.

41. Pascual E, Batlle-Gualda E, Martínez A, et al. Synovial fluid analysis for diagnosis of intercritical gout. Ann Intern Med 1999;131:756–9.

42. Grassi W, Menga G, Pascual E, et al. "Crystal Clear"-sonographic assessment of gout and calcium pyrophosphate deposition disease. Semin Arthritis Rheum 2006;36:197–202.

43. Wright SA, Filippucci E, McVeigh C, et al. High-resolution ultrasonography of the first metatarsal phalangeal joint in gout: a controlled study. Ann Rheum Dis 2007;66:859–64.

44. Baker JF, Synnott KA. Clinical images: gout revealed on arthroscopy after minor injury. Arthritis Rheum 2010;62:895.

45. Sivera F, Aragón R, Pascual E. First metatarsophalangeal joint aspiration using a 29-gauge needle. Ann Rheum Dis 2008;67:273–5.

46. Pascual E, Doherty M. Aspiration of normal or asymptomatic pathological joints for diagnosis and research: indications, technique and success rate. Ann Rheum Dis 2009;68:3–7.

47. Simkin PA, Bassett JE, Lee QP. Not water, but formalin, dissolves urate crystals in tophaceous tissue samples. J Rheumatol 1994;21:2320–1.

48. Galvez J, Saiz E, Linares LF, et al. Delayed examination of synovial fluid by ordinary and polarized light microscopy to detect and identify crystals. Ann Rheum Dis 2002;61:444–7.

49. Selvi E, DeStefano R, Lorenzini S, et al. Arthritis induced by corticosteroid crystals. J Rheumatol 2004;31:622.

50. McCarty DJ, Hogan JM. Inflammatory reaction after intrasynovial injection of microcrystalline adrenocorticosteroid esters. Arthritis Rheum 1964;7:359–67.

51. Gordon GV, Schumacher HR. Electron microscopic study of depot corticosteroid crystals with clinical studies after intra-articular injection. J Rheumatol 1979;6:7–14.

52. Kahn CB, Hollander JL, Schumacher HR. Corticosteroid crystals in synovial fluid. JAMA 1970;211:807–9.

53. Ettlinger RE, Hunder CG. Synovial effusions containing cholesterol crystals report of 12 patients and review. Mayo Clin Proc 1979;54:366–74.

54. Fam AG, Pritzker KPH, Cheng P, et al. Cholesterol crystals in osteoarthritis joint effusions. J Rheumatol 1981;8:273–80.

55. Lazarevic MB, Skosey JL, Vitc J, et al. Cholesterol crystals in synovial and bursal fluid. Semin Arthritis Rheum 1993;23:99–103.

56. Berthekit JM, Huguet D, Gouin F, et al. Multiple rheumatoid burstitis with migrating cylous cysts. Report of a case in a European woman and review of the literature. Rev Rheumatol Engl Educ 1999;66:354–8.

57. Riordan JW, Dieppe PA. Cholesterol crystals in shoulder synovial fluid. Br J Rheumatol 1987;23:430–2.

58. Ho S, Srinivasan U, Bevan M. Cholesterol crescents and plates in shoulder effusion of a rheumatoid patient. Rheumatology 2008;47:377–8.

59. DeMarco PJ, Keating RM. Cholesterol crystals. N Engl J Med 1995;333:1325.

60. Pritzker KP, Fam AG, Omar SA, et al. Experimental cholesterol crystal arthropathy. J Rheumatol 1981;8:281–90.

60a. Duewell P, Kono H, Rayner KJ, Sirois CM, Vladimer G, Bauernfeind FG, Abela GS, Franchi L, Nuñez G, Schnurr M, Espevik T, Lien E, Fitzgerald KA, Rock KL, Moore KJ, Wright SD, Hornung V, Latz E: NLRP3 inflammasomes are required for atherogenesis and activated by cholesterol crystals, Nature 464(7293):1357–1361, 2010 Apr 29.

61. Reginato AJ, Ferreiro Seoane JL, Barbazan Alvarez C, et al. Arthropathy and cutaneous calcinosis in hemodialysis oxalosis. Arthritis Rheum 1986;29:1387–96.

62. Rosenthal A, Ryan LM, McCarty DJ. Arthritis associated with calcium oxalate crystals in an anephric patient treated with peritoneal dialysis. JAMA 1988;260:1280–2.

63. Verbruggen LA, Bourgain C, Verbeelen D. Late presentation and microcrystalline arthropathy in primary hyperoxaluria. Clin Exp Rheumatol 1989;7:631–3.

64. Maldonado I, Prasad V, Reginato AJ. Oxalate crystal deposition disease. Curr Rheumatol Rep 2002;4:257–64.

65. Hoffman GS, Schumacher HR, Paul H, et al. Calcium oxalate microcrystalline-associated arthritis in end-stage renal disease. Ann Intern Med 1982;97:36–42.

66. Tate GA, Schumacher HR, Reginato AJ, et al. Synovial fluid crystals derived from erythrocyte degradation products. J Rheumatol 1992;19:1111–4.

67. Atanes A, Fernandez V, Nuñez R, et al. Idiopathic eosinophilic synovitis. Case report and review of the literature. Scand J Rheumatol 1996;25:183–5.

68. Menard HA, de Medicis R, Lessier A, et al. Charcot-Leyden crystals in synovial fluid. Arthritis Rheum 1981;24:1591–3.

69. Dougados M, Benhamou L, Amor B. Charcot-Leyden crystals in synovial fluid. Arthritis Rheum 1983;26:1416–6.

70. Rodriguez-Paez AC, Seetharaman M, Brent LH. Cryoglobulin crystal arthropathy in a patient with multiple myeloma. J Clin Rheumatol 2009;15:238–40.

71. Papo T, Musset L, Bardin T, et al. Cryocrystalglobulinemia as a cause of systemic vasculopathy and widespread erosive arthropathy. Arthritis Rheum 1996;39:1441–6.

72. Reginato AJ, Schumacher HR, Allan DA, et al. Acute monoarthritis associated with lipid liquid crystals. Ann Rheum Dis 1985;44:537–43.

73. Lawrence C, Seife B. Bone marrow in joint fluid: clue to fracture. Ann Intern Med 1971;74:740–2.

74. Jadhav KB, Gupta N, Ahmed MB. Maltese cross: starch artifact in oral cytology, divulged through polarized microscopy. J Cytol 2010;27:40–1.

75. Levison DA, Crocker PR, Jones S, et al. The varied appearances of starch particles in smears and paraffin sections. Histopathology 1988;13:667–74.
76. Reginato AJ, Schumacher HR, Allan DA, et al. Acute monoarthritis associated with lipid liquid crystals. Ann Rheum Dis 1985;44:537–43.
77. Hackeng CM, de Bruijn LAM, Douw CM, et al. Presence of birefringent, Maltese-cross-appearing spherules in synovial fluid in a case of acute monoarthritis. Clin Chem 2000;46:1861–3.
78. Oliviero F, Frallonardo P, Peruzzo L, et al. Evidence of silicon dioxide crystals in synovial fluid of patients with osteoarthritis. J Rheumatol 2008;35:1092–5.

Section II

Gout

Chapter **3**

Purine Metabolism in the Pathogenesis of Hyperuricemia and Inborn Errors of Purine Metabolism Associated With Disease

Rosa Torres Jiménez and Juan García Puig

KEY POINTS

- Purine nucleotide synthesis and degradation form a crucial metabolic pathway for cell integrity and reproduction.
- Phosphoribosyl pyrophosphate synthetase superactivity, a rare X chromosome–linked disorder, causes juvenile gout.
- Clinical features of hypoxanthine-guanine phosphoribosyltransferase (HPRT) deficiency include uric acid overproduction–related symptoms, neurologic manifestations, and hematologic disturbances including megaloblastic anemia.
- A continuous spectrum of neurologic involvement is present in HPRT-deficient patients.
- Compulsive self-injurious behavior is only present in patients with the complete HPRT enzyme defect.
- Uric acid overproduction in patients with Lesch-Nyhan disease is effectively controlled with allopurinol.
- Xanthinuria is suspected on the basis of a diminished serum urate and urinary uric acid excretion, and most of the patients with classic xanthinuria are asymptomatic.
- The 2,8-dihydroxyadenine stones are caused by adenine phosphoribosyltransferase deficiency, a rare autosomal recessive disorder.
- The association of hypouricemia, recurrent infections, neurologic symptoms, and autoimmune disease prompts the diagnosis of purine-nucleoside phosphorylase deficiency.

Human Purine Metabolism

Purines are molecules with diverse functions in cell physiology. They are essential compounds for nucleic acid synthesis, energy-requiring reactions, cofactor reactions, and intercellular and intracellular signaling. The pathways for purine synthesis, metabolism, and degradation are shown in Figure 3-1. Purine metabolism synthesizes the ribonucleotides adenosine monophosphate, inosine monophosphate, xanthosine monophosphate, and guanosine monophosphate (AMP, IMP, XMP, and GMP, respectively), which produce the deoxyribonucleotides, key elements for nucleic acid synthesis (DNA and RNA).

Three different processes yield an adequate cellular purine concentration: de novo purine synthesis from smaller organic molecules, salvage of preformed purine bases, and purine uptake from the extracellular medium.[1]

Purine Synthesis and Regulation

The *de novo purine synthesis* occurs through a multistep process regulated at different points (see Fig. 3-1).

The first step is the synthesis of phosphoribosyl pyrophosphate (PRPP) from ribose-5-phosphate, glycine, and adenosine triphosphate (ATP) (see Fig. 3-1). This reaction is catalyzed by the enzyme phosphoribosylpyrophosphate synthetase (PRS). PRPP offers the "phosphoribosyl" skeleton on which several atoms are incorporated through 10 reactions leading to the synthesis of inosinic acid (IMP). The last two reactions are catalyzed by a dual-action enzyme termed AICAR transformylase/IMP cyclohydrolase (ATIC). De novo purine synthesis is mainly regulated by the enzyme amidophosphoribosyltransferase (AMPRT; see Fig. 3-1). This enzyme is stimulated by increased substrate concentrations (PRPP) and is subject to feedback inhibition by the purine nucleotides IMP, AMP, and GMP (see Fig. 3-1, broken lines). Most cells are capable of synthesizing purines de novo, although this is metabolically expensive: the synthesis of one molecule of IMP requires the consumption of four amino acids, two folates, one PRPP molecule, and three ATP molecules.

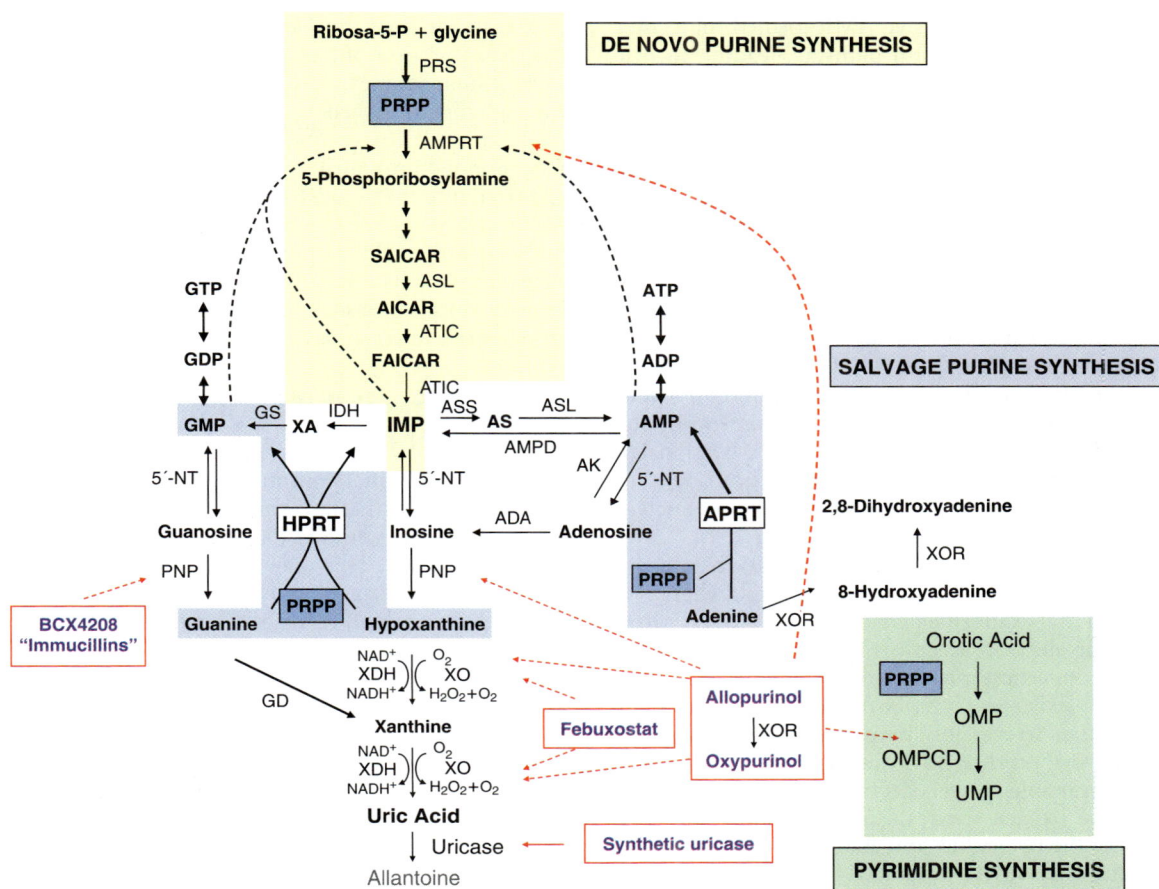

Figure 3-1 Purine synthesis de novo, purine nucleotide degradation, and salvage of preformed purine bases. *ADA,* Adenosine deaminase; *ADP,* adenosine diphosphate; *AICAR,* amidoimidazole carboxamide ribotide; *AK,* adenosine kinase; *AMP,* adenosine monophosphate; *AMPD,* AMP deaminase or myoadenilate deaminase; *AMPRT,* amidophosphoribosyltransferase; *APRT,* adenine phosphoribosyltransferase; *AS,* adenylsuccinate; *ASL,* adenine succinate lyase; *ASS,* adenine succinate synthase; *ATIC,* AICAR transformylase/IMP cyclohydrolase; *ATP,* adenosine triphosphate; *FAICAR,* formamidoimidazole carboxamide ribotide; *GD,* guanine deaminase; *GDP,* guanosine diphosphate; *GMP,* guanosine monophosphate; *GS,* GMP synthetase; *GTP,* guanosine triphosphate; *HPRT,* hipoxanthine-guanine phosphoribosyltransferase; *IDH,* IMP dehydrogenase; *IMP,* inosine monophosphate; *5′-NT,* 5′-nucleotidases; *OMP,* orotidine-5′-monophosphate; *OMPDC,* orotidine-5′-monophosphate decarboxylase; *PNP,* purine nucleotide phosphorylase; *PRPP,* phosphoribosylpyrophosphate; *PRS,* phosphoribosylpyrophosphate synthetase; *Ribose-5-P,* ribose-5-phosphate; *SAICAR,* S-amidoimidazole carboxamide ribotide; *UMP,* uridine monophosphate; *XA or XMP,* xanthinilic acid; *XOR,* xanthine oxidoreductase. The *broken lines* indicate an inhibitory effect. At de novo purine synthesis, the enzyme AMPRT is inhibited by purine nucleotides (IMP, AMP, and GMP). At the purine nucleotide degradation pathway, allopurinol, oxypurinol, and febuxostat inhibit the enzyme xanthine oxidoreductase (XOR). Allopurinol and its active metabolite, oxypurinol, inhibit mainly the reduced form xantine dehydrogenase (XDH). In addition, allopurinol and oxypurinol inhibit the enzyme orotidine-5′-monophosphate decarboxylase (OMPDC), causing orotic acid accumulation. Allopurinol is transformed by HPRT in allopurinol and oxypurinol nucleotides, consuming PRPP substrate. Allopurinol and oxypurinol nucleotides suppress amidotransferase activity via allosteric negative regulation (*broken line*). The inhibitory action on PNP by allopurinol is weak (*broken line*) and probably due to hypoxanthine and xanthine accumulation. Febuxostat is a potent inhibitor of both the oxidized and the reduced (XO and XDH) forms of the enzyme xanthine oxidoreductase (XOR). Febuxostat does not inhibit PNP and OMPDC. *Yellow shadow,* de novo purine synthesis pathway; *blue shadow,* salvage purine synthesis pathway; *green shadow,* pyrimidin synthesis pathway.

Purine nucleotide interconversion is also a complex, multistep process, under feedback control. The conversion of IMP to xanthinilic acid (XA or XMP) by the enzyme IMP dehydrogenase (IDH; see Fig. 3-1) is the first step leading to guanine nucleotides and is inhibited by GTP. XMP is further converted into GMP via amination by GMP synthetase (GS). Similarly, the conversion of IMP to adenylsuccinate (AS or S-AMP) by the enzyme adenylsuccinate synthetase (ASS; see Fig. 3-1) is the first step leading to adenine nucleotide synthesis (AMP, ADP, ATP; see Fig. 3-1). Adenylsuccinate is further converted to AMP by the enzyme adenylsuccinate lyase (ASL, see Fig. 3-1). This enzyme catalyzes also the synthesis of AICAR in the de novo purine pathway. The congenital absence of this

enzyme causes AS accumulation and a severe neurologic disease. AMP is converted into IMP through the enzyme AMP deaminase (AMPD; see Fig. 3-1). Adenylate kinase (ADK) catalyzed the reversible reaction AMP + ATP ↔ 2ADP.

Conditions that increase ATP degradation (i.e., ischemia with hypoxia that limits ATP regeneration from both ADP and AMP) or enhance ATP consumption (i.e., ingestion of ethanol, which is metabolized in the liver to form acetate) promote hyperuricemia. Each mole of ethanol consumes two moles of high-energy phosphate and can increase AMP formation. Most of the AMP formed is used for ATP synthesis (see Fig. 3-1), provided an adequate oxygen supply. However, if this is not the case and the increased amount of AMP is not recycled back to ATP, the excessive AMP formed may enter the purine nucleotide degradation pathway, leading to uric acid synthesis. The administration of ethanol has been shown to increase the adenine nucleotide pool turnover (i.e., hyperuricemia associated with alcohol consumption),[2] although lactate production from ethanol metabolism also increases renal urate reabsorption.

Purine nucleotide degradation is initiated by nucleotide dephosphorylation and nucleoside formation (adenosine, inosine, and guanosine) (see Fig. 3-1). This reaction is catalyzed by 5′-nucleotidases (5′-NT; see Fig. 3-1) and unspecific phosphatases. Inosine and guanosine, through the action of purine-nucleoside phosphorylase (PNP; see Fig. 3-1), are transformed into the purine bases hypoxanthine and guanine, respectively. Adenosine is converted into inosine by the enzyme adenosine deaminase (ADA; see Fig. 3-1). Finally, the purine bases hypoxanthine and xanthine (oxipurines) are oxidized to uric acid by the enzyme xanthine oxidoreductase (XOR; see Fig. 3-1).

XOR was isolated in its xanthine oxidase (XO) form using oxygen as the electron acceptor from cow's milk, whereas it has been purified in its xanthine dehydrogenase (XDH) form, with NAD^+ as the electron acceptor. Both enzymes, XO and XDH, are interconvertible products of the same gene. The enzyme originally exists in its XDH form but is readily converted to XO either irreversibly by proteolysis or reversibly by oxidation of Cys residues to form disulfide groups. The reversible or irreversible conversion of XDH to the XO form generates reactive oxygen species (i.e., H_2O_2 and O_2^-). The main product of the reversible conversion of XDH to its XO form is O_2^-, and that of XO to its XDH form is H_2O_2. Both have a relevant role in a myriad of physiologic and pathologic mechanisms such as reduction of cytochrome *c*, defense against infectious pathogens, or in the pathology of post ischemia-reperfusion injury.

Guanine, on the other hand, is converted to xanthine by guanine deaminase or guanase (GD; see Fig. 3-1). In general, the activity of these enzymes is regulated by substrate availability. In humans and primates, uric acid is the final product of purine metabolism, but in other animals, uric acid is degraded to allantoin by the enzyme uricase (uricase; see Fig. 3-1).

Salvage of preformed purine bases: Purine recycling in humans is mediated by three different enzymes: hypoxanthine-guanine phosphoribosyltransferase (HPRT), adenine-phosphoribosyltransferase (APRT), and adenosine kinase (AK; see Fig. 3-1). It is estimated that 90% of the free purines generated in the intracellular metabolism are recycled rather than degraded or excreted. This allows for a very efficient functioning with respect to purine metabolism. HPRT recycles hypoxanthine and guanine into IMP and GMP, respectively (see Fig. 3-1). Xanthine is also a substrate of HPRT, but the affinity of HPRT for xanthine is much lower than that for hypoxanthine. APRT, structurally and functionally similar to HPRT, recycles free adenine into AMP (see Fig. 3-1). HPRT and APRT need the cosubstrate PRPP for purine base recycling. AK (see Fig. 3-1) phosphorylates adenosine to generate AMP. AK prevents the diffusion of free adenosine from the cell or its degradation into inosine by adenosine deaminase (ADA; see Fig. 3-1). Thus, AK is a very important enzyme that contributes to maintain the purine nucleotide pool.

Maintenance of the purine nucleotide pool is also due to the incorporation of free purine bases and nucleosides from extracellular sources. Dietary vegetables and animal products, through digestion, generate purines following DNA and RNA degradation. These compounds are absorbed from the gut and incorporated into purines by the liver. These purine bases are exported into the bloodstream to be used by other tissues. The salvage enzymes are crucial to incorporate preformed purine bases into the cellular purine pool. Thus, a salvage enzyme deficiency results not only in an inability to salvage intracellular purines but also in an inability to incorporate purines from extracellular sources.

Drugs That Inhibit Purine Nucleotide Degradation

Uric acid is the final compound of purine nucleotide degradation and is synthesized through the enzyme XOR (see Fig. 3-1). Uric acid synthesis may be enhanced when cell turnover is increased. This may occur in a myriad of pathologic processes, including enzyme overactivities, proliferative diseases, glycogen storage disease, malignancies, and hematologic disorders. The first drug clinically used to inhibit purine nucleotide degradation was allopurinol.[3] Allopurinol was synthesized in 1950 to inhibit the oxidative degradation of 6-mercaptopurine (an antileukemic agent only active when converted into its cytotoxic nucleotide [thioinosinic acid] by HPRT). Detailed metabolic studies in patients with chronic myeloid leukemia showed that 5% to 7% of a given dose of mercaptopurine was excreted into the urine as the free compound and 25% to 30% was oxidized to the inert thiouric acid. At that time, there seemed to be no feasible way to increase the rate of nucleotide synthesis and attention was given to inhibit the oxidative degradation of 6-mercaptopurine. Among the purine and pyrimidine derivatives studied, 4-hydroxy-(3,4d)-pyrazolopyrimidine (4-HPP or allopurinol) was not only an inhibitor but a substrate for the enzyme XOR that did not affect tumor growth. Allopurinol given concomitantly with 6-mercaptopurine markedly reduced thioinosinic acid and increased 6-mercaptopurine efficacy. The continued administration of allopurinol markedly decreased serum urate concentrations and urinary uric acid excretion.

Since approved in 1964, allopurinol has been a cornerstone in the treatment of hyperuricemic conditions and processes with increased uric acid production, typically identified by increased urinary uric acid excretion.[4] Allopurinol competitively inhibits XOR (see Fig. 3-1) and thus reduces uric acid synthesis. In normal conditions, allopurinol increases the reutilization of hypoxanthine for nucleotide and nucleic acid synthesis, via HPRT activity, and thereby consumes substrate (PRPP). The resultant increase in allopurinol nucleotide concentration leads to feedback inhibition of de novo purine synthesis at the level of allosteric regulation of amidotransferase activity.

In patients with HPRT deficiency, allopurinol increases mean xanthine excretion 10-fold and has been associated with xanthine urolithiasis.[5] The long-lived active metabolite of allopurinol is oxypurinol, which normally is predominantly renally cleared and has a 24-hour half-life but its half-life is increased by renal impairment. Oxypurinol is also a competitive inhibitor of XOR (see Fig. 3-1). Both allopurinol and oxypurinol are substrates of HPRT. Their corresponding nucleotides exert an inhibitory effect on AMPRT activity and decrease de novo purine synthesis (see Fig. 3-1). This explains the fact that the reduction in uric acid synthesis is not replaced by a stoichiometric replacement by hypoxanthine and xanthine.[6]

A new potent inhibitor of XOR has been recently approved for the treatment of gout. Febuxostat (2-[3-cyano-4-isobutoxyphenyl]-4-methyl-5-thiazolecarboxylic acid), unlike allopurinol, is not a purine analogue and inhibits both the oxidized and reduced forms of the enzyme XOR (see Fig. 3-1) in a noncompetitive way, by interfering with access of substrate to the active site of the enzyme.[7] This difference has been postulated to account for the higher potency and long-lasting action of febuxostat compared to allopurinol. Importantly, and contrary to allopurinol, febuxostat is not a substrate of purine and pyrimidine metabolic enzymes, such as HPRT or orotate phosphoribosyltransferase, and it does not inhibit purine nucleoside phosphorylase and orotidine-5′-monophosphate decarboxylase (see Fig. 3-1, green area).

On a milligram orally administered basis, febuxostat inhibitory effect appears to be superior to that of allopurinol (febuxostat 40 mg equals allopurinol 300 mg) and does not require dosage adjustment in patients with mild to moderate renal impairment (creatinine clearance, 30 to 89 ml/min).[7] The precise indications, dosing, effectiveness, and side effect profile of febuxostat in the treatment of hyperuricemia in gout and other conditions are discussed in Chapter 15.

Disorders of Purine Metabolism: Classification

Most disorders of purine metabolism are expressed by a considerable variation in serum urate concentration and urinary uric acid excretion, since uric acid is the final product of purine metabolism in human beings (see Fig. 3-1). A detailed clinical study from a given patient may disclose whether he or she has a congenital or an acquired disease. This chapter will focus on congenital disorders of purine metabolism that cause hyperuricemia and hypouricemia. Purine metabolism congenital diseases may compromise the following enzymes: (1) purine synthesis de novo—PRS, adenylatosuccinate lyase, and ATIC; (2) salvage purine synthesis—HPRT and APRT; and (3) purine interconversion and degradation pathway—XOR, PNP, ADA, adenylate kinase, and myoadenilate deaminase. On the other hand, certain drugs may also inhibit enzymes of the purine nucleotide degradation pathway or may modify renal uric acid excretion. Enzymopathies may be classified into two main groups: overactivity and deficiency, the last being, by far, the most frequent. From a clinical point of view, purine disorders may be classified according to the clinical syndromes they determine: hyperuricemia and gout (Table 3-1), nephrolithiasis, immunodeficiency, anemia, diseases of the peripheral and central nervous systems, and myopathies (Table 3-2).

Some enzyme defects of carbohydrate metabolism (glycogen storage diseases) have been associated with hyperuricemia and gout[8] (Fig. 3-2). Type I glycogenosis, due to glucose-6-phosphate deficiency, compromises glucose dephosphorylation and may increase serum urate concentrations via a dual mechanism: increased lactate production, which may interfere with urinary uric acid excretion.[9] On the other hand, hyperuricemia in type I glycogenosis may also be the result of increased hypoxanthine, xanthine, and uric acid synthesis

Table 3-1 Clinical Disorders Associated With Alteration of Purine Metabolism and Hyperuricemia

HYPERURICEMIA AND GOUT

- Primary hyperuricemia
  - Increased urinary uric acid excretion ("uric acid overproduction," ~5-10%)
  - Normal or decreased urinary uric acid excretion ("relative uric acid underexcretion," ~90-95%)
- Secondary hyperuricemia (normal synthesis of uric acid and decreased uric acid excretion)
  - Common
    Hypertension
    Metabolic syndrome
    Chronic kidney disease
    Extracellular volume contraction and volume depletion
    Acidosis
    Drugs: thiazides and loop diuretics, salicylates (low doses), niacin, pyrazinamide
  - Rare
    Lead intoxication
    Analgesic neuropathy
    Polycystic kidney disease
    Medullary cystic kidney disease
    Other familial interstitial nephropathies (i.e., uromodulin deposits)
    Endocrinopathies (i.e., hyperparathyroidism, hypothyroidism)
- Secondary hyperuricemia (increased synthesis of uric acid and increased uric acid excretion)
  - Common
    Purine overingestion
    Increased ATP catabolism (i.e., ethanol, exhausting exercise, tissue ischemia, glycogenosis)
    Psoriasis
    Paget's disease of bone
    Hematologic and neoplastic diseases with increased cell turnover
    Drugs: cytotoxic chemotherapy (including tumor lysis syndrome)
  - Rare
    Phosphoribosylpyrophosphate synthetase (PRPPs)* overactivity
    Hypoxanthine-guanine phosphoribosyltransferase (HPRT) deficiency
    Glucose-6-phosphate dehydrogenase deficiency (Von Gierke disease)

*PRPPs is also called PRS overactivity.

due to enhanced ATP breakdown and increased AMP production.[10] In glycogenosis types III, V and VII, acetyl-CoA synthesis is impaired leading to poor citric cycle efficiency with diminished ATP production.[10] To compensate this, the adenine nucleotide cycle overproduces fumarate to fuel the activity of the Krebs cycle. The overactivity of the adenine nucleotide cycle leads to increased IMP formation from AMP that may enter the purine nucleotide degradation pathway, leading to increased uric acid synthesis[10] (see Fig. 3-2).

Congenital Disorders of Purine Metabolism Causing Hyperuricemia

The synthesis of uric acid may be viewed as the result of two main processes: (1) de novo purine synthesis (i.e., the formation of purines from nonpurine compounds) leading to the

Table 3-2 Other Clinical Disorders of Purine Metabolism

NEPHROLITHIASIS

- Uric acid
- Phosphoribosylpyrophosphate synthetase (PRPPs) overactivity*
- Hypoxanthine-guanine phosphoribosyltransferase deficiency (HPRT) deficiency
- Glucose-6-phosphate dehydrogenase deficiency
- Xanthine
- Xanthine oxidoreductase deficiency (hereditary xanthinuria)
- Drugs: allopurinol, febuxostat
- 2,8-Dihydroxyadenine
- Adenine phosphoribosyltransferase deficiency (APRT)

INMUNODEFICIENCIES

- Adenosine deaminase (ADA) deficiency
- Purine nucleoside phosphorylase (PNP) deficiency

ANEMIA

- Hemolytic
- Adenylate kinase deficiency
- ADA overactivity
- PNP deficiency
- Megaloblastic
- PRPPs overactivity*
- HPRT deficiency
- PNP deficiency

DISEASES OF THE PERIPHERAL AND CENTRAL NERVOUS SYSTEMS

- PRPPs overactivity*
- HPRT deficiency
- Adenylosuccinate lyase deficiency
- ADA deficiency
- PNP deficiency
- Guanine deaminase deficiency
- PRPPs deficiency*

MYOPATHIES

- Myoadenylate deaminase deficiency (Fig. 3-1, also called AMPD)
- Xanthine oxidoreductase deficiency
- Metabolic myopathies (i.e., mitochondrial myopathies)

*PRPPs is also called PRS overactivity.

nucleotides IMP, AMP, GMP, and XMP, and (2) the catabolism of these nucleotides (purine nucleotide degradation) (see Fig. 3-1). Two main enzyme defects have been described that markedly increase uric acid synthesis. One is located at de novo purine synthesis (PRS overactivity), and the second at the salvage pathway (HPRT deficiency) (see Fig. 3-1).

Phosphoribosylpyrophosphate Synthetase Superactivity

PRS superactivity (OMIM 300661) (also known as PRPP synthetase superactivity) is a rare X chromosome–linked disorder causing juvenile gout. PRS catalyzes the synthesis of phosphoribosylpyrophosphate (PRPP), which is a main substrate in the synthesis of purine, pyridine, and pyrimidine nucleotides (see Fig. 3-1). The disorder is characterized by hyperuricemia and gout, which are accompanied, in the most severe phenotype, by neurologic manifestations. To date, about 30 patients have been reported with this enzyme defect, which was described for the first time in 1972.[11]

Clinical Description

PRS superactivity results in two different phenotypes. The mild phenotype is characterized by gout and uric acid urolithiasis with late-juvenile or early-adult onset.[11,12] Gout arthritis is severe and is accompanied by tophi. About 75% of patients present with recurrent uric acid stones. Uric acid urolithiasis is usually the first manifestation of the disease. Blood and urine levels of uric acid are particularly increased. Acute renal failure presentation is not as common as it is in HPRT deficiency, but it has been described in a patient presenting with a uric acid renal excretion of 2400 mg/24 hr. Recurrent uric acid stone complications such as urinary tract infection, pyelonephritis, hypertension, and renal failure may develop. Heterozygous females carrying the defect do not present clinical manifestations.

The severe phenotype is usually diagnosed in early childhood or infancy due to neurologic impairment and uric acid overproduction manifestations. Sensorineural deafness, mental retardation, hypotonia, ataxia, and progressive axonal neuropathy with demyelination have been described.[13-16] Heterozygous females can also present with uric acid overproduction, with uric acid lithiasis and juvenile gout, and in some cases with sensorineural deafness.[17]

Pathophysiology

PRS catalyzes the PRPP synthesis from Mg-ATP and ribose-5-phosphate in a reaction that requires Mg^{2+} and inorganic phosphate (P_i) as activators.[18] P_i enzymatic activation involves two mechanisms: P_i stabilizes the enzyme loop involved in the binding of ATP, facilitating the substrate binding of Mg-ATP complex, and P_i is also an allosteric competitor of the enzyme inhibitor ADP. PRS reaction is subject to inhibition in a feedback mechanism by purine nucleotides as ADP and GDP. PRPP is substrate of three enzymes of purine metabolic pathway: PRPP amidotransferase, in de novo synthesis pathway, which serves specifically as the rate-limiting reaction for the purine synthesis, and HPRT and APRT in the salvage pathway. In addition to de novo synthesis of purine, PRPP is used in the pyrimidine and pyridine nucleotide synthesis. PRPP is cofactor for uridine monophosphate synthetase (UMPS), which converts orotic acid into UMP, the precursor of all other pyrimidine nucleotides. Finally, PRPP is utilized for pyridine nucleotide synthesis by nicotinate phosphoribosyl transferase (NAPRT) and nicotinamide phosphoribosyl transferase (NAMPT) for the nicotinamide adenine dinucleotide (NAD) and nicotinamide adenine dinucleotide phosphate (NADP) synthesis.

PRS overactivity causes an increase in intracellular PRPP, which in turn is the cause of increased purine synthesis and uric acid overproduction. However, the pathophysiology of the neurologic dysfunction remains unclear.

Although PRS activity is coded by three different genes—*PRPS1*, *PRPS2*, and *PRPS3* or *PRPS1L1*, to date, PRS overactivity is caused exclusively by an alteration in *PRPS1* (MIM 311850), which codes for PRS-I or ribose-phosphate pyrophosphokinase 1. PRPS1 is located in chromosome X, and mutations in this gene have been also associated with three syndromes in which PRS-I activity is decreased: Arts syndrome (MIM 301835),[19] Charçot-Marie-Tooth disease-5 (MIM 311070),[20] and X-linked nonsyndromic sensorineural

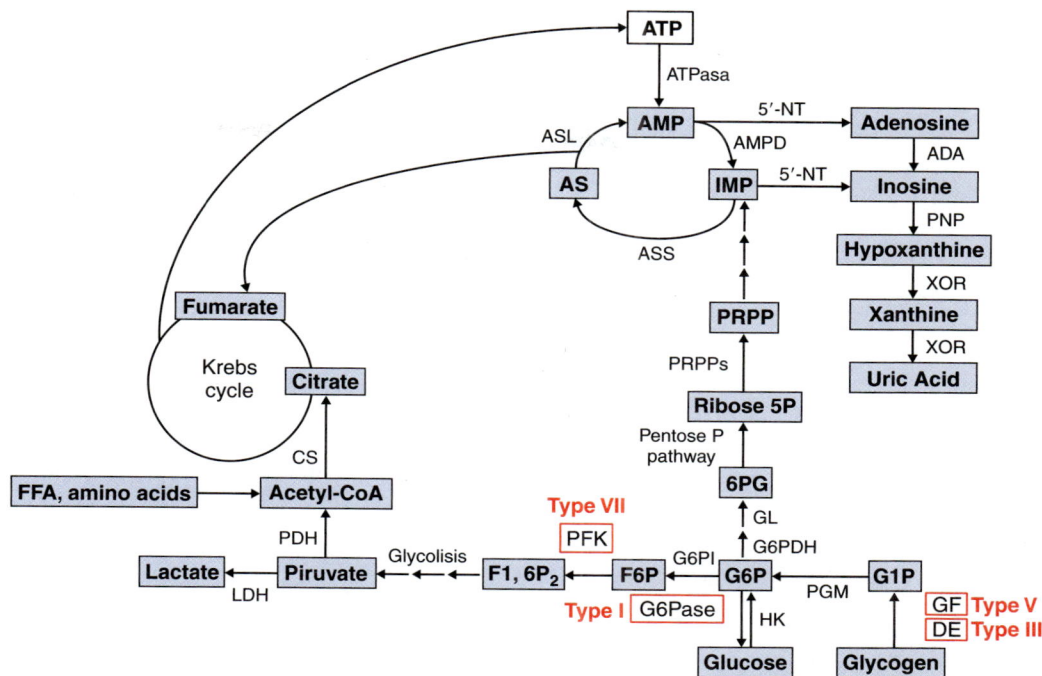

Figure 3-2 Biochemical mechanisms leading to increased uric acid synthesis in certain glycogen storage diseases (type III, debrancher deficiency [Cori-Forbes disease]; type V, muscle glycogen phosphorylase deficiency [McArdle disease]; and type VII, phosphofructokinase deficiency [Tauri disease]). These three enzyme defects diminish glucose phosphorylation and reduce acetyl-CoA synthesis. This impairs ATP (adenosine triphosphate) production at the Krebs cycle. Increased fumarate production by the adenine nucleotide cycle compensates the citric acid cycle activity to restore the ATP pool. However, the increased activity of the adenine nucleotide cycles renders an increased adenosine monophosphate (AMP) production, which may fuel the adenine nucleotide degradation pathway, leading to increased uric acid synthesis. Type I glycogenosis (von Gierke disease) is due to glucose-6-phosphatase deficiency, and increased serum urate concentration has been related to a dual mechanism—increased lactate production, which competes with uric acid for a common tubular transporter, and increased availability of liver 6-phosphogluconate (G6P), which fuels the pentose phosphate pathway, leading to increased NADPH and phosphoribosylpyrophosphate (PRPP) production. *ADA*, adenosine deaminase; *AMPD*, AMP deaminase; *AS*, adenylsuccinate; *ASL*, adenine succinate lyase; *ASS*, adenine succinate synthase; *CS*, citrate synthase; *DE*, Debrancher enzyme; *F6P*, fructose 1-phosphate; *F1,6P2*, fructose 1,6-diphosphate; *GF*, glycogen fosforilase; *GL*, gluconolactonase; *G6PDH*, glucose-6-phosphate dehydrogenase; *G1P*, glucose 1-phosphate; *G6P*, glucose 6-phosphate; *G6Pase*, glucose 6-phosphatase; *G6PI*, glucose 6-phosphate isomerase; *FFA*, free fatty acids; *HK*, hexokinase; *IMP*, inosine monophosphate; *PDH*, piruvate dehydrogenase; *PFK*, phosphofructokinase; *PGM*, phosphoglucomutase; *PNP*, purine nucleotide phosphorylase; *LDH*, lactate dehydrogenase; *5′-NT*, 5′-nucleotidase; *Pentose P pathway*, pentose phosphate pathway; *PRPPs*, phosphoribosylpyrophosphate synthetase; *Ribose 5P*, ribose 5-phosphate; *XOR*, xanthine oxidoreductase.

deafness or DFN2[21] (MIM 304500). Clinical manifestations of these syndromes include sensorineural deafness, mental retardation, hypotonia, peripheral neuropathy with demyelination, ataxia, and optic atrophy.

Severe PRS superactivity phenotype is caused by point mutations in the *PRPS1* gene.[11,13,22] These mutations result in an alteration in the enzyme regulation with decreased inhibition by purine nucleotides and a higher P_i affinity and activation (Fig. 3-3). Mutations causing PRS-I superactivity are located by disturbing the allosteric sites, directly or by altering the homodimer interface (see Fig. 3-3). This fact explains the loss of feedback inhibition but may also result in a decrease protein stability.[23] Thus, in these patients, PRS activity determined in hemolysate is usually decreased due to the instability of the mutant protein in erythrocytes. Nucleotide levels are also low in erythrocytes. These facts suggest that PRS activity could be also decreased in neuronal cells, causing neurologic symptoms that develop only in the severe phenotype. However, a mild phenotype is caused by an increased PRPS1 expression of unknown mechanism.[24] In these patients, a higher V_{max} is present due to a higher protein concentration and PRS activity is high in all cells tested.[24,25]

Diagnosis

All patients show an elevated serum urate and urinary uric acid excretion rate. Diagnosis is confirmed by enzyme activity determinations in erythrocytes, fibroblasts, or lymphocytes. In addition of enzyme activity, the kinetics of enzyme activation by P_i or inhibition by nucleotides need to be tested. The enzyme activity in erythrocytes of patients with the severe phenotype is usually decreased, due to abnormal enzyme stability; however, enhanced enzyme affinity for P_i and reduced inhibition of the activity by ADP and GDP are observed in cultured fibroblasts and lymphoblasts. In the mild phenotype, PRS-I activity is increased at all P_i concentrations with normal inhibition by nucleotides and normal K_m for P_i inhibition.

Molecular Diagnosis

In patients with the severe phenotype, molecular diagnosis can be made by sequencing PRPS1 exons or PRPS1 cDNA. To date, seven different point mutations have been described. Carrier females are heterozygous for the mutation. No mutations can be found in patients with the mild phenotype in either the coding region or in the promoter or 3′-untranslated

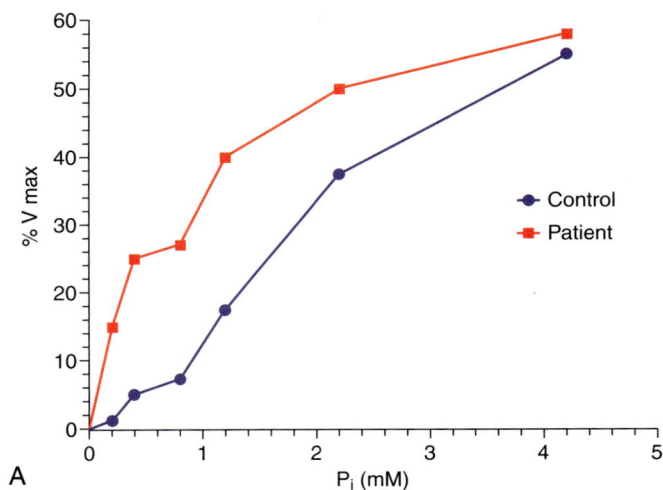

A

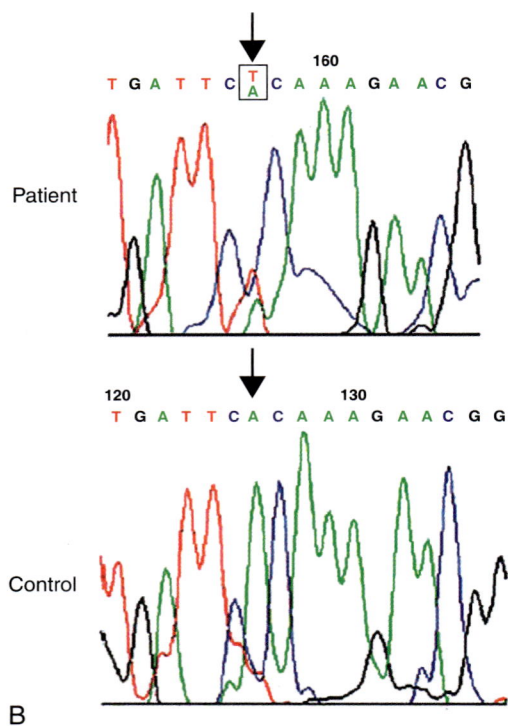

B

Figure 3-3 Severe phosphoribosylpyrophosphate synthetase (PRS) superactivity phenotype. **A,** PRS activity was determined in the hemolysate from a patient with PRS superactivity and a control subject. Note that activation by P_i, expressed as the percentage of the maximum velocity of enzyme reaction (V_{max}), is higher in the hemolysate from the patient. **B,** DNA sequencing from a patient with PRS overactivity and a control subject. PRS superactivity in this patient was caused by a point mutation in the *PRPS1* gene.[17] PRS superactivity in a female patient heterozygous for point mutation 570 A>T in exon 5 from the *PRS1* gene. Spherograms from automated sequencing of patient PRS1 exon 5 showed a double signal for A and T in position 570. This change causes a substitution of Leu (CTC) for His (CAC) in the PRS protein at the aminoacid position 192.

regions. In these patients, an increased PRPS1 mRNA expression can be found.

Treatment

Uric acid overproduction is managed by inhibiting XO with allopurinol, at an initial dosage of 5 to 10 mg/kg/day, and colchicine prophylaxis to avoid gout flares. To prevent uric acid or xanthine urolithiasis, allopurinol should be given together with adequate hydration and urine alkalinization.

Hypoxanthine-Guanine Phosphoribosyltransferase Deficiency

In 1964, Lesch and Nyhan reported the cases of two brothers with a disorder of uric acid metabolism and neurologic dysfunction.[26] The first Lesch-Nyhan disease (OMIM 300322) clinical description included hyperuricemia, mental retardation, self-injurious behavior, and motor abnormalities such as spasticity and choreathetosis. In 1967, Seegmiller et al.[27] reported the complete deficiency of the enzyme HPRT activity as the cause of Lesch-Nyhan disease. HPRT is a key enzyme in the salvage of purine metabolism (see Fig. 3-1). Also in 1967, Kelley et al.[28] described a partial deficiency of HPRT activity associated with gout and no neurologic involvement. This partial deficiency was termed Kelley-Seegmiller syndrome or HPRT-related gout (OMIM 300323). It is currently considered that a continuous spectrum of neurologic involvement is present in HPRT-deficient patients.[29,30] The term "Lesch-Nyhan variants" has been introduced to include patients with HPRT-related gout and varying degrees of neurologic involvement but without the complete clinical features of Lesch-Nyhan disease.

Clinical Description

Clinical features of HPRT deficiency include uric acid overproduction–related symptoms, neurologic manifestations, and hematologic disturbances including megaloblastic anemia.[31] Hyperuricemia-related renal and articular symptoms (acute arthritis, tophi, nephrolithiasis or urolithiasis, and renal disease) are present in all HPRT-deficient patients and are not related to the severity of the enzyme defect.[29] One of the first signs of the disease, which may appear in the first months of life, is the observation of orange crystals in the diapers, crystalluria with obstruction of the urinary tract, or renal failure.

A continuum spectrum of neurologic manifestations, which depends on the severity of the defect, may be present in HPRT-deficient patients. Neurologic symptoms affect the motor sphere, cognitive, and behavioral aspects.[30] In the complete Lesch-Nyhan syndrome, patients are normal at birth. Psychomotor delay becomes evident within 3 to 6 months with a delay in the acquisition of sitting and head support with hypotonia. Self-mutilation, in the form of lip biting or finger chewing, can appear as soon as teeth are present. The motor syndrome evolves to a severe action dystonia, superimposed on a baseline hypotonia.[32] Its severity leads to an inability to stand up and walk, and patients are confined to a wheelchair. Involuntary movements, such as choreoathetosis and ballismus, are usually associated with voluntary movements and increase with excitement and anxiety (Fig. 3-4).

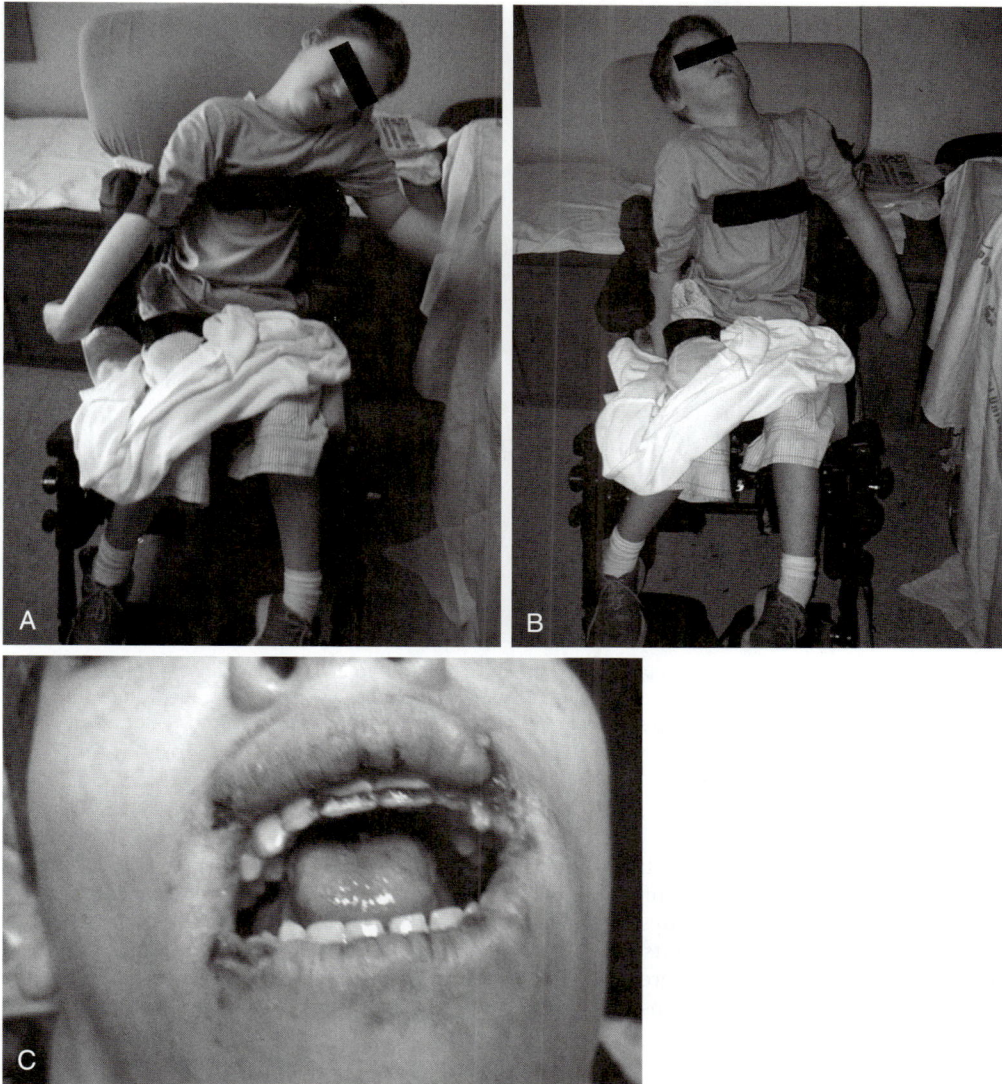

Figure 3-4 Lesch-Nyhan disease. **A** and **B,** Severe generalized dystonia in a patient with the complete form of Lesch-Nyhan disease. Dystonia leads to an inability to stand up and walk; patients are confined to a wheelchair. Involuntary movements, such as choreoathetosis and ballismus, are usually associated with voluntary movements and increase with excitement and anxiety. **C,** Compulsive self-injurious behavior: multiple lip erosions due to biting.

Dysarthria and dysphagia are always present and opisthotonus is frequently reported. Corticospinal tract signs such as spasticity, hyperreflexia, and extensor plantar reflex are generally reported in later years and may reflect an acquired defect.[32] The first Lesch-Nyhan description included mental retardation as a characteristic of the disease. However, complete HPRT-deficient patients, when evaluated with specific tests for motor difficulties, show mild to moderate mental retardation.[33]

Compulsive self-injurious behavior, the most striking feature of Lesch-Nyhan syndrome, is only present in patients with the complete enzyme defect. The patients bite their lips, tongue, or fingers, causing important automutilating lesions (see Fig. 3-4). In some instances, the aggressive behavior is also directed against their family and friends, with patients spitting or using abusive language. The mutilation is not the result of a lack of sensation (the patients

feel pain and are relieved when protected from themselves), and recently it has been ascribed to an obsessive-compulsive behavior. Self-mutilation may start between 2 and 16 years of age and evolves with periods of different intensity. Generally it is associated with or aggravated by psychological stress (adolescence, familial conflicts) or concomitant diseases. Despite their periodic aggressive behavior, Lesch-Nyhan patients are frequently happy and engaging children when they are restrained. In our experience with 40 HPRT-deficient patients diagnosed at our institution since 1984, the neurobehavioral disorder may be markedly modulated by numerous environmental factors, among which education is one of the most relevant.

In Lesch-Nyhan variants, a complete motor syndrome may be present in the most severe forms, but self-injurious behavior is always absent.[30] In these cases, involuntary movements are present and generalized dystonia precludes to stand up

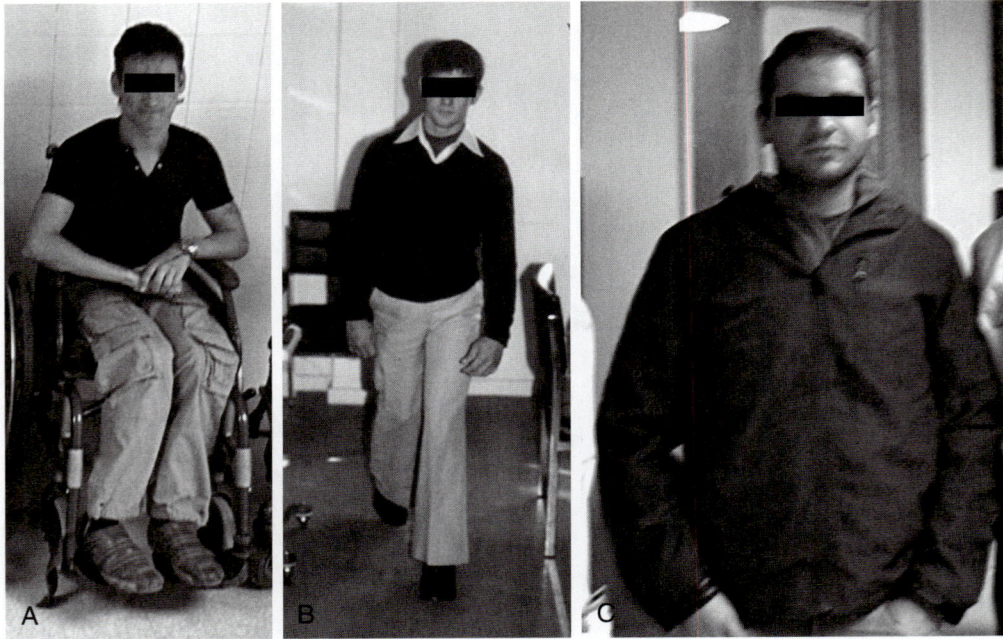

Figure 3-5 The continuum spectrum of Lesch-Nyhan variants. **A,** In the most severe form of Lesch-Nyhan "variants," a complete motor syndrome is present, but self-injurious behavior is always absent. In this patient, generalized dystonia precludes the patient from standing up and walking and involuntary movements are present, but he never showed self-injurious behavior. **B,** In other variant patients, the grade of dystonia is less severe and appears in the form of a dystonic gait and speech difficulties. **C,** In the less-affected patients, the motor syndrome is unapparent, and hypoxanthine-guanine phosphoribosyltransferase activity residual activity is measurable in the hemolysate.

and walk (Fig. 3-5, *A*). In other variant patients, the grade of dystonia is less severe and appears in the form of a dystonic gait, speech difficulties, or exercised-induced dystonia or is unapparent (Fig. 3-5, *B* and *C*).[29] These patients may carry independent lives. They can present varying degrees of mental retardation or normal intelligence, but they usually show attention deficits.

Pathophysiology

HPRT catalyzes the salvage synthesis of IMP and GMP from the purine bases hypoxanthine and guanine, respectively, using 5′-phosphoribosyl-1-pyrophosphate (PRPP) as a cosubstrate (see Fig. 3-1). HPRT deficiency results in the accumulation of the substrates hypoxanthine, guanine, and PRPP. Hypoxanthine is converted into uric acid by means of XOR, and the increased availability of PRPP for PRPP amidotransferase increases purine synthesis de novo. On the other hand, there is a decrease in IMP and GMP, which are PRPP amidotransferase feedback inhibitors. This dual mechanism results in an increased de novo synthesis of purine nucleotides.[34]

The connection between the aberrant purine metabolism and the neurologic and behavioral characteristics remains unknown. Image studies and postmortem examination of brains from Lesch-Nyhan patients have not disclosed any characteristic morphologic abnormality; thus a functional instead of a morphologic alteration is postulated. Clinical data suggest a basal ganglia alteration. Both extrapyramidal motor syndrome, with involuntary movements and dystonia, and behavioral disturbances are signs of basal ganglia damage.[35] Several neurotransmitter changes seem to be implicated in Lesch-Nyhan syndrome pathophysiology. Neurochemistry analysis of postmortem tissues and cerebrospinal fluid analysis showed a decreased level of dopamine and the dopamine metabolite homovanillic acid, whereas serotonin and 5-hydroxyindoleacetic levels show discrepant results.[35] Studies with positron-emission tomography and ligands that bind to dopamine-related proteins have confirmed an alteration of the dopaminergic system in Lesch-Nyhan patients.[35] Dopamine deficiency in the striatum has been confirmed in animal models of HPRT deficiency.[35] Alterations in other neurotransmitter systems, such as adenosine, have also been implicated.[36] As a consequence of HPRT deficiency, Lesch-Nyhan patients' cerebrospinal fluid shows an increased hypoxanthine concentration.[37] Toxic effects of this metabolite have been implicated in the pathogenesis of neurologic dysfunction by means of an alteration in adenosine transport, Na^+,K^+-ATPase activity, serotonin content, and neuronal development.[38] The possible deficit of other purine compounds due to the enzyme defect is controversial, and altered nucleotide concentrations have been postulated as a possible cause of changes in G protein–mediated signal transduction. Finally, a defective developmental process of dopaminergic neurons is thought to be implicated in Lesch-Nyhan neurologic manifestations.

Lesch-Nyhan patients present with megaloblastic anemia,[39] which has been associated with megaloblastic findings in the bone marrow. Ineffective erythropoiesis has been postulated as the cause of anemia in the Lesch-Nyhan patients. In addition, increased folic acid consumption, due to enhanced de novo purine synthesis, has been implicated in its pathogenesis. Nevertheless, anemia is not corrected by folate therapy.

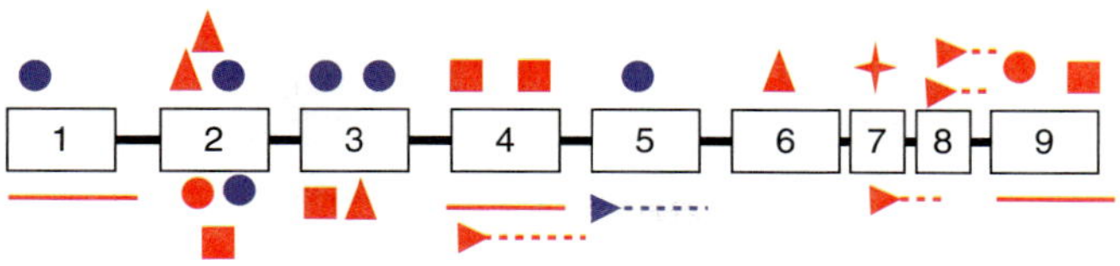

Figure 3-6 Mutations in *HPRT1* gene found in Spanish hypoxanthine-guanine phosphoribosyltransferase (HPRT)-deficient patients. *HPRT1* gene presents 9 exons (*gray boxes*) separated for intronic sequences (*black line*). We have found 26 different mutations from 7 Lesch-Nyhan variant patients (*blue*) and 19 Lesch-Nyhan patients (*red*). Type of mutations included eight missense point mutations (*circle*), one nonsense point mutation (*star*), three deletions of the complete exon (*gross line*), five splicing mutations causing exon exclusion splicing (*intermittent line*), five small deletions (*square*), and four small insertion (*triangle*).

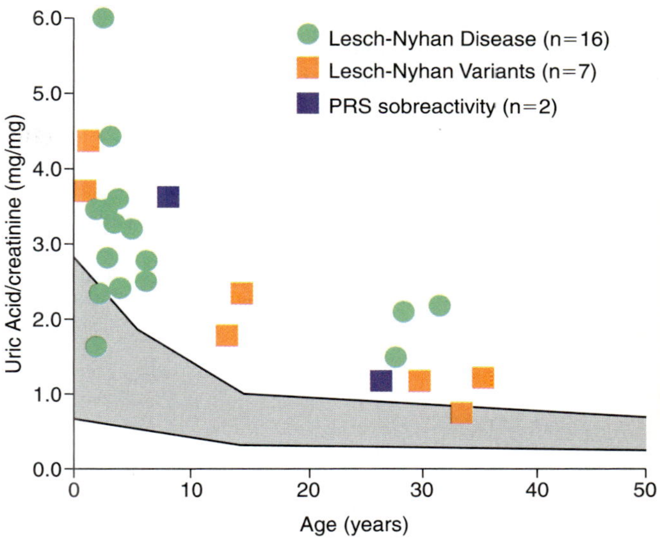

Genetics

Human HPRT is encoded by a single structural gene spanning approximately 45 kb on the long arm of the X chromosome at Xq26. It consists of nine exons with a coding sequence of 654 bp. HPRT deficiency is inherited as a recessive X-linked trait. Thus, males are generally affected and women are generally asymptomatic carriers. At least five women with Lesch-Nyhan syndrome due to a variety of molecular mechanisms have been described in the literature.[31] Although most heterozygotes are clinically asymptomatic, some have evidenced elevated serum urate levels, increased urinary uric acid excretion, or a moderate increase in the rate of purine synthesis de novo. In a study designed to ascertain whether heterozygotes for HPRT deficiency exhibit an increased purine synthesis that may be useful for carrier testing,[40] a large group of women at risk of being carriers of the enzyme defect, both premenopausal and postmenopausal, were examined. Purine metabolism was thoroughly assessed by determining hypoxanthine, xanthine, and uric acid metabolism. The results show that female heterozygotes for HPRT deficiency showed a mean plasma concentration of hypoxanthine, xanthine, and uric acid similar to control subjects but significantly increased urinary excretion rates of these purines, which suggests an increased purine synthesis in carrier women for HPRT deficiency.

HPRT mutations accounting for HPRT deficiency are heterogeneous in type and localization (Fig. 3-6). More than 300 disease-associated mutations (deletions, insertions, duplications, and point mutations) have been found dispersed within the gene.[41]

Diagnosis

The diagnosis of HPRT deficiency must be supported by clinical, biochemical, enzymatic, and molecular data. Hyperuricemia with hyperuricosuria is the biochemical hallmark that prompts an enzymatic diagnosis. HPRT deficiency should be suspected in patients with hyperuricemia and elevated uric acid excretion in urine, with or without neurologic impairment. During the first year of life, serum and urine uric acid determinations should be included in the differential diagnosis of psychomotor delay. Nephrolithiasis and obstructive nephropathy are common early manifestations in patients with HPRT deficiency. Neuroimaging testing such as computed tomography (CT), magnetic resonance imaging (MRI), and electroencephalography is not diagnostic.

Figure 3-7 Urinary uric acid–to–creatinine ratio in the diagnosis of purine disorders. The urinary uric acid–to–creatinine ratio can be used as a screening test for inherited disorders of purine metabolism but the values should be evaluated based on the age of the patient. *Shadow area* represents normal values of urinary uric acid–to–creatinine ratio relating to age.

A high serum urate concentration is usually the biochemical finding that prompts the search for a specific diagnosis, although some patients, particularly young infants, may have borderline serum urate levels due to increased uric acid renal clearance. Normal values for serum urate levels depend on the patient's age and sex. Similarly, the urinary uric acid–to–creatinine ratio can be used as a screening test for inherited disorders of purine metabolism, but the values should be evaluated based on the age of the patient (Fig. 3-7). Normal values for the urinary uric acid–to–creatinine ratio are below 1.0 after the age of 3 years. Mean plasma concentrations of urate, hypoxanthine, and xanthine, and their urinary excretion rates, are markedly elevated in HPRT-deficient patients. However, there is a non–statistically significant difference in these biochemical variables between partially and fully expressed Lesch-Nyhan syndrome patients, except for xanthine urinary excretion, which appears to be increased in Lesch-Nyhan patients compared to variant patients.[29]

HPRT deficiency must be confirmed with enzymatic determinations. Patients present with low or undetectable HPRT activity in hemolysates, with increased APRT activity. Lesch-Nyhan patients present with undetectable HPRT activity. In contrast, in HPRT-deficient variant patients, the enzyme activity ranges from 0% to 10% in the hemolysate.[31] To better characterize HPRT deficiency, enzyme activity can be measured in intact cells (erythrocytes or fibroblasts) (information about diagnostic testing in the United States and other countries can be found at www.lesch-nyhan.com). A correlation has been found between residual HPRT activity in intact erythrocytes and fibroblasts and the neurologic involvement, although values may overlap for patients with very different phenotypes. Female carriers cannot be detected without laboratory testing since they are usually asymptomatic. In our experience, most female carriers for HPRT deficiency can be differentiated from noncarriers when 24-hour urine samples are analyzed after a 5-day purine-restricted diet: carriers show significantly higher mean urinary excretion rates of hypoxanthine and xanthine compared to noncarrier females from the same families.[41] HPRT activity is most often normal in the hemolysate of female carriers due to selection against HPRT-deficient erythrocyte precursors. Enzymatic diagnosis of the carrier state can be performed by identification of HPRT-deficient hair follicles or cultured fibroblasts because of their mosaicism in terms of HPRT activity, although such diagnosis is not infallible. HPRT-deficient cells from carrier females can be selected based on their 6-thioguanine resistance. Proliferation assay of peripheral blood T-lymphocytes in the presence of 6-thioguanine is diagnostic in most cases.[42]

Molecular Diagnosis

Most HPRT-deficient patients show HPRT mRNA expression, and molecular diagnosis can be accomplished with HPRT cDNA sequencing. In some cases, genomic DNA sequencing may be necessary. Documented mutations in HPRT deficiency show a high degree of heterogeneity in type and location within the gene: deletions, insertions, duplications, and point mutations have been described as the cause of HPRT deficiency. The molecular diagnosis of HPRT deficiency requires analysis of the HPRT coding region by reverse transcription–polymerase chain reaction or genomic analysis of the HPRT gene, to find the particular mutation in each patient. In some cases, the HPRT coding region is normal and the patients present with decreased HPRT mRNA expression of unknown origin.[43] Single-point mutations are the main cause of partial deficiency of the enzyme, whereas Lesch-Nyhan syndrome is caused mainly by mutations that modify the size of the predicted protein.[29] However, patients in the same family, with the same mutation, may show present a markedly different phenotype (Fig. 3-8). HPRT deficiency is inherited as an X-linked recessive trait. However, about 30% of the patients' mothers are not somatic carriers, and these patients probably carry de novo mutations due to a germinal cell mutation. Molecular diagnosis in HPRT-deficient patients allows faster and more accurate carrier and prenatal diagnosis. When the HPRT mutation has been characterized in the family, faster and more accurate carrier diagnosis can be performed with molecular methods. Prenatal diagnosis for Lesch-Nyhan syndrome can be performed in the amniotic cells obtained by amniocentesis at about 15 to 18 weeks' gestation or chorionic villus cells obtained at about 10 to 12 weeks' gestation. Both HPRT enzymatic assay and molecular analysis for the known disease-causing mutation can be performed.

Treatment

Uric acid overproduction is effectively controlled with the XOR inhibitor allopurinol, which blocks the conversion of xanthine and hypoxanthine into uric acid. Allopurinol has no effect on behavioral and neurologic symptoms, but it should be administered as soon as the enzyme deficiency has been diagnosed, to avoid renal damage. In adults, or when there are great tissue urate deposits, combined treatment with colchicine prophylaxis is required to avoid gout flares. The optimal allopurinol dose for HPRT-deficient patients has not been established, but, in our experience, when serum urate is maintained close to its solubility threshold, urate deposition

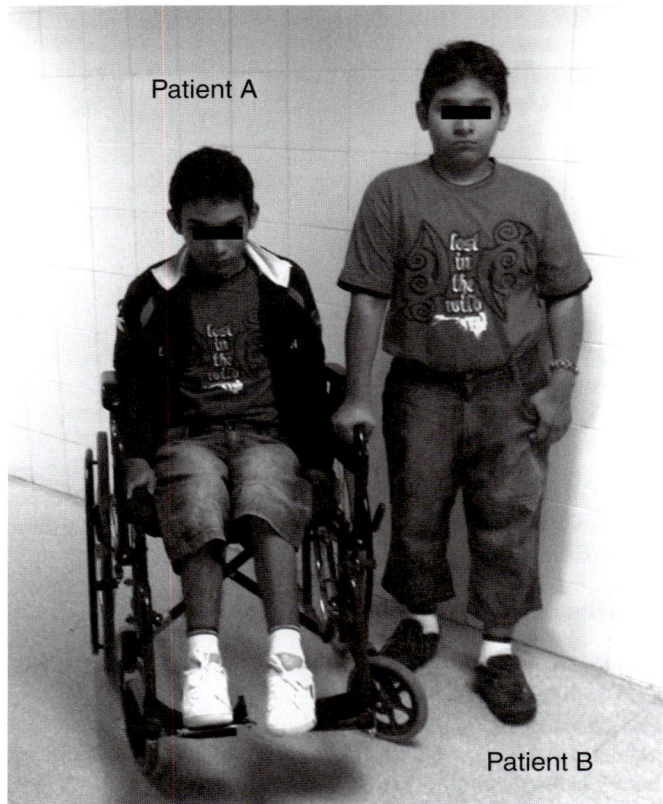

Figure 3-8 Phenotype variability in hypoxanthine-guanine phosphoribosyltransferase (HPRT) deficiency. Two brothers with HPRT deficiency, and the same mutation, show a markedly different phenotype. Patient A is unable to stand up and walk. His younger brother (patient B) has a dystonic gait but can walk without help.

does not occur and the incidence of xanthine lithiasis may be diminished.[44] The initial dosage of allopurinol is 5 to 10 mg/kg/day, and it should be adjusted to maintain high-normal serum uric acid levels and a urinary uric acid–to–creatinine ratio lower than 1.0. In our experience, treatment with allopurinol normalized serum urate level in all HPRT-deficient patients and resulted in a mean reduction of serum urate of about 50% and a 74% reduction in urinary uric acid–to–creatinine ratio. However, allopurinol inhibition of XOR in these patients accounts for increased hypoxanthine and xanthine urinary excretion rates of about 5- and 10-fold, respectively, compared to baseline levels. Under normal conditions, allopurinol increases the reutilization of hypoxanthine for nucleotide and nucleic acid synthesis, via HPRT activity. The resultant increase in nucleotide concentration leads to feedback inhibition of de novo purine synthesis (see Fig. 3-1). However, in HPRT-deficient patients, hypoxanthine cannot be reutilized and there is a markedly increased purine production. In these circumstances, the absolute concentration of xanthine could rise to a level at which deposition in the urinary tract may occur and xanthine lithiasis may develop as a consequence of allopurinol therapy, In our experience, xanthine lithiasis may be prevented by sequential determination of urinary oxypurines, which should be at a certain balance with uric acid excretion, and by titrating allopurinol doses to maintain high-normal serum uric acid levels.[44]

Allopurinol should be administered with adequate hydration to achieve maximum diuresis. Alkalinization, of considerable benefit in relation to urate stones, may be less so in relation to xanthine stones. Allopurinol treatment reduces serum urate and urine uric acid levels, preventing uric acid crystalluria, nephrolithiasis, gouty arthritis, and tophi in Lesch-Nyhan patients. With adequate allopurinol doses and compliance, renal function usually remains stable or even improves.

Allopurinol hypersensitivity has been described in 0.4% of patients receiving this treatment. The higher incidence of hypersensitivity in patients with decreased renal function has prompted the adjustment of allopurinol doses according to the creatinine clearance. However, this procedure does not always prevent allopurinol hypersensitivity. To our knowledge, no hypersensitivity reactions have been described in Lesch-Nyhan patients despite impaired renal function. Use of the new XOR inhibitor febuxostat has not yet been described in HPRT-deficient patients, but it appears to be a useful alternative to allopurinol.

In most mammals, the hepatic enzyme uricase or urate oxidase transforms uric acid into the more soluble compound allantoin (see Fig. 3-1). In humans, due to mutations in the uricase gene, uric acid is the last product of purine metabolism. Rasburicase, a uricase purified from *Aspergillus flavus*, is used to prevent tumor lysis syndrome in hematologic malignancies. It is administered intravenously at doses of 0.20 mg/kg/day during a short period of 5 to 7 days. In HPRT-deficient patients, xanthine lithiasis could be avoided by uricase treatment. However, there is no long-term evidence of rasburicase treatment safety, which is known to be antigenic. Its short half-life (18 hours) and its form of administration (injection) are inconvenient for chronic therapy. However, rasburicase may be effective in infants with acute kidney injury.[45] We share the experience of two Lesch-Nyhan patients who presented with renal failure in the first months of life and were treated with rasburicase during a short period of time at established doses, followed by allopurinol treatment. In both patients, renal function improved with rasburicase treatment.

A genetically engineered, recombinant, polyethylene glycol (PEG)–conjugated mammalian uricase (pegloticase) has been developed and approved by the U.S Food and Drug Administration (FDA). This agent has the potential to reduce immunogenicity and be present for a longer half-life. This uricase is approved by the FDA to be administered intravenously every 2 weeks to patients with treatment-failure gout to maintain serum urate levels within normal limits and promote resolution of tophi. Results of phase III studies showed that anti-Pegloticase antibodies commonly develop over months, with such antibodies associated with reduced circulating half-life of Pegloticase in some patients, loss of pharmacodynamic effects on serum urate, and infusion reactions, often appearing at the time of loss of serum urate normalization. Pegloticase represents a useful potential option for Lesch-Nyhan and PRS hyperuricemia syndromes. It will present the advantage in respect to allopurinol of avoiding the increase of urinary excretion of hypoxanthine and xanthine and the appearance of xanthine lithiasis

As in many generalized dystonic syndromes, the lack of precise understanding of the cause of the neurologic dysfunction has precluded the development of useful therapies in HPRT deficiency. Rigorous placebo-controlled studies have

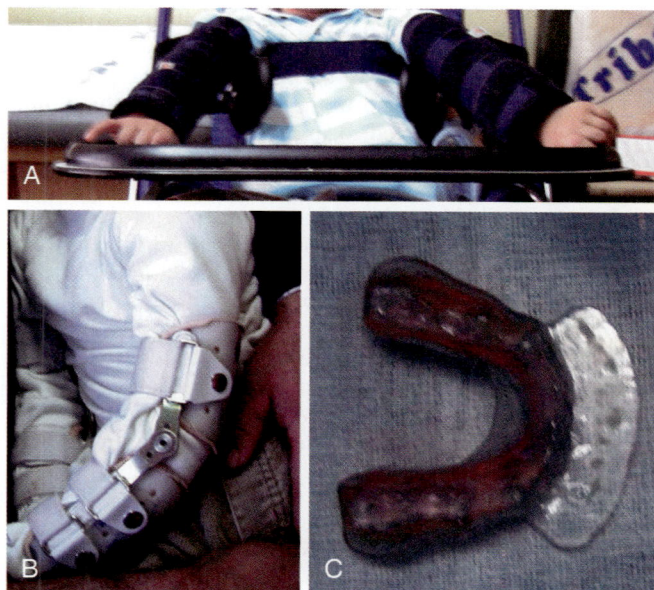

Figure 3-9 Different devices to manage Lesch-Nyhan self-injurious behavior. **A** and **B,** Arm protection to avoid finger biting. **C,** Dental protection to avoid lip damage due to biting.

not been conducted in Lesch-Nyhan patients. Spasticity and dystonia can be managed with benzodiazepines and gamma-amino butyric acid inhibitors such as baclofen. No medication has been found to effectively control the extrapyramidal manifestations of the disease. Dopamine replacement therapy in Lesch-Nyhan patients has been reported in a few noncontrolled studies with very heterogeneous responses. Most of the treated patients presented with intolerable side effects.

Physical rehabilitation, including management of dysarthria and dysphagia, special devices to enable hand control of objects, appropriate walking aids, and a program of posture management to prevent deformities, is key for the management of the motor manifestations of Lesch-Nyhan syndrome. Self-injurious behavior must be managed with a combination of physical restraints (Fig. 3-9) and behavioral and pharmaceutical treatments. Benzodiazepines and carbamazapine are sometimes useful for ameliorating behavioral manifestations and anxiety.[31] Stress increases self-injurious behavior. Thus, stressful situations should be avoided and aversive techniques should not be used. Instead, behavioral extinction methods have proved to be partially efficacious in a controlled setting. Some reports have suggested that the antiepileptic drug gabapentin may improve self-injurious behavior, and no side effects have been associated with its use. However, no controlled trials have been conducted in Lesch-Nyhan patients. Also, the atypical antipsychotic drug risperidone, a nonselective antagonist of both serotonin type 2A and dopamine D2 receptors, has been found to reduce self-injurious behavior in some Lesch-Nyhan patients. Other treatments under investigation for the management of self-injurious behavior include local injections of botulin toxin. Several authors have reported the use of repeated botulin toxin A injections into the bilateral masseters or into the facial muscles to prevent tongue- and lip-biting in Lesch-Nyhan patients. In our patients, botulin toxin injection is usually efficacious for a limited period of time. When injecting into the masseters, the toxin could spread to pharyngeal muscles, causing dysphagia. As self-injurious intensity varies within periods of time, this procedure could be useful in the most aggressive periods to avoid tissue damage. Deep brain stimulation at the globus pallidus has been reported to improve self-injurious behavior in few Lesch-Nyhan patients. This therapy needs to demonstrate its efficacy and safety in the long-term management of these patients. Nowadays, the cornerstone of day-to-day management of Lesch-Nyhan syndrome self-injurious behavior is still adapted physical restraint to protect patients from themselves. For instance, elbow restraints allow hand use without the possibility of finger mutilation, and dental guards prevent cheek biting. Patients frequently request restrictions and become anxious if they are unrestrained. Some restraints that would appear to be ineffective, such as a pair of gloves to prevent finger biting, are very useful and children turn quiet as they are "protected."

Congenital Disorders of Purine Metabolism Causing Hyporuricemia

Xanthinuria

Xanthinuria is a descriptive term for excess urinary excretion of the purine base xanthine. Xanthine is a highly insoluble purine that precipitates in renal excretory system when its urinary concentration is elevated. The urinary elevation of xanthine can be inherited or acquired. Hereditary xanthinuria is an autosomal recessive disorder principally resulting from a deficiency of the enzyme XOR (see Fig. 3-1), which is the enzyme responsible for degrading hypoxanthine and xanthine to uric acid. Deficiency of XOR results in plasma accumulation and excess urinary excretion of xanthine, which may lead to arthropathy, myopathy, crystal nephropathy, urolithiasis, or renal failure. Hypoxanthine does not accumulate to an appreciable degree because it is recycled through a salvage pathway by the enzyme HPRT (see Fig. 3-1). Xanthine continues to accumulate, despite the recycling of hypoxanthine, because of the metabolism of guanine to xanthine by the enzyme guanase.[46,47]

Clinical Manifestations

Acquired xanthinuria is generally iatrogenic. Allopurinol treatment, administered to block XOR and prevent uric acid overproduction, leads to the accumulation of xanthine. Rarely, in the setting of aggressive chemotherapy with rapid tumor lysis or in patients with HPRT deficiency on allopurinol therapy, complications of renal failure can develop from xanthine crystal nephropathy.

There are two forms of hereditary xanthinuria: classic xanthinuria is caused by XOR deficiency alone (type I) (OMIM 278300) or combined with aldehyde oxidase deficiency (type II) (OMIM 603592). About 70% of the patients with classic xanthinuria are asymptomatic. A casual laboratory test with a serum urate concentration below 2 mg/dl (120 μmol/L) usually prompts the diagnosis. Some patients may report symptomatic xanthine nephrolithiasis with radiolucent stone formation. Myopathy and arthropathy are rare clinical manifestations of xanthinuria, attributed to xanthine crystal deposition. Xanthine crystals have been found in muscle fibers but not in synovial fluid.

The other inherited form of xanthinuria is termed molybdenum cofactor deficiency (OMIM 252150), and it is caused by a congenital defect of a molybdenum-containing cofactor essential for the function of three distinct enzymes: XOR, aldehyde oxidase, and sulfite oxidase. This defect presents in the neonatal period with untreatable neonatal epilepsy, microcephaly, hyperreflexia, severe metabolic acidosis, and intracranial hemorrhage. Death in the first year of life is caused by the deficiency of sulfite oxidase, which is the final step in cysteine metabolism.

Genetics

Classic xanthinuria type I is due to mutations in the *XOR* gene located in chromosome 2p22-23. Type II is caused by mutations in the molybdenum cofactor sulfurase gene located in chromosome 18q12. Both XOR and aldehyde oxidase enzymatic activity are dependent of the molybdenum cofactor sulfuration, but sulfite oxidase activity is independent of that reaction. Molybdenum cofactor deficiency is due to mutations in several genes implicated in cofactor biosynthesis (*MOCS1*, *MOCS2*, and *GEPH* located in chromosome 6, 5, and 14, respectively).

Diagnosis

Classic xanthinuria is suspected by a diminished serum urate and urinary uric acid excretion (less than 80 mg/day). Diagnosis can be confirmed by elevated levels of xanthine and hypoxanthine in plasma and urine with a hypoxanthine-to-xanthine ratio of 4:1. XOR activity can be measured by obtaining a liver or intestinal biopsy sample. As aldehyde oxidase activity oxidizes allopurinol to oxypurinol, type II xanthinuria can be differentiated from type I by an allopurinol load test. Type II patients are unable to convert allopurinol to oxypurinol. In molybdenum cofactor deficiency, there is also an elevation of urinary sulfite.

Several inborn errors of purine metabolism may be associated with nephrolithiasis of various composition and pathophysiology. Nephrolithiasis may develop in phosphoribosylpyrophosphate synthetase (PRPPs) superactivity, HPRT deficiency, xanthinuria, and APRT deficiency.

APRT deficiency (OMIM 102600) is a rare autosomal recessive disorder causing 2,8-dihydroxyadenine stones and renal failure due to intratubular crystalline precipitation.[48,49] Most patients present with recurrent urolithiasis during infancy, although in some cases the defect is asymptomatic. Renal failure has been described as the primary APRT-deficiency manifestation. APRT deficiency leads to the accumulation of adenine, which is sequentially oxidized to 8-hydroxyadenine and 2,8-dihydroxyadenine by XOR (see Fig. 3-1). Diagnosis is made by infrared spectroscopy analysis of the calculi and/or by APRT enzymatic determination in hemolysate or intact erythrocytes. Patients usually present an elevated urinary excretion of adenine, 8-hydroxyadenine, and 2,8-dihydroxyadenine. Molecular diagnosis implies sequencing of the *APRT* gene in chromosome 16q24. Allopurinol is used to avoid conversion of adenine to its oxidized forms.

Treatment

There is no specific treatment for classic xanthinuria. High fluid intake and purine dietary restriction are recommended. XOR and aldehyde oxidase metabolize certain medications, and the enzyme-deficient or inhibited state can lead to toxic accumulation of the parent drug. XOR is involved in the degradation of azathioprine or 6-mercaptopurine, and aldehyde oxidase metabolizes allopurinol, cyclophosphamide, methotrexate, and quinine. Substitution therapy with purified cyclic pyranopterin monophosphate has demonstrated efficacy in a molybdenum cofactor–deficiency patient.

PNP Deficiency

In 1975, Eloise Giblett reported the case of a child with a specific T-cell immunodeficiency and traced the biochemical defect to a genetic deficiency of PNP.[50] PNP deficiency (OMIM 613179) is an autosomal recessive disorder characterized by severe combined immunodeficiency associated in most cases with neurologic deficit and autoimmune disease.

Clinical Manifestations

Initial symptoms are usually recurrent infections in the first year of life. Patients with PNP deficiency develop a combined immunodeficiency particularly affecting T-cell function, while B-cell function may be preserved longer. This disorder accounts for about 4% of severe combined immunodeficiencies. Immunodeficiency is associated with autoimmune diseases, such as hemolytic anemia, thrombocytopenic purpura, or lupus in 30% of the patients. Most patients (60%) present with heterogeneous neurologic symptoms including development delay, ataxia, spasticity, tremor, and mental retardation. Patients usually die in the first or second decade of life due to recurrent infections. The diagnosis can be suspected by low levels of uric acid in the serum and especially in urine.[51]

Pathophysiology

PNP reversibly catalyzes dephosphorylation of guanosine, deoxyguanosine, inosine, and deoxyinosine (see Fig. 3-1). The biochemical link between PNP and T-cell deficiency is the failure to degrade deoxyguanosine and its conversion to dGTP in activated T cells. Although studies on the neuropathology of PNP deficiency are rare, intracellular accumulation of toxic purines is the probable cause of brain damage.

Genetics

The *PNP* gene is located in chromosome 14q13. To date, various mutations have been identified as the cause of the disease.

Diagnosis

Association of hypouricemia (typical serum urate level being undetectable) with recurrent infections, neurologic deficit, and autoimmune disease prompts the diagnosis of PNP deficiency. This has to be confirmed by determining PNP activity in erythrocytes. Inosine, guanosine, desoxyguanosine, and desoxyinosine are also elevated in urine. Homozygous PNP-deficient patients show less than 5% of the normal activity in erythrocytes, and heterozygous subjects present about 50% of normal PNP activity without immune dysfunction.

ADA deficiency (OMIM 102700) is an autosomal recessive inborn error of purine metabolism also causing severe combined immunodeficiency.[52,53] Immunodeficiency affects both T- and B-cell function and it is not accompanied by neurologic deficits. ADA deficiency accounts for about 15% of severe combined immunodeficiency syndromes. As in the case of PNP deficiency, toxic accumulation of the enzyme substrate deoxyadenosine and, secondarily, of dATP is the cause of lymphocyte damage. Increased plasma and urine levels of deoxyadenosine and decreased or absent ADA activity in erythrocyte confirmed the diagnosis. Uric acid levels are not pathologic in these patients.

Treatment

The only curative treatment is bone marrow transplantation. This treatment has corrected the metabolic abnormality and the immunodeficiency in several patients. However, neurologic abnormalities usually persist, although the treatment may prevent further neurologic deterioration.

PNP inhibitors, termed immucillins (see Fig. 3-1), are currently under study as therapeutic agents, primarily for selective suppression of cellular immunity without compromising humoral immunity. Immucillins have been used in malignant lymphoproliferative diseases, in suppression of host-versus-graft responses following organ and bone marrow transplantation, and to counter autoimmune diseases, such as rheumatoid arthritis, psoriasis, multiple sclerosis, etc. Since an additional symptom of PNP deficiency is a decrease in plasma and urine levels of urate, PNP inhibitors may be useful in hyperuricemic states. A second generation of immucillins called DADMe-IMMH (BCX4208) are being developed for gout treatment and are following the clinical trial phase.

Acknowledgments

We acknowledge grants from the Fondo de Investigaciones Sanitarias (FIS 08/0009) and from CIBERER (Centro de Investigaciones Biomedicas en Red para el Estudio de las Enfermedades Raras). We are grateful to the specialists and family physicians belonging to the network Grupo MAPA-MADRID, supported by the Red Española de Atención Primaria (REAP, 2009/70) and by RECAVA (RD06/0014/0026) Grupo Clínico Asociado, for referring their patients. We are indebted to the nursing staff (G. Santas Camino, I. Narillos Sánchez, and A. Sánchez Martín) for excellent patient care of our HPRT-deficient patients. We gratefully acknowledge Dr. Carolina Velasco García as the general manager of the Metabolic and Vascular Research Unit and Dr. Almudena Ligos for her superb work as our research secretarial assistant.

References

1. Jinnah HA, Friedmann T. Lesch-Nyhan disease and its variants. In: Scriver CR, Beaudet AL, Sly WS, Valle D, editors. The Metabolic and Molecular Basis of Inherited Disease. 8th ed. New York, NY: McGraw-Hill; 2001:2537–70.
2. Puig JG, Fox IH. Ethanol-induced activation of adenina mucelotide turnover. Evidence for a role of acetate. J Clin Invest 1984;74:936–41.
3. Rundles WR. The development of allopurinol. Arch Intern Med 1985;145:1492–503.
4. Scout JT. Symposium on allopurinol. Ann Rheum Dis 1966;25(suppl):599–718.
5. Torres RJ, Prior C, Puig JG. Efficacy and safety of allopurinol in patients with hypoxanthine-guanine phosphoribosyltransferase deficiency. Metabolism 2007;56:1179–86.

6. Edwards NL, Recaer D, Airozo D, et al. Enhanced purine salvage during allopurinol therapy: an important pharmacologic property in humans. J Lab Cli Med 1981;98:673–83.

7. Ernst ME, Fravel MA. Febuxostat: a selective xanthine-oxidase/xanthine dehydrogenase inhibitor for the management of hyperuricemia in adults with gout. Clin Ther 2009;31:2503–18.

8. Holling HE. Gout and glycogen storage disease. Ann Intern Med 1963;58:654–63.

9. Howell RR. The interrelationship of glycogen storage disease and gout. Arthritis Rheum 1965;8:780–5.

10. Mineo I, Kono N, Hara N, et al. Myogenic hyperuricemia: a common pathophysiologic feature of glycogenosis types III, V, and VII. N Eng J Med 1987;317:75–80.

11. Sperling O, Boer P, Persky-Brosh S, et al. Altered kinetic property of erythrocyte phosphoribosylpyrophosphate synthetase in excessive purine production. Rev Eur Etud Clin Biol 1972;17:703–6.

12. Zoref E, De Vries A, Sperling O. Mutant feedback-resistant phosphoribosylpyrophosphate synthetase associated with purine overproduction and gout. Phosphoribosylpyrophosphate and purine metabolism in cultured fibroblasts. J Clin Invest 1975;56:1093–9.

13. Becker MA, Puig JG, Mateos FA, et al. Inherited superactivity of phosphoribosylpyrophosphate synthetase: association of uric acid overproduction and sensorineural deafness. Am J Med 1988;85:383–90.

14. Nyhan WL, James JA, Teberg AJ, et al. A new disorder of purine metabolism with behavioral manifestations. J Pediatr 1969;74:20–7.

15. Simmonds HA, Webster DR, Wilson J, et al. An X-linked syndrome characterised by hyperuricaemia, deafness, and neurodevelopmental abnormalities. Lancet 1982:68–70.

16. Christen HJ, Hanefeld F, Duley JA, et al. Distinct neurological syndrome in two brothers with hyperuricaemia. Lancet 1992;340:1167–8.

17. García-Pavía P, Torres RJ, Rivero M, et al. Phosphoribosylpyrophosphate synthetase overactivity as a cause of uric acid overproduction in a young woman. Arthritis Rheum 2003;48:2036–41.

18. Fox IH, Kelley WN. Human phosphoribosylpyrophosphate synthetase. Distribution, purification, and properties. J Biol Chem 1971;246:5739–48.

19. de Brouwer AP, Williams KL, Duley JA, et al. Arts syndrome is caused by loss-of-function mutations in PRPS1. Am J Hum Genet 2007;81:507–18.

20. Kim HJ, Sohn KM, Shy ME, et al. Mutations in PRPS1, which encodes the phosphoribosyl pyrophosphate synthetase enzyme critical for nucleotide biosynthesis, cause hereditary peripheral neuropathy with hearing loss and optic neuropathy (cmtx5). Am J Hum Genet 2007;81:552–8.

21. Liu X, Han D, Li J, et al. Loss-of-function mutations in the PRPS1 gene cause a type of nonsyndromic X-linked sensorineural deafness, DFN2. Am J Hum Genet 2010;86:65–71.

22. Becker MA, Smith PR, Taylor W, et al. The genetic and functional basis of purine nucleotide feedback-resistant phosphoribosylpyrophosphate synthetase superactivity. J Clin Invest 1995;96:2133–41.

23. de Brouwer AP, van Bokhoven H, Nabuurs SB, et al. PRPS1 mutations: four distinct syndromes and potential treatment. Am J Hum Genet 2010;86:506–18.

24. Becker MA, Taylor W, Smith PR, et al. Overexpression of the normal phosphoribosylpyrophosphate synthetase 1 isoform underlies catalytic superactivity of human phosphoribosylpyrophosphate synthetase. J Biol Chem 1996;271:19894–9.

25. Becker MA, Losman MJ, Itkin P, et al. Gout with superactive phosphoribosylpyrophosphate synthetase due to increased enzyme catalytic rate. J Lab Clin Med 1982;99:495–511.

26. Lesch M, Nyhan WL. A familial disorder of uric acid metabolism and central nervous system function. Am J Med 1964;36:561–70.

27. Seegmiller JE, Rosenbloom FM, Kelley WN. Enzyme defect associated with a sex-linked human neurological disorder and excessive purine synthesis. Science 1967;155:1682–4.

28. Kelley WN, Rosenbloom FM, Henderson JF, et al. A specific enzyme defect in gout associated with overproduction of uric acid. Proc Natl Acad Sci USA 1967;57:1735–9.

29. García Puig J, Torres Jiménez R, Mateos F, et al. The spectrum of hypoxanthine-guanine phosphoribosyltransferase (HPRT) deficiency. Clinical experience based on 22 patients from 18 Spanish families. Medicine (Balt) 2001;80:102–12.

30. Jinnah HA, Ceballos-Picot I, Torres RJ, et al. Attenuated variants of Lesch-Nyhan disease. Brain 2010;133:671–89.

31. Torres RJ, Puig JG. Hypoxanthine-guanine phosphoribosyltransferase (HPRT) deficiency: Lesch-Nyhan syndrome. Orphanet J Rare Dis 2007;2:48.

32. Jinnah HA, Visser JE, Harris JC, et al. Delineation of the motor disorder of Lesch-Nyhan disease. Brain 2006;129:1201–17.

33. Matthews WS, Solan A, Barabas G, et al. Cognitive functioning in Lesch-Nyhan syndrome: a 4-year follow-up study. Dev Med Child Neurol 1999;41:260–2.

34. Rosenbloom FM, Henderson JF, Caldwell IC, et al. Biochemical bases of accelerated purine biosynthesis de novo in human fibroblasts lacking hypoxanthine-guanine phosphoribosyltransferase. J Biol Chem 1968;243:1166–73.

35. Visser JE, Bar PR, Jinnah HA. Lesch-Nyhan disease and the basal ganglia. Brain Res Rev 2000;32:449–75.

36. Torres RJ, Deantonio I, Prior C, et al. Adenosine transport in peripheral blood lymphocytes from Lesch-Nyhan patients. Biochem J 2004;377:733–9.

37. Prior C, Torres RJ, Puig JG. Hypoxanthine decreases equilibrative type of adenosine transport in lymphocytes from Lesch-Nyhan patients. Eur J Clin Invest 2007;37:905–11.

38. Harkness RA, McCreanor GM, Watts RW. Lesch-Nyhan syndrome and its pathogenesis: purine concentrations in plasma and urine with metabolite profiles in CSF. J Inherit Metab Dis 1988;11:239–52.

39. van der Zee SP, Schretlen ED, Monnens LA. Megaloblastic anaemia in the Lesch-Nyhan syndrome. Lancet 1968;1:1427.

40. Puig JG, Mateos FA, Torres RJ, et al. Purine metabolism in female heterozygotes for hypoxanthine-guanine phosphoribosyltransferase (HPRT) deficiency. Eur J Clin Invest 1998;28:950–7.

41. Official website of the Lesch-Nyhan Disease Study Group. www.lesch-nyhan.org.

42. O'Neill JP. Mutation carrier testing in Lesch-Nyhan syndrome families: HPRT mutant frequency and mutation analysis with peripheral blood T lymphocytes. Genet Test 2004;8:51–64.

43. García MG, Torres RJ, Prior C, et al. Normal HPRT coding region in complete and partial HPRT deficiency. Mol Genet Metab 2008;94:167–72.

44. Torres RJ, Prior C, Puig JG. Efficacy and safety of allopurinol in patients with hypoxanthine-guanine phosphoribosyltransferase deficiency. Metabolism 2007;56:1179–86.

45. Roche A, Pérez-Dueñas B, Camacho JA, et al. Efficacy of rasburicase in hyperuricemia secondary to Lesch-Nyhan syndrome. Am J Kidney Dis 2009;53:677–80.

46. Dent CE, Philpot GR. Xanthinuria, an inborn error (or deviation) of metabolism. Lancet 1954;266:182–5.

47. Simmomds HA, Reiter S, Nishino T. Hereditary xanthinuria. In: Beaudet AL, Sly WS, Valle D, editors. The Metabolic and Molecular Basis of Inherited Disease. 7th ed. New York, NY: McGraw-Hill; 1995:1781–97.

48. Emmerson BT, Gordon RB, Thompson L. Adenine phosphoribosyltransferase deficiency: its inheritance and occurrence in a female with gout and renal disease. Aust N Z J Med 1975;5:440–6.

49. Bollée G, Dollinger C, Boutaud L, et al. Phenotype and genotype characterization of adenine phosphoribosyltransferase deficiency. J Am Soc Nephrol 2010;21:679–88.

50. Giblett ER, Ammann AJ, Wara DW, et al. Nucleoside-phosphorylase deficiency in a child with severely defective T-cell immunity and normal B-cell immunity. Lancet 1975;1:1010–3.

51. Markert ML. Purine nucleoside phosphorylase deficiency. Immunodefic Rev 1991;3:45–81.

52. Giblett ER, Anderson JE, Cohen F, et al. Adenosine-deaminase deficiency in two patients with severely impaired cellular immunity. Lancet 1972;2:1067–9.

53. Hershfield MS, Mitchell BS. Immunodeficiency diseases caused by adenosine deaminase deficiency and purine nucleoside phosphorylase deficiency. In: Scriver CR, Beaudet AL, Sly WS, Valle D, editors. The Metabolic and Molecular Bases of Inherited Disease. 8th ed. New York, NY: McGraw-Hill; 2001:2585–625.

Renal Basis of Hyperuricemia

Naohiko Anzai and Hitoshi Endou

KEY POINTS

- Approximately 90% of cases of hyperuricemia are caused by uric acid underexcretion from the kidneys. In addition, renal hypouricemia is caused by increased renal uric acid excretion. Thus, renal urate anion handling plays a major role in determination of serum urate level.

- The proximal tubule is the major site of renal urate anion transport, and this process is bidirectional, with reabsorption being predominant, and multiple transporters at apical and basolateral membranes playing significant roles.

- We propose that urate reabsorption in human proximal tubules is mainly performed by the "exchanger" URAT1 (*SLC22A12*) at the apical membrane and the "facilitator" URATv1/GLUT9 (*SLC2A9*) at the basolateral membrane in tandem, because there is in vivo evidence from human patient analysis that hypouricemia of renal origin has been caused by loss-of-function mutations of either transporter genes.

- Estrogen and androgens (via transcriptional effects), salicylates and nicotinate (niacin), and multiple potent uricosuric drugs (e.g., probenecid, benzbromarone) all influence specific mechanisms of renal urate anion transport in the proximal tubule.

Introduction

Humans have higher serum levels of urate, the ionized form of uric acid, than do other mammalian species due to evolutionary loss of the hepatic enzyme uricase that metabolizes relatively insoluble urate to ultimately generate highly soluble allantoin.[1,2] Although uricase loss may have been beneficial to early primate survival by possibly providing antioxidant defense in the human body, sustained hyperuricemia has pathogenetic roles in gout and renal diseases as well as putative roles in hypertension and cardiovascular diseases.[3] Since human serum urate (SUA) levels are largely determined by the balance between reabsorption and secretion of urate anion in the kidney, it is important to understand the molecular mechanism of renal urate handling.[4] Although molecular identification of the kidney-specific urate/anion exchanger, *SLC22A12* (URAT1), in 2002 paved the way for successive characterization of the physiologic roles of several urate transport-related proteins,[5] the entire picture of effective renal urate handling in humans has not yet been clarified. Recently, several genomewide association studies (GWAS) have revealed substantial association between uric acid concentration and single nucleotide polymorphisms (SNPs) in at least 10 genetic loci related to uric acid metabolism including *SLC2A9* (GLUT9/URATv1), *ABCG2* (BCRP), and *SLC17A3* (NPT4).[6,7] In 2008, we functionally characterized the facilitatory glucose transporter family member *SLC2A9* (GLUT9), one of the candidate genes for urate handling, as a voltage-driven urate transporter, URATv1, at the basolateral side of renal proximal tubules, which constitutes the main route of the urate reabsorption pathway, in tandem with URAT1 at the apical side.[8] Recently, we found that the orphan transporter *SLC17A3* (NPT4) functions as an apical exit path for both urate and drugs in renal proximal tubules with voltage-driven transport properties.[9] Recent advances in research on renal urate transport and its significance in understanding SUA disorders are reviewed here. Reviews in the pre-GWAS era covered detailed information on renal urate transport.[10-13] Several reviews that cover part of the present theme have also been published recently.[14-17]

Urate Handling in the Kidney and Hyperuricemia

Uric acid is a breakdown product of ingested and endogenously synthesized purine nucleotides in humans and higher primates. Serum urate level is determined by interplay between the rates of production and elimination.[4] Urate is produced primarily in the liver by xanthine oxidase, and two-thirds of it is excreted via the kidneys with the remaining third excreted into the gut.[1] Therefore, in humans, increased uric acid production and/or reduced uric acid elimination causes hyperuricemia. Approximately 90% of hyperuricemia cases are caused by uric acid underexcretion from the kidneys.[4] In addition, renal hypouricemia is caused by increased renal uric acid excretion. Thus, renal urate handling plays an important role in the determination of SUA level.

Urate is freely filtered through the glomerulus and it is almost completely reabsorbed, normally resulting in excretion of about 10% of its filtered load in humans.[1] Thus, the presence of an effective renal urate reabsorption system in addition to the absence of uricase contributes to much higher basal SUA levels (about 300 μmol/L; about 5 mg/ml) in humans than in other mammals.[4] The majority of studies indicate that the proximal tubule is the major site of renal urate transport.[18] Bidirectional transport of urate, reabsorption being predominant, in proximal tubules was demonstrated by in vitro micropuncture and microperfusion studies in "urate reabsorber" species such as the rat, dog, and the Cebus monkey.[19] In humans, it was suggested that urate is not only reabsorbed but also secreted as in other urate reabsorbers with a predominant reabsorption.[19]

Historically, "the four-component model" (Figure 4-1) was proposed for the mechanism of urate transport in human proximal tubules based on the hypothesis that pyrazinoate (PZA), an active metabolite of pyrazinamide, inhibits urate secretion.[19] Since *trans*-stimulation of urate uptake via urate/anion exchanger *SLC22A12* by PZA was demonstrated by

Enomoto et al.,[5] the four-component model seems incomplete or inaccurate. Here, we propose a simple "three factor model" to explain renal urate handling related to the onset of hyperuricemia as shown in Figure 4-2. We propose that urate reabsorption in human proximal tubules is mainly performed by the "exchanger" *SLC22A12* (URAT1)[5] at the apical membrane and the "facilitator" *SLC2A9* (URATv1/GLUT9)[8] at the basolateral membrane in tandem because there is in vivo evidence from patient analysis that renal hypouricemia was caused by loss-of-function mutations of either transporter genes. Recently, Kamatani et al. reported strong GWAs with urate to SNPs in *SLC22A12* ($p = 2.34 \times 10^{-31}$) and *SLC2A9* ($p = 7.09 \times 10^{-24}$) from about 14,700 Japanese individuals,[20] replicating associations previously identified by GWA studies in European populations.[6,7] In addition, luminal "facilitator" *SLC17A3* (NPT4),[9] which was also reported its association to hyperuricemia,[7] has been proposed to function as exit pathways for urate reabsorbed by *SLC22A12* because urate exit from the basolateral side is limited by the gatekeeper of urate, *SLC2A9*. In this model, increased *SLC2A9* function and/or decreased *SLC17A3* function may induce hyperuricemia (see Figure 4-2, *B* and *C*).

Renal Urate Transporters

Urate Transporter/Channel *LGALS9* (UAT)

The research group of Ruth Abramson screened rat cDNA using antibodies to pig liver uricase and isolated a protein comprising 322 amino acid residues.[21] This protein, termed UAT (urate transporter/*LGALS9*), was found in renal proximal tubules. When recombinant *LGALS9* protein was reconstituted in planar lipid bilayers, membrane potential-dependent, channel-like currents evoked by urate were recorded. *LGALS9* is for this reason regarded as a channel (urate channel) rather than a transporter. However, transport of urate by *LGALS9* was not confirmed in a tracer experiment (RI-labeled urate), and at present it is unclear whether *LGALS9* actually contributes to transmembrane transport of

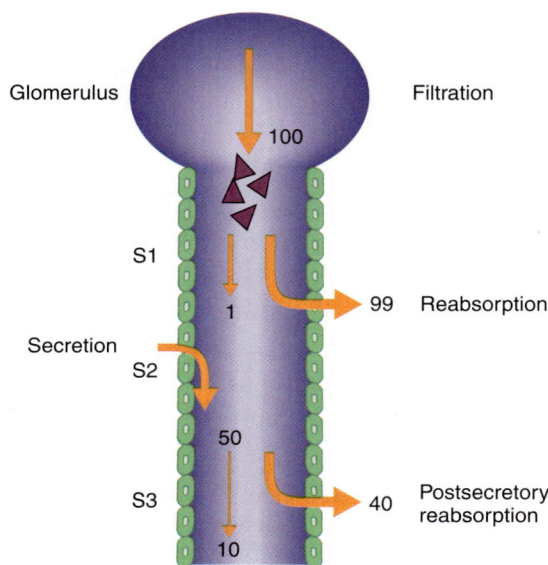

Figure 4-1 Classic "four-component model" for renal urate transport. Reabsorption, secretion, and postsecretory reabsorption in S1, S2, and S3 segments of renal proximal tubules as well as glomerular filtration were "components" for uric acid handling in the kidneys. *(Modified from Sica DA, Schoolwerth AC. Renal handling of organic anions and cations: Excretion of uric acid. In: Brenner BM, editor. The Kidney. 6th ed. Philadelphia, PA: WB Saunders; 2000:680-700.)*

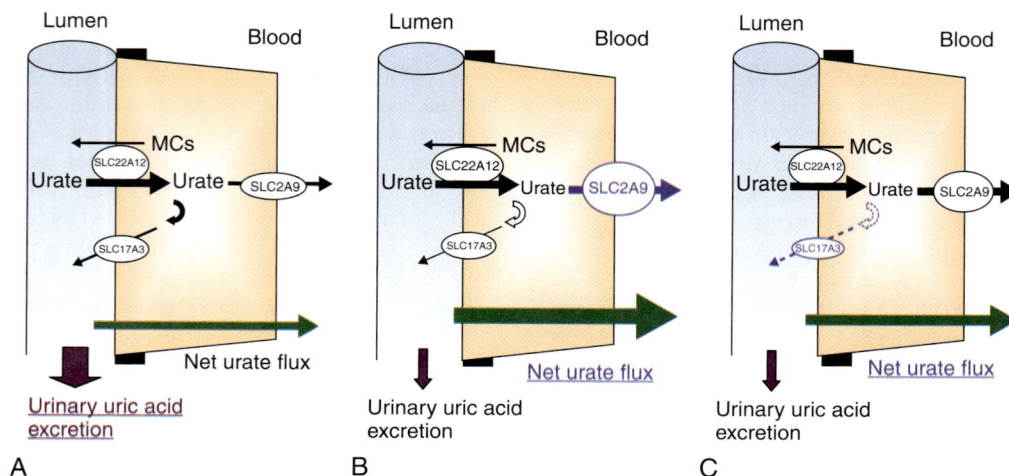

Figure 4-2 Three-factor model for renal urate transport. Reabsorption of urate is mainly performed by apical exchanger *SLC22A12* (URAT1) and basolateral facilitator *SLC2A9* (URATv1) in tandem. Apical leak for urate is performed by another facilitator, *SLC17A3* (NPT4). **A,** Normal case. **B,** Increased function of *SLC2A9* may drive net urate flux, thereby diminishing urinary uric acid excretion leading to hyperuricemia. **C,** Decreased function of *SLC17A3* may also drive net urate flux, thereby diminishing urinary uric acid excretion and leading to hyperuricemia. *MCs,* Monocarbolates.

urate. *LGALS9* is also hypothesized as being a 4-transmembrane domain protein, but this structure differs substantially from a typical transporter with 12-transmembrane domains.[21] *LGALS9* is expressed ubiquitously, not only in the kidney, and is hypothesized to efflux urate, produced by intracellular purine metabolism, outside cells.

Organic Anion Transporter (OAT) Family SLC22

Uric acid is a weak organic acid that dissociates H⁺ under physiologic conditions and is present in the blood in the form of urate. This fact has encouraged speculation that urate may be transported by an organic anion/drug transporter. Excretion of organic anions and drugs via the kidneys is carried out by multispecific organic anion transporters (OATs) expressed in the renal tubules.[22-24] Beginning with *SLC22A6* (OAT1), the first organic anion transporter identified in the rat kidney by our research group in 1997, four isoforms of human organic anion transporter—*SLC22A6* (OAT1), *SLC22A7* (OAT2), *SLC22A8* (OAT3), and *SLC22A11* (OAT4)—were identified in the kidneys.[24] These isoforms are expressed variously at the basolateral (*SLC22A6* to *SLC22A8*) or luminal (*SLC22A11*) membranes in the proximal-to-distal tubules and serve to transport endogenous or exogenous (e.g., drug) organic anions. *Oat1*- and *Oat3*-null mice demonstrated decreased secretion rather than reabsorption, suggesting that OAT1 and/or OAT3 is involved in urate secretion in vivo.[25] Kolz et al.[6] conducted a meta-analysis of GWAS with a total of 28,141 participants of European descent and reported that *SLC22A11* is one of the five new loci that influence uric acid concentrations. Hagos et al.[26] reported that *SLC22A11* (OAT4) takes up urate by exchanging OH⁻ and suggested an involvement of *SLC22A11* as a cause of hydrochlorothiazide-induced hyperuricemia, because urate uptake increases when cells are pretreated with thiazide diuretics. However, there has been no in vivo evidence that OAT4 is involved in renal urate transport—for example, no *SLC22A11* mutation was found in renal hypouricemia patients and further analysis is necessary.

SLC22A12 (URAT1; urate transporter 1) is a member of the OAT family and is localized in the apical membrane of proximal tubular epithelial cells.[5] Functional studies using a *Xenopus* oocyte expression system showed that URAT1 mediates the transport of urate in a time- and concentration-dependent manner (K_m about 370 μmol/L). The driving force for urate transport via URAT1 was shown to be exchange of luminal urate and intracellular inorganic (Cl⁻) and organic anions (lactate, nicotinate [niacin], PZA),[5] indicating that intracellularly accumulated organic anions will favor the uphill reabsorption of urate in exchange for these anions, which move down their electrochemical gradients into the lumen. Administration of benzbromarone for patients with hereditary renal hypouricemia caused by *SLC22A12* mutation failed to show a stimulating effect, indicating that URAT1 is the site of action for an in vivo effect of benzbromarone.[27]

Transport function of a mouse ortholog of *SLC22A12* (mUrat1), or renal-specific transporter (RST), was also characterized.[28] mUrat1 transports urate (K_m 1.2 mmol/L) and is *cis*-inhibited by probenecid, benzbromarone, and lactate. The fact that there are higher mRNA and protein levels of mUrat1 in male kidneys than in female kidneys may explain why the SUA level is higher in males than in females.[28]

Facilitated Glucose Transporter Family SLC2A9

In 2007, Li et al.[29] first reported that the glucose transporter family GLUT9 (*SLC2A9*) is a gene correlated with the SUA level based on the results from a GWAS of a genetically isolated population in Sardinia. Similar results have been reported from several facilities.[6,7,30-33] Vitart et al.[30] also reported that *SLC2A9* (GLUT9), initially reported as a fructose transporter, mediates the transport of urate. Human GLUT9 has two isoforms (GLUT9 and GLUT9ΔN) depending on the splicing of the intracellular part of the N-terminal region. When artificially expressed in polarized MDCK cells, GLUT9 (or long form) is expressed at the basal side, and GLUT9ΔN (or short form) is expressed at the apical side.[34]

After the report by Li et al., we also evaluated the urate transport activity of *SLC2A9* using a *Xenopus* oocyte expression system. We found that the *SLC2A9* gene product is URATv1, a voltage-driven bidirectional urate transporter, which transports urate in a potential-dependent manner.[8] In addition, since *SLC2A9* is mainly expressed on the basolateral membrane of proximal tubular epithelial cells in the human kidney in vivo,[34] we suggested that *SLC2A9* (URATv1) is involved in the efflux of urate toward the blood side.[16,17] Recently, we confirmed the voltage-dependent property of *SLC2A9*-mediated urate transport by using the two-electrode voltage clamp method,[35] since another facility had also shown that mouse Glut9 is involved in voltage-dependent urate transport.[36] In 2009, Dinour et al.[37] reported that homozygous *SLC2A9* mutations (L75R) cause severe renal hypouricemia leading to exercise-induced acute renal failure. It is concluded that renal hypouricemia can be induced by mutation of not only *SLC22A12* (URAT1), an apical influx transporter of urate, but also *SLC2A9* (URATv1), a basolateral efflux transporter of urate.[16,17] Therefore, at least two types of renal hypouricemia (i.e., *SLC22A12* and *SLC2A9* types) are likely to exist.

To investigate the effects of URATv1 gene overexpression in the kidney, we constructed *SLC2A9* (human *URATv1*) transgenic (Tg) mice, in which the transgene was under the control of mouse Urat1 promoter that induces transgene expression in renal proximal tubules. We confirmed exogenous expression of human URATv1 only at the basolateral side of renal proximal tubules and found that *SLC2A9* Tg mice showed reduced urinary urate secretion compared with that in wild-type mice, although SUA levels showed no change.[38] In contrast, there is no phenotype in apical Urat1 Tg mice.[38] Since almost all GWA studies have demonstrated that *SLC2A9* has a strong association with SUA concentration,[6,7,30-33] it is likely that the basolateral *SLC2A9* is a gatekeeper to determine net urate transport in renal proximal tubules in vivo.

ATP-Binding Cassette ABC Transporters ABCC4 and ABCG2

MRP4 (multidrug resistance-associated protein 4; *ABCC4*), which exists at the apical membrane of renal proximal tubules, was reported to perform ATP-dependent urate anion excretion (K_m 1.5 mmol/L).[39] MRP4 is proposed to function as another exit pathway for urate in urate secretion, although there is no clear in vivo evidence for these functions.

As mentioned earlier, Dehghan et al.[7] proposed that, in addition to *SLC2A9* (URATv1/GLUT9), *ABCG2* (BCRP) and *SLC17A3* (NPT4) are candidates for genetic causes of hyperuricemia. BCRP, breast cancer resistance protein (*ABCG2*), a member of the same ABC transporter family to which *ABCC4* (MRP4) belongs, was reported recently to transport uric acid.[40] In addition, the finding that Q141K polymorphism associated with gout leads to decreased uric acid excretion capacity suggests that ABCG2 contributes to urate anion excretion at the apical membrane of renal proximal tubules and/or at the luminal membrane of the intestine.[40] Although the human kidney is known to express many drug efflux pumps at the apical side of proximal tubules such as *ABCB1* (P-glycoprotein/MDR1), *ABCC2* (MRP2), and *ABCC4* (MRP4),[41] evidence for *ABCG2* (BCRP) expression in the kidney has been somewhat confusing: according to one report, a moderate level of *ABCG2* protein expression was detected despite no mRNA expression in the human kidney.[42] Given its expression pattern (i.e., high levels in the liver and intestine), it is likely that the hypoactive variant of ABCG2 leads to decreased urate excretion into the intestine rather than (or as well as?) decreased uric acid excretion from the kidney.

Type I Na+-Dependent Phosphate Transporter Family SLC17A1 and SLC17A3

In 2000, Uchino et al.[43] showed that human sodium-dependent phosphate transporter type 1 (NPT1) in the SLC17 family, present in renal apical membrane, mediates the transport of urate. Considering its chloride ion sensitivity, *SLC17A1* (NPT1) was expected to function for secretion of organic anions from renal proximal tubular cells. Although Iharada et al.[44] reported that *SLC17A1* functions as a Cl−-dependent urate exporter only in proteoliposomes, we could not observe a voltage-dependency property for urate transport via *SLC17A1* in *Xenopus* oocytes or in mammalian cell expression systems to date (P. Jutabha, N. Anzai, et al., unpublished observation).

In a genomewide study to determine genetic causes of hyperuricemia, Dehghan et al.[7] found that *SLC17A3* (NPT4) as well as *ABCG2* (BCRP) are candidates in addition to *SLC2A9* (URATv1/GLUT9). Human NPT4 (hNPT4) has two splice variants: hNPT4_L (long isoform) and hNPT4_S (short isoform). It has been reported that hNPT4_S lacking the fourth exon shows intracellular localization when expressed in COS cells.[45] Recently, we found that the long isoform of the orphan transporter hNPT4 (hNPT4_L), expressed in the plasma membrane of *Xenopus* oocytes, mediated low-affinity transport of organic anions such as *para*-aminohippurate (PAH), estrone sulfate and urate in a voltage-sensitive manner.[9] *SLC17A3* mRNA expression was detected in the kidneys and liver. *SLC17A3* was found to be localized at the apical side of renal tubules by immunohistochemistry, indicating that *SLC17A3* functions as a voltage-driven urate efflux transporter. An in vivo role of *SLC17A3* was suggested by two missense mutations in *SLC17A3* with reduced urate efflux in vitro from hyperuricemia patients. These findings will complete a model of urate secretion in renal proximal tubular cells, in which intracellular urate taken up via *SLC22A6*/*SLC22A8* from the blood exits from the cells into the lumen via *SLC17A3*.[46]

Urate Transportsome (Urate-Transporting Molecular Complex)

In the C-terminal intracellular portion, *SLC22A12* has a specific amino acid sequence (T-Q-F) for protein–protein interaction, termed a PDZ motif.[47] We hypothesized that some proteins bind to this site and regulate urate transport function of *SLC22A12*. We performed yeast two-hybrid screening against a human kidney cDNA library using *SLC22A12* C-terminus as "bait." We found that the multivalent PDZ-domain protein PDZK1 is a binding partner for urate transporter *SLC22A12* and confirmed that the interaction of PDZK1 enhances *SLC22A12*-mediated urate transport in vitro.[48] Recently, Kolz et al.[6] also reported from results of their GWA scans that PDZK1 is one of the five new loci that influence uric acid concentrations.

Since PDZK1 is expressed at the apical side of renal proximal tubules and this protein also binds to several other transporters,[49] we proposed the possibility that membrane transport proteins manifesting their function, while maintaining a relationship with intracellular signaling systems and other regulatory molecules, are bundled by PDZ proteins such as PDZK1 and NHERFs and other scaffolding proteins to form a "membrane transport molecular complex (transportsome)" that makes up functional units of in vivo transmembrane substrate transport.

Accordingly, we proposed a model of urate-transporting molecular complex (urate transportsome) at the apical membrane of renal proximal tubules (Figure 4-3). This model not only clarifies the role of *SLC22A12* in renal urate reabsorption

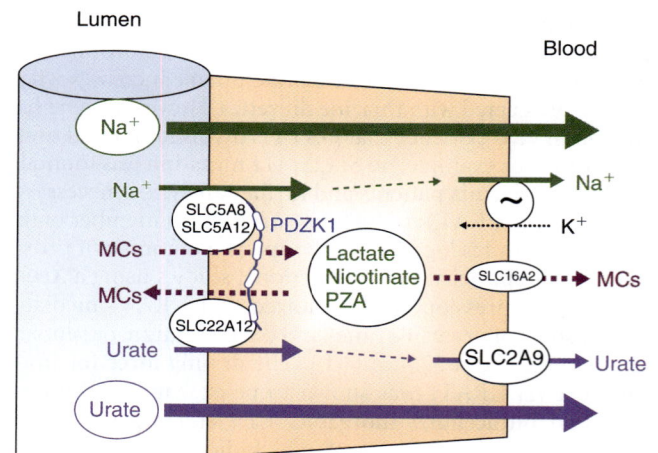

Figure 4-3 Proposed model of "urate transportsome" in renal proximal tubules. Apical urate-transporting multimolecular complex (urate transportsome) is composed of *SLC22A12* (URAT1) and *SLC5A8* (SMCT1)/*SLC5A12* (SMCT2), each of which has a PDZ motif at their C-terminus, scaffolded by PDZ-domain protein PDZK1 underneath the plasma membrane. A model of indirect coupling of sodium and urate transport via *SLC22A12* is illustrated. Coupling of anions to sodium uptake along the luminal membrane and later exchange of the anions for urate by *SLC22A12* in the proximal tubule. This model focuses on the functional coupling between *SLC22A12* and SMCTs; therefore, other urate transporters such as *SLC22A11* (OAT4)/*SLC22A13* (OAT10) are not included on the apical side in order to avoid confusion. *SLC16A2*, Monocarboxylate transporter 2 (MCT2); *MCs*, monocarboxylates; *PZA*, pyrazine carboxylate. *(Modified from Anzai N, Jutabha P, Kimura T, et al. Urate transport: relationship with serum urate disorder. Curr Rheumatol Rev, 2011;7:123-31.)*

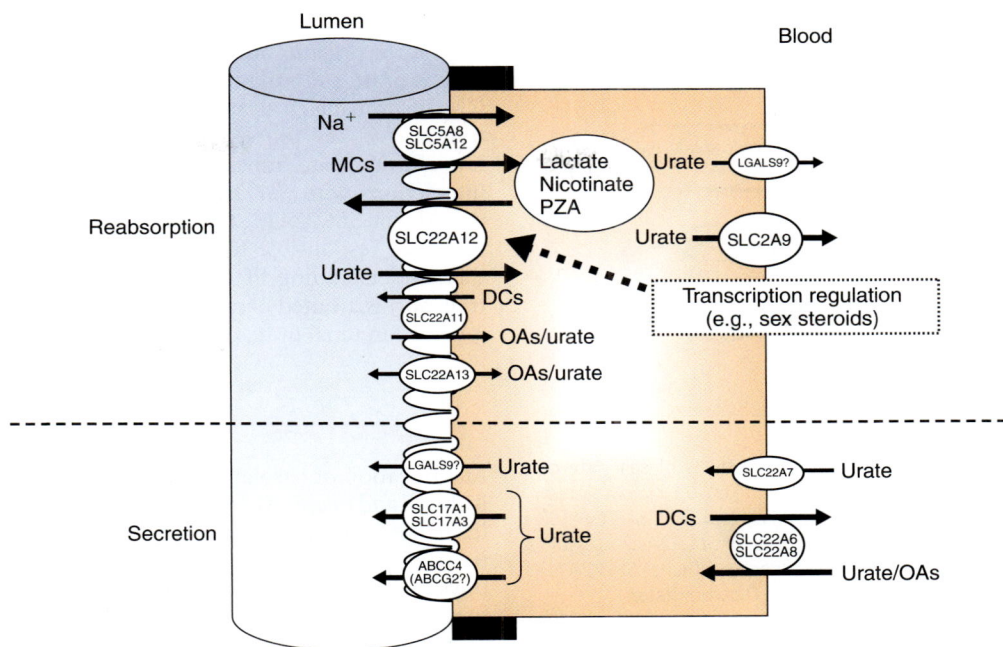

Figure 4-4 Models of transcellular urate transport in the proximal tubule. *DCs,* dicarboxylates; *MCs,* monocarboxylates; *OAs,*Organic anions; *PZA,* pyrazinoate, metabolite of pyrazinamide. *(Modified from Anzai N, Jutabha P, Kimura T, et al. Urate transport: relationship with serum urate disorder. Curr Rheumatol Rev, 2011;7:123-31.)*

but also contributes to an understanding of renal urate handling as a supramolecular phenomenon provided by functional units comprising *SLC22A12* and other interacting molecules mediated by the PDZ scaffold. Since our yeast two-hybrid screening revealed that Na+-dependent monocarboxylate transporters *SLC5A8* (SMCT1) and *SLC5A12* (SMCT2) ("SMCTs") bind with PDZK1,[50] we suggest that the link between URAT1 and SMCTs through common transport substrates such as lactate in the vicinity, as Thangaraju et al.[51] demonstrated using c/ebpdelta−/− mice, is supported by PDZK1 and it may demonstrate one of the physiologic roles of "urate transportsome" (see Figure 4-3). For example, the concept of "urate transportsomes" may explain a long-hypothesized "Na+-dependent urate transport" mechanism that affects SUA levels in several pathophysiologic conditions. Figure 4-4 depicts the known urate transport–related molecules in renal proximal tubules.

Renal Urate Transporters as Causes of Drug-Induced Hyperuricemia

Diuretics

Common diuretics such as loop diuretics (furosemide and bumetanide) and thiazide reduce urinary uric acid excretion and increase SUA levels[52] (Figure 4-5). Although acute administration of diuretics increases the fractional excretion of uric acid (FE_{UA}), chronic administration decreases FE_{UA}, leading to hyperuricemia. In addition to contraction of extracellular fluid volume, diuretics that are secreted into the urine tend to compete with the tubular secretion of urate and contribute further to reduction of renal excretion of uric acid.[1] Since *SLC17A3* is likely to act as a common secretion route for both drugs and urate, this protein may play an important role in

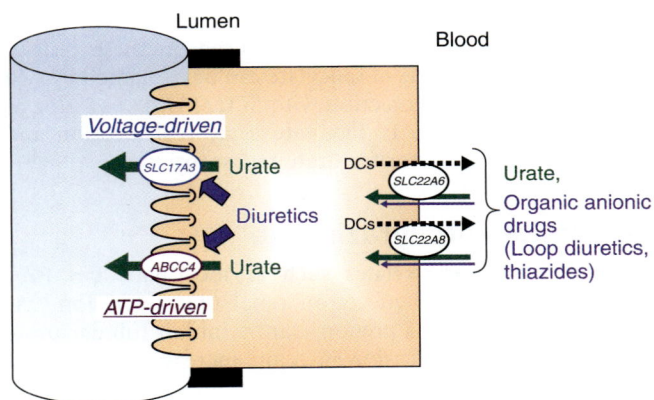

Figure 4-5 Putative model of diuretic-induced hyperuricemia. Urate, as well as organic anionic drugs such as diuretics, are taken up by basolateral transporters *SLC22A6* (OAT1) and/or *SLC22A8* (OAT3) in exchange for intracellular dicarboxylates (DCs). Then, diuretics may share the same substrate binding site for urate in voltage-driven transporter *SLC17A3* (NPT4) and/or ATP-driven transporter *ABCC4* (MRP4). This diuretic–urate interaction at the apical exit pathway may promote diuretic-induced hyperuricemia.

diuretic-induced hyperuricemia.[9] Besides *SLC17A3*, El-Sheikh et al.[53] reported inhibitory effects of furosemide and thiazide on *ABCC4*-mediated urate transport and they suggested that *ABCC4* is the site of action for diuretic-induced hyperuricemia.

Salicylate

Salicylic acid derivatives are the most widely prescribed analgesic-antipyretic and antiinflammatory agents (Figure 4-6). Salicylate is known to have "paradoxical effects" on renal

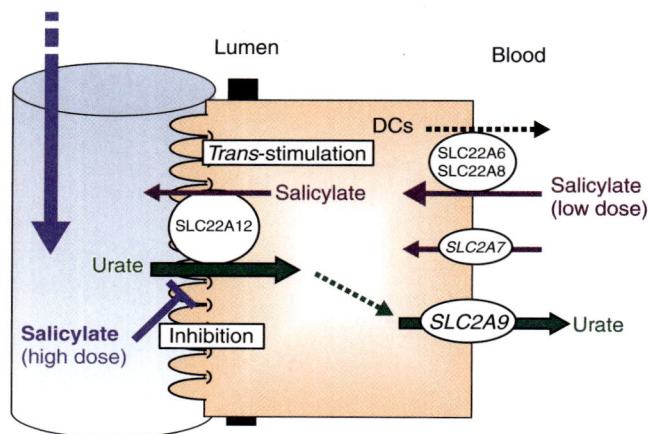

Figure 4-6 Putative model for the paradoxical effects of salicylate on renal urate disposition. Low-dose salicylate is taken up by basolateral transporters *SLC22A6* (OAT1), *SLC22A7* (OAT2), and *SLC22A8* (OAT3), then it becomes an exchange substrate for urate at *SLC22A12* (URAT1). Glomerular filtrated high-dose salicylate directly inhibits *SLC22A12*-mediated urate uptake from luminal side. *DCs,* Dicarboxylates.

urate transport: at low concentrations (5 to 10 mg/dl), it inhibits renal uric acid excretion and thereby increases SUA levels, but at high concentrations (15 mg/dl or higher), it inhibits renal urate reabsorption in renal tubules leading to decrease in SUA levels.[1] Recently, we found that salicylate is not only an inhibitor of *SLC22A12*-mediated urate transport but also its transport substrates.[54] Based on these results, such paradoxical effects of salicylate can be explained by two modes of salicylate interaction with *SLC22A12*: (1) acting as an exchange substrate to facilitate urate reabsorption and (2) acting as an inhibitor for urate reabsorption.

Nicotinate and Pyrazinoate

Aromatic monocarboxylates such as nicotinate and PZA also have paradoxical effects on renal urate secretion.[1] At low doses, these agents predominantly inhibit tubular urate secretion, thereby decreasing FE_{UA} and increasing SUA levels, whereas tubular urate reabsorption is inhibited at high doses, leading to an increase in FE_{UA} and reduction in SUA levels. These phenomena can be explained by in vitro transport properties of *SLC22A12*: preloading with nicotinate and PZA *trans*-stimulated urate uptake via *SLC22A12* and the efflux of nicotinate injected into oocytes was *trans*-stimulated when urate was added to the extracellular solution.[5] These results also indicate that nicotinate and PZA act as exchange substrates to facilitate *SLC22A12*-mediated urate reabsorption and they act as inhibitors for its reabsorption.

Cyclosporine A

Cyclosporine A (CsA) is used as a common immunosuppressant for management of organ transplantation and various autoimmune diseases. One of the well-known side effects of CsA treatment is hyperuricemia,[55] but there is no convincing evidence that hyperuricemia is due to CsA-induced impairment of tubular urate handling. Bahn et al.[56] analyzed *SLC22A13*, an orphan transporter expressed mainly in the kidney and weakly in the brain, heart, and intestine, using a

Xenopus oocyte expression system and found that *SLC22A13* transports organic anions such as nicotinate and PAH as well as urate and renamed the transporter OAT10. Since the IC_{50} of nonlabeled urate on *SLC22A13*-mediated nicotinate transport is 759 μmol/L, they reported that *SLC22A13* is a low-affinity urate transporter. Since CsA showed substantial interactions with *SLC22A13*, of which CsA enhanced urate uptake via *SLC22A13*, they suggested that *SLC22A13* is the molecule responsible for CsA-induced hyperuricemia. Further understanding of the role of *SLC22A13* in renal urate transport is awaited because there is also no evidence that it is involved in renal urate transport in humans in vivo.

Perspectives

Identification of basolateral urate efflux transporter URATv1 in 2008[8] and of apical organic anion efflux transporter hNPT4[9] led to the proposal of the "three-factor model" for transepithelial transport of urate in renal proximal tubules. However, the physiologic and pathophysiologic roles of molecules related to renal urate handling have not been completely clarified yet; we must continue to investigate their precise roles in vivo.

Discussion of the renal pathogenesis of hyperuricemia in a variety of nephropathies (including polycystic and medullary cystic kidney diseases and analgesic nephropathy) and in lead intoxication was beyond the scope of this review. The linkage of uromodulin (*UMOD*) mutations to hyperuricemia does warrant brief mention.[57] UMOD-related kidney diseases include medullary cystic kidney disease type 2 (MCKD2) and familial juvenile hyperuricemic nephropathy (FJHN), and inheritance is autosomal dominant. In these conditions, decreased renal fractional excretion of uric acid develops, and precocious hyperuricemia and gout can occur, and tubulointerstitial nephropathy can be progressive. Medullary cysts also can develop but may be a late finding, and age of onset and age of end-stage renal disease are variable. *UMOD* encodes for Tamm-Horsfall protein (THP), and increased THP deposition in the kidney has been observed in this spectrum of disorders. It is not yet clear how mutants of THP, which is synthesized in the thick ascending limb of the nephron, cause hyperuricemia, and THP does not appear to bind uric acid, which argues against an effect on uric acid disposition in the distal nephron.

Throughout this review, we emphasized the importance of the kidneys in urate metabolism in the human body. However, we think that, in addition to the kidneys, clarification of urate metabolism in extrarenal tissues such as the intestine and the liver is also important. For example, recent GWAS (see Chapter 8) have revealed eight transporter-coding genes related to SUA level.[6,7] Although some gene products have not been functionally confirmed yet as urate transporters, it seems likely that multiple transporter genes are involved in urate handling in humans—not only in the kidney but also in other tissues.

In the liver, urate is synthesized from its precursors by the enzyme xanthine oxidase (XO).[58] XO catalyzes both the process by which hypoxanthine is converted to xanthine and the process by which xanthine is converted to uric acid. Precursors of uric acid production such as inosine and guanosine, as well as hypoxanthine and xanthine, may enter hepatocytes via membrane transporters whose molecular identities are still unknown. Furthermore, how urate produced in the liver is secreted into the blood is also not known. These processes may be mediated by transporters that will be potential targets for novel therapeutics.

In the intestine, one third of the daily production of urate is excreted into the gut by biliary, gastric, and intestinal secretions.[1] The intestine is another important organ for uric acid production because XO has also been identified in the intestine as well as in the liver.[58] Thus, the transporters responsible for membrane permeation of urate need to be clarified because both absorption and secretion of urate were observed in the intestine.[59] Enhanced intestinal excretion of urate occurring as a compensatory mechanism was found in chronic renal disease with compromised renal uric acid excretion. *ABCG2* (BCRP) seems to be the most probable candidate for urate excretion in the luminal side of the intestine.

The macromolecular structure-function of URAT1 and other urate transporters, including assembly of functional "protein scaffolds," exemplified by URAT1 and NPT1 interaction with PZDK1 protein, is important for understanding therapeutic "handles" in renal urate anion transport, let alone some genetic associations with hyperuricemia (see Chapter 8). In human studies to date, *SLC2A9* effects on SUA were much greater in women. Androgens and estrogens, let alone age, are among the regulatory factors for expression of specific urate transporters in the proximal tubule, and at least one study suggested URAT1 to be a "male-dominant" urate transporter.[60] Further elucidation of how hypertension, the renin-angiotensin axis, and various forms of chronic kidney disease modulate renal urate transporters could help in personalization of urate-lowering treatment strategies. Already noteworthy, in a translational sense, is the knowledge that multiple uricosurics, including probenecid, benzbromarone fenofibrate, losartan, and the experimental drug RDEA594, act on URAT1.

Finally, an understanding of urate transport in the kidneys as well as in extrarenal tissues will advance not only the understanding of urate metabolism in humans but also clarification of the physiologic role of urate itself in the human body.

Acknowledgments

This work was supported in part by grants from JSPS (KAKENHI 21390073, 21659216), Takeda Science Foundation, Gout Research Foundation of Japan, and the Nakatomi Foundation to N.A.

References

1. Sica DA, Schoolwerth AC. Renal handling of organic anions and cations: excretion of uric acid. In: Brenner BM, editor. The Kidney. 6th ed. Philadelphia, PA: WB Saunders; 2000:680–700.
2. Burckhardt G, Pritchard JB. Organic anion and cation antiporters. In: Seldin DW, Giebisch G, editors. The Kidney: Physiology and Pathophysiology. 3rd ed. Philadelphia, PA: Lippincott Williams & Wilkins; 2000. p. 193–222.
3. Kutzing MK, Firestein BL. Altered uric acid levels and disease states. J Pharmacol Exp Ther 2008;324:1–7.
4. Anzai N, Endou H. Drug discovery for hyperuricemia. Exp Opin Drug Discov 2007;2:1251–61.
5. Enomoto A, Kimura H, Chairoungdua A, et al. Molecular identification of a renal urate anion exchanger that regulates blood urate levels. Nature 2002;417:447–52.
6. Kolz M, Johnson T, Sanna S, et al. Meta-analysis of 28,141 individuals identifies common variants within five new loci that influence uric acid concentrations. Plos Genet 2009;5:1–0.
7. Dehghan A, Köttgen A, Yang Q, et al. Association of three genetic loci with uric acid concentration and risk of gout: a genome-wide association study. Lancet 2008;372:1953–61.
8. Anzai N, Ichida K, Jutabha P, et al. Plasma urate level is directly regulated by a voltage-driven urate efflux transporter URATv1 (SLC2A9) in humans. J Biol Chem 2008;283:26834–8.
9. Jutabha P, Anzai N, Kitamura K, et al. Human sodium-phosphate transporter 4 (hNPT4/SLC17A3) as a common renal secretory pathway for drugs and urate. J Biol Chem 2010;285:35123–32.
10. Rafey MA, Lipkowitz MS, Leal-Pinto E, et al. Uric acid transport. Curr Opin Nephrol Hypertens 2003;12:511–6.
11. Anzai N, Enomoto A, Endou H. Renal urate handling: clinical relevance of recent advances. Curr Rheumatol Rep 2005;7:227–34.
12. Anzai N, Kanai Y, Endou H. New insights into renal transport of urate. Curr Opin Rheumatol 2007;19:151–7.
13. Taniguchi A, Kamatani N. Control of renal uric acid excretion and gout. Curr Opin Rheumatol 2008;20:192–7.
14. Choi HK, Zhu Y, Mount DB. Genetics of gout. Curr Opin Rheumatol 2010;22:144–51.
15. Ichida K. What lies behind serum urate concentration? Insights from genetic and genomic studies.
16. Anzai N, Jutabha P, Endou H. Renal solute transporters and their relevance to serum urate disorder. Curr Hypertens Rev 2010;6:148–54.
17. Anzai N, Jutabha P, Kimura T, et al. Urate transport: regulators of with serum urate levels in human. Curr Rheumatol Rev 2011;7:123-31.
18. Kahn AM, Weinman EJ. Urate transport in the proximal tubule: in vivo and vesicle studies. Am J Physiol 1985;249:F789–98.
19. Roch-Ramel F, Guisan B. Renal transport of urate in humans. News Physiol Sci 1999;14:80–4.
20. Kamatani Y, Matsuda K, Okada Y, et al. Genome-wide association study of hematological and biochemical traits in a Japanese population. Nat Genet 2010;42:210–5.
21. Lipkowitz MS, Leal-Pinto E, Rappoport JZ, et al. Functional reconstitution, membrane targeting, genomic structure, and chromosomal localization of a human urate transporter. J Clin Invest 2001;107:1103–15.
22. Ahn SY, Bhatnagar V. Update on the molecular physiology of organic anion transporters. Curr Opin Nephrol Hypertens 2008;17:499–505.
23. El-Sheikh AA, Masereeuw R, Russel FG. Mechanisms of renal anionic drug transport. Eur J Pharmacol 2008;585:245–55.
24. Anzai N, Kanai Y, Endou H. Organic anion transporter family: current knowledge. J Pharmacol Sci 2006;100:411–26.
25. Eraly SA, Vallon V, Rieg T, et al. Multiple organic anion transporters contribute to net renal excretion of uric acid. Physiol Genom 2008;33:180–92.
26. Hagos Y, Stein D, Ugele B, et al. Human renal organic anion transporter 4 operates as an asymmetric urate transporter. J Am Soc Nephrol 2007;18:430–9.
27. Ichida K, Hosoyamada M, Hisatome I, et al. Clinical and molecular analysis of patients with renal hypouricemia in Japan: influence of URAT1 gene on urinary urate excretion. J Am Soc Nephrol 2004;15:164–73.
28. Hosoyamada M, Ichida K, Enomoto A, et al. Function and localization of urate transporter 1 in mouse kidney. J Am Soc Nephrol 2004;15:261–8.
29. Li S, Sanna S, Maschio A, et al. The GLUT9 gene is associated with serum uric acid levels in Sardinia and Chianti cohorts. PLoS Genet 2007;3:e194.
30. Vitart V, Rudan I, Hayward C, et al. SLC2A9 is a newly identified urate transporter influencing serum urate concentration, urate excretion and gout. Nat Genet 2008;40:437–42.
31. Caulfield MJ, Munroe PB, O'Neill D, et al. SLC2A9 is a high-capacity urate transporter in humans. PLoS Med 2008;5:e197.
32. Wallace C, Newhouse SJ, Braund P, et al. Genome-wide association study identifies genes for biomarkers of cardiovascular disease: serum urate and dyslipidemia. Am J Hum Genet 2008;82:139–49.
33. Döring A, Gieger C, Mehta D, et al. SLC2A9 influences uric acid concentrations with pronounced sex-specific effects. Nat Genet 2008;40:430–6.
34. Augustin R, Carayannopoulos MO, Dowd LO, et al. Identification and characterization of human glucose transporter-like protein-9 (GLUT9): alternative splicing alters trafficking. J Biol Chem 2004;279:16229–36.
35. Anzai N, Jutabha P, Kaneko S, et al. Voltage-dependent urate transport on a urate efflux transporter URATv1 expressed in *Xenopus* oocytes [abstract]. J Pharmacol Sci 2010;112:202P.
36. Bibert S, Hess SK, Firsov D, et al. Mouse GLUT9: evidences for a urate uniporter. Am J Physiol Renal Physiol 2009;297:F612–9.
37. Dinour D, Gray NK, Campbell S, et al. Homozygous SLC2A9 mutations cause severe renal hypouricemia. J Am Soc Nephrol 2010;21:64–72.

38. Kimura T, Tsukada A, Amonpatumrat S, et al. Elucidation of urate transport mechanism by analysis of renal urate transporters transgenic mice [abstract]. J Pharmacol Sci 2010;112:66.

39. van Aubel RA, Smeets PH, van den Heuvel JJ, et al. Human organic anion transporter MRP4 (ABCC4) is an efflux pump for the purine end metabolite urate with multiple allosteric substrate binding sites. Am J Physiol Renal Physiol 2005;288:F327–33.

40. Woodward OM, Köttgen A, Coresh J, et al. Identification of a urate transporter, ABCG2, with a common functional polymorphism causing gout. Proc Natl Acad Sci USA 2009;106:10338–42.

41. Huls M, Brown CD, Windass AS, et al. The breast cancer resistance protein transporter ABCG2 is expressed in the human kidney proximal tubule apical membrane. Kidney Int 2008;73:220–5.

42. Krishnamurthy P, Schuetz JD. Role of ABCG2/BCRP in biology and medicine. Annu Rev Pharmacol Toxicol 2006;46:381–410.

43. Uchino H, Tamai I, Yamashita K, et al. p-Aminohippuric acid transport at renal apical membrane mediated by human inorganic phosphate transporter NPT1. Biochem Biophys Res Commun 2000;270:254–9.

44. Iharada M, Miyaji T, Fujimoto T, et al. Type 1 sodium-dependent phosphate transporter (SLC17A1 protein) is a Cl(-)-dependent urate exporter. J Biol Chem 2010;285:26107–13.

45. Melis D, Havelaar AC, Verbeek E, et al. NPT4, a new microsomal phosphate transporter: mutation analysis in glycogen storage disease type Ic. J Inherit Metab Dis 2004;27:725–33.

46. Anzai N, Endou H. Urate transporters: an evolving field. Semin Nephrol, in press.

47. Lamprecht G, Seidler U. The emerging role of PDZ adapter proteins for regulation of intestinal ion transport. Am J Physiol Gastrointest Liver Physiol 2006;291:G766–77.

48. Anzai N, Miyazaki H, Noshiro R, et al. The multivalent PDZ domain-containing protein PDZK1 regulates transport activity of renal urate-anion exchanger URAT1 via its C terminus. J Biol Chem 2004;279:45942–50.

49. Gisler SM, Pribanic S, Bacic D, et al. PDZK1: I. a major scaffolder in brush borders of proximal tubular cells. Kidney Int 2003;64:1733–45.

50. Srivastava S, Anzai N, Miyauchi S, et al. Identification of the multivalent PDZ protein PDZK1 as a binding partner of sodium-coupled monocarboxylate transporter SMCT1 (SLC5A8) and SMCT2 (SLC5A12) by yeast two-hybrid assay [abstract]. J Pharmacol Sci 2009;109:68P.

51. Thangaraju M, Ananth S, Martin PM, et al. c/ebpdelta Null mouse as a model for the double knock-out of slc5a8 and slc5a12 in kidney. J Biol Chem 2006;281:26769–73.

52. Reyes AJ. Cardiovascular drugs and serum uric acid. Cardiovasc Drugs Ther 2003;17:397–414.

53. El-Sheikh AA, van den Heuvel JJ, Koenderink JB, et al. Effect of hypouricaemic and hyperuricaemic drugs on the renal urate efflux transporter, multidrug resistance protein 4. Br J Pharmacol 2008;155:1066–75.

54. Ohtsu N, Anzai N, Fukutomi T, et al. Human renal urate transporter URAT1 mediates the transport of salicylate [in Japanese]. Nippon Jinzo Gakkai Shi 2010;52:499–504.

55. Zürcher RM, Bock HA, Thiel G. Hyperuricaemia in cyclosporin-treated patients: GFR-related effect. Nephrol Dial Transplant 1996;11:153–8.

56. Bahn A, Hagos Y, Reuter S, et al. Identification of a new urate and high affinity nicotinate transporter, hOAT10 (SLC22A13). J Biol Chem 2008;283:16332–41.

57. Gersch MS, Sautin YY, Gersch CM, et al. Does Tamm-Horsfall protein-uric acid binding play a significant role in urate homeostasis? Nephrol Dial Transplant 2006;21(10):2938–42.

58. Berry CE, Hare JM. Xanthine oxidoreductase and cardiovascular disease: molecular mechanisms and pathophysiological implications. J Physiol 2004;555:589–606.

59. Sorensen LB, Levinson DJ. Origin and extrarenal elimination of uric acid in man. Nephron 1975;14:7–20.

60. Cheng X, Klaassen CD. Tissue distribution, ontogeny, and hormonal regulation of xenobiotic transporters in mouse kidneys. Drug Metab Dispos 2009;37(11):2178–85.

Tophus Biology and Pathogenesis of Monosodium Urate Crystal–Induced Inflammation

Ru Liu-Bryan and Robert Terkeltaub

KEY POINTS

- Tophi are macroaggregates of monosodium urate (MSU) crystals and in most tissues are formed as granulomas with cellular content that includes phagocytes, mast cells, B- and T-lymphocytes, and plasma cells.
- MSU crystals induce a plethora of inflammatory mediators. Although the precise factors by which gouty inflammation is triggered via changes in previously quiescent or smoldering urate crystal deposits remain poorly understood, the physical characteristics of MSU crystals, tophus stability, and systemic triggers from outside the joint likely play a substantial role.
- MSU crystals drive gouty inflammation by directly or indirectly inducing or using multiple mediators of extracellular and intracellular innate immunity, such as C5b-9 complement assembly, TLR signaling, NLRP3 inflammasome and caspase-1 activation, and induction of interleukin-1β and -8.
- The effects of urate crystals and/or crystal-induced mediators of inflammation on endothelial cells, synovial lining cells, mast cells, and monocyte-derived macrophages orchestrate the course of gouty inflammation. Subsequent neutrophil influx into the joint space appears to execute and amplify gouty arthritis.
- Macrophage uptake of apoptotic neutrophils is a major mechanism involved in the spontaneous resolution of gouty inflammation.

Overview of Gouty Inflammation and Tophus Dynamics

Acute gouty arthritis is characteristically a roaring inflammatory reaction that develops in association with microscopic or macroscopic tophaceous deposits of monosodium urate (MSU) crystals. Since the establishment, in the modern era of science, of the inflammatory potential in vivo of synthetic

Supported by the VA Research Service.

MSU crystals approximately 50 years ago, there has been an accelerating evolution of understanding how MSU crystals can trigger inflammation. Initial studies described the capacity of MSU crystals to activate complement and the contact system of coagulation; stimulate a variety of cells, including platelets and neutrophils; and promote degranulation and activation of prostaglandin synthesis.

The primary focus of much early work in the field was neutrophil activation and degranulation directly by MSU crystals, since the findings of MSU crystals phagocytosed by neutrophils in synovial fluid, and neutrophil influx into the joint, are central in diagnosis of acute gout. Moreover, animal model studies by Phelps and McCarty[1] indicated the importance of neutrophils to experimental gouty arthritis. Schumacher and colleagues[2] described intense neutrophil infiltration into the synovial membrane in acute gout. In addition, neutrophils phagocytosing MSU crystals were observed to release a small peptide neutrophil chemotaxin abundant in granules, termed crystal-induced chemotactic factor (CCF). The CCF molecule was isolated and characterized by Spilberg and colleagues[3] and likely represented the first description of the calgranulin heterodimer S100A8/9.[4,5]

A stunning discovery in the 1980s was that serum coating reduced MSU crystal inflammatory potential, and that low-density lipoprotein (LDL), and the very large, cationic LDL constituent apolipoprotein (apo) B by itself, mediated this effect and potently inhibited the capacity of MSU crystals to physically interact with cells.[6,7] Some tophi in the synovial membrane had been described as "walled off" in a thick layer of protein.[2] A concept emerged of MSU crystals constitutively rendered passive by protein coating prior to and in the resolution of gouty inflammation as large serum proteins had more readily entered the joint space. This model still fits well with the notion that remodeling or ruptured synovial tophi, or MSU crystal macroaggregates deposited at or near the surface of articular cartilage (see Chapter 2), shed small "naked" MSU crystals with heightened inflammatory potential to trigger gout. This theoretically occurs at times such as in the early phases of intense urate-lowering therapy (or when walls of tophi or urate crystal masses at the cartilage surface are compromised by trauma, or when there is a phase of rapid, disorganized increase in MSU crystal deposition in tophi or at the cartilage surface at times of abrupt increases in serum urate). However, we now recognize that synovial and bursal tophi are not simple, passively walled-off structures but instead are dynamic granulomas,[8] with mononuclear leukocyte traffic in and out of the tophi, and apoptosis and matrix metalloproteinase expression.[9]

The cytokine era of MSU crystal inflammation biology was marked by the discovery of the ability of MSU crystals and a variety of other crystals and particulates (including calcium pyrophosphate dihydrate [CPPD]) to induce interleukin (IL)-1β, tumor necrosis factor-alpha (TNFα), IL-6, and chemokine IL-8 (CXCL8) and GROα (CXCL1) expression by cells including mononuclear phagocytes.[10-14] Molecular and translational biology implications of these findings have become substantial. In particular, selective IL-1 antagonism has emerged in the clinic as a novel and effective biologic strategy for gout attack prophylaxis (see Chapter 16) and, in some cases, treatment of acute gout (see Chapter 11) and chronic gouty arthritis.[15] The particularly profound contribution of chemokine ligands of CXCR2 (e.g., IL-8/CXCL8 and GROα/CXCL1) to experimental gouty inflammation[14] indicates the potential of biologic antagonism of CXCR2 and its ligands for gouty inflammation. One suspects that the priming of many gout attacks, for example in association with intercurrent medical or surgical illness, or spreading polyarticular attacks, may be mediated by arousal of smoldering inflammation in tophi driven by systemic release of IL-1, TNFα, and other cytokines.

Starting in the 1990s, attention also began to be paid to how MSU crystals induce cell activation by triggering proinflammatory signal transduction and transcriptional activation involving several Src family kinases, proline-rich tyrosine kinase 2 (Pyk2), spleen tyrosine kinase (Syk), mitogen-activated protein kinases, phosphatidylinositol-3-kinase (PI3K), mitogen-activated protein kinases (including p38), and necrosis factor (NF)-κB and AP-1 transcription factor activity.[16-25] These findings also helped explain many of the therapeutic effects in gout of colchicine, nonsteroidal antiinflammatory drugs (NSAIDs), and corticosteroids.

The last decade has seen remarkable discovery and evolution in the definition of the roles of extracellular and intracellular innate immunity in gouty inflammation.[26-29] In particular, there has been implication of Toll-like receptors (TLRs) 2 and 4 and their shared adaptor protein CD14[27-29] and of the direct involvement of the NLRP3 (formerly known as NALP3) inflammasome, and caspase-1–mediated and various other modes of pro-IL-1β cleavage leading to release of mature, active IL-1β.[30-35] In addition, elegant studies have further defined the cellular dynamics of gouty inflammation, highlighting early roles of mast cell and monocyte ingress, maturation, and macrophage activation, and the orchestration of the natural upward and downward course of the process by alternatively differentiated monocyte-derived macrophages and their interactions with not only MSU crystals but also apoptotic neutrophils.[36-38]

Tophus Biology

Tophi are not only macroaggregates of MSU crystals but also, in most tissues, are formed as granuloma with cellular content. The "corona" and "fibrovascular" zones, surrounding packed crystals, includes phagocytes, mast cells, and, surprisingly, B- and T-lymphocytes, as well as plasma cell[8] (Fig. 5-1). Moreover, an adaptive immunity component in urate crystal deposition, mediated by IgG and IgM, has been theorized, originally via studies in rabbits "immunized" repeatedly by

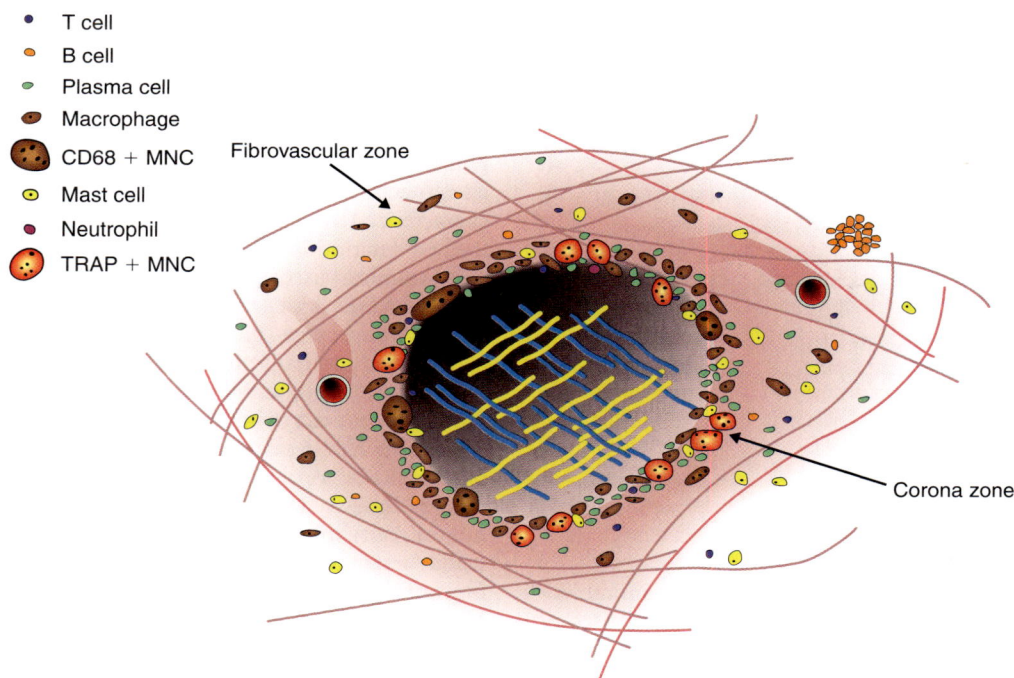

Figure 5-1 Cellular model of the gouty tophus. Cells depicted in corona and fibrovascular zones based on type and number of cells identified by immunohistochemistry. *MNC,* Mononuclear cells; *TRAP,* tartrate-resistant acid phosphatase. *(From Dalbeth N, Pool B, Gamble GD, et al. Cellular characterization of the gouty tophus: a quantitative analysis. Arthritis Rheum 2010;62(5):1549-56. Used with permission.)*

injection of synthetic MSU crystals,[39] and this is discussed in detail later. Mononuclear phagocytes do not always surround larger urate deposits,[40] and olecranon bursa tophi contain small acini of macrophages surrounding necrotic tissues. Some have hypothesized[40] that cells play an active role in urate deposition by the transport (and perhaps centripetal sequestration) of organic anions.[41] One strongly suspects a specific role of expression of urate transporters (see Chapter 27), likely modulated by inflammation, in concentrating urate at the core of macroaggregates of urate crystals. It is noted, as an example, that chondrocytes express the major urate transporter GLUT9/SLC2A9.[42]

Gout can develop, although quite uncommonly, in individuals without preexisting hyperuricemia,[43] but this phenomenon appears too rare to offer significant opportunities to better understand the mechanisms of tophus development. Perhaps the markedly hyperuricemic uricase knockout mice may present further opportunities to understand MSU crystal deposition in vivo, but these mice, unless given serum urate–lowering treatment such as with xanthine oxidase inhibition, succumb to massive uric acid urolithiasis and renal failure apparently before they develop any detectable gross tophi.[44]

Nucleation and Growth of Urate Crystals in Tissues

At physiologic pH in supersaturated tissue fluids, uric acid crystallizes as its MSU salt. De novo precipitation of MSU may be indicated in some instances by development of urate spherulites,[45] not simply the formation of needle-shaped MSU crystals. It is unclear why a minority with sustained hyperuricemia develop clinical tophi and gout. However, results of recent high-resolution ultrasound studies suggest that MSU crystal deposition at the articular cartilage in patients with asymptomatic, sustained hyperuricemia may be much more common than previously suspected (see Chapter 27).[46] Specifically, on arthroscopic and high-resolution ultrasound examinations, the earliest MSU crystal deposits appear to be not only in the synovium as "microtophi" seen as white furuncles with an erythematous base but also in articular cartilage, as detected at the cartilage surface by the "double contour" sign of high-resolution ultrasound (see Chapter 27).

Effects of Temperature, pH, and Specific Solutes

Listed in Table 5-1 are major factors believed to regulate MSU crystal deposition. MSU is clearly less soluble at the lower temperatures of peripheral, poorly vascularized soft tissues and distal joints, such as the first metatarsophalangeal (MTP) joint. The predilection for MSU crystal deposition in the first MTP joint may not reflect simply low temperature but also the repetitive biomechanical injury to this joint, since the rate of diffusion of urate molecules from the synovial space to plasma is only half that of water.[47] This situation promotes focal urate concentration after trauma. A similar mechanism could also mediate rapid tophus formation at the site of burns ("blister tophi").[48]

Solubility of sodium urate, in contrast to that of uric acid, increases as pH decreases from 7.4 to 5.8. However, measurements of both pH and buffering capacity in gouty joints have

failed to demonstrate significant acidosis. Acidification may enhance urate nucleation in vitro via the formation of protonated solid phases. However, acute pH changes are unlikely to significantly influence intraarticular MSU crystal formation.

A relative lack of tophi in gout secondary to the hyperuricemia of advanced renal disease is a long-recognized clinical observation. In this context, critical urate supersaturation levels in vitro can be altered by several other solutes, with sodium and calcium as examples. Lead excess also can promote nucleation of MSU crystals in normal saline in which there is already a high concentration (10 mg/dl) of urate,[49] but the physiologic significance of this effect, relative to promotion of hyperuricemia and nephropathy by lead, is not clear.

Effects of Extracellular Matrix Components on MSU Crystal Deposition

Chapter 2 describes some of the relationships between urate crystals and extracellular matrix. However, specific effects of extracellular matrix constituents and turnover on tophus development are not well understood. We do know that urate is more soluble in the presence of aggregated than nonaggregated proteoglycans, and the levels of insoluble collagen and chondroitin sulfate also appear to influence urate crystal formation in vitro.[50,51] Moreover, Katz and Schubert[52] observed 3-fold elevations of serum uronic acid in patients with articular gout but not in patients with hyperuricemia or with other inflammatory diseases; these changes were normalized by conventional doses of colchicine, a drug with some effects on extracellular matrix metabolism. Importantly, tophi and acute gout can develop in small hand joints at sites of nodal osteoarthritis.[53] The capacity of chondrotin sulfate to promote MSU crystal nucleation could be of particular interest with respect to the known linkage of gout to antecedent osteoarthritis.

Effects of Plasma Proteins and of Lipids on MSU Crystal Deposition

A partial deficiency of a uric acid–binding α-globulin was described in familial gout[54], but the role plasma proteins play in MSU crystal nucleation and growth in vivo remains highly controversial. In fact, soluble uric acid binds weakly and

Table 5-1 Factors that have been Proposed to Regulate Monosodium Urate (MSU) Crystal Deposition in Tissues

- Decreased temperature (such as in cool, distal joints)
- pH
- Glycosaminoglycans (e.g., chondroitin sulfate) and connective tissue composition, integrity, and turnover
- Trauma or tissue injury promoting local urate supersaturation (e.g., "blister tophi")
- Osteoarthritis (e.g., tophi in Bouchard and Heberden nodes)
- Nonspecific effects of binding of certain plasma proteins (e.g., IgG, albumin)
- Effects of IgM and IgM specifically induced by immunogenicity of MSU crystals
- Concentrations of certain solutes (e.g., lead, calcium, sodium)
- Urate transport and sequestration within macrophage acini
- Innate immune inflammation (?)
- Adaptive immunity (?) (including effects of plasma cells and B and T cells in tophi)

reversibly to plasma proteins, and plasma proteins exert only minimal effects on uric acid distribution in equilibrium dialysis.[55] Although several plasma proteins other than immunoglobulins have been observed to promote MSU crystallization from supersaturated uric acid solutions in vitro,[51,56] such effects have largely failed to be reproducible and appear dependent on the heat stability of individual proteins and on the pH of the experimental system. As a prime example, albumin, which appears to interact selectively with one of the hydrophilic faces of urate crystals, promotes MSU crystal nucleation at pH above 7.5, yet effects of albumin are minimal at a pH of 7.0, putatively due to a need for available albumin hydroxylate groups.[56]

IgG, which binds anionic MSU crystals via the cationic F(ab′)2 antibody binding domain, has been suggested to promote MSU crystal nucleation in patients with gout.[51,57] For example, in several studies, IgG from gouty synovial fluids, but not other diseases, increased the rate of MSU crystal nucleation from urate-supersaturated fluid in vitro.[51,57] It is not clear that such effects are due to increased MSU crystal nucleation or an artefactual increase in the rate of MSU crystal growth, due to the likelihood of exceedingly small "seed" microcrystals of MSU in gouty synovial fluids.

In a seminal study, injection of rabbits with MSU crystals (once a week for 8 weeks) was linked with subsequent emergence of serum IgG that increased the rate of nucleation of MSU crystals in vitro,[57] an effect that gradually resolved without "booster" doses of MSU crystals injected into the rabbits. In this study, control weekly injections with crystallized allopurinol or, surprisingly, with MSU crystals in adjuvant failed to induce the same effect on crystallization of MSU.[57] It is a provocative concept that MSU crystal nucleation is triggered by IgG adsorbed to neoantigens intrinsic to the surface of MSU crystals (or absorbed to the crystal surface, with MSU crystals serving as a hapten). This model is short of being established but is supported by another study demonstrating that mouse serum contains IgM antibodies that bind to MSU crystals and promote nucleation of MSU crystals in uric acid solutions.[58] These antibodies were much greater in serum of mice "immunized" with MSU crystals and the antibodies did not bind xanthine crystals.[58]

Lipid debris could be an innocent bystander, a byproduct, or an active mediator of MSU crystal deposition. Lipid debris, in varying amounts, has been observed in the extracellular matrix between crystals of tophi, and lipids also have been associated with cartilage deposits of CPPD crystals, although they could represent phospholipids from cartilage matrix vesicles in that circumstance. The effects of lipids and lipoproteins (free fatty acids, LDL, and VLDL) on experimental MSU crystal–associated inflammation (discussed later) are more clear than effects of the same moieties on MSU crystal deposition.

Fundamental Components of Gouty Inflammation

Tophus Remodeling and Loosening of MSU Crystals From Tophi and Cartilage Crystal Macroaggregates as Triggers for Gouty Inflammation

As reviewed in detail in Chapter 2, in gout, MSU crystals are deposited into tophaceous, granuloma-like synovial microenvironments, and in macroaggregates at or near the articular

cartilage surface, that can remain quiescent prior to and following attacks of acute gout. It appears that tophi dynamically recruit monocytes that differentiate to macrophages, which is consistent with hypothesized active remodeling of tophi.[9] The capacity of different subsets of macrophages to exert proinflammatory or antiinflammatory effects transduced by uptake of MSU crystals[59-61] likely mediates the inflammatory potential of tophi. The adaptive immune cells in tophi[8] also may favor tophi being undervascularized and quiescent in an inflammatory sense, with the result that nascent tophi can grow with sustained hyperuricemia. In this context, adaptive T-cell immunity suppresses the activation of the NLRP3 inflammasome central to acute gouty inflammation.[62]

Chronic, silent tophi, and tophi remodeled in response to urate-lowering therapy are directly associated with bone and, to a lesser degree, cartilage erosion, indicative of chronic inflammation.[63] However, some microscopic tophi in the synovium were previously described as a macrophage-rich and fibroblast-rich "holding tank" for MSU crystals lined by a ring of fibrinogen and other proteins.[2] The predominant effect of whole serum protein binding to MSU crystals is physical suppression of crystal–cell interaction and consequent crystal inflammatory potential, mediated in large part by avid binding to the negatively charged MSU crystal surface of highly cationic apo B in large molecules of LDL.[6,7] Among likely factors that ignite acute gouty arthritis are not only crystal shedding but also dissociation of such antiinflammatory crystal surface proteins. Decrease in the large size of MSU crystals via remodeling or mechanical disruption of tophi (or cartilage surface crystal macroaggregates) is probably involved. Triggering of gouty arthritis by these changes reflects events such as rapid rise or decrease in ambient urate concentrations levels (e.g., due to changes in urate-lowering therapy, hydration, diet, or alcohol consumption), mechanical trauma to the joint, or priming effects of systemic cytokine release driven by intercurrent illness or surgery.

Acute Gout Inflammatory Process as a Paradigm of the "Early Induced" Innate Immune Response

Acute gout is classically a recurrent, paroxysmal disease and is mediated by differentiated "professional" phagocytes. In this context, the completed spectrum of acute gouty arthritis is characterized by the influx into both the synovium and synovial fluid of neutrophils, which are normally absent from the joint. These neutrophils aggregate and degranulate in the synovium and its microvasculature,[2] as well as joint fluid, and they take up MSU crystals as one of the central diagnostic features of gout.

Similar to many types of innate immune encounters with microbial pathogens, there is extracellular innate immune alternative complement pathway activation; expression of inflammatory cytokines such as IL-1β, TNFα, and chemokines; and uptake of the offending pathogen by resident and recruited "professional phagocytes" in a rapid mobilization to eliminate the noxious agent. This classic innate immune "early induced" response is quite distinct from adaptive immune responses, since there is no clear induction of "immunologic memory" or enduring protective immunity. However, there is a possible exception of some of those gout patients who develop chronic, rheumatoid arthritis–like proliferative synovitis linked with gross, tophaceous disease. Systematic study of the immunopathology of synovium in such cases would be informative.

Innate Immune Engagement of the Naked MSU Crystal Surface and Effects of TLRs and the NLRP3 Inflammasome in Gouty Inflammation

Naked MSU crystals have a negatively charged and highly reactive surface that nonspecifically binds many plasma proteins[64] and also engages cell surface proteins, including the Fc receptor CD16 and platelet[65] and leukocyte integrins (e.g., leukocyte CD11b/CD18).[24] Both the negativity of crystal surface charge and surface irregularity appear to be important determinants of the inflammatory potential of MSU crystals. Mandel and colleagues[66] describe that the surfaces of more inflammatory membranolytic crystals (e.g., MSU and CPPD) are irregular and possess a high density of charged groups. This is in contrast to the smooth surfaces of noninflammatory crystals such as diamond dust. Significantly, the potent binding of MSU crystals to plasma membrane cholesterol, and membrane lipid rearrangement, does not require membrane protein binding to induce Syk kinase activation in leukocytes.[67]

We implicated innate immune inflammatory responses to the naked MSU crystal surface in pathogenesis of acute gout.[27-29] In this work, we determined that TLR2 and TLR4 in macrophage lineage cells, and TLR2 in chondrocytes (like macrophages, an NLRP3 inflammasome–expressing cell), are critical for capacity of inert MSU crystals to turn on inflammatory pathways. TLR2 and TLR4 expression also promotes macrophage capacity for phagocytosis of pyrogen-free naked MSU crystals, and consequent inflammatory cytokine expression in vitro. Deficient expression of either TLR2 or TLR4 partially inhibited MSU crystal-induced inflammation and expression of IL-1β and the chemokine CXCL1 (and also antiinflammatory crystal-induced transforming growth factor [TGF]β expression) in the MSU crystal–induced mouse subcutaneous air pouch model of gouty synovitis.[28]

Subsequently, we discovered that expression of the shared TLR2 and TLR4 adaptor protein CD14, a nonsignaling GPI-anchored cell surface protein, was necessary to convert macrophage ingestion of MSU crystals from a noninflammatory event to an inflammatory event in vitro.[29] Furthermore, coating of MSU crystals with CD14 partially reconstituted proinflammatory potential of naked MSU crystals for CD14 knockout macrophages, and in so doing induced NLRP3 inflammasome activation and activation of IL-1β.[29] CD14 knockout mice had a significantly decreased inflammatory response to MSU crystals in the air pouch synovitis model in vivo.[29] We, and subsequently others, demonstrated that acute MSU crystal–induced inflammation in vivo was dependent on myeloid differentiation factor-88 (MyD88) expression and signaling.[28,68] Moreover, MyD88 expression played a major role in the capacity of macrophages to phagocytose MSU crystals in vitro.[28] MyD88 transduces TLR2 responses, some TLR4 responses, and signaling by IL-1 and certain other cytokines that is essential for these mediators to activate cells.

It was elegantly demonstrated that IL-1 receptor signaling at the level of resident cells, but not bone marrow–derived cells, was essential for MSU crystal–induced peritonitis.[68]

Subsequent corroborative studies by others demonstrated that TLR2 and TLR4 together are required for urate crystals to induce lung inflammation[32] and that hydroxyapatite particles require TLR4 to activate TNFα expression.[69] MSU crystals have been observed to induce triggering receptor expressed on myeloid cells-1 (TREM-1) in phagocytes in vitro and in vivo.[70,71] TREM-1 is a cell surface–expressed Ig superfamily protein, which signals using the adapter protein DAP12. TREM-1 induction depends on TLR2, TLR4, and MyD88. TREM-1 amplifies a variety of inflammatory responses, including those to MSU crystals.[70]

Mechanistically (Fig. 5-2), on one hand, functional complexes of TLR2 or TLR4, CD14, and leukocyte β2 integrins could mediate TLR dimerization, as reviewed previously.[72] This could optimize how macrophages engage and respond to MSU crystals (see Fig. 5-2). Alternatively, TLR2 and TLR4 signaling prime a variety of NLRP3 inflammasome-driven inflammatory responses, some with additional involvement of P2X7 purinergic receptor signaling.[73-75] In this context, TLR2 and TLR4 expression promote caspase-1 and IL-1β mRNA expression[73,74] and prime the ability of monocyte-macrophage lineage cells to optimally carry out phagocytosis of a variety of particulates,[72] including MSU crystals,[28] as well as priming effector functions of the NLRP3 inflammasome in response to MSU crystals (see Fig. 5-2). CD14[29] also modulates proinflammatory differentiation of macrophages.[76]

Significantly, one set of studies, using a model of injection into mouse joints of relatively low concentrations of MSU crystals for relatively short time periods, suggests that TLR2 (but not TLR4) plays a major role in gouty inflammation via priming effects of TLR2 ligand free fatty acids[74] (see Fig. 5-2). Such findings conceivably contribute diet and alcohol triggers of gout attacks.

NLRP3 Inflammasome and IL-1β Release in MSU Crystal–Induced Inflammation

The NLRP3 inflammasome, central to several autoinflammatory syndromes, is a multiprotein cytosolic complex assembled and activated in response to a large variety of soluble and particulate ligands.[77-79] These include elevated concentrations of extracellular ATP (partly mediated by signaling via P2X7[75]), crystals of MSU and CPPD, as first described in the pioneering work of Jurg Tschopp and coworkers,[30-35] cholesterol crystals that promote atherogenesis,[80] alum used as an adjuvant in vaccines,[81] and, mediated in some conditions by TLR2, "wear particles" from prosthetic materials used in joint replacement.[82,83] In addition, the NLRP3 inflammasome can be activated by sensing of reactive oxygen species that are released during cell stress.[77-79] Caspase-1 is recruited and activated (via proteolytic cleavage) by the NLRP3 inflammasome, and activated caspase-1 proteolytically cleaves and activates the inactive proform of IL-1β, facilitating secretion of the active cytokine.[77-79] It should be noted that this mechanism is not universal in crystal-induced inflammation, since octacalcium crystals (a form of basic calcium phosphates) activate IL-1–dependent but NLRP3-independent mechanisms in stimulating peritoneal inflammation, likely involving rapid phagocyte death.[84]

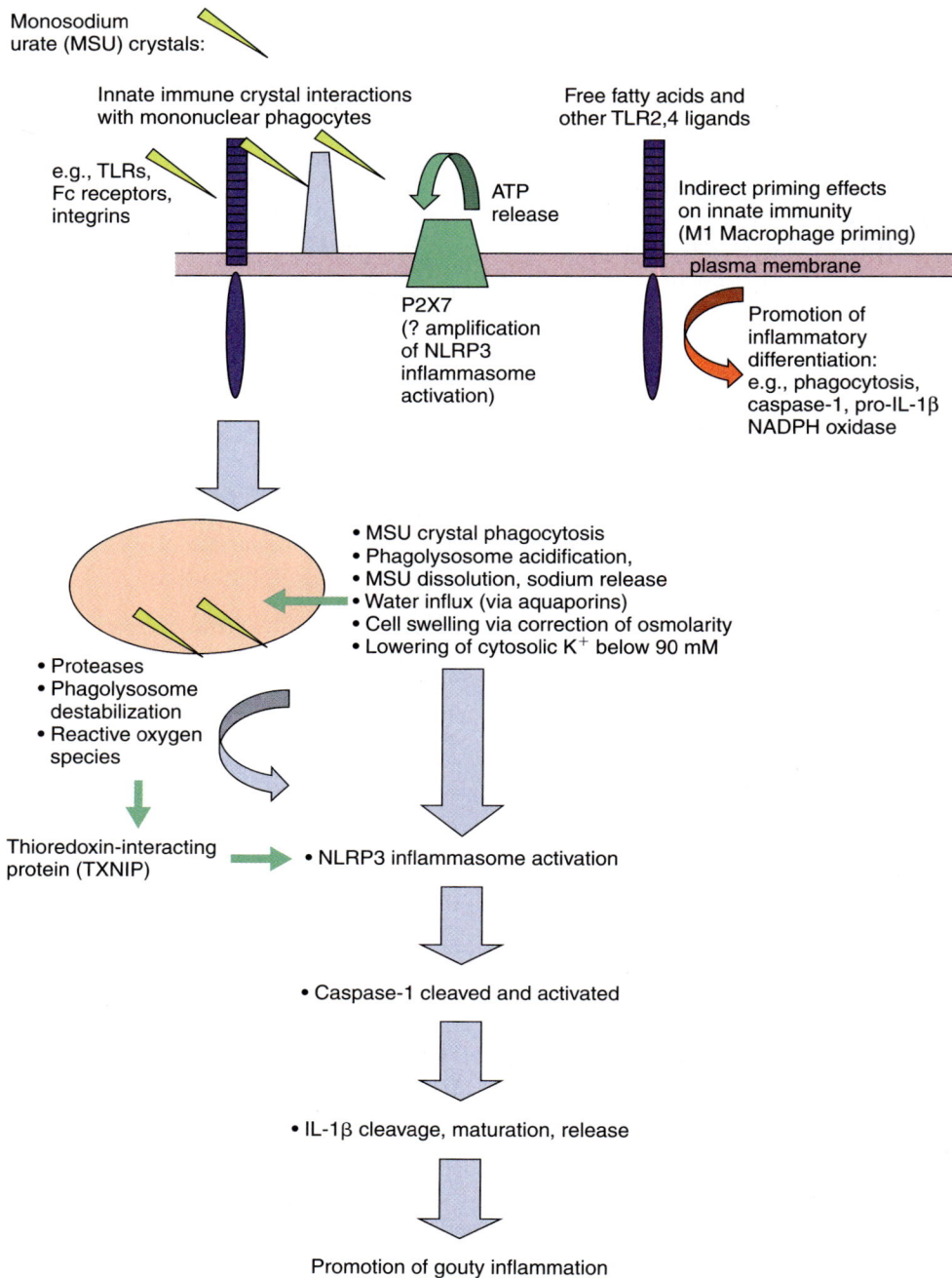

Figure 5-2 Innate immune activation of inflammation by monosodium urate (MSU) crystals: NLRP3 (cryopyrin) inflammasome and interleukin (IL)-1β processing and secretion in crystal-induced inflammation. Depicted here are different innate immune aspects of MSU crystal interaction with mononuclear phagocytes, which express NLRP3 and the other components of the NLRP3 inflammasome. In this model, MSU crystals perturb membranes and engage and cluster mobile membrane proteins at the macrophage surface, mediated by Fc receptors, integrins, as well as the Toll-like receptors TLR2 and TLR4 and associated MyD88 signaling. Priming of MSU crystal–induced macrophage activation by TLR2 ligand free fatty acids also is illustrated. Crystal uptake, and associated reactive oxygen species generation, protease release from phagolysosomes, sodium release from MSU crystal dissolution in phagolysosomes (and lowering of cytosolic calcium via consequent water influx, as well as P2X7-mediated K+ efflux), and recruitment of TXNIP, synergistically promote activation of the NLRP3 inflammasome, as illustrated. Consequent endoproteolytic activation of caspase-1 stimulates pro-IL-1β maturation, and results in secretion of mature IL-1β. This is a major mechanism that stimulates model gouty inflammation, and it also appears to be implicated in acute and chronic human gouty arthritis, as reviewed in the text. *MyD88,* Myeloid differentiation primary response gene 88; *NLRP,* Nacht domain, leucine-rich repeat-, and PYD-containing protein; *TLR,* Toll-like receptor.

Multiple studies of mice with knockout of IL-1β, caspase-1, and the NLRP3 inflammasome constituent ASC, as well as NLRP3 itself, and the NLRP3 mutant mice with deletion of the entire leucine-rich repeat region have revealed a central role of the NLRP3 inflammasome in experimental gouty inflammation and MSU crystal–induced lung inflammation.[30-34] MSU crystal–induced ATP release also has been suggested to amplify experimental gouty inflammation via P2X7 signaling.[75] Activated P2X7, a ligand-gated ion channel, induces cytosolic K^+ release, and lowering of cytosolic K^+ clearly promotes NLRP3 inflammasome activation.[85] One study has suggested that signaling of the purinergic receptor P2Y2 by ATP, released in response to MSU crystals in leukocytes, could also promote gouty inflammation.[86]

Recently, NLRP3 has been shown to interact with thioredoxin (TRX)-interacting protein (TXNIP), and MSU crystals induced the dissociation of TXNIP from thioredoxin in a reactive oxygen species–sensitive manner and allowed binding to NLRP3[87] (see Fig. 5-2). In addition, TXNIP deficiency impaired NLRP3 inflammasome activation and IL-1β release in macrophages in response to MSU crystals.[87] Conversely, the tripartite-motif protein 30 (TRIM30) is a constitutive suppressor of NLRP3 inflammasome activation, including by MSU crystals, and functions to limit MSU crystal–induced peritonitis in vivo.[88]

Effects of Sodium Release From Dissolved MSU Crystals in the Phagolysosome in Gouty Inflammation

A new model of MSU crystal–induced NLRP3 inflammasome activation[35] provides a molecular follow-up to the MSU crystal–induced "suicide sac" observations of Weissmann and coworkers of the 1970s.[89] Specifically, endosomes containing ingested MSU crystals in macrophages, following fusion with acidified lysosomes, induce sodium release via MSU crystal dissolution in the phagolysosome that raises intracellular osmolarity.[35] Compensatory water influx through aquaporins then causes cell swelling that dilutes intracellular K^+ below the threshold of 90 mmol/L known to activate the NALP3 inflammasome, without requirement for net loss of cytoplasmic K^+ ions. Important support for this model is that ingested monopotassium urate crystals do not induce NLRP3 inflammasome activation,[90] although a distinct crystal structure of potassium urate might contribute, in theory. Moreover, suppression of lysosomal acidification (using ammonium chloride and chloroquine) and of aquaporins (using mercury chloride and phloretin) all significantly decreased the production of IL-1β by human monocytes in response to MSU crystals. A limiting issue of this work to clinical gout may be that the concentrations of MSU crystals in vivo sufficient to raise intracellular osmolarity via Na^+ release are often going to be less than the 1 mg/ml used in this study.[35] Nevertheless, in vivo, chloroquine significantly reduced the IL-1β response to MSU crystals,[35] suggesting translational significance for clinical trials needed to study potential use of hydroxychloroquine, for example, for antiinflammatory management of refractory gout.

Controversial Aspects of Innate Immune Pathogenesis of MSU Crystal–Induced Inflammation

Notably, there has been one exception to results regarding the essential nature of the NLRP3 inflammasome in MSU crystal–induced inflammation.[74] Furthermore, study of MSU crystal–induced peritonitis suggested greater inflammation in dual TLR2/4 knockout mice,[68] which we speculate is possibly related to decreased MSU crystal–induced release of TGFβ,[28] a known inhibitor of gouty inflammation.[91] The reasons for discrepancies in results related to TLR2, TLR4, and NLRP3 in MSU crystal–induced inflammation are likely complex.

Commercial uric acid* used to make synthetic MSU crystals is typically loaded with the endogenous pyrogen lipopolysaccharide (LPS), and generation of synthetic crystals is best done when the uric acid is first baked adequately (e.g., 2 hours at 200°C) to remove LPS. Many studies have not done so and had inadequate control validation of the LPS-free nature of the crystals, such as use of a uricase control to dissolve the crystals. This issue is notable in part because LPS uses TLR4 signaling to turn on cells and also because MSU crystals enhance responses to LPS.[92]

Differences in MSU crystal size and surface properties among various studies could be substantial, since MSU crystals larger than the diameter of most phagocytes (i.e., greater than 15 µm) are less inflammatory, and crystals have been made in nonstandardized ways for published work in the area. For example, synthesis of MSU crystals using borate as opposed to the conventional use of sodium hydroxide imposes a variable in the characteristics of MSU crystals between studies. Last, there are substantial differences in MSU crystal inflammation model systems (e.g., injection of crystals into joints, synovium-like subcutaneous air pouches peritoneum, lung tissue). It is possible that different types of resident cells in these models (e.g., tissue macrophages or serosal surface fibroblasts) have differential requirements for activation and/or local factors (e.g., proteins) bound to crystals may modify the cellular responses.

Concept of Uric Acid as an Endogenous "Danger Signal"

The provocative notion has emerged, primarily from the work of Rock and colleagues,[93,94] that uric acid released from degraded nucleotides of dying cells is a danger signal that serves a proinflammatory function in injury of the liver, lung, and other tissues and also mediates adaptive immunity, as well as immune responses to tumor cells. It has also been proposed that such a danger signal mechanism of uric acid is involved in progression of osteoarthritis.[95] The collective evidence, which is principally from studies in mice, indicates that uric acid reaches supersaturated concentrations in and around necrotic cells, and includes elegant experiments on the potentiation of the inflammatory response to cell necrosis in mice transgenic for intracellular and extracellular uricase.[94] However, there has not yet been a morphologic demonstration that MSU crystallizes (i.e., forms tiny "ultramicrocrystals") in lymphatics or in injured liver, lung, or other warm (37°C), well-vascularized central organs and tissues. On the other hand, absence of evidence is not evidence of absence.

---

*The use of the term "uric acid crystals" in many of the recent studies of MSU crystals and innate immunity is inappropriate.

It is also possible (although not yet clearly established) that soluble urate exerts inflammation-modulating effects.[96] The most likely mechanism would be via myeloperoxidase-catalyzed oxidation of urate to reactive oxygen radicals, dependent on the presence of peroxide and superoxide.[97] Studies on the proinflammatory effects of soluble urate that use uricase and xanthine oxidase as controls to lower serum urate also have limitations, since uricase generates hydrogen peroxide and allopurinol effects are nonspecific to purine metabolism. For example, xanthine oxidase (xanthine oxidoreductase) generates superoxide, and it is proinflammatory in macrophages, in part through modulation of peroxisome proliferator-activated receptor γ (PPAR γ) and chemokine expression.[98] Since xanthine oxidase tissue distribution appears more limited in humans than in mice, the biologic significance of some of the aforementioned findings in humans is not yet clear.

Other Signal Transduction Mechanisms by Which MSU Crystals Activate Cells to Promote Inflammation

MSU crystals induce functional responses such as degranulation, reactive oxygen species generation, and inflammatory gene expression in a huge variety of cells. MSU crystals can physically perturb cell membranes and increase membrane permeability through membranolytic effects first characterized in erythrocytes. However, plasma membrane activation by MSU crystals is far more complex and involves engagement and clustering of membrane proteins (e.g., CD11b/Cd18, Fc receptor CD16) and effects such as activation of membrane G proteins (including Giα2) in neutrophils.[99] The rapid induction by MSU crystals of cytosolic calcium mobilization is modulated by phosphatidylinositol-4,5-bisphosphate (PIP2) hydrolysis and inositol-1,4,5-trisphosphate (IP3) generation.[100] These effects of MSU crystals develop slowly relative to the effects of chemotactic factors in neutrophils and do not require pertussis toxin–sensitive G protein activation.[99,100] Plasma membrane phospholipid remodeling also includes activation of phospholipases A2 and D.[23,101]

The activation by MSU crystals of the focal adhesion mediating kinase Pyk2 supports the importance of point adhesion of the crystal to the plasma membrane.[17] MSU crystals also induce activation of Src family tyrosine kinases, which is necessary for activation of several other kinases, including phospholipase C, conventional protein kinase C (PKC), Syk, Tec, and PI3K, which play a major role in numerous inflammatory responses.[16] IL-8 induction is an example of a well-studied response. MSU crystals activate Src family tyrosine kinases that lead to activation of downstream mitogen-activated protein kinases (MAPKs) ERK1/ERK2, JNK, and p38 in monocytic lineage cells to induce IL-8.[18] In particular, activation of the ERK1/2 pathway mediates activation of transcription factors NF-κB and AP-1, an essential set of signals for induction of IL-8 mRNA in response to MSU crystals.[19]

Effects of MSU Crystal–Bound Proteins on Cell Activation

It is not clear if cell adhesion to MSU crystals is crystal face specific.[102] In our experience, opsonization of MSU crystals is not required for cell activation (e.g., Liu-Bryan et al.[28] and

Onello et al.[100]). However, it has been reported that heat-labile serum factors and divalent cations are involved in ingestion of MSU crystals by phagocytes.[103] That said, synthetic MSU crystals (and MSU crystals from tophi) are actually rendered markedly less stimulatory for cells via preincubation with whole serum.[100] The major MSU crystal–bound antiinflammatory factors in serum are apo B–containing lipoproteins.[6] LDL, the predominant apo B–containing lipoprotein, suppresses multiple responses to MSU by binding to the crystal surface, and it thereby physically limits interaction with cells and uptake of the crystals.[6,104] Apo B, a huge cationic protein that avidly binds the negatively charged surface of MSU crystals, mediates this activity of LDL.[6,7] MSU crystals have been shown to bind LDL in vivo.[105,106] LDL only enters joint fluids in a robust way when permeability is increased by inflammation, and this could help limit gouty attacks.

Apolipoprotein (apo) E, a component of VLDL and high-density lipoprotein (HDL), also binds MSU crystals in vivo, and MSU crystal–bound apo E suppresses crystal-induced neutrophil activation in vitro.[107] Unlike apo B, apo E is synthesized in joints by monocyte/macrophage lineage cells[107] and could be a local factor in MSU crystal quiescence in joints.

The surface coat of MSU crystals undergoes dynamic alteration during acute gout and experimental gouty inflammation.[105,106] MSU crystal–bound IgG increases the capacity of the crystals to stimulate a variety of cells and generally becomes less abundant on the crystal surface with time.[105] In contrast, MSU crystal–bound apo B increases as gouty inflammation starts to resolve.[105] It should be noted that oxidation of LDL lipids, known to occur in inflammatory synovial fluids, transforms LDL into a molecule that induces IL-8 and many other inflammatory mediators.[108]

Pathogenic Cascades in the Initiation and Amplification of Acute Gouty Inflammation

Figure 5-3 schematizes major events in gouty inflammation, including the pathologic hallmark of neutrophil influx into both synovium and joint fluid[2] and the robust cycle of neutrophil recruitment and activation whose interruption appears intrinsic to the effectiveness of antiinflammatory treatments such as NSAIDs, corticosteroids, and colchicine in acute gout. Direct and indirect activation of resident cells such as synovial lining cells,[2] mast cells, and tissue macrophages by free MSU crystals promotes monocyte and then neutrophil ingress,[36] with the recruited monocytes differentiating over a few days into proinflammatory macrophages (M1 type) in experimental gout.[37,38] Neutrophil influx is promoted by the capacity of IL-1β and TNFα to turn on activation of the endothelium and E-selectin expression,[109,110] a primary target of low (nanomolar) concentrations of colchicines.[111] The additional chemotactic activities of IL-8/CXCL8 and closely related chemokine ligands of the CXCR2 receptor such as CXCL1 are essential for gouty inflammation.[13,14] Other chemokines involved in acute gouty inflammation include CXCL16, a ligand of CXCR6 that chemoattracts neutrophils, as shown in an elegant model using human synovium grafted into SCID mice.[112] Furthermore, a variety of monocyte chemotactic chemokines are induced by MSU crystals, and these include MCP-1.[22]

Local generation and systemic release of IL-1β, TNFα, and IL-6 contribute to fever and the hepatic acute phase response in acute gout and can promote bone erosion in chronic gout. In this pathogenic scheme, C5 cleavage on the MSU crystal surface and consequent C5b-9 membrane attack complex assembly play a major role in endothelial activation, IL-8 expression, and neutrophil influx, as supported in studies of C6-deficient rabbits.[26] Furthermore, proteases released from mast cells (e.g., chymase) and neutrophils (e.g., proteinase 3, elastase) provide important alternative modes to caspase-1 for the maturation and activation of IL-1β and amplification and perpetuation of gouty inflammation[113-116] (see Fig. 5-3).

Neutrophils entering the joint are exposed to a soup of soluble inflammatory mediators, as well as MSU crystals, and these encounters amplify the acute gout attack. Only a small fraction of neutrophils in the joint space are seen to ingest MSU crystals, but crystal uptake induces mediators such as superoxide, IL-1β, leukotriene B4, some chemokines, and S100A8 and S100A9. The calgranulins S100A8 and S100A9[4,5] are small calcium-binding polypeptides that heterodimerize and are highly abundant in the cytosol of the resting neutrophil. S100A8/S100A9 are ligands of TLR4 and certain other receptors, and exert a variety of proinflammatory effects.

The model depicted in Figure 5-3 does not feature an assessment of the net role of TNFα in acute gouty inflammation, and this remains unclear, but it is likely substantially less than the role of IL-1β. Also, the model does not take into consideration potential effects of NK cells,[117] T- and B-lymphocytes, and platelets[66] on the course of acute gouty inflammation. Acute gout can be ignited in joints manifesting subclinical inflammation,[118] and it should be noted that the model illustrated in Figure 5-3 is derived from experiments in small animals in which there was injection of substantial amounts of MSU crystals into noninflamed loci of animals naïve to MSU crystals.

Other mediators induced by MSU crystals not depicted in Figure 5-3 may not be essential to human gouty inflammation yet are likely to play roles in pain and swelling. These include kallikrein, bradykinin, plasmin, and other products of activation of Hageman factor and the contact coagulation system.

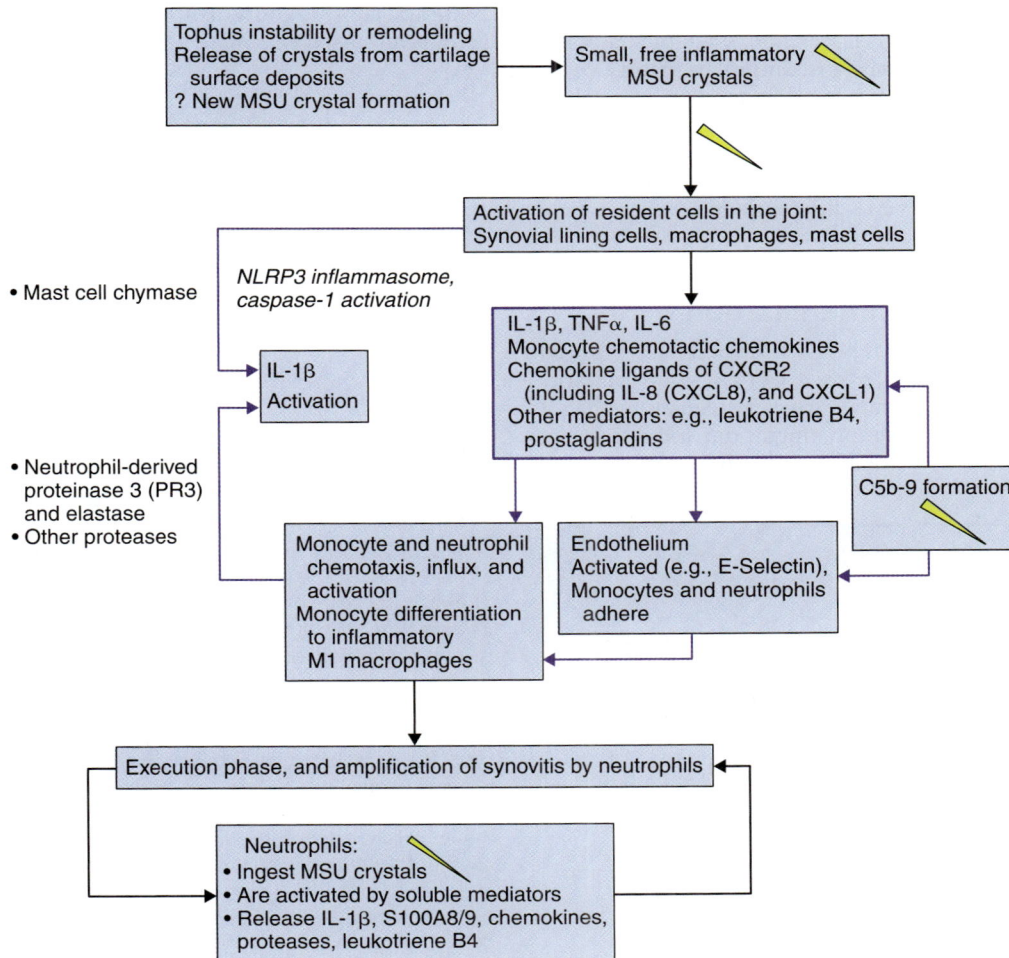

Figure 5-3 Inflammatory systems that drive initiation and amplification of acute gouty arthritis. The figure schematizes mechanisms for acute gouty arthritis that are reviewed in the text. These include monosodium urate (MSU)–induced complement activation by C5 cleavage on the crystal surface, activation of monocytes/macrophages and of synovial lining cells in the joint, activation of vascular endothelium, and complementary mechanisms for proteolytic activation of interleukin (IL)-1β maturation, including the NLRP3 inflammasome mechanism illustrated in Figure 5-2, and release of proteases from mast cells and neutrophils. Monocyte recruitment and maturation to inflammatory macrophages help to orchestrate and perpetuate gouty inflammation, and the vicious cycle of neutrophil influx and activation illustrated in the figure is a central "execution phase" of gouty arthritis.

They also include histamine derived from mast cells[119] and the effects of prostaglandins. It is conceivable that pain signals of substance P, which exerts several proinflammatory functions, also mediate gouty inflammation.

Mechanisms Involved in Spontaneous Limitation of Acute Gouty Inflammation

Natural mechanisms clearly limit gouty inflammation, as recognized since the time of Hippocrates. Major factors in self-limitation of gout attacks are cited in Table 5-2. As discussed earlier, MSU crystal–bound proteins may influence their inflammatory potential. MSU crystal dissolution by oxidants is not the primary reason for spontaneous resolution of gout, since free MSU crystals typically remain in synovial fluid even as and after acute gout attacks resolve. Lipoxins, PPARγ induction,[120] and tachyphylaxis to some inflammatory mediators are likely involved, but a major mechanism appears to be via mature, polarized antiinflammatory macrophages (likely the M2 macrophage subtype involved in tissue repair) that ingest both apoptotic neutrophils and MSU crystals, thereby promoting antiinflammatory TGFβ and IL-1 receptor antagonist release and decreased TNFα expression.[121-124] Macrophage transglutaminase 2 (TG2)[124] and other mediators at the "apoptotic synapse" involved in antiinflammatory clearance of apoptotic cells ("efferocytosis") are centrally involved in resolution of experimental gouty inflammation (Fig. 5-4). PPAR signaling promotes M2 macrophage differentiation, whereas ethanol and high fat feeding are among the factors that promote inflammatory M1 differentiation.

Perspectives on Effects of Commonly Used Therapies on Gouty Inflammation

This chapter reviewed mechanisms of MSU crystal–induced inflammation. Drugs currently used to treat gout primarily act on these mechanisms, as cited earlier, by regulating phagocyte signal transduction, adhesion, migration, and activation, including expression of cytokines and other inflammatory mediators. A full review of the molecular sites at which the major antiinflammatory therapeutics act in gout is beyond the scope of this discussion. Colchicine mechanism of action and clinical pharmacology are reviewed in Chapter 16; neutrophil adhesion, migration, and activation are major targets of colchicine. NSAIDs and COX-2–selective inhibitors clearly act on both phagocyte-mediated inflammation and pain as primary targets in gout.

Corticosteroid therapeutic actions are driven by four distinct mechanisms of action, as recently reviewed in exquisite detail.[125] These are genomic effects via activation of the cytosolic glucocorticoid receptor (cGR); secondary nongenomic effects driven by the cGR; membrane-bound GR–mediated nongenomic actions; and nonspecific, nongenomic effects arising from interactions with cellular membranes. Major suppressive effects on cytokine expression are a hallmark of corticosteroid action for gout. In addition, corticosteroids promote M2 macrophage differentiation. Phagocyte melanocortin 3 receptor agonism mediates rapid antiinflammatory actions of ACTH in gout,[126,127] with adrenal corticosteroid induction by ACTH mediating further therapeutic actions.

IL-1 antagonism as an emerging modality for treatment of acute and chronic gouty arthritis, and as gouty attack prophylaxis, is discussed elsewhere in this book (see Chapters 11, 16,

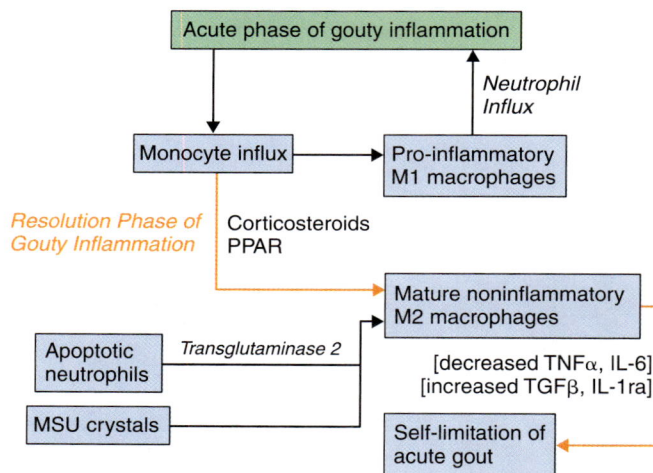

Figure 5-4 Macrophage-driven switching mechanisms between the inflammatory and resolution phases of acute gouty inflammation. The schematic summarizes mechanisms of macrophage differentiation and function switches that play a central role in the spontaneous (and therapy-assisted) self-limitation of gouty inflammation, as discussed in the text. The influx into the joint of monocytes is linked with further monocyte differentiation to inflammatory macrophages (termed M1 macrophages by some) that further turn on the acute phase of gouty arthritis. In this model, the alternative switch of macrophage differentiation to the antiinflammatory tissue repair M2 macrophage subtype alters the course of acute gouty inflammation by stimulating resolution of acute arthritis. This occurs via uptake of apoptotic neutrophils, mediated partly by transglutaminase 2 (TG2), and consequent release of transforming growth factor (TGF)β. In addition, the nature of macrophage encounters with MSU crystals in the joint space is antiinflammatory in M2 type macrophages, also being linked to induction of TGFβ release, and M2 macrophages also express interleukin (IL)-1 receptor antagonist. Factors that promote M1 macrophage differentiation include alcohol and high fatty acid intake. Factors that promote M2 macrophage differentiation include PPAR signaling (known to be induced in the course of gouty inflammation), STAT transcription factor signaling, and corticosteroids.

Table 5-2 Potential Mechanisms of Spontaneous Resolution of Acute Inflammation in Clinical Gout

- Macrophage ingestion of apoptotic neutrophils ("efferocytosis") mediated by transglutaminase 2 (TG2) and other molecules of the "apoptotic synapse," with associated antiinflammatory effects, including increased antiinflammatory transforming growth factor β (TGFβ) release
- Monosodium urate (MSU) crystal clearance by antiinflammatory M2 macrophages involved in tissue repair, with associated effects that suppress gouty inflammation, including TGFβ and interleukin (IL)-1 receptor antagonist release
- Decreased MSU crystal inflammatory potential secondary to large, bound apolipoprotein B and apolipoprotein E–containing lipoproteins (low- and very low-density lipoproteins)
- Change in the balance of, and responses to, proinflammatory and antiinflammatory mediators, such as:
  o Native IL-1 receptor antagonist
  o Lipoxins
  o Effects of peroxisome proliferator activated receptor (PPAR) subtypes α and γ
  o Shedding of soluble TNF and Fc receptors

17, and 28). There are no consistent therapeutic benefits yet described for TNFα antagonism in gout.

The development of selective biologics targeting IL-1 and other cytokines for gout will lead to improvements in care and outcomes. However, nonselective antiinflammatory therapies retain a strong rationale in gout, given the plethora of important inflammatory mediators at different phases of the acute gouty attack and in chronic gouty arthritis, let alone the relatively low cost of the well-established agents. Combination drug treatment strategies, and analgesic benefits of regimens using NSAIDs or COX-2 inhibitors, are valuable considerations.

In the future, chemokines such as IL-8, and potentially monocyte chemoattractant chemokines, represent attractive targets for selective therapeutics in gout, although attention to decreased host defense is a concern with many chemokine inhibitors. Hydroxychloroquine merits consideration for clinical investigation in resistant cases of chronic gouty inflammation.[35] Last, the therapeutic potentials of natural substances such as tart cherry extracts, gamma linolenic acid and eicosapentaenoic acid, and milk constituents have been proposed for gouty inflammation[128-130] but warrant more detailed and direct clinical study in human gout.

References

1. Phelps P, McCarty Jr DJ. Crystal-induced inflammation in canine joints. II. Importance of polymorphonuclear leukocytes. J Exp Med 1966;124(1):115–26.
2. Schumacher Jr HR. Pathology of crystal deposition diseases. Rheum Dis Clin North Am 1988;14:269–88.
3. Bhatt A, Spilberg I. Purification of crystal induced chemotactic factor from human neutrophils. Clin Biochem 1988;21(6):341–5.
4. Ryckman C, McColl SR, Vandal K, et al. Role of S100A8 and S100A9 in neutrophil recruitment in response to monosodium urate monohydrate crystals in the air-pouch model of acute gouty arthritis. Arthritis Rheum 2003;48(8):2310–20.
5. Ryckman C, Gilbert C, de Medicis R, et al. Monosodium urate monohydrate crystals induce the release of the proinflammatory protein S100A8/A9 from neutrophils. J Leukoc Biol 2004;76(2):433–40.
6. Terkeltaub R, Curtiss LK, Tenner AJ, et al. Lipoproteins containing apoprotein B are a major regulator of neutrophil responses to monosodium urate crystals. J Clin Invest 1984;73(6):1719–30.
7. Terkeltaub R, Martin J, Curtiss L, et al. Apolipoprotein B mediates the capacity of low density lipoprotein to suppress neutrophil stimulation by particulates. J Biol Chem 1986;261(33):15662–7.
8. Dalbeth N, Pool B, Gamble GD, et al. Cellular characterization of the gouty tophus: a quantitative analysis. Arthritis Rheum 2010;62(5):1549–56.
9. Schweyer S, Hemmerlein B, Radzun HJ, et al. Continuous recruitment, co-expression of tumour necrosis factor-alpha and matrix metalloproteinases, and apoptosis of macrophages in gout tophi. Virchows Arch 2000;437(5):534–9.
10. Di Giovine FS, Malawista SE, Nuki G, et al. Interleukin-1 (IL-1) as a mediator of crystal arthritis: stimulation of T cell and synovial fibroblast mitogenesis by urate crystal-induced IL-1. J Immunol 1987;138(10):3213–8.
11. Guerne PA, Terkeltaub R, Zuraw B, et al. Inflammatory microcrystals stimulate interleukin-6 production and secretion by human monocytes and synoviocytes. Arthritis Rheum 1989;32(11):1443–52.
12. di Giovine FS, Malawista SE, Thornton E, et al. Urate crystals stimulate production of tumor necrosis factor alpha from human blood monocytes and synovial cells: cytokine mRNA and protein kinetics, and cellular distribution. J Clin Invest 1991;87(4):1375–81.
13. Terkeltaub R, Zachariae C, Santoro D, et al. Monocyte-derived neutrophil chemotactic factor/IL-8 is a potential mediator of crystal-induced inflammation. Arthritis Rheum 1991;34(7):894–903.
14. Terkeltaub R, Baird S, Sears P, et al. The murine homolog of the interleukin-8 receptor CXCR2 is essential for the occurrence of neutrophilic inflammation in the air pouch model of acute urate crystal-induced gouty synovitis. Arthritis Rheum 1998;41(5):900–9.
15. Neogi T. Interleukin-1 antagonism in acute gout: is targeting a single cytokine the answer? Arthritis Rheum 2010;62(10):2845–9.
16. Popa-Nita O, Naccache PH. Crystal-induced neutrophil activation. Immunol Cell Biol 2010;88(1):32–40.
17. Liu R, Lioté F, Rose DM, et al. Proline-rich tyrosine kinase 2 and Src kinase signaling transduce monosodium urate crystal-induced nitric oxide production and matrix metalloproteinase 3 expression in chondrocytes. Arthritis Rheum 2004;50(1):247–58.
18. Liu R, Aupperle K, Terkeltaub R. Src family protein tyrosine kinase signaling mediates monosodium urate crystal-induced IL-8 expression by monocytic THP-1 cells. J Leukoc Biol 2001;70(6):961–8.
19. Liu R, O'Connell M, Johnson K, et al. Extracellular signal-regulated kinase 1/extracellular signal-regulated kinase 2 mitogen-activated protein kinase signaling and activation of activator protein 1 and nuclear factor kappaB transcription factors play central roles in interleukin-8 expression stimulated by monosodium urate monohydrate and calcium pyrophosphate crystals in monocytic cells. Arthritis Rheum 2000;43(5):1145–55.
20. Popa-Nita O, Marois L, Paré G, et al. Crystal-induced neutrophil activation: X. Proinflammatory role of the tyrosine kinase Tec. Arthritis Rheum 2008;58(6):1866–76.
21. Popa-Nita O, Rollet-Labelle E, Thibault N, et al. Crystal-induced neutrophil activation. IX. Syk-dependent activation of class Ia phosphatidylinositol 3-kinase. J Leukoc Biol 2007;82(3):763–73.
22. Jaramillo M, Godbout M, Naccache PH, et al. Signaling events involved in macrophage chemokine expression in response to monosodium urate crystals. J Biol Chem 2004;279(50):52797–805.
23. Marcil J, Harbour D, Houle MG, et al. Monosodium urate-crystal-stimulated phospholipase D in human neutrophils. Biochem J 1999;337 (Pt 2):185–92.
24. Barabé F, Gilbert C, Liao N, et al. Crystal-induced neutrophil activation VI. Involvement of FcgammaRIIIB (CD16) and CD11b in response to inflammatory microcrystals. FASEB J 1998;12(2):209–20.
25. Naccache PH, Bourgoin S, Plante E, et al. Crystal-induced neutrophil activation. II. Evidence for the activation of a phosphatidylcholine-specific phospholipase D. Arthritis Rheum 1993;36(1):117–25.
26. Tramontini N, Huber C, Liu-Bryan R, et al. Central role of complement membrane attack complex in monosodium urate crystal-induced neutrophilic rabbit knee synovitis. Arthritis Rheum 2004;50(8):2633–9.
27. Liu-Bryan R, Pritzker K, Firestein GS, et al. TLR2 signaling in chondrocytes drives calcium pyrophosphate dihydrate and monosodium urate crystal-induced nitric oxide generation. J Immunol 2005;174(8):5016–23.
28. Liu-Bryan R, Scott P, Sydlaske A, Terkeltaub R. Innate immunity conferred by Toll-like receptors 2 and 4 and myeloid differentiation factor 88 expression is pivotal to monosodium urate monohydrate crystal-induced inflammation. Arthritis Rheum 2005;52(9):2936–46.
29. Scott P, Ma H, Viriyakosol S, Terkeltaub R, Liu-Bryan R. Engagement of CD14 mediates the inflammatory potential of monosodium urate crystals. J Immunol 2006;177(9):6370–8.
30. Martinon F, Pétrilli V, Mayor A, et al. Gout-associated uric acid crystals activate the NALP3 inflammasome. Nature 2006;440(7081):237–41.
31. Pétrilli V, Papin S, Dostert C, et al. Activation of the NALP3 inflammasome is triggered by low intracellular potassium concentration. Cell Death Differ 2007;14(9):1583–9.
32. Gasse P, Riteau N, Charron S, et al. Uric acid is a danger signal activating NALP3 inflammasome in lung injury inflammation and fibrosis. Am J Respir Crit Care Med 2009;179(10):903–13.
33. Zhou R, Tardivel A, Thorens B, et al. Thioredoxin-interacting protein links oxidative stress to inflammasome activation. Nat Immunol 2010;11(2):136–40.
34. Hoffman HM, Scott P, Mueller JL, et al. Role of the leucine-rich repeat domain of cryopyrin/NALP3 in monosodium urate crystal-induced inflammation in mice. Arthritis Rheum 2010;62(7):2170–9.
35. Schorn C, Frey B, Lauber K, et al. Sodium overload and water influx activate the NALP3 inflammasome. J Biol Chem 2011;286(1):35–41.
36. Schiltz C, Lioté F, Prudhommeaux F, et al. Monosodium urate monohydrate crystal-induced inflammation in vivo: quantitative histomorphometric analysis of cellular events. Arthritis Rheum 2002;46(6):1643–50.
37. Martin WJ, Walton M, Harper J. Resident macrophages initiating and driving inflammation in a monosodium urate monohydrate crystal-induced murine peritoneal model of acute gout. Arthritis Rheum 2009;60(1):281–9.
38. Martin WJ, Shaw O, Liu X, et al. MSU crystal-recruited non-inflammatory monocytes differentiate into M1-like pro-inflammatory macrophages in a peritoneal murine model of gout. Arthritis Rheum 2011;in press.
39. Kam M, Perl-Treves D, Caspi D, et al. Antibodies against crystals. FASEB J 1992;6(8):2608–13.

40. Palmer DG, Highton J, Hessian PA. Development of the gouty tophus: an hypothesis. Am J Clin Pathol 1989;91(2):190–5.

41. Steinberg TH, Newman AS, Swanson JA, et al. Macrophages possess probenecid-inhibitable organic anion transporters that remove fluorescent dyes from the cytoplasmic matrix. J Cell Biol 1987;105(6Pt1):2695–702.

42. Mobasheri A, Dobson H, Mason SL, et al. Expression of the GLUT1 and GLUT9 facilitative glucose transporters in embryonic chondroblasts and mature chondrocytes in ovine articular cartilage. Cell Biol Int 2005;29(4):249–60.

43. McCarty DJ. Gout without hyperuricemia. JAMA 1994;271(4):302–3.

44. Wu X, Wakamiya M, Vaishnav S, et al. Hyperuricemia and urate nephropathy in urate oxidase-deficient mice. Proc Natl Acad Sci U S A 1994;91(2):742–6.

45. Fiechtner JJ, Simkin PA. Urate spherulites in gouty synovia. JAMA 1981;245(15):1533–6.

46. American College of Rheumatology Musculoskeletal Ultrasound Task Force. Ultrasound in American rheumatology practice: report of the American College of Rheumatology musculoskeletal ultrasound task force. Arthritis Care Res (Hoboken) 2010;62(9):1206–19.

47. Simkin PA. Concentration of urate by differential diffusion: a hypothesis for initial urate deposition. Adv Exp Med Biol 1974;41:547–50.

48. Schumacher HR. Bullous tophi in gout. Ann Rheum Dis 1977;36(1):91–3.

49. Tak HK, Wilcox WR, Cooper SM. The effect of lead upon urate nucleation. Arthritis Rheum 1981;24(10):1291–5.

50. Burt HM, Dutt YC. Growth of monosodium urate monohydrate crystals: effect of cartilage and synovial fluid components on in vitro growth rates. Ann Rheum Dis 1986;45(10):858–64.

51. McGill NW, Dieppe PA. The role of serum and synovial fluid components in the promotion of urate crystal formation. J Rheumatol 1991;18(7): 1042–5.

52. Katz WA, Schubert M. The interaction of monosodium urate with connective tissue components. J Clin Invest 1970;49(10):1783–9.

53. Lally EV, Zimmerman B, Ho Jr G, et al. Urate-mediated inflammation in nodal osteoarthritis: clinical and roentgenographic correlations. Arthritis Rheum 1989;32(1):86–90.

54. Alvsaker JO. Genetic studies in primary gout. Investigations on the plasma levels of the urate-binding alpha 1-alpha 2-globulin in individuals from two gouty kindreds. J Clin Invest 1968 Jun;47(6):1254–61.

55. Hardwell TR, Manley G, Braven J, et al. The binding of urate plasma proteins determined by four different techniques. Clin Chim Acta 1983;133(1):75–83.

56. Perl-Treves D, Addadi L. A structural approach to pathological crystallizations: gout: the possible role of albumin in sodium urate crystallization. Proc R Soc Lond 1988;235(1279):145–59.

57. Kam M, Perl-Treves D, Caspi D, et al. Antibodies against crystals. FASEB J 1992;6(8):2608–13.

58. Kanevets U, Sharma K, Dresser K, Shi Y. A role of IgM antibodies in monosodium urate crystal formation and associated adjuvanticity. J Immunol 2009;182(4):1912–8.

59. Yagnik DR, Hillyer P, Marshall D, et al. Noninflammatory phagocytosis of monosodium urate monohydrate crystals by mouse macrophages. Implications for the control of joint inflammation in gout. Arthritis Rheum 2000;43(8):1779–89.

60. Landis RC, Yagnik DR, Florey O, et al. Safe disposal of inflammatory monosodium urate monohydrate crystals by differentiated macrophages. Arthritis Rheum 2002;46(11):3026–33.

61. Yagnik DR, Evans BJ, Florey O, et al. Macrophage release of transforming growth factor beta1 during resolution of monosodium urate monohydrate crystal-induced inflammation. Arthritis Rheum 2004;50(7):2273–80.

62. Guarda G, Dostert C, Staehli F, et al. T cells dampen innate immune responses through inhibition of NLRP1 and NLRP3 inflammasomes. Nature 2009;460(7252):269–73.

63. McCarthy GM, Barthelemy CR, Veum JA, et al. Influence of antihyperuricemic therapy on the clinical and radiographic progression of gout. Arthritis Rheum 1991;34(12):1489–94.

64. Terkeltaub R, Tenner AJ, Kozin F, et al. Plasma protein binding by monosodium urate crystals: analysis by two-dimensional gel electrophoresis. Arthritis Rheum 1983;26(6):775–83.

65. Jaques BC, Ginsberg MH. The role of cell surface proteins in platelet stimulation by monosodium urate crystals. Arthritis Rheum 1982; 25(5):508–21.

66. Mandel NS. The structural basis of crystal-induced membranolysis. Arthritis Rheum 1976 May-Jun;19(Suppl. 3):439–45.

67. Ng G, Sharma K, Ward SM, et al. Receptor-independent, direct membrane binding leads to cell-surface lipid sorting and Syk kinase activation in dendritic cells. Immunity 2008;29(5):807–18.

68. Chen CJ, Shi Y, Hearn A, et al. MyD88-dependent IL-1 receptor signaling is essential for gouty inflammation stimulated by monosodium urate crystals. J Clin Invest 2006;116(8):2262–71.

69. Grandjean-Laquerriere A, Tabary O, Jacquot J, et al. Involvement of toll-like receptor 4 in the inflammatory reaction induced by hydroxyapatite particles. Biomaterials 2007;28(3):400–4.

70. Pessler F, Mayer CT, Jung SM. Identification of novel monosodium urate crystal regulated mRNAs by transcript profiling of dissected murine air pouch membranes. Arthritis Res Ther 2008;10(3):R64:Epub 2008 Jun 3.

71. Murakami Y, Akahoshi T, Hayashi I. Induction of triggering receptor expressed on myeloid cells 1 in murine resident peritoneal macrophages by monosodium urate monohydrate crystals. Arthritis Rheum 2006;54(2): 455–62.

72. Liu-Bryan R, Terkeltaub R. Evil humors take their toll as innate immunity makes gouty joints TREM-ble. Arthritis Rheum 2006;54(2):383–6.

73. Babelova A, Moreth K, Tsalastra-Greul W, et al. Biglycan, a danger signal that activates the NLRP3 inflammasome via toll-like and P2X receptors. J Biol Chem 2009;284(36):24035–48.

74. Joosten LA, Netea MG, Mylona E, et al. Engagement of fatty acids with Toll-like receptor 2 drives interleukin-1β production via the ASC/caspase 1 pathway in monosodium urate monohydrate crystal-induced gouty arthritis. Arthritis Rheum 2010;62(11):3237–48.

75. Piccini A, Carta S, Tassi S, et al. ATP is released by monocytes stimulated with pathogen-sensing receptor ligands and induces IL-1beta and IL-18 secretion in an autocrine way. Proc Natl Acad Sci U S A 2008;105(23): 8067–72.

76. Merino A, Buendia P, Martin-Malo A, et al. Senescent CD14+CD16+ monocytes exhibit proinflammatory and proatherosclerotic activity. J Immunol 2010 Dec 29:[Epub ahead of print].

77. Schroder K, Tschopp J. The inflammasomes. Cell 2010;140(6):821–32.

78. Tschopp J, Schroder K. NLRP3 inflammasome activation: the convergence of multiple signalling pathways on ROS production? Nat Rev Immunol 2010;10(3):210–5.

79. Schroder K, Zhou R, Tschopp J. The NLRP3 inflammasome: a sensor for metabolic danger? Science 2010;327(5963):296–300.

80. Duewell P, Kono H, Rayner KJ, et al. NLRP3 inflammasomes are required for atherogenesis and activated by cholesterol crystals. Nature 2010;464(7293):1357–61.

81. Spreafico R, Ricciardi-Castagnoli P, Mortellaro A. The controversial relationship between NLRP3, alum, danger signals and the next-generation adjuvants. Eur J Immunol 2010;40(3):638–42.

82. St Pierre CA, Chan M, Iwakura Y, et al. Periprosthetic osteolysis: characterizing the innate immune response to titanium wear-particles. J Orthop Res 2010;28(11):1418–24.

83. Maitra R, Clement CC, Scharf B, et al. Endosomal damage and TLR2 mediated inflammasome activation by alkane particles in the generation of aseptic osteolysis. Mol Immunol 2009;47(2-3):175–84.

84. Narayan S, Pazar B, Ea HK, et al. Octacalcium phosphate (OCP) crystals induce inflammation in vivo through IL-1 but independent of the NLRP3 inflammasome. Arthritis Rheum 2010 Nov 15:[Epub ahead of print].

85. Pétrilli V, Papin S, Dostert C, et al. Activation of the NALP3 inflammasome is triggered by low intracellular potassium concentration. Cell Death Differ 2007;14(9):1583–9.

86. Kobayashi T, Kouzaki H, Kita H. Human eosinophils recognize endogenous danger signal crystalline uric acid and produce proinflammatory cytokines mediated by autocrine ATP. J Immunol 2010;184(11):6350–8.

87. Zhou R, Tardivel A, Thorens B, et al. Thioredoxin-interacting protein links oxidative stress to inflammasome activation. Nat Immunol 2010;11(2): 136–40.

88. Hu Y, Mao K, Zeng Y, et al. Tripartite-motif protein 30 negatively regulates NLRP3 inflammasome activation by modulating reactive oxygen species production. J Immunol 2010 Dec 15;185(12):7699–705.

89. Hoffstein S, Weissmann G. Mechanisms of lysosomal enzyme release from leukocytes. IV. Interaction of monosodium urate crystals with dogfish and human leukocytes. Arthritis Rheum 1975;18(2):153–65.

90. Schorn C, Janko C, Munoz L, et al. Sodium and potassium urate crystals differ in their inflammatory potential. Autoimmunity 2009;42(4):314–6.

91. Lioté F, Prudhommeaux F, Schiltz C, et al. Inhibition and prevention of monosodium urate monohydrate crystal-induced acute inflammation in vivo by transforming growth factor beta1. Arthritis Rheum 1996;39(7):1192–8.

92. Giamarellos-Bourboulis EJ, Mouktaroudi M, Bodar E, et al. Crystals of monosodium urate monohydrate enhance lipopolysaccharide-induced release of interleukin 1 beta by mononuclear cells through a caspase 1-mediated process. Ann Rheum Dis 2009;68(2):273–8.

93. Kono H, Chen CJ, Ontiveros F, Rock KL. Uric acid promotes an acute inflammatory response to sterile cell death in mice. J Clin Invest 2010;120(6):1939–49.

94. Shi Y, Evans JE, Rock KL. Molecular identification of a danger signal that alerts the immune system to dying cells. Nature 2003;425(6957):516–21.

95. Denoble AE, Huffman KM, Stabler TV, et al. Uric acid is a danger signal of increasing risk for osteoarthritis through inflammasome activation. Proc Natl Acad Sci U S A 2011 Jan 18:[Epub ahead of print].

96. Convento MS, Pessoa E, Dalboni MA, et al. Pro-inflammatory and oxidative effects of noncrystalline uric acid in human mesangial cells: contribution to hyperuricemic glomerular damage. Urol Res 2010 Jun 4:[Epub ahead of print].

97. Meotti FC, Jameson GN, Turner R, et al. Urate as a physiological substrate for myeloperoxidase: implications for hyperuricemia and inflammation. J Biol Chem 2011 Jan 25:[Epub ahead of print].

98. Gibbings S, Elkins ND, Fitzgerald H, et al. Xanthine oxidoreductase promotes the inflammatory state of mononuclear phagocytes through effects on chemokine expression, peroxisome proliferator-activated receptor-{gamma} sumoylation, and HIF-1{alpha}. J Biol Chem 2011;286(2):961–75.

99. Terkeltaub R, Sklar LA, Mueller H. Neutrophil activation by inflammatory microcrystals of monosodium urate monohydrate utilizes pertussis toxin-insensitive and sensitive pathways. J Immunol 1990;144(7):2719–24.

100. Onello E, Traynor-Kaplan A, Sklar L, et al. Mechanism of neutrophil activation by an unopsonized inflammatory particulate: monosodium urate crystals induce pertussis toxin-insensitive hydrolysis of phosphatidylinositol 4,5-bisphosphate. J Immunol 1991;146(2):4289–99.

101. Bomalaski JS, Baker DG, Brophy LM, et al. Monosodium urate crystals stimulate phospholipase A2 enzyme activities and the synthesis of a phospholipase A2-activating protein. J Immunol 1990;145(10):3391–7.

102. Hanein D, Geiger B, Addadi L. Differential adhesion of cells to enantiomorphous crystal surfaces. Science 1994;263(5152):1413–6.

103. Schorn C, Strysio M, Janko C, et al. The uptake by blood-borne phagocytes of monosodium urate is dependent on heat-labile serum factor(s) and divalent cations. Autoimmunity 2010;43(3):236–8.

104. Terkeltaub R, Smeltzer D, Curtiss LK, et al. Low density lipoprotein inhibits the physical interaction of phlogistic crystals and inflammatory cells. Arthritis Rheum 1986;29(3):363–70.

105. Ortiz-Bravo E, Sieck M, Schumacher R. Changes in the proteins coating monosodium urate crystals during active and subsiding inflammation. Arthritis Rheum 1993;9(9):1274–85.

106. Ortiz-Bravo E, Schumacher HR. Components generated locally as well as serum alter the phlogistic effect of monosodium urate crystals in vivo. J Rheumatol 1993;20(7):1162–6.

107. Terkeltaub R, Dyer C, Martin J, et al. Apolipoprotein E (apo E) inhibits the capacity of monosodium urate crystals to stimulate neutrophils: characterization of intraarticular apo E and demonstration of apo E binding to urate crystals in vivo. J Clin Invest 1991;87(1):20–6.

108. Terkeltaub R, Banka C, Solan J, et al. Oxidized LDL induces the expression by monocytic cells of IL-8, a chemokine with T lymphocyte chemotactic activity. Arterioscler Thromb Vasc Biol 1994;14(1):47–53.

109. Chapman PT, Yarwood H, Harrison AA, et al. Endothelial activation in monosodium urate monohydrate crystal-induced inflammation: in vitro and in vivo studies on the roles of tumor necrosis factor alpha and interleukin-1. Arthritis Rheum 1997;40(5):955–65.

110. Chapman PT, Jamar F, Harrison AA, et al. Characterization of E-selectin expression, leucocyte traffic and clinical sequelae in urate crystal-induced inflammation: an insight into gout. Br J Rheumatol 1996;35(4):323–34.

111. Cronstein BN, Molad Y, Reibman J, et al. Colchicine alters the quantitative and qualitative display of selectins on endothelial cells and neutrophils. J Clin Invest 1995;96(2):994–1002.

112. Ruth JH, Arendt MD, Amin MA, et al. Expression and function of CXCL16 in a novel model of gout. Arthritis Rheum 2010;62(8):2536–44.

113. Guma M, Ronacher L, Liu-Bryan R, et al. Caspase 1-independent activation of interleukin-1beta in neutrophil-predominant inflammation. Arthritis Rheum 2009;60(12):3642–50.

114. Joosten LA, Netea MG, Fantuzzi G, et al. Inflammatory arthritis in caspase 1 gene-deficient mice: contribution of proteinase 3 to caspase 1-independent production of bioactive interleukin 1beta. Arthritis Rheum 2009;60(12):3651–62.

115. Netea MG, Simon A, van de Veerdonk F, et al. IL-1beta processing in host defense: beyond the inflammasomes. PLoS Pathog 2010;6(2):e1000661.

116. Stehlik C. Multiple interleukin-1beta-converting enzymes contribute to inflammatory arthritis. Arthritis Rheum 2009;60(12):3524–30.

117. Empson VG, McQueen FM, Dalbeth N. The natural killer cell: a further innate mediator of gouty inflammation? Immunol Cell Biol 2010;88(1):24–31.

118. Pascual E, Castellano JA. Treatment with colchicine decreases white cell counts in synovial fluid of asymptomatic knees that contain monosodium urate crystals. J Rheumatol 1992;19(4):600–3.

119. Getting SJ, Flower RJ, Parente L, et al. Molecular determinants of monosodium urate crystal-induced murine peritonitis: a role for endogenous mast cells and a distinct requirement for endothelial-derived selectins. J Pharmacol Exp Ther 1997;283(1):123–30.

120. Akahoshi T, Namai R, Murakami Y, et al. Rapid induction of peroxisome proliferator-activated receptor gamma expression in human monocytes by monosodium urate monohydrate crystals. Arthritis Rheum 2003;48(1):231–9.

121. Yagnik DR, Hillyer P, Marshall D, et al. Noninflammatory phagocytosis of monosodium urate monohydrate crystals by mouse macrophages. Implications for the control of joint inflammation in gout. Arthritis Rheum 2000;43(8):1779–89.

122. Landis RC, Yagnik DR, Florey O, et al. Safe disposal of inflammatory monosodium urate monohydrate crystals by differentiated macrophages. Arthritis Rheum 2002;46(11):3026–33.

123. Yagnik DR, Evans BJ, Florey O, et al. Macrophage release of transforming growth factor beta1 during resolution of monosodium urate monohydrate crystal-induced inflammation. Arthritis Rheum 2004;50(7):2273–80.

124. Rose DM, Sydlaske AD, Agha-Babakhani A, et al. Transglutaminase 2 limits murine peritoneal acute gout-like inflammation by regulating macrophage clearance of apoptotic neutrophils. Arthritis Rheum 2006;54(10):3363–71.

125. Buttgereit F, Burmester GR, Straub RH, et al. Exogenous and endogenous glucocorticoids in rheumatic diseases. Arthritis Rheum 2011;63(1):1–9.

126. Getting SJ, Christian HC, Flower RJ, et al. Activation of melanocortin type 3 receptor as a molecular mechanism for adrenocorticotropic hormone efficacy in gouty arthritis. Arthritis Rheum 2002;46(10):2765–75.

127. Getting SJ, Gibbs L, Clark AJ, et al. POMC gene-derived peptides activate melanocortin type 3 receptor on murine macrophages, suppress cytokine release, and inhibit neutrophil migration in acute experimental inflammation. J Immunol 1999;162(12):7446–53.

128. Tate G, Mandell BF, Laposata M, et al. Suppression of acute and chronic inflammation by dietary gamma linolenic acid. J Rheumatol 1989;16(6):729–34.

129. Tate GA, Mandell BF, Karmali RA, et al. Suppression of monosodium urate crystal-induced acute inflammation by diets enriched with gamma-linolenic acid and eicosapentaenoic acid. Arthritis Rheum 1988;31(12):1543–51.

130. Dalbeth N, Gracey E, Pool B, et al. Identification of dairy fractions with anti-inflammatory properties in models of acute gout. Ann Rheum Dis 2010;69(4):766–9.

Chapter **6**

Gout: Epidemiology and Risk Factors

Eswar Krishnan

KEY POINTS

- Unlike osteoarthritis and rheumatoid arthritis, gout is typically an episodic arthritis. The intervals between attacks can be as long as decades with complete absence of symptoms between attacks. These factors, and errors in diagnosis, intrinsically complicate assessment of gout epidemiology.

- The case definitions used for epidemiologic studies of gout are seldom as rigorous as those used for clinical diagnosis. For example, investigators in the Sudbury Study[1] could validate only 44% of self-reported cases using Rome or New York criteria, and in a study of health professionals,[2] only 70% of cases could be validated by ACR criteria. However, in one study of physicians,[3] it was reported that 100% of self-reported cases could be validated by ACR criteria and medical record review. The variable magnitude and direction of this measurement error mean that all statistical conclusions about gout epidemiology need to be carefully scrutinized.

- A large proportion of people with gout have relatively minor and self-limiting forms of the disease; these patients seldom require medical attention, and the diagnosis is often not confirmed.

- The appropriate utilization of gout medications in primary care is notoriously poor; those on gout medications do not necessarily have gout, unlike diagnostic certainty in patients treated with chemotherapy for cancer or insulin for diabetes, as common examples.

- There is no way to reliably distinguish the many possible health outcomes of gout from those of concurrent osteoarthritis and other comorbid conditions.

- Although several authors have defined "primary" gout as the disease occurring in the absence of other causes such as diuretics, this definition is difficult to apply in epidemiologic studies.

Introduction

Gouty arthritis (gout) is common in industrialized nations. Gout is a complex disease involving the metabolic, renal, cardiovascular and immunologic systems; advances in clinical care of the disease have followed the lava-lamp model (Figure 6-1).

Epidemiologic Principles

The building blocks of epidemiologic inferences are incidence rates.[4] Accurate measurement of incidence of any disease is, to some extent, dependent on case definition and classification criteria used. The primary epidemiologic risk factors for gout include increasing age, male gender, menopausal status among women, renal dysfunction, hypertension and other comorbidities that decrease renal uric acid excretion such as metabolic syndrome and obesity, use of diuretics (which increase renal urate reabsorption), diet and alcohol factors (see Chapter 12), comorbidities that increase purine turnover such as psoriasis, rare single-gene disorders such as HPRT deficiency, and dietary risk factors. The relationships among these risk factors are complex, and for a nuanced understanding of the epidemiology of gout, it is critical to recognize the first principles of gout epidemiology cited in the Key Points at the head of this chapter.

Descriptive Epidemiology

The two metrics used to characterize the frequency of chronic diseases in a population are incidence and prevalence. Incidence rates represent the number of newly diagnosed cases in a well-defined population in a specified time, usually number per 1000 individuals per year. The prevalence proportion represents the proportion of individuals alive with a specific condition at a given time. In case of episodic arthritis syndromes like gout, one needs to differentiate between 1-year prevalence (i.e., had an attack in the past 1 year) versus lifetime prevalence (i.e., ever had a gout attack). For chronic diseases with low mortality rate, the prevalence rates can be expected to increase with age even with steady incidence rates.

Prevalence of gout

Table 6-1 summarizes all the relevant studies of prevalence in the United States. The prevalence figures vary substantially among studies because some authors used period prevalence and some used lifetime prevalence; in other studies, the definition used was not clearly stated. In the most recent NHIS survey on gout (1996), the prevalence for the 1-year period was 940 per 100,000 adults aged 18 years or older in the United States. In 2008, the prevalence proportion of self-reported gout in the United States was estimated to be approximately 2

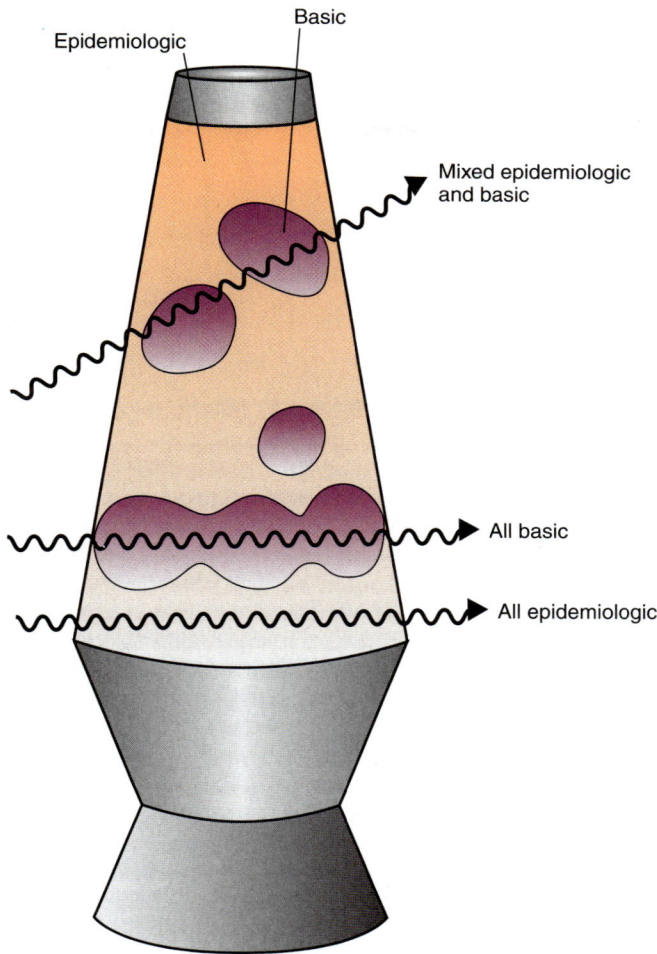

Figure 6-1 The lava lamp model of clinical advances. Clinical advances are represented as traversing the lamp. The liquid (*tan*) and the denser material (*red*) in the lamp represent epidemiologic and "basic" science, respectively. Advances can occur by several trajectories, and there is no one path to a useful solution. Some solutions will involve just clinical science, and others will involve a mixture of basic science and epidemiology. Importantly, the definitions of basic science and epidemiology, and their relative positions, may change with time. Rate limiting is the ability to see through the lamp and then traverse it. *(Modified from Rees J. Complex disease and the new clinical sciences. Science 2002;296(5568):698-700.)*

Table 6-1 Prevalence of Gout in the United States[a]

Source and year of study/gout definition[b]	Age, y	Prevalence per 100,000		
		Male	**Female**	**Total**
REGIONAL POPULATION STUDIES				
Tecumseh Community Health Study, 1960/"Rome"[d]	≥20	720	480	ND[c]
Framingham Heart Study, 1964/arbitrary[e]	≥42 (mean 58)	2850	390	1480
Sudbury Study, 1972/Rome and New York	≥15	660	100	370
NATIONAL SURVEY STUDIES				
NHIS, 1988/self-report (1-year prevalence)[f]	≥18	ND	ND	850
	18–44	290	90	310
	45–64	3350	950	2100
	≥65	4110	1700	2700
NHIS, 1992/self-report (1-year prevalence)[f]	≥18	ND	ND	840
	18–44	440	30	380
	45–64	2630	810	1680
	≥65	4410	1820	2900
NHIS, 1996/self-report (1-year prevalence)[f]	≥18	ND	ND	940
	18–44	340	20	180
	45–64	3350	1200	2240
	≥65	4640	1950	3080
NHANES III, 1988-1994/self-report (lifetime prevalence)[g]	≥20	3,800	1,600	2,600
	≥20-29	200	500	400
	30-39	2,100	100	1,100
	40-49	2,600	900	1,700
	50-59	5,600	2,300	3,900
	60-69	9,400	3,200	6,100
	70-79	11,600	5,200	8,000
	≥80	7,100	5,300	5,900

[a]Data from Lawrence RC, Felson DT, Helmick CG, et al. Estimates of the prevalence of arthritis and other rheumatic conditions in the United States. Part II. Arthritis Rheum 2008;58(1):26-35.
[b]NHIS, National Health Interview Survey; NHANES III, National Health and Nutrition Examination Survey III.
[c]ND = no data.
[d]Rome = Rome criteria used "insofar as possible."
[e]Arbitrary indicated at least two of the following three features: a typical attack of arthritis, an attack of arthritis with a prompt response to colchicine therapy and/or hyperuricemia.
[f]One-year prevalence of gout was ascertained by the question, "Have you or any member of your household had gout within the past year?"
[g]Lifetime prevalence of gout ascertained by the question, "Has a doctor ever told you that you had gout?" Interviewers were instructed to emphasize the word "doctor." If the respondent stated that it was another health professional who gave the diagnosis of gout, the answer was coded as "no."

to 3 million adults.[5] Managed care data (based on claims data codes) suggests that the prevalence rates have increased over time, especially among older adults (older than 65 years) as shown in Figure 6-2.[6]

The unadjusted prevalence of gout in the U.K. population has been estimated to be 1.4%.[7,8] A general practice–based study with a smaller sample size reported an unadjusted prevalence rate of 1%.[9] Almost all the recent national data from the United Kingdom come from general practice–based registers. These include smaller consortia , the General Practice Research Database (GPRD), and the Royal College of General Practitioners Weekly Returns Service sentinel general practice network in England and Wales.[10] The second and fourth U.K. National Morbidity Studies demonstrated a threefold increase in gout prevalence between 1971 and 1991.[10] In a study using the large GPRD, the unadjusted prevalence of gout in 1999

was 1.4%, with the highest rate of 7.3% observed in men aged 75 to 84 years.[8] A more recent study in Germany and the United Kingdom showed the same 1.4% prevalence of gout in both countries over the period 2000 to 2005.[7] The yearly incidence rates for the United Kingdom derived from the GPRD for 1990 through 1999 showed modest increases in the early 1990s in older men and women but a return toward 1990 values by the end of the decade. However, such trends were not observed in the Royal College of General Practitioners study (Figure 6-3).[10]

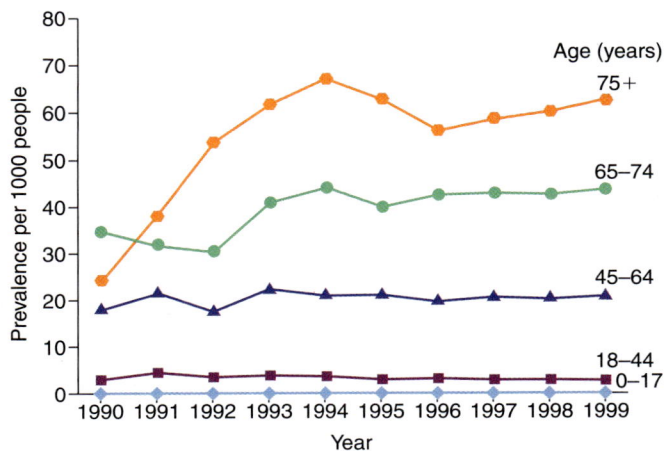

Figure 6-2 Prevalence of gout in U.S. men, 1990–1999. *(From Wallace KL, Riedel AA, Joseph-Ridge N, et al. Increasing prevalence of gout and hyperuricemia over 10 years among older adults in a managed care population. J Rheumatol 2004;31(8):1582-7.)*

Incidence

There have been relatively few studies that have examined the incidence of gout. Methodologically, the most rigorous was a population-based study from Rochester, Minnesota, that compared incidence rates of new cases of gout using American College of Rheumatology Classification Criteria between 1977/1978 and 1995/1996. The authors of this study concluded that the unadjusted incidence rate of gout doubled from 45 per 100,000 to 62 per 100,000.[11] Such increases would have contributed to the increasing prevalence of gout over time. The U.S. hospitalization data are also consistent with this theory (Figure 6-4).

Epidemiology of Tophaceous Gout

The population epidemiology of tophi is harder to study than that for other clinical manifestations of gout since visible tophi tend to be asymptomatic and diagnosis during a physical examination requires some degree of sophistication. The proportion of tophaceous disease among those with gout varies substantially, with the Sudbury study[1] reporting that about 23% of patients with gout had tophaceous gout, the Framingham Study reporting[12] about 7%,[13] and the study on the Hmong reporting 31%.[14]

Menopausal Women and Gout

As can be expected from differences in the distribution of serum urate concentrations, women in general have lower prevalence of gout than do men (Figure 6-5). This disparity is evident through all age groups. There is a belief that women are protected from gout in the premenopausal age group and that in the postmenopausal period, the rates "catch up" with those among men. This is an inherently difficult hypothesis to test in epidemiologic studies since age, age at menopause, and menopausal status are highly correlated with each other. The prevalence of gout among premenopausal women is low compared to that among men of the same age range but the relative prevalence remains lower in older age groups as well.

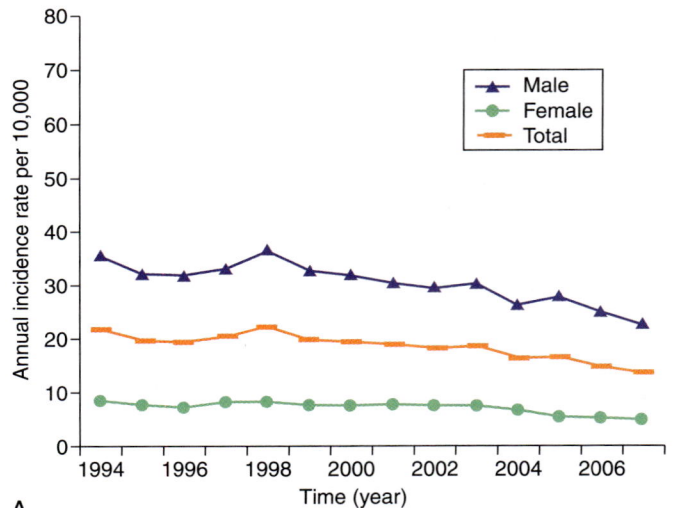

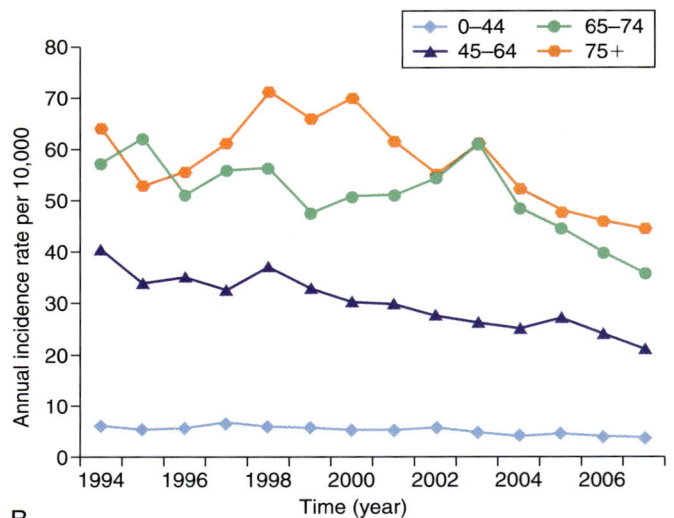

Figure 6-3 Incidence of gout in the United Kingdom (1994–2007). **A,** Annual incidence of acute attacks of gout per 10,000 population (1994–2007); data are shown for all ages (total) and for males and females. **B,** Age-specific annual incidence of acute attacks of gout per 10,000 population (1994–2007). *(From Elliot AJ, et al. Seasonality and trends in the incidence and prevalence of gout in England and Wales 1994-2007. Ann Rheum Dis 2009;68:1728-33.)*

In the NHANES III surveys, the lifetime prevalence of gout among men increased from 2600 per 10,000 in the 40- to 49-year-old age groups to 9400 per 10,000 in the 60- to 69-year-old age group—a 3.6-fold increase. The corresponding figures among women were 900 and 3200, respectively—a similar 3.5-fold increase. Such a proportional increase was also observed in the data from the U.K. GPRD data (see Figure 6-5). These data suggest that increases in prevalence of gout among menopausal women are merely a reflection of age-related changes and are unrelated to menopause. On the other hand, a cross-sectional study of the U.S. population reported a definite but modest (about 0.30 mg/dl) increase in serum urate concentration associated with menopause, compared to age- and other risk-adjusted premenopausal women. [15] In this study as well as in others, postmenopausal women who used hormones had an about 0.2 mg/dl lower serum urate level

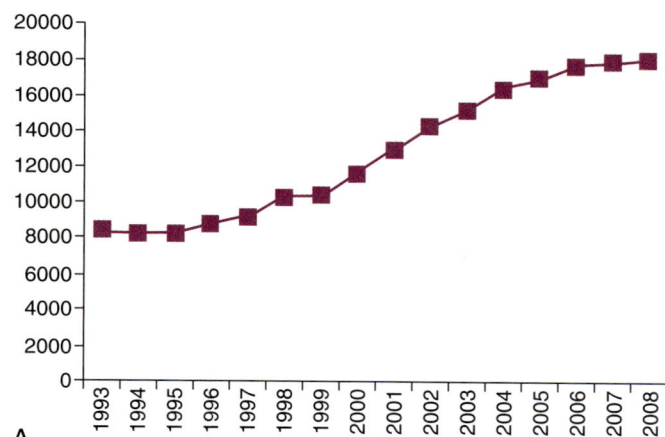

A

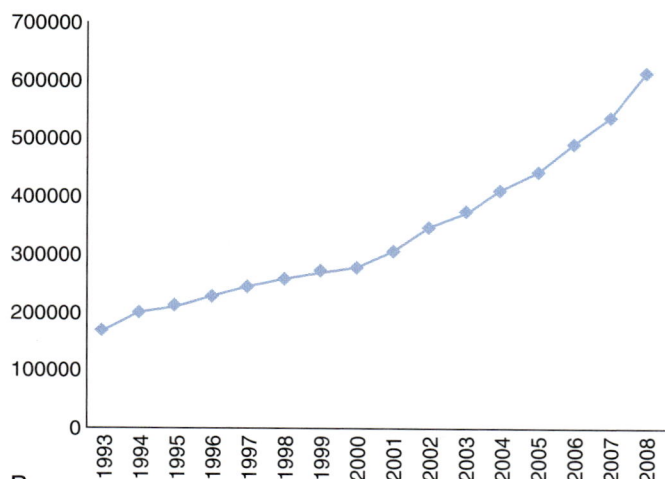

B

Figure 6-4 Trends in hospitalizations with gout as a principal diagnosis (**A**) and the presence of gout as a comorbid diagnosis in the United States over time (**B**). The data are weighted national estimates from the Healthcare Cost and Utilization Project (HCUP) Nationwide Inpatient Sample (NIS), Agency for Healthcare Research and Quality (AHRQ), based on data collected by individual states and provided to AHRQ.

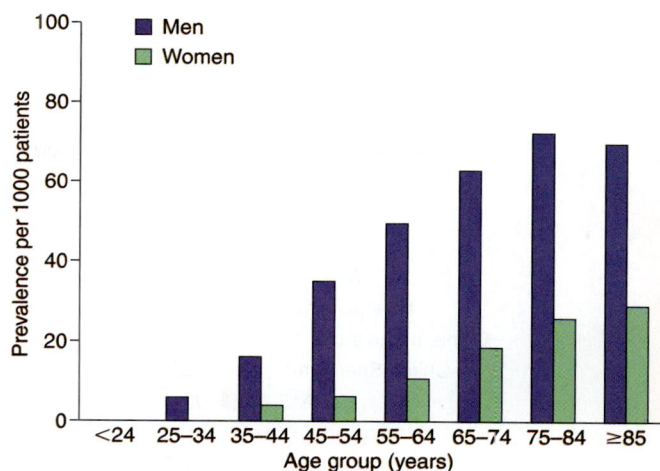

Figure 6-5 Prevalence of gout by age and gender. The proportionate increase with age is similar in men and women. *(From Mikuls TR, Farrar JT, Bilker WB, et al. Gout epidemiology: results from the UK. General Practice Research Database, 1990-1999. Ann Rheum Dis 2005;64(2):267-72.)*

compared to nonusers; one interpretation is that the "estrogen attributable fraction" of hyperuricemia may be too modest to be of any clinical utility.[15-17] Interestingly, data on gout incidence reported from the Nurses Health Study report an approximately 20% increase in the risk for gout attributable to menopause and an approximately 20% decrease in risk with hormone replacement.[18] The significance of this investigation is in the implications for the prevention of gout.

Seasonality of Gout

There is some evidence of seasonality for gout incidence and flares, but the relative magnitude of such seasonality is negligible compared to those of other seasonal illnesses such as hay fever and flu. Gout has been described in the popular literature as the "scourge of the holiday season" (November-December), presumably because of dietary indiscretions.[19] However, this is not supported by data. Schlesinger et al.[20] reported that in patients from Pennsylvania, crystal gout flares were the lowest in the winter and highest in the spring. There was no

consistent correlation between gout flares and temperature or humidity. These observations were confirmed in a study of patients from Ferrara, Italy; in these patients, the peak incidence of flares was in April.[21] It is notable that these studies defined *flares* as those with crystal demonstration in synovial fluid and that the pattern of diagnosis might be influenced by performance of arthrocentesis over different months of the year. Another Italian study examined the first-ever attack of gout in a cohort of 73 patients and concluded that June, July, and December were the peak incidence months.[22] The largest study to date confirmed that new diagnoses of gout peak between late-April and mid-September.[10]

Geography, Ethnicity, and Gout

Wide variations in the incidence, prevalence, and severity of gout among various ethnicities have been observed as illustrated by Figure 6-6.[23,24] Most notable is the high prevalence of gout among Pacific Islanders. Maoris in particular have greater severity of gout as manifested by hospitalization rates 6 times greater than that of the New Zealand general population.[25] Asian/Pacific Islanders in the United States (especially Filipinos, Tongans, and Samoans) have an almost threefold higher frequency than the age- and gender-adjusted white population.[26] The proposed explanation is an underlying inability of people of these ethnicities to clear uric acid by the kidneys when challenged with a high-purine diet.[27] This hypothesis is supported by the observation that the rates of gout among the Maoris have increased with increasing adoption of European diet and lifestyle.[28] Heterogeneity of methodology explains some but not all of this variation; most is likely due to complex gene–environment interactions. Whether Western dietary amounts of fructose consumption is a factor is not yet clear. (See also Chapter 11.)

Risk Factors and Causality

In most epidemiologic studies, the true objective is to detect and measure the *effects* of an etiologic factor or an intervention. Sometimes the effect is not directly observable and we

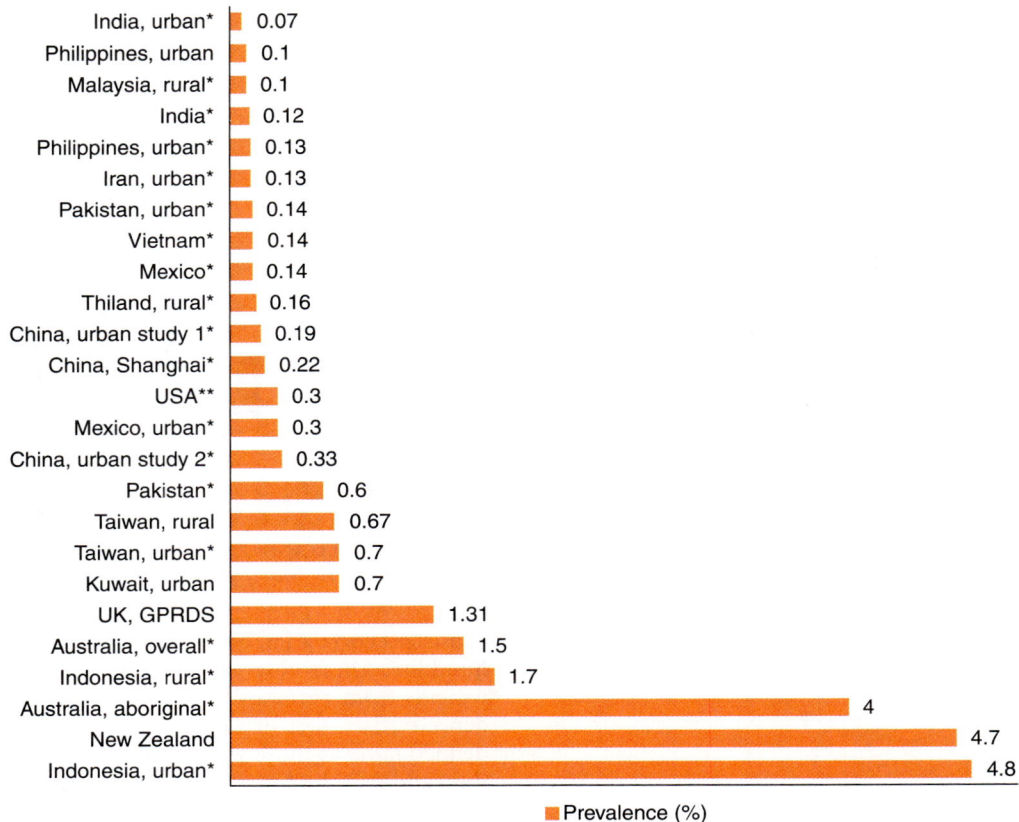

Figure 6-6 Geography, ethnicity and prevalence rates of gout. An asterisk indicates that prevalence of gout was assessed by the COPCORD group of investigators.[4] The rates are not necessarily directly comparable to each other, but the markedly high rates in indigenous people of Australia are consistent with observations in other indigenous Pacific Islanders. The mean U.S. prevalence rate (indicated by **) was calculated from the National Institutes of Health estimates of 6 million lifetime prevalent cases in a population of 250 million. *Data for the United Kingdom were obtained from GPRDS (United Kingdom General Practice Research Data).*

have to settle for the observation of the *association* of that specific factor or intervention. The measurement of a substitute may work well in cases where the association does not equal the effect. For example, the effect of caffeine consumption and arthritis is difficult to measure but the association between self-reported coffee consumption and arthritis risk is not difficult to assess. However, the latter may or may not be the true effect of caffeine. On the other hand, use of moonshine whiskey as a surrogate for lead-toxicity–related gout may provide a good reflection of the effect of lead on gout incidence.

The term *risk factor* denotes a factor associated with an increased risk of disease or other poor outcomes. Risk factors are correlations and correlation does not imply causation. For example, watching more than 5 hours of television every day may be a risk factor for gout but it is not causal. It is the association with a lifestyle characterized by low physical activity, obesity, and insulin resistance that is the real pathway to gout.

Causality is a subject of perennial discussion among professional philosophers. In the context of epidemiologic research, causal relationships have a narrower interpretation and the features that "upgrade" a risk factor to a causal factor have been well accepted (Table 6-2). In the case of gout, few risk factors have successfully passed through the "filter of truth" (Figure 6-7).

Multiple Causation

Within an individual patient, barring certain genetic syndromes, gout is likely to be caused by several factors. "Multiple causation" is the canon of contemporary epidemiology, and its metaphor and model is the "web of causation."[29] Several of these causes facilitate gout but are not sufficient to cause gout individually (Figure 6-8). The most important categories of risk factors include (1) the metabolic "six-pack" of obesity, diet, inactivity, shared genes, hypertension, and hyperlipidemia (discussed later); (2) other comorbidities that increase uric acid production or decrease uric acid excretion; (3) other genetic factors; and (4) medications. All of these influence the risk for gout by affecting serum urate concentration (see Figure 6-8).

Hyperuricemia: A Necessary but Not Sufficient Cause of Gout

The U.S. Veterans Normative Aging Study reported that among those with serum urate concentrations greater than 79 mg/dl, the cumulative 5-year incidence of gout was 22%, whereas the incidence rate for those with a lower serum urate concentration (7.0 to 8.9 mg/dl) was about 3%.[30] The annual incidence rates were about 5% in the former group compared to 0.5% in the latter and 0.1% among those with serum urate concentration less than 7.0 mg/dl. In the Framingham Study, the 12-year cumulative incidence rates were 36% among

Table 6-2 Characteristics Distinguishing Causal Relationships From Correlative Observations

TEMPORALITY

There is a time relationship between cause and effect in that the effect occurs after the cause. If some delay is expected between cause and effect, then that delay should be observed.

STRENGTH AND ASSOCIATION

Cause and effect may be observed by statistical correlation between strength of response and consistently strong of result in repeated events or experiments. Full strength correlation has a correlation coefficient of 1. A weaker association between cause and effect will see greater variation.

BIOLOGICAL GRADIENT (DOSE-RESPONSE)

In treatment, there might be expected to be a relationship between the dose given and the reaction of the patient. This may not be a simple linear relationship and may have minimum and maximum thresholds.

CONSISTENCY

One apparent success does not prove a general cause and effect in wider contexts. For example, to prove a treatment is useful, it must give consistent results in a wide range of circumstances.

PLAUSIBILITY

The apparent cause and effect must make sense in the light of current theories and results. If a causal relationship appears to be outside of current science then significant additional hypothesizing and testing will be required before a true cause and effect can be found.

SPECIFICITY

A specific relationship is found if there is no other plausible explanation. This is not always the case in medicine where any given symptoms may have a range of possible causing conditions.

EVIDENCE

A very strong proof of cause and effect comes from the results of experiments, where many significant variables are held stable to prevent them interfering with the results. Other evidence is also useful but cause and effect cannot be as readily determined as in controlled experiments.

ANALOGY

When something is suspected of causing an effect, then other factors similar or analogous to the supposed cause should also be considered and evaluated as a possible cause or otherwise eliminated from the investigation.

COHERENCE

If laboratory experiments in which variables are controlled and external everyday evidence are in alignment, then it is said that there is coherence.

those with serum urate concentration greater than 8 mg/dl and 1.8% for those with serum urate concentration less than 6.0 mg/dl. Such stark differences in the risk rates are likely to be an exaggeration, as those with higher urate concentrations are more likely to be older and male, whereas those with lowest serum urate concentrations are likely to be younger and female.

Although urate concentration is clearly a risk factor, there are other clues that suggest that the link between hyperuricemia and gout may not be linear. Several studies have documented the presence of intraarticular urate crystals without clinical inflammatory manifestations.[31] This is instructive because urate crystals are strong stimulants of innate immunity, and lack of gout in some but not others may signify heterogeneity of immune responses to crystals.[32]

Web of Causation of Gout

All known risk factors for new-onset gout are linked through hyperuricemia (see Figure 6-8). The metabolic six-pack is composed of six overlapping factors that lead to hyperinsulinemia and other related effects (putatively including increased leptin in obesity) that in turn reduce the renal clearance of uric acid. These include the factors of the metabolic syndrome—hypertension, hyperlipidemia, obesity (especially truncal obesity), and lifestyle factors such as poor physical activity and high-risk diet. The latter risk factors are discussed separately.

The risk factors for *incidence* of gout (i.e., gout for the first time in a person) may be different from those for *recurrent* gout flares. A novel case-crossover study has examined these factors and observed that the chronicity of gout and comorbid factors are the two major determinants of recurrence of gout flares in addition to alcohol and diuretic use.[33-35]

It is notable that hyperuricemia was included as a criterion for metabolic syndrome when the term was coined by Haller in 1977.[29] Two often-used sets of criteria for metabolic syndrome are shown in Table 6-3. The World Health Organization (WHO) criteria require the presence of dysglycemia, whereas the NCEP criteria does not; the presence of renal dysfunction is included in the WHO criteria but not in the NCEP criteria. Nevertheless, these two sets identify populations with existing or imminent insulin resistance and subclinical renal dysfunction—factors that lead to reduced renal clearance of uric acid.[36,37]

Comorbidities that increase urate production and reduce excretion are also correlated with the presence of gout. These conditions are typically those that involve increased cell turnover. For example, a common comorbidity is psoriasis. Hemoglobinopathy, including sickle cell disease or trait, might be thought of as a risk factor that could contribute to the relatively high incidence of gout among African Americans,

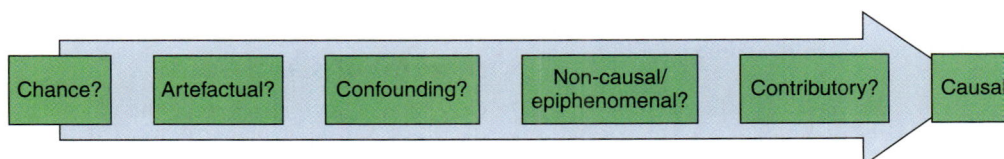

Figure 6-7 Association to causality: Epidemiologic truth filters weed out misleading associations from true causative factors. These filters are critical for identification of points of intervention that can be used to successfully reduce the burden of illness for the individual and the population.

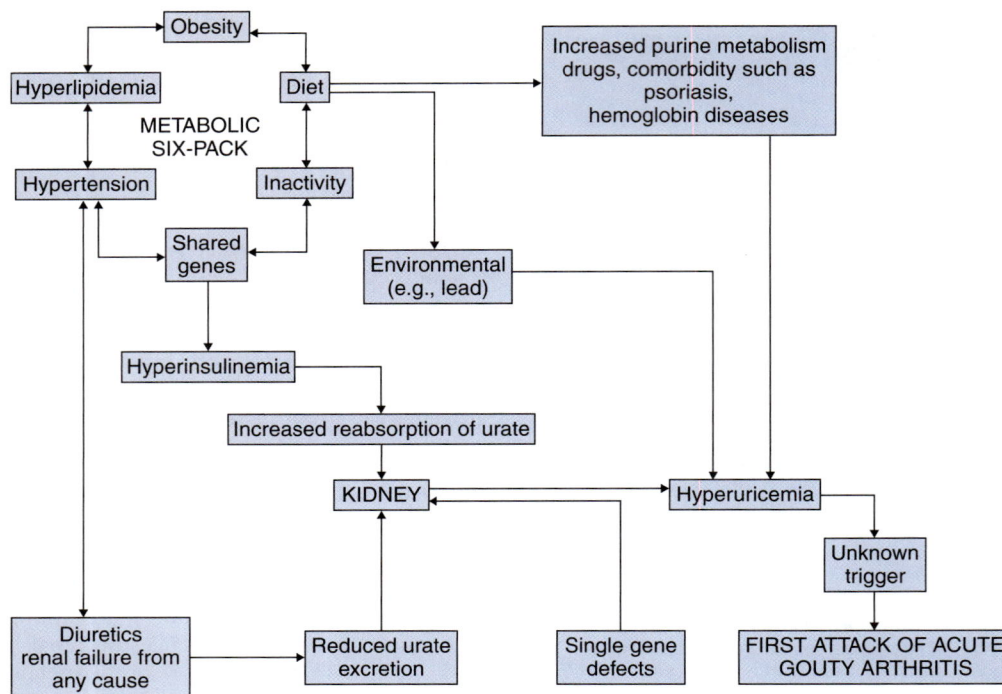

Figure 6-8 Web of causation in gout. All known risk factors for gout are linked through hyperuricemia. Notably, lifestyle and metabolic factors are tightly correlated and possibly act on the kidney through hyperinsulinemia.

Table 6-3 Criteria for Metabolic Syndrome

ATP criteria require at least three of the following:
- Central obesity: waist circumference ≥ 102 cm or 40 inches (male); ≥ 88 cm or 36 inches (female)
- Dyslipidemia: triglycerides (TG) ≥1.7 mmol/L (150 mg/dl)
- Dyslipidemia: high-density lipoprotein cholesterol (HDL-C) <40 mg/dl (male); < 50 mg/dl (female)
- Blood pressure: ≥130/85 mm Hg
- Fasting plasma glucose: ≥6.1 mmol/L (110 mg/dl)

The World Health Organization criteria (1999) require presence of diabetes mellitus, impaired glucose tolerance, impaired fasting glucose or insulin resistance, AND two of the following:
- Blood pressure: ≥140/90 mm Hg
- Dyslipidemia: TG ≥1.695 mmol/L and HDL-C ≤0.9 mmol/L (male), ≤1.0 mmol/L (female)
- Central obesity: waist:hip ratio >0.90 (male); > 0.85 (female) or body mass index >30 kg/m²
- Microalbuminuria: urinary albumin excretion ratio ≥20 μg/min or albumin:creatinine ratio ≥30 mg/g

From Third Report of the National Cholesterol Education Program (NCEP) Expert Panel on Detection, Evaluation, and Treatment of High Blood Cholesterol in Adults (Adult Treatment Panel III) final report. Circulation 2002;106:3143-421.

but hypertension is much more likely. Renal insufficiency (chronic kidney disease [CKD]) can decrease renal uric acid clearance substantially, especially in the context of end-stage renal disease.

The topic of genetics of gout has been addressed in Chapter 8. Gout is known to cluster in families. A tiny fraction of these cases are related to genetically driven overproduction of uric acid stemming from abnormally high purine turnover (e.g., HPRT enzyme deficiency). Some genetic factors can be protective. For example, the G774A mutation in *SLC22A12* is associated with low serum urate levels.[38] In 2002, Enomoto et al.[39] reported the identification of the urate transporter in the human kidney. URAT1, encoded by *SLC22A12*, is one of the members of the organic anion transporter (OAT) family and is a urate–anion exchanger localized on the apical side of the proximal tubule. Other mutations have been linked with increased gout risk as well.[40] Renal handling of urate can also explain some of the familial clusters of gout. A study of 21 cases of early onset (mean age 28 years) showed that uric acid clearance relative to creatinine was subnormal in 15 cases, including all of the women.[41]

Most of these studies were performed in relatively small numbers of selected patients with gout. The relative importance of heritable and environmental factors has been examined in a unique twin study[12] of 508 twin pairs, in whom the cumulative incidence of gout did not differ between monozygotic twins and dizygotic twins (11.1% and 10.9%, respectively). The concordance of hyperuricemia, however, was 56% in monozygotic twins and 31% in dizygotic twin pairs ($p < .001$). Multivariable analyses confirmed that hyperuricemia has a significant heritability component, whereas gout does not.[12] Larger studies will determine if there is a heritability component smaller in magnitude than can be assessed in a twin study of this size.

Medications and Gout

Certain medications increase the risk of gout. Diuretics are the most common class of drugs that can increase serum urate concentration (Figure 6-9) and ultimately increase gout risk (Table 6-4). Epidemiologic data suggest a 70% increase in the risk for gout among diuretic users. However, the use

n = 11
Mean, SEM

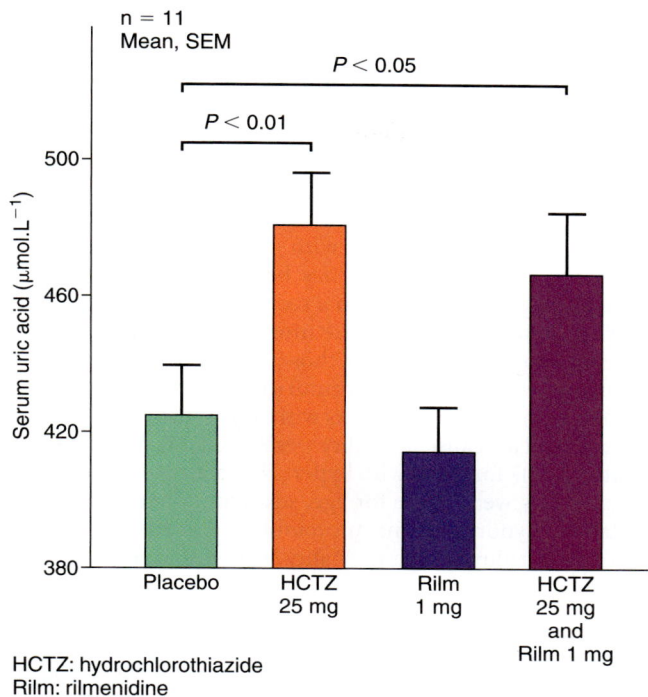

HCTZ: hydrochlorothiazide
Rilm: rilmenidine

Figure 6-9 Diuretics increase serum uric acid concentration and gout risk. Healthy subjects received once-daily oral doses of placebo or one of three active-medication formulations at 8:00 a.m. during four separate single-treatment periods of 4 days each. An individually randomized, crossover, and double-blind design was followed. The values depicted were derived from the individual averages of assessments made in blood samples withdrawn just before and 6 and 24 hours after dosing on day 4. ANOVA for repeated measures: $p < .0001$. Active-medication mean values were compared with the placebo mean by Dunnett's test. *(Data from Reyes AJ. Cardiovascular drugs and serum uric acid. Cardiovasc Drugs Ther 2003;17(5-6):397-414.)*

Table 6-4 Changes in Serum Urate Concentration During Effective Antihypertensive Pharmacotherapy With Low-Dose Diuretics[a]

No. of Patients	Treatment (Diuretic Drug and Once-Daily Dose)	Serum Uric Acid Concentration, µmol/L	
		Baseline	% Change
50	Bendrofluazide 1.25 mg[b]	314	6% (weeks 10–12)[d]
31	Bendrofluazide 1.25 mg	254	19% (week 16)[e]
12	Bendrofluazide 1.25 mg	330	12% (week 8)[e]
12	Chlorthalidone 12.5[b]	278	15% (week 12)[e]
162	Chlorthalidone 12.5[c]	309	10% (week 9)[e]
298	Chlorthalidone 25 mg	274	15% (week 4)[e]
118	Hydrochlorothiazide 12.5 mg	349	9% (week 12)[f]
46	Indapamide 1 mg	327	9% (week 6)[e]

[a]Data from Reyes AJ. Cardiovascular drugs and serum uric acid. Cardiovasc Drugs Ther 2003;17(5-6):397-414.
[b]Plus potassium chloride.
[c]The dose was increased from 12.5 to 25 mg once daily in 34% of patients at the end of week 4.
[d]Significantly different from the corresponding change in the placebo group of 52 patients (baseline serum uric acid mean value 300 µmol/L, mean change –1.6%).
[e]Significant change vs. baseline.
[f]Significantly different from corresponding change in the placebo group of 111 patients (baseline serum uric acid mean value; 331 µmol/L, mean change –0.2%).

of diuretics in the context of hypertension did not appear to increase serum urate concentration among those who are already hyperuricemic (mean serum urate 7.7 mg/dl) compared to those at the lowest quartile (mean serum urate 4.9 mg/dl).[42] Further, the number of cases of diuretic-induced gout that necessitated discontinuation of diuretics in the hypertension detection and follow-up program has been few (15 of 3693 participants).[42] A recent prospective study showed that, after adjusting for alcohol consumption and purine intake, the odds ratio for recurrent gout attacks from all diuretic use over the previous 48 hours was 3.6. The odds ratios of recurrent gout attacks were 3.2 and 3.8 for use of thiazide and loop diuretics, respectively.[35]

Drugs used in the context of posttransplant immunosuppression are a major cause of iatrogenic gout. Cyclosporine and, to a lesser extent, tacrolimus can cause hyperuricemia and increase the risk for gout about eightfold.[8,43,44] This risk is likely significantly elevated among those with other risk factors for gout such as renal insufficiency, gender, and insulin resistance. It is not clear what the immunomodulatory and certain other biologic effects of these agents have on the incidence and clinical features of the clinical disease. Gout develops in more than 10% of patients within a few years of transplantation and is often severe and polyarticular.[45,46] Among renal transplant recipients, the prevalence of gout has been estimated to range from 2% to 28%.[47] The pretransplant hyperuricemia status appears to be an important predictor of posttransplant gout. In a study from Mexico City, Mexico, the incidence of gout was 19.7 per 1000 and 2.67 per 1000 patient-years in the groups with and without hyperuricemia pretransplant, respectively.[48]

Other drugs that act on urate transporters in the kidneys and decrease plasma urate levels are high-dose aspirin (greater than 3 g/day), benzbromarone, probenecid, sulfinpyrazone, and losartan, whereas other agents such as pyrazinoate (the active metabolite of pyrazinamide), nicotinate (niacin), and low-dose aspirin (about 75 mg/day) have the opposite effect,[49] as does lactate. Not all these substances have been directly linked to clinical incidence of gouty arthritis. New research on non-URAT1 transporters of uric acid is ongoing, with the identification of multidrug resistance protein MRP4 as a luminal efflux transporter for urate in the proximal tubule—this, and the effects of OAT4 on urate–thiazide diuretic exchange by renal proximal tubule epithelial cells , may be a pathway of action of diuretics.[50,51]

Lead and Gout

Sequestration of lead from daily activities has reduced exposure and toxicity from lead (typical blood lead levels [BLL] > 80 µg/dl) in industrialized countries. Nevertheless, the world production of lead has increased by about 50% over the past 50 years. Lead is primarily used to make batteries, and lead contamination of the environment remains a problem. Lead becomes a part of the food chain because certain plants are avid retainers of lead. Tobacco plants in particular accumulate lead, which is later transferred to the smoker. Lead exposure can lead to renal failure (lead nephropathy), which in turn can increase retention of ingested lead, hyperuricemia, and gout. Some data suggest that gout among individuals with lead nephropathy is a mild disease.[52] Among those without clinical evidence of renal failure, the highest quartile of BLL (mean about 3 μg/dl) was associated with an eightfold increase in the prevalence of gout—an association that remained significant after adjustment of the effects of age, gender, adiposity, race, diabetes, diuretic use, and creatinine clearance.[53]

Morbidity and Mortality of Gout

Over the past decade, there have been numerous reports of high rates of morbidity and mortality associated with gout—rates higher than would be expected from the existing risk factors. It is thought that such excess morbidity and mortality

might be due to gout itself. This section describes the links between gout and comorbidities (Table 6-5). The role of hyperuricemia is addressed in Chapter 19.

Coronary Artery Disease

The link between gout and cardiovascular diseases has been observed anecdotally and in several studies. Of the cardiovascular diseases, the link with coronary artery disease/acute myocardial infarction has been well characterized in large prospective studies.[54] In a recent study, one of the largest studies so far, the all-cause mortality rates for gout were observed to be higher than those with hyperuricemia and about twice that among normouricemic individuals (Figure 6-10). Compared with subjects with normouricemia, the hazard ratios of all-cause mortality were 1.46 for individuals with gout and 1.07 for those with hyperuricemia, respectively, after adjustments were made for age, sex, component number of metabolic syndrome, and proteinuria. The adjusted hazard ratios of cardiovascular mortality were 1.97 for individuals

Table 6-5 Studies of Gout, CVD, and Mortality

Study	Population	Study Design	No. of Subjects With Gout (Total)	Follow-up, y	Outcomes[a]	No. of Subjects With Outcome of Gout (Total)	Adjusted Effect Size (95% CI)
Yu, 1980 (USA)	A gout research clinic	Case Series	2000	30	Mortality	382	N/A (Descriptive Data)
Nishioka, 1981 (Japan)	Gout patients	Case Series	104	8	CVD	28	N/A (Descriptive Data)
Darlington, 1983 (UK)	A rheumatology institute	Case Series	180	6	CVD mortality	5	N/A (O/I ratio, *ns*)
Abbot 1988 (USA) [b]	Framingham cohort	Cohort	94 (1858)	32	CHD	37(509)	1.60(1.10-2.50)*s*
Gelber, 1997 (USA)	Meharry-Hopkins cohort	Cohort	93 (1624)	30	CHD	7(182)	0.59(0.24-1.46)*ns*
Janssens, 2003 (Netherlands) [c]	Continuous Morbidity Registration cohort	Case Control	170 (510)	11	CVD	44(114)	0.98(0.65-1.47)*ns*
Krishnan, 2006 (USA)	Multiple Risk Factor Intervention Trial Cohort	Cohort	1123 (12,866)	6.5	a. Fatal MI b. All MI	22(246) 118(1108)	a. 0.96(0.66-1.44)*ns* b. *1.26(1.14-1.40)s*
Chen, 2007 (Taiwan)	Ho-Ping Gout database	Cross-sectional	22,572	N/A	QWMI	393	1.18(1.01-1.38)*s*[d]
Choi, 2007 (USA)	Health professionals Follow-up cohort	Cohort	2773 (51,297)	12	a. All-cause mort. b. CVD mortality c. CVD mortality	645(5825) 304(2132) 238(1576)	a. 1.28(1.15-1.41)*s* b. 1.38(1.15-1.66)*s* c. 1.55(1.24-1.93)*s*
Krishnan, 2008 (USA)	Multiple Risk Factor Intervention Trial cohort	Cohort	655 (9105)	17	a. Fatal MI b. CHD Mortality d. CVD Mortality	36(360) 78(833) 110(1241)	a. 1.35(0.94-1.93)*ns* b. 1.35(1.06-1.72)*s* c. 1.21(0.99-1.49)*ns*
Cohen, 2008 (USA)	US Renal Data System dialysis patients	Cohort	24,415 (234,794)	5	a. All-cause mort. b. CVD mortality	Not reported	a. 1.49(1.43-1.55)*s* b. 1.47(1.26-1.59)*s*

From Kim SY, De Vera MA, Choi HK. Gout and mortality. Clin Exp Rheumatol 2008;26(5 suppl 51):S115-9.
[a]*CHD*, coronary disease; *CVD*, Cardiovascular disease; *MI*, myocardial infarction; *ns*, gout is not independent predictor of outcome; *O/I ratio*, ratio of observed vs. expected deaths; *QWMI*, Q-wave myocardial infarction; *s*, gout is independent predictor of outcome.
[b]Results reported for males only.
[c]Results reported for gout cases with no prevalent CVD.
[d]Effect size for frequency of gout attack on outcome.

MORTALITY RATES PER 1000 PERSON-YEARS

■ Cardiovascular   ■ All-cause

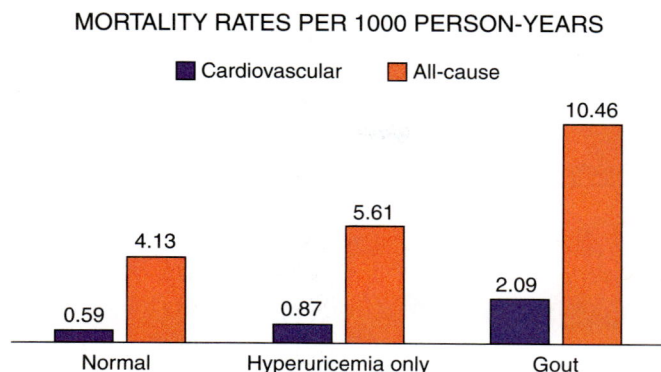

Figure 6-10 Mortality for hyperuricemia and gout. From 2000 to 2006, data on 61,527 individuals were analyzed [men: 34,126 (55.5%); women: 27,401 (44.5%)]. The study population was an average of 49.1 (11.0) years old for males and 50.8 (10.8) years old for females. Among them, 78.1% (n =48,021) of the subjects were normouricemic, 19.8% (n =12,195) had hyperuricemia, and 2.1% (n =1311) had gout. The mean serum urate level was 6.9 (1.5) mg/dl in males and 5.4 (1.4) mg/dl in females. A total of 1383 deaths (198 cardiovascular deaths) were identified. Log-rank test revealed that gout and hyperuricemia were associated with a greater all-cause ($p < .001$) and cardiovascular mortality ($p < .001$) than normouricemic subjects. Of the 1383 deaths, 198 (14.3%) were attributed to the circulatory system in the study population. More cardiovascular deaths were found among subjects with gout [n = 12 (20.0%); $p < .001$] and hyperuricemia (n =57; 17.1%; $p < .001$). Stroke, coronary heart disease, heart failure, and hypertensive heart diseases accounted for 83 (41.9%), 62 (31.3%), 13 (7.1%), and 10 (5.1%) deaths, respectively. *(Data from Kuo CF, See LC, Luo SF, et al. Gout: an independent risk factor for all-cause and cardiovascular mortality. Rheumatology (Oxf) 2010;49(1):141-146.)*

with gout and 1.08 for those with hyperuricemia.[55] Taken together, these data suggest that gout might have an independent link with mortality outcomes, especially from cardiovascular causes. Importantly, lowering serum (e.g., through the use of allopurinol or benzbromarone) has been suggested to mitigate some of this excess risk,[56-58] but this is not yet directly established.

Chronic Kidney Disease

The presence of CKD in patients with gout is often considered a poor prognostic factor, since CKD aggravates hyperuricemia and renders more difficult the aggressive dosing of urate-lowering therapies. On the other hand, extreme CKD, end-stage renal disease, is reported to be associated with fewer gout attacks, possibly due to concomitant immunosuppression.[59] Two small retrospective studies of patients with gout undergoing maintenance dialysis documented fewer gout attacks after the initiation of dialysis.[60,61] In a claims-based analysis performed using commercial health insurance datasets in the United States, the prevalence of any CKD was 39% (Figure 6-11). Over time, the proportion of patients with gout and renal failure can be expected to rise.

Pharmacoepidemiology and Economics of Gout Medications

The most common medications prescribed for gout taken from the 2002 U.S. National Ambulatory Medical Care Survey data, which included information from private practices and

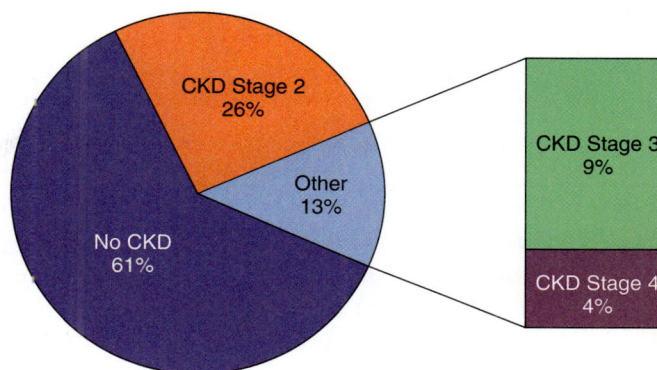

Figure 6-11 Prevalence of chronic kidney disease among patients with gout. From commercial health plan data in the United States, 3929 subjects were identified with gout based on the presence of at least two claims, including a medical claim with an *ICD-9* code of 274 and at least one for gout medication (allopurinol, probenecid, colchicines, and/or sulfinpyrazone). Estimated glomerular filtration rate was calculated using the formula used in the Modification of Diet in Renal Disease (MDRD) Study. Chronic kidney disease was staged using the National Kidney Foundation Kidney Disease Outcomes Quality Initiative (NKF-KDOQI). *(Data presented at the Annual Meeting of the European League against Rheumatism [2008].)*

Table 6-6 Medications Prescribed for Gout in Ambulatory Care in 2002.

- 2.8 Million prescriptions (95% CI 1.9–3.7 million) for allopurinol
- About 8000 prescriptions (95% CI 0–25,511) for probenecid
- 381,000 (95% CI 81,000–681,000) prescriptions for colchicine
- 4.6% patients were co-prescribed colchicine (95% CI 2%–12%)
- 341,000 prescriptions (95% CI 44,700–638,000) for prednisone
- 700,000 (95% CI 300,000–1.1 million) prescriptions for NSAIDs over 18% of visits (95% CI 11%–28%)

Data from Krishnan E, Lienesch D, Kwoh CK. Gout in ambulatory care settings in the United States. J Rheumatol 2008;35(3):498-501.

hospital-based clinics, are shown in Table 6-6. Just over 1% of all outpatient visits to rheumatologists are for gout (Table 6-7).

Allopurinol is an inhibitor of the xanthine oxidoreductase system; this system is a major component of free radical metabolism. Allopurinol is currently the most commonly used urate-lowering therapy in patients with gout. The use of allopurinol is associated with improved cardiovascular condition and all-cause mortality outcomes.[62]

Allopurinol is a relatively inexpensive generic medication. In a study of costs associated with gout among the elderly (aged 65 and older), it was estimated that all-cause health care costs for patients with gout were about US$3000 per year. Among those with gout, the presence of gout or documentation of uncontrolled serum urate concentration was associated with the highest costs.[63,64] The main components of these costs are hospital utilization (64.4%), medications (23.1%), and physician visits (12.5%).[65] Optimal management of gout remains elusive for a majority of patients.[66,67] One study found that physician consultation for an attack was associated with about twofold increased risk of inappropriate therapy.[68] Another study found that inappropriate physician prescribing

Table 6-7 Distribution of Visits to Specialists Among Patients With a Gout Visit (None Were Seen by Pediatricians, Neurologists, or Psychiatrists)

Specialty	Visits for Non–Gout-Related Reasons	Visits for Gout-Related Reasons	Proportion of All Gout-Related Visits to This Specialty, %	Overall Number of Visits
General/family practice	213,965,547	1,500,425	38.34	215,465,972
Internal medicine	155,488,884	1,203,310	30.75	156,692,194
Orthopedic surgery	38,018,169	9,710	0.25	38,027,879
Cardiovascular diseases	20,430,843	390,774	9.99	20,821,617
Dermatology	32,207,648	19,450	0.5	32,227,098
Rheumatology	3,437,744	46,019	1.18	3,483,763
Other specialties	103,586,205	388,049	8.74	100,490,491
Unknown/not available	83,103,414	235,656	6.02	83,339,070
Total	969,406,505	3,913,056	100	973,319,561

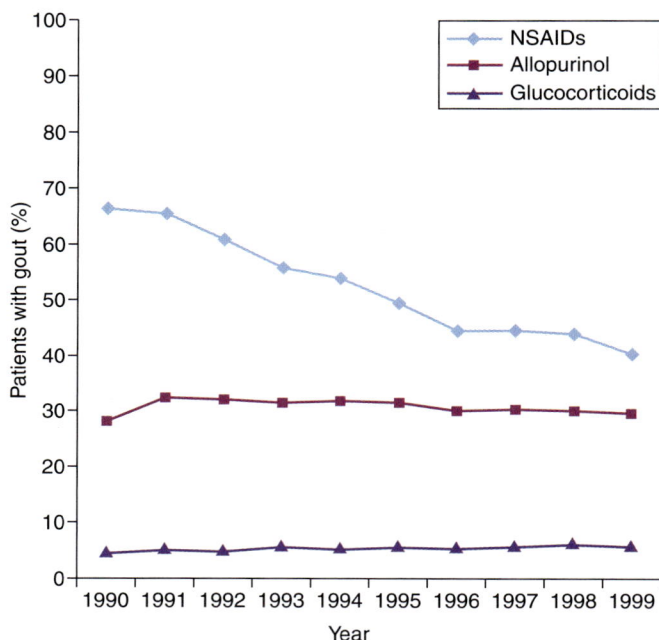

Figure 6-12 Annual frequency of NSAID, allopurinol, and glucocorticoid use among patients with gout. In this study of 63,105 patients enrolled in the U.K. GPRD, 1990–1999, frequency of use included any prescription received within the same calendar year. Colchicine (range 0.9%–3.4%) and uricosuric (range 0.8%–1.0%) use are not shown. NSAID use among patients with gout declined significantly over this period (*p* < .001) and use among osteoarthritis patients also declined during the period of observation (data not shown) from a high of 63.7% in 1990 to a low of 39.0% in 1999 (*p* < .001 for trend). (*From Mikuls TR, Farrar JT, Bilker WB, et al. Gout epidemiology: results from the UK. General Practice Research Database, 1990-1999. Ann Rheum Dis 2005;64(2):267-272.*)

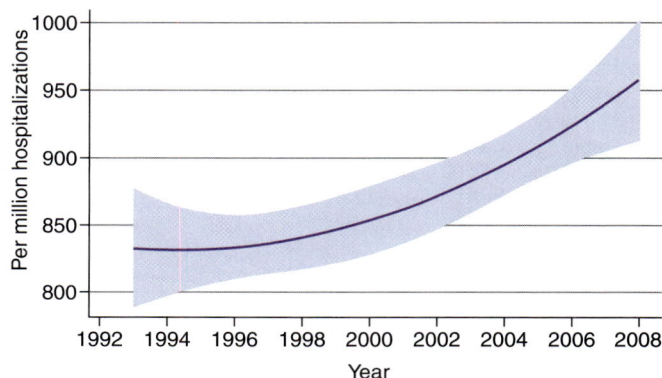

Figure 6-13 Trends in use of arthrocentesis. During the 15-year period from 1993 to 2008, there were an estimated 588 million hospitalizations in the United States, of which arthrocentesis was performed in 514,460 hospitalizations. In 2008, 75,000 arthrocentesis procedures were performed. Of these, 38,000 were documented to be the primary hospital procedure performed. The data are weighted national estimates from Healthcare Cost and Utilization Project (HCUP) Nationwide Inpatient Sample (NIS), Agency for Healthcare Research and Quality (AHRQ), based on data collected by individual states and provided to AHRQ by the states.

Epidemiology of Arthrocentesis

Arthrocentesis, in the hands of a trained professional, is an important tool that not only helps diagnose gout but also enables pain relief via the relief of pressure and injection of corticosteroids. This procedure can be performed in an outpatient setting or an emergency department. Little is known about the epidemiology of utilization, indications, and complications of arthrocentesis. National U.S. data suggest that arthrocentesis is being used more frequently (Figure 6-13).

Concluding Remarks

Gout is perhaps the only curable arthritis. Effective medications are available, and more are on the way; yet the management of this disease is poor, and the culprit is poor physician

practices accounted for as many as one fourth of all gout medication errors.[69] The low rates of utilization of probenecid and sulfinpyrazone (less than 1%) were evident in Nova Scotia and the United Kingdom as well.[8] Over the years, the utilization of nonsteroidal antiinflammatory drugs (NSAIDs) for the treatment of gout appears to be declining, probably because of safety concerns with this class of drugs (Figure 6-12).

education (coupled with poor patient education). As the description of epidemiologic features indicates, much more is unknown about this condition than is known. The interplay of risk factors that leads to causation is nuanced and not linear. Future research will shed light on the relative roles of genes and environment in the etiology of gout.

References

1. O'Sullivan JB. Gout in a New England town. A prevalence study in Sudbury, Massachusetts. Ann Rheum Dis 1972;31(3):166–9.
2. Choi HK, Atkinson K, Karlson EW, et al. Purine-rich foods, dairy and protein intake, and the risk of gout in men. N Engl J Med 2004;350(11):1093–103.
3. Gelber AC, Klag MJ, Mead LA, et al. Gout and risk for subsequent coronary heart disease. The Meharry-Hopkins Study. Arch Intern Med 1997;157(13):1436–40.
4. Rothman KJGS. The emergence of modern epidemiology. In: Rothman KJ GS, editor. Modern Epidemiology. Philadelphia, PA: Lippincott Williams & Wilkins; 1998:4.
5. Lawrence RC, Felson DT, Helmick CG, et al. Estimates of the prevalence of arthritis and other rheumatic conditions in the United States. Part II. Arthritis Rheum 2008;58(1):26–35.
6. Wallace KL, Riedel AA, Joseph-Ridge N, et al. Increasing prevalence of gout and hyperuricemia over 10 years among older adults in a managed care population. J Rheumatol 2004;31(8):1582–7.
7. Annemans L, Spaepen E, Gaskin M, et al. Gout in the UK and Germany: prevalence, comorbidities and management in general practice 2000-2005. Ann Rheum Dis 2008;67(7):960–6.
8. Mikuls TR, Farrar JT, Bilker WB, et al. Gout epidemiology: results from the UK General Practice Research Database, 1990-1999. Ann Rheum Dis 2005;64(2):267–72.
9. Harris CM, Lloyd DC, Lewis J. The prevalence and prophylaxis of gout in England. J Clin Epidemiol 1995;48(9):1153–8.
10. Elliot AJ, Cross KW, Fleming DM. Seasonality and trends in the incidence and prevalence of gout in England and Wales 1994-2007. Ann Rheum Dis 2009;68(11):1728–33.
11. Arromdee E, Michet CJ, Crowson CS, et al. Epidemiology of gout: is the incidence rising? J Rheumatol 2002;29(11):2403–6.
12. Krishnan E, Lessov-Schlaggar CN, Fries J, et al. Hyperuricemia and gout: nature versus nurture. Arthritis Rheum 2010;62(Suppl. 10):S364.
13. Hall AP, Barry PE, Dawber TR, et al. Epidemiology of gout and hyperuricemia. A long-term population study. Am J Med 1967;42(1):27–37.
14. Wahedduddin S, Singh JA, Culhane-Pera KA, et al. Gout in the Hmong in the United States. J Clin Rheumatol 2010;16(6):262–6.
15. Hak AE, Choi HK. Menopause, postmenopausal hormone use and serum uric acid levels in US women: the Third National Health and Nutrition Examination Survey. Arthritis Res Ther 2008;10(5):R116.
16. Gaffo AL, Saag KG. Serum urate, menopause, and postmenopausal hormone use: from eminence to evidence-based medicine. Arthritis Res Ther 2008;10(5):120.
17. Nicholls A, Snaith ML, Scott JT. Effect of oestrogen therapy on plasma and urinary levels of uric acid. Br Med J 1973;1(5851):449–51.
18. Hak AE, Curhan GC, Grodstein F, et al. Menopause, postmenopausal hormone use and risk of incident gout. Ann Rheum Dis 2010;69(7):1305–9.
19. The gout: scourge of the holiday season. http://www.huffingtonpost.com/dr-rock-positano/the-gout-scourge-of-the-h_b_72896.html.
20. Schlesinger N, Gowin KM, Baker DG, et al. Acute gouty arthritis is seasonal. J Rheumatol 1998;25(2):342–4.
21. Gallerani M, Govoni M, Mucinelli M, et al. Seasonal variation in the onset of acute microcrystalline arthritis. Rheumatology (Oxf) 1999;38(10):1003–6.
22. Zampogna G, Andracco R, Parodi M, et al. [Clinical features of gout in a cohort of Italian patients]. Reumatismo 2009;61(1):41–7.
23. Muirden KD. Community oriented program for the control of rheumatic diseases: studies of rheumatic diseases in the developing world. Curr Opin Rheumatol 2005;17(2):153–6.
24. Sopoaga F, Buckingham K, Paul C. Causes of excess hospitalizations among Pacific peoples in New Zealand: implications for primary care. J Prim Health Care 2010;2(2):105–10.
25. Sopoaga F, Buckingham K, Paul C. Causes of excess hospitalizations among Pacific peoples in New Zealand: implications for primary care. J Prim Health Care 2010;2(2):105–10.
26. Krishnan E, Lienesch D, Kwoh CK. Gout in ambulatory care settings in the United States. J Rheumatol 2008;35(3):498–501.
27. Nugent CA, Tyler FH. The renal excretion of uric acid in patients with gout and in nongouty subjects. J Clin Invest 1959;8:1890–8.
28. Lennane GA, Rose BS, Isdale IC. Gout in the Maori. Ann Rheum Dis 1960;9:120–5.
29. Krieger N. Epidemiology and the web of causation: has anyone seen the spider? Soc Sci Med 1994;39(7):887–903.
30. Campion EW, Glynn RJ, DeLabry LO. Asymptomatic hyperuricemia. Risks and consequences in the Normative Aging Study. Am J Med 1987;82(3):421–6.
31. Bomalaski JS, Lluberas G, Schumacher Jr HR. Monosodium urate crystals in the knee joints of patients with asymptomatic nontophaceous gout. Arthritis Rheum 1986;29(12):1480–4.
32. Terkeltaub RA. Gout and mechanisms of crystal-induced inflammation. Curr Opin Rheumatol 1993;5(4):510–6.
33. Zhang Y, Chaisson CE, McAlindon T, et al. The online case-crossover study is a novel approach to study triggers for recurrent disease flares. J Clin Epidemiol 2007;60(1):50–5.
34. Zhang Y, Woods R, Chaisson CE, et al. Alcohol consumption as a trigger of recurrent gout attacks. Am J Med 2006;119(9):800:e813.
35. Hunter DJ, York M, Chaisson CE, et al. Recent diuretic use and the risk of recurrent gout attacks: the online case-crossover gout study. J Rheumatol 2006;33(7):1341–5.
36. Laws A, Reaven GM. Insulin resistance and risk factors for coronary heart disease. Baillieres Clin Endocrinol Metab 1993;7(4):1063–78.
37. Facchini F, Chen YD, Hollenbeck CB, et al. Relationship between resistance to insulin-mediated glucose uptake, urinary uric acid clearance, and plasma uric acid concentration. JAMA 1991;266(21):3008–11.
38. Taniguchi A, Urano W, Yamanaka M, et al. A common mutation in an organic anion transporter gene, SLC22A12, is a suppressing factor for the development of gout. Arthritis Rheum 2005;52(8):2576–7.
39. Enomoto A, Kimura H, Chairoungdua A, et al. Molecular identification of a renal urate anion exchanger that regulates blood urate levels. Nature 2002;417(6887):447–52.
40. Taniguchi A, Kamatani N. Control of renal uric acid excretion and gout. Curr Opin Rheumatol 2008;20(2):192–7.
41. Calabrese G, Simmonds HA, Cameron JS, et al. Precocious familial gout with reduced fractional urate clearance and normal purine enzymes. Q J Med 1990;75(277):441–50.
42. Langford HG, Blaufox MD, Borhani NO, et al. Is thiazide-produced uric acid elevation harmful? Analysis of data from the Hypertension Detection and Follow-up Program. Arch Intern Med 1987;147(4):645–9.
43. Marcen R, Gallego N, Orofino L, et al. Impairment of tubular secretion of urate in renal transplant patients on cyclosporine. Nephron 1995;70(3):307–13.
44. Abdelrahman M, Rafi A, Ghacha R, et al. Hyperuricemia and gout in renal transplant recipients. Ren Fail 2002;24(3):361–7.
45. Burack DA, Griffith BP, Thompson ME, et al. Hyperuricemia and gout among heart transplant recipients receiving cyclosporine. Am J Med 1992;92(2):141–6.
46. Lin HY, Rocher LL, McQuillan MA, et al. Cyclosporine-induced hyperuricemia and gout. N Engl J Med 1989;321(5):287–92.
47. Stamp L, Searle M, O'Donnell J, et al. Gout in solid organ transplantation: a challenging clinical problem. Drugs 2005;65(18):2593–611.
48. Hernandez-Molina G, Cachafeiro-Vilar A, Villa AR, et al. Gout in renal allograft recipients according to the pretransplant hyperuricemic status. Transplantation 2008;86(11):1543–7.
49. So A, Thorens B. Uric acid transport and disease. J Clin Invest 2010;120(6):1791–9.
50. El-Sheikh AA, van den Heuvel JJ, Koenderink JB, et al. Effect of hypouricaemic and hyperuricaemic drugs on the renal urate efflux transporter, multidrug resistance protein 4. Br J Pharmacol 2008;155(7):1066–75.
51. Stark K, Reinhard W, Grassl M, et al. Common polymorphisms influencing serum uric acid levels contribute to susceptibility to gout, but not to coronary artery disease. PLoS One 2009;4(11):e7729.
52. Emmerson BT. The clinical differentiation of lead gout from primary gout. Arthritis Rheum 1968;11(5):623–34.
53. Krishnan E, Lingala B, Fries J, et al. Lead and gout–going, going…not gone! Arthritis Rheum 2010;62(10):S802.
54. Krishnan E. Gout and coronary artery disease: epidemiologic clues. Curr Rheumatol Rep 2008;10(3):249–55.
55. Kuo CF, See LC, Luo SF, et al. Gout: an independent risk factor for all-cause and cardiovascular mortality. Rheumatology (Oxf) 2010;49(1):141–6.

56. Wei L, Fahey T, Struthers AD, et al. Association between allopurinol and mortality in heart failure patients: a long-term follow-up study. Int J Clin Pract 2009;63(9):1327–33.

57. Luk AJ, Levin GP, Moore EE, et al. Allopurinol and mortality in hyperuricaemic patients. Rheumatology (Oxf) 2009;48(7):804–6.

58. Chen J-H, Pan W. Effects of urate lowering therapy on cardiovascular mortality: a Taiwanese cohort study [abstract 2088]. American College of Rheumatology Annual Meeting: Atlanta GA; 2010.

59. Schreiner O, Wandel E, Himmelsbach F, et al. Reduced secretion of proinflammatory cytokines of monosodium urate crystal-stimulated monocytes in chronic renal failure: an explanation for infrequent gout episodes in chronic renal failure patients? Nephrol Dial Transplant 2000;15(5):644–9.

60. Ohno I, Ichida K, Okabe H, et al. Frequency of gouty arthritis in patients with end-stage renal disease in Japan. Intern Med 2005;44(7):706–9.

61. Ifudu O, Tan CC, Dulin AL, et al. Gouty arthritis in end-stage renal disease: clinical course and rarity of new cases. Am J Kidney Dis 1994;23(3):347–51.

62. Smith CR. Possible cardioprotective effects of allopurinol. Am J Prev Med 1988;4(Suppl. 2):33–8.

63. Wu EQ, Patel PA, Yu AP, et al. Disease-related and all-cause health care costs of elderly patients with gout. J Manag Care Pharm 2008;14(2):164–75.

64. Wu EQ, Patel PA, Mody RR, et al. Frequency, risk, and cost of gout-related episodes among the elderly: does serum uric acid level matter? J Rheumatol 2009;36(5):1032–40.

65. Hanly JG, Skedgel C, Sketris I, et al. Gout in the elderly: a population health study. J Rheumatol 2009;36(4):822–30.

66. Singh JA, Hodges JS, Toscano JP, et al. Quality of care for gout in the US needs improvement. Arthritis Rheum 2007;57(5):822–9.

67. Mikuls TR, Farrar JT, Bilker WB, et al. Suboptimal physician adherence to quality indicators for the management of gout and asymptomatic hyperuricaemia: results from the UK General Practice Research Database (GPRD). Rheumatology (Oxf) 2005;44(8):1038–42.

68. Neogi T, Hunter DJ, Chaisson CE, et al. Frequency and predictors of inappropriate management of recurrent gout attacks in a longitudinal study. J Rheumatol 2006;33(1):104–9.

69. Mikuls TR, Curtis JR, Allison JJ, et al. Medication errors with the use of allopurinol and colchicine: a retrospective study of a national, anonymous Internet-accessible error reporting system. J Rheumatol 2006;33(3):562–6.

Genetics of Gout

Philip L. Riches

KEY POINTS

- Serum urate levels are highly heritable and principally determined by the fractional excretion of uric acid in the kidney. The heritability of gout remains to be properly established.
- Genetic association studies have identified many common variants that contribute to both the variation of serum urate and gout risk. These variants are predominantly expressed in the proximal renal tubule epithelium, where they mediate urate anion transport.
- Marked differences in the frequency of predisposing genetic variants exist between populations.
- Genetic studies do not support the conclusion that elevated serum urate causes cardiovascular disease. Comparative genetic studies suggest there has been evolutionary advantage in having high serum urate levels.
- The absolute contribution of genetic variants to levels of serum urate is relatively small in clinical terms. The most important gene identified to date, *SLC2A9,* accounts for 3.5% of the variation of serum urate.
- Recent advances allow the evaluation of existing and novel uricosuric therapies. Future discoveries may identify novel pathways in the pathogenesis of gout.

Introduction

Humans have high basal levels of serum urate due to mutations of the uricase gene, which render it inactive; consequently, humans, almost uniquely among mammalian species, are prone to gout. Over and above this specieswide increased baseline level of serum urate, a familial clustering of gout cases has long been recognized, although this reflects the importance of shared environmental influence as much as heritability. Initial progress in identifying genetic variants predisposing to gout came from linkage studies performed in rare lineages with monogenic disorders associated with gout and led to advances in the understanding of purine formation and metabolism. Subsequent studies established the control of serum urate to be highly heritable and largely determined by the fractional renal excretion of uric acid. More recently, genomewide association studies of quantitative traits have succeeded in identifying common variants in the general population that are implicated in the renal regulation of urate. It is not surprising that many of these variants have in turn been associated with the development of gout. This chapter will review the evidence for a genetic contribution to hyperuricemia and gout and discuss the approaches that have been used to find the underlying genes. The specific variants identified will be discussed in detail as well as the general insights that genetic studies have given into the role of urate transport in health and disease.

Heritability of Serum Urate and Gout

Initial studies into the heritability of serum urate drew conflicting conclusions on the pattern of inheritance observed, perhaps due to the heterogeneity in serum urate that is observed between populations. One approach to attempt to control for environmental factors has been an analysis of the strength of correlation between identical (monozygotic [MZ]) or nonidentical (dizygotic [DZ]) twins. If stronger correlation is observed between MZ twins than between DZ twins, then this allows an estimate to be made of the inherited contribution to a given trait. Such studies have demonstrated serum urate and subsequently also the renal fractional excretion of urate (FE_{UA}) to be significantly influenced by genetic factors. A correlation of 85% in the FE_{UA} was observed between MZ twins compared to 66% in DZ twins with the overall heritability estimated at 87%, although with broad confidence intervals.[1,2] Subsequently, segregation analysis in families, attempting to control for known environmental factors, has also shown that serum urate has a significant heritable component (heritability 0.4) with the overall pattern of inheritance seen best explained by a complex model incorporating interaction between more than one major gene, several modifying genes, and further environmental factors.[3] This conclusion is broadly supported by the results of genomewide association studies, which have identified multiple genes influencing serum urate.

Many of the genes associated with hyperuricemia, as well as further candidate genes, have in turn been established as contributing to the risk of gout. Estimating the overall size of gout heritability, however, remains difficult, with a dearth of published information. One recent attempt to measure this using a twin study found no evidence of a genetic contribution to incident gout, although the study was not powered to detect a small effect.[4] That serum urate might be the predominant heritable trait, rather than gout itself, might seem counterintuitive, yet a similar phenomenon is observed in the field of osteoporosis; the heritabililty of bone mineral density is well established, yet that of the clinically relevant endpoint of hip fracture has proved difficult to ascertain. This paradox appears to have been resolved by studies showing high heritability of fracture in those under the age of 65 but almost no heritable component after the age of 80, presumably reflecting the major influence of environmental risk factors for falling in the elderly.[5] In gout, establishing the relative importance of genetic and environmental influence remains a major challenge.

Methods of Identifying Susceptibility Genes

Linkage Studies

Initial success in the identification of contributory genes came from the analysis of rare syndromes of hyperuricemia and gout using linkage analysis. In these studies, markers spread across the genome are analyzed in families harboring a disease, and loci common only to those individuals carrying the disease are sought. This approach has proved most useful in identifying rare genetic variants with powerful effect, although it has not been able to identify common genetic variation affecting the general population. The genes involved were often associated with the overproduction of urate. New methods have been required to identify more common variants of modest to weak effects, namely a candidate gene approach or genomewide association studies (GWAS).

Candidate Gene Studies

In candidate gene studies, polymorphic variants in a gene with a putative role in regulation of urate or gout are analyzed. Typically, a case-control design is used for a categorical trait such as gout, and statistical analysis of variance (ANOVA) is used between genotypes for quantitative traits such as serum urate. Although such studies are relatively straightforward to perform, there is an inherent risk of identifying spurious associations. This is particularly true where the samples size is small, but it can also be caused by mistakes in the study design, such as where different populations are recruited as cases and controls. Better design and power of such studies will help reduce these problems, but confirmation of any result requires replication of the finding in independent cohorts. Alternatively, where only a few variants have been assessed in a gene of interest, it is possible to miss a true association caused by further variant at an unrelated part of the gene. While better understanding of conserved genetic regions now allows the comprehensive coverage of variance throughout a gene with analysis of relatively few polymorphisms, it is salutary to note that regulatory variants may be far removed from the gene itself.

Genomewide Association Studies

The availability of mass genotyping technology has allowed the analysis of common genetic variation across the entire genome in large populations. Simultaneous measurement of quantitative traits allows the identification of discrete genomic regions in which greater than expected genetic variation correlates with increased levels of the trait under study, such as serum urate. To date, no GWAS have been performed in a gout population specifically. A major advantage of this approach is that it is hypothesis-free and so allows the identification of entirely unexpected genes or regions of interest and, consequently,

novel pathogenic pathways. Powerful, mass genotyping techniques also have the potential to produce spurious results due to the inherent risk of chance observations caused by multiple testing or, again, through unrecognized population stratification. The solution is to look for replication in different populations or, where available, meta-analysis of such studies.

Overview

A large number of genes involved in the pathogenesis of hyperuricemia and gout have been identified through these approaches, which are discussed in detail later and illustrated in Figure 7-1. Although the precise role of many of the common variants remains to be established, the majority appear to be involved in controlling the renal excretion of uric acid.[6] This is to be expected given that reduced FE_{UA} is the primary mechanism of hyperuricemia in more than 90% of patients with gout.[7]

While there have been great advances in understanding as a result of these approaches, the variants thus far described collectively account for only a small proportion of the observed variance in serum urate, let alone the risk of gout. Performing GWAS in gout may uncover variants involved in novel pathways that contribute to crystal deposition or the subsequent florid inflammation observed. Already, the astonishing advances in mass genotyping techniques mean that GWAS are being replaced by whole exome or indeed genome sequencing. These techniques offer great promise in identifying novel, probably rare, variants; however, there will be new challenges in the rigorous analysis of such large volumes of data. Of course, there will always remain the need to perform the painstaking work of demonstrating the functional consequences of suggested mutations.

Single Gene Disorders Associated With Gout

A number of rare disorders have been described that are typically complicated by hyperuricemia and gout. Such diseases are frequently caused by mutations in a single gene and have demonstrated that both overproduction of urate and diminished renal excretion of urate can result in hyperuricemia and clinical gout (Table 7-1).

Lesch-Nyhan Syndrome

Inactivating mutations in the hypoxanthine-guanine phosphoribosyl transferase (*HPRT*) gene, an enzyme involved in the purine salvage pathway, can cause hyperuricemia and gout in the form of Lesch-Nyhan syndrome.[8] As discussed in detail in Chapter 3, this is an X-linked recessive disorder associated with overproduction of serum urate, neurologic dysfunction, and behavioral disturbance. The neurologic deficits appear unrelated to hyperuricemia and are more likely explained by disturbance of purine-mediated neurotransmission.[9]

Uromodulin-Associated Kidney Diseases

Both autosomal dominant and recessive syndromes of progressive nephropathy and early-onset gout have been described associated with mutations of the uromodulin gene.

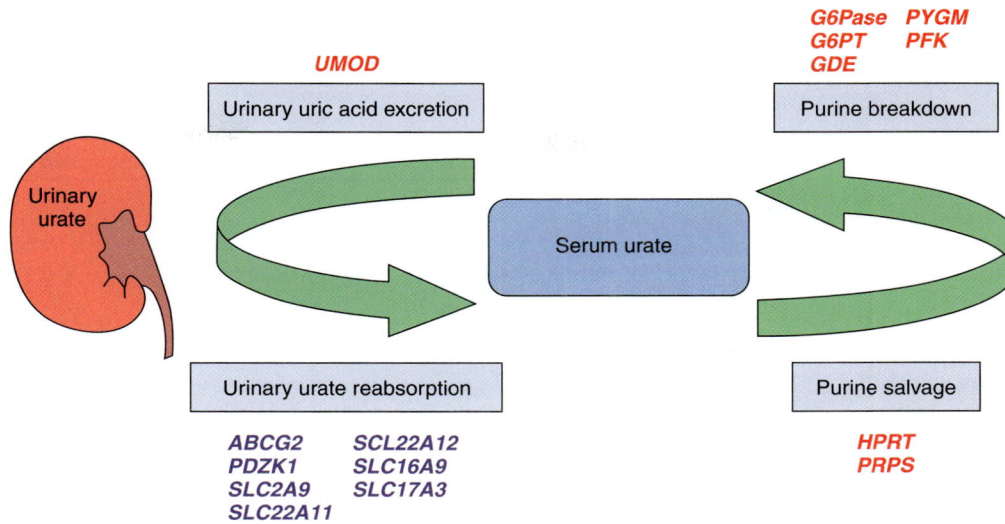

Figure 7-1 Role of genetic variants so far identified in urate homeostasis. Early studies identified rare variants with strong effects (shown in *red*). *UMOD* (uromodulin) mutations result in medullary cystic kidney disease and hyperuricemic nephropathy with associated renal impairment and diminished urate excretion. Glycogen storage diseases are associated with increased cell breakdown and production of urate: G6Pase (glucose-6-phosphatase), G6PT (glucose-6-phosphate transporter), GDE (glycogen debranching enzyme), PYGM (muscle glycogen phosphorylase), and PFK (phosphofructokinase). Disorders of the purine salvage pathway are caused by mutations of *HPRT* (hypoxanthine guanine phosphoribosyl transferase) and *PRPS* (phosphoribosyl pyrophosphate synthetase). Common variants (shown in *blue*) predominantly increase the reabsorption of urate from the kidney: ABCG2 (ATP binding cassette family), SLC family members (solute carrier proteins), and PDZK1 (postsynaptic density protein 95/*Drosophila* Disks large/Zona occludens-1).

Table 7-1 Mendelian Syndromes Associated With Hyperuricemia and Gout

Disease	Locus	Inheritance	Gene	Phenotype
SYNDROMES OF ALTERED PURINE METABOLISM				
HPRT related	Xq26-q27.2	XD	Hypoxanthine guanine phosphoribosyl transferase (*HPRT 1*)	Hyperuricemia, gout, neurologic dysfunction
PRPS related	Xq22-q24	XD	Phosphoribosyl pyrophosphate synthetase 1 (*PRPS 1*)	Hyperuricemia, gout
SYNDROMES OF EXCESSIVE CELL DEATH AND URATE GENERATION				
Glycogen storage disease type Ia	17q21	AR	Glucose-6-phosphatase	Growth retardation, hypoglycemia, hepatomegaly, hyperuricemia, gout, lactic acidosis
Glycogen storage disease type Ib	11q23	AR	Glucose 6 phosphate transporter	Growth retardation, hypoglycemia, hepatomegaly, hyperuricemia, gout, lactic acidosis
Glycogen storage disease type III	1q21	AR	Glycogen debranching enzyme	Early-onset hyperuricemia, gout
Glycogen storage disease type V	11q13	AR	Muscle glycogen phosphorylase	Early-onset hyperuricemia, gout
Glycogen storage disease type VII	12q13.3	AR	Muscle phosphofructokinase	Early-onset hyperuricemia, gout
SYNDROMES OF REDUCED RENAL EXCRETION OF URIC ACID				
Medullary cystic kidney disease, type 1	1q21	AD	Unknown	Variable penetrance: renal dysfunction, hypertension, gout
Medullary cystic kidney disease, type 2	16p12.3	AD/AR	Uromodulin	Progressive renal dysfunction, variable hyperuricemia, early-onset gout
Familial juvenile hyperuricemic nephropathy	16p12.3	AD	Uromodulin	Progressive renal dysfunction, variable hyperuricemia, early-onset gout

A variety of mutations lead to the defective transport and apical membrane expression of uromodulin, a protein expressed abundantly in the thick ascending limb of the loop of Henle.[10] An early feature of these diseases is reduced fractional excretion of uric acid. Defective uromodulin secretion caused by protein misfolding correlates directly with decreased urine osmolarity and decreased urinary uric acid excretion, although the mechanism remains uncertain.[11,12] It is interesting to note that a polymorphism associated with diminished uromodulin secretion is associated with a reduced risk of hypertension.[13]

Other Monogenic Disorders

As reviewed in Chapter 3, X-linked dominant inheritance of primary hyperuricemia and gout is seen with activating mutations in phosphoribosyl pyrophosphatase synthetase,[14] an enzyme involved in urate synthesis. Gout and hyperuricemia can also complicate glycogen storage diseases[15] and some other rare inborn errors of metabolism through the overproduction of serum urate induced by cell breakdown (see Table 7-1).

Candidate Genes Regulating Hyperuricemia and Gout

Great progress has been made in understanding the pathogenesis of hyperuricemia and gout through genetic association studies. The genes identified are listed alphabetically and summarized in Table 7-2. The majority of genes identified in the regulation of serum urate are expressed in the renal proximal convoluted tubule epithelium, as illustrated in Figure 7-2, emphasizing the importance of this region in the regulation of serum urate. *ABCG2* may also act by mediating urate efflux into the small intestine, where urate can ultimately be degraded by uricase expressed in colonic bacterial flora. Similarly, extrarenal effects of *SLC2A9* appear to be important given that variants of *SLC2A9* associated more closely with the serum level of urate, rather than the FE_{UA}.[16]

ABCG2

Polymorphisms in the *ABCG2* gene have been consistently associated with serum urate by GWAS and replicated in cases of clinical gout from Caucasian, African, and Asian populations.[17-20] The strongest association across these populations is with a coding single nucleotide polymorphism (SNP) in exon 5 of the gene (rs2231142), which leads to a glutamine-to-lysine amino acid substitution (Q141 K). This SNP also emerged as the strongest predictor of urate levels after *SLC2A9* in a meta-analysis of genomewide studies accounting for 0.57% of the variation of serum urate.[6] A stronger effect size was seen in men than in women. The *ABCG2* gene encodes a transporter of the ATP-binding cassette (ABC) family, which is expressed in the apical plasma membrane of human kidney proximal tubule epithelial cells, and has been shown to transport urate. Introduction of the glutamine-to-lysine substitution in vitro has been shown to cause a 53% reduction in urate transport by *ABCG2*, suggesting that this is the pathologic variant and that *ABCG2* functions as an efflux transporter of urate.[21] The consistent identification of this variant across diverse populations with distinctive haplotype structures also supports this conclusion.

Table 7-2 Common Genetic Variants Associated With Serum Urate

Gene	Explained Variability Serum Urate	Effect Size in Gout	Populations in Whom Association With Gout Shown
ABCG2	0.57%	1.7–2.0	African American, Caucasian, Chinese, Japanese, Polynesian
GCKR	0.13%	...	...
LRRC16A	0.12%	...	...
PDZK1	0.19%	...	...
SLC2A9	3.53%	1.3–5.0	Caucasian, Chinese, Polynesian
SLC16A9	0.17%	...	...
SLC17 locus	0.19%	1.2–1.9	Caucasian, Japanese
SLC22A11	0.19%	...	...
SLC22A12	0.13%	1.2–1.8	Chinese, Mexican American, Solomon Island

The estimates of explained variability in serum urate are derived from a meta-analysis of genomewide association studies in Caucasian individuals.[6] These estimates are based on the strongest single nucleotide polymorphism from each locus. Those loci that have had a confirmed effect in gout are shown with the effect size (odds ratio) for single copy of the risk variant shown.[63]

Polymorphisms of *ABCG2* appear to be a particularly strong risk factor for gout in Asian populations, in whom the frequency of the Q141 K risk allele has been reported to be as high as 32%.[18,22] By contrast, the allele frequency in Caucasian populations has been reported to be approximately 12%.[20] An independent nonsynonymous polymorphism of *ABCG2*, Q126X, that is associated with hyperuricemia and gout has also been described in a Japanese population although the functional effect of this variant is not yet fully characterised.[23] A final insight into the importance of differences between populations comes from an analysis of Polynesians. Surprisingly, although both Maoris and Pacific Islanders are known to be at a greatly increased risk of gout, the Q141 K variant is only significantly associated with gout in western Polynesians, presumably due to the chance depletion of this allele during eastward migrations.[24]

SLC2A9

The *SLC2A9* gene has been consistently identified as an important regulator of serum urate and urine uric acid excretion by GWAS in diverse populations.[20,25-27] In addition, variants of *SLC2A9* have shown significant association with cohorts of clinical gout in Caucasian, Chinese, and Pacific Island populations.[20,27-29] The effect of variation in *SLC2A9* is most pronounced in females, in whom it accounts for approximately 6% of the variance of serum urate, compared with 2% in males. The overall effect for both genders is 3.5%.[6,25] The *SLC2A9* gene encodes a membrane spanning protein from the major facilitator transporter superfamily and includes elements of sugar transporters—indeed, it was initially assumed to be a fructose transporter.[30] Functional studies in *Xenopus* oocytes have shown that *SLC2A9* encodes a highly efficient transporter of urate anion, with a capacity far higher than the only

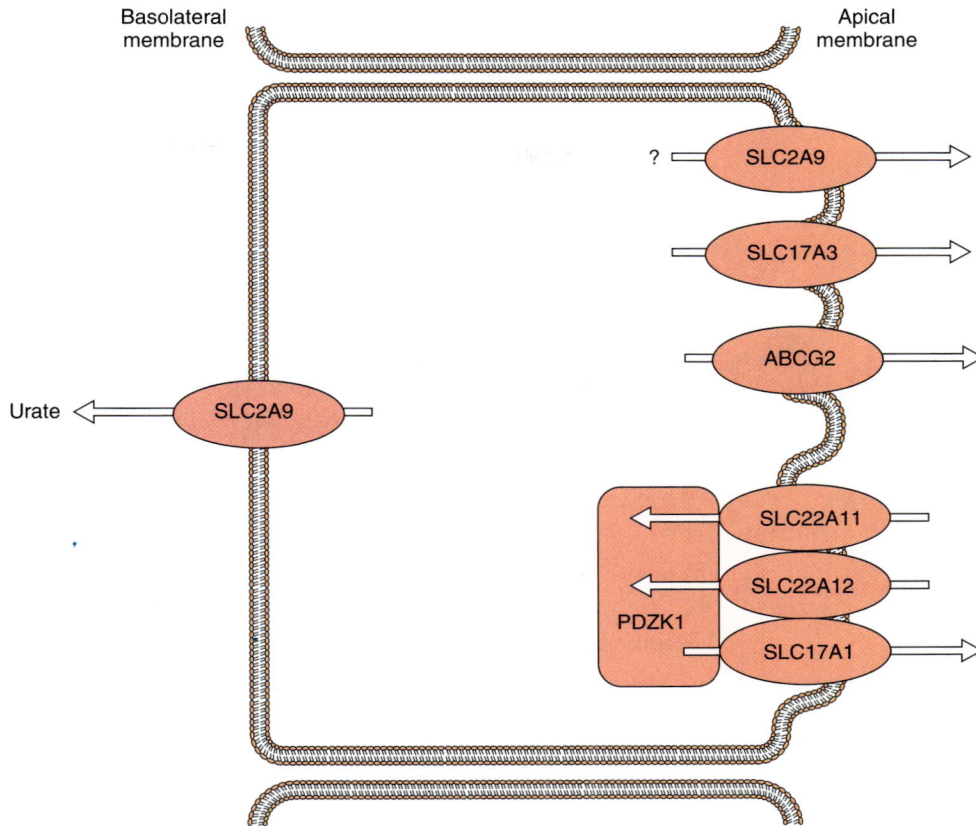

Figure 7-2 Genes associated with hyperuricemia expressed in the proximal renal tubule. The likely direction of transport or urate anion is indicated by *plain arrows*. *ABCG2* is a unidirectional transporter expressed on the apical membrane. *SLC2A9* is a voltage-driven urate transporter whose dominant effect is to mediate urate reabsorption via its basolaterally expressed form. The direction of transport of the apical form is not yet established. *SLC22A12* encodes URAT1, the first established urate transporter, and *SLC22A11* encodes OAT4. *SLC17A1* encodes NPT1 and *SLC17A3* encodes NPT4, which appear to mediate urate efflux, although due to significant linkage disequilibrium, it is not clear which gene has the predominant effect. PDZK1 is a scaffolding protein involved in the assembly of a transporter complex in the apical membrane.

previously described urate transporter URAT1.[27] Although capable of transporting sugars in vitro, it is approximately 50 times more effective as a urate transporter.[31] There is no evidence to support a direct inhibitory interaction between sugars and urate transport, although exogenous glucose has been shown to trans-stimulate urate efflux from cells.[27,31]

The *SLC2A9* gene has two major transcript variants, and, importantly, the long isoform of *SLC2A9* is expressed on the basolateral membrane of proximal renal tubular epithelial cells, with loss of function resulting in hypouricemia,[32,33] suggesting it is the dominant mediator of urate movement from renal tubular epithelial cells back into the bloodstream. A shorter isoform localizes to the apical membrane of proximal renal tubular cells,[34] and it has been assumed that this mediates absorption of urate from the renal tubule. Certainly both isoforms of *SLC2A9* have urate transporter activity[31] although this has been shown to be voltage dependent, favoring efflux from the cell. This suggests that apical *SLC2A9* physiologically might secrete urate back into the renal tubule,[35] but it should be noted that hepatic *SLC2A9* in dogs is a key promoter of urate influx into hepatocytes, where the urate is degraded by hepatic peroxisomal uricase.

Although five polymorphisms of *SLC2A9* have been reported that result in nonsynonymous amino acid substitutions, these have typically shown less significant associations with serum urate than noncoding variants. Only one study has found the strongest association with a coding polymorphism (V253I),[20] and this finding has not been replicated nor have any functional consequences of this variant been reported. In view of this, the many coding polymorphisms are most likely to be in linkage disequilibrium with causal variations in promoter or enhancer sequences that predispose to gout by altering levels of gene expression. Supporting this, there is evidence that expression levels of *SLC2A9* may play a greater role in determining serum urate levels than functional variants.[25]

Rare homozygous loss-of-function mutations of *SLC2A9* have been reported in individuals with hypouricemia, nephrolithiasis, or exercise-induced acute renal failure (EIARF). These patients have very low residual urate transport activity (19% to 38% of normal), high fractional excretion of uric acid (greater than 150%), and very low serum urate concentrations (mean 0.17 mg/dl).[32] A less severe phenotype is seen in patients with heterozygous mutations in *SLC2A9*, which is associated with partial reductions in urate transport activity (about 50% to 75% of normal activity), and most of whom were asymptomatic but some of whom developed nephrolithiasis or EIARF.[27,33,35] Whether the occurrence of EIARF is mediated entirely by abnormalities in renal uric acid

SLC17 locus

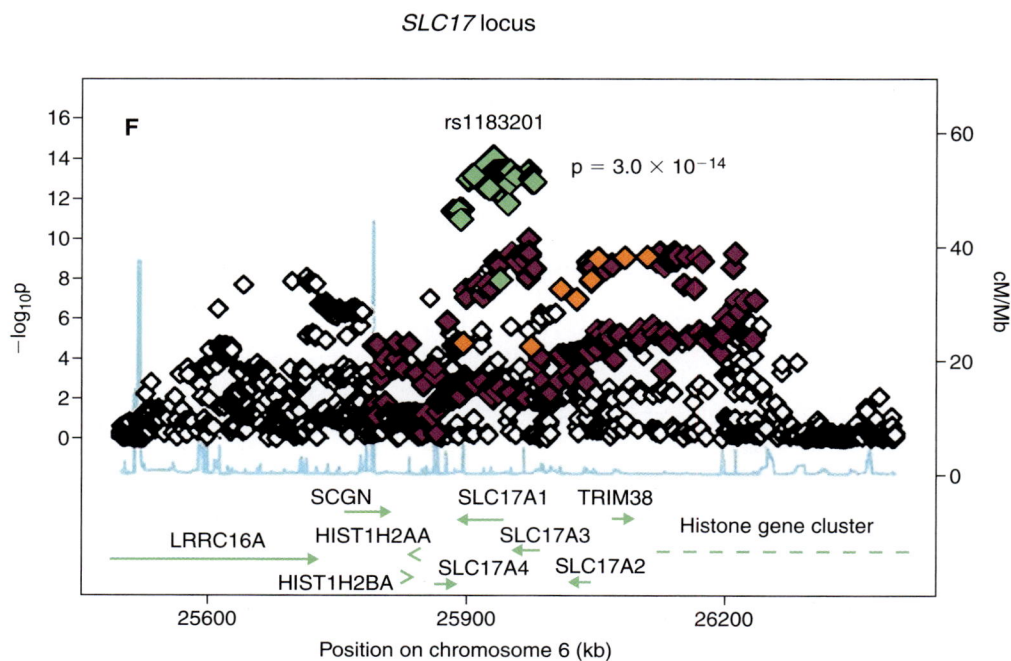

Figure 7-3 Linkage disequilibrium in the *SLC17* locus. Regional association plot showing extensive linkage disequilibrium in the region surrounding single nucleotide polymorphism (SNP) rs1183201.[6] Diamonds in *green* indicate the most significant SNP in the region, while other SNPs in the region are given as color-coded smaller *diamonds*. Green diamonds indicate high correlation with the lead SNP ($r^2 > 0.8$), *orange diamonds* indicate moderate correlation with the most significant SNP ($0.5 < r^2 < 0.8$), *purple* indicates markers in weak correlation with the most significant SNP ($0.2 < r^2 < 0.5$), *white* indicates no correlation with the most significant SNP ($r^2 < 0.2$). Estimated recombination rates (HapMap Phase II) are given in *light blue*, genes as well as the direction of transcription (NCBI) are displayed by *green bars*. Further fine mapping will be required to identify any causal variant(s) within this region. http://en.wikipedia.org/wiki/File:Xanthin_-_Xanthine.svg. *ABC*, ATP binding cassette; *EIARF*, exercise-induced acute renal failure; *G6Pase*, glucose-6-phosphatase; *G6PT*, glucose-6-phosphate transporter; *GDE*, glycogen debranching enzyme; *GWAS*, genomewide association study; *HPRT*, hypoxanthine guanine phosphoribosyl transferase; *LD*, linkage disequilibrium; *PRPS*, phosphoribosyl pyrophosphatase synthetase; *PYGM*, muscle glycogen phosphorylase; *PFK*, phosphofructokinase; *PDZK1*, postsynaptic density protein 95/*Drosophila* Disks large/Zona occludens-1; *SLC*, solute carrier; *SNP*, single nucleotide polymorphism; *UMOD*, uromodulin.

deposition or also in processes such as reduced blood antioxidant capacity and oxygen free radical–induced renal vasoconstriction[32,36] remains unclear. However, it is known that urate accounts for about 60% of the antioxidant capacity in human plasma.[37]

SLC2A9 is known to be expressed in human articular chondrocytes,[38] and cartilage is a site of urate deposition in gout; synovial tissue itself also has been shown to express urate transporters. The extent to which this transport is coordinated and regulated is currently not known but it is of great interest in understanding the pathogenesis of tophus formation in gout.

SLC17 Locus

Polymorphisms in a locus on 6p21 that contains three members of the *SLC17* gene family (*SLC17A3, SLC17A1,* and *SLC17A4*) were identified as significant predictors of serum urate levels and gout by GWAS in Caucasian populations.[20] The strongest association was with rs1165205 within intron 1 of *SLC17A3*, but several other SNPs within the locus reached genomewide significance. The *SLC17A3* gene encodes a sodium phosphate transporter (*NPT4*), which is expressed at the apical plasma membrane of renal proximal tubule epithelial cells. Functional studies have confirmed *NPT4* to be

capable of urate transport, and patients with hyperuricemia and missense mutations of *NPT4* have been reported, suggesting that it secretes urate from the apical membrane of the proximal tubule.[39] To complicate matters, a subsequent meta-analysis identified a different SNP (rs1183201) within *SLC17A1* as the strongest predictor of serum urate within this locus[6] (Figure 7-3). The *SLC17A1* gene lies immediately downstream of *SLC17A3* and encodes *NPT1*, which is expressed in the human kidney and has been shown to be a voltage-driven urate anion transporter in vitro.[40] A missense SNP was identified in *SLC17A1* (T269I) that reached genomewide significance in the Framingham study but was in strong linkage disequilibrium with rs116205 within *SLC17A3*. Because of the strong linkage disequilibrium in this locus, further studies will be required to identify the causal SNP that regulates serum urate levels and susceptibility to gout.

SLC22A12

As reviewed in Chapter 4, *SLC22A12*, encoding URAT1, was the first confirmed urate transporter and was identified by its homology to the organic anion transporter family. It is expressed on the apical plasma membrane of renal tubular epithelial cells, and loss-of-function mutations identified in Japanese patients are associated with hypouricemia, suggesting that it plays an important role in the renal uptake of urinary urate.[41] Variation of *SLC22A12* has also been associated with clinical gout in non-Caucasian populations.[42] By contrast, no mutations of *SLC22A12* were found in a small population of Caucasian patients with hypouricemia,[43] nor has it been associated with clinical gout.[44] *SLC22A12* has not emerged as a major determinant of serum urate levels in recent GWAS, although the coverage of URAT1 in most panels of SNPs is poor.[25] In mice, the loss of URAT1 has a relatively minor effect on urate metabolism, suggesting that other transporters are at least as important.[45] Although polymorphisms of *SLC22A12* have been associated with raised serum urate levels and decreased fractional urate excretion in Caucasians,[46] the functional mechanisms that underlie these associations remain unclear. Overall, a recent meta-analysis of studies in populations of European descent suggested *SLC22A12* contributed only 0.13% of variance in SUA, although even this effect remains difficult to interpret due to close linkage disequilibrium with the low-affinity urate transporter *SLC22A11*.[6]

Tumor Necrosis Factor-α

A polymorphism in the gene encoding tumor necrosis factor (TNF)-α has been associated with gout in a small study of 106 male Taiwanese patients and 159 control subjects[47] but not replicated in a similarly sized Chinese cohort.[48] Although this is of interest because of the well-recognized role of TNF-α in inflammatory arthritis, this finding must remain in doubt until it is replicated in an adequately powered study.

Transforming Growth Factor-β1

The inflammation suppressor cytokine transforming growth factor (TGF)-β1 has been shown to be expressed in gouty tophi and appears likely to play a role in reducing leukocyte infiltration and hence arthritic attacks and/or tophus formation.[49] A polymorphism in the TGF-β1 gene has been associated with tophus formation in a small cohort of 73 Taiwanese gout patients, although not with the development of gout itself or with other severity markers such as age of onset or frequency of attacks.[50] Once again, this is potentially of great interest, but the result requires to be replicated in an adequately powered study.

Additional Candidate Genes Associated With Hyperuricemia

Meta-analysis of 14 GWAS with a total of 28,141 European participants have identified five additional loci as being associated with serum urate levels. These loci are *SLC22A11*, the glucokinase regulatory protein (*GCKR*) gene, *SLC16A9*, the *LRRC16A* gene coding for Carmil, and near PDZ domain containing 1 (*PDZK1*) gene.[6]

The *SLC22A11* gene encodes OAT4, a solute transporter in the same family as URAT1, which has been shown to be a low-affinity urate transporter.[51] The scaffolding proteins PDZK1 and Na+/H+ exchange regulatory factor-1 (NHERF1) have been reported to interact directly with several key transporters including OAT4, URAT1, and NPT1 and appear to be involved in the assembly of a transporter complex.[52] Potentially this would allow the balanced secretion (NPT1) and

reabsorption (URAT1) of urate in the apical membrane of the renal proximal tubule epithelial cells, along with other anions. The *GCKR* gene is predominantly expressed in liver, where it stabilizes and regulates glucokinase, and mice with targeted inactivation of *CGKR* have impaired glucose tolerance.[53] It has been suggested that *GCKR* variants may cause hyperuricemia by causing insulin resistance.[6] The *SLC16A9* gene encodes monocarboxylic acid transporter MCT9, which is expressed in the kidney and appears likely to indirectly influence urate reabsorption. The *LRRC16A* gene product Carmil has been shown to be expressed in kidney and epithelial tissues and is a key inhibitor of actin capping protein, regulating polymerization.[54] The mechanisms by which variants at this gene locus regulate serum urate remain unclear.

Variation in the *ADRB3* gene encoding the β3-adrenergic receptor has been associated with the development of hyperuricemia in a prospective cohort from Spain, presumably via induction of insulin resistance. This finding awaits replication and functional characterization.

MTHFR gene variants (methylene tetrahydrofolate reductase) have also been associated with hyperuricemia in several small Asian cohorts.[55] The mechanism has yet to be established. The same variant CT677 has been extensively studied in relation to homocysteine levels and cardiovascular disease, although it remains uncertain whether there is any significant association.[56]

Genetic Insights Into Urate Transport

Insights From Other Mammalian Species

Clues to the role of urate transport in health and disease have emerged through genetic studies in both human and other mammalian species. Humans and other primates have uniquely high basal levels of serum urate due to mutations of the uricase gene, which render it inactive. Although there is a common mutation shared by humans, chimpanzees, and orangutans, an independent deletion event is found in gibbons suggesting that survival advantage in hominid species accrues from this loss of uricase activity.[57] Numerous potential benefits of normal serum urate levels of humans (i.e, approximately 5 to 6 mg/dL) have been proposed including neuroprotective effects as well as the adjuvant effects of urate crystals.[58,59] The identification of genetic variants associated with hyperuricemia allows these hypotheses to be tested. To date, variants associated with hyperuricemia have been associated with a later age of onset of Alzheimer disease[60] and improvement in memory function.[61]

By an unhappy coincidence for their breed, a founder inactivating mutation in the orthologue of *SLC2A9* is found in all Dalmatian dogs. This appears to result in functional loss of uricase activity due to loss of *SLC2A9* mediated hepatic uptake, as the liver is the major site of uricase activity. As a consequence, Dalmatians suffer from hyperuricemia. In humans, the long isoform of *SLC2A9* remains strongly expressed in the liver,[34] and although the relevance of this is uncertain, the liver is, of course, the major site of purine synthesis. Dalmatians also suffer from hyperuricosuria and urinary tract uric acid stones due to their inability to reabsorb urinary urate,[62] in a fashion similar to humans with loss-of-function mutations of *SLC2A9*.

Gene–Environment Interaction

Effects of genetic variation may be unmasked by changes in lifestyle. This is demonstrated dramatically by a rapid rise in incidence of gout in New Zealand Maori, who now have one of the highest prevalences of gout worldwide (affecting 15% of men) yet in whom gout was reportedly rare prior to Westernization.[63] Examination of genetic influence on gout and hyperuricemia is complicated greatly by the extent and variability of environmental influence, and a major challenge is improving the measurement and recording of such influences in future studies.

These same lifestyle issues in Western populations are associated with the epidemic of metabolic syndrome, which comprises the association of obesity, insulin resistance, hypertension, and dyslipidemia with a consequently increased risk of cardiovascular disease. Elevated serum urate has long been associated with the metabolic syndrome, although it remains unclear whether it is a cause or a consequence of cardiovascular risk factors and/or disease.[64] As a result, serum urate has variously been considered an inert end product, a beneficial antioxidant, or, more recently, a harmful mediator of endothelial damage. The role of serum urate has been reexamined using the genetic variants associated with hyperuricemia to strip out the confounding influences in the metabolic syndrome, and overall these results do not support a causative role for elevated serum urate in cardiovascular disease. An additive score of the eight strongest loci for serum urate has been analyzed in a meta-analysis of GWAS involving 28,283 individuals, with the results replicated in a further large cohort of 22,054 women. No association between the genetic urate score and coronary heart disease, glucose, blood pressure, or renal impairment was observed.[65] Similarly, no association has been found between variants of *SLC2A9* and metabolic syndrome or blood pressure.[27,31] A large case-control study analyzing the GCKR rs780094 polymorphism found it to be associated with dyslipidemia but a reduced risk of type 2 diabetes.[66] Consistent with all these findings, a "Mendelian randomization" approach has found the weight of evidence to be against a causal relationship between urate levels and the metabolic syndrome.[67]

Clinical Implications

At the present time, asymptomatic hyperuricemia is not considered to be an indication for urate-lowering therapy,[68] and in clinical practice, urate-lowering treatment for gout is currently advised only in patients with specific indications, as discussed elsewhere in this book. The identification of alleles that increase the risk of gout could in the future be used in targeting high-risk patients for earlier intervention with urate-lowering therapy. However, the relative contribution of the currently identified genes to serum urate variability has been estimated at between 0.12% and 3.53% only (see Table 7-2), and so, at present, genetic profiling seems unlikely to affect clinical decision making. This may well change as new variants are identified by whole genome sequencing technologies or through identification of novel genetic variation such as methylation pattern or copy number.

Another potential application of these genetic studies lies in the development of therapeutics. The identification of the key transporters of urate anion in the proximal convoluted tubule makes possible the intelligent screening of compound libraries for novel uricosuric therapeutics, as well as the reassessment of existing therapies.[69]

In future a better understanding of the pathogenesis of crystal deposition and inflammation may enable entirely new therapeutic strategies to be developed.

References

1. Boyle JA, Greig WR, Jasani MK, et al. Relative roles of genetic and environmental factors in the control of serum uric acid levels in normouricaemic subjects. Ann Rheum Dis 1967;26:234–8.
2. Emmerson BT, Nagel SL, Duffy DL, et al. Genetic-control of the renal clearance of urate: a study of twins. Ann Rheum Dis 1992;51:375–7.
3. Wilk JB, Djousse L, Borecki I, et al. Segregation analysis of serum uric acid in the NHLBI Family Heart Study. Hum Genet 2000;106:355–9.
4. Krishnan E, Lessov-Schlaggar CN, Fries JF, et al. Hyperuricemia and gout: nature versus nurture. Arthritis Rheum 2010;62:S364.
5. Ralston SH, Uitterlinden AG. Genetics of osteoporosis. Endocrine Rev 2010;31:629–62.
6. Kolz M, Johnson T, Sanna S, et al: for the EUROSPAN Consortium, for the ENGAGE Consortium, for the PROCARDIS Consortium, for the KORA Study, and for the WTCCC. Meta-analysis of 28,141 individuals identifies common variants within five new loci that influence uric acid concentrations. PLoS Genet 2009;5:e1000504.
7. Choi HK, Mount DB, Reginato AM. Pathogenesis of gout. Ann Intern Med 2005;143:499–516.
8. Jinnah HA, De Gregorio L, Harris JC, et al. The spectrum of inherited mutations causing HPRT deficiency: 75 new cases and a review of 196 previously reported cases. Mutat Res 2000;463:309–26.
9. Deutsch SI, Long KD, Rosse RB, et al. Hypothesized deficiency of guanine-based purines may contribute to abnormalities of neurodevelopment, neuromodulation, and neurotransmission in Lesch-Nyhan syndrome. Clin Neuropharmacol 2005;28.
10. Vyletál P, Stiburková B, Kublová M, et al. Alterations of uromodulin biology: a common denominator of the genetically heterogeneous FJHN/MCKD syndrome. Kidney Int 2006;70:1155–69.
11. Williams SE, Reed AAC, Galvanovskis J, et al. Uromodulin mutations causing familial juvenile hyperuricaemic nephropathy lead to protein maturation defects and retention in the endoplasmic reticulum. Hum Mol Genet 2009.
12. Scolari F, Caridi G, Rampoldi L, et al. Uromodulin storage diseases: clinical aspects and mechanisms. Am J Kidney Dis 2004;44:987–99.
13. Padmanabhan S, Melander O, Johnson T, et al. Global BPgen Consortium. Genome-wide association study of blood pressure extremes identifies variant near UMOD associated with hypertension. PLoS Genet 2010;6:e1001177.
14. Ahmed M, Taylor W, Smith PR, et al. Accelerated transcription of PRPS1 in X-linked overactivity of normal human phosphoribosylpyrophosphate synthetase. J Biol Chem 1999;274:7482–8.
15. Reginato AM, Olsen BR. Genetics and experimental models of crystal-induced arthritis. Lessons learned from mice and men: is it crystal clear? Curr Opin Rheumatol 2007;19:134–45.
16. Rule AD, de Andrade M, Matsumoto M, et al. Association between SLC2A9 transporter gene variants and uric acid phenotypes in African American and white families. Rheumatology 2010. doi:10.1093/rheumatology/keq425.
17. Stark K, Reinhard W, Grassl M, et al. Common polymorphisms influencing serum uric acid levels contribute to susceptibility to gout, but not to coronary artery disease. PLoS ONE 2009;4:e7729.
18. Yamagishi K, Tanigawa T, Kitamura A, et al. The rs2231142 variant of the ABCG2 gene is associated with uric acid levels and gout among Japanese people. Rheumatology 2010;49:1461–5.
19. Wang B, Miao Z, Liu S, et al. Genetic analysis of *ABCG2* gene C421A polymorphism with gout disease in Chinese Han male population. Hum Genet 2010;127:245–246.
20. Dehghan A, Kottgen A, Yang Q, et al. Association of three genetic loci with uric acid concentration and risk of gout: a genome-wide association study. Lancet 2008;372:1953–61.
21. Woodward OM, Kottgen A, Coresh J, et al. Identification of a urate transporter, ABCG2, with a common functional polymorphism causing gout. Proc Natl Acad Sci U S A 2009;106:10338–42.
22. Wang B, Miao Z, Liu S, et al. Genetic analysis of ABCG2 gene C421A polymorphism with gout disease in Chinese Han male population. Hum Genet 2010;127:245–6.

23. Matsuo H, Takada T, Ichida K, et al. Common defects of ABCG2, a high-capacity urate exporter, cause gout: a function-based genetic analysis in a Japanese population. Science Transl Med 2009;1:5ra11.
24. Phipps-Green AJ, Hollis-Moffatt JE, Dalbeth N, et al. A strong role for the ABCG2 gene in susceptibility to gout in New Zealand Pacific Island and Caucasian, but not Maori, case and control sample sets. Hum Mol Genet.
25. Doring A, Gieger C, Mehta D, et al. SLC2A9 influences uric acid concentrations with pronounced sex-specific effects. Nat Genet 2008;40:430–6.
26. Wallace C, Newhouse SJ, Braund P, et al. Genome-wide association study identifies genes for biomarkers of cardiovascular disease: serum urate and dyslipidemia. Am J Hum Genet 2008;82:139–49.
27. Vitart V, Rudan I, Hayward C, et al. SLC2A9 is a newly identified urate transporter influencing serum urate concentration, urate excretion and gout. Nat Genet 2008;40:437–42.
28. Stark K, Reinhard W, Neureuther K, et al. Association of common polymorphisms in GLUT9 gene with gout but not with coronary artery disease in a large case-control study. PLoS ONE 2008;3:e1948.
29. Hollis-Moffat JE, Xu X, Dalbeth N, et al. Role of the urate transporter SLC2A9 gene in susceptibility to gout in New Zealand Maori, Pacific Island, and Caucasian case-control sample sets. Arthritis Rheum 2009;60:3485–92.
30. Manolescu AR, Augustin R, Moley K, et al. A highly conserved hydrophobic motif in the exofacial vestibule of fructose transporting SLC2A proteins acts as a critical determinant of their substrate selectivity. Mol Membr Biol 2007;24:455–63.
31. Caulfield MJ, Munroe PB, O'Neill D, et al. SLC2A9 is a high-capacity urate transporter in humans. PLoS Med 2008;5:1509–23.
32. Dinour D, Gray NK, Campbell S, et al. Homozygous SLC2A9 mutations cause severe renal hypouricemia. J Am Soc Nephrol 2010;21:64–72.
33. Matsuo H, Chiba T, Nagamori S, et al. Mutations in glucose transporter 9 gene SLC2A9 cause renal hypouricemia. Am J Hum Genet 2008;83:744–51.
34. Augustin R, Carayannopoulos MO, Dowd LO, et al. Identification and characterization of human glucose transporter-like protein-9 (GLUT9): alternative splicing alters trafficking. J Biol Chem 2004;279:16229–36.
35. Anzai N, Ichida K, Jutabha P, et al. Plasma urate level is directly regulated by a voltage-driven urate efflux transporter URATv1 (SLC2A9) in humans. J Biol Chem 2008;283:26834–8.
36. Sperling O. Hereditary renal hypouricemia. Mol Genet Metab 2009;89:14–8.
37. Waring WS, McKnight JA, Webb DJ, et al. Uric acid restores endothelial function in patients with type 1 diabetes and regular smokers. Diabetes 2006;55:3127–32.
38. Richardson S, Neama G, Phillips I, et al. Molecular characterization and partial cDNA cloning of facilitative glucose transporters expressed in human articular chondrocytes; stimulation of 2-deoxyglucose uptake by IGF-I and elevated MMP-2 secretion by glucose deprivation. Osteoarthritis Cartilage 2003;11:92–101.
39. Jutabha P, Anzai N, Kitamura K, et al. Human sodium phosphate transporter 4 (hNPT4/SLC17A3) as a common renal secretory pathway for drugs and urate. J Biol Chem 2010;285:35123–32.
40. Uchino H, Tamai I, Yamashita K, et al. p-Aminohippuric acid transport at renal apical membrane mediated by human inorganic phosphate transporter NPT1. Biochem Biophys Res Commun 2000;270:254–9.
41. Enomoto A, Kimura H, Chairoungdua A, et al. Molecular identification of a renal urate anion exchanger that regulates blood urate levels. Nature 2002;417:447–52.
42. Vazquez-Mellado J, Jimenez-Vaca AL, Cuevas-Covarrubias S, et al. Molecular analysis of the SLC22A12 (URAT1) gene in patients with primary gout. Rheumatology 2007;46:215–9.
43. Tzovaras V, Chatzikyriakidou A, Bairaktari E, et al. Absence of SLC22A12 gene mutations in Greek Caucasian patients with primary renal hypouricaemia. Scand J Clin Lab Investig 2007;67:589–95.
44. Stark R, Andre C, Thierry D, et al. The expression of cytokine and cytokine receptor genes in long-term bone marrow culture in congenital and acquired bone marrow hypoplasias. Br J Haematol 1993;83:560–6.
45. Eraly SA, Vallon V, Rieg T, et al. Multiple organic anion transporters contribute to net renal excretion of uric acid. Physiol Genom 2008;33:180–92.
46. Graessler J, Graessler A, Unger S, et al. Association of the human urate transporter 1 with reduced renal uric acid excretion and hyperuricemia in a German Caucasian population. Arthritis Rheum 2006;54:292–300.
47. Chang SJ, Tsai PC, Chen CJ, et al. The polymorphism -863C/A in tumour necrosis factor gene contributes an independent association to gout. Rheumatology 2007;46:1662–6.
48. Chen ML, Tsai FJ, Tsai CH, et al. Tumor necrosis factor-alpha and interleukin-4 gene polymorphisms in Chinese patients with gout. Clin Exp Rheumatol 2007;25:385–9.
49. Dalbeth N, Pool B, Gamble GD, et al. Cellular characterization of the gouty tophus: a quantitative analysis. Arthritis Rheum 2010;62:1549–56.
50. Chang SJ, Chen CJ, Tsai FC, et al. C. Associations between gout tophus and polymorphisms 869T/C and 509C/T in transforming growth factor +¦1 gene. Rheumatology 2008;47:617–21.
51. Hagos Y, Stein D, Ugele B, et al. Human renal organic anion transporter 4 operates as an asymmetric urate transporter. J Am Soc Nephrol 2007;18:430–9.
52. Miyazaki H, Anzai N, Ekaratanawong S, et al. Modulation of renal apical organic anion transporter 4 function by two PDZ domain-containing proteins. J Am Soc Nephrol 2005.
53. Grimsby J, Coffey JW, Dvorozniak MT, et al. Characterization of glucokinase regulatory protein-deficient mice. J Biol Chem 2000;275:7826–31.
54. Uruno T, Remmert K, Hammer III JA. CARMIL is a potent capping protein antagonist: identification of a conserved CARMIL domain that inhibits the activity of capping protein and uncaps capped actin filaments. J Biol Chem 2006;281:10635–50.
55. Dalbeth N, Merriman T. Crystal ball gazing: new therapeutic targets for hyperuricaemia and gout. Rheumatology 2009;48:222–6.
56. Wald DS, Wald NJ, Morris JK, et al. Folic acid, homocysteine, and cardiovascular disease: judging causality in the face of inconclusive trial evidence. Br Med J 2006;333:1114–7.
57. Wu X, Muzny DM, Chi Lee C, et al. Two independent mutational events in the loss of urate oxidase during hominoid evolution. J Mol Evol 1992;34:78–84.
58. Shi Y, Evans JE, Rock KL. Molecular identification of a danger signal that alerts the immune system to dying cells. Nature 2003;425:516–21.
59. Kutzing MK, Firestein BL. Altered uric acid levels and disease states. J Pharmacol Exp Ther 2008;324:1–7.
60. Facheris M, Hicks A, Minelli C, et al. Variation in the uric acid transporter gene SLC2A9 and its association with AAO of Parkinson's disease. J Mol Neurosci 2010:1–5.
61. Houlihan LM, Wyatt ND, Harris SE, et al. Variation in the uric acid transporter gene (SLC2A9) and memory performance. Hum Mol Genet 2010;19:2321–30.
62. Bannasch D, Safra N, Young A, et al. Mutations in the SLC2A9 gene cause hyperuricosuria and hyperuricemia in the dog. PLoS Genet 2008;4:e1000246.
63. Merriman TR, Dalbeth N. The genetic basis of hyperuricaemia and gout. Joint Bone Spine 2010. doi:10.1016/j.jbspin.2010.02.027.
64. Feig DI, Kang D-H, Johnson RJ. Uric acid and cardiovascular risk. N Engl J Med 2008;359:1811–21.
65. Yang Q, Kottgen A, Dehghan A, et al. Multiple genetic loci influence serum urate and their relationship with gout and cardiovascular disease risk factors. Circ Cardiovasc Genet 2010. doi:10.1161.
66. Sparso T, Andersen G, Nielsen T, et al. The GCKR rs780094 polymorphism is associated with elevated fasting serum triacylglycerol, reduced fasting and OGTT-related insulinaemia, and reduced risk of type 2 diabetes. Diabetologia 2008;51:70–5.
67. McKeigue PM, Campbell H, Wild S, et al. Bayesian methods for instrumental variable analysis with genetic instruments (Mendelian randomization): example with urate transporter SLC2A9 as an instrumental variable for effect of urate levels on metabolic syndrome. Int J Epidemiol 2010;39:907–18.
68. Zhang W, Doherty M, Bardin T, et al. EULAR evidence based recommendations for gout. Part II: Management. Report of a task force of the EULAR standing committee for international clinical studies including therapeutics (ESCISIT). Ann Rheum Dis 2006;65:1312–24.
69. Anzai N, Jin CJ, Jutabha P, et al. Interaction of a novel urate efflux transporter URATv1 (SLC2A9) with uricosuric agents. FASEB J 2009;23:797.

Chapter **8**

Diagnosis of Gout

Angelo L. Gaffo

KEY POINTS

- The aspiration of a joint with undiagnosed arthritis, or analysis of a tissue biopsy with subsequent visualization of monosodium urate (MSU) crystals, is considered the diagnostic standard for gout.
- Elements of the history and physical examination that have been found to be useful when making an evidence-based diagnosis of a gout flare include a rapid onset of symptoms, a first metatarsophalangeal or tarsal joint location, characteristics of the joint involvement (redness and swelling associated), and prior episodes of arthritis with similar characteristics to the one being experienced by the patient.
- The confirmation of subcutaneous or other tissue masses found on physical examination as tophi through MSU crystal identification can establish a diagnosis of gout, although this is rarely a presenting symptom of the disease.
- Serum urate levels should not be used to confirm or rule out the presence of acute gouty arthritis.
- The role of conventional radiography in patients suspected of having gout is limited by the relatively late development of radiographic changes in the disease.
- Ultrasound is a valuable tool in the assessment of patients with very early phases of gout, including initial gout attacks and even asymptomatic hyperuricemia.
- Conditions commonly prominent in the differential diagnosis of gout attacks include septic arthritis, pseudogout, trauma, and rheumatoid arthritis. For chronic gout, the differential diagnosis usually includes rheumatoid arthritis, osteoarthritis, and calcium pyrophosphate deposition disease.
- Classification criteria and diagnostic rules published for gout have not been properly validated and should be used with caution.

Introduction

The aspiration of a suspicious joint, or analysis of a tissue biopsy, with subsequent visualization of monosodium urate (MSU) crystals is considered the diagnostic standard for gout. Unfortunately, this deceivingly simple process is plagued with challenges for primary care providers, researchers, and even rheumatologists. Common challenges for primary care providers stem from their experience level in accessing the affected joint, as well as this provider having access to rapid identification of crystals by an experienced examiner.

In addition, primary care providers and rheumatologists alike face diverse forms of presentation provided by the setting of the clinical encounter (e.g., office versus hospital) and the disease stage (gout attack versus intercritical period versus chronic gout), which add considerable heterogeneity to the diagnostic approach. For researchers trying to recruit new patients with gout or gather large numbers of existing patients for epidemiologic studies, the difficulties are multiple, as problems with clinical diagnosis of gout usually translate into large proportions of diagnostic misclassification that can jeopardize the validity of any obtained results.

Because of these challenges, alternative or complementary approaches to gout diagnosis have been used, including adding a role for serum urate, radiographs or other imaging, the use of diagnostic rules or classification criteria, and the use of administrative diagnostic codes. With the objective of providing the reader with a comprehensive view of the diagnostic approach to gout, this chapter will review the role of the clinical history and physical examination, laboratory studies, imaging, and MSU crystal examination. In addition, the value of administrative diagnostic codes, past and current diagnostic rules, and classification criteria will be analyzed.

History and Physical Examination

Diagnosis of Gout

For a complete discussion of the clinical features of gout, refer to Chapter 9. A careful history and physical examination will be important when attempting to establish a gout diagnosis. However, different aspects of this process will acquire more relevance depending on which gout disease stage is encountered. Patients with gout can go through different stages, including (1) asymptomatic hyperuricemia, (2) gout flares, (3) intercritical periods, and (4) chronic and usually tophaceous gout.[1] By definition, asymptomatic hyperuricemia does not have clinical manifestations related to gout (although other disease associations are described; see Chapter 19). On the other hand, gout attacks ("flares"), intercritical periods, and chronic gout can have clues that offer an insight into the diagnosis.

Diagnosis of Gout Flares

Even though the concept of a gout flare is familiar to both rheumatologists and primary care providers, there is a paucity of studies addressing the relevance of different clinical features when trying to make a diagnosis of gout. Preliminary classification criteria for acute gout (flares) published by

Table 8-1 Items Selected for a Gout Flare Definition and Endorsement by a Group of 20 Gout Patients

Item	Patients Endorsing, %
Affected joint is swollen	84
Affected joint is red	84
Affected joint is extremely tender to touch	100
The pain is at its worst very quickly (4-12 hours)	95
The pain is much worse than usual	95
The affected joint is the knee, ankle, foot, or toe	95
It stops me from doing usual activities	96
I can't walk during the attack	96
It gets better within 3-14 days	79
It was very similar to other attacks of gout	96

Data from Taylor WJ, Shewchuk R, Saag KG, et al. Toward a valid definition of gout flare: results of consensus exercises using Delphi methodology and cognitive mapping. Arthritis Rheum 2009;61(4):535-43.

Table 8-2 Multivariable Analysis of Clinical Elements Significantly Associated With a Crystal-Proved Diagnosis of Gout in Patients With Acute Monoarthritis

Variable	Odds Ratio (95% Confidence Interval)
Male sex	6.7 (3.3-13.7)
Previous patient-reported arthritis attack	4.1 (2.2-7.8)
First metatarsophalangeal involvement	6.5 (3.4-12.5)
Hypertension or more than one cardiovascular disease	3.2 (1.8-5.7)

Clinical elements not associated with a diagnosis of gout after multivariable analysis included joint redness, onset within 1 day, medication use, family history of gout, body mass index, and presence of diabetes.
Data from Janssens HJ, Fransen J, van de Lisdonk EH, et al. A diagnostic rule for acute gouty arthritis in primary care without joint fluid analysis. Arch Intern Med 2010;170(13):1120-6.

the American College of Rheumatology (formerly American Rheumatism Association) (ACR) identified history and physical examination criteria, such as maximum inflammation within 1 day, monoarthritis, joint redness, first metatarsophalangeal or tarsal joint involvement, presence of tophus, and recurrent attacks of monoarthritis as relevant.[2] The European League Against Rheumatism (EULAR) conducted a systematic review of the literature as part of its evidence-based recommendations for diagnosis, finding two elements pertaining to the history as being associated with a high strength of recommendation: these were a rapid onset of the flare (within 6 to 12 hours) and typical presentations for gout (the example of podagra in the setting of hyperuricemia is given).[3] As part of the process of identifying response domains in acute gout (flares) and chronic gout developed by the Outcomes Measures in Rheumatology Group (OMERACT),[4] a Delphi exercise and cognitive mapping process were performed among nine gout experts, which yielded a list of elements associated with the presence of a gout flare.[5] Most of these elements are easy to obtain from a simple history of joint complaints (presence of swollen, tender, and warm joints), patient self-report of pain and global assessment, time to maximum pain, and complete resolution of pain. More than 80% of gout patients surveyed as part of the same study endorsed these elements as representative of a gout flare experience (Table 8-1). An additional element added by the patients as representative of the gout flare experience was a similarity between the current experience and previous gout attacks.

As part of the process of creating a rule to aid physicians in diagnosing gout among episodes of acute monoarthritis, Dutch investigators assessed multiple history and physical examination elements for their performance in predicting gout as the cause of monoarthritis[6] (Table 8-2). Male sex, a previous attack of arthritis, involvement of the first metatarsophalangeal joint, and the presence of hypertension or other cardiovascular comorbidities were associated with gout as a diagnosis.

In conclusion, elements of the history and physical examination that have been consistently found to be useful when making an evidence-based diagnosis of a gout flare include a rapid onset of symptoms, the location (first metatarsophalangeal joint) characteristics of the joint involvement (redness and swelling more associated), and prior episodes of arthritis with similar characteristics to the one being experienced by the patient.

Diagnosis of Intercritical and Chronic Gout

The assessment of risk factors for the metabolic syndrome (obesity, hyperglycemia, hyperlipidemia, hypertension) is important to establish pretest probabilities for gout.[3,6] These elements apply to patients in intercritical or chronic phases of gout, in addition to patients going through flares. Pain levels may not completely subside as patients move from the intercritical phase of the disease into chronic gouty arthritis. The confirmation of subcutaneous or other tissue masses found on physical examination as tophi through MSU crystal identification can establish a diagnosis of gout, although this is rarely a presenting symptom of the disease. In some cases, gout can cause a chronic arthritis with deformities that can mimic rheumatoid arthritis.

Laboratory Studies Relevant for Gout Diagnosis

Serum Urate in the Diagnosis of Acute Gout

Many studies have attempted to define the role of serum urate measurements in episodes of acute arthritis suspected of being a gout flare. The most common mistake is to negate the diagnosis of gout in a patient with a serum urate below the in vitro urate saturation level of 6.8 mg/dl. Investigations with groups of patients undergoing gout flares have described frequencies of normouricemia at 14% to 49%.[7,8] An important caveat with these studies is the wide variability in the definition of what constitutes a normal serum urate, with ranges between 6.0 and 8.0 mg/dl. The latter threshold is usually based on a statistical definition (2 standard deviations above mean serum urate for a population) but has no physiologic basis and leads to different definitions for men and women. The threshold of 6.0 mg/dl is closer to the saturation point for urate and has been embraced as a goal for therapy by published guidelines.[3] Regardless of the definition, it is well established that gout flares can occur while serum urate is at subsaturation levels and that serum urate during acute episodes of arthritis should not be used to rule out gout as an etiology. Physiologic explanations and clinical scenarios for this phenomenon have been postulated and include (1) that patients could have been recently initiated in urate-lowering therapy without effective gout flare prophylaxis and—having already achieved a normal serum urate—are still undergoing urate deposit removal from tissues, (2) increased urate diuresis (driven by inflammatory mediators including interleukin [IL]-6) during an acute gout flare leading to normouricemia,[8] and (3) patients with a modifiable factor explaining the hyperuricemia (alcohol intake, obesity) could develop gout and still have flares after this factor is removed and they are normouricemic.[9] Many of these explanations arise from the fact that serum urate is not always representative of the total body uric acid pool.[10,11]

Classification and diagnostic criteria have incorporated hyperuricemia as a supportive element for the diagnosis or classification of gout. High serum urate values are elements of the Rome[12] and ACR preliminary classification criteria.[2] In a diagnostic rule for diagnosis of gout in patients with monoarthritis patients with a serum urate greater than 5.88 mg/dl were 9.8 times more likely to have gout against other diagnoses after multivariable adjustment.[6] Epidemiologic data support this way of thinking, given the observation that individuals without a prior diagnosis of gout and serum urate levels greater than 9.0 mg/dl have a risk of incident gout of 20% per year.[13] Despite these arguments, the role of hyperuricemia in the diagnosis of gout should be considered merely supportive and not confirmatory, given its high prevalence in the general population.[14] In addition, patients with high serum urate values also tend to have comorbidities (cardiovascular and renal disease, metabolic syndrome, and diabetes) that place them at high risk for conditions in the differential diagnosis of gout, such as infectious arthritis and other crystal arthropathies.

In conclusion, serum urate levels should not be used to confirm or rule out the presence of gout flares and their role in this context should be only marginal, possibly to establish a pretest probability for gout.

Serum Urate in the Diagnosis of Chronic and Intercritical Gout

There are no studies assessing the role of serum urate in patients suspected of having gout while not having a flare. The role of serum urate in this context should be supportive, as in the case of acute flares. Hyperuricemia can support a consideration of gout in undiagnosed patients going through the chronic or tophaceous stages, but this argument must be weighted in the context of the high prevalence of hyperuricemia in the general population.

Patients in which gout is suspected but who have normal serum urate levels could, as in the case of gout flares, have had a modifiable factor associated with hyperuricemia (obesity, alcohol intake) removed or have been chronically exposed to a uricosuric agent, such as losartan, ascorbic acid, or large doses of acetylsalicylic acid. However, these factors would be unlikely to bring to a markedly high serum urate level to normal. Normal serum urate levels could support ruling out gout in suspected cases not undergoing a flare, but other considerations, like a strong clinical suspicion based on a past clinical presentation, compelling physical findings, or radiologic findings, should carry a larger diagnostic weight.

Inflammatory Markers in the Diagnosis of Gout

Serum levels of inflammatory markers, including C-reactive protein (CRP) and sedimentation rate, are elevated during gout flare episodes.[8] Associated inflammatory cytokines, such as IL-6, have also been found to be elevated during gout flares. An elevation in inflammatory markers is correlated with an increase in renal uric acid excretion and is possibly the mechanism behind a normal serum urate in some patients undergoing gout flares.

Increases in inflammatory markers are in part a consequence of NLRP3 inflammasome-mediated mechanisms behind gout flares. Activation of the NLRP3 inflammasome leads to IL-1–mediated induction of CRP and IL-6, similar to other conditions such as certain autoinflammatory syndromes.[15] Given the lack of specificity of inflammatory markers, these are rarely used to confirm the presence of a gout flare. Inflammatory markers could also be affected by interventions such as glucocorticoids, and the absence of an elevation in these should also be interpreted with caution.

Crystal and Synovial Fluid Analysis in the Diagnosis of Gout

Chapter 2 provides a complete description of MSU and calcium pyrophosphate dihydrate (CPPD) crystal analysis in joint fluids. Visualization of MSU in synovial fluid or tissues remains the standard practice for the diagnosis of gout. However, its performance faces many challenges in daily clinical practice, and it is performed in a minority of patients who carry the diagnosis of gout. In an epidemiologic study based on patients from the Health Professionals Study, it was found that only 118 of 730 carried a diagnosis of gout based on a crystal analysis or presence of tophi.[16]

Despite its accepted role as the standard for the diagnosis of gout, there is a paucity of studies examining the diagnostic performance of microscopic examination for MSU crystals. As reviewed in Chapter 2, there is considerable variability in the reported performances, with sensitivities ranging from 69% to 98% and specificities greater than 90%.[17-20] Sources of variation in the diagnostic performance included the experience level of the examiner as well as heterogeneity in sample processing.[20] The performance of the test has been reported to be consistent among well-trained and experienced examiners.[17]

Synovial fluid analysis with crystal identification may also play an important role in the diagnosis of patients in the intercritical period of gout, as demonstrated by a study in which knees and first metatarsophalangeal (MTP) joints of patients with gout who were not going through an acute flare were aspirated and examined. All of the synovial fluid of patients who were not on urate-lowering therapy (most of whom were hyperuricemic) was positive for the identification of MSU crystals. Of the patients on urate-lowering therapy, 70% had a positive test for MSU crystals.[21] This study demonstrated that synovial fluid analysis could be helpful for establishing diagnosis even outside the gout flare stage. In addition, it conveyed the argument that patients with an established diagnosis of gout presenting with acute arthritis of etiologies other than gout could have a false-positive test for MSU crystals. An open differential diagnosis should be maintained in patients with gout when they present with acute arthritides resembling a flare.

Other characteristics of synovial fluid in patients with gout include a translucent to cloudy appearance, low viscosity, cells counts ranging from 200 to 50,000/mm^2, and proportions of polymorphonuclear leukocytes among the nucleated cells of greater than 90%. Unfortunately, there is a wide overlap with the fluid characteristics of pseudogout and septic arthritis, not allowing for a clear differentiation based on these additional features only.

Imaging Studies in the Diagnosis of Gout

For a complete discussion on the different radiologic and ultrasound modalities used for gout diagnosis and management, refer to Chapters 26 and 28. Imaging studies are useful for the assessment of severity, follow-up, and outcome measure studies of gout. The role of imaging in the diagnosis of gout is complementary to that of the clinical examination and compensated polarized light microscopic examination. In addition, data describing the diagnostic performance of imaging studies are, for the most part, scarce.

Conventional Radiography

The diagnostic usefulness of plain radiography is limited by the fact that radiographic changes are relatively late features of the disease, with changes noticeable only years after onset of gout flares (5 years on average in typical patients) or when the disease has progressed to the chronic or tophaceous stages.[22,23] Changes that are suggestive of gouty arthritis include an erosive arthropathy without periarticular osteopenia and with overhanging erosions or sclerotic margins, soft tissue opacifications, and marginal osteophytes.[22] These changes are most commonly found in the feet.

A study in which radiographic findings for gout were compared with clinical diagnosis of gout and other arthropathies found that having at least one radiologic finding of gout was 31% sensitive and 93% specific[24] (Table 8-3). This was in accordance with a previous report from a large cohort that showed that 45% of patients with confirmed gout did not show any radiographic changes.[22]

As a consequence, the role of conventional radiography in patients suspected of having gout and who are undergoing their initial episodes of acute arthritis is limited to support in exploring considerations in the differential diagnosis (e.g., septic or rheumatoid arthritis). For undiagnosed patients in the chronic or tophaceous stages of the disease, radiographic findings confer reasonable specificity and positive predictive value, providing valuable support for the diagnosis.

Computed Tomography

Computed tomography (CT) has been described as a useful tool for the assessment of erosions and tophi. The latter application is the one that has gained more attention, as CT has been found to be valuable in differentiating tophaceous subcutaneous nodules or intraarticular deposits as a result of other etiologies,[25] although studies evaluating its diagnostic performance in this setting are lacking. Dual-energy CT scans

Table 8-3 Diagnostic Performance of Conventional Radiography and High-Resolution Ultrasonographic Findings in Patients With Gout

	Sensitivity (%)	Specificity (%)	Positive Predictive Value (%)	Negative Predictive Value (%)	Accuracy (%)
CONVENTIONAL RADIOLOGY					
Soft tissue opacifications	26	97			
Bone erosions	20	95			
Marginal osteophytes at erosions or tophi sites	5	100			
Presence of any radiographic sign	31	93	89	44	63
ULTRASONOGRAPHY					
Bright stippled foci	80	75			
Hyperechoic areas	79	95			
Bone erosions	24	69			
Hypoechoic streaks	80	49			
Hypervascularization by Doppler	94	53			
Presence of any ultrasonographic findings	96	73	86	91	88

Data from Rettenbacher T, Ennemoser S, Weirich H, et al. Diagnostic imaging of gout: comparison of high-resolution US versus conventional X-ray. Eur Radiol 2008;18(3):621-30.

offer excellent visualization of tophi deposits,[26] but their use has been primarily limited to estimation of tophi burden, and not diagnosis.

Ultrasound

Ultrasonography is rapidly gaining wide adoption as a sensitive way of evaluating multiple musculoskeletal conditions, including soft tissue disorders and arthritides of inflammatory and degenerative nature.[27] In addition, its usefulness in guiding invasive procedures is considerable. These characteristics, along with its relatively low cost compared with other techniques, portability, "patient-friendliness," and absence of ionizing radiation exposure have contributed to its progressive acceptance in the rheumatology community.

Ultrasonographic findings have been described at very early stages of gout, even in patients with asymptomatic hyperuricemia.[28] In these very early stages, small tophaceous deposits and increased power-Doppler signal could be demonstrated in at least a third of subjects in some studies, suggesting active subclinical tophus formation. In established gout, high-resolution ultrasonographic findings include a double-contour sign (deposition of urate over the hyaline cartilage), hyperechoic and bright dotted foci, erosions, hypervascularization, and visualization of tophi.[29]

The diagnostic performance of ultrasonographic findings in patients with gout and other arthritides was evaluated in a study that described a sensitivity of 96% and a specificity of 73% for any ultrasonographic finding in patients with the disease[24] (see Table 8-3). A second smaller study confirmed a superiority of ultrasound compared with conventional radiographs and clinical findings.[30]

Ultrasound can play a valuable supportive role in the assessment of patients with very early phases of gout, including initial gout attacks and even asymptomatic hyperuricemia. It can also provide support in patients with established gout who are undiagnosed. The main challenge to ultrasonography is its marked operator-dependency, although this should improve as the technique gains more acceptance and training becomes more standardized. More studies are necessary to reevaluate its diagnostic performance in the different gout clinical stages. Its utilization in diagnostic rules for gout flares or chronic gout has not been assessed yet, but the perspective appears promising.

Magnetic Resonance Imaging

Magnetic resonance imaging (MRI) is a useful technique for early detection of tophi, bony erosions, and synovial involvement.[29] Its performance in differentiating tophi from other soft-tissue masses has been reported as lower than CT,[25] but performance evaluation in other scenarios related to diagnosis of gout is lacking. MRI is limited by its higher cost and limited portability, and it has not been adopted as a standard measure in the diagnostic workup of gout.

Administrative Databases in the Diagnosis of Gout

The use of administrative databases for diagnosis of medical conditions based on the International Classification of Diseases (ICD) codes pertains mainly to research and has no application in patient care. Its utilization is wide in epidemiologic and clinical research. In rheumatology, it has been applied to conditions such as osteoarthritis, spondyloarthritides, and rheumatoid arthritis.[31-33] In the case of gout, two studies have been performed in the United States comparing information obtained through ICD-9 codes against investigators' criteria and ACR, Rome, and New York criteria for gout.

The first study used administrative claims data from four large health care plans in the United States. A random sample of 200 patients yielded 121 patients with probable of definitive gout by the investigators' consensus. When comparing the presence of two or more diagnostic codes for gout with the investigators opinion, the diagnostic codes yielded a positive predictive value of only 61%. The agreement between the diagnostic codes and accepted diagnostic criteria was poor with concordance rates (kappa) of only 0.16 to 0.20.[34] An additional study evaluated data from the Veterans Affairs medical system in the United States. In this case, records of 281 patients with two or more diagnostic codes for gout were compared against diagnostic criteria. Depending on the specific rule applied, only 18% to 36% of patients fulfilled the standardized definition.[35] It is important to mention that many more patients met the definition when a rheumatologist followed them.

In conclusion, current evidence reveals that the accuracy of administrative diagnoses for gout is insufficient to confidently establish a diagnosis of gout in the research setting. Additional steps should confirm these diagnoses to have a reliable representation of gout patients.

Differential Diagnosis of Gout

Gout flares can be mimicked by other inflammatory, degenerative, and infectious conditions. The clinical differentiation between these conditions can be difficult in the immunosuppressed, elderly, or patients with multiple comorbidities. The differential diagnosis could be divided into conditions that can mimic gout flares and those that could mimic chronic or intercritical gout (Table 8-4). Some conditions, like CPPD crystal deposition disease, could mimic both phases of the disease. A discussion about the most important conditions in the differential diagnosis follows.

Septic Arthritis

In all patients in whom a gout flare is suspected, even those with well-established gout, the possibility of an alternative or concurrent diagnosis of septic arthritis should be considered. The prior statement is especially true in immunosuppressed patients, transplant recipients, those with end-stage renal disease or undergoing dialysis, or those with multiple medical comorbidities. The possibility of having septic arthritis has been analyzed in a systematic review of the literature that assessed the diagnostic performance of clinical and laboratory findings in this regard[36] (Table 8-5). Relevant among these factors when considering the differential against gout are age (older age carries a greater risk for septic arthritis), presence of diabetes mellitus, recent joint surgery, fever, and synovial fluid findings. Acute gout (and pseudogout) can sometimes be associated with synovial fluid leukocyte counts higher than the "inflammatory synovial fluid" range of 50,000/mm³;

conversely, white blood cell counts in synovial fluid in the 20,000 to 50,000/mm^3 range (but typically with 90% or more neutrophils) are frequently seen with septic arthritis. However, white blood cell counts in synovial fluid greater than 50,000/mm^3 were found to be highly sensitive for septic arthritis, and in this setting, clinicians might avoid fully committing to only a diagnosis of gout until further confirmation with a negative culture is available.

When considering a differential diagnosis of gout (or pseudogout) against septic arthritis, it is also very important to emphasize that the two conditions can coexist in the same joint, since abnormal joints such as those in chronic crystal arthropathy (not just rheumatoid arthritis) have heightened susceptibility to infection. In a systematic review of random cases found to have positive aspirates for MSU crystals in an urban emergency department, 0.5% were found to have concurrent septic arthritis.[37] In a systematic review of 30 cases of concomitant gouty and septic arthritis, one third of patients

were afebrile at presentation, 30% had normal leukocyte counts in peripheral blood, and 10% had a synovial leukocyte count of less than 6000. Most patient had long-standing disease, tophi, and 50% had medical comorbidities. *Staphylococcus aureus* was the causative agent in half of the cases, followed by *Streptococcus* spp.[38]

In conclusion, it is very challenging to differentiate gout flares from septic arthritis. Risk factors and clinical and laboratory findings should be carefully integrated when trying to differentiate these two conditions.

CPPD Crystal Deposition Disease

For a complete discussion of the clinical features of CPPD deposition disease, refer to Chapter 21. CPPD arthropathy could simulate gout when it presents in the form of acute pseudogout or chronic painful arthritis in its form of pseudo-rheumatoid arthritis or pseudo-osteoarthritis. Acute pseudogout attacks usually involve large joints such as the knees, which are also commonly affected in gout flares. Other affected joints in pseudogout include the wrists and ankles. It is important to emphasize that first MTP involvement is not exclusive to gout, as the involvement of this joint by CPPD arthropathy (pseudo-podagra) is described, although it is not overly common.[39] Features that could help in differentiating gout flares and pseudogout are presented in Table 8-6.[40]

The pseudo-rheumatoid arthritis or pseudo-osteoarthritis presentations of CPPD can involve joints such as metacarpophalangeals, wrists, knees, and ankles that also could be painful in chronic gout. Besides the clinical presentation, features that can be used to differentiate chronic CPPD arthropathies and chronic gout include a cautious interpretation of serum urate levels, differences in radiographic features of CPPD arthropathy and chronic gout, and synovial fluid analysis findings.

Table 8-4 Differential Diagnosis of Gout

Gout Attacks	Chronic Gout
Septic arthritis	Rheumatoid arthritis
Pseudogout and other crystal arthritides	Osteoarthritis
Trauma	Calcium pyrophosphate deposition disease (pseudo-rheumatoid arthritis)
Rheumatoid arthritis	Psoriatic arthritis
Acute spondyloarthropathy	Polymyalgia rheumatica
Other: e.g., stress fracture, avascular necrosis, neuropathic arthritis	

Table 8-5 Sensitivity, Specificity, and Likelihood Ratios of Selected Clinical and Laboratory Elements for the Diagnosis of Septic Arthritis

	Sensitivity (%)	Specificity (%)	Likelihood Ratio Positive (%)	Likelihood Ratio Negative (%)
Age >80 y	19	95	3.5	0.86
Diabetes mellitus	12	96	2.7	0.93
Rheumatoid arthritis	68	73	2.5	0.45
Recent joint surgery	24	96	6.9	0.78
Hip or knee prosthesis	35	89	3.1	0.73
Skin infection	32	88	2.8	0.76
HIV-1 infection	79	50	1.7	0.47
Fever	46	31	0.67	1.7
Peripheral white blood cell count >10,000/mm^3	90	36	1.4	0.28
Erythrocyte sedimentation rate >30 mm/h	95	29	1.3	0.17
C-reactive protein >100 mg/L	77	53	1.6	0.44
Synovial fluid white blood cell count >50,000/mm^3	62	92	7.7	0.42
Synovial fluid white blood cell count >100,000/mm^3	29	99	28	0.71
Polymorphonuclear cells >90% in synovial fluid	73	79	3.4	0.34

Data from Margaretten ME, Kohlwes J, Moore D, et al. Does this adult patient have septic arthritis? JAMA 2007;297(13):1478-88.

Table 8-6 Comparison of Clinical, Laboratory, and Radiologic Features That Can Help Differentiate Gout and Calcium Pyrophosphate Deposition Disease (CPPD) Arthropathy

	Gout	CPPD Arthropathy
Age group	Middle-aged and elderly men, postmenopausal women	Elderly men and women
Gender distribution characteristics	Strong preference for men that narrows considerably after menopause Extremely rare in women before menopause	Approximately equal sex ratio
Joints involved	Preference for lower extremities: first metatarsophalangeal, ankles, knees Upper extremities involved later in disease	Large joint predominance Wrists and knees involved early in disease
First metatarsophalangeal involvement	First metatarsophalangeal is classic	First metatarsophalangeal is reported, but rare
Tophi	Present	Absent
Conventional radiography	Erosions with overhanging edges, tissue opacification	Chondrocalcinosis, degenerative changes in non–weight-bearing areas
Ultrasonography	Brightly stippled deposits over cartilage	Hyperechoic signals within cartilage (chondrocalcinosis)
Crystals	Needle shaped and strongly negative birefringent	Small, romboid-shaped or irregular, and weakly positive birefringent

Adapted from Schlesinger N. Diagnosis of gout: clinical, laboratory, and radiologic findings. Am J Manag Care 2005;11(15 suppl):S443-50; quiz S465-8.

The coexistence of MSU crystal and calcium pyrophosphate crystals in the same patients has been reported and is not at all rare in clinical practice, especially in settings where there are many elderly patients. A review of six such cases found all to be affecting the knee joints,[41] with no differences in serum urate, synovial white cell counts, or age of the patients affected when comparing with cases of isolated gout.[42]

Rheumatoid Arthritis

Chronic gouty arthritis can simulate gout with polyarticular involvement, and rheumatoid nodules could be confused with tophi. A careful history and clinical examination should suffice for the differentiation between the two conditions. A history of intense flares of disease followed by almost complete resolution of pain and swelling is more suggestive of gout and atypical for rheumatoid arthritis. Furthermore, rheumatoid nodules are usually firm, rubbery, and nontender as opposed to the harder and tenderer tophi. Both can be localized in similar areas in the body, such as extensor surfaces and points of contact. Aspiration of the nodules with visualization of MSU crystals and the characteristic radiologic features of chronic gout and rheumatoid arthritis can be used as additional features that differentiate these conditions. The concurrent presence of rheumatoid arthritis and gouty arthritis, once considered very rare,[43] is now reported more frequently.[44]

Classification Criteria and Diagnostic Rules

Efforts have been made to aid in the diagnosis and classification of gout through classification criteria and diagnostic rules. As should be the case with all classification criteria, their application should be to enroll patients in clinical studies (epidemiologic or clinical trials) in a uniform manner. Classification criteria should not be applied to the diagnosis of individual patients without a validation exercise in the specific population where they will be applied.[45] One diagnostic rule has been published with the aim of diagnosing gout in patients with monoarthritis.

Rome and New York Criteria

The first criteria for the classification of gout to be published were presented at Rome during the Symposium at Population Studies in the Rheumatic Diseases in 1963[12] (Table 8-7). These criteria were evaluated in a population of 82 U.S. veterans who had synovial fluid aspiration as a gold standard. Applying a modified version of the criteria (presence of two of three elements, given that MSU crystal positivity in synovial fluid was the gold standard), these were found to be 67% sensitive and 89% specific and to have a positive predictive value of 77%.[46] The main limitation recognized with these criteria is having a serum urate component, when it has been demonstrated that gout flares can occur in the context of normal serum urate levels (see earlier).

These criteria were modified in 1966 in an international symposium held in New York[47] (Table 8-8). The main modifications were the removal of the serum urate component, the addition of podagra, and a favorable response to colchicine. When tested in a population of U.S. veterans,[46] these were found to be 70% sensitive and 82% specific and to have a positive predictive value of 77%.

American College of Rheumatology Preliminary Criteria for Acute Gouty Arthritis

In 1977, the ACR Subcommittee on Classification Criteria for Gout analyzed data from 706 patients with gout and other acute arthritides, leading to the publication of preliminary criteria for the classification of the acute arthritis of primary gout[2] (Table 8-9). The objective of these classification criteria is to separate from all cases of acute arthritis those that can be considered to be secondary to gout. Presence of MSU crystals in synovial fluid or tophi was sufficient to classify an acute

Table 8-7 Rome Criteria for the Classification of Gout (1963)

Two of the following four criteria had to be present to make a diagnosis of gout:	Authors' comments on selected criteria
• Serum urate level >7.0 mg/dl in men or >6.0 mg/dl in women	• Serum urate levels are normal in important proportions of gout patients undergoing flares or during the intercritical period[7,8,10]
• Tophi	• Highly specific finding; however, is a late occurrence in a majority of patients
• Urate crystals in synovial fluid or tissues	• Considered as standard practice for diagnosis of gout
• History of attacks of painful joint swelling of abrupt onset with remission within 2 weeks	• These symptoms have been endorsed by a majority of patients as representative of a gout flare experience[5]

Table 8-8 New York Criteria for the Classification of Gout (1968)

To classify a case as gout it is necessary:	Authors' comments on selected criteria
• To find uric acid crystals in synovial fluid or tissue (tophi)	• Considered as standard practice for diagnosis of gout
OR the presence of two or more of the following criteria:	
• History or observation of at least two attacks of painful limb swelling with remission within 1 to 2 weeks	• These symptoms have been endorsed by a majority of patients as representative of a gout flare experience[5]
• History or observation of podagra	• Highly sensitive and specific location for gout flares.[3] However, involvement of this joint by other arthropathies (e.g., calcium pyrophosphate deposition disease) can rarely occur
• Presence of tophus	• Highly specific finding. However, is a late occurrence in a majority of patients
• History or observation of a good response to colchicine (major reduction in objective signs of inflammation within 24 hours of onset of therapy)	• Major response to colchicine is not present in a majority of gout patients according to most recent randomized controlled trial[50]

Table 8-9 American College of Rheumatology Preliminary Criteria for the Classification of the Acute Arthritis of Primary Gout (1977)

In Order to Be Classified as Gout, a Case Must Present:	Authors' Comments on Selected Criteria
• Urate crystals in joint fluid	• Considered as standard practice for diagnosis of gout
OR	
• Tophus (proven by microscopic evaluation or tissue biopsy)	• Highly specific finding; however, is a late occurrence in a majority of patients
OR at least six of the following:	
• More than one attack of acute arthritis	• Most patients with gout have more than one attack in their lifetimes; however, this criteria will not consider patients with new onset of gout
• Maximal inflammation developed within 1 day	• Presentation endorsed by a majority of patients with gout[5]
• Monoarthritis attack	• Presentation of gout is most commonly polyarticular in the elderly and hospitalized patients
• Redness observed over joints	• Symptom endorsed by most patients with gout[5]
• First metatarsophalangeal joint painful or swollen	• Highly sensitive and specific location for gout flares.[3] However, involvement of this joint by other arthropathies (e.g., calcium pyrophosphate deposition disease) can rarely occur
• Unilateral first metatarsophalangeal joint attack	
• Unilateral tarsal joint attack	
• Suspected tophus	
• Hyperuricemia	• Serum urate levels are normal in important proportions of gout patients undergoing flares or during the intercritical period[7,8,10]
• Asymmetric swelling within a joint on radiograph • Subcortical cysts without erosions on radiograph	• Radiographic changes occur relatively late (average of 5 years) in the course of the disease.[22,23] Asymmetric swelling and subcortical cysts are not among the most characteristic findings in systematic reviews.[22]
• Joint fluid culture negative for organisms during attacks	

arthritis as gout. If none of these were present, 6 of 12 criteria needed to be satisfied to achieve a sensitivity of 85% and a specificity of 93%.

These classification criteria remain preliminary, as no formal validation exercise has been undertaken since its publication. Two publications have evaluated the performance of these criteria in different clinical settings. When applied to adults with acute monoarthritis in a primary care clinic in the Netherlands, and with MSU crystal demonstration in synovial fluid as a gold standard, the presence of 6 of 12 criteria was found to be 80% sensitive and 64% specific. The positive and negative predictive values were 80% and 64%, respectively.[48] In a population of U.S. veterans attending a rheumatology clinic the presence of 6 of 12 criteria yielded a sensitivity of 70%, a specificity of 79%, and a positive predictive value of 66%.[46]

Despite its broad utilization, these criteria apply to a specific clinical scenario: differentiating gout from other conditions in patients with acute arthritis. Their lack of validation and limited applicability to other clinical contexts emphasize the need to better classify gout and its specific clinical scenarios.

European League Against Rheumatism Evidence-Based Recommendations for the Diagnosis of Gout

In 2006, a group of 19 rheumatologists with expertise in gout and 1 expert in evidence-based medicine on behalf of the European League Against Rheumatism published evidence-based guidelines for the diagnosis of gout.[3] After following a Delphi methodology considering published evidence until 2006 as well as expert consensus, 10 key propositions for the diagnosis of gout were elaborated (Table 8-10). Information available from the literature allowed the group to estimate diagnostic characteristics for each proposition and to develop a diagnostic model ("ladder") for gout (Fig. 8-1). This diagnostic model has not been validated.

Table 8-10 European League Against Rheumatism Evidence-Based Recommendations for the Diagnosis of Gout (2006)

Proposition	Strength of Recommendation (0 to 100)*	Percentage of Participants That Strongly or Fully Recommended	Authors' Comments on Selected Propositions
In acute attacks the rapid development of severe pain, swelling, and tenderness that reaches its maximum within just 6 to 12 hours, especially with overlying erythema, is highly suggestive of crystal inflammation though not specific for gout	88	93	Rapid symptom onset and joint redness is endorsed by a majority of patients with gout.[5] However, specificity is limited and other conditions can mimic this presentation
For typical presentations of gout (such as recurrent podagra with hyperuricemia) a clinical diagnosis alone is reasonably accurate but not definitive without crystal confirmation	95	100	The combination of podagra (highly sensitive and specific) with hyperuricemia is highly suggestive of a gout diagnosis. However, most clinical presentations of gout will require crystal confirmation
Demonstration of MSU crystals in synovial fluid or tophus aspirates permits a definitive diagnosis of gout	96	100	Considered as standard practice for diagnosis of gout
A routine search for MSU crystals is recommended in all synovial fluid samples obtained from undiagnosed inflamed joints	90	87	
Identification of MSU crystals from asymptomatic joints may allow definite diagnosis in intercritical periods	84	93	Patients with hyperuricemia and inflammatory arthritides other than gout could be falsely diagnosed as gout
Gout and sepsis may coexist, so when septic arthritis is suspected Gram stain and culture of synovial fluid should still be performed even if MSU crystals are identified	93	93	
While being the most important risk factor for gout, serum urate levels do not confirm or exclude gout as many people with hyperuricemia do not develop gout, and during acute attacks serum levels may be normal	95	93	Serum urate levels should only play a marginal role in gout diagnosis, and should not be used to confirm or exclude the condition
Renal uric acid excretion should be determined in selected gout patients, especially those with a family history of young onset gout, onset of gout under age 25, or with renal calculi	72	60	Should not be a part of an initial diagnostic workup for gout flares or chronic gout. It could be helpful with therapeutic decisions

Table 8-10 European League Against Rheumatism Evidence-Based Recommendations for the Diagnosis of Gout (2006)—cont'd

Proposition	Strength of Recommendation (0 to 100)*	Percentage of Participants That Strongly or Fully Recommended	Authors' Comments on Selected Propositions
Although radiographs may be useful for differential diagnosis and may show typical features in chronic gout, they are not useful in confirming the diagnosis of early or acute gout	86	93	Radiographic changes occur relatively late (average of 5 years) in the course of the disease.[22, 23]
Risk factors for gout and associated comorbidities should be assessed, including features of the metabolic syndrome (obesity, hyperglycemia, hyperlipidemia, hypertension)	93	100	These risk factors can be useful in establishing a pretest probability for gout and their ascertainment is a component of any careful history necessary to establish the diagnosis of gout

MSU, Monosodium urate.

*Based on a 0-100 visual analog scale by participating rheumatologists with expertise in gout.

Adapted from Zhang W, Doherty M, Pascual E, et al. EULAR evidence based recommendations for gout. Part I: Diagnosis. Report of a task force of the Standing Committee for International Clinical Studies Including Therapeutics (ESCISIT). Ann Rheum Dis 2006;65(10):1301-11.

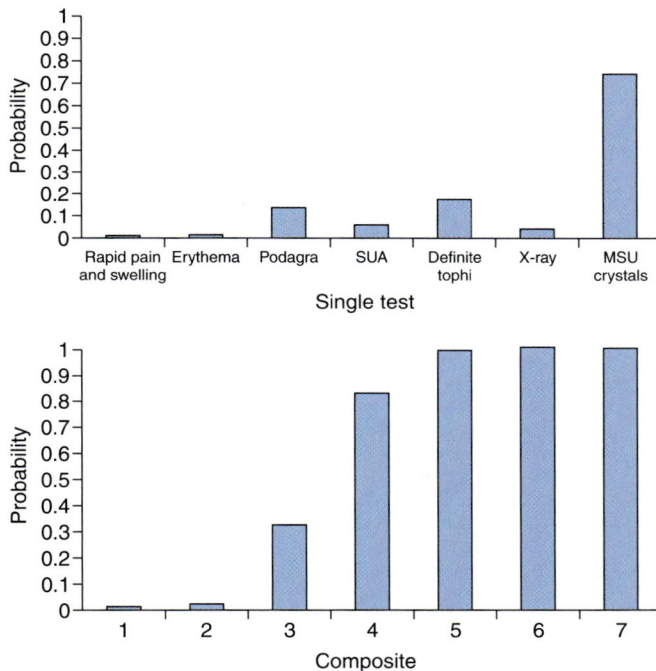

Table 8-11 Diagnostic Rule to Calculate Prevalence of Gout Among Patients Presenting With Acute Monoarthritis in a Primary Care Setting

Variable	Clinical Score
Male sex	2.0
Previous patient-reported arthritis attack	2.0
Onset within 1 day	0.5
Joint redness	1.0
First metatarsophalangeal involvement	2.5
Hypertension or more than one cardiovascular diseases: angina pectoris, myocardial infarction, heart failure, cerebrovascular accident, transient ischemic attack, or peripheral vascular disease	1.5
Serum urate >5.88 mg/dl	3.5

A score <4 translates into a prevalence of gout of 2.8%, for a score between 4 and <8, the prevalence is 27%, and for a score of ≥8, the prevalence is 80.4%. Data from Janssens HJ, Fransen J, van de Lisdonk EH, et al. A diagnostic rule for acute gouty arthritis in primary care without joint fluid analysis. Arch Intern Med 2010;170(13):1120-6.

Figure 8-1 Diagnostic "ladder" model for gout. Diagnostic ladder of gout: composite 1, rapid pain and swelling; composite 2, composite 1 plus erythema; composite 3, composite 2 plus podagra; composite 4, composite 3 plus hyperuricemia; composite 5, composite 4 plus tophi; composite 6, composite 5 plus x-ray changes; composite 7, composite 6 plus MSU crystals. *MSU,* Monosodium urate; *SUA,* serum urate. *(From Zhang W, Doherty M, Pascual E, et al. EULAR evidence based recommendations for gout. Part I: Diagnosis. Report of a task force of the Standing Committee for International Clinical Studies Including Therapeutics (ESCISIT). Ann Rheum Dis 2006;65(10):1301-11.)*

Other Diagnostic Rules

In 2010, a group of Mexican rheumatologists proposed a novel rule that combined features from the ACR classification criteria and the EULAR guidelines into one unified diagnostic rule for chronic gout, and they tested its performance against the ACR criteria in a group of 549 patients with gout.[49] The rule determined that the diagnosis of chronic gout should be considered in patients when four or more of the following elements are present currently or as part of the history: one or more attack of acute arthritis, monoarthritis or oligoarthritis attacks, rapid onset of pain and swelling, podagra, erythema, unilateral tarsitis, possible tophi, and hyperuricemia. This rule identified patients with gout at similar rates to the ACR criteria, but no specific data about its diagnostic performance were provided in the publication.

In the same year, investigators from the Netherlands published a rule for the diagnosis of gout in patients with episodes of acute monoarthritis without need for synovial fluid analysis.[6] The rule was generated from and oriented toward patients seen in primary care settings, Elements from the history, physical examination, and serum urate levels were combined into a point score system for the final rule (Table 8-11). At different thresholds in the clinic scores, the prevalence of gout could be calculated. A score of 4 or less essentially ruled out gout (prevalence of 2.8%). The area under the curve for the model was 0.89.

References

1. Edwards NL. Gout. Clinical features. In: Klippel JH, editor. Primer on the Rheumatic Diseases. 13th ed. New York, NY: Springer; 2008.
2. Wallace SL, Robinson H, Masi AT, et al. Preliminary criteria for the classification of the acute arthritis of primary gout. Arthritis Rheum 1977;20(3):895–900.
3. Zhang W, Doherty M, Pascual E, et al. EULAR evidence based recommendations for gout. Part I: diagnosis. Report of a task force of the Standing Committee for International Clinical Studies Including Therapeutics (ESCISIT). Ann Rheum Dis 2006;65(10):1301–11.
4. Taylor WJ, Schumacher Jr HR, Baraf HS, et al. A modified delphi exercise to determine the extent of consensus with omeract outcome domains for studies of acute and chronic gout. Ann Rheum Dis 2008;67(6):888–91.
5. Taylor WJ, Shewchuk R, Saag KG, et al. Toward a valid definition of gout flare: results of consensus exercises using Delphi methodology and cognitive mapping. Arthritis Rheum 2009;61(4):535–43.
6. Janssens HJ, Fransen J, Van De Lisdonk EH, et al. A diagnostic rule for acute gouty arthritis in primary care without joint fluid analysis. Arch Intern Med 2010;170(13):1120–6.
7. Logan JA, Morrison E, Mcgill PE. Serum uric acid in acute gout. Ann Rheum Dis 1997;56(11):696–7.
8. Urano W, Yamanaka H, Tsutani H, et al. The inflammatory process in the mechanism of decreased serum uric acid concentrations during acute gouty arthritis. J Rheumatol 2002;29(9):1950–3.
9. McCarty DJ. Gout without hyperuricemia. JAMA 1994;271(4):302–3.
10. Schlesinger N, Baker DG, Schumacher Jr HR. Serum urate during bouts of acute gouty arthritis. J Rheumatol 1997;24(11):2265–6.
11. Schlesinger N, Norquist JM, Watson DJ. Serum urate during acute gout. J Rheumatol 2009;36(6):1287–9.
12. Kellgren J, Jeffrey M, Ball J. The Epidemiology of Chronic Rheumatism. Oxford, UK: Blackwell; 1963.
13. Campion EW, Glynn RJ, Delabry LO. Asymptomatic hyperuricemia. Risks and consequences in the Normative Aging Study. Am J Med 1987;82(3):421–6.
14. Fang J, Alderman MH. Serum uric acid and cardiovascular mortality The NHANES I Epidemiologic Follow-Up Study, 1971-1992. National Health and Nutrition Examination Survey. JAMA 2000;283(18):2404–10.
15. Martinon F. Mechanisms of uric acid crystal-mediated autoinflammation. Immunol Rev 2010;233(1):218–32.
16. Choi HK, Atkinson K, Karlson EW, et al. Alcohol intake and risk of incident gout in men: a prospective study. Lancet 2004;363(9417):1277–81.
17. Lumbreras B, Pascual E, Frasquet J, et al. Analysis for crystals in synovial fluid: training of the analysts results in high consistency. Ann Rheum Dis 2005;64(4):612–5.
18. Schumacher Jr HR, Sieck MS, Rothfuss S, et al. Reproducibility of synovial fluid analyses. a study among four laboratories. Arthritis Rheum 1986;29(6):770–4.
19. Gordon C, Swan A, Dieppe P. Detection of crystals in synovial fluids by light microscopy: sensitivity and reliability. Ann Rheum Dis 1989;48(9):737–42.
20. Swan A, Amer H, Dieppe P. The value of synovial fluid assays in the diagnosis of joint disease: a literature survey. Ann Rheum Dis 2002;61(6):493–8.
21. Pascual E, Batlle-Gualda E, Martinez A, et al. Synovial fluid analysis for diagnosis of intercritical gout. Ann Intern Med 1999;131(10):756–9.
22. Bloch C, Hermann G, Yu TF. A radiologic reevaluation of gout: a study of 2,000 patients. AJR Am J Roentgenol 1980;134(4):781–7.
23. Nakayama DA, Barthelemy C, Carrera G, et al. Tophaceous gout: a clinical and radiographic assessment. Arthritis Rheum 1984;27(4):468–71.
24. Rettenbacher T, Ennemoser S, Weirich H, et al. Diagnostic imaging of gout: comparison of high-resolution us versus conventional x-ray. Eur Radiol 2008;18(3):621–30.
25. Gerster JC, Landry M, Dufresne L, et al. Imaging of tophaceous gout: computed tomography provides specific images compared with magnetic resonance imaging and ultrasonography. Ann Rheum Dis 2002;61(1):52–4.
26. Johnson TR, Weckbach S, Kellner H, et al. Clinical image: dual-energy computed tomographic molecular imaging of gout. Arthritis Rheum 2007;56(8):2809.
27. Kane D, Grassi W, Sturrock R, et al. Musculoskeletal ultrasound: a state of the art review in rheumatology. Part 2: clinical indications for musculoskeletal ultrasound in rheumatology. Rheumatology (Oxford) 2004;43(7):829–38.
28. Puig JG, De Miguel E, Castillo MC, et al. Asymptomatic hyperuricemia: impact of ultrasonography. Nucleosides Nucleotides Nucl Acids 2008;27(6):592–5.
29. Perez-Ruiz F, Dalbeth N, Urresola A, et al. Imaging of gout: findings and utility. Arthritis Res Ther 2009;11(3):232.
30. Wright SA, Filippucci E, McVeigh C, et al. High-resolution ultrasonography of the first metatarsal phalangeal joint in gout: a controlled study. Ann Rheum Dis 2007;66(7):859–64.
31. Singh JA, Holmgren AR, Krug H, et al. Accuracy of the diagnoses of spondylarthritides in Veterans Affairs Medical Center databases. Arthritis Rheum 2007;57(4):648–55.
32. Singh JA, Holmgren AR, Noorbaloochi S. Accuracy of Veterans Administration databases for a diagnosis of rheumatoid arthritis. Arthritis Rheum 2004;51(6):952–7.
33. Harrold LR, Yood RA, Andrade SE, et al. Evaluating the predictive value of osteoarthritis diagnoses in an administrative database. Arthritis Rheum 2000;43(8):1881–5.
34. Harrold LR, Saag KG, Yood RA, et al. Validity of gout diagnoses in administrative data. Arthritis Rheum 2007;57(1):103–8.
35. Malik A, Dinnella JE, Kwoh CK, et al. Poor validation of medical record icd-9 diagnoses of gout in a Veterans Affairs database. J Rheumatol 2009;36(6):1283–6.
36. Margaretten ME, Kohlwes J, Moore D, et al. Does this adult patient have septic arthritis? JAMA 2007;297(13):1478–88.
37. Shah K, Spear J, Nathanson LA, et al. Does the presence of crystal arthritis rule out septic arthritis? J Emerg Med 2007;32(1):23–6.
38. Yu KH, Luo SF, Liou LB, et al. Concomitant septic and gouty arthritis: an analysis of 30 cases. Rheumatology (Oxford) 2003;42(9):1062–6.
39. Goupille P, Valat JP. Hydroxyapatite pseudopodagra in young men. AJR Am J Roentgenol 1992;159(4):902.
40. Schlesinger N. Diagnosis of gout: clinical, laboratory, and radiologic findings. Am J Manag Care 2005;11(Suppl. 15):S443–50; quiz S465–8.
41. Jaccard YB, Gerster JC, Calame L. Mixed monosodium urate and calcium pyrophosphate crystal-induced arthropathy. A review of seventeen cases. Rev Rhum Engl Ed 1996;63(5):331–5.
42. Robier C, Neubauer M, Quehenberger F, et al. Coincidence of calcium pyrophosphate and monosodium urate crystals in the synovial fluid of patients with gout determined by the cytocentrifugation technique. Ann Rheum Dis 2011;70(6):1163-4.
43. Rizzoli AJ, Trujeque L, Bankhurst AD. The coexistence of gout and rheumatoid arthritis: case reports and a review of the literature. J Rheumatol 1980;7(3):316–24.
44. Kuo CF, Tsai WP, Liou LB. Rare copresent rheumatoid arthritis and gout: comparison with pure rheumatoid arthritis and a literature review. Clin Rheumatol 2008;27(2):231–5.
45. Yazici H. Diagnostic versus classification criteria: a continuum. Bull NY Hosp Jt Dis 2009;67(2):206–8.
46. Malik A, Schumacher HR, Dinnella JE, et al. Clinical diagnostic criteria for gout: comparison with the gold standard of synovial fluid crystal analysis. J Clin Rheumatol 2009;15(1):22–4.
47. Bennett P, Wood P. Presented at the Population Studies of the Rheumatic Diseases: Proceedings of the Third International Symposium; June 5-10, 1968; New York.
48. Janssens HJ, Janssen M, Van De Lisdonk EH, et al. Limited validity of the American College of Rheumatology criteria for classifying patients with gout in primary care. Ann Rheum Dis 2010;69(6):1255–6.
49. Pelaez-Ballestas I, Hernandez Cuevas C, Burgos-Vargas R, et al. Diagnosis of chronic gout: evaluating the American College of Rheumatology proposal, European League Against Rheumatism recommendations, and clinical judgment. J Rheumatol 2010;37(8):1743–8.
50. Terkeltaub RA, Furst DE, Bennett K, et al. High versus low dosing of oral colchicine for early acute gout flare: twenty-four-hour outcome of the first multicenter, randomized, double-blind, placebo-controlled, parallel-group, dose-comparison colchicine study. Arthritis Rheum 2010; 62(4):1060–8.

Clinical Features of Gout

William J. Taylor and Rebecca Grainger

KEY POINTS

- The key clinical features of acute gouty arthritis have been recognized for hundreds of years and include podagra (inflammatory arthritis of the first metatarsophalangeal joint), rapid rise to maximal symptoms, and complete resolution over 7 to 10 days.

- Few patients have a single isolated attack of gout and most will experience recurrent episodes, albeit with very variable frequency.

- Over decades, chronic gouty arthritis often with tophaceous disease can develop with very frequent attacks of arthritis or persisting symptoms between attacks of acute arthritis.

- Tophi are most commonly observed as subcutaneous lumps overlying joints or bony prominences but have rarely been reported in many anatomical locations including the spine, conjunctiva, larynx, bowel, cardiac valves, and pancreas.

- Gout may affect the kidney in a variety of ways, including uric acid nephrolithiasis, interstitial urate nephopathy in the absence of overt lithiasis, familial juvenile hyperuricemic nephropathy and hypoxanthine-guanine phosphoribosyltransferase deficiency, acute uric acid–related nephropathy due to tumor lysis and possibly soluble urate may have a direct pathogenic effect as a renal and vascular toxin.

- Elderly women with gout often present with tophi in nodal osteoarthritis of the hands, frequently in the context of diuretic medication use.

- Gout is the most common inflammatory arthritis following solid organ transplantation, occurring in up to one fourth of renal and cardiac recipients, and can progress more quickly to polyarticular disease. Management is facilitated by changing immunosuppression with cyclosporine-A or azathioprine to other regimens.

A Historical Perspective on the Clinical Features of Gout

Gout is clearly an ancient disease. The Egyptians had first written about it by ca. 2640 BC, and archeological skeletal remains at Philae, Upper Egypt, were discovered in 1910 that clearly document an advanced stage of the disease.[1] In the Ebers and Edwin Smith Papyri (ca. 1552 BC), gout is described and reference is made to much earlier medical writing by Imhotep (ca. 2650 to 2600 BC), the great luminary of Egyptian medicine, engineering, and architecture. Imhotep is credited with being the father of medicine, having been the first named physician who wrote about disease in nonmagical ways.[2,3]

One thousand years after the Ebers and Edwin Smith Papyri were written, Hippocrates (ca. 460 BC to 370 BC), who had studied at the temple of Imhotep at Memphis, separated gout from rheumatism, developing the term "podagra" from *pous* (ποῦς) meaning "foot" and *agra* (ἄγρα) meaning "prey" (a "foot-trap") for severe pain and swelling in the first metatarsophalangeal joint.[4] This important clinical feature remains a key pointer toward the diagnosis of gout. Hippocrates' observations on the relationship between an intemperate lifestyle and gout set the scene for an interesting centuries-long concept of the disease as a badge of the rich and powerful. Five aphorisms of Hippocrates on gout continue to describe the general epidemiology fairly well (Table 9-1).

The typical clinical phenomenon of gout (which shall be described in detail in this chapter) has been known for thousands of years. In the first century, Arataeus of Cappadocia (ca. 120) perfectly describes gout as:

Pain seizes the great toe, then the forepart of the heel on which we rest; next it comes into the arch of the foot … the ankle joint swells last of all … no pain is more severe than this, not iron screws, nor cords, not the wound of a dagger, nor burning fire.

He also gives an excellent example of the fact of complete clinical remission between episodes of gout:

This disease remits sometimes for long periods … hence a person subject to the gout has been known to win the race in the Olympic Games during an interval of the disease.[5]

The Romans were also well aware of gout. Galen (ca. 129 to 199/217) was the first to describe tophi and also the hereditary nature of gout, although the important environmental predisposing factors tended to overshadow this aspect for centuries. The first inherited specific purine enzyme deficiency to be associated with gout was described only in 1967[6] in the condition that came to be known as Lesch-Nyhan syndrome.[7]

The actual term "gout" to describe the disease that we know as gout was not used until medieval times, when the Dominican monk Randolfus of Bocking described it as "the gout which is called podagra or arthritis" [*gutta quam podagram vel artiticam vocant*].[5,8] Apparently Randolfus considered that the condition could be cured by wearing the boots belonging to Saint Richard of Wyche, Bishop of Chichester. The term *gutta* ("drop") refers to the belief that disease was caused by imbalance in the four humors, so that under certain circumstances

Table 9-1	**Five Aphorisms of Hippocrates on Gout**
VI-28	Eunuchs do not take gout, nor become bald
VI-29	A woman does not take gout, unless her menses be stopped
VI-30	A youth does not get gout before sexual intercourse
VI-40	In gouty affectations, inflammation subsides within 40 days
VI-55	Gouty affectations become active in spring and autumn

From Nuki G, Simkin PA. A concise history of gout and hyperuricemia and their treatment. Arthritis Res Ther 2006;8.

an excess of one of these humors would "drop" or flow into a joint, causing pain and inflammation.

Sydenham (1624 to 1689) particularly emphasized the association of gout with debauchery, although this had also been recognized in Roman times:

> Gout attacks such old men as, after passing the best part of their life in ease and comfort, indulging freely in high living, wine, and other generous drinks, at length, from inactivity, the usual attendant of advanced life, have left off altogether the bodily exercises of their youth.[9]

Sydenham, who had gout himself, described most of the important clinical features of gout that we would recognize. For example, he also noted the hereditability of the disease (many sufferers "have received the ill seeds of the disease from their parents by inheritance"); that gout can be extremely destructive ("sometimes distorting one or more fingers, making them look like a bunch of parsnips"); the eventual appearance of tophi ("stony concretions of the ligaments of the joints"), and renal stones ("it breeds the stone in the kidney" and "the stone is made of a part of the same kind of matter" as the rest of the gout).[8]

The association with dietary excess has led to gout being used as a literary device by Shakespeare and others, offering insights into the public perception of this condition over the past 400 years. In *The Adventure of the Missing Three-quarter*, Arthur Conan Doyle vividly described the appearance of tophi: "Yes, he was his heir, and the old boy is nearly eighty—cram full of gout, too. They say he could chalk his billiard-cue with his knuckles."[10]

Gout has sometimes been used as a means to moral exhortation to lead a more temperate, God-fearing life.

> "What a man gout makes! Devout, morally pure, temperate, circumspect," Cardano said, adding, "No one is so mindful of God as the man who is in the clutches of the pain of gout. He who suffers gout cannot forget that he is mortal."[11]

As a result, there remains a stigma associated with gout that implies it is largely self-inflicted. Like many victim-blaming approaches, this belief is probably unhelpful and can lead to poorer treatment outcomes. On the other hand, the association between a rich lifestyle and gout has sometimes led to gout being an almost desirable condition. Even in modern times, an association between intelligence or behavioral characteristics associated with high performance, and serum urate levels was documented.[12] These factors may further discourage adequate treatment of clinical gout.

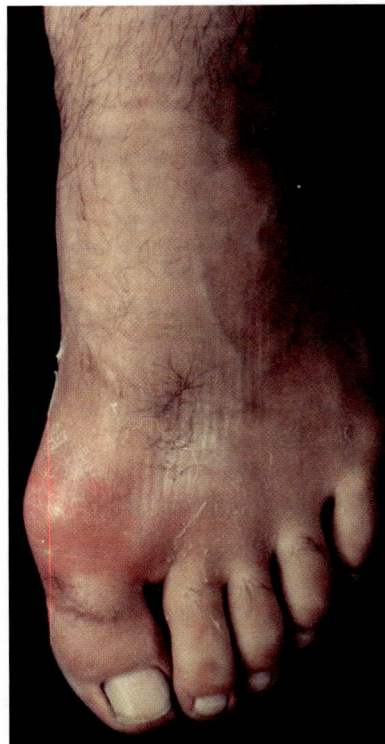

Figure 9-1 A metatarsophalangeal joint of the great toe with underlying mild hallux valgus affected by acute gout with redness and swelling. *(From Slide Atlas of Rheumatology. London, UK: Gower Medical Publishing Ltd.; 1984.)*

Acute Gouty Arthritis

The initial manifestation of gout is usually an acute attack of gouty arthritis. This is characterized by abrupt onset of severe pain and swelling, usually in a single joint in the lower limb. Maximal inflammation typically occurs within 4 to 12 hours. The classic presentation is that of an acute arthritis of the metatarsophalangeal joint (MTPJ) of the great toe, called podagra (Fig. 9-1). In this and other superficial joints, erythema and soft tissue edema may also be observed. Other areas commonly involved in initial attacks of gout can include mid-tarsal joints and the hindfoot, including the ankle. The pain experienced during an attack of gout is almost always severe with patients protecting the affected joint from any use. The pain interrupts sleep, can prevent walking, and interferes with daily activities. Without treatment, the gouty inflammation in a single joint characteristically subsides over 7 to 10 days. Desquamation of the erythematous skin overlying the joint can occur in superficial joints. After repeated attacks, many patients can recognize a prodrome in the hours leading up to an attack, describing an ill-defined discomfort or tingling in the joint.

Pattern of Joint Involvement

Hospital-based case series have reported monoarticular onset of gout in 70% to 90% of individuals,[13,14] with the MTPJ of the great toe affected in more than 50% of individuals.[15,16] Acute gout predominantly affects the joints of the lower limb, including the first MTPJ, mid foot, ankle, and knee.[15,17,18] Common

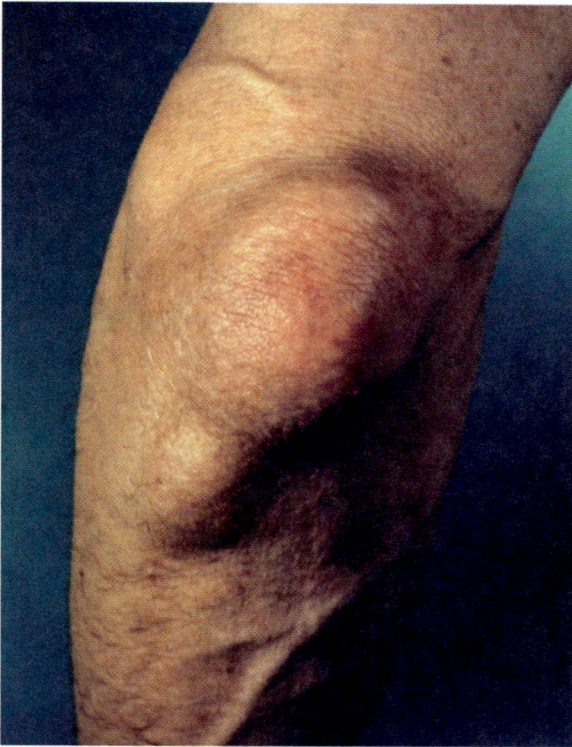

Figure 9-2 An inflamed olecranon bursa. Aspirate confirmed the presence of monosodium urate crystals. *(From Slide Atlas of Rheumatology. London, UK: Gower Medical Publishing Ltd.; 1984.)*

Table 9-2 Joint Involvement by Percentage Over Duration of Gout in Published Case Series

Study	Grahame, 1970	Currie, 1978	Roddy, 2007
Type of practice	Hospital	Primary care	Primary care
Country	United Kingdom	United Kingdom	United Kingdom
Diagnosis of gout	Clinical	Clinical	Clinical
Number of cases	354	604	164
Great toe	76%	70%	66%
Ankle/foot	50%	34%	35%
Knee	32%	20%	12%
Finger	25%	12%	7%
Wrist	10%	7%	4%
Elbow	10%	7%	4%
Other	4%	17%	1%
Extra-articular	3%	3%	Not specified

sites of acute gout in the upper limb include the small joints of the fingers, elbows, and wrists. The shoulder joint and hip joint are rarely involved but can be affected, along with spinal joints, in particularly severe cases, and in major organ transplant recipients, it is linked with cyclosporine use. Gout in the wrist and elbow is usually associated with longer duration of disease.[15,17] Bursae that are near or communicate with affected joints may also become acutely inflamed during an attack of gout. The prepatellar and olecranon bursae are common sites of extra-articular involvement[19] (Fig. 9-2).

Polyarticular gout occurs in the first attack of gout in 11% to 28% of patients in hospital-based series.[13,20] This is likely to be a much higher proportion than would be seen in the community or in primary care; however, there are no published data on joint involvement at gout onset in community series. Fewer than four joints are involved at onset when gout develops into a polyarticular attack.[21] Resolution of inflammation in polyarticular gout may take a number of weeks. Table 9-2 summarizes the pattern of joint involvement from published case series.

The pattern of joint involvement in gout is probably explained by the physicochemical and local factors influencing the deposition of monosodium urate (MSU) crystals. A prerequisite for MSU crystal formation is hyperuricemia; however, de novo MSU crystal formation may be facilitated by other factors[22] (see Chapter 5). Situations that may favor change in serum urate or tophus remodeling, such as vigorous exercise and joint trauma, have been suggested as possible precipitants to attacks of gout.[17,23]

The intense local inflammation in gout can be associated with a systemic inflammatory response, including fever, neutrophilia, and elevation of acute phase reactants. Fever occurs more frequent in polyarticular gout, but there is no correlation between severity of fever or neutrophilia and the number of involved joints.[21,24]

Precipitants

Precipitating factors for gouty attacks are reviewed in detail in the discussion on attack prophylaxis in Chapter 15. Acute gout appears to occur more frequently in the spring or summer months.[25-27] In hospital practice, acute gout is often seen during other acute illnesses, postoperatively, or following trauma. In this context, dehydration, fasting, change in medication (particularly introduction of diuretics), and changes in alcohol intake can all contribute to rapid changes in serum urate concentration linked to promotion of gout attacks. Cessation or introduction of urate-lowering medications can also precede an attack of gout.[28-30]

Individuals with gout report a variety of activities and events that may precipitate an attack of gout, most often dietary. Data from the Health Professionals Follow-Up Study have confirmed that higher intakes of meat, seafood, and alcohol, particularly beer and spirits, are associated with a higher risk of the onset of gout.[31,32] Patients will often report dietary indiscretion or heavy alcohol intake in the days preceding the onset of an attack of gout.

Differential Diagnosis

Diagnosis of gout is reviewed in Chapter 7. In brief, spontaneous onset of an acute, severe monoarthritis affecting the MTPJ of the great toe in a middle-aged man with hyperuricemia is most commonly gout. The differential for an acute monoarthritis or oligoarthritis is very broad and includes pseudogout, septic arthritis, and spondyloarthritis. The differential for an acute

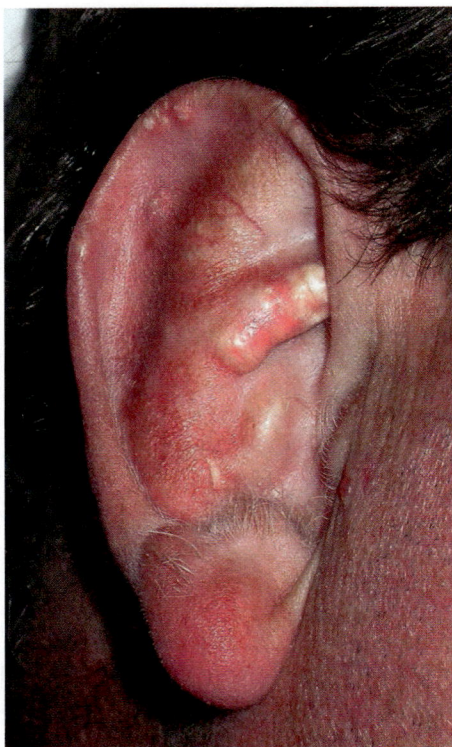

Figure 9-3 Small tophi in the classical location of the helix of the pinnae, with a large tophus on the anthelix. (*Photograph courtesy of Louise Goossens, Photographic Unit, University of Otago, Wellington.*)

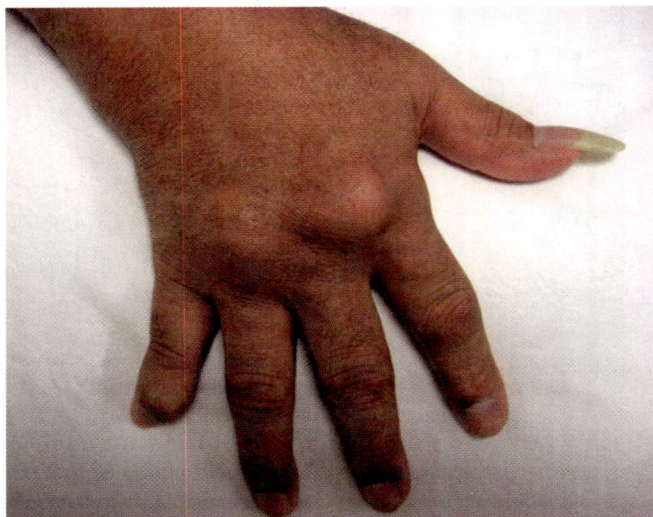

Figure 9-4 Large tophi overlying the dorsal aspect of the hand between the index and middle finger and middle finger and ring finger metocarpophalangeal joints. Swelling of the proximal and distal interphalangeal joints is due to intra- and periarticular tophi. (*Images courtesy of Rebecca Grainger, taken with permission from the patient.*)

polyarthritis also includes the systemic immune arthritides. The critical diagnostic investigation is joint arthrocentesis with demonstration of MSU crystals in synovial fluid. This should be performed in all instances of a possible diagnosis of gout, to confirm the diagnosis and exclude septic arthritis. Careful examination for the presence of tophi may assist in diagnosis but should not preclude examination of synovial fluid.

Chronic Gout

If hyperuricemia persists, gout may evolve from a sporadic acute monoarthritis to a pattern of more frequent acute attacks, which may affect multiple joints simultaneously (polyarticular gout) or in rapid succession. Macroscopic deposits of MSU crystals, known as tophi, may accumulate in the joints, tendon sheaths, over bony prominences, and in subcutaneous tissues. Clinically, tophi are recognized as asymmetric white to yellow firm swellings under the skin. Common soft tissue locations of subcutaneous tophi include the ear pinnae, olecranon or prepatella bursae, the distal interphalangeal joints, and overlying the dorsum of the MTPJ and metacarpophalangeal joint (MCPJ) (Figs. 9-3 and 9-4).

Microscopically tophi are deposits of MSU crystal surrounded by a chronic inflammatory infiltrate consisting of macrophages, lymphocytes, and occasional neutrophils.[33] Tophi can be accompanied by persistent low-grade inflammation causing chronic pain, tenderness, swelling, and redness of affected tophi or joints. This presentation may resemble the widespread small and large joint synovitis of rheumatoid arthritis or psoriatic arthritis.

Complications of Chronic Gout

Articular and periarticular tophi can be associated with bone erosions and significant joint deformities. Articular and periarticular tophi can cause marked swelling at the proximal and distal interphalangeal joints and the MCPJs. Hand deformities can include swan neck, boutonniere, and flexion deformities, virtually indistinguishable from those seen in rheumatoid arthritis (Figs. 9-4 and 9-5). Tophi may erode the overlying soft tissue and cause ulcerating lesions that discharge a chalk-like material consisting of MSU crystals (Fig. 9-6). The deformities, mechanical impact of tophi, and ulceration all contribute to loss of joint and limb function and are often cosmetically unappealing. Patients often are unable to wear normal footwear and resort to sandals or cutting holes in shoes to accommodate tophi. Tophi overlying the olecranon are frequently traumatized during daily activity or employment, becoming inflamed and painful. In the hand, the number of tophi overlying joints is the best predictor of hand function with greater number of tophi associated with worse hand function.[34] The frequency and impact of other direct complications of tophi have not been formally quantified but undoubtedly have impacts on health-related quality of life and health care costs for individuals with tophaceous gout.

Tophi that ulcerate the skin can become secondarily infected, causing cellulitis or infections of the deep tissues including septic arthritis and osteomyelitis. As ulcerated tophi often already have local inflammation in response to the MSU crystal, a high index of suspicion must be maintained for coexistent infection. Increasing pain, purulent discharge, enlarging area of erythema, or systemic illness may all suggest secondary infection.

Surgery for Tophi

Occasionally, tophi may require surgical excision or debridement if the tophus is frequently injured, painful, becomes infected, or interferes with limb function, footwear, or ability

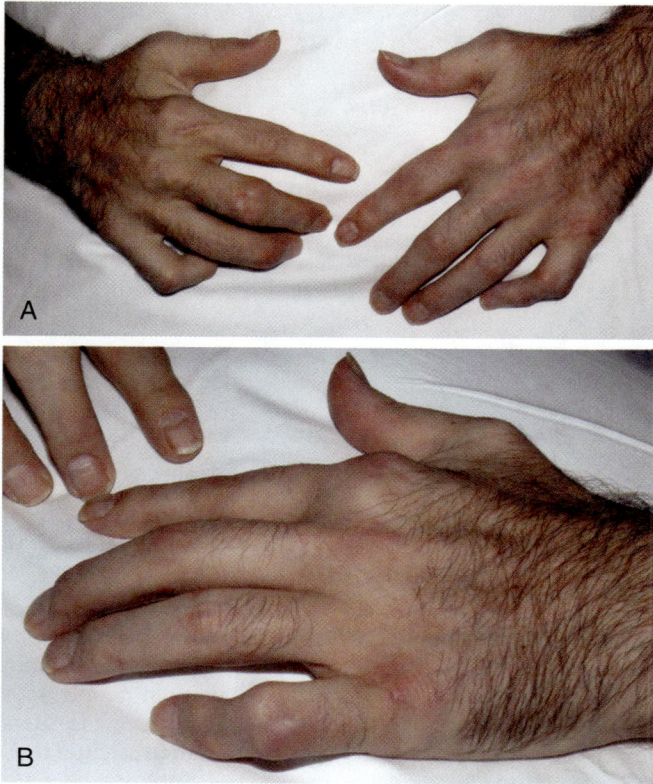

Figure 9-5 This man with tophaceous gout has swelling of the proximal and distal interphalangeal joints. There are flexion deformities affecting both little fingers with pearly white subcutaneous visible at the distal interphalangeal joint. *(Photograph courtesy of Louise Goossens, Photographic Unit, University of Otago, Wellington.)*

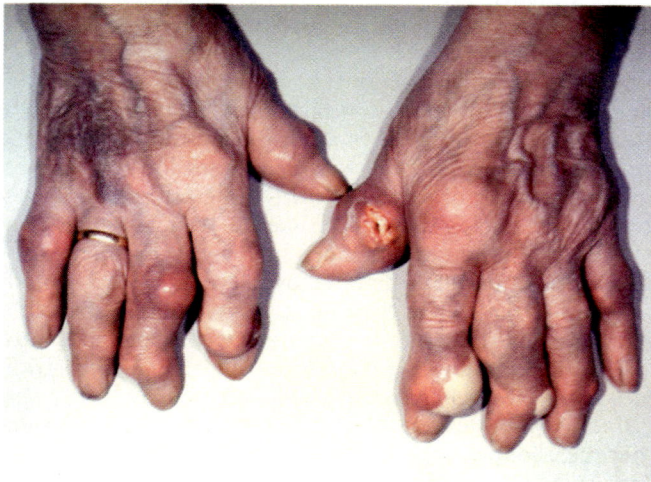

Figure 9-6 Severe, advanced tophaceous gout of the hands with prominent superficial tophi visible is overlying the left index and middle finger distal interphalangeal joints and an ulcerated tophus over the interphalangeal joint of the left thumb. *(From Slide Atlas of Rheumatology. London, UK: Gower Medical Publishing Ltd.; 1984.)*

to complete daily activities. Ulcerated tophi can become secondarily infected and surgical debridement is often necessary prior to curative treatment with antibiotics. In the largest case series reporting 45 cases requiring surgical management of tophi in gout, indications for surgery were control of sepsis

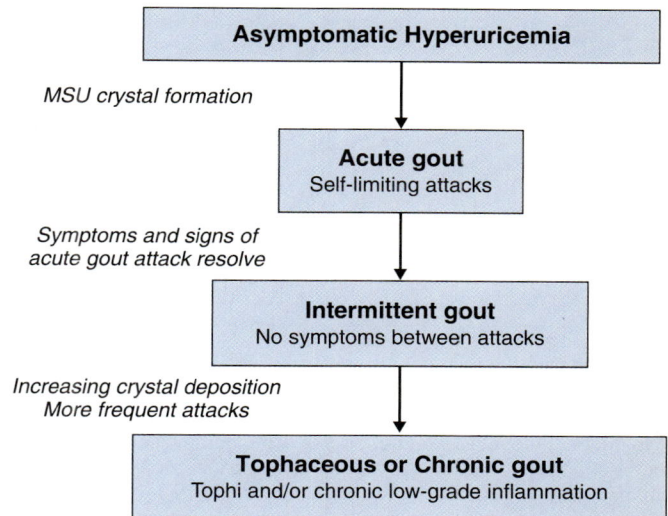

Figure 9-7 The clinical stages of gout. There are limited data describing the natural history of gout; however most clinicians recognize progression through the clinical stages if hyperuricemia remains untreated.

(51%), mechanical problems in hand, foot, or elbow (27%), and pain (4%).[35] The remaining 18% of procedures were for excision of a soft tissue mass of unknown etiology, with subsequent demonstration of MSU crystals within the excised tophaceous deposit. Delayed wound healing (longer than 1 week) occurred in just over half of cases, within delayed healing twice as common in surgery to the lower limb than to the upper limb. Factors contributing to impaired wound healing included preceding local infection, inadequate debridement of tophi, and unrecognized vascular disease. Newer techniques such as hydrosurgical debridement may offer improved debulking of large subcutaneous tophi with improved wound healing.[36,37] Optimal perioperative care of individuals undergoing surgery on tophi must include assessment and optimization of vascular supply, aggressive control of sepsis, control of blood glucose in coexisting diabetes, and meticulous wound management. Optimization of urate-lowering medication is imperative for all patients with complicated tophi.

Natural History of Gout

After resolution of the first acute attack of gout, an individual is asymptomatic and this period between attacks is referred to as "intercritical gout." Following a initial attack of gout, it is estimated that 60% of individuals will experience a further attack within 1 year and 80% within 3 years.[38] With subsequent attacks and increasing duration of gout, the frequency of polyarticular attacks increases and there is more frequent involvement of the upper limb.[13,15,16]

There are few useful longitudinal data on the natural history of gout, but the generally accepted dogma is that if the underlying hyperuricemia remains untreated, there is evolution, usually over many years, from acute, sporadic monoarticular or polyarticular gout (acute gout) to recurrent polyarthritis and formation of tophi, known as chronic tophaceous gout (Fig. 9-7). Chronic tophaceous gout can manifest with persistent, mild to moderate joint and peritophaceous inflammation, which causes chronic pain (Fig. 9-8).

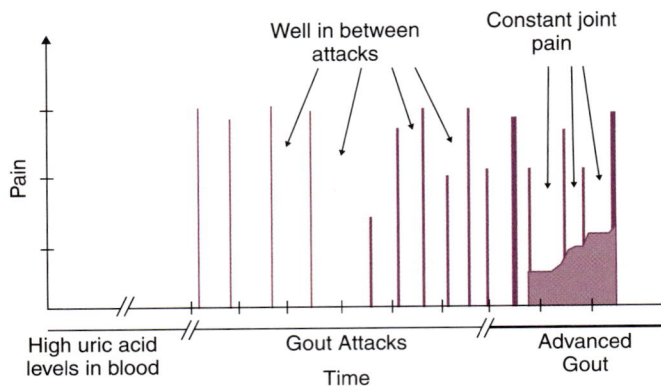

Figure 9-8 The natural history of gout is progression from asymptomatic hyperuricemia to intermittent attacks of acute gout, with no symptoms between attacks. In chronic tophaceous gout, patients often experience chronic daily joint pain and swelling, punctuated by acute attacks of gout. (Adapted from Klippel et al, eds. Primer on the Rheumatic Diseases. 12th ed. Arthritis Foundation; 2001:313.)

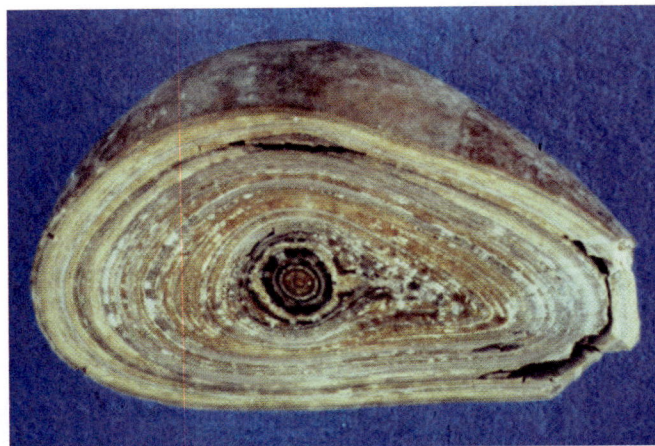

Figure 9-9 A uric acid stone. (From Slide Atlas of Rheumatology. London, UK: Gower Medical Publishing Ltd.; 1984.)

The natural history of progression through these three stages is highly variable. Before the use of urate-lowering therapy, chronic polyarticular gout or tophi developed 3 to 42 years after a first attack of gout, with an average of 11.6 years.[39] More recent data in untreated gout have shown tophi develop in 12% of patients within 5 years and 55% of patients in 20 years.[40] In certain circumstances, tophi may develop very rapidly, after one or two acute attacks, particularly in women with osteoarthritis in the small joints of the hands who are treated with diuretics[41,42] and in patients with organ transplantation treated with cyclosporine.[43] Other risk factors for progression to tophaceous gout are not well defined but one study has identified an increased incidence of tophi in individuals with younger age at onset, longer duration of gout, delay in commencement of urate-lowering therapy, and history of polyarticular or upper limb involvement.[44]

Renal Manifestations of Gout

In the majority of people with gout, the principal reason for hyperuricemia is relative underexcretion of filtered urate.[45] In this sense, gout could be considered a primary renal disease.[46] The renal defects that underlie this metabolic abnormality are described more fully elsewhere in this textbook (see Chapter 4).

However, in addition to the most common cause of gout being located in the kidney, the consequences of gout and hyperuricemia are also manifest in the kidney and comprise a number of clinical syndromes that will be the focus of this section. These may be considered in the order in which they appeared historically: uric acid nephrolithiasis, urate nephropathy in the absence of overt lithiasis, recognition of familial juvenile hyperuricemic nephropathy (FJHN) and complete or partial hypoxanthine-guanine phosphoribosyltransferase (HPRT) deficiency (Lesch-Nyhan and Kelley-Seegmiller syndromes, respectively), acute uric acid–related nephropathy due to tumor lysis with the introduction of cytotoxic chemotherapy, and, most recently, the notion that soluble urate may have a direct pathogenic effect as a renal and vascular toxin.[47]

Uric Acid Nephrolithiasis

Uric acid was first identified as a component of kidney stones (Fig. 9-9) in 1776 and now accounts for around 10% of nephrolithiasis in the United States. Uric acid stones are the main reason for the higher rate of nephrolithiasis in people with type 2 diabetes mellitus and obesity. Uric acid stone formers tend to be older and more likely to be obese than calcium oxalate stone formers.[48]

Nephrolithiasis presents in much the same way regardless of the chemical nature of the kidney stone, with the classic symptoms of renal colic and hematuria. Uric acid stones are radiopaque but are well demonstrated on computed tomography (CT), and dual-energy CT (DECT) identifies uric acid stones with higher specificity than other modalities.[49] The risk of recurrence is not greatly affected by the chemical nature of the stone and is 27% over 7.5 years.[50]

Although people with gout are at higher risk of uric acid stone formation compared with nongout populations (with a multivariate relative risk of 2.12 in men of incident kidney stones[51]), most patients with uric acid stones do not have gout or hyperuricemia or even necessarily hyperuricosuria.[52] Men with nephrolithiasis are no more likely to have gout than men without nephrolithiasis.[51] Among men with gout, the prevalence of nephrolithiasis detected by helical CT was 27% but over half of these were clinically asymptomatic.[53] Men with gout and nephrolithiasis are more likely to be obese. Symptomatic nephrolithiasis was observed in 15% of men with gout in the Health Professionals Follow-Up Study.[51]

Calcium oxalate stones are more common in people with gout than are uric acid stones and pure uric acid stones are distinctly uncommon, being present in 16 of 163 (10%) stone-formers with gout from a stone registry.[54] The major metabolic characteristics of calcium oxalate stone formers are greater urinary calcium excretion and lower urinary citrate excretion leading to higher urinary saturation of calcium oxalate. Urinary calcium levels following an oral calcium load are also greater, suggesting increased gastrointestinal absorption of calcium.[54] The mechanism for these observations is unclear.

The major metabolic abnormality that underpins uric acid lithiasis is excessive urinary acidity since urine pH is the major determinant of uric acid crystallization. In most

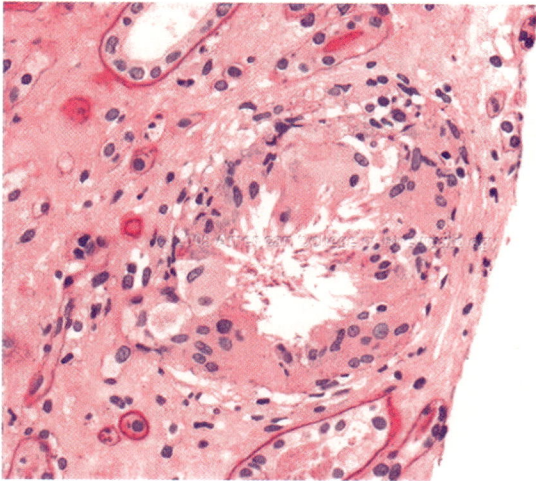

Figure 9-10 Urate nephropathy. There is chronic tubulointerstitial nephritis. Note the tubule distended by a collection of needle-like spaces, originally containing urate deposits, associated with multinucleated giant cells (PAS stain, magnification ×40). (© 2011 American College of Rheumatology. Available online at Rheumatology Image Bank: http://images.rheumatology.org/viewphoto.php?albumId=75676&;imageId=2862276.)

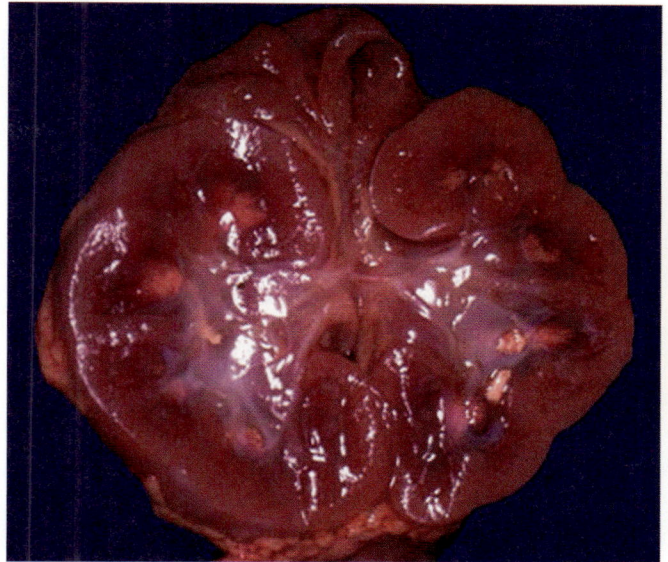

Figure 9-11 This is chronic urate nephropathy with pale yellowish tan tophaceous deposits in the medulla. (Image © Edward C. Klatt, MD, Savannah, Georgia, USA. All rights reserved. Available at http://library.med.utah.edu/WebPath/RENAHTML/RENAL121.html.)

cases, this is idiopathic. Acidic urine is observed in people with gout, even in the absence of renal stones, but is worse in stone formers,[52] and this is associated with a deficit of ammonium excretion.[55]

Although hyperuricosuria is a very important factor in leading to uric acid stones in some patient groups, this is not present in most people with uric acid nephrolithiasis. Hyperuricosuria may occur in rare metabolic conditions such as Lesch-Nyhan syndrome, Kelley-Seegmiller syndrome, some glycogen storage diseases, or rare cases of URAT1 (*SLC22A12*)[56] or GLUT9 (*SLC2A9*)[57] mutations associated with severe hypouricemia (see Chapter 4).

Recently, an association between the metabolic syndrome and uric acid nephrolithiasis has been identified. This association appears not to be due to the known association of hyperuricemia and the metabolic syndrome but rather an association between an unduly acidic urinary pH and the metabolic syndrome. The principal mechanisms of urinary acidity in uric acid nephrolithiasis are increased net acid excretion and impaired buffering caused by inadequate ammonium excretion. Urinary pH and ammonium excretion are directly correlated with the number of metabolic syndrome features, with more features being associated with a more acidic urine and lower ammonium excretion. In studies using the hyperinsulinemic euglycemic clamp technique, insulin resistance was shown to be associated with excessive urinary acidity.[58]

Urate Nephropathy

The extent to which hyperuricemia causes rather than is caused by renal impairment has long been a subject for discussion and is reviewed in Chapter 19. It is important to clarify terminology. Urate interstitial nephropathy is urate crystal deposition in the physiologic pH of renal medulla, as opposed to tubular lumen obstruction due to uric acid urolithiasis seen in tumor lysis syndrome or uricase knockout mice.

With specific respect to urate nephropathy ("gouty nephropathy"), Sydenham[9] describes "morbific matter" in what may be an early account of gouty nephopathy:

The viscera in time are so much injured, from the stagnation of the morbific matter therein, that the organs of secretion no longer perform their functions, whence the blood, overcharged with vitiated humours, stagnates, and the gouty matter ceases to be thrown upon the extremities as formerly, so that at length death frees him from his misery.

In the middle of the 20th century, it was well recognized that patients with gout could frequently develop renal impairment.[59] In that era prior to the widespread introduction of effective urate-lowering therapy or antihypertensive therapy, renal failure in patients with primary gout was not rare. For example, a case series of approximately 300 patients with mainly untreated gout from the 1950s observed significant renal disease in 18% to 25% of cases, and renal histologic changes, in 1960, were observed in the large majority of people with gout.[59] However, whether these observations were due to hyperuricemia directly or to hypertension that is often coexistent with gout is difficult to determine. Pathologically, the kidneys of people with gout are characterized mainly by changes typically associated with hypertensive renal disease: advanced arteriosclerosis, glomerulosclerosis, and interstitial fibrosis (Figs. 9-10 and 9-11). Urate crystal deposition is observed, but the focal nature of that feature seems inconsistent with the diffuse nature of the renal disease.[60] Furthermore, perhaps analogous to the fact that most people with hyperuricemia do not develop gout, 86% of postmortem cases with renal medullary urate deposits did not have gout in life.[61]

In people with elevated serum urate, it has been postulated that hyperuricemia itself is directly nephrotoxic, even prior to the development of the clinical syndrome of gout, and may be a mechanism for the increased rate of hypertension, cardiovascular disease and renal impairment that is observed (see Chapters 6 and 19).[62,63] On the other hand, some authors have called this a "non-disease" based on the infrequency of the combination of chronic hyperuricemic nephropathy and renal failure not otherwise explained that was observed in a large series of postmortem examinations[64] or in longitudinal cohort studies.[65] Similarly, serum urate levels have not always been found to be an independent risk factor for renal progression, especially when baseline renal impairment is taken into account.[66] In a longitudinal study that followed people with gout over a decade, it was observed that only those with associated hypertension had progressive renal impairment but control of hyperuricemia appeared to have no significant association with progressive renal impairment.[67]

In contrast, studies of patients with immunoglobulin A (IgA) nephropathy have shown that hyperuricemia was an independent risk factor for progressive renal dysfunction, having adjusted for proteinuria, hypertension, diabetes, age, gender, and obesity.[68] In addition, a large study of male railway workers showed that baseline hyperuricemia of greater than 8.5 mg/dL was associated with an 8.5-fold increased rate of death with renal failure at 5 years.[69] This latter study did not appear to adjust for important comorbidities.

Although earlier Framingham Study data did not support the notion that serum urate was independently associated with cardiovascular morbidity,[70] there is now evidence from large epidemiologic studies, including the MRFIT study,[71] Framingham study,[72] and the Health Professionals Follow-Up Study,[73] that several cardiovascular outcomes are independently associated with gout in men. The risk of coronary heart disease is independently increased (odds ratio [OR] 1.6, 95% confidence interval [CI] 1.1 to 2.5[72]; OR 1.26, 95% CI 1.14 to 1.40[71]). And the risk of all cardiovascular death (OR 1.38, 95% CI 1.15 to 1.66) and fatal coronary heart disease is also increased (OR 1.55, 94% CI 1.04 to 2.41).[73]

The analytic difficulty with determining the connection between serum urate, hypertension, and renal outcomes is the close association of renal function itself with uric acid levels and the association of hyperuricemia with other causes of renal impairment (especially hypertension), confounding the interpretation of direction or mechanism of the association. One way to resolve the difficulty would be experimental—directly testing the notion that a reduction in uric acid levels leads to improvement in renal function. While there are some experiments in animals that support this idea, for example,[74,75] there is limited evidence that reduction of serum urate with allopurinol reduces progression of renal function in patients with renal impairment and no history of gout. In one study, creatinine rose by 21% in allopurinol-treated patients compared to a 55% increase in patients allocated to placebo. However, the small numbers of patients and variability in renal function progression meant that this apparent difference was not statistically significant at the conventional 5% level.[76] Another small, nonrandomized, study of allopurinol treatment in people with asymptomatic hyperuricemia and normal renal function showed that renal function improved significantly in allopurinol-treated patients but there was no change in normal control subjects.[77] This study is difficult to interpret because the control subjects were normouricemic and there was no random allocation. There remains a need for a large, properly designed study to test the notion that urate-lowering therapy improves renal outcomes.

Familial Juvenile Hyperuricemic Nephropathy (FJHN, OMIM 162000)

This condition is an autosomal dominant disease characterized by end-stage renal failure at a young age, reduced fractional excretion of urate, renal interstitial urate deposits, and sporadic gouty arthritis. In one Polynesian family, two sisters and a child of the propositus (who presented with gout and end-stage renal failure) had renal failure and hyperuricemia but not gout.[78] More than 50 families with FJHN have been described in various ethnic groups since the original description in 1960.[79] The condition is genetically heterogeneous and can be caused by mutations in the *UROMODULIN* (*UMOD*) gene located on chromosome 16p12.3 to p13.11.[80] The *UMOD* gene encodes uromodulin, also known as the Tamm-Horsfall glycoprotein. It has been suggested that the disease is associated with abnormalities in protein folding, maturation, and trafficking of uromodulin rather than deficiency.[80]

Acute Hyperuricemic Nephropathy

This condition is not usually associated with gout but is a disorder of sudden, massive urate load caused by tumor lysis, often in children with hematopoietic malignancies. Dehydration and low urinary pH may be associated features. Due to a sudden oversaturation of uric acid in the urine, uric acid precipitates as crystals or sludge in tubules and collecting ducts leading to urinary obstruction. Interstitial fibrosis or tophi are not generally observed.

Unusual Clinical Features

Although gout has a characteristic presentation that helps with recognition and diagnosis in clinical practice, there are a large number of less common presentations of which the practitioner should be aware. These typically relate to an unusual distribution of joint involvement, such as the acromioclavicular joint,[81] or an unusual location of a tophaceous deposit, such as the odontoid process.[82] It is suggested that a high index of suspicion be entertained in people with severe tophaceous disease. Tophi have been described in diverse locations, typically in regions with relatively poor blood supply. Interestingly, the brain appears to be protected from tophaceous disease since there has never been a case report of intracranial tophi, although tophaceous bony destruction of the base of the skull has been described in relation to extension from the temporomandibular joint.[83]

Although not exclusively, these rare complications generally represent extremely severe gout with very high urate load. In earlier years, such gout was termed "malignant." For example, a patient with extremely severe gout that developed at the age of 18 years and led to early mortality from renal failure and ileus was described (Fig. 9-12). At postmortem, multiple small tophi were found throughout the small intestine.[84]

Skin Disease

While subcutaneous tophi ulcerating through the skin overlying joints are commonly observed in severe tophaceous gout, other less typical manifestations of cutaneous tophi have been

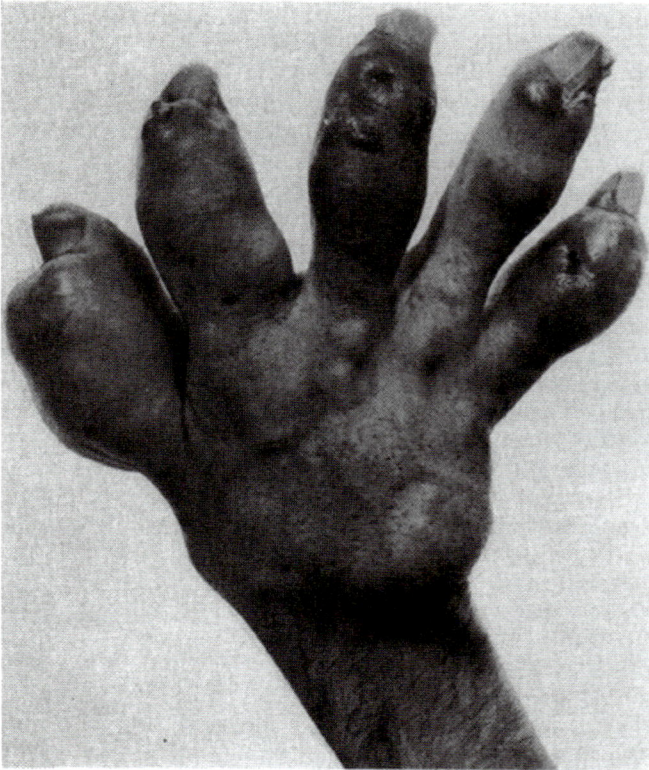

Figure 9-12 Very severe gout producing an appearance similar to a "bunch of parsnips" in a patient with "malignant gout." *(From Hawkins CF, Ellis HA, Rawson A. Malignant gout with tophaceous small intestine and megaloblastic anaemia. Ann Rheum Dis 1965;34.)*

described. Panniculitis in which subcutaneous tophi lead to chronic inflammatory changes in tissue distant from joints is one example.[85-87] An acute pustular eruption on the palm and sole was also described in a patient, in which a biopsy of a pustule showed uric acid crystals to be present, presumably causing this particular inflammatory response.[88] Cutaneous gout may arise without a history of arthritis.[89]

Laryngeal Involvement

Gouty laryngitis has been described since Garrod found urate deposits on the arytenoid cartilage of a man who had severe tophaceous gout at postmortem examination.[90] Ewart mentions previous descriptions of sputum containing uric acid and speculates that these arise from ulcerating laryngeal tophi.[91] Laryngeal tophi have been excised in life,[92] and the most recent review of this topic notes its apparent rarity (only 12 reported cases) and clinical presentations that can include a neck lump, hoarseness, odynophagia, dysphagia, dysphonia, stridor, and airway obstruction.[93] Lack of diagnostic awareness may contribute to its apparent rarity.

Saturnine Gout

Lead toxicity may cause gout via incompletely understood mechanisms. The term "saturnine" derives from the use of lead goblets to drink large quantities of wine during the Roman festival of Saturn. In modern times, the risk appears to be greatest for occupations that have significant lead exposure such as battery manufacture, exposure to lead-containing paint, and potters. Lead poisoning has been reported to affect renal tubular reabsorption of uric acid, leading to decreased fractional urate excretion and urinary uric acid–to–creatinine ratio.[94] Lead-urate complexes in the serum of people with saturnine gout have also been reported.[95]

Saturnine gout is usually preceded by other features of lead toxicity such as anemia (with basophilic stippling), abdominal pain, and nerve palsies. Acute arthritis typical of primary gout may not occur despite the development of a chronic gouty arthropathy. The knee tends to be more commonly affected than the first MTPJ, but otherwise the clinical presentation is similar to that of primary gout. One other important difference is that renal impairment frequently precedes the development of saturnine gout, rather than being a late complication.[96]

Spinal Gout

This topic was recently examined by Konatalapalli et al.[97] These authors note that axial gout can present with pain, stiffness, radiculopathy, and spinal cord compression or may be asymptomatic. Both tophaceous deposits and gouty arthritis of spinal joints, including sacroiliac joints, have been reported.[98] CT was recommended over magnetic resonance imaging (MRI) to help confirm the diagnosis. In the series of patients reported by Konatalapalli et al., 9 of 64 patients (14%) with gout who had undergone CT imaging for a variety of reasons (not because of suspicion of axial gout) showed features of axial gout, and this most frequently affected the lumbar spine.

Visceral Gout

Renal disease is described elsewhere in this chapter but there are many case reports of other visceral tophi deposition–mimicking conditions such as pancreatic tumor,[99] endocarditis or other heart valve disease,[100,101] breast mass, or intestinal tumor.

For example, a case was reported of a man with longstanding, poorly controlled gout presenting with abdominal pain and imaging findings that suggested pelvic abscess.[102] The MRI findings included rim-enhancing cystic lesions along the left psoas and iliacus muscles and soft tissue swelling around these muscles (Fig. 9-13). Only direct aspiration of the lesion under CT guidance confirmed that the lesion represented a tophus.

Ocular Gout

Conjunctival gouty tophi have been reported in a woman with severe, longstanding, poorly treated gout[103] (Fig. 9-14). Other ocular manifestations include uveitis, band keratopathy, glaucoma, asteroid hyalosis,[104] and periocular tophi (Fig. 9-15).[105] Red eye related to conjunctival and episcleral hyperemia was the most common ocular abnormality observed in a series of 69 patients with gout. The mechanism of this association is not clear but presumably relates to precipitated urate crystals.

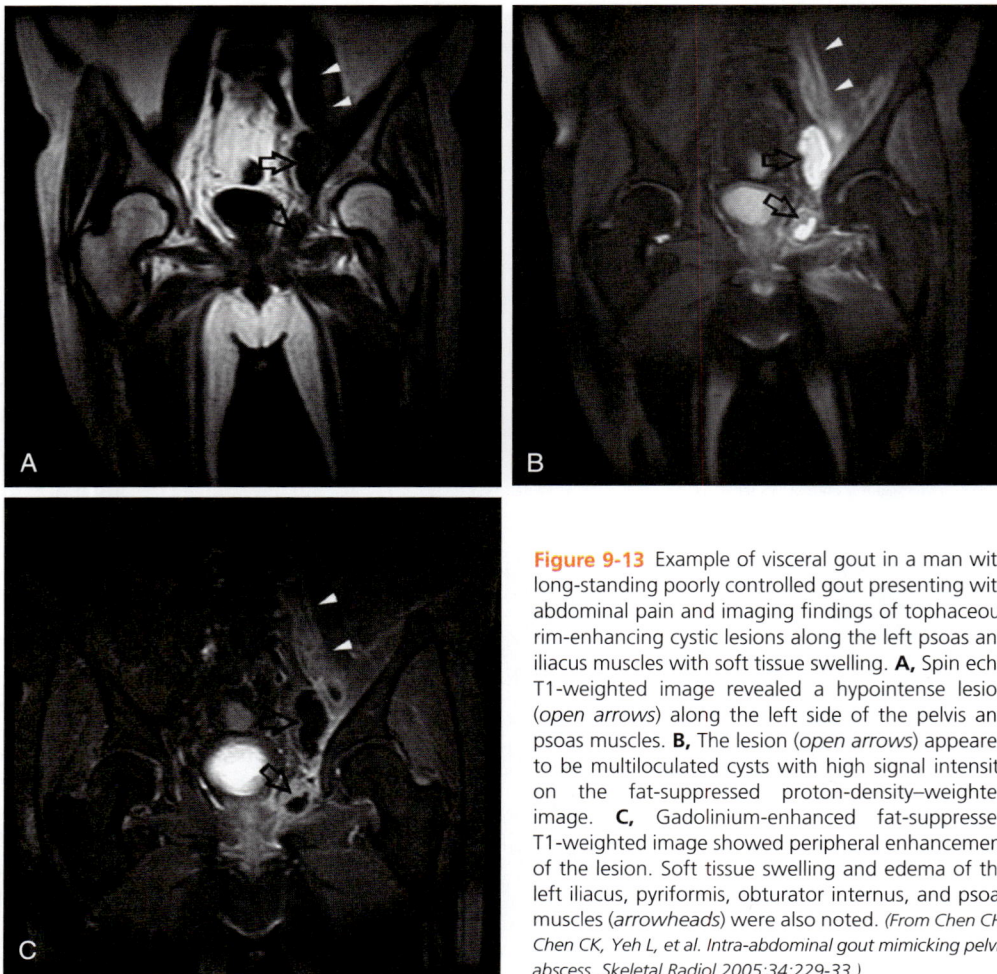

Figure 9-13 Example of visceral gout in a man with long-standing poorly controlled gout presenting with abdominal pain and imaging findings of tophaceous rim-enhancing cystic lesions along the left psoas and iliacus muscles with soft tissue swelling. **A,** Spin echo T1-weighted image revealed a hypointense lesion (*open arrows*) along the left side of the pelvis and psoas muscles. **B,** The lesion (*open arrows*) appeared to be multiloculated cysts with high signal intensity on the fat-suppressed proton-density–weighted image. **C,** Gadolinium-enhanced fat-suppressed T1-weighted image showed peripheral enhancement of the lesion. Soft tissue swelling and edema of the left iliacus, pyriformis, obturator internus, and psoas muscles (*arrowheads*) were also noted. *(From Chen CH, Chen CK, Yeh L, et al. Intra-abdominal gout mimicking pelvic abscess. Skeletal Radiol 2005;34:229-33.)*

Tenosynovitis and Entrapment Neuropathies

Tenosynovitis caused by gout can mimic infection and requires histologic studies to distinguish.[106,107] Carpal tunnel syndrome and other entrapment neuropathies caused by flexor tenosynovitis and tophaceous deposits have been reported.[108,109] Tophaceous infiltration of tendon can lead to rupture.[110]

Classification Criteria

Although classification criteria are not designed to be diagnostic criteria, they usually contain cardinal features of the disease that might be useful for diagnosis. There are no clinical features that are completely specific for gout. Nevertheless, there are several clinical features that are very typical that form part of the recent European League Against Rheumatism (EULAR) consensus statement on the diagnosis of gout (Table 9-3). Other diagnostic considerations are discussed elsewhere, but this section focuses on the clinical features that can help identify gouty arthritis.

These include the distribution of joint involvement (especially the first MTPJ involvement) but other lower limb joints are frequently involved (knee, ankle, tarsal). The abrupt

onset, rapid rise to maximal pain, and extreme tenderness that form the classic description by Sydenham are very accurately observed:

> The victim goes to bed and sleeps in good health. About two o'clock in the morning he is awakened by a severe pain in the great toe; more rarely in the heel, ankle or instep.... He cannot bear the weight of bedclothes nor the jar of a person walking in the room....[9]

Spontaneous resolution of the acute episode by 10 to 14 days is also typical—persistent symptoms during the intercritical period is a clue toward chronic gouty arthropathy or an alternative diagnosis. The patient with gout will often have fairly stereotypical episodes that characterize an acute attack, which can be easily identified as such without the need for repeated synovial fluid analysis. Patient self-report was the most accurate clinical means of identifying a gout attack in a cohort study of patients with known gout.[111]

A consensus study to identify the features that best characterized an attack of gout (in people known to have gouty arthritis) found that the most important features were marked tenderness of the affected joint, swelling of the affected joint, maximum pain within 4 to 12 hours, acute onset, similarity to previous flares, redness of the affected joint, moderate response to standard antiinflammatory gout therapy, and

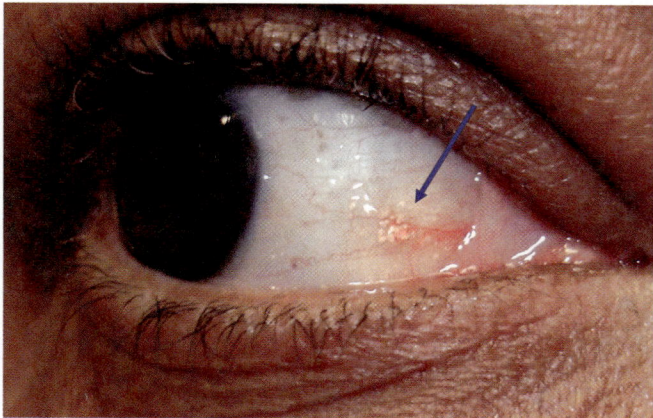

Figure 9-14 External photograph of bulbar conjunctiva in patient with tophaceous gout. Many distinct granular deposits of chalky white material are present in conjunctiva (*arrow*). *(From Lo WR, Broocker G, Grossniklaus HE. Histopathologic examination of conjunctival tophi in gouty arthritis. Am J Ophthalmol 2005;140(6):1152-4, Figure 1.)*

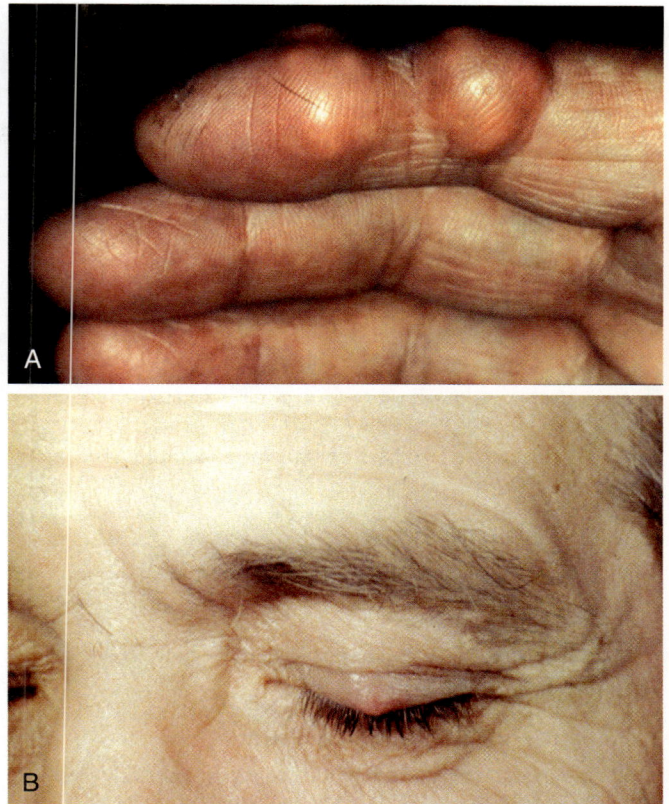

Figure 9-15 Tophus occurring on the upper eyelid in a patient with tophaceous gout. *(From Slide Atlas of Rheumatology. London, UK: Gower Medical Publishing Ltd.; 1984.)*

recurrent pattern of attacks. These are generally also endorsed by patients with gout as indicating key features of a gout attack.[112] While these are features that characterize attacks in people known to have gout, they can be somewhat helpful pointers toward a diagnosis of gout in those not yet diagnosed.

In many situations, the pathologic gold standard for case definition is not available. This is particularly true of epidemiologic studies of gout where it is impractical to require synovial fluid analysis of every participant. It may also be true for clinical trials and in some clinical situations where access to polarizing light microscopy is limited or where it is impractical to aspirate joints. While it may appear that the problem is the same for each of the situations, the appropriate solution is quite different.

It is very important to understand the difference in case definition between research studies (clinical trials or epidemiology) and clinical work. The purpose in the former is to apply a standardized (restricted) set of criteria that most closely mimic the pathologic gold standard (MSU crystals in synovial fluid). In the latter situation, the objective is to use all available information, including the intuition and experience of the physician, to make as accurate a diagnosis as possible for a particular individual. Elements of standardized classification criteria will usually be part of the informational database used by a physician, but he or she is not restricted to these elements and may consider many other data to help form a judgment. Thus, unless the classification criteria *perfectly* mimics the pathologic gold standard (in which case it *is* the gold standard), criteria should never be used for diagnosis in an individual-clinician encounter but only as an aid to recalling important parts of the informational database.

Unbiased classification criteria have several requirements that need to be met in their development[113]: a development cohort of unselected cases and controls is assembled that are similar to the population in which the criteria will be used (this is especially true of the controls), the pathologic gold standard (or proxy) is available for each subject, a comprehensive list of potential items of the criteria is compiled independently of the "gold standard" definition of *case-ness* (this is especially important when the "gold standard" is physician judgment),

and the derived criteria are also tested in an independent cohort of controls and cases to determine its performance.

There have been three published classification criteria for gout but only one is usually cited.[114] The criteria from the Rome symposium in 1961[115] and New York in 1966[116] criteria are shown in Table 9-4. These criteria identify key features of gout but were not developed through observed data and have been tested only to a limited extent.

A study of 22 patients with gout in Sudbury, Massachusetts, found that 8 patients satisfied the Rome criteria only, 4 the New York criteria only, and 10 satisfied both sets (yields a sensitivity of 0.82 and 0.64 for the Rome and New York criteria, respectively).[117] A much larger second study of consecutive rheumatology clinic attendees from six European centers (59 patients with gout and 761 patients with other rheumatic diseases) showed that the specificity of both sets was very high (0.99 for both Rome and New York) but the sensitivity was not (0.64 and 0.80 for the Rome and New York sets, respectively).[118] The requirement for tophi may limit the sensitivity of these criteria since only 31% of patients with gout had a definite tophus in the larger second study.

The 1977 American Rheumatism Association (ARA) criteria (Table 9-5), now over 30 years old, were informed by data to identify the acute arthritis of primary gout—how adequately were they developed and how well do they perform? The case and control participants were drawn from 706 patients submitted by 38 rheumatologists across the United States. How the cases and controls were selected was not specified but only patients with rheumatoid arthritis, pseudogout,

Table 9-3 Recommendations From the EULAR Task Force of the Standing Committee for International Clinical Studies Including Therapeutics (ESCISIT) Concerning the Diagnosis of Gout

	Proposition	Strength of Recommendation (95% Confidence Interval)
1	In acute attacks, the rapid development of severe pain, swelling, and tenderness that reaches its maximum within just 6-12 hours, especially with overlying erythema, is highly suggestive of crystal inflammation although not specific for gout.	88 (80-96)
2	For typical presentations of gout (such as recurrent podagra with hyperuricemia), a clinical diagnosis alone is reasonably accurate but not definitive without crystal confirmation.	95 (91-98)
3	Demonstration of MSU crystals in synovial fluid or tophus aspirates permits a definitive diagnosis of gout.	96 (93-100)
4	A routine search for MSU crystals is recommended in all synovial fluid samples obtained from undiagnosed inflamed joints.	90 (83-97)
5	Identification of MSU crystals from asymptomatic joints may allow definite diagnosis in intercritical periods.	84 (78-91)
6	Gout and sepsis may coexist, so when septic arthritis is suspected Gram stain and culture of synovial fluid should still be performed even if MSU crystals are identified.	93 (87-99)
7	While being the most important risk factor for gout, serum urate levels do not confirm or exclude gout as many people with hyperuricemia do not develop gout, and during acute attacks serum levels may be normal.	95 (92-99)
8	Renal uric acid excretion should be determined in selected gout patients, especially those with a family history of young onset gout, onset of gout under age 25, or with renal calculi.	72 (62-81)
9	Although radiographs may be useful for differential diagnosis and may show typical features in chronic gout, they are not useful in confirming the diagnosis of early or acute gout.	86 (79-94)
10	Risk factors for gout and associated comorbidity should be assessed, including features of the metabolic syndrome (obesity, hyperglycemia, hyperlipidemia, hypertension).	93 (88-98)

MSU, Monosodium urate .
From Zhang W, Doherty M, Pascual E, et al. EULAR evidence based recommendations for gout. Part I: Diagnosis. Report of a Task Force of the Standing Committee for International Clinical Studies Including Therapeutics (ESCISIT). Ann Rheum Dis 2006;65:1301-11.

Table 9-4 The Rome and New York Classification Criteria for Gout

ROME	
1	Serum urate >7 mg/dL in men and >6 mg/dL in women
2	Presence of tophi
3	Monosodium urate crystals in synovial fluid or tissue
4	History of attacks of painful joint swelling with abrupt onset and resolution within 2 weeks
Diagnosis:	Two or more of any criteria

NEW YORK	
1	At least two attacks of painful joint swelling with complete resolution with 2 weeks
2	A history or observation of podagra
3	Presence of tophi
4	Rapid response to colchicine treatment, defined as a major reduction in the objective signs of inflammation within 48 hours
Diagnosis:	Two or more of any criteria OR presence of monosodium urate crystals in synovial fluid or on deposition.

Table 9-5 American Rheumatism Association Preliminary Survey Classification Criteria for Acute Gout

1	More than one attack of acute arthritis
2	Maximum inflammation developed within one day
3	Oligoarthritis attack
4	Redness observed over joints
5	First metatarsophalangeal joint painful or swollen
6	Unilateral first metatarsophalangeal joint attack
7	Unilateral tarsal joint attack
8	Tophus (suspected or proven)
9	Hyperuricemia (more than 2 SD greater than the normal population average)
10	Asymmetric swelling within a joint on x-ray
11	Complete termination of an attack
Diagnosis: 6 of 11 criteria required	

From Wallace SL, Robinson H, Masi AT, et al. Preliminary criteria for the classification of the acute arthritis of primary gout. Arthritis Rheum 1977;20:895-900.

and acute septic arthritis were accepted as controls. So even from the earliest stage of the design of this criteria development study, there are problems. Many other rheumatic diseases and even population normals may be among the group of patients or respondents for whom such classification criteria for gout need to be applied. Importantly, for epidemiologic population studies where the frequency of gout among people with hyperuricemia is an important question, the criteria need to be constructed with a general population control group in addition to a clinical population control group. As it is, the existing criteria are also not designed for use in people with possible osteoarthritis or psoriatic arthritis, both conditions that may mimic gout. In particular, psoriatic arthritis can cause oligoarthritis or monoarthritis of the lower limb joints and be associated with hyperuricemia. It is questionable whether persons with septic arthritis represent an appropriate control group, since the diagnosis of septic arthritis relies on the results of synovial fluid analysis—a procedure for which the criteria aim to mimic.

The gold standard chosen for the classification criteria was physician diagnosis. In this way, the performance of such features such as synovial fluid analysis could be examined. Only in 76 of 90 (84%) patients in whom synovial fluid was examined were MSU crystals identified. This is difficult to understand when it is generally considered that identification of MSU crystals in synovial fluid is the defining characteristic of gout. It is possible that excellent treatment of some patients led to clearance of irate crystals, but the lower than expected sensitivity of synovial fluid analysis raises questions about the physician diagnosis (did the crystal-negative patients really have gout?) and the quality of the synovial fluid analysis.

Many patients had incomplete data. For example, half of the cases and a little over half of the controls did not have synovial fluid analysis. This was particularly problematic in controls with rheumatoid arthritis, in whom only around one quarter had synovial fluid analysis. Other important data elements that were missing were suspicion of tophus (39% of cases and 5% of controls) and hyperuricemia (6% of cases and 32% of controls). Missing data were input randomly in proportion to the presence or absence of the feature in those with nonmissing data. However, the extent of missing data in this study does significantly increase the likelihood of bias, whereby those tested (for example, serum urate) may differ systematically from those not tested (more likely to be abnormal).

Two sets of criteria were proposed. The observed performance of the proposed criteria that do not require joint or tophus aspiration (6 or more of 11 features; see Table 9-5) was sensitivity of 84.8% and specificity of 97%.

External validation of the ARA criteria has only recently been reported.[119] In this study of 80 patients who had undergone synovial fluid analysis, the performance of classification criteria was assessed against the presence of MSU acid crystals in synovial fluid (the gold standard). The clinical features of the ARA preliminary classification criteria had only 70% sensitivity and 78.8% specificity. These results underscore the need for better criteria and that the gold standard for diagnosis remains identification of MSU crystals in synovial fluid. In a more recent study of patients suspected of having gout in primary care, the ARA criteria had a sensitivity of 80% and a specificity of 64% when tested against the presence of MSU crystals in synovial fluid.[120]

Notwithstanding the problems of classification for acute gouty arthritis, there is also a need for classification criteria for intercritical or chronic gout. In most clinical research settings, participants will not have acute gout at the time of evaluation so that it is clearly necessary to develop classification criteria that do not require current evidence of active joint inflammation.

It will be difficult to undertake a robust criteria development study that uses synovial fluid analysis as the gold standard for case definition. An approach that retrospectively identifies patients for whom existing synovial fluid samples have been submitted for microscopy will be biased and limited by the extent of missing data. It may be possible to collect complete (historical) data from such patients prospectively, subsequent to their synovial fluid analysis, but this will depend on the stability of the clinical population following the index synovial fluid collection and will be limited by recall bias. Another approach would be to collect synovial fluid from consecutive patients with untreated gout, consecutive controls with arthritis and normal individuals, but this also poses difficulties (potential adverse events associated with arthrocentesis of normal joints). A worldwide collaborative effort, perhaps based around the OMERACT Gout Special Interest Group, should be pursued.

Gout in Special Populations

There are a number of clinical situations in which gout can present with atypical features. These can include a demographic group not usually affected by gout, specific patterns of joint involvement or patients with a rapidly progressing or aggressive natural history: inherited enzyme abnormalities of purine metabolism, postmenopausal women, and solid organ transplantation. HPRT deficiency and PRPP synthetase superactivity are reviewed in Chapter 3.

Gout in Women

Gout is often considered a disease of men, and this is reflected in the reported larger case series of gout, in which women make up less than 25% of the total gout cases.[15,121] In subjects younger than 65 years, the prevalence of gout is 4-fold higher in men than in women[122]; however, in older age groups, the relative prevalence of gout in women increases. Individuals older than 75 years have gout prevalence ratio of 3:1 for males to females, and in the over 80 group, this ratio falls to 2:1[122,123] (Table 9-6). Small cross-sectional studies have suggested that in the overwhelming majority of women, the onset of gout occurs after the menopause.[26,42,124] A large population-based study has confirmed that menopause is an independent risk factor for gout, probably due to the increase in the serum urate seen in women after the menopause.[125,126] The increase in serum urate postmenopausal women is attributed to the drop in circulating estrogen. Furthermore, estrogen administration after the menopause lowers serum urate, probably by promoting more efficient renal clearance of urate.[127,128]

In clinical practice, elderly women with gout often present with tophi in nodal osteoarthritis of the hands, frequently in the context of diuretic medication use. A systematic review of case series comparing clinical features of gout in men and women identified four studies reporting location of joint

Table 9-6 Estimated Prevalence of Gout in Men and Women in the United States by Age Category in a Population-Based Study in the U.S. Adult Population

Gender	Age Category (y)	Population Prevalence (%)
Male	20-29	0.2
	30-39	2.1
	40-49	2.2
	50-59	5.7
	60-69	9.1
	70-79	10.8
	>80	8.6
Women	20-29	0.6
	30-39	0.1
	40-49	0.6
	50-59	2.3
	60-69	3.5
	70-79	4.6
	>80	5.6

Estimates from the Third National Health and Nutrition Examinations Survey on self-report of doctor diagnosis of gout.
Data from Kramer HM, Curhan G. The association between gout and nephrolithiasis: the National Health and Nutrition Examination Survey III, 1988-1994. Am J Kidney Dis 2002;40:37-42.

frequency in men than in women and that women more often have gout in the ankle and upper limb joints, particularly the fingers.[129] In hospital-based case series including patients with aspirate-proved gout, women with gout are more commonly using diuretics than men (57% to 85% versus 14% to 47%),[42,124] perhaps reflecting the higher prevalence of renal insufficiency and hypertension among women with gout in these series.

Gout in Transplantation

Gout is the most common inflammatory arthritis following solid organ transplantation, occurring in up to one quarter of kidney and heart recipients.[130-132] Gout is less common after liver transplantation, despite similar rates of hyperuricemia.[131] Risk factors for gout include preexisting hyperuricemia or gout, use of cyclosporine-A, and diuretic use.[130,133] As in the general population, gout is more common in men, and in renal transplantation the risk is increased with increasing body mass index and age.[132] The initial episode of gout is often the classic presentation with podagra; however, rapid progression to tophi and polyarticular gout can occur within 3 to 5 years, compared to more than 10 years in the general population for the natural history of gout.[134,135]

Joint aspiration for diagnosis of acute and chronic arthritis is important in this immunosuppressed population because septic arthritis must be excluded, particularly as joints unusual for gout may be involved, such as the hip, and chronic indolent arthritis develops in some without typical acute attacks. Treatment of gout in renal and cardiac transplantation can be challenging due to coexistent conditions and medications.[136]

Nonsteroidal antiinflammatory drugs must be used with extreme caution with renal impairment or compensated heart failure. Colchicine use is associated with a higher risk of colchicine neuromyopathy or myelosuppression when used with concomitant cyclosporine-A, as the latter inhibits colchicine metabolism via CYP3A4 and multidrug-resistant glycoprotein transport pump. If colchicine is used in prophylaxis, colchicine dose reduction is recommended, with specifics as discussed in Chapter 15. Increasing the maintenance dose of oral glucocorticoids for 7 to 10 days or in the setting of monoarthritis, where septic arthritis has been excluded, is effective treatment in this population. Urate-lowering therapy is indicated after the first episode of gout and may be indicated if cyclosporine-A (or tacrolimus) needs to be continued and hyperuricemia is severe. Allopurinol inhibits the metabolism of azathioprine and increases cyclosporine-A trough levels, mandating substitution of mycophenolate mofetil for azathioprine and dose reduction with increased monitoring of cyclosporine-A.

References

1. Schwartz SA. Disease of distinction. Explore J Sci Healing 2006;2:515–9.
2. Osler W. The Evolution of Modern Medicine. Whitefish, MT: Kessinger Publishing; 1904.
3. Shehata M. The father of medicine. A historical reconsideration. Turkiye Klinikleri J Med Ethics 2004;12:171–6.
4. Nuki G, Simkin PA. A concise history of gout and hyperuricemia and their treatment. Arthritis Res Ther 2006:8.
5. Copeman WSC. A short history of the Gout and the Rheumatic Diseases. Los Angeles, CA: University of California Press; 1964.
6. Seegmiller JE, Rosenbloom FM, Kelley WN. Enzyme defect associated with a sex-linked human neurological disorder and excessive purine synthesis. Science 1967;155:1682–4.
7. Lesch M, Nyhan WL. A familial disorder of uric acid metabolism and central nervous system function. Am J Med 1964;36:561–70.
8. Hartung EF. Symposium on Gout: Historical considerations. Metab Clin Exp 1957;6:196–208.
9. Sydenham T. The Works of Thomas Sydenham, MD. London: Sydenham Society; 1848.
10. Conan Doyle A. The return of Sherlock Holmes. London: George Newnes; 1905.
11. Potter R, Rousseau GS. Gout: The Patrician Malady. New Haven: Yale University Press; 1998.
12. Brooks QW, Mueller E. Serum urate concentrations among university professors: relation to drive, achievement and leadership. JAMA 1966;195:415–8.
13. Lawry 2nd GV, Fan PT, Bluestone R. Polyarticular versus monoarticular gout: a prospective, comparative analysis of clinical features. Medicine (Baltimore) 1988;67:335–43.
14. Nishioka N, Mikanagi K. Clinical features of 4,000 gouty subjects in Japan. Adv Exp Med Biol 1980;122A:47–54.
15. Grahame R, Scott JT. Clinical survey of 354 patients with gout. Ann Rheum Dis 1970;29:461–8.
16. Currie WJ. The gout patient in general practice. Rheumatol Rehabil 1978;17:205–17.
17. Roddy E, Zhang W, Doherty M. Are joints affected by gout also affected by osteoarthritis? Ann Rheum Dis 2007;66:1374–7.
18. Currie WJ. Prevalence and incidence of the diagnosis of gout in Great Britain. Ann Rheum Dis 1979;38:101–6.
19. Dawn B, Williams JK, Walker SE. Prepatellar bursitis: a unique presentation of tophaceous gout in an normouricemic patient. J Rheumatol 1997;24:976–8.
20. Raddatz DA, Mahowald ML, Bilka PJ. Acute polyarticular gout. Ann Rheum Dis 1983;42:117–22.
21. Hadler NM, Franck WA, Bress NM, et al. Acute polyarticular gout. Am J Med 1974;56:715–9.
22. Tak HK, Cooper SM, Wilcox WR. Studies on the nucleation of monosodium urate at 37 degrees c. Arthritis Rheum 1980;23:574–80.

23. Knochel JP, Dotin LN, Hamburger RJ. Heat stress, exercise, and muscle injury: effects on urate metabolism and renal function. Ann Intern Med 1974;81:321–8.
24. Ho Jr G, DeNuccio M. Gout and pseudogout in hospitalized patients. Arch Intern Med 1993;153:2787–90.
25. Schlesinger N, Gowin KM, Baker DG, et al. Acute gouty arthritis is seasonal. J Rheumatol 1998;25:342–4.
26. Gallerani M, Govoni M, Mucinelli M, et al. Seasonal variation in the onset of acute microcrystalline arthritis. Rheumatology (Oxford) 1999;38:1003–6.
27. Elliot AJ, Cross KW, Fleming DM. Seasonality and trends in the incidence and prevalence of gout in England and Wales 1994-2007. Ann Rheum Dis 2009;68:1728–33.
28. Paulus HE, Schlosstein LH, Godfrey RG, et al. Prophylactic colchicine therapy of intercritical gout. A placebo-controlled study of probenecid-treated patients. Arthritis Rheum 1974;17:609–14.
29. Borstad GC, Bryant LR, Abel MP, et al. Colchicine for prophylaxis of acute flares when initiating allopurinol for chronic gouty arthritis. J Rheumatol 2004;31:2429–32.
30. Hollingworth P, Reardon JA, Scott JT. Acute gout during hypouricaemic therapy: prophylaxis with colchicine. Ann Rheum Dis 1980;39:529.
31. Choi HK, Atkinson K, Karlson EW, et al. Alcohol intake and risk of incident gout in men: a prospective study. Lancet 2004;363:1277–81.
32. Choi HK, Atkinson K, Karlson EW, et al. Purine-rich foods, dairy and protein intake, and the risk of gout in men. N Engl J Med 2004;350:1093–103.
33. Schumacher HR. Pathology of the synovial membrane in gout. Light and electron microscopic studies. Interpretation of crystals in electron micrographs. Arthritis Rheum 1975;18:771–82.
34. Dalbeth N, Collis J, Gregory K, et al. Tophaceous joint disease strongly predicts hand function in patients with gout. Rheumatology (Oxford) 2007;46:1804–7.
35. Kumar S, Gow P. A survey of indications, results and complications of surgery for tophaceous gout. N Z Med J 2002;115:U109.
36. Lee SS, Lin SD, Lai CS, et al. The soft-tissue shaving procedure for deformity management of chronic tophaceous gout. Ann Plast Surg 2003;51:372–5.
37. Vanwijck R, Kaba L, Boland S, et al. Immediate skin grafting of sub-acute and chronic wounds debrided by hydrosurgery. J Plast Reconstr Aesthet Surg 2010;63:544–9.
38. Ferraz MB, O'Brien B. A cost effectiveness analysis of urate lowering drugs in nontophaceous recurrent gouty arthritis. J Rheumatol 1995;22:908–14.
39. Hench PS. The diagnosis of gout and gouty arthritis. J Lab Clin Med 1936;22:48–55.
40. Wallace SL, Singer JZ. Therapy in gout. Rheum Dis Clin North Am 1988;14:441–57.
41. Macfarlane DG, Dieppe PA. Diuretic-induced gout in elderly women. Br J Rheumatol 1985;24:155–7.
42. Puig JG, Michan AD, Jimenez ML, et al. Female gout. Clinical spectrum and uric acid metabolism. Arch Intern Med 1991;151:726–32.
43. Clive DM. Renal transplant-associated hyperuricemia and gout. J Am Soc Nephrol 2000;11:974–9.
44. Nakayama DA, Barthelemy C, Carrera G, et al. Tophaceous gout: a clinical and radiographic assessment. Arthritis Rheum 1984;27:468–71.
45. Terkeltaub R, Bushinsky D, Becker M. Recent developments in our understanding of the renal basis of hyperuricemia and the development of novel antihyperuricemic therapeutics. Arthritis Res Ther 2006;8:S4.
46. Avram Z, Krishnan E. Hyperuricaemia: where nephrology meets rheumatology. Rheumatology (Oxford) 2008;47:960–4.
47. Cameron JS. Uric acid and renal disease. Nucleosides Nucleotides Nucl Acids 2006;25:1055–64.
48. Negri AL, Spivacow R, Del Valle E, et al. Clinical and biochemical profile of patients with "pure" uric acid nephrolithiasis compared with "pure" calcium oxalate stone formers. Urol Res 2007;35:247–51.
49. Choi HK, Al Arfaj AM, et al. Dual energy computed tomography in tophaceous gout. Ann Rheum Dis 2009;68:1609–12.
50. Trinchieri A, Ostini F, Nespoli R, et al. A prospective study of recurrence rate and risk factors for recurrence after a first renal stone. J Urol 1999;162:27–30.
51. Kramer HJ, Choi HK, Atkinson K, et al. The association between gout and nephrolithiasis in men: The Health Professionals' Follow-Up Study. Kidney Int 2003;64:1022–6.
52. Cameron MA, Sakhaee K. Uric acid nephrolithiasis. Urol Clin North Am 2007;34:335–46.
53. Shimizu T, Hori H. The prevalence of nephrolithiasis in patients with primary gout: a cross-sectional study using helical computed tomography. J Rheumatol 2009;36:1958–62.
54. Pak CY, Moe OW, Sakhaee K, et al. Physicochemical metabolic characteristics for calcium oxalate stone formation in patients with gouty diathesis. J Urol 2005;173:1606–9.
55. Gibson T, Highton J, Potter C, et al. Renal impairment and gout. Ann Rheum Dis 1980;39:417–23.
56. Tanaka M, Itoh K, Matsushita K, et al. Two male siblings with hereditary renal hypouricemia and exercise-induced ARF. Am J Kidney Dis 2003;42:1287–92.
57. Dinour D, Gray NK, Campbell S, et al. Homozygous SLC2A9 mutations cause severe renal hypouricemia. J Am Soc Nephrol 2010;21:64–72.
58. Sakhaee K, Maalouf NM. Metabolic syndrome and uric acid nephrolithiasis. Semin Nephrol 2008;28:174–80.
59. Talbott JH, Terplan KL. The kidney in gout. Medicine (Baltimore) 1960;39:405–7.
60. Feig DI, Kang D, Johnson RJ. Uric acid and cardiovascular risk. N Engl J Med 2008;359:1811–21.
61. Linnane JW, Burry AF, Emmerson BT. Urate deposits in the renal medulla. Nephron 1981;29:216–22.
62. Johnson RJ, Kivlighn SD, Kim Y, et al. Reappraisal of the pathogenesis and consequences of hyperuricemia in hypertension, cardiovascular disease, and renal disease. Am J Kidney Dis 1999;33:225–34.
63. Feig DI. Uric acid: a novel mediator and marker of risk in chronic kidney disease? Curr Opin Nephrol Hypertens 2009;18:526–30.
64. Nickeleit V, Mihatsch M. Uric acid nephropathy and end-stage renal–review of a non-disease. Nephrol Dial Transplant 1997;12:1832–8.
65. Beck LH. Requiem for gouty nephropathy. Kidney Int 1986;30:280–7.
66. Meier-Kriesche HU, Schold JD, et al. Uric acid levels have no significant effect on renal function in adult renal transplant recipients: evidence from the symphony study. Clin J Am Soc Nephrol 2009;4:1655–60.
67. Berger L, Yu T. Renal function in gout, IV. An analysis of 524 gouty subjects including long-term follow-up studies. Am J Med 1975;59:605–13.
68. Ohno I, Hosoya T, Gomi H, et al. Serum uric acid and renal prognosis in patients with IgA nephropathy. Nephron 2001;87:333–9.
69. Tomita M, Mizuno S, Yamanaka H, et al. Does hyperuricemia affect mortality? A prospective cohort study of Japanese male workers. J Epidemiol 2000;10:403–9.
70. Culleton BF, Larson MG, Kannel WB, et al. Serum uric acid and risk for cardiovascular disease and death: the Framingham Heart Study. Ann Intern Med 1999;131:7–13.
71. Krishnan E, Baker JF, Furst DE, et al. Gout and the risk of acute myocardial infarction. Arthritis Rheum 2006;54:2688–96.
72. Abbott RD, Brand FN, Kannel WB, et al. Gout and coronary heart disease: the Framingham Study. J Clin Epidemiol 1988;41:237–42.
73. Choi HK, Curhan G. Independent impact of gout on mortality and risk for coronary heart disease. Circulation 2007;116:894–900.
74. Kosugi T, Nakayama T, Heinig M, et al. Effect of lowering uric acid on renal disease in the type 2 diabetic db/db mice. Am J Physiol Renal Physiol 2009;297:F481–8.
75. Sánchez, Lozada LG, Tapia E, et al. Effect of febuxostat on the progression of renal disease in 5/6 nephrectomy rats with and without hyperuricemia. Nephron Physiol 2008;108:69–78.
76. Siu Y, Pong, Leung K, et al. Use of allopurinol in slowing the progression of renal disease through its ability to lower serum uric acid level. Am J Kidney Dis 2006;47:51–9.
77. Kanbay M, Ozkara A, Selcoki Y, et al. Effect of treatment of hyperuricemia with allopurinol on blood pressure, creatinine clearance, and proteinuria in patients with normal renal functions. Int Urol Nephrol 2007;39:1227–33.
78. Reiter L, Brown MA, Edmonds J. Familial hyperuricemic nephropathy. Am J Kidney Dis 1995;25:235–41.
79. Stiburkova B, Majewski J, Hodanova K, et al. Familial juvenile hyperuricaemic nephropathy (FJHN): linkage analysis in 15 families, physical and transcriptional characterisation of the FJHN critical region on chromosome 16p11.2 and the analysis of seven candidate genes. Eur J Hum Genet 2002;11:145–54.
80. Williams SE, Reed AAC, Galvanovskis J, et al. Uromodulin mutations causing familial juvenile hyperuricaemic nephropathy lead to protein maturation defects and retention in the endoplasmic reticulum. Hum Mol Genet 2009;18:2963–74.
81. Musgrave DS, Ziran BH. Monoarticular acromioclavicular joint gout: a case report. Am J Orthop 29:544-7.
82. Fraser JF, Anand VK, Schwartz TH. Endoscopic biopsy sampling of tophaceous gout of the odontoid process. Case report and review of the literature. J Neurosurg Spine 2007;7:61–4.

83. Ballhaus S, Mees K, Vogl T. [Infratemporal gout tophus–a rare differential diagnosis in primary parotid gland disease]. Laryngorhinootologie 1989;68:638–41.

84. Hawkins CF, Ellis HA, Rawson A. Malignant gout with tophaceous small intestine and megaloblastic anaemia. Ann Rheum Dis 1965;34.

85. Snider AA, Barsky S. Gouty panniculitis: a case report and review of the literature. Cutis 2005;76:54–6.

86. Dahiya A, Leach J, Levy H. Gouty panniculitis in a healthy male. J Am Acad Dermatol 2007;57:S52–4.

87. Niemi KM. Panniculitis of the legs with urate crystal deposition. Arch Dermatol 1977;113:655–6.

88. Apibal Y, Jirasuthus S, Puavilai S. Abruption pustular gouty tophi of palm and sole. J Med Assoc Thai 2009;92:979–82.

89. Kurita Y, Tsuboi R, Numata K, et al. A case of multiple urate deposition, without gouty attacks, in a patient with systemic lupus erythematosus. Cutis 1989;43:273–5.

90. Garrod AB. Nature and Treatment of Gout and Rheumatic Gout. 2nd ed. London: Walton and Maberly; 1863.

91. Ewart W. Gout and Goutiness. New York: William Wood and Co; 1896.

92. Lefkovits AM. Gouty involvement of the larynx. Report of a case and review of the literature. Arthritis Rheum 1965;8:1019–26.

93. Tsikoudas A, Coatesworth AP, Martin-Hirsch DP. Laryngeal gout. J Laryngol Otol 2002;116:140–2.

94. Poór G, Mituszova M. The occurrence of hyperuricemia and gout in workers exposed to lead. Hung Rheumatol 1988;29:69–76.

95. Tak HK, Wilcox WR, Cooper SM. The effect of lead upon urate nucleation. Arthritis Rheum 1981;24:1291–5.

96. Poór G, Mituszova M. Saturnine gout. Balliéres Clin Rheumatol 1989;3:51–61.

97. Konatalapalli RM, Demarco PJ, Jelinek JS, et al. Gout in the axial skeleton. J Rheumatol 2009;36:609–13.

98. Jajic I. Gout in the spine and sacro-iliac joints: radiological manifestations. Skeletal Radiol 1982;8:209–12.

99. Gupta S, McMahan Z, Patel PC, et al. Pancreatic gout masquerading as pancreatic cancer in a heart transplant candidate. J Heart Lung Transpl 2009;28:1112–3.

100. Curtiss EI, Miller TR, Shapiro LS. Pulmonic regurgitation due to valvular tophi. Circulation 1983;67:699–701.

101. Gawoski JM, Balogh K, Landis WJ. Aortic valvular tophus: identification by X-ray diffraction of urate and calcium phosphates. J Clin Pathol 1985;38:873–6.

102. Chen CH, Chen CK, Yeh L, et al. Intra-abdominal gout mimicking pelvic abscess. Skeletal Radiol 2005;34:229–33.

103. Lo WR, Broocker G, Grossniklaus HE. Histopathologic examination of conjunctival tophi in gouty arthritis. Am J Ophthalmol 2005;140:1152–4.

104. Ferry AP, Safir A, Melikian HE. Ocular abnormalities in patients with gout. Ann Ophthalmol 1985;17:632–5.

105. Jordan DR, Belliveau MJ, Brownstein S, et al. Medial canthal tophus. Ophthalmic Plast Reconstr Surg 2008;24:403–4.

106. Aslam N, Lo S, McNab I. Gouty flexor tenosynovitis mimicking infection: a case report emphasising the value of ultrasound in diagnosis. Acta Orthop Belg 2004;70:368–70.

107. Weniger FG, Davison SP, Risin M, et al. Gouty flexor tenosynovitis of the digits: report of three cases. J Hand Surg Am 2003;28:669–72.

108. Patil VS, Chopra A. Watch out for 'pins and needles' in hands: it may be a case of gout. Clin Rheumatol 2007;26:2185–7.

109. Akizuki S, Matsui T. Entrapment neuropathy caused by tophaceous gout. J Hand Surg Br 1984;9:331–2.

110. De Yoe BE, Ng A, Miller B, et al. Peroneus brevis tendon rupture with tophaceous gout infiltration. J Foot Ankle Surg 1999;38:359–62.

111. Gaffo AL, Schumacher Jr HR, Saag KG, et al. Developing American College of Rheumatology and European League Against Rheumatism criteria for definition of a flare in patients with gout. Arthritis Rheum 2009;60:S563.

112. Taylor WJ, Shewchuk R, Saag KG, et al. Toward a valid definition of gout flare: results of consensus exercises using delphi methodology and cognitive mapping. Arthritis Care Res 2009;61:535–43.

113. Sindhu RJ, Oemer, Necmi G, et al. Classification criteria in rheumatic diseases: a review of methodologic properties. Arthritis Care Res 2007;57:1119–33.

114. Wallace SL, Robinson H, Masi AT, et al. Preliminary criteria for the classification of the acute arthritis of primary gout. Arthritis Rheum 1977;20:895–900.

115. Kellgren JH, Jeffery MR, Ball JF, editors. The Epidemiology of Chronic Rheumatism. Oxford: Blackwell Scientific; 1963.

116. Decker JL. Report from the Subcommittee on Diagnostic Criteria for Gout. In: Bennett PH, Wood PHN, editors. Population Studies of the Rheumatic Diseases: Proceedings of the Third International Symposium New York, June 5-10, 1966. Amsterdam: Excerpta Medica Foundation; 1968:385–7.

117. O'Sullivan JB. Gout in a New England town. A prevalence study in Sudbury, Massachusetts. Ann Rheum Dis 1972;31:166–9.

118. Rigby AS, Wood PHN. Serum uric acid levels and gout: what does this herald for the population? Clin Exp Rheumatol 1994;12:395–400.

119. Malik A, Schumacher HR, Dinnella JE, et al. Clinical diagnostic criteria for gout: comparison with the gold standard of synovial fluid crystal analysis. JCR J Clin Rheumatol 2009;15:22–4.

120. Janssens HJEM, Janssen M, van de Lisdonk EH, et al. Limited validity of the American College of Rheumatology criteria for classifying patients with gout in primary care. Ann Rheum Dis 2009.

121. Kuzell WC, Schaffarzick RW, Naugler WE, et al. Some observations on 520 gouty patients. J Chronic Dis 1955;2:645–69.

122. Wallace KL, Riedel AA, Joseph-Ridge N, et al. Increasing prevalence of gout and hyperuricemia over 10 years among older adults in a managed care population. J Rheumatol 2004;31:1582–7.

123. Choi H. Epidemiology of crystal arthropathy. Rheum Dis Clin North Am 2006;32:255–73.

124. Lally EV, Ho Jr G, Kaplan SR. The clinical spectrum of gouty arthritis in women. Arch Intern Med 1986;146:2221–5.

125. Hak AE, Curhan GC, Grodstein F, et al. Menopause, postmenopausal hormone use and risk of incident gout. Ann Rheum Dis 2010;69:1305–9.

126. Hak AE, Choi HK. Menopause, postmenopausal hormone use and serum uric acid levels in US women: the Third National Health and Nutrition Examination Survey. Arthritis Res Ther 2008;10:R116.

127. Sumino H, Ichikawa S, Kanda T, et al. Reduction of serum uric acid by hormone replacement therapy in postmenopausal women with hyperuricaemia. Lancet 1999;354:650.

128. Simon JA, Lin F, Vittinghoff E, et al. The relation of postmenopausal hormone therapy to serum uric acid and the risk of coronary heart disease events: the Heart and Estrogen-Progestin Replacement Study (HERS). Ann Epidemiol 2006;16:138–45.

129. Dirken-Heukensfeldt KJ, Teunissen TA, van de Lisdonk H, et al. Clinical features of women with gout arthritis. A systematic review. Clin Rheumatol 2010;29:575–82.

130. Stamp L, Ha L, Searle M, et al. Gout in renal transplant recipients. Nephrology (Carlton) 2006;11:367–71.

131. Shibolet O, Elinav E, Ilan Y, et al. Reduced incidence of hyperuricemia, gout, and renal failure following liver transplantation in comparison to heart transplantation: a long-term follow-up study. Transplantation 2004;77:1576–80.

132. Abbott KC, Kimmel PL, Dharnidharka V, et al. New-onset gout after kidney transplantation: incidence, risk factors and implications. Transplantation 2005;80:1383–91.

133. Hernandez-Molina G, Cachafeiro-Vilar A, Villa AR, et al. Gout in renal allograft recipients according to the pretransplant hyperuricemic status. Transplantation 2008;86:1543–7.

134. Baethge BA, Work J, Landreneau MD, et al. Tophaceous gout in patients with renal transplants treated with cyclosporine A. J Rheumatol 1993;20:718–20.

135. Burack DA, Griffith BP, Thompson ME, et al. Hyperuricemia and gout among heart transplant recipients receiving cyclosporine. Am J Med 1992;92:141–6.

136. Schwab P, Lipton S, Kerr GS. Rheumatologic sequelae and challenges in organ transplantation. Best Pract Res Clin Rheumatol 2010;24:329–40.

137. Kramer HM, Curhan G. The association between gout and nephrolithiasis: the National Health and Nutrition Examination Survey III, 1988-1994. Am J Kidney Dis 2002;40:37–42.

138. Zhang W, Doherty M, Pascual E, et al. EULAR evidence based recommendations for gout. Part I: Diagnosis. Report of a task force of the Standing Committee for International Clinical Studies Including Therapeutics (ESCISIT). Ann Rheum Dis 2006;65:1301–11.

Treatment of Acute Gout

Naomi Schlesinger

KEY POINTS

- Nonsteroidal antiinflammatory drugs (NSAIDs) (or cyclooxygenase-2–selective coxibs), systemic oral corticosteroids (prednisone or prednisolone), and colchicine are the primary therapy options for an acute gout attack. However, there remains no single standard of therapy for an acute gout attack.
- Selection of treatment should be individualized by taking into consideration comorbidities, potential drug-drug interactions, and duration and severity of the gout attack.
- Indomethacin, starting at 50 mg orally three times daily, is effective in acute gout but gastrointestinal and central nervous system side effects are limitations. Many NSAIDs are effective alternatives, but high doses of aspirin (acetylsalicylic acid) or nonacetylated salicylates are not recommended for acute gout.
- When prednisone or prednisolone is used to treat acute gouty arthritis, the starting dose should be at least 0.5 mg of prednisone or prednisolone/kg per day.
- The use of prednisone for acute gout attack is associated with the potential for rebound attacks of acute gout, and colchicine gout attack prophylaxis can be added as an adjunctive therapy.
- Oral colchicine appears most effective when given promptly in the first 12 to 36 hours of an acute gout attack.
- The dosing regimen of colchicine for treating an acute early attack of gout (defined as within 12 hours of onset) should be limited on day 1 to 1.2 mg orally followed by 0.6 mg 1 hour later. Twelve to 24 hours later, low-dose colchicine gout attack prophylaxis can be commenced. Higher colchicine doses do not add efficacy and increase toxicity.

Introduction

Acute gout is characteristically an intensely painful inflammatory arthritis. A quote from the English poet John Milton published in Samuel Johnson's *Lives of the Poets* series (1779–1781) illustrates this: "Was he free from the pain the gout gave him, his blindness would be tolerable." The goal of therapy in acute gout is prompt and safe termination of the acute attack. To terminate the acute gout attack, pharmacotherapy needs to be rapidly initiated and an appropriate dose be given for a sufficiently long duration. This chapter summarizes the main treatment options for acute gout, how commonly each is used in practice, and the clinical trials supporting use of each option. Importantly, substantially more detail on strategically choosing between these options is provided in Chapter 16.

Without pharmacotherapy, the extreme pain of acute gout may resolve within a few days, but in many it may last longer, even up to several weeks. Using no medication for acute gout appears inappropriate and inhumane. Bellamy et al.[1] evaluated the natural course of acute gout. This study serves as a benchmark for comparing the efficacy of treatments for acute gout. In this 7-day study, 2 of 11 patients withdrew because of severe persistent pain after 4 days. All of the remaining patients showed some improvement in pain by day 5 and in swelling by day 7. Tenderness improved in 7 of the 9 remaining patients; however, full resolution of pain was observed in only 3 patients. It is therefore necessary to give the patient with acute gout prompt treatment with antiinflammatory therapy.

The primary options available for the treatment of acute gout are nonsteroidal antiinflammatory drugs (NSAIDs), colchicine, systemic corticosteroids (CSs), intraarticular CSs, and adrenocorticotropic hormone (ACTH). It is important to note that in a growing number of patients, one or more of the available treatments for acute gout are contraindicated (relative or absolute contraindication), largely due to the presence of comorbidities. Indeed, hypertension, cardiovascular disease including congestive heart failure, diabetes and renal impairment, peptic ulcer disease, the metabolic syndrome, and liver disease are all highly prevalent in individuals with gout and may lead to standard treatments being inappropriate. It is important to consider these comorbidities when treating acute gout. In this chapter, the new and the old treatments for acute gout, as well as drugs in development, are discussed.

Nonpharmacologic Treatment

Joint motion may increase inflammation in experimentally induced gout, whereas rest of affected joint(s) may aid in its resolution.[2] Less medication is needed if the patient can rest the afflicted joint for 1 to 2 days.[3]

Topical ice applications should be used as an adjunct to pharmacologic treatment of acute gout. In a prospective randomized trial,[4] patients with acute gout in whom topical ice treatments were added to pharmacologic antiinflammatory treatment had a greater reduction in pain ($p = .021$), joint circumference, and synovial fluid volume compared with the control group. In a study in dogs, heat application to inflamed joints exacerbated urate-induced synovitis.[5]

Pharmacologic Treatment

There are few guidelines for the treatment of acute gout and only a few randomized controlled trials have evaluated the efficacy of the various treatments for acute gout. A task force of the European League Against Rheumatism (EULAR) Standing Committee for International Clinical Studies Including Therapeutics (ESCISIT) published recommendations for gout management. These recommendations are based on 19 rheumatologists and one evidence-based medicine experts' Delphi consensus approach for different propositions. Research evidence was searched systematically for each proposition. The following recommendations for acute gout management were published[6]: oral colchicine and/or NSAIDs are first-line agents for the systemic treatment of acute gout. In the absence of contraindications, an NSAID is a convenient and well-accepted option; high doses of colchicine lead to side effects and low doses may be sufficient for some patients with acute gout; and intraarticular aspiration and injection of long-acting steroid provide an effective and safe treatment for an acute attack. The American College of Rheumatology (ACR) is developing practice guidelines for the treatment of gout so as to reduce inappropriate care, minimize geographic variations in practice patterns, and enable the effective use of health care resources.

Suboptimal prescribing practices may have an impact on the effectiveness of gout management.[7] Neogi et al.[7] reported an online prospective case-crossover study of 211 patients meeting ACR preliminary criteria for gout. They reported inappropriate therapy (not using antiinflammatory therapy) for acute gout in 26% of patients for some or all of their acute gout attacks. Prevalence of types of therapies among study participants with gout who had inappropriate treatment included (1) analgesia alone (22% of patients), (2) starting urate-lowering therapy (allopurinol 12%; probenecid 3%) acutely without having used it chronically, and (3) no medication given for the acute attack (60% of patients). In another study, 41% of 630 primary care physicians reported that they started allopurinol during the acute attack.[8] In a recent Australian study,[9] 9% of hospitalized patients with acute gout received no pharmacotherapy. This is surprising and concerning because pharmacotherapy should have been readily available for these hospitalized patients.

Combination Therapy to Treat Acute Gout

Most American rheumatologists use combination therapy to treat acute gout. In an American survey study evaluating the treatment of gout,[10] most American rheumatologists (64%) were found to use combination therapy for acute gout, whereas American internists tended to use monotherapy (p = .0005). The first three most frequently used combination therapies for acute gout in an otherwise healthy patient were NSAIDs with intraarticular CS (43%), NSAIDs with oral CSs (33%), and NSAIDs with oral colchicine (32%). NSAIDs alone were used in 27%. This was confirmed by a study evaluating the treatment of hospitalized patients with acute gout that found combination therapy was used in more than 50% of these patients.[11] In a recent Australian study,[9] combination therapy was used in 43% of patients with acute gout. The most frequently used combination therapies for acute gout included colchicine with oral CSs (35%), oral colchicine with an NSAID (39%), oral colchicine, NSAID, and oral CSs (16%), and NSAIDs with oral CSs (10%).[12]

Colchicine and its metabolites are excreted through the urinary and biliary tracts, and the presence of renal or liver disease impairs clearance of colchicines,[13,14] as reviewed in detail in Chapter 15. It is well known that NSAIDs also should be used with caution in patients with renal disease to avoid renal toxicity. Gutman[15] suggested in 1965 that there is some advantage to combining NSAID treatment with colchicine 2.0 mg daily in divided doses for the first 2 days of the attack and then tapering off. However, there still is little literature to support the use of such combination therapy in acute gout.[12] Most studies in acute gout have evaluated monotherapy despite the regular use of combination therapy in clinical practice. This common practice merits study.

Monotherapy

Colchicine and NSAIDs are the most commonly used drugs in the treatment of acute gout.[12] In the American survey study,[16] NSAIDs were reported to be the most commonly used monotherapy (77%). Interestingly, in this study, intraarticular CS injections (47%) and oral prednisone (42%) were more commonly reported to be used to treat acute gout than was oral colchicine (37%). Triamcinolone intramuscularly (11%) and ACTH intramuscularly (5%) were also reported to be used uncommonly. In the United States, oral CSs were reported to be the most commonly used monotherapy by rheumatologists in patients with chronic kidney disease, which is a common comorbidity seen in patients with gout.

In an American study, monotherapy was used in 58% of hospitalized patients with acute gout. In the patients who were prescribed monotherapy, colchicine use (76%) exceeded NSAID (14%) and oral CS (10%) use. A recent Australian study[9] found similar findings. Colchicine was the most common monotherapy (75%), followed by NSAIDs (32%) and oral CSs (28%). Oral CSs were used to treat acute gout in approximately 10% of patients. Interestingly, a recent Malaysian study[17] of primary care physicians found oral CSs were used to treat acute gout in approximately 10% of patients, as was suggested by the two other studies.

NSAIDs were the most commonly used drugs in acute gout in other survey studies, too. Among Canadian physicians, only 11% of family physicians and 6% of rheumatologists would use colchicine in the acute situation.[18] A similar preference for NSAIDs has been noted in Australia,[19] New Zealand,[20] and Malaysia.[17] In contrast, in a French survey study evaluating the treatment of gout,[21] colchicine was found to be the most commonly used drug as monotherapy. The most widely prescribed treatments for acute gout were colchicine alone (63%), colchicine with an NSAID (31.7%), and an NSAID alone (5.2%).

As shown in Table 10-1, in survey studies, many clinicians claim to use NSAIDs, colchicines, or CSs alone or in combination therapy. Table 10-2 lists the mainstay therapeutic options for acute gout.

Table 10-1 Treatment of Acute Gout: Survey Studies

Study Reference	Country	No. of Physicians	Colchicine as Primary Agent	Colchicine Plus NSAIDs	NSAIDs Alone	Corticosteroids
19	Canada	71	6%	?	?	
20	New Zealand	26	12%	25%	Indomethacin used in 73%	
22	Brazil		57%			
21	France	750	63%	32%	5%	0
23	USA	100		69%	33%	27%
12	USA	518	37%	32%	27%	42% (71% if CKD)
24	China	82	77%		17%	1% (48% if CKD)
17	Malaysia	128 Primary care physicians	10.2%		68%	10%

CKD, Chronic kidney disease; *NSAID,* nonsteroidal antiinflammatory drug.

Table 10-2 Acute Gout: Mainstays of Treatment

- NSAIDs (nonselective or selective COX-2 inhibitors) for 5-10 days. Most NSAIDs in clinical trials compared with indomethacin have been of equivalent efficacy in clinical trials, and this also has been the case for some selective COX-2 inhibitors tested (e.g., etoricoxib and high-dose celecoxib).
- Systemic corticosteroids—*Oral:* prednisone taper 30-40 mg daily for 2-3 days followed by 7-10 day taper, or prednisolone 35 mg for 5 days; *intravenous:* methylprednisolone 50-150 mg once a day for 1-3 days followed if needed by a corticosteroid taper); or *intramuscular* (triamcinolone 40-80 mg; repeat injection if recurrence of pain).
- Colchicine given within 36 hours of the initial flare. (Oral colchicine 1.2 mg initially to be followed 1 hour later with 0.6 mg is the FDA-approved regimen for early acute gout flare, defined as onset in the last 12 hours; EULAR recommendations are for colchicine 0.5 mg PO tid for acute gout.)
- Intraarticular corticosteroid (preferably medium to long acting) when one or two joints are involved.

NSAID, nonsteroidal antiinflammatory drug.
Tables 10-3 and 10-4 highlight evidence on which these recommendations are based. ACTH is rarely used (see Table 10-5). In clinical trials, IL-1 inhibitors have been assessed for acute gout (see Table 10-6).

Colchicine

Colchicine is an alkaloid derived from the autumn crocus (also known as meadow saffron; *Crocus autoimmale*). Colchicum in the form of extracts from the bulb of *C. autoimmale* has been known since antiquity, although it came into widespread use only around 1800.[25] As reviewed in Chapter 15, colchicine disrupts cytoskeletal functions through inhibition of β-tubulin polymerization into microtubules[26] and, consequently, at low (nanomolar) concentrations, interferes with many neutrophil functions, including adhesion to endothelium and chemotaxis. At higher concentrations, colchicine globally suppresses neutrophil functions.[27]

Absorption of oral colchicine is rapid but incomplete (time to maximum is 2 hours; bioavailability is 25% to 50%). Colchicine is excreted in the urine and via the biliary tract after it is metabolized in the liver. However, absorption can be highly variable. The half-life of colchicine after an oral dose in patients with normal renal and hepatic functions is approximately 9 hours, whereas in patients with renal failure, it is 2 to 3 times normal (about 24 hours), and in cirrhotic patients with renal failure, it is 10 times normal (approximately 4 days).[28] Hemodialysis does not remove colchicine.[29]

Until recently, only one placebo-controlled trial of colchicine treatment in acute gout was reported.[30] All other data reported were accumulated through review rather than through prospective studies. In this placebo-controlled study, Ahern et al. studied 43 patients (40 men, 3 women); 22 patients received colchicine 1 mg then 0.5 mg every 2 hours until complete response or toxicity and 21 patients were in the placebo group. No NSAIDs were used during the study. All participants had monosodium urate (MSU) crystal–proved gout. In this placebo-controlled study, two thirds of the colchicine-treated patients improved after 48 hours but only one third of the patients receiving placebo demonstrated similar improvement. Oral colchicine was shown to be efficacious in two thirds of patients presenting with acute gout. It was more effective when used within 24 hours of an acute attack. Importantly, more than 80% of patients experienced nausea, vomiting, diarrhea, and abdominal pain after oral administration before full clinical improvement.[30]

Despite the widespread use of oral colchicine, it did not have U.S. Food and Drug Administration (FDA) approval until recently. It did not have FDA-approved prescribing information, dosage recommendations, or drug interaction warnings until August 2009. In the AGREE trial,[31] a randomized, double-blind placebo-controlled study in which 184 patients with acute gout were treated for an acute attack within 12 hours of the onset of the attack, low-dose colchicine (1.2 mg then 0.6 mg 1 hour later for a total of 1.8 mg) was found to be equally effective and better tolerated than high-dose colchicine (1.2 mg then 0.6 mg hourly × 6 hours for a total of 4.8 mg). There was a significantly higher incidence of gastrointestinal adverse events (diarrhea, nausea/vomiting) with high-dose colchicine than with either low-dose colchicine or placebo. If needed on day 2 of early gout attack treatment, the patient can be started on gout attack prophylactic doses of colchicine (e.g., 0.6 mg PO twice daily if renal function and hepatobiliary function are preserved and there are no significant drug-drug interactions).

Previous recommendations for treatment of acute gout that involved repeated dosing of colchicine over multiple hours for acute gout until toxicity or pain relief developed[32] are no longer tenable. To lessen colchicine side effects, Morris et al.[33] suggested that in a patient with acute gout, colchicine should be used at lower doses: 500 mcg three times a day or less frequently, especially in those with renal impairment. However, the recommended dosage of colchicine depends on the patient's age, renal function, hepatic function, and use of coadministered drugs. For treatment of acute gout attacks in patients with mild (glomerular filtration rate [GFR] of 50 to 80 ml/min) to moderate (GFR of 30 to 50 ml/min) kidney disease, adjustment of this recommended dose is not required. For patients with acute gout requiring repeated courses of colchicine, consideration should be given to alternate therapy. For patients undergoing dialysis, the total recommended dose for the treatment of acute gout should be reduced to a single dose of 0.6 mg (1 tablet). For these patients, the treatment course should not be repeated more often than once every 2 weeks. Treatment of gout attacks with colchicine is not recommended in patients with renal impairment who are receiving colchicine prophylaxis.[31]

There has been little information on colchicine drug-drug interactions until recently (as reviewed in detail in Chapter 15). Colchicine was found to be a substrate for both the CYP3A4 enzyme and P-glycoprotein (P-gp) transporter. Therefore, coadministration with drugs known to inhibit CYP3A4 and/or P-gp increases the risk of colchicine-induced toxic effects. These drugs include cyclosporine, erythromycin, and calcium channel antagonists such as verapamil and diltiazem. Other examples of P-gp and strong CYP3A4 inhibitors include telithromycin, ketoconazole, itraconazole, HIV protease inhibitors, and nefazodone.[34] The FDA required patients treated with P-gp or strong CYP3A4 inhibitor drugs within 14 days of colchicine use for acute gout to have a dose reduction in or interruption of colchicine treatment.

Colchicine appears most effective for acute gout when started in the first 1 to 2 days of the onset of the gout attack. It is important to note that a clinical response to colchicine is not pathognomonic for acute gout. A clinical response can be seen in patients with pseudogout, sarcoid arthropathy, psoriatic arthritis, and calcific tendonitis.

Oral Nonsteroidal Antiinflammatory Drugs

Currently, approximately 50 different NSAID preparations are available and, as a class, they are among the most commonly prescribed drugs worldwide.[35] NSAIDs are structurally diverse and differ in pharmacokinetic and pharmacodynamic properties but share the same mode of action. NSAIDs exert their antiinflammatory action by inhibiting cyclooxygenase (COX), an enzyme that transforms phospholipid-derived arachidonic acid into prostaglandins. NSAIDs may be nonselective, inhibiting both COX-1 and COX-2 (e.g., ibuprofen and naproxen), or may be more COX-1 (e.g., aspirin) or COX-2 (e.g., celecoxib) selective.

There are no randomized controlled trials comparing colchicine to NSAIDs. Even so, NSAIDs are the drugs of choice in patients with gout without underlying comorbidities. The most important determinant of therapeutic success is not which NSAID is chosen but rather how soon NSAID therapy is initiated—that proper dosages be given at the onset of symptoms or at the time of diagnosis and continued for a sufficiently long period (e.g., at least several days after complete resolution of the acute attack).

Unfortunately, the use of NSAIDs is limited by side effects.[35] The gastrointestinal adverse effects of traditional NSAIDs are well known. Clinically important NSAID-related gastrointestinal side effects may lead to bleeding, hospitalization, and death. The gastrointestinal side effects of NSAIDs may be lessened by coadministration of a proton pump inhibitor. In addition, the use of NSAIDs confers increased cardiovascular risk in patients with known heart disease or those thought to be at high risk of heart disease. This is commonly the case in our patients with gout. All patients taking NSAIDs should be carefully monitored for the development of high blood pressure, worsening heart disease, worsening renal function, fluid retention, gastrointestinal bleeding, and elevations in liver enzymes.

A number of head-to-head controlled studies, including randomized controlled trials, in acute gout show equivalence between the different NSAIDs. Most were small trials[12] (Table 10-3). Most of these studies compared indomethacin with another NSAID. Indomethacin 50 mg orally three times daily has been held to be a gold standard for acute gout treatment, but the gastrointestinal and central nervous system side effects of indomethacin are often limiting. Naproxen 500 mg orally twice daily is one of the effective alternatives, and sulindac 150 or 200 mg orally twice daily also is FDA approved for the treatment of gout. High-dose salicylates are not advised for acute gout treatment, since the time to buildup of analgesic efficacy can be slow with acetylsalicylic acid and all high-dose salicylates lower serum urate via uricosuric effects, which has the potential to worsen the acute gout attack.

With respect to selective COX-2 inhibitor therapy in gout, lumiracoxib and etoricoxib (which are not available in the United States) and celecoxib have been observed to be effective in studies of acute gout. A relatively large set of trials compared etoricoxib versus indomethacin.[47,48] In these two studies, etoricoxib 120 mg once daily was comparable to indomethacin 50 mg three times daily when used as treatment for acute gout. Also in clinical trials is the comparison of celecoxib versus indomethacin (50 mg three times daily) for 8 days. Initial results showed equivalence in efficacy for acute gout between the 800 mg at onset/400 mg twice daily celecoxib and the indomethacin groups, with a superior overall side effect profile of the high-dose celecoxib group.[49]

Systemic Corticosteroids

The immunomodulatory actions of CSs are exerted in part by interfering with induction of multiple proinflammatory signaling processes.[50] An important antiinflammatory effect of CSs occurs through direct inhibition of transcription factor activity by transrepression. CSs inhibit expression of several proinflammatory cytokines involved in gouty arthritis, such as interleukin (IL)-1, IL-6, IL-8, and tumor necrosis factor-alpha (TNF-α) and also interfere with phospholipase A_2 and eicosanoid production. CS therapeutic effects pertinent to gout are discussed briefly in Chapter 5.

Table 10-3 Treatment of Acute Gout With Nonsteroidal Antiinflammatory Drugs

Study Reference	Study	No. of Patients	Days of Treatment/ Regimen	Qualifiers/ Diagnosis	Assessment Criteria
36	Placebo only	11	7 days no treatment	Acute podagra (1-5 days) with prior attacks and hyperuricemia No treatment	Improvement within 7 days without NSAIDs Resolution Day 7: pain = 3, tenderness = 0, swelling = 9, erythema = 9 2 withdraw day 4
37	Double-blind, Indomethacin (I) versus phenylbutazone (P)	28 (31 attacks)	I 200, 150, 100 P 800, 600, 400	Clinical	Subjective: pain Objective: Heat, erythema swelling ESR (P) $p < .001$
38	Comparative double-blind, Indomethacin (I) versus proquazone (P)	18	10 days of P 300 mg tid, bid versus I 50 mg tid, bid	SU Crystals in some radiographs	Improvement in 2-3 days
39	Open study suldinac (S)	12	S: 200 mg bid When improvement, dose reduced	Onset <48 hr prior to screening Age 30-65	Improvement within 24 hr. Complete recovery 5 days (average)
40	Open study naproxen (N)	20	12 patients 600 mg initial, followed by 300 mg q8h or tapered 3-4 days; 8 patients 750 mg initially followed by q8h 500 mg, then 250 mg q8h for 48-72 hr tapering dose	Acute arthritis Hyperuricemia (17 patients) with or without crystals	15/20 Clearing of inflammatory changes 24-48 hr Higher dose more rapid clearing of attack
41	Open study naproxen (N)	12	Initial 48 hr 600 mg N, followed by 300 q8h	Monoarticular with hyperuricemia and/or MSU crystals	Majority of patients treated within 48hrs did well: reduction pain, tenderness, heat, swelling
42	Open study piroxicam (P) (Feldene)	34	17 P 40 mg for 7 days versus 17 P 40 mg first day followed by 20 mg daily for 6 days	MSU crystals	Pin score 0-3, tenderness score 0-3. Improvement of pain and tenderness scores days 3 and 7. No difference between groups
43	Double-blind comparative ketoprofen (K) versus indomethacin (I)	59	29 K 100 mg versus 30 I 50 mg tid	MSU crystals or clinical criteria	More than 90% pain relief in both groups. Complete relief day 5: 7 patients K, 6 I group
44	Double-blind fenoprofen (F) versus phenylbutazone (P)	30	4 days 15 F: 3.6 g first day then 3 g qd 15 P: 700 mg first day then 400 mg qd	MSU crystals	Both as effective. Reduction in pain, heat, swelling, redness Day 4 77% in F, 81% in P
45	Double-blind IM ketorolac (K) versus indomethacin (I) PO	20	10 days 60 mg K IM and oral placebo versus 10 days 50 mg I tid for 2 days then 50 mg bid for 5 days and IM placebo	Wallace criteria	2 hr decreased pain 50% (except in 2 patients in each group). I group 24 hr. No change in pain score; K after 6 hr rebound pain
46	Double-blind etodolac (E) versus naproxen (N)	61	7 days		No statistical difference between the groups
47	Double-blind etoricoxib (E) Prospective randomized controlled trial versus indomethacin (I)	150	14 days 120 mg E vs 150 mg tid	Wallace criteria	No statistical difference between the groups

Continued

Table 10-3 Treatment of Acute Gout With Nonsteroidal Antiinflammatory Drugs—cont'd

Study Reference	Study	No. of Patients	Days of Treatment/ Regimen	Qualifiers/ Diagnosis	Assessment Criteria
48	Double-blind prospective randomized controlled trial Etoricoxib (E) versus indomethacin (I)	189	14 days 120 mg E vs 150 mg tid	Wallace criteria	No statistical difference between the groups
49	Double-blind prospective randomized controlled trial Celebrex (C) versus indomethacin (I)	400	8-day C: 50 mg bid C: 400, 200 mg followed by 200 mg bid for 7 days C: 800, 400 mg followed by 400 mg bid for 7 days I: 50 mg tid	Wallace criteria Onset <48 hr prior to screening	No statistical difference between the C 400 mg, 800 mg and I groups

Systemic CSs have been used for the treatment of acute gout since 1952. CSs can be given to those patients who cannot use NSAIDs or colchicine. CSs can be given orally, intravenously, intramuscularly, and intraarticularly. A CS is often preferred for treatment of polyarticular gout. Prednisone (or prednisolone) should be initiated in acute gout at a dosage of at least 0.5 mg/kg per day. In clinical practice in the USA, prednisone is typically given at a starting dosage of 30 to 60 mg for 1 to 3 days and then tapered over 1 to 2 weeks. Tapering more rapidly can result in a rebound flare. It is unclear whether parenteral CS confers any advantage unless the patient cannot take oral medications.

In a prospective trial using systemic CS treatment for acute gout in patients who had contraindications to the use of NSAIDs, Groff et al.[51] noted improvement within 12 to 48 hours. Here, 13 patients with 15 episodes of acute gout were treated with systemic CSs. Eight of the 13 had MSU-proved gout. In 11 of 13 attacks, complete resolution of the signs and symptoms occurred within 7 days, and resolution occurred within 10 days in the remainder. Patients with more than five involved joints required longer courses of therapy (mean 17 days). Nine patients received an initial dosage of 20 to 50 mg/day with a tapering dose over a mean time of 10.5 days (4 to 20 days). Three patients with more than five joints involved and longer duration of symptoms and one with multiple myeloma received either intravenous prednisolone or a prolonged prednisone taper over a mean of 17 days. Comparison of different dosing regimens has not been done.

Alloway et al.[52] reported 27 patients presenting within 5 days of onset of an acute gout attack. They noted that resolution of all symptoms occurred at an average of 8 days for indomethacin-treated patients (50 mg PO three times daily) and 7 days for patients treated with triamcinolone (60 mg IM). The difference in response was not statistically significant.

In a controlled nonblinded study, Siegel et al.[53] prospectively compared patients receiving a single dose of 40 IU ACTH IM (n = 16) with patients receiving 60 mg triamcinolone acetonide IM (n = 15) in acute gout. The two groups had similar mean times to complete resolution (7.9 and 7.6 days, respectively); however, the triamcinolone group required fewer repeat injections compared with the ACTH group.

In a recently published prospective randomized controlled trial comparing prednisolone 35 mg daily with naproxen 500 mg twice daily for 5 days in acute gout, 120 patients with monoarthritis referred by their family physicians within 24 hours of initial presentation were enrolled. All patients had MSU crystal–proved gout. Ninety-six patients with MSU crystal–proved gout were excluded, mostly because of the current use of NSAIDs or colchicine or contraindications to NSAIDs. Janssens et al.[54] found oral prednisolone to be comparably effective to naproxen 500 mg twice daily in treating acute gout. At 90 hours, mean reductions in pain (assessed on a visual analog scale [VAS]) were similar in the naproxen and prednisolone groups. Adverse effects during treatment were minor and comparable between groups. At 3-week follow-up, all patients reported complete resolution of pain and disability.

A summary of these trials is seen in Table 10-4. Further randomized controlled trials are needed. Comparison of different dosing regimens and modes of administration (oral, intramuscular, and intravenous) needs to be further studied.

Intraarticular Corticosteroids

Intraarticular CSs are currently accepted as beneficial when one or two joints are actively inflamed. Patients with polyarticular gout who demonstrate suboptimal or delayed response to oral NSAIDs or who have contraindications to usual NSAIDs may also benefit from adjunctive CS injections into joints with persistent synovitis. This approach is less favored when more than two joints are involved or the involved joint is not easily amenable to aspiration. Ensuring that the joint is not infected prior to injecting intraarticular CSs is particularly important. Systemic and intraarticular steroids should be avoided if septic arthritis is suspected.

This modality has not been well studied, but in an uncontrolled trial,[55] small intraarticular doses of triamcinolone acetonide (10 mg in knees and 8 mg in small joints) helped resolve 20 attacks of acute gout in 19 men. Joints involved were 11 knees, 4 metatarsophalangeal joints, 3 ankles, and 2 wrists. All had an MSU crystal–proved diagnosis. After intraarticular injection of triamcinolone acetonide in 11 joints (55%), the acute gout attack had resolved at 24 hours, and in 9 joints (45%), there was resolution at 48 hours. All acute gout attacks in the 19 patients receiving intraarticular CS injections improved within 48 hours.

Future studies are needed to compare different intraarticular CS preparations and dosages to further our understanding of their efficacy and safety in treating acute gout.

Table 10-4 **Treatment of Acute Gout With Corticosteroids**					
Study Reference	Study	No. of Patients	Days of Treatment/ Regimen	Qualifiers/ Diagnosis	Assessment Criteria
52	Prospective case series IV methylpredniso-lone, oral prednisone	13	9 patients initial dose: 20-50 mg/day tapering 5-10 days 4 patients: More than 5 joints involved IV prednisolone treatment 17-20 days	Contraindication to NSAIDs	Mean time to improve-ment: 12-48 hr Complete resolution 11/13: 7 days, 2/13: 10 days
53	Prospective indo-methacin (I) versus triamcinolone (T)	27	I 50 mg tid vs T 60 mg IM	Within 5 days of attack onset	Complete resolution: 8 days: I 7 days T
54	Prospective ACTH vs triamcinolone (T)	31	ACTH 40 IU IM vs T 60 mg IM		Fewer repeat injections in T group (9/15 vs 5/16)
55	Prospective random-ized controlled trial Prednisolone (P) versus naproxen (N)	120	P 35 mg daily vs N 500 mg bid for 5 days	Monoarthritis Within 24 hr of onset of attack	At 90 hr VAS scale reductions in pain similar in both groups

Adrenocorticotropic Hormone

ACTH is a hormone secreted by the pituitary gland that stimulates the production of cortisol, corticosterone, and androgens by the pituitary gland. The exact mechanism of action of ACTH on the inflammatory process in gout is not well understood. The use of ACTH was believed to exert its main beneficial effect via adrenal CS release, but new evidence shows that ACTH could be responsible, at least in part, for its rapid efficacy in acute gout, peripherally by activation of a melanocortin receptor: the melanocortin type 3 recep-tor (MC3R).[56] Getting et al.[57] demonstrated that smaller fragments of α- and β-melanocyte stimulating hormones could inhibit MSU crystal–induced neutrophil migration and release of proinflammatory cytokines and chemokines. These antiinflammatory effects occurred in a corticosterone-independent manner; hence, no reflex stimulation of the hypothalamic-pituitary-adrenal axis was observed.

A retrospective study of 33 patients who received ACTH for their acute gout attack or their acute pseudogout attack[58] found the most common regimen (90%) to be 40 IU adminis-tered intramuscularly every 8 hours. Duration of therapy was 1 to 14 days. A 97% resolution rate was reported. The mean time to complete resolution was 5.5 days. A relapse rate of 11% (n = 4) was noted.

A prospective controlled, nonblinded study involving 76 patients with MSU crystal–proved gout who presented within 24 hours of onset of an acute gout attack[59] compared paren-tal ACTH (40 IU administered IM) versus oral indomethacin 50 mg four times daily and found that the mean pain interval from administration of the study drug to complete pain relief was 3 ± 1 hour with corticotropin and 24 ± 10 hours with indomethacin (p < .0001). They concluded that the patients who received ACTH experienced a quicker onset of pain relief than those who received oral indomethacin.

There is no convincing evidence that ACTH is superior to CS treatment in acute gout. No randomized controlled trials have been conducted comparing ACTH to other modalities (Table 10-5). Future studies are needed to compare ACTH treatment to other therapies used in acute gout treatment.

Interleukin 1 Inhibitors (Anakinra, Rilonacept, Canakinumab)

Interleukin (IL)-1β has an important role in experimental and clinical gouty inflammation. MSU crystals stimulate IL-1 release by phagocytes[60] mediated by the cryopyrin (NLRP3) inflammasome, an intracellular, multiprotein complex. Cryo-pyrin regulates the protease caspase-1 and controls the acti-vation of IL-1β. Once caspase-1 becomes active, it cleaves pro-IL-1β to release the mature p17 form of IL-1β resulting in active, secreted IL-1β.[61,62] IL-1 inhibition has now been shown to have a beneficial effect in gouty inflammation in clinical research studies.

Anakinra is a nonglycosylated recombinant human IL-1 receptor antagonist (IL-1ra). IL-1ra is an endogenous recep-tor antagonist for the IL-1 receptor (IL-1RI). It binds to IL-1RI and prevents it from associating with its accessory pro-tein, IL-1RAcP, thus preventing signal transduction. Due to its short plasma half-life of approximately 4 to 6 hours follow-ing subcutaneous administration, anakinra is administered daily. Adults receive 100 mg/day subcutaneously. Anakinra significantly relieved the pain following acute gout in patients who could not tolerate or had failed standard antiinflamma-tory therapies.[63] So et al.[63] assessed anakinra in an open-label pilot study of 10 patients with gout (some of whom had acute gout and others who had subacute gout) the response to IL-1Ra: anakinra 100 mg daily subcutaneously for 3 days. They reported a 78% response in their pilot study of 10 patients. A retrospective study looked at the efficacy of anakinra in the treatment of acute gout[64] in 15 hospitalized patients who had failed CS treatment or had comorbid limitations to the use of CSs. The dose given in these patients was anakinra 100 mg daily subcutaneously for 3 days. In 19 of 22 anakinra courses, substantial pain reduction was reported. Anakinra was reported as successful in resolving the acute gout attack in all patients who had failed CS treatment, and anakinra treatment was reported as effective in prophylaxis of recurrent acute gout attacks in this same uncontrolled, retrospective analysis.

Another IL-1 inhibitor is rilonacept. Rilonacept binds to IL-1α and IL-1β with high affinity, thus preventing IL-1 from

Table 10-5 Treatment of Acute Gout With ACTH

Study Reference	Study	No. of Patients	Days of Treatment/ Regimen	Qualifiers/ Diagnosis	Assessment Criteria
58	Retrospective ACTH IM, IV, SC 40 IU vs 80 IU	33 patients; 38 attacks	1-14 days; IV (n = 27), IM (n = 6), SC (n = 5) 34: 40 IU ACTH q8-12h to daily; 4: 80 IU ACTH q8h Prophylactic colchicine in 79% (n = 30)	MSU (n = 11)	Mean time to resolution: 5.5 days Relapse n = 4 (11%)
59	Prospective Quasi-randomized (patients alternately assigned) Single-blind ACTH vs indomethacin (I)	76	ACTH 40 IU IM vs I 50 mg q6h	MSU in all Within 24 hr of attack No tophi No CRF No probenecid/ allopurinol/colchicine	Complete resolution 3±1 ACTH; 24±10 for I ACTH (n = 36) resolution in 4 hr
54	Prospective ACTH versus triamcinolone (T)	31	ACTH 40 IU IM vs T 60 mg IM		Fewer repeat injections in T group (9/15 vs 5/16)

binding to the IL-1 receptor. The plasma half-life of rilonacept is 67 hours. When rilonacept was administered as 160 mg subcutaneously once a week, it decreased the disease activity and pain in patients with chronic active gouty arthritis in a small, pilot, controlled crossover study.[65] However, preliminary results of an acute gout trial comparing indomethacin alone versus rilonacept with indomethacin versus rilonacept alone (initial phase 3 studies results for rilonacept in the treatment of patients for of an acute gout attack[66]) suggest that rilonacept, when combined with indomethacin and when used alone, failed to significantly improve pain relative to indomethacin during acute gout.

Another IL-1 inhibitor currently in trials, canakinumab, a fully human monoclonal anti-human IL-1β antibody that binds to human IL-1β and thus blocks the interaction of this cytokine with its receptors. It does not bind IL-1α or IL-1ra. Canakinumab has a long plasma half-life of 21 to 28 days and is effective in the picomolar range. Recently, canakinumab completed phase II adaptive dose-ranging, multicenter, single-blind, double-dummy, active-controlled study to determine the target dose of canakinumab in the treatment of acute gout attacks (of up to 5 days duration) in patients who are refractory to or have a contraindication to NSAIDs and/or colchicine.[67] Canakinumab 150 mg as a single injection was found to provide rapid pain relief. In this study, a statistically significant dose response was observed at 72 hours for canakinumab 150 mg given subcutaneously. It was superior, starting at 24 hours, in providing pain relief compared to the active comparator 40 mg of triamcinolone acetonide given intramuscularly as a single dose. The median time to 50% reduction in pain was reached at 1 day with canakinumab 150 mg versus 2 days for the triamcinolone acetonide group ($p = .0006$).[67]

A summary of studies evaluating IL-1 inhibitors is given in Table 10-6.

Treatment of Acute Gout: Summary

There are few guidelines for the treatment of acute gout and only a few randomized controlled trials evaluating the efficacy of the various treatments for acute gout. Adverse events,

Table 10-6 Treatment of Acute Gout With Interleukin (IL)-1 Antagonists

Study Reference	Drug	Mechanism	Status
63, 64	Anakinra	IL-1 receptor antagonist	Pilot data
65, 66	Rilonacept	Soluble IL-1 blockade	Phase III trial
67	Canakinumab	Fully humanized IL-1β monoclonal antibody	Phase III trial
68	Xoma 052	Human engineered IL-1β IgG2 antibody	Preclinical development

comorbidities, and clinical preferences have dictated drug choices. However, a task force of the EULAR recently published recommendations for gout management, and the ACR is developing practice guidelines for the treatment of gout. It is hoped that these will reduce inappropriate care.

The current options for the treatment of acute gout are NSAIDs, colchicine, and systemic and intraarticular CSs as well as ACTH. Many rheumatologists use combination therapy to treat acute gout, a practice that merits study. In a patient without comorbidities, NSAIDs are the preferred therapy. CSs are often used in patients who failed NSAID or colchicine treatment or have contraindications to the use of NSAIDs. The most important determinant of therapeutic success is dependent on how soon therapy is initiated and whether the patient receives an adequate dose and for a sufficiently long period. On the horizon are new treatment options for patients with acute gout who cannot tolerate, who have contraindications, or who are not responsive to current treatments. IL-1 inhibition has been shown to have a beneficial effect on gouty inflammation and several new IL-1 blockers are currently in clinical trials for acute gout. We appear headed to changes and improvement in the treatment of acute gout.

References

1. Bellamy N, Downie WW, Buchanan WW. Observations on spontaneous improvement in patients with podagra: implications for therapeutic trials of nonsteroidal anti-inflammatory drugs. Br J Clin Pharmacol 1987;24:33–6.
2. Agudelo CA, Schumacher Jr HR, Phelps P. Effect of exercise on urate crystal-induced inflammation in canine joints. Arthritis Rheum 1972;15:609–16.
3. Schumacher Jr HR. Crystal induced arthritis: An overview. Am J Med 1996;100(Suppl. 2A):46–52.
4. Schlesinger N, Baker DG, Beutler AM, et al. Local ice therapy during bouts of acute gouty arthritis. J Rheumatol 2002;29:331–4.
5. Dorwart BB, Hansell JR, Schumacher Jr HR. Effects of cold and heat on urate-induced synovitis in dog. Arthritis Rheum 1974;17:563–71.
6. Zhang W, Doherty M, Bardin T, et al. EULAR Standing Committee for International Clinical Studies Including Therapeutics. EULAR evidence based recommendations for gout. Part II, management. Report of a task force of the EULAR Standing Committee for International Clinical Studies Including Therapeutics (ESCISIT). Ann Rheum Dis 2006;65:1312–24.
7. Neogi T, Hunter DJ, Chaisson CE, et al. Frequency and predictors of inappropriate management of recurrent gout attacks in a longitudinal study. J Rheumatol 2006;33:104–9.
8. Weaver AL, Cheh MA, Kennison RH. How PCP education can impact gout management: the gout essentials. J Clin Rheumatol 2008;14:S42–6.
9. Gnanenthiran SR, Hassett GM, Gibson KA, et al. Acute gout management during hospitalisation: a need for a protocol. Intern Med J 2010:(Epub ahead of print).
10. Schlesinger N, Moore DF, Sun JD, et al. A survey of current evaluation and treatment of gout. J Rheumatol 2006;33:2050–2.
11. Petersel D, Schlesinger N. Treatment of acute gout in hospitalized patients. J Rheumatol 2007;34:1566–8.
12. Schlesinger N. Management of acute and chronic gouty arthritis: present state-of-the-art. Drugs 2004;64(21):2399–416.
13. Ben-Chetrit E, Levy M. Colchicine: 1998 update. Semin Arthritis Rheum 1998;28:48–59.
14. Schlesinger N, Schumacher R, Catton M, et al. Colchicine for acute gout. Cochrane Database Syst Rev 2006;4:CD006190.
15. Gutman AB. Treatment of primary gout: the present status. Arthritis Rheum 1965;8:911–20.
16. Schlesinger N, Moore DF, Sun JD, et al. A survey of current evaluation and treatment of gout. J Rheumatol 2006;33:2050–2.
17. Yeap SS, Goh EML, Gun SC. A survey on the management of gout in Malaysia. Int J Rheum Dis 2009;12:329–35.
18. Bellamy N, Gilbert JR, Brooks PM, et al. A survey of current prescribing practices of anti-inflammatory and urate lowering drugs in gouty arthritis in the Province of Ontario. J Rheumatol 1988;15:1841–71.
19. Bellamy N, Brooks PM, Gilbert RJ, et al. Survey of current prescribing practices of anti-inflammatory and urate lowering drugs in gouty arthritis in New South Wales and Queensland. Med J Austral 1989;151:537–51.
20. Stuart RA, Gow PJ, Bellamy N, et al. A survey of current prescribing practices of anti-inflammatory and urate-lowering drugs in gouty arthritis. N Z Med J 1991;104(908):115–7.
21. Rozenberg S, Lang T, Laatar A, et al. Diversity of opinions on the management of gout in France. A survey of 750 rheumatologists. Rev Rheum Engl Educ 1996;63:255–61.
22. Ferraz MB, Sato EI, Nishie IA, et al. A survey of current prescribing practices in gouty arthritis and symptomatic hyperuricemia in San Paulo, Brazil. J Rheumatol 1994;21(2):374–5.
23. Schlesinger N, Johanson Jr WG, Jyoti Rao, et al. A survey of current evaluation and treatment of gout. Arthritis Rheum 1999;42(Suppl. 9):S536.
24. Fang W, Zeng X, Li M, et al. The management of gout at an academic healthcare center in Beijing: a physician survey. J Rheumatol 2006;33:2041–9.
25. Weede RP. Poison in the Pot: The Legacy of Lead. Carbondale and Edwardsville, IL: Southern Illinois University Press; 1984:83.
26. Katzung BG. Basic and Clinical Pharmacology. Norwalk, CT: Appleton and Lange; 1995:536-559.
27. Martinon F, Petrilli V, Mayor A, et al. Gout-associated uric acid crystals activate the NALP3 inflammasome. Nature 2006;440:237–41.
28. Levy, et al. Colchicine: a state-of-the-art review. Pharmacotherapy 1991;11:196–211.
29. Yang LPH. Oral colchicine (Colcrys®) in the treatment and prophylaxis of gout. Drugs 2010;70(12):1603–13.
30. Ahern MJ, Reid C, Gordon TP. Does colchicine work? Results of the first controlled study in gout. Austr N Z J Med 1987;17:301–4.
31. Terkeltaub RA, Furst DE, Bennett K, et al. High versus low dosing of oral colchicine for early acute gout flare: twenty-four–hour outcome of the first multicenter, randomized, double-blind, placebo-controlled, parallel-group, dose-comparison colchicine study. Arthritis Rheum 2010;63:1050–8.
32. British Medical Association (BMA). Royal Pharmaceutical Society (RPS) of Great Britain. British national formulary. London, UK: BMA, RPS; 2002, 500 (No. 44).
33. Morris I, Varughese G, Mattingly P. Colchicine in acute gout. BMJ 2003;327:1275–6.
34. www.fda.gov/.../DrugSafetyInformationforHeathcareProfessionals/ucm174315.htm.
35. Vonkeman HE, van de Laar MAFJ. Nonsteroidal anti-inflammatory drugs: adverse effects and their prevention. Semin Arthritis Rheum 2010;39(4):294–312.
36. Bellamy N, Downie WW, Buchanan WW. Observations on spontaneous improvement in patients with podagra: implications for therapeutic trials of non-steroidal anti-inflammatory drugs. Br Clin Pharm 1987;24(1):33–6.
37. Smythe CJ, Percy JS. Comparison of indomethacin and phenylbutazone in acute gout. Ann Rheum Dis 1973;32(4):351–3.
38. Rousti A, Vainio U. Treatment of acute gouty arthritis with proquazone and indomethacin. A comparative double-blind trial. Scand J Rheumatol 1978(Suppl. 21):15–7.
39. Zollner N, Adam O, Wolfram G. Suldinac, a new anti-inflammatory agent, in the treatment of acute gout. Treat Rheum Dis 1976:175–81.
40. Willkens RF, Case JB, Huix FJ. The treatment of acute gout with naproxen. J Clin Pharmac 1975:363–6.
41. Willkens RF, Case JB. Treatment of acute gout with naproxen. Scand J Rheumatol 1973;2:69–71.
42. Tumrasvin T, Deesomchok U. Piroxicam in treatment of acute gout high dose versus low dose. J Med SS Thailand 1985;68(3):111–6.
43. Altman RD, Honig S, Levin JM, et al. Ketoprofen versus indomethacin in patients with acute gouty arthritis: a multicenter, double blind comparative study. J Rheumatol 1988;15:1422–6.
44. Weiner GI, White SR, Weitzner RI, et al. Double blind study of phenoprofen versus phenylbutazone in acute gouty arthritis. Arthritis Rheum 1979;22:425–6.
45. Shrestha M, Morgan DL, Moreden JM, et al. Randomized double-blind comparison of the analgesic efficacy of intramuscular ketorolac and oral indomethacin in the treatment of acute gouty arthritis. Ann Emerg Med 1995;26:682–6.
46. Macagno A, Di Giorgio E, Romanowicz A. Effectiveness of etodolac (Lodine) compared with naproxen in patients with acute gout. Curr Med Res Opin 1991;12:423–9.
47. Schumacher HR, Boice J, Dahikh DI, et al. Randomized double blind trial of etoricoxib and indomethacin in treatment of acute gouty arthritis. BMJ 2002;324:1488–92.
48. Rubin BR, Burton R, Navarra S, et al. Efficacy and safety profile of treatment with etoricoxib 120 mg once daily compared with indomethacin 50 mg three times daily in acute gout: a randomized controlled trial. Arthritis Rheum 2004;50:598–606.
49. Schumacher HR, Berger M, Li-Yu J, et al. Efficacy and tolerability of celecoxib in the treatment of moderate to extreme pain associated with acute gouty arthritis: a randomized controlled trial. Arthritis Rheum 2010;60 (Suppl. 9):S151.
50. Riccardi C, Bruscoli S, Migliorati G. Molecular mechanisms of immunomodulatory activity of glucocorticoids. Pharmacol Res 2002;45:361–8.
51. Groff GD, Franck WA, Raddatz DA. Systemic steroid therapy for acute gout: a clinical trial and review of the literature. Semin Arthritis Rheum 1990;19:329–36.
52. Alloway JA, Moriarty MJ, Hoogland YT, et al. Comparison of triamcinolone acetonide with indomethacin in the treatment of acute gouty arthritis. J Rheumatol 1993;20:111–3.
53. Siegel LB, Alloway JA, Nashel DJ. Comparison of adrenocorticotropic hormone and triamcinolone acetonide in the treatment of gouty arthritis. J Rheumatol 1994;21:1325–7.
54. Janssens HJ, Janssen M, van de Lisdonk EH, et al. Use of oral prednisolone or naproxen for the treatment of gout arthritis: a double-blind, randomized equivalence trial. Lancet 2008;371:1854–60.
55. Fernandez C, Noguera R, Gonzalez JA, et al. Treatment of acute attacks of gout with small doses of intraarticular triamcinolone acetonide. J Rheumatol 1999;26:2285–6.
56. Getting SJ, Christian HC, Flower RJ, et al. Activation of melanocortin type 3 receptor as a molecular mechanism for adrenocorticotropic hormone efficacy in gouty arthritis. Arthritis Rheum 2002;46(10):2765–75.

57. Getting SJ, Gibbs L, Clark AJL, et al. POMC gene derived peptides activate MC3R on murine macrophages, suppress cytokine release and inhibit neutrophil migration in acute experimental inflammation. J Immunol 1999;162:7446–53.

58. Ritter J, Kerr LD, Valeriano-Marcet J, et al. ACTH revisited: effective treatment for acute crystal induced synovitis in patients with multiple medical problems. J Rheumatol 1994;21:696–9.

59. Axelrod D, Preston S. Comparison of parenteral adrenocorticotropic hormone with oral indomethacin in the treatment of acute gout. Arthritis Rheum 1988;31:803–56.

60. Di Giovine FS, Malawista SE, Nuki G, et al. Interleukin 1 (IL 1) as a mediator of crystal arthritis. Stimulation of T cell and synovial fibroblast mitogenesis by urate crystal-induced IL 1. J Immunol 1987;138:3213–8.

61. Martinon F, Petrilli V, Mayor A, et al. Gout-associated uric acid crystals activate the NALP3 inflammasome. Nature 2006;440:237–41.

62. Cronstein RN, Terkeltaub R. The inflammatory process of gout and its treatment. Arthritis Res Ther 2006;8(Suppl. 1):S3.

63. So A, De Smedt T, Revaz S, et al. A pilot study of IL-1 inhibition by anakinra in acute gout. Arthritis Res Ther 2007;12:9:R28.

64. Cho M, Ghosh P, Hans G, et al. The safety and efficacy of Anakinra in the treatment of acute gout in hospitalized patients. Arthritis Rheum 2010;60 (Suppl. 9):S163.

65. Terkeltaub R, Sundy JS, Schumacher HR, et al. The IL-1 inhibitor rilonacept in treatment of chronic gouty arthritis: results of a placebo-controlled, monosequence crossover, nonrandomized, single-blind pilot study. Ann Rheum Dis 2009;68(10):1613–7.

66. Investor teleconference: June 9, 2010. http://files.shareholder.com/downloads/REGN/941483174x0x380925/e99d3c78-f180-4597-a98d-fc1ce20abe49/REGN_Rilonacept_Call_Presentation.pdf

67. So A, De Meulemeester M, Pikhlak A, et al. Canakinumab for treatment of acute flares in difficult-to-treat gouty arthritis. Arthritis Rheum 2010;62(10):3064–76.

68. XOMA. http://www.xoma.com

Diet, Alcohol, Obesity, Hyperuricemia, and Risk of Gout

Hyon K. Choi

KEY POINTS

- Lifestyle and dietary modifications can influence serum urate levels and the risk of gout and are the only acceptable options when urate-lowering medications are not yet indicated or are successfully terminated after durable remission of gout.

- Lifestyle modifications should continue as an adjunct measure to aid pharmacologic urate-lowering therapy regardless of the stage of gout, which is analogous to how hypertensive patients should continue lifestyle modifications in all stages of hypertension.

- Lifestyle modifications for gout patients should take into account both associated benefits and risks in a holistic manner, since gout is often associated with many important comorbidities including the metabolic syndrome and an increased future risk of cardiovascular disease and mortality.

- Reducing weight with daily exercise and limiting intake of red meat and sugary beverages would help reduce uric acid levels, the risk of gout, insulin resistance, and comorbidities.

- While heavy drinking should be avoided, moderate drinking, sweet fruits, and seafood intake, particularly oily fish, should be tailored to the individual, considering their anticipated health benefits against cardiovascular disease.

- Dairy products, vegetables, nuts, legumes, fruits (less sugary ones), and whole grains are healthy dietary choices for the comorbidities of gout and would likely help prevent gout by reducing insulin resistance and thus inducing urinary uric acid excretion.

- Coffee (regular or decaffeinated) and vitamin C supplementation may be considered as long-term preventive measures as they can lower urate levels as well as the risk of gout and some associated comorbidities.

Introduction

Historical descriptions of gout, including typical demographics, secular trends, and anecdotal observations, have all suggested that lifestyle factors substantially influence the risk of gout.[1,2] Previous short-term purine feeding studies and the observed urate-lowering response associated with purine-restrictive diets have indicated a significant impact of dietary purine intake on serum urate levels. A less recognized but important point to consider is that long-term effects of lifestyle factors for insulin resistance syndrome are likely to have a considerable role in the risk of hyperuricemia and gout as well.[1] Increasing trends in these lifestyle risk factors may help explain the increasing disease burden of gout that has been observed during the past several decades.[1] Recent large-scale studies have confirmed some of the long-purported dietary risk factors for hyperuricemia and gout, including meat, seafood, beer, liquor, adiposity, and weight gain[1] (Fig. 11-1). Other putative risk factors, such as protein and purine-rich vegetables, were exonerated, and a potential protective effect of dairy products was newly identified.[3,4] Furthermore, several other factors that had not been included in traditional lifestyle recommendations have been identified, including offending factors like fructose- and sugar-sweetened soft drinks[5-8] and protective factors such as coffee[9,10] and vitamin C supplements.[11-13] Moreover, recent studies have identified the substantial comorbidity burden of cardiovascular-metabolic conditions among patients with hyperuricemia and gout.

Lifestyle and dietary recommendations are the only acceptable option when urate-lowering medications are not yet indicated or are successfully terminated after durable remission of gout (Fig. 11-2). Furthermore, these recommendations should continue as an adjunct measure to aid pharmacologic urate-lowering therapy (ULT) regardless of the stage of gout, which is analogous to how hypertensive or diabetic patients should not give up lifestyle modifications in any stage of hypertension[14] or type 2 diabetes.[15] The application of scientific knowledge on the risk factors for hyperuricemia and gout into practice requires consideration of the health impact of these factors on the frequent comorbidities of hyperuricemia and gout. This is particularly relevant because a number of major cardiovascular-metabolic conditions often co-occur in these patients.[16-23] In an extreme scenario, if a certain lifestyle modification can reduce the risk of gout but could also contribute to an increased risk of a major health outcome such as acute myocardial infarction or premature death, it would be difficult to justify its long-term implementation. Thus, it is important to consider holistic lifestyle recommendations that take into account both the impact on gout and relevant

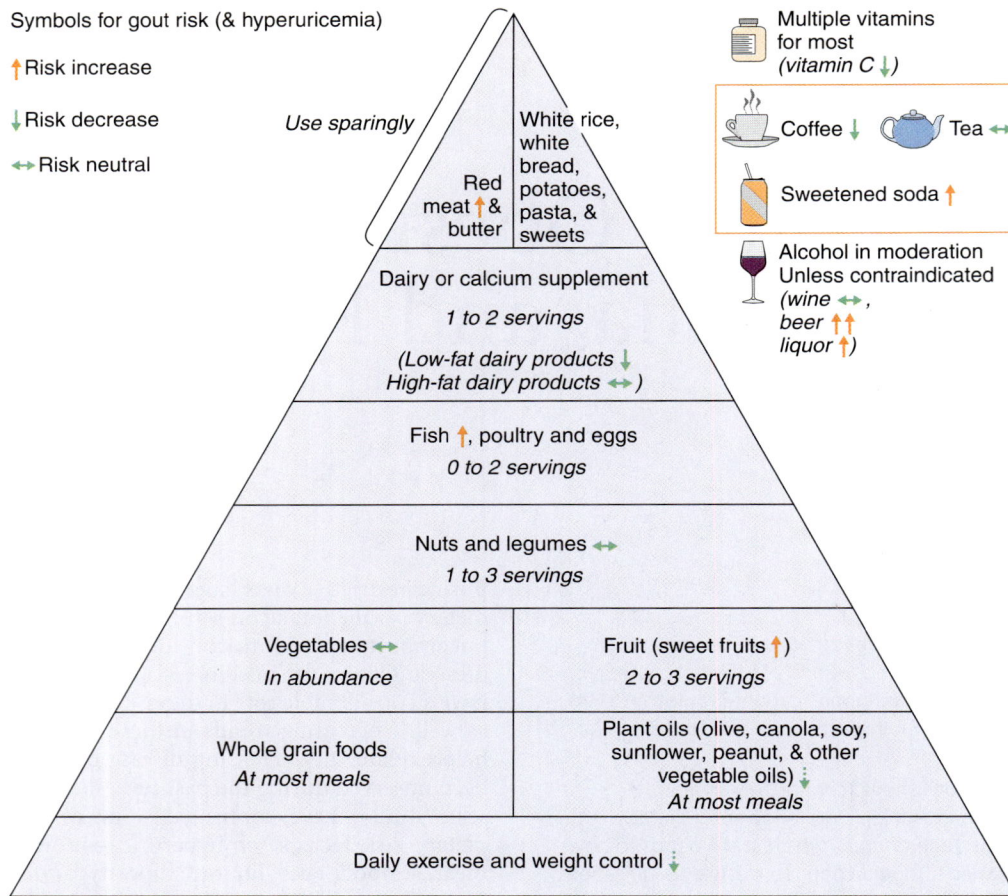

Figure 11-1 Lifestyle impacts on the risk of gout and their implications within a healthy eating guideline pyramid. The references on the relation between diet and the risk of gout are listed in Tables 11-1 and 11-2. *Up arrows* denote an increased risk of gout, whereas *down arrows* denote a decreased risk. *Horizontal arrows* denote no influence on the risk of gout. *Dotted arrows* denote a potential effect but without prospective evidence for the outcome of gout. *(Modified from Willett WC, Stampfer MJ. Rebuilding the food pyramid. Sci Am 2003;288:64-71.)*

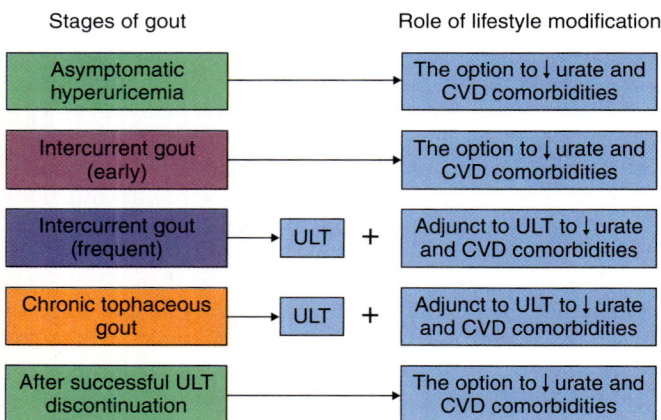

Figure 11-2 Role of lifestyle modification according to stages of gout. *ULT*, Urate-lowering therapy.

other relevant health outcomes, particularly cardiovascular-metabolic comorbidities of gout.

This chapter reviews the lifestyle risk factors for hyperuricemia and gout and attempts to provide holistic recommendations, considering both their impacts on the risk of gout and other potential health implications.

Historical Perspectives of Lifestyle Factors and Gout

Once known as a "disease of kings and king of diseases," gout has affected important figures such as Alexander the Great, Charlemagne, Henry VIII, the Emperor Charles V, Benjamin Franklin, Alexander Hamilton, Tennyson, Coleridge, Voltaire, Isaac Newton, Charles Darwin, and Leonardo da Vinci.[2,24,25] Also described by Hippocrates during the Golden Age of Greece, gout was previously considered a disease of the affluent, primarily observed in middle-aged men of the wealthy upper class ("the Patrician malady").[24-26] During the days of the Roman Empire, Seneca remarked that even women were getting gout, for "in this age, women now rival men in every kind of lasciviousness."[2] As is appreciable in these historical descriptions, gout had often afflicted the wealthy and the educated, and particularly those who not only could afford the comforts of life but also enjoyed its excesses, with habits that bordered on overindulgence, gluttony, and intemperance.[25] As these lifestyles have become affordable and prevalent in the general public in the modern era, particularly in Western society with abundantly available foods and a strong tendency toward sedentary lifestyle, gout has changed its epidemiology from a "disease of kings" to a "disease of commoners."

These historical observations and trends are consistent with the long-hypothesized notion about the links between excessive ingestion of purine-rich foods and alcohol and the development of gout. They are also in line with the conventional approach of limiting these factors in the lifestyle recommendations for gout management. Historically, other dietary approaches have also been proposed to help prevent gout. For example, a diet low in meat and high in dairy products was proposed as a means to prevent gout by the philosopher John Locke (1632-1704), who encouraged milk drinking and "eating very little flesh but abundance of herbs"; similar diets were proposed by George Cheyne in the 1700s and by Alexander Haig in the late 1800s.[25] Also in the late 1800s, Sir William Osler prescribed diets low in fructose as means to prevent gout as he wrote in his 1892 textbook, *The Principles and Practice of Medicine*, that "The sugar should be reduced to a minimum. The sweeter fruits should not be taken."[27,28] These approaches have been supported by recent large-scale studies,[3,7,29] which are discussed in detail later in this chapter.

Species Differences, Westernization, and Gout Trends

Humans are the only mammals that are known to develop gout spontaneously, probably because hyperuricemia commonly develops only in humans.[1,25] In most fish, amphibians, and nonprimate mammals, uric acid generated from purine metabolism undergoes oxidative degradation via the uricase enzyme, which produces the more soluble compound allantoin.[1] Thus, it is difficult to induce serum urate levels in rats unless an inhibitor of uricase is administered,[25,30] whereas feeding meat to birds and many reptiles induces a substantial increase in serum urate levels as these species lack uricase, like humans. For example, gout has been observed in turkeys that were fed horse meat.[31]

The impact of diet on the uric acid levels in species that lack uricase may also provide insight into why the serum urate levels in the great apes (1.5 to 3.0 mg/dl)[25] are substantially lower than those in humans in the modern era (4.8 mg/dl among women and 6.1 mg/dl among men in the U.S. general population, 1999-2008). The great apes primarily consume fruit and vegetation while their animal protein intake is minimal.[25] Early humans in indigenous scavenging and gathering societies who lived on traditional diets primarily derived from fruits and vegetables with sporadic additions of fish and game likely had serum urate levels similar to those of the great apes.[25]

A number of epidemiologic studies from a diverse range of countries suggest that gout has increased in prevalence and incidence in the last few decades. This increase is likely explained in large part by trends in lifestyle factors associated with Westernization.[1,32] For example, since the introduction of Western culture and dietary habits, gout has become an epidemic among some native peoples, such as the Maori of New Zealand.[25,33,34] After the introduction of a diet high in fatty meats and carbohydrates and low in dairy products in the early 1900s, an epidemic of obesity and gout developed.[25,33,34] Similarly, gout was rare among blacks in Africa, especially in rural areas where traditional agricultural and dairy-based diets were common, but its frequency has been increasing, particularly in urban communities.[25] Gout was considered rare among African Americans in the early 1900s,

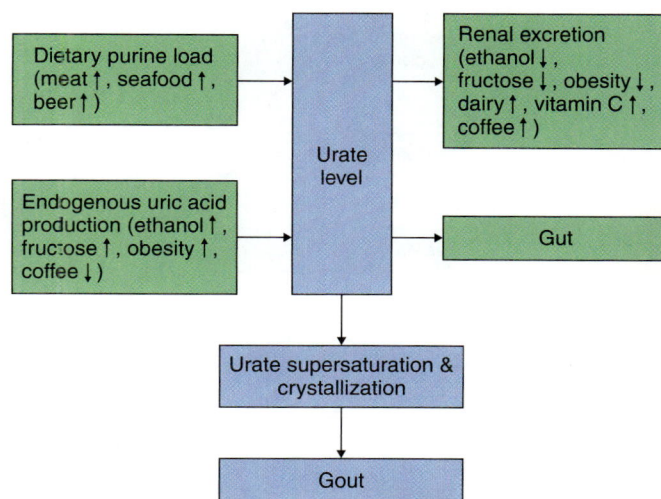

Figure 11-3 Determinants of serum uric levels and their pathogenetic action sites. Directions of arrows denote the direction of influence. *Up arrows* denote hazardous influence contributing to increasing serum uric acid levels, whereas *down arrows* denote benefits contributing to decreasing serum uric acid levels.

but changes in diet have led to a rapid development of obesity, diabetes, and hypertension. Today, the mean serum urate levels are higher and gout is more common among African Americans than among whites.[25,35] Furthermore, ecologic studies of Japanese[36] and Filipino[37] populations have found that U.S. immigrants from these countries had increases in serum urate levels, the incidence of gout, or both, compared with their offshore counterparts.

Pathophysiologic Considerations in Lifestyle Recommendations for Gout

The amount of urate in the body, the culprit in the causation of gout, depends on the balance among dietary intake, synthesis, and excretion.[1] Hyperuricemia results from the underexcretion of uric acid in the vast majority of cases (90%), overproduction of uric acid, or a combination of the two.[1] Thus, while lifestyle factors such as oral purine load can contribute to uric acid burden and the risk of gout to a certain extent, factors that can affect renal uric acid excretion or both production and excretion would likely have a substantial impact on uric acid burden and risk of gout. The purine-loading lifestyle factors (e.g., meat, seafood, alcohol, fructose-rich food) that affect serum urate levels can acutely increase the risk of urate crystal formation and gout attacks (Fig. 11-3). In comparison, the factors that affect insulin resistance (e.g., adiposity, dairy intake, coffee) and the renal excretion of urate can improve urate levels[38-40] and the risk of gout in a long-term manner (Fig. 11-4). Traditional lifestyle approaches have almost exclusively focused on acute gout prevention with the purine-loading risk factors. However, since the insulin resistance syndrome is a highly prevalent comorbidity among gout patients[16] and has cardiovascular-metabolic consequences,[17-23] it is important to consider the factors that can improve insulin resistance, particularly in long-term lifestyle recommendations.

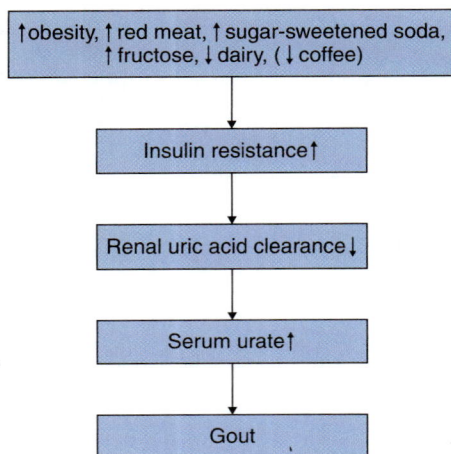

↑obesity, ↑ red meat, ↑ sugar-sweetened soda, ↑ fructose, ↓ dairy, (↓ coffee)

↓

Insulin resistance↑

↓

Renal uric acid clearance↓

↓

Serum urate↑

↓

Gout

Figure 11-4 Lifestyle factors and their influence on insulin resistance, serum uric acid levels, and the risk of gout. Directions of arrows denote the direction of exposure levels of lifestyle factors or influence of involved pathogenetic steps.

Gout Is a Metabolic Disorder Associated With Multiple Associated Comorbidities and Cardiovascular-Metabolic Sequelae

Although the cardinal feature of gout is inflammatory arthritis, it is a metabolic condition associated with elevated uric acid burden.[1,41] A number of associated cardiovascular-metabolic conditions have been identified, including increased adiposity,[16,23] hypertension,[23,42] dyslipidemia,[16] insulin resistance,[16,22] hyperglycemia,[16,22] certain renal conditions,[22,43] and atherosclerotic cardiovascular disorders.[17-20] Recent studies have quantified the magnitude of associations with these comorbid conditions. For example, in a representative sample of U.S. adult men and women (NHANES III), the prevalence of the metabolic syndrome, as defined by the revised National Cholesterol Education Program Adult Treatment Panel III (NCEP/ATP III), was 63% among individuals with gout and 25% among individuals without gout.[16] Previous hospital-based case series reported that the prevalence of the metabolic syndrome was 82% in Mexican men[44] and 44% in Korean men[45] with gout. These quantitative population data indicate that the prevalence of the metabolic syndrome is remarkably high among individuals with hyperuricemia and gout. Correspondingly, the prevalence of the metabolic syndrome has been found to increase substantially with increasing levels of serum urate, from 19% for serum urate levels less than 6 mg/dl to 71% for levels of 10 mg/dl or greater.[46] While more than 50% of gout patients have hypertension,[16,23,42] coronary artery disease (CAD) has been observed in 25% of gout patients in the United Kingdom[47] and in 18% of U.S. male health professionals with gout.[19] Overweight and obese statuses have been observed in 71% and 14% of U.S. health professional men with gout,[23] respectively, whereas obesity has been reported to be as high as 27.7% in a U.K. general practitioners' population.[47] The association with diabetes is generally weak, with a prevalence of 6% of gout patients in the United Kingdom[48] and 5% among male health professionals with gout.[19] The prevalence of kidney stones is 15% among male health professionals with

gout[49] and renal insufficiency was found to be 5% in the U.S. general population.[50]

These cross-sectional associations have been consistently translated into increased future risk of relevant cardiovascular-metabolic sequelae. For example, the Framingham Heart Study found that gout was associated with a 60% increased risk of CAD in men, which was not explained by clinically measured risk factors.[17] Also, in the Multiple Risk Factor Intervention Trial (MRFIT), participants with a history of gout had a 26% increased independent risk of myocardial infarction,[18] a 33% increased risk of peripheral arterial disease,[51] and a 35% increased risk of coronary heart disease (CHD) mortality.[52] Similarly, the Health Professionals Follow-Up Study (HPFS) cohort showed a 59% increased risk of nonfatal myocardial infarction and a 55% increased risk of fatal myocardial infarction.[19] Furthermore, in the HPFS, men with gout had a 28% higher risk of death from all causes, a 38% higher risk of death from cardiovascular disease (CVD), and a 55% higher risk of death from CHD.[19] Finally, an analysis based on the MRFIT data showed that men with gout had a 41% increased risk of incident type 2 diabetes.[20]

These comorbidities of gout and independent associations with future risks of CVD and mortality add to the overall burden of gout and provide strong support for serious consideration of these issues in determining appropriate lifestyle recommendations for gout patients.

Low-Purine Diet Versus a Dietary Approach Against the Metabolic Syndrome

The conventional dietary approach to gout management limits food or drinks that are known to potentially precipitate an acute gouty attack, such as large servings of meat and heavy beers.[41] However, a rigid purine-restricted diet has been thought to be of dubious therapeutic value and can rarely be sustained for long.[41] Furthermore, low-purine foods are often rich in both refined carbohydrates (including fructose) and saturated fat.[41,53] These tend to further decrease insulin sensitivity, leading to higher plasma levels of insulin, glucose, triglycerides, and low-density lipoprotein cholesterol (LDL-C) levels and decreased levels of high-density lipoprotein cholesterol (HDL-C), thereby furthering the risk of the metabolic syndrome and its complications in these patients.[41,53] In contrast, a diet aimed to lower insulin resistance can not only improve uric acid levels[53] but also improve insulin sensitivity and decrease plasma glucose, insulin, and triglyceride levels, which would lead to a reduction in the incidence and mortality of CVD.[41] Of note, the HPFS data on incident gout are largely consistent with the lifestyle recommendations against insulin resistance. For example, measures that are known to reduce insulin resistance like weight loss,[23] higher dairy intake,[3] lower fructose intake,[7] and higher coffee intake[10] have all been found to be protective against the risk of developing new cases of gout (Fig. 11-4, Table 11-1).

Furthermore, the fact that previously forbidden items such as purine-rich vegetables, nuts, legumes, and vegetable protein are, despite their high purine content, not associated with an increase in gout risk[23] also supports their overall beneficial effects in gout patients, likely through lowering insulin resistance. (In fact, individuals who consumed a larger amount of

Table 11-1 Lifestyle Risk Factors of Hyperuricemia and Gout

Risk Factors	Direction of Risk		
	Risk of Hyperuricemia	Risk of Gout	References
Adiposity			23, 68, 206
Body mass index	↑	↑	
Waist-to-hip ratio	↑	↑	
Weight gain	↓	↓	
Weight loss	↓	↓	
Purine-rich foods			3, 4
Meats	↑	↑	
Seafoods	↑	↑	
Purine-rich vegetables/nuts		↔	
Alcohol	↑	↑	109, 110
Fructose	↑	↑	5-8, 29
Sugar-sweetened beverages	↑	↑	
Sweet fruits/fruit juices	↑	↑	
Coffee/ decaffeinated coffee	↓	↓	9, 10, 77, 157
Dairy products			3, 4
Low-fat dairy products	↓	↓	
High-fat dairy products		↔	
Vitamin C supplements	↓	↓	11, 12, 179, 180, 209

vegetable protein [the highest quintile] had a 27% lower risk of gout compared with the lowest quintile.[3]) These approaches could not only reduce uric acid levels and the risk of gout in the long run but could also lower the major consequences of insulin resistance.[16-23] In other words, the overall risk-benefit ratio of the diet approach against the metabolic syndrome would likely yield a more favorable net outcome in the long run than the traditional low-purine diet. Furthermore, as compared with the less palatable low-purine diet,[54] a dietary approach against the metabolic syndrome may achieve higher long-term compliance. A formal comparison of these dietary approaches would be valuable.

Long-term Versus Short-term Implications of Lifestyle Interventions

Certain lifestyle interventions may have differential short-term versus long-term effects on the risk of gout, similar to the paradoxical short-term flares versus long-term benefits of ULT. For example, the more potent and immediate the urate-lowering effect of a certain lifestyle factor, the more likely it is that these paradoxical flares are expected, just as with potent pharmacologic ULTs. This means that if a certain lifestyle factor is associated with short-term flares but long-term benefits, physicians and patients should be aware of such effects, and its initiation among gout patients may require a gradual introduction, similar to ULT. Regardless, since ULTs are continued beyond the initial phase of paradoxical flares when indicated, lifestyle modifications may also be appropriately sustained beyond this initial phase in order to lower uric acid levels. The advantage of lifestyle modifications over ULT use is that one needs not consider adverse events and costs of drugs, as lifestyle approaches are generally healthy and affordable.

A similar analogy can be found in the use of exercise as a preventive measure against the risk of myocardial infarction. Although acute exertion associated with exercise can lead to a short-term increased risk of myocardial infarction, individuals who exercise regularly have a lower risk of developing myocardial infarction, and thus regular exercise is recommended as a CVD prevention measure. This is because the long-term benefits of exercise outweigh the short-term risk, particularly when the exercise regimen is gradually initiated. In the case of gout, a similar example might be that a burst of high consumption of caffeinated beverages may induce a short-term gout attack by promoting a decrease in both serum urate and hydration, but the long-term effects of steady consumption may be beneficial by lowering uric acid levels and the risk of developing gout. Thus, if a patient with gout chooses to try regular coffee intake to help reduce serum urate levels, its initiation may need to be similar to that of gradually implementing an exercise program in CVD prevention or initiating ULT. Alternatively, decaffeinated coffee may be considered without risking paradoxical flares associated with initiation.

Short-term Feeding Studies for Serum Uric Acid Levels

The long-suspected role of purine-rich food of animal origin on the risk of gout had been supported by metabolic experiments in animals and humans that examined the impact of artificial short-term loading of purified purine on the serum uric acid level (not gouty arthritis per se).[55-58] While these studies provided a basis for the potential long-term effects of purine-rich food items, such as red or organ meat, on hyperuricemia and, conceivably, on the eventual development of gout in the long run, several hurdles existed before such a conclusion could be drawn. First, little has been known about the precise identity and quantity of individual purines in most foods, especially when cooked or processed.[59] Additionally, the bioavailability of various purines contained in different foods varies substantially. For example, dietary substitution-addition experiments showed that RNA has a greater effect than an equivalent amount of DNA,[58] ribomononucleotides have a greater effect than nucleic acid,[60] and adenine has a greater effect than guanine.[55] Finally, the outcome of interest in these studies was hyperuricemia, rather than gout,[55-58,60] and a substantial proportion of hyperuricemic patients do not develop gouty arthritis.[21,61] Thus, these short-term feeding studies are informative, but based on these studies alone, it is difficult to conclude whether a certain "purine-rich" food or food group actually affects the risk of gout per se.

Long-term, Prospective Cohort Studies of Lifestyle Factors for Gout

The limitations of short-term feeding studies can be addressed by long-term, prospective studies that collect dietary and other lifestyle information and track the development of gout among individuals without existing gout at baseline. These studies can examine the relation between actual foods or food groups (as opposed to purified purines) and the risk of developing gout on a long-term basis and can provide practical information. While the data from these studies are directly relevant to prevention of new cases of gout, these observations are likely applicable to patients with preexisting gout as well. In fact, the effects could be even more exaggerated as absorption of dietary purines causes a steeper rise in blood urate levels in these patients than in normouricemic individuals due to the relative impairment of renal uric acid clearance in the majority of these patients.[62,63]

Several earlier prospective cohort studies that examined the risk factors for gout had a relatively small number of incident cases of gout (range of 60 to 102) and lacked comprehensive dietary information, including The Johns Hopkins Precursor Study,[21] the Normative Aging Study,[61] and the Framingham Heart Study.[17] Thus, their ability to detect risk factors was somewhat limited to more obvious and common factors such as increased adiposity. More recently, two large prospective studies comprehensively gathered dietary and lifestyle information and had a large number of incident cases of gout during follow-up (730 men and 889 women with gout by 1998 and 2006, respectively).[3,29] As the substantial amount of the data discussed in this chapter are based on these two prospective studies, relevant study specifics are summarized next, before individual risk factors are discussed.

Health Professionals Follow-Up Study

The HPFS is an ongoing longitudinal study of 51,529 male dentists, optometrists, osteopaths, pharmacists, podiatrists, and veterinarians who were 40 to 75 years of age in 1986. While there were no exclusions by race, 1% were African American and 2% were Asian. The participants returned a mailed questionnaire in 1986 concerning diet, medical history, and medications. To assess dietary intake, a validated food-frequency questionnaire was used to inquire about the average use of more than 130 foods and beverages during the previous year.[64,65] The baseline dietary questionnaire was completed in 1986 and was updated every 4 years. Nutrient intake was computed from the reported frequency of consumption of each specified unit of food or beverage and from published data on the nutrient content of the specified portions.[65] Food and nutrient intakes assessed by this dietary questionnaire have been validated previously against two 1-week diet records in this cohort.[64,66] At baseline, and every 2 years thereafter, the participants provided information on weight, regular use of medications (including diuretics), and medical conditions (including hypertension and chronic renal failure). The follow-up for this cohort has exceeded 90%.

Beginning in 1986, biennial questionnaires asked whether participants had ever received a physician diagnosis of gout and, if so, the date of first occurrence. If the participant

reported that gout had been diagnosed in 1986 (when dietary information was first collected) or later, we mailed a supplementary questionnaire to confirm the diagnosis according to the American College of Rheumatology (ACR) survey gout criteria,[67] the age of occurrence, family history of gout, and other relevant information including treatment for gout. The response rate to the supplementary questionnaire was approximately 80%. To confirm the validity of the ACR survey gout criteria in this cohort, two board-certified rheumatologists reviewed the medical records of a sample of 76 men who had reported having gout and had consented to the release of their medical records. Of these 76 men, 26 did not have relevant and complete records. Among the remaining 50 men, the rate of concordance between the diagnosis of gout according to the ACR criteria[67] and the diagnosis of gout according to our review of the medical records was 94%. Of note, the incidence rate in this cohort[3] was very close to that of male physicians in the Johns Hopkins Precursor Study that used the same ACR gout definition.[68]

Nurses' Health Study (NHS) Cohorts

In 1976, 121,700 female U.S. registered nurses between the ages of 30 and 55 years, residing in 11 large U.S. states, completed an initial NHS questionnaire.[29] The NHS population is predominantly white, reflecting the ethnic background of women entering nursing in the United States in the 1950s and 1960s. The 1992 questionnaire indicated the following ethnic composition: 1.2% African American, 0.6% Hispanic, 0.8% Asian, 17% southern European or Mediterranean, 7% Scandinavian, 60% other white, and 4% other ancestry. Similar to HPFS, the NHS cohort has been followed by mailed questionnaires sent every 2 years to update exposure information and to ascertain incident diseases. The participation rate has been very high. The follow-up for this cohort has exceeded 90% as well.

In 1982, 1984, 1986, 1988, 2002, and thereafter, biennial questionnaires asked whether participants had received a physician diagnosis of gout and, if so, the date of first occurrence.[29] If the participant reported that gout had been diagnosed in 1980 (when dietary information was first collected) or later, a supplementary questionnaire was mailed to confirm the diagnosis according to the ACR survey gout criteria,[67] the age of occurrence, family history, the type of symptoms, other relevant medical conditions, and treatment. The overall response rate for the supplementary gout questionnaire was 81%, similar to that observed in the HPFS. The concordance rate between the ACR criteria and medical records was greater than 90% based on 56 medical records.[29]

The restriction to registered health professionals and nurses in these cohorts is both a strength and a limitation. The cohort of well-educated individuals minimizes potential for confounding associated with socioeconomic status, and investigators were able to obtain high-quality data with minimal loss to follow-up. Although the absolute rates of health outcomes and distribution of respective exposure intake may not be representative of a random sample of U.S. adults, their biological effects should be similar. These two prospective cohorts have provided a series of studies regarding lifestyle factors for the risk of gout, and those factors are discussed in detail next.

Individual Dietary and Lifestyle Factors and the Risk of Gout

Meat Intake

Meat intake could contribute to an increased risk of gout,[3] likely because its high purine content raises serum urate levels, as was demonstrated by short-term metabolic experiments of purine loading in animals and humans.[55-58] Furthermore, red meat is a key source of saturated fats, which are positively associated with insulin resistance,[69,70] which reduces the renal excretion of uric acid.[38,39,53,71] Indeed, a nationally representative sample of U.S. men and women indicated that higher levels of meat were associated with higher serum urate levels.[4]

The HPFS showed that men in the highest quintile of meat intake had a 41% higher risk of gout compared with the lowest quintile.[3] Specifically, the intake of two or more weekly servings of beef, pork, or lamb as a main dish was associated with a 50% increased risk of gout compared with less than one serving per month (*p* for trend = .01).[3] Saturated fats in red meat also increase LDL cholesterol levels more than HDL cholesterol, adding to a negative net health effect. Higher levels of these fats and red meat consumption have been linked to major disorders such as CAD, type 2 diabetes, and certain types of cancer. Thus, it would be beneficial for patients with gout to limit red and organ meat intake to help reduce the risk of both gout and associated major comorbidities[72] (see Fig. 11-4).

Seafood and Omega-3 Fatty Acids

Seafood intake can also increase the risk of gout[3] through its high purine content, despite not being associated with increased insulin resistance like red meat. The same nationally representative study showed higher levels of seafood consumption were associated with higher serum urate levels.[4] The HPFS found that men in the highest quintile of seafood intake had a 51% higher risk compared with the lowest quintile.[3] Increased intakes of tuna, dark fish, other fish; and shrimp, lobster, or scallops were all associated with an increased risk of gout (*p* for trend <.05 for all items).[3]

The recommendation regarding seafood in prevention of gout is not as straightforward as that for meat intake, because oily fish and omega-3 fatty acids reduce the incidence of cardiovascular disorders, according to many studies and clinical trials.[73] Based on these data, the American Heart Association (www.americanheart.org) concludes that omega-3 fatty acids benefit the hearts of healthy people and those at high risk of—or who suffer from—CVD and currently recommends eating fish (particularly oily fish) at least twice weekly.[73] Prospective secondary prevention studies suggest that eicosapentaenoic acid (EPA) and docosahexaenoic acid (DHA) supplementation ranging from 0.5 to 1.8 g/d (either as fatty fish or supplements) significantly reduces subsequent cardiac and all-cause mortality.[73] Similarly, total intakes of 1.5 to 3 g/d of α-linolenic acid seem beneficial.[73] These apparent cardiovascular benefits from fish products make it difficult to justify a long-term recommendation to avoid all fish intake, considering the risk of gouty flares only. Cardiovascular prevention is likely more relevant among gouty patients, since the associated comorbidities of gout (e.g., insulin resistance syndrome, hypertension) or gout itself may pose an increased risk of CVD.[17]

Patients with gout or hyperuricemia could consider the use of plant-derived omega-3 fatty acids or supplements of EPA and DHA in the place of fish consumption, for their cardiovascular prevention effects. This approach would provide the benefit of omega-3 fatty acids and avoid the increased risk of gout from the purine load contained in seafood. Further, diets enriched in both linolenic acid and EPA significantly suppress urate crystal–induced inflammation in a rat model,[41,74] raising an intriguing potential protective role of these fatty acids against gout flares.

Dairy Intake

Dairy products may exert their urate-lowering effects without the concomitant purine load contained in other animal protein sources such as meat and seafood.[75-77] Ingestion of milk proteins (casein and lactalbumin) has been shown to decrease serum urate levels in healthy subjects via the uricosuric effect of these proteins.[75] Furthermore, a recent randomized trial has shown that milk intake has an acute urate-lowering effect via its low purine content in combination with increased excretion of uric acid in response to a protein load.[77] Conversely, a previous 4-week randomized clinical trial showed a significant increase in uric acid level was induced by a dairy-free diet.[76] In terms of nationally representative data on this link, dairy consumption was inversely associated with serum urate levels.[4]

For the risk of gout, men in the highest quintile of dairy intake in the HPFS had a 44% lower risk compared with the lowest quintile, and the inverse association was limited to low-fat dairy consumption.[3] Men in the highest quintile of dairy protein intake had a 48% lower risk of gout compared with the lowest quintile.[3] The absence of the inverse association with high-fat dairy products could result from the counteracting effect of saturated fats contained in high-fat dairy products. Studies have suggested that low-fat dairy foods are associated with several potential health benefits, including a lower incidence of CHD,[78] premenopausal breast cancer,[79] colon cancer,[80] and type 2 diabetes.[81] Further, low-fat dairy foods have been one of the main components of the Dietary Approaches to Stop Hypertension (DASH) diet, which has been shown to substantially lower blood pressure.[82] However, dairy consumption, including low-fat dairy foods, has been implicated in possible increases in prostate cancer.[83] Weighing these benefits and risks, the recent healthy lifestyle pyramid recommends one to two daily servings of dairy products[72] (see Fig. 11-1). This recommendation could be readily extended to patients with gout or hyperuricemia, perhaps with added benefits against comorbidities such as hypertension, diabetes, and cardiovascular disorders.[78,81,82]

Purine-Rich Vegetables and Vegetable Protein

Contrary to popular belief and conventional practice, the consumption of purine-rich vegetables was found not to be associated with the risk of incident gout.[3] Correspondingly, intake of individual purine-rich vegetable items was not associated with the risk of gout, including nuts, legumes, spinach, mushrooms, oatmeal, and cauliflower. Men in the highest quintile of vegetable protein consumption actually had a 27% lower risk of gout compared with the lowest quintile.[3] While these findings may be explained by insufficient amounts or bioavailability of purine content in these food items,[55-60] other major constituents of these items (fiber or healthy fat) may contribute to lowering insulin resistance and help reduce uric acid levels and eventually the risk of gout.[84]

These findings have important long-term implications for patients with hyperuricemia and gout, as there are virtually no other protein sources for macronutrients, other than vegetables, once animal protein sources such as meat and seafood are reduced or eliminated from gout patients' diets. Furthermore, these vegetables (especially nuts and legumes) are excellent sources of protein, fiber, vitamins, and minerals. Studies have suggested that nut consumption is associated with several important health benefits, including a lower incidence of CHD,[85,86] sudden cardiac death,[87] gallstones,[88,89] and type 2 diabetes.[90] Many kinds of nuts contain healthy fats, and controlled feeding studies have shown that nuts improve blood cholesterol ratios.[72] Legumes or dietary patterns with increased legume consumption have been linked to a lower incidence of CHD,[91-93] stroke,[94] certain types of cancer,[95,96] and type 2 diabetes.[97] The recent healthy eating pyramid recommends once- to three-times daily consumption of nuts and legumes (see Fig. 11-1),[72] which is also readily applicable to patients with gout or hyperuricemia.

Alcoholic Beverages

Alcohol can induce hyperuricemia, likely through both decreased uric acid excretion[98-101] and increased production.[102,103] The former is via conversion of alcohol to lactic acid, which reduces renal uric acid excretion by inhibiting urate anion secretion into the tubule lumen in the renal proximal tubule.[41,59,104,105] The confounding effect of fasting often associated with heavy drinking has also been implicated as the culprit of decreased urinary excretion via inducing acetoacetic and beta-hydroxybutyric acidemia.[59,106] Additionally, ethanol administration was shown to increase uric acid production by increasing adenosine triphosphate (ATP) degradation to adenosine monophosphate (AMP), a uric acid precursor.[102] This process was later shown to involve acetate conversion to acetyl coenzyme A (CoA) in the metabolism of ethanol.[103] Factors not directly related to uric acid implicated in the pathogenesis of gout include the frequent coexistence in heavy drinkers of other provocative factors, such as trauma and hypothermia of the lower extremities.[41,100] These factors may explain why alcoholic gouty patients tend to have significantly lower serum urate levels than nonalcoholics during acute attacks of gout.[100]

Prior to the HPFS, several cohort studies attempted to evaluate the association between alcohol intake and gout, but these studies were limited by small sample size and lack of relevant dietary variables.[17,61,68,107,108] Subsequently, the HPFS showed that increasing alcohol intake was associated with increasing risk of gout in a dose-response relationship.[109] Specifically, as compared with abstinence, daily alcohol consumption of 10 to 14.9 g increased the risk of gout by 32%, 15 to 29.9 g by 49%, 30 to 49.9 g by 96%, and 50 or more g by 153% (*p* for trend <.001). Beer consumption showed the strongest independent association with the risk of gout (multivariate risk ratio [RR] per 12-oz serving per day 1.49; 95% CI 1.32-1.70). Consumption of liquor was also significantly associated with gout (multivariate RR per drink or shot per day 1.15; 95%

CI 1.04-1.28); however, wine consumption was not associated with an increased risk of gout in this study (multivariate RR per 4-oz serving per day 1.04; 95% CI, 0.88-1.22).[109] Correspondingly, a U.S. national survey study demonstrated corresponding associations between these individual alcoholic beverages and serum urate levels.[110]

These findings confirmed the long-held belief of an association between alcohol intake and the risk of gout. In addition, they suggest that certain nonalcoholic components that vary among these alcoholic beverages may play a role in the incidence of gout. Beer is the only alcoholic beverage acknowledged to have a large purine content, which is predominantly guanosine, a readily absorbable nucleoside.[59,111] The effect of ingested purine in beer on serum urate may be sufficient to augment the hyperuricemic effect of alcohol itself, producing a greater risk of gout than liquor or wine.[109] There may be other nonalcoholic offending factors, particularly in beer. Wine is known to contain a number of nonalcohol components including antioxidants,[112-114] vasorelaxants,[115] and stimulants to antiaggregatory mechanisms.[116] Since uric acid is considered an indicator for increased oxidative stress, nonalcoholic components in wine (e.g., polyphenols with antioxidant properties[112-114]) may potentially play a role in mitigating the impact of alcohol on serum urate.

The health benefits of moderate drinking likely outweigh the risks, especially among those within the demographics of the peak prevalence of gout (e.g., middle-aged men). More than 60 prospective studies consistently demonstrated that moderate alcohol consumption is associated with a 25% to 40% reduced risk of CHD.[117] Also, a number of prospective studies also suggest a similar degree of protective effect against ischemic stroke, peripheral vascular disease, sudden cardiac death, and death from all cardiovascular causes.[117] The benefits of moderate drinking appear to go beyond the heart. For example, moderate drinking has been linked to a decreased risk of gallstones[118] and type 2 diabetes[119] compared with abstinence. Based on these data, the recent Healthy Eating guideline for the general public allows moderate alcohol consumption[72] (see Fig. 11-1), especially if one already drinks alcohol. The key is to keep the consumption in the moderate range (i.e., one to two drinks per day for men, and no more than one drink per day for women[120]). However, starting drinking is not generally recommended, as similar benefits could be alternatively sought via exercise or healthier eating.[120]

These other health effects of moderate drinking may be considered in advising about alcohol intake to patients with existing gout or at a high risk of developing gout. For example, if you are a middle-aged man with no history of alcoholism who is at moderate to high risk for heart disease and gout, allowing a daily drink of wine may be acceptable, as it could bring associated health benefits perhaps without substantially increasing the risk of gout attacks. This approach may be especially relevant if the patient has low HDL-cholesterol that is not responsive to diet and exercise therapy, because moderate amounts of alcohol raise levels of HDL-cholesterol.[121]

Sugar-Sweetened Sodas and Fructose-Rich Foods

The doubling of the prevalence[122] and incidence[123] of gout over the last few decades in the United States has coincided with a substantial increase in soft drink and fructose

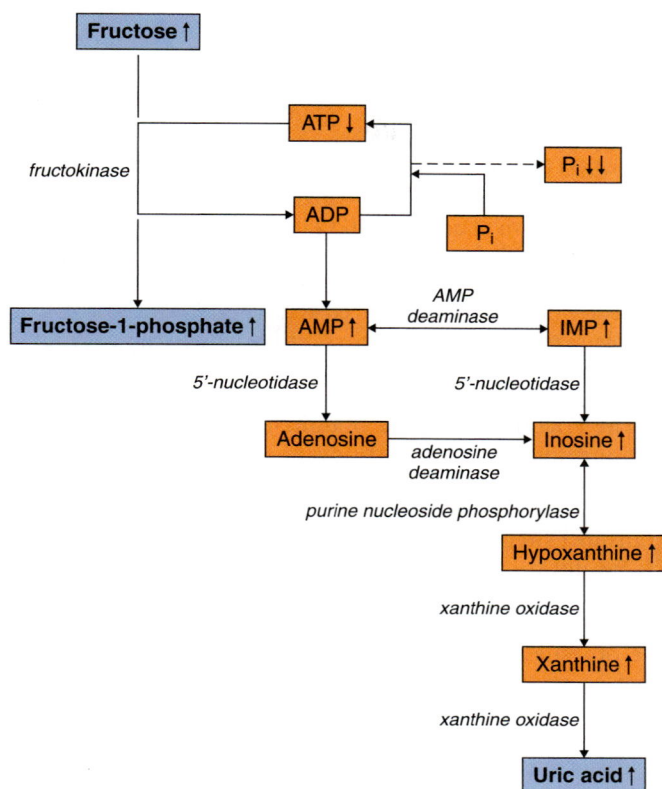

Figure 11-5 Mechanism of fructose-induced hyperuricemia. Fructose induces hepatic uric acid production by increasing adenosine triphosphate (ATP) degradation to adenosine monophosphate (AMP), a uric acid precursor. The phosphorylation of fructose to fructose-l-phosphate causes ATP to be degraded to adenosine diphosphate (ADP). Fructose-l-phosphate traps inorganic phosphate, and ADP is converted back to ATP by using inorganic phosphate (P_i). The net result is reduced levels of intracellular ATP and P_i combined with a buildup of AMP, which also leads to increased IMP concentration. Elevated AMP and IMP levels activate the catabolic pathways leading to increased synthesis of uric acid, accounting for hyperuricemia.

consumption.[124] Fructose consumption has also increased dramatically since the introduction of commercially produced high-fructose corn syrup in 1967,[125] while ingestion of naturally occurring fructose consumption has remained relatively stable.[126] Fructose intake can raise serum urate levels by increasing hepatic ATP degradation to AMP, prompting activation of the pathway of purine degradation to uric acid[127,128] (Fig. 11-5). In contrast, glucose and other simple sugars do not have this effect.[28] Furthermore, fructose intake is associated with serum insulin levels and insulin resistance[126] and could, therefore, indirectly increase serum urate levels and the risk of gout.[38,39,71]

Two large cohort studies, the HPFS in men and the NHS in women, have found that consumption of sugar-sweetened soft drinks and fructose is associated with an increased risk of gout in both genders.[7,29] The risk for incident gout was 85% higher among men who consumed two servings or more of sugar-sweetened soft drinks per day compared with those who consumed less than one per month. In contrast, diet soft drinks were not associated with a risk for gout. Consistent associations have been observed in women.[29]

The risk for gout increased as fructose consumption rose. Other major contributors to fructose intake such as total fruit juice or fructose-rich fruits (i.e., apples and oranges) were associated with a modestly increased risk for gout among men[7] but not among women.[29] Correspondingly, in a nationally representative sample of U.S. men and women (NHANES III), serum urate concentration increased with intake of sugar-sweetened soft drinks, whereas diet soft drink consumption was not associated with serum urate concentration.[6] In men, added sugar intake was also associated with serum urate concentration[5] and a similar association was observed in adolescents.[8]

Regarding other potential health impacts, increased fructose consumption can lead to a positive energy balance,[129,130] which may contribute to the high prevalence of insulin resistance and adiposity.[125,131,132] Fructose intake may also be associated with an increased risk of pancreatic,[133] breast,[134] colorectal cancer,[135] and symptomatic gallstone disease.[136] However, a modest inverse association with the risk of prostate cancer has been suggested.[137]

Conventional dietary recommendations for gout focus on restriction of purine intake, although low-purine diets are often high in carbohydrates, including fructose-rich foods and refined carbohydrates.[41] However, if the risk posed by fructose and sugar intake could be as large as that posed by purine-rich foods such as total meat consumption (RR between extreme quintiles—1.41[3]) as per the prospective data,[7,29] the conventional dietary approach carries the potential to worsen the overall net health outcome in gout patients, including gout attacks. Reducing sugar intake in dietary recommendations for hyperuricemia and gout may be important in order to reduce the risk of gout and to improve overall long-term outcomes, as higher sugar consumption is also associated with excess adiposity and risk for type 2 diabetes.[138,139]

Although certain fructose-rich fruits (i.e., apples and oranges) may also increase the risk of gout in men,[3] higher consumption of fruits and vegetables is associated with other relevant health benefits. For example, higher consumption of fruits and vegetables is one of the main components of the DASH diet, which has been shown to substantially lower blood pressure,[140] and is associated with a modest reduction in the development of major chronic disease, mainly CVDs.[141] These relevant health benefits and risks associated with individual food items should be carefully considered in the potential application of these findings to dietary recommendations for hyperuricemic or gouty individuals (see Fig. 11-1).

Coffee, Teas, and Caffeine

Coffee is one of the most widely consumed beverages in the world. For example, more than 50% of Americans drink coffee, and the average per capita intake is about two cups per day.[142,143] Given this widespread use, the potential health effects of coffee are important for public health as well as for helping an individual make an informed choice regarding coffee consumption. Coffee consumption may reduce the risk of gout via various mechanisms, including reducing serum urate levels[144,145] and influencing insulin resistance.[143,146-152] For example, caffeine (1,3,7-trimethyl-xanthine) is a methylxanthine and may be a competitive inhibitor of xanthine oxidase as demonstrated in rats.[145] This potential property of caffeine may exert a protective effect against gout similar to that of allopurinol. Higher long-term coffee intake has been associated with lower insulin levels[151] and increased insulin sensitivity.[153] Because there is a strong positive relation between serum insulin resistance and hyperuricemia[1,22,40,41,154], and insulin reduces the renal excretion of urate,[38-40] decreased insulin resistance and insulin levels associated with coffee consumption may lead to a lower risk of hyperuricemia and gout.[10]

Indeed, cross-sectional studies based on Japanese adults[144,155] and U.S. adults[156] showed a significant inverse association between coffee consumption and serum urate levels. Correspondingly, increasing coffee intake was inversely associated with the risk of gout in both men[10] and women.[157] The risk of gout was 40% lower with coffee intake of four to five cups daily and 59% lower with six cups daily or more, compared with no use among men,[10] whereas the risk of gout was 22% lower with coffee intake of one to three cups daily and 57% lower with four cups daily or more, compared with no use among women.[157] Furthermore, a modest inverse association was found for decaffeinated coffee in both genders.[10,157] However, tea intake was not associated with risk of gout in either gender.[10,157] Interestingly, cross-sectional studies based on Japanese men[144] and U.S. adults[156] also found that serum urate level was not associated with tea intake.

The absence of associations between serum urate levels and tea intake suggests that the presence of components in coffee other than caffeine that may contribute to the inverse association with intake of coffee (both regular and decaffeinated). As mentioned, the mechanism behind this decreased risk of gout may be through the effect of coffee on insulin sensitivity, as higher long-term coffee intake is associated with lower insulin levels[151] and improved insulin sensitivity[153] and renal uric acid clearance is inversely related to the degree of insulin resistance.[38,39,71] Furthermore, coffee (both regular and decaffeinated) is the major source of the phenol chlorogenic acid, a strong antioxidant. Plasma glucose concentrations may be reduced by chlorogenic acid,[158] which acts as a competitive inhibitor of glucose absorption in the intestine[159] and may combine with other antioxidants in coffee to decrease oxidative stress.[151] Antioxidants may improve insulin sensitivity[160] and decrease insulin levels.[161] Tea also has many different types of antioxidants; however, the antioxidant capacity per serving and total contributions are substantially higher in coffee than in tea.[151,162,163]

Regular coffee drinking also reduces the risk of incident type 2 diabetes,[143,164,165] kidney stones,[166,167] symptomatic gallstone disease,[168,169] and Parkinson disease.[170] There is no evidence that coffee consumption increases the risk for CVD,[171-173] with the potential exception of high consumption of unfiltered boiled coffee (e.g., Scandinavian-style boiled coffee), which increases both plasma total and LDL cholesterol.[174] Furthermore, caffeine tends to promote urinary calcium excretion, and drinking coffee in excess of four or more cups per day may increase the risk of fracture.[175-178] The inverse associations between coffee intake (regular and decaffeinated) and the risk of gout suggest that continued coffee drinking can be allowed if the patient is already drinking coffee regularly but that this recommendation should be considered in conjunction with other health effects of coffee (see Fig. 11-1).

Vitamin C (Ascorbate)

The suspicion for a potential protective effect of vitamin C intake against gout originally stemmed from metabolic experiments that examined the impact of short-term loading of high-dose vitamin C on the serum urate levels. For example, ingestion of a single dose of 4 g vitamin C doubled the fractional excretion of uric acid and a daily ingestion of 8 g of vitamin C for 3 to 7 days reduced serum urate by 2.0 to 3.1 mg/dl as a result of uricosuria.[179] Furthermore, a double-blinded placebo-controlled randomized trial (N = 184) showed that supplementation with vitamin C as low as 500 mg daily for 2 months reduced serum urate by 0.5 mg/dl, compared to no change in the placebo group.[11]

The uricosuric effect of vitamin C is likely due to a competition for renal reabsorption of uric acid via an anion-exchange transport system at the proximal tubule.[179,180] Recent advances in molecular mechanisms of renal urate transport suggest that the uricosuric effect may be through *cis*-inhibition of *URAT1* (urate transporter 1, the key target of typical uricosurics),[181] Na$^+$-dependent anion cotransporter (e.g., *SLC5A8/A12*), or both in the proximal tubules.[1] Furthermore, a recent randomized trial showed vitamin C supplements (500 mg/d) significantly increased glomerular filtration rate, providing another potential mechanism for the uricosuric effect of vitamin C intake.[11] It remains speculative whether the antioxidant action of vitamin C may have a protective effect against gouty inflammation, as was suggested for reducing the risk of inflammatory polyarthritis according to a recent prospective study.[182]

A retrospective Taiwanese case-control study (91 gout cases and 91 controls) reported an inverse association between vitamin C intake and the presence of gout (unadjusted OR between the extreme tertiles, 0.31; 95% CI, 0.15 to 0.35), although no multivariate adjustment for the link was reported.[84] In the HPFS, the risk of gout was 17% lower with total vitamin C intake 500 to 999 mg/d, 34% lower with 1000 to 1499 mg/d, and 45% lower with 1500 mg/d or more (p for trend <.001) compared with vitamin C intake less than 250 mg/d among men.[10] While these data suggest that total vitamin C intake of 500 mg/d or more is associated with a reduced risk, the potential benefit of lower intake is not clear.

According to a recent analysis of nine prospective studies, compared with subjects who did not take supplemental vitamin C, those who took greater than 700 mg supplemental vitamin C/d had a 25% lower risk of CHD (95% CI, 7% to 40%; p for trend <.001).[183] The same study found that supplemental vitamin E intake was not significantly related to reduced CHD risk.[183] This potential cardiovascular benefit of vitamin C may be particularly relevant among gout patients given their increased risk of cardiovascular morbidity and mortality.[19,52] However, vitamin C intake has been associated with an increased risk of nephrolithiasis, similar to the typical property of uricosuric drugs.[184] Given the general safety profile associated with vitamin C intake, particularly, within the generally consumed ranges as in our study (e.g., tolerable upper intake level of vitamin C less than 2000 mg in adults according to the Food and Nutrition Board, Institute of Medicine),[185] vitamin C may provide a useful option in the prevention of gout.

Adiposity and the Risk of Gout

Increased adiposity is associated with hyperuricemia via both increased production and decreased renal excretion of urate.[41,186] Conversely, weight loss likely decreases urate levels by increasing renal excretion of uric acid and in part by decreasing urate production.[41,186,187] For example, an intervention study of 27 obese individuals found that fractional excretion of uric acid was significantly reduced (4% in men and 5% in women compared with 11% and 12% in normal controls, respectively).[188] Interestingly, urinary uric acid excretions were also lower in obese subjects than in controls, suggesting that hyperuricemia in these obese individuals was mainly attributed to an impaired renal clearance of uric acid rather than overproduction. Furthermore, weight reduction by a low-calorie diet and exercise therapy resulted in the normalization of fractional excretion of uric acid.[188] This is likely through decreasing insulin resistance and insulin levels, which lead to decreased renal excretion of uric acid and hyperuricemia. For example, exogenous insulin has been shown to reduce the renal excretion of uric acid in both healthy and hypertensive subjects.[38-40] Renal clearance of uric acid has been shown to have an inverse relation with both the degree of insulin resistance[71] and visceral fat area, as measured by abdominal computed tomography.[189] Insulin may enhance renal urate reabsorption via stimulation of urate-anion exchanger and/or the Na^+-dependent anion cotransporter in brush border membranes of the renal proximal tubule.[1] Additionally, since serum levels of leptin and urate tend to rise together,[190,191] some investigators have suggested that leptin may affect renal reabsorption.[1] Finally, in the insulin resistance syndrome, impaired oxidative phosphorylation may increase systemic adenosine concentrations by increasing the intracellular levels of CoA esters of long-chain fatty acids.[1] Increased adenosine, in turn, can result in renal retention of sodium, urate, and water.[192-194] Some have speculated that chronically increased extracellular adenosine concentrations may also contribute to hyperuricemia by increasing urate production.[192] Factors not related to uric acid such as chronic joint trauma due to excess weight have been proposed as an additional explanation for the association between obesity and gout.[21,41]

Prospective cohort studies have consistently found the association between increased adiposity and gout,[17,61,68,108] although the lack of data and small number of gout cases limited the comprehensive adjustment of relevant covariates in earlier studies. The Johns Hopkins Precursor Study (60 cases of incident gout) found that increased body mass index at age 35, but not at baseline (mean age, 22 years), was associated with the risk of gout (12% increased risk of gout unit increase in body mass index).[68] The Normative Aging Study showed body mass index at baseline (mean age, 52 years) was significantly associated with hyperuricemia or gout, although the study had similar limitations.[61] In the Framingham Study, there was a significantly higher body mass index among gout patients after adjusting for age but no multivariate adjustment results were presented.[17] In the HPFS where substantial number of covariates were adjusted for including dietary risk factors, higher adiposity and weight gain are strong risk factors for gout in men, while weight loss is protective.[23] Specifically, compared to men with body mass index 21 to 22.9 kg/m², the risk of gout was 95% higher for men with body mass index 25 to 29.9 kg/m², 233% higher for 30 to 34.9 kg/m², and 297%

higher for greater than 35 kg/m² (p for trend <.001).[23] The risk of gout among men in the highest waist-to-hip ratio quintile (0.98 to 1.39) was 82% higher than among men in the lowest quintile (0.70 to 0.88). Further, compared with men who maintained their weight (−4 to +4 lb) since age 21, the risk of gout for men who gained 30 lb or more was 99% higher. In contrast, the risk of gout for men who lost 10 lb or more since the study baseline was 39% lower.[23] Correspondingly, a recent analysis of the MRFIT data showed that as compared with no weight change (−0.9 to 0.9 kg), the multivariate odds ratios of achieving normouricemia (i.e., serum uric acid level 6 mg/dl or less) for a weight loss of 1 to 4.9, 5 to 9.9, and 10 kg or greater were 1.43 (95% CI, 1.33 to 1.54), 2.17 (1.95 to 2.40), and 3.90 (3.31 to 4.61), respectively.[195] The corresponding serum urate level changes were −7, −19, and −37 µmol/L (−0.12, −0.31, and −0.62 mg/dl). Furthermore, a recent multivariate analysis of the Framingham Heart Study found consistent associations between obesity and the risk of gout.[196]

The impact of adiposity on gout adds to the already substantial hazards associated with the obesity epidemic in the United States. The 2007-2008 National Health and Nutrition Examination Survey estimated that the age-adjusted prevalence of obesity (body mass index 30 kg/m² or greater) among U.S. adults is 33.8%.[197] The prevalence of class 3 obesity (body mass index 40 kg/m² or greater) among adults has more than doubled in 10 years, with an estimated prevalence of 5.7% in the year 2007-2008.[197] Obesity is associated with at least as much morbidity as are poverty, smoking, and problem drinking[198] and leads to approximately 300,000 deaths per year in the United States.[199] For example, weight gain has been linked to increased risks of CHD,[200,201] hypertension,[202] type 2 diabetes,[119,203] kidney stones,[204] and gallstones.[205] As the healthy lifestyle guidelines strongly recommend daily exercise and weight control by placing them at the foundation of the pyramid (see Fig. 11-1), equal emphasis can be placed on lifestyle modifications for gout patients.[72] A comprehensive effort to reduce adiposity would contribute to substantially reducing the disease burden of gout and associated morbidities.[53]

A Prescription for Lifestyle Change in Patients With Hyperuricemia and Gout

The goals of lifestyle modifications are to help prevent both gout attacks and complications of gout and its comorbidities, including cardiovascular-metabolic sequelae and premature deaths. Thus, if certain factors can help prevent both recurrent gout attacks and other major health consequences, such measures would be highly desirable. In contrast, if certain factors can reduce the risk of recurrent gout but can increase the risk of major health outcomes such as CVDs, type 2 diabetes, or cancer, it would be difficult to justify their long-term implementation among gout patients, particularly among those with comorbidities. A simple pharmacologic analogy of this would be the use of low-dose aspirin. Even though low-dose aspirin can increase the risk of gout, it is difficult to justify stopping this medication given its cardioprotective benefits. The same holistic risk-benefit consideration would be needed in determining appropriate lifestyle recommendations for gout patients.

This leads us to consider the identified lifestyle risk factors of gout within a healthy lifestyle paradigm geared to prevent other common major disorders such as CVD, type 2 diabetes, and certain types of cancers.[72] Figure 11-1 summarizes this integration of the impacts of identified risk factors for gout into recommended dietary guidelines for the general public (i.e., Healthy Eating Pyramid).[72] As discussed, most of the identified factors affect the risk of gout in the same direction as other major health outcomes, while the potential exceptions include seafood, sugary fruits, and alcoholic beverages. Each identified risk factor is discussed, as well as summarized in Table 11-2, with a holistic risk-benefit recommendation considering both the risk of gout and other major health outcomes.[72]

- *Exercise daily and reduce weight with gradual calorie reduction,* as increased adiposity is associated with higher uric acid levels and an increased future risk of gout, whereas weight loss is associated with lower uric acid levels and a decreased risk of gout.[23,68,206] The healthy eating pyramid strongly recommends daily exercise and weight control by placing them at the foundation of the pyramid, as obesity is associated with many important health outcomes, including CHD,[200,201] hypertension,[202] type 2 diabetes,[119,203] kidney stones,[204] and gallstones.[205] Many patients with gout are overweight or obese, and weight reduction through gradual caloric restriction and exercise can substantially help lower uric acid levels and the risk of gout attacks,[53] in addition to its beneficial effects on associated cardiovascular-metabolic commodities and sequelae.

- *Limit red meat intake,* as it is associated with higher uric acid levels and increased future risk of gout.[3,4] The mechanism behind this increased risk may be multifactorial. The urate-raising effect of artificial short-term loading of purified purine has been well demonstrated by metabolic experiments in animals and humans.[55-58] Further, red meat is the main source of saturated fats, which are positively associated with insulin resistance,[69,70] which in turn reduces renal excretion of uric acid.[38,39,53,71] These fats also increase LDL-C levels more than HDL-C, creating a negative net effect. Higher levels of these fats or red meat consumption have been linked to major disorders such as CAD, type 2 diabetes, and certain types of cancer.

- *Tailor seafood intake to the individual taking into account cardiovascular comorbidities, and consider omega-3 fatty acid supplements.* Seafood intake has been linked to higher serum uric acid levels and increased future risk of gout, which is likely due to its high purine content.[3,4] Increased intakes of oily fish, other fish, and shellfish are all associated with an increased risk of gout. However, given the apparent cardiovascular benefits from fish products,[73] particularly oily fish that are rich in omega-3 fatty acids, it would be difficult to justify a recommendation to avoid all fish intake considering only the risk of gouty flares. Oily fish[73] may be allowed while implementing other lifestyle measures, particularly among gouty patients with cardiovascular comorbidities.

- *Consume skim milk or other low-fat dairy products, up to two servings daily.* Low-fat dairy consumption has been inversely associated with serum uric acid levels as well as future risk of gout.[3,4] Furthermore, low-fat dairy foods have been linked to a lower incidence of CHD,[78] premenopausal breast cancer,[79] colon cancer,[80] and type 2 diabetes.[81] Finally, low-fat dairy foods have been one of the main components of the DASH diet that has been shown to substantially lower blood pressure.[82]

- *Consume vegetable protein, nuts, legumes, and purine-rich vegetables,* as they do not increase the risk of gout[3] and these food items (especially nuts and legumes) are excellent sources of protein, fiber, vitamins, and minerals. In fact, individuals who consumed vegetable protein in the highest quintile of intake actually had a 27% lower risk of gout compared to the lowest quintile.[3] Furthermore, nut consumption is associated with several important health benefits including a lower incidence of CHD,[85,86] sudden cardiac death,[87] gallstones,[88,89] and type 2 diabetes.[90] Legumes or dietary patterns with increased legume consumption have been linked to a lower incidence of CHD,[91-93] stroke,[94] certain types of cancer,[95,96] and type 2 diabetes.[97] The recently developed healthy eating pyramid recommends one to three daily servings of nuts and legumes (Fig. 11-X),[72] which appears readily applicable to patients with gout or hyperuricemia.

- *Reduce alcoholic beverages, particularly if you are drinking more than a moderate level* (i.e., one to two drinks per day for men, and no more than one drink per day for women), as these beverages, particularly beer and liquor, have been associated with higher uric acid levels and an increased risk of gout.[109,110] The overall health benefits of sensible moderate drinking (one to two drinks per day for men and one drink or less per day for women) likely outweigh the risks, as allowed by dietary guidelines by the U.S. Department of Agriculture (www.healthierus.gov/dietaryguidelines), the American Heart Association,[207] and our recent food pyramid[208] (see Fig. 11-1). More than 60 prospective studies have consistently indicated that moderate alcoholic consumption is associated with a 25% to 40% reduced risk of CHD.[207,208] Also, prospective studies suggest a similar protective effect against other CVDs and death.[207] These benefits are particularly relevant to middle-aged men,[207,208] the demographic in whom gout occurs most often. However, it is not generally recommended to start drinking alcohol, since similar benefits can be achieved with exercise or healthier eating.[120] These other health effects of moderate drinking may be considered in advising about alcohol intake to patients with existing gout or at a high risk of developing gout.

- *Reduce sugar-sweetened soft drinks and beverages,* as fructose contained in these beverages increases serum urate levels and the risk of gout.[5-8] Furthermore, fructose intake has been linked to increased insulin resistance,[126] a positive energy balance,[129,130] weight gain, obesity,[125,131,132] type 2 diabetes,[138,139] an increased risk of certain cancers,[133-135] and symptomatic gallstone disease.[136] Thus, unlike alcoholic beverages, which are associated with cardioprotective benefits when consumed moderately, no health benefits are anticipated from sugary soft drinks. Sweet fruits (i.e., apples and oranges) have also been linked to hyperuricemia and the risk of gout.[5-8] However, given the other health benefits of these food items,[140,141] it appears difficult to justify restricting these items among gout patients.

- *Allow coffee drinking if already drinking coffee* as both regular and decaffeinated coffee drinking have been associated

Table 11-2 Evidence-Based Prescription for Lifestyle Change in Patients With Hyperuricemia and Gout

Recommendations	Expected Health Benefits	Expected Health Hazards
Exercise daily and reduce weight with gradual calorie reduction	↓ Uric acid levels and the risk of gout[23,68,206] ↓ Risk of comorbidities including coronary heart disease,[200,201] hypertension,[202] type 2 diabetes,[119,203] kidney stones,[204] and gallstones[205]	None
Limit red meat intake	↓ Uric acid levels and the risk of gout[3,4] ↓ Risk of insulin resistance,[69,70] coronary artery disease, type 2 diabetes, and certain types of cancer[72]	None
Tailor seafood intake to the individual taking CV comorbidities into account, and consider omega-3 fatty acid supplements	↓ Seafood intake → ↓ uric acid levels and the risk of gout[3,4] Omega-3 fatty acids or supplements of eicosapentaenoic acid and docosahexaenoic acid → CV benefits without ↑ uric acid levels and the risk of gout	Reduced intake of oily fish could limit CV benefits from omega-3 fatty acids.[73]
Consume skim milk or other low-fat dairy products up to two servings daily	↓ Uric acid levels and the risk of gout[3,4] ↓ Risk of coronary heart disease,[78] premenopausal breast cancer,[79] colon cancer,[80] hypertension,[82] and type 2 diabetes[81]	Dairy consumption including low-fat dairy foods has been implicated in possible increases in prostate cancer[83]
Consume vegetable protein, nuts, legumes, and purine-rich vegetables	No ↑ in risk of gout[3] (Actually, vegetable protein may be associated with ↓ risk of gout[3]) ↓ Risk of coronary heart disease,[85,86,91-93] sudden cardiac death,[87] stroke,[94] gallstones,[88,89] type 2 diabetes,[90,97] and certain types of cancer [95,96]	None
Reduce alcoholic beverages, particularly if currently drinking more than a moderate level	↓ Uric acid levels and the risk of gout[3,4]	Moderate alcohol consumption is associated with a 25% to 40% reduced risk for coronary heart disease[207,208] and a similar protective effect against other CVDs and death[207]
Reduce sugar-sweetened soft drinks and beverages	↓ Uric acid levels and the risk of gout[5-8] ↓ Risk of insulin resistance,[126] a positive energy balance,[129,130] weight gain, obesity,[125,131,132] type 2 diabetes,[138,139] risk of certain cancers,[133,134,135] and symptomatic gallstone disease[136]	None Sweet fruits (i.e., apples and oranges) have also been linked to hyperuricemia and the risk of gout.[5-8] However, given the other health benefits of these food items,[140,141] it appears difficult to justify restricting these items among gout patients
Allow coffee drinking if already drinking coffee or consider drinking decaffeinated coffee	↓ Uric acid levels and the risk of developing gout[3,4] ↓ Risk of CVD[183]	Four or more cups per day may increase the risk of fractures among women.[178] Intermittent use of caffeinated beverages or acute introduction of large quantities of caffeinated beverages may trigger gout attacks as does allopurinol introduction. Avoid initiating caffeinated drinks or introduce gradually, if pursued.
Consider vitamin C supplements	↓ Uric acid levels and the risk of gout[11,12,179,180,209] ↓ Risk of type 2 diabetes,[143,164,165] kidney stones,[166,167] symptomatic gallstone disease,[168,169] and Parkinson disease[170]	Similar to pharmacologic uricosuric agents, vitamin C intake has been associated with an increased risk of nephrolithiasis[184]

with lower uric acid levels and a decreased risk of gout.[9,10] In addition, coffee drinking has been linked to a lower risk of type 2 diabetes,[143,164,165] kidney stones,[166,167] symptomatic gallstone disease,[168,169] and Parkinson disease.[170] However, caffeine tends to promote calcium excretion in urine, and drinking a lot of coffee, about four or more cups per day, may increase the risk of fractures among women.[178] Caffeine, being a xanthine (i.e., 1,3,7-trimethyl-xanthine) likely exerts a protective effect against gout similar to allopurinol through xanthine oxidase inhibition.[11,145] This means that intermittent use of coffee or acute introduction of a large amount coffee may trigger gout attacks as does allopurinol introduction. Thus, if a patient with gout chooses to try coffee intake to help reduce uric acid levels and the risk of gout, it may need to be initiated in a similar manner to allopurinol.

■ *Consider taking vitamin C supplements* as vitamin C has been found to reduce serum uric acid levels in clinical trials[11,179,180,209] and has recently been linked to a reduced future risk of gout.[12] While these data suggest that total vitamin C intake of 500 mg/d or more is associated with a reduced risk, the potential benefit of smaller quantities remains unclear. This potential cardiovascular benefit of vitamin C[183] may also be of particular relevance among gout patients, because of their increased risk of cardiovascular morbidity and mortality.[19,52] Given the general safety profile associated with vitamin C intake, particularly within the generally consumed ranges as in our study (e.g., tolerable upper intake level of vitamin C less than 2000 mg in adults according to the Food and Nutrition Board, Institute of Medicine),[185] vitamin C may provide a useful option in the prevention of gout.

Conclusion

Lifestyle and dietary recommendations for gout patients should consider a variety of other health benefits and risks, since gout is often associated with major chronic disorders such as the metabolic syndrome and an increased risk for CVD and mortality. Reducing weight with daily exercise and limiting intake of red meat and sugary beverages would help reduce uric acid levels, the risk of gout, insulin resistance, and comorbidities. While heavy drinking should be avoided, moderate consumption of alcohol, sweet fruits, and seafood intake, particularly oily fish, should be tailored to the individual, considering their anticipated health benefits against CVD. Alternatively, the use of plant-derived omega-3 fatty acids or supplements of EPA and DHA could be considered instead of fish consumption. Vegetable and dairy protein, nuts, legumes, fruits (less sugary ones), and whole grains are healthy choices against various comorbidities of gout that do not increase the risk of gout, and indeed may even help lower the risk of gout by reducing insulin resistance. Coffee can be allowed if it is already being consumed, and vitamin C supplementation can be considered, as both can lower serum urate levels, as well as the risk of gout and some of its comorbidities.

References

1. Choi HK, Mount DB, Reginato AM. Pathogenesis of gout. Ann Intern Med 2005;143:499–516.
2. Nuki G, Simkin PA. A concise history of gout and hyperuricemia and their treatment. Arthritis Res Ther 2006;8(Suppl. 1):S1.
3. Choi HK, Atkinson K, Karlson EW, et al. Purine-rich foods, dairy and protein intake, and the risk of gout in men. N Engl J Med 2004;350:1093–103.
4. Choi HK, Liu S, Curhan G. Intake of purine-rich foods, protein, dairy products, and serum uric acid level: the Third National Health and Nutrition Examination Survey. Arthritis Rheum 2005;52:283–9.
5. Gao X, Qi L, Qiao N, et al. Intake of added sugar and sugar-sweetened drink and serum uric acid concentration in US men and women. Hypertension 2007;50:306–12.
6. Choi JW, Ford ES, Gao X, et al. Sugar-sweetened soft drinks, diet soft drinks, and serum uric acid level: the Third National Health and Nutrition Examination Survey. Arthritis Rheum 2008;59:109–16.
7. Choi HK, Curhan G. Soft drinks, fructose consumption, and the risk of gout in men: prospective cohort study. BMJ 2008;336:309–12.
8. Nguyen S, Choi HK, Lustig RH, et al. Sugar-sweetened beverages, serum uric acid, and blood pressure in adolescents. J Pediatr 2009;154:807–13.
9. Choi HK, Curhan G. Coffee, tea, and caffeine consumption and serum uric acid level: the Third National Health and Nutrition Examination survey. Arthritis Rheum 2007;57:816–21.
10. Choi HK, Willett W, Curhan G. Coffee consumption and risk of incident gout in men: a prospective study. Arthritis Rheum 2007;56:2049–55.
11. Huang HY, Appel LJ, Choi MJ, et al. The effects of vitamin C supplementation on serum concentrations of uric acid: results of a randomized controlled trial. Arthritis Rheum 2005;52:1843–7.
12. Choi HK, Gao X, Curhan G. Vitamin C intake and the risk of gout in men: a prospective study. Arch Intern Med 2009;169:502–7.
13. Gao X, Curhan G, Forman JP, et al. Vitamin C intake and serum uric acid concentration in men. J Rheumatol 2008;35:1853–8.
14. August P. Initial treatment of hypertension. N Engl J Med 2003;348:610–7.
15. Kasper DL, Braunwald E, Fauci AS, et al. Harrison's Principles of Internal Medicine. New York, NY: McGraw-Hill Professional Publishing; 2004.
16. Choi HK, Ford ES, Li C, et al. Prevalence of the metabolic syndrome in patients with gout: the Third National Health and Nutrition Examination Survey. Arthritis Rheum 2007;57:109–15.
17. Abbott RD, Brand FN, Kannel WB, et al. Gout and coronary heart disease: the Framingham Study. J Clin Epidemiol 1988;41:237–42.
18. Krishnan E, Baker JF, Furst DE, et al. Gout and the risk of acute myocardial infarction. Arthritis Rheum 2006;54:2688–96.
19. Choi HK, Curhan G. Independent impact of gout on mortality and risk for coronary heart disease. Circulation 2007;116:894–900.
20. Choi HK, De Vera MA, Krishnan E. Gout and the risk of type 2 diabetes among men with a high cardiovascular risk profile. Rheumatology (Oxford) 2008;47:1567–70.
21. Roubenoff R. Gout and hyperuricemia. Rheum Dis Clin North Am 1990;16:539–50.
22. Rathmann W, Funkhouser E, Dyer AR, et al. Relations of hyperuricemia with the various components of the insulin resistance syndrome in young black and white adults: the CARDIA study. Coronary Artery Risk Development in Young Adults. Ann Epidemiol 1998;8:250–61.
23. Choi HK, Atkinson K, Karlson EW, et al. Obesity, weight change, hypertension, diuretic use, and risk of gout in men: the health professionals follow-up study. Arch Intern Med 2005;165:742–8.
24. Copeman WSC. A Short History of the Gout and the Rheumatic Diseases. Los Angeles, CA: University of California Press; 1964.
25. Johnson RJ, Rideout BA. Uric acid and diet: insights into the epidemic of cardiovascular disease. N Engl J Med 2004;350:1071–3.
26. Porter R, Rousseau GS. Gout: The Patrician Malady. New Haven, CT: Yale University Press; 1998.
27. Osler W. Gout. The Principles and Practice of Medicine. New York, NY: Appleton; 1893:287–295.
28. Nakagawa T, Tuttle KR, Short RA, et al. Hypothesis: fructose-induced hyperuricemia as a causal mechanism for the epidemic of the metabolic syndrome. Nat Clin Pract Nephrol 2005;1:80–6.
29. Choi HK, Willett W, Curhan G. Fructose-rich beverages and risk of gout in women. JAMA 2010;304:2270–8.
30. Mazzali M, Kanellis J, Han L, et al. Hyperuricemia induces a primary renal arteriolopathy in rats by a blood pressure-independent mechanism. Am J Physiol Renal Physiol 2002;282:F991–7.
31. Bollman JL, Schlotthauer CF. Experimental gout in turkeys. Am J Dig Dis 1936;3:133–88.
32. Lawrence RC, Felson DT, Helmick CG, et al. Estimates of the prevalence of arthritis and other rheumatic conditions in the United States: part II. Arthritis Rheum 2007;58:26–35.
33. Lennane GA, Rose BS, Isdale IC. Gout in the Maori. Ann Rheum Dis 1960;19:120–5.
34. Klemp P, Stansfeld SA, Castle B, et al. Gout is on the increase in New Zealand. Ann Rheum Dis 1997;56:22–6.
35. Fang J, Alderman MH. Serum uric acid and cardiovascular mortality the NHANES I epidemiologic follow-up study, 1971-1992. National Health and Nutrition Examination Survey. JAMA 2000;283:2404–10.
36. Kagan A, Harris BR, Winkelstein Jr W, et al. Epidemiologic studies of coronary heart disease and stroke in Japanese men living in Japan, Hawaii and California: demographic, physical, dietary and biochemical characteristics. J Chronic Dis 1974;27:345–64.
37. Torralba TP, Bayani-Sioson PS. The Filipino and gout. Semin Arthritis Rheum 1975;4:307–20.
38. Ter Maaten JC, Voorburg A, Heine RJ, et al. Renal handling of urate and sodium during acute physiological hyperinsulinaemia in healthy subjects. Clin Sci (Lond) 1997;92:51–8.
39. Muscelli E, Natali A, Bianchi S, et al. Effect of insulin on renal sodium and uric acid handling in essential hypertension. Am J Hypertens 1996;9:746–52.
40. Emmerson B. Hyperlipidaemia in hyperuricaemia and gout. Ann Rheum Dis 1998;57:509–10.
41. Fam AG. Gout, diet, and the insulin resistance syndrome. J Rheumatol 2002;29:1350–5.

42. Wallace KL, Riedel AA, Joseph-Ridge N, et al. Increasing prevalence of gout and hyperuricemia over 10 years among older adults in a managed care population. J Rheumatol 2004;31:1582–7.

43. Hsu CY, Iribarren C, McCulloch CE, et al. Risk factors for end-stage renal disease: 25-year follow-up. Arch Intern Med 2009;169:342–50.

44. Vazquez-Mellado J, Conrado GG, Vazquez SG, et al. Metabolic syndrome and ischemic heart disease in gout. J Clin Rheumatol 2004;10:105–9.

45. Rho YH, Choi SJ, Lee YH, et al. The prevalence of metabolic syndrome in patients with gout: a multicenter study. J Korean Med Sci 2005;20:1029–33.

46. Choi HK, Ford ES. Prevalence of the metabolic syndrome in individuals with hyperuricemia. Am J Med 2007;120:442–7.

47. Annemans L, Spaepen E, Gaskin M, et al. Gout in the UK and Germany: prevalence, comorbidities and management in general practice 2000-2005. Ann Rheum Dis 2008;67:960–6.

48. Mikuls TR, Farrar JT, Bilker WB, et al. Gout epidemiology: results from the UK General Practice Research Database, 1990-1999. Ann Rheum Dis 2005;64:267–72.

49. Kramer HJ, Choi HK, Atkinson K, et al. The association between gout and nephrolithiasis in men: The Health Professionals' Follow-Up Study. Kidney Int 2003;64:1022–6.

50. Kramer HM, Curhan G. The association between gout and nephrolithiasis: the National Health and Nutrition Examination Survey III, 1988-1994. Am J Kidney Dis 2002;40:37–42.

51. Baker JF, Schumacher HR, Krishnan E. Serum uric acid level and risk for peripheral arterial disease: analysis of data from the multiple risk factor intervention trial. Angiology 2007;58:450–7.

52. Krishnan E, Svendsen K, Neaton JD, et al. Long-term cardiovascular mortality among middle-aged men with gout. Arch Intern Med 2008;168:1104–10.

53. Dessein PH, Shipton EA, Stanwix AE, et al. Beneficial effects of weight loss associated with moderate calorie/carbohydrate restriction, and increased proportional intake of protein and unsaturated fat on serum urate and lipoprotein levels in gout: a pilot study. Ann Rheum Dis 2000;59:539–43.

54. Bieber JD, Terkeltaub RA. Gout: on the brink of novel therapeutic options for an ancient disease. Arthritis Rheum 2004;50:2400–14.

55. Clifford AJ, Riumallo JA, Young VR, et al. Effects of oral purines on serum and urinary uric acid of normal, hyperuricaemic and gouty humans. J Nutr 1976;106:428–50.

56. Clifford AJ, Story DL. Levels of purines in foods and their metabolic effects in rats. J Nutr 1976;106:435–42.

57. Zollner N. Influence of various purines on uric acid metabolism. Bibl Nutr Dieta 1973;34–43.

58. Zollner N, Griebsch A. Diet and gout. Adv Exp Med Biol 1974;41:435–42.

59. Gibson T, Rodgers AV, Simmonds HA, et al. A controlled study of diet in patients with gout. Ann Rheum Dis 1983;42:123–7.

60. Griebsch A, Zollner N. Effect of ribomononucleotides given orally on uric acid production in man. Adv Exp Med Biol 1974;41:443–9.

61. Campion EW, Glynn RJ, DeLabry LO. Asymptomatic hyperuricemia. Risks and consequences in the Normative Aging Study. Am J Med 1987;82:421–6.

62. Nugent CA. Renal urate excretion in gout studied by feeding ribonucleic acid. Arthritis Rheum 1965;8:671–85.

63. Gibson T, Highton J, Potter C, et al. Renal impairment and gout. Ann Rheum Dis 1980;39:417–23.

64. Rimm EB, Giovannucci EL, Stampfer MJ, et al. Reproducibility and validity of an expanded self-administered semiquantitative food frequency questionnaire among male health professionals. Am J Epidemiol 1992;135:1114–26.

65. Willett WC, Sampson L, Stampfer MJ, et al. Reproducibility and validity of a semiquantitative food frequency questionnaire. Am J Epidemiol 1985;122:51–65.

66. Feskanich D, Rimm EB, Giovannucci EL, et al. Reproducibility and validity of food intake measurements from a semiquantitative food frequency questionnaire. J Am Diet Assoc 1993;93:790–6.

67. Wallace SL, Robinson H, Masi AT, et al. Preliminary criteria for the classification of the acute arthritis of primary gout. Arthritis Rheum 1977;20:895–900.

68. Roubenoff R, Klag MJ, Mead LA, et al. Incidence and risk factors for gout in white men. JAMA 1991;266:3004–7.

69. Christiansen E, Schnider S, Palmvig B, et al. Intake of a diet high in trans monounsaturated fatty acids or saturated fatty acids. Effects on postprandial insulinemia and glycemia in obese patients with NIDDM. Diabetes Care 1997;20:881–7.

70. Feskens EJ, Kromhout D. Habitual dietary intake and glucose tolerance in euglycaemic men: the Zutphen Study. Int J Epidemiol 1990;19:953–9.

71. Facchini F, Chen YD, Hollenbeck CB, et al. Relationship between resistance to insulin-mediated glucose uptake, urinary uric acid clearance, and plasma uric acid concentration. JAMA 1991;266:3008–11.

72. Willett WC, Stampfer MJ. Rebuilding the food pyramid. Sci Am 2003;288:64–71.

73. Kris-Etherton PM, Harris WS, Appel LJ. Fish consumption, fish oil, omega-3 fatty acids, and cardiovascular disease. Circulation 2002;106:2747–57.

74. Tate GA, Mandell BF, Karmali RA, et al. Suppression of monosodium urate crystal-induced acute inflammation by diets enriched with gamma-linolenic acid and eicosapentaenoic acid. Arthritis Rheum 1988;31:1543–51.

75. Garrel DR, Verdy M, PetitClerc C, et al. Milk- and soy-protein ingestion: acute effect on serum uric acid concentration. Am J Clin Nutr 1991;53:665–9.

76. Ghadirian P, Shatenstein B, Verdy M, et al. The influence of dairy products on plasma uric acid in women. Eur J Epidemiol 1995;11:275–81.

77. Dalbeth N, Wong S, Gamble GD, et al. Acute effect of milk on serum urate concentrations: a randomised controlled crossover trial. Ann Rheum Dis 69:1677-82.

78. Hu FB, Stampfer MJ, Manson JE, et al. Dietary saturated fats and their food sources in relation to the risk of coronary heart disease in women. Am J Clin Nutr 1999;70:1001–8.

79. Shin MH, Holmes MD, Hankinson SE, et al. Intake of dairy products, calcium, and vitamin D and risk of breast cancer. J Natl Cancer Inst 2002;94:1301–11.

80. Kampman E, Slattery ML, Caan B, et al. Calcium, vitamin D, sunshine exposure, dairy products and colon cancer risk (United States). Cancer Causes Control 2000;11:459–66.

81. Choi HK, Willett WC, Stampfer M, et al. Dairy consumption and risk of type 2 diabetes mellitus in men: a prospective study. Arch Intern Med 2005;165:997–1003.

82. Sacks FM, Svetkey LP, Vollmer WM, et al. Effects on blood pressure of reduced dietary sodium and the Dietary Approaches to Stop Hypertension (DASH) diet. DASH-Sodium Collaborative Research Group. N Engl J Med 2001;344:3–10.

83. Chan JM, Giovannucci EL. Dairy products, calcium, and vitamin D and risk of prostate cancer. Epidemiol Rev 2001;23:87–92.

84. Lyu LC, Hsu CY, Yeh CY, et al. A case-control study of the association of diet and obesity with gout in Taiwan. Am J Clin Nutr 2003;78:690–701.

85. Hu FB, Stampfer MJ, Manson JE, et al. Frequent nut consumption and risk of coronary heart disease in women: prospective cohort study. BMJ 1998;317:1341–5.

86. Hu FB, Stampfer MJ. Nut consumption and risk of coronary heart disease: a review of epidemiologic evidence. Curr Atheroscler Rep 1999;1:204–9.

87. Albert CM, Gaziano JM, Willett WC, et al. Nut consumption and decreased risk of sudden cardiac death in the Physicians' Health Study. Arch Intern Med 2002;162:1382–7.

88. Tsai CJ, Leitzmann MF, Hu FB, et al. Frequent nut consumption and decreased risk of cholecystectomy in women. Am J Clin Nutr 2004;80:76–81.

89. Tsai CJ, Leitzmann MF, Hu FB, et al. A prospective cohort study of nut consumption and the risk of gallstone disease in men. Am J Epidemiol 2004;160:961–8.

90. Jiang R, Manson JE, Stampfer MJ, et al. Nut and peanut butter consumption and risk of type 2 diabetes in women. JAMA 2002;288:2554–60.

91. Bazzano LA, He J, Ogden LG, et al. Legume consumption and risk of coronary heart disease in US men and women: NHANES I Epidemiologic Follow-up Study. Arch Intern Med 2001;161:2573–8.

92. Fung TT, Willett WC, Stampfer MJ, et al. Dietary patterns and the risk of coronary heart disease in women. Arch Intern Med 2001;161:1857–62.

93. Hu FB, Rimm EB, Stampfer MJ, et al. Prospective study of major dietary patterns and risk of coronary heart disease in men. Am J Clin Nutr 2000;72:912–21.

94. Fung TT, Stampfer MJ, Manson JE, et al. Prospective study of major dietary patterns and stroke risk in women. Stroke 2004;35:2014–9.

95. Fung T, Hu FB, Fuchs C, et al. Major dietary patterns and the risk of colorectal cancer in women. Arch Intern Med 2003;163:309–14.

96. Kolonel LN, Hankin JH, Whittemore AS, et al. Vegetables, fruits, legumes and prostate cancer: a multiethnic case-control study. Cancer Epidemiol Biomarkers Prev 2000;9:795–804.

97. Fung TT, Schulze M, Manson JE, et al. Dietary patterns, meat intake, and the risk of type 2 diabetes in women. Arch Intern Med 2004;164:2235–40.

98. Sharpe CR. A case-control study of alcohol consumption and drinking behaviour in patients with acute gout. Can Med Assoc J 1984;131:563–7.

99. Drum DE, Goldman PA, Jankowski CB. Elevation of serum uric acid as a clue to alcohol abuse. Arch Intern Med 1981;141:477–9.

100. Vandenberg MK, Moxley G, Breitbach SA, et al. Gout attacks in chronic alcoholics occur at lower serum urate levels than in nonalcoholics. J Rheumatol 1994;21:700–4.

101. Eastmond CJ, Garton M, Robins S, et al. The effects of alcoholic beverages on urate metabolism in gout sufferers. Br J Rheumatol 1995;34:756–9.

102. Faller J, Fox IH. Ethanol-induced hyperuricemia: evidence for increased urate production by activation of adenine nucleotide turnover. N Engl J Med 1982;307:1598–602.

103. Puig JG, Fox IH. Ethanol-induced activation of adenine nucleotide turnover. Evidence for a role of acetate. J Clin Invest 1984;74:936–41.

104. Yu TF, Sirota JH, Berger L. Effect of sodium lactate infusion on urate clearance in man. Proc Soc Exp Biol Med 1957;96:809–13.

105. Beck LH. Clinical disorders of uric acid metabolism. Med Clin North Am 1981;65:401–11.

106. Machlachlan MJ, Rodnan GP. Effects of food, fast and alcohol on serum uric acid and acute attacks of gout. Am J Med 1967;42:38–57.

107. Shadick NA, Kim R, Weiss S, et al. Effect of low level lead exposure on hyperuricemia and gout among middle aged and elderly men: the Normative Aging Study. J Rheumatol 2000;27:1708–12.

108. Hochberg MC, Thomas J, Thomas DJ, et al. Racial differences in the incidence of gout. The role of hypertension. Arthritis Rheum 1995;38:628–32.

109. Choi HK, Atkinson K, Karlson EW, et al. Alcohol intake and risk of incident gout in men: a prospective study. Lancet 2004;363:1277–81.

110. Choi HK, Curhan G. Beer, liquor, wine, and serum uric acid level: the Third National Health and Nutrition Examination Survey. Arthritis Rheum 2004;51:1023–9.

111. Gibson T, Rodgers AV, Simmonds HA, et al. Beer drinking and its effect on uric acid. Br J Rheumatol 1984;23:203–9.

112. Maxwell S, Cruickshank A, Thorpe G. Red wine and antioxidant activity in serum. Lancet 1994;344:193–4.

113. Frankel EN, Waterhouse AL, Kinsella JE. Inhibition of human LDL oxidation by resveratrol. Lancet 1993;341:1103–4.

114. Booyse FM, Parks DA. Moderate wine and alcohol consumption: beneficial effects on cardiovascular disease. Thromb Haemost 2001;86:517–28.

115. Fitzpatrick DF, Hirschfield SL, Coffey RG. Endothelium-dependent vasorelaxing activity of wine and other grape products. Am J Physiol 1993;265:H774–8.

116. Rimm EB, Klatsky A, Grobbee D, et al. Review of moderate alcohol consumption and reduced risk of coronary heart disease: is the effect due to beer, wine, or spirits. BMJ 1996;312:731–6.

117. Goldberg IJ, Mosca L, Piano MR, et al. AHA Science Advisory: Wine and your heart: a science advisory for healthcare professionals from the Nutrition Committee, Council on Epidemiology and Prevention, and Council on Cardiovascular Nursing of the American Heart Association. Circulation 2001;103:472–5.

118. Leitzmann MF, Giovannucci EL, Stampfer MJ, et al. Prospective study of alcohol consumption patterns in relation to symptomatic gallstone disease in men. Alcohol Clin Exp Res 1999;23:835–41.

119. Conigrave KM, Hu BF, Camargo Jr CA, et al. A prospective study of drinking patterns in relation to risk of type 2 diabetes among men. Diabetes 2001;50:2390–5.

120. Dietary Guidelines for Americans. US Department of Health and Human Services and US Department of Agriculture. www.healthierus.gov/dietaryguidelines2005.

121. Camargo Jr CA, Stampfer MJ, Glynn RJ, et al. Prospective study of moderate alcohol consumption and risk of peripheral arterial disease in US male physicians. Circulation 1997;95:577–80.

122. Lawrence RC, Helmick CG, Arnett FC, et al. Estimates of the prevalence of arthritis and selected musculoskeletal disorders in the United States. Arthritis Rheum 1998;41:778–99.

123. Arromdee E, Michet CJ, Crowson CS, et al. Epidemiology of gout: is the incidence rising? J Rheumatol 2002;29:2403–6.

124. Apovian CM. Sugar-sweetened soft drinks, obesity, and type 2 diabetes. JAMA 2004;292:978–9.

125. Gross LS, Li L, Ford ES, et al. Increased consumption of refined carbohydrates and the epidemic of type 2 diabetes in the United States: an ecologic assessment. Am J Clin Nutr 2004;79:774–9.

126. Wu T, Giovannucci E, Pischon T, et al. Fructose, glycemic load, and quantity and quality of carbohydrate in relation to plasma C-peptide concentrations in US women. Am J Clin Nutr 2004;80:1043–9.

127. Fox IH, Kelley WN. Studies on the mechanism of fructose-induced hyperuricemia in man. Metabolism 1972;21:713–21.

128. Fox IH. Metabolic basis for disorders of purine nucleotide degradation. Metabolism 1981;30:616–34.

129. Anderson JW, Story LJ, Zettwoch NC, et al. Metabolic effects of fructose supplementation in diabetic individuals. Diabetes Care 1989;12:337–44.

130. Tordoff MG, Alleva AM. Effect of drinking soda sweetened with aspartame or high-fructose corn syrup on food intake and body weight. Am J Clin Nutr 1990;51:963–9.

131. Thorburn AW, Storlien LH, Jenkins AB, et al. Fructose-induced in vivo insulin resistance and elevated plasma triglyceride levels in rats. Am J Clin Nutr 1989;49:1155–63.

132. Bray GA, Nielsen SJ, Popkin BM. Consumption of high-fructose corn syrup in beverages may play a role in the epidemic of obesity. Am J Clin Nutr 2004;79:537–43.

133. Michaud DS, Liu S, Giovannucci E, et al. Dietary sugar, glycemic load, and pancreatic cancer risk in a prospective study. J Natl Cancer Inst 2002;94:1293–300.

134. Romieu I, Lazcano-Ponce E, Sanchez-Zamorano LM, et al. Carbohydrates and the risk of breast cancer among Mexican women. Cancer Epidemiol Biomarkers Prev 2004;13:1283–9.

135. Michaud DS, Fuchs CS, Liu S, et al. Dietary glycemic load, carbohydrate, sugar, and colorectal cancer risk in men and women. Cancer Epidemiol Biomarkers Prev 2005;14:138–47.

136. Tsai CJ, Leitzmann MF, Willett WC, et al. Dietary carbohydrates and glycaemic load and the incidence of symptomatic gall stone disease in men. Gut 2005;54:823–8.

137. Giovannucci E, Rimm EB, Wolk A, et al. Calcium and fructose intake in relation to risk of prostate cancer. Cancer Res 1998;58:442–7.

138. Ludwig DS, Peterson KE, Gortmaker SL. Relation between consumption of sugar-sweetened drinks and childhood obesity: a prospective, observational analysis. Lancet 2001;357:505–8.

139. Schulze MB, Manson JE, Ludwig DS, et al. Sugar-sweetened beverages, weight gain, and incidence of type 2 diabetes in young and middle-aged women. JAMA 2004;292:927–34.

140. Appel LJ, Moore TJ, Obarzanek E, et al. A clinical trial of the effects of dietary patterns on blood pressure. DASH Collaborative Research Group. N Engl J Med 1997;336:1117–24.

141. Hung HC, Joshipura KJ, Jiang R, et al. Fruit and vegetable intake and risk of major chronic disease. J Natl Cancer Inst 2004;96:1577–84.

142. Lundsberg LS. Caffeine consumption. Caffeine. Boca Raton, FL: CRC Press; 1998:199-224.

143. Salazar-Martinez E, Willett WC, Ascherio A, et al. Coffee consumption and risk for type 2 diabetes mellitus. Ann Intern Med 2004;140:1–8.

144. Kiyohara C, Kono S, Honjo S, et al. Inverse association between coffee drinking and serum uric acid concentrations in middle-aged Japanese males. Br J Nutr 1999;82:125–30.

145. Kela U, Vijayvargiya R, Trivedi CP. Inhibitory effects of methylxanthines on the activity of xanthine oxidase. Life Sci 1980;27:2109–19.

146. Petrie HJ, Chown SE, Belfie LM, et al. Caffeine ingestion increases the insulin response to an oral-glucose-tolerance test in obese men before and after weight loss. Am J Clin Nutr 2004;80:22–8.

147. Greer F, Hudson R, Ross R, et al. Caffeine ingestion decreases glucose disposal during a hyperinsulinemic-euglycemic clamp in sedentary humans. Diabetes 2001;50:2349–54.

148. Keijzers GB, De Galan BE, Tack CJ, et al. Caffeine can decrease insulin sensitivity in humans. Diabetes Care 2002;25:364–9.

149. Thong FS, Derave W, Kiens B, et al. Caffeine-induced impairment of insulin action but not insulin signaling in human skeletal muscle is reduced by exercise. Diabetes 2002;51:583–90.

150. Thong FS, Graham TE. Caffeine-induced impairment of glucose tolerance is abolished by beta-adrenergic receptor blockade in humans. J Appl Physiol 2002;92:2347–52.

151. Wu T, Willett WC, Hankinson SE, et al. Caffeinated coffee, decaffeinated coffee, and caffeine in relation to plasma C-peptide levels, a marker of insulin secretion, in U.S. women. Diabetes Care 2005;28:1390–6.

152. van Dam RM, Hu FB. Coffee consumption and risk of type 2 diabetes: a systematic review. JAMA 2005;294:97–104.

153. Arnlov J, Vessby B, Riserus U. Coffee consumption and insulin sensitivity. JAMA 2004;291:1199–201.

154. Lee J, Sparrow D, Vokonas PS, et al. Uric acid and coronary heart disease risk: evidence for a role of uric acid in the obesity-insulin resistance syndrome. The Normative Aging Study. Am J Epidemiol 1995;142:288–94.

155. Pham NM, Yoshida D, Morita M, et al. The relation of coffee consumption to serum uric acid in Japanese men and women aged 49-76 years. J Nutr Metab 2010.

156. Choi HK, Curhan G. Coffee, tea, and caffeine consumption and serum uric acid level: the Third National Health and Nutrition Examination Survey. Arthritis Rheum (in press).

157. Choi HK, Curhan G. Coffee consumption and risk of incident gout in women: the Nurses' Health Study. Am J Clin Nutr 2010;92:922–7.

158. Arion WJ, Canfield WK, Ramos FC, et al. Chlorogenic acid and hydroxynitrobenzaldehyde: new inhibitors of hepatic glucose 6-phosphatase. Arch Biochem Biophys 1997;339:315–22.

159. Johnston KL, Clifford MN, Morgan LM. Coffee acutely modifies gastrointestinal hormone secretion and glucose tolerance in humans: glycemic effects of chlorogenic acid and caffeine. Am J Clin Nutr 2003;78:728–33.
160. Bruce CR, Carey AL, Hawley JA, et al. Intramuscular heat shock protein 72 and heme oxygenase-1 mRNA are reduced in patients with type 2 diabetes: evidence that insulin resistance is associated with a disturbed antioxidant defense mechanism. Diabetes 2003;52:2338–45.
161. Thirunavukkarasu V, Anuradha CV. Influence of alpha-lipoic acid on lipid peroxidation and antioxidant defence system in blood of insulin-resistant rats. Diabetes Obes Metab 2004;6:200–7.
162. Richelle M, Tavazzi I, Offord E. Comparison of the antioxidant activity of commonly consumed polyphenolic beverages (coffee, cocoa, and tea) prepared per cup serving. J Agric Food Chem 2001;49:3438–42.
163. Svilaas A, Sakhi AK, Andersen LF, et al. Intakes of antioxidants in coffee, wine, and vegetables are correlated with plasma carotenoids in humans. J Nutr 2004;134:562–7.
164. van Dam RM, Willett WC, Manson JE, et al. Coffee, caffeine, and risk of type 2 diabetes: a prospective cohort study in younger and middle-aged U.S. women. Diabetes Care 2006;29:398–403.
165. van Dam RM, Feskens EJ. Coffee consumption and risk of type 2 diabetes mellitus. Lancet 2002;360:1477–8.
166. Curhan GC, Willett WC, Speizer FE, et al. Beverage use and risk for kidney stones in women. Ann Intern Med 1998;128:534–40.
167. Curhan GC, Willett WC, Rimm EB, et al. J. Prospective study of beverage use and the risk of kidney stones. Am J Epidemiol 1996;49:240–7.
168. Leitzmann MF, Stampfer MJ, Willett WC, et al. Coffee intake is associated with lower risk of symptomatic gallstone disease in women. Gastroenterology 2002;123:1823–30.
169. Leitzmann MF, Willett WC, Rimm EB, et al. A prospective study of coffee consumption and the risk of symptomatic gallstone disease in men. JAMA 1999;281:2106–12.
170. Hernan MA, Takkouche B, Caamano-Isorna F, et al. A meta-analysis of coffee drinking, cigarette smoking, and the risk of Parkinson's disease. Ann Neurol 2002;52:276–84.
171. Grobbee DE, Rimm EB, Giovannucci E, et al. Coffee, caffeine, and cardiovascular disease in men. N Engl J Med 1990;323:1026–32.
172. Willett WC, Stampfer MJ, Manson JE, et al. Coffee consumption and coronary heart disease in women. A ten-year follow-up. JAMA 1996;275:458–62.
173. Lopez-Garcia E, van Dam RM, Willett WC, et al. Coffee consumption and coronary heart disease in men and women: a prospective cohort study. Circulation 2006;113:2045–53.
174. Jee SH, He J, Appel LJ, et al. Coffee consumption and serum lipids: a meta-analysis of randomized controlled clinical trials. Am J Epidemiol 2001;153:353–62.
175. Kiel DP, Felson DT, Hannan MT, et al. Caffeine and the risk of hip fracture: the Framingham Study. Am J Epidemiol 1990;132:675–84.
176. Hernandez-Avila M, Colditz GA, Stampfer MJ, et al. Caffeine, moderate alcohol intake, and risk of fractures of the hip and forearm in middle-aged women. Am J Clin Nutr 1991;54:157–63.
177. Meyer HE, Pedersen JI, Loken EB, et al. Dietary factors and the incidence of hip fracture in middle-aged Norwegians. A prospective study. Am J Epidemiol 1997;145:117–23.
178. Hallstrom H, Wolk A, Glynn A, et al. Coffee, tea and caffeine consumption in relation to osteoporotic fracture risk in a cohort of Swedish women. Osteoporos Int 2006;17:1055–64.
179. Stein HB, Hasan A, Fox IH. Ascorbic acid-induced uricosuria. A consequence of megavitamin therapy. Ann Intern Med 1976;84:385–8.
180. Berger L, Gerson CD, Yu TF. The effect of ascorbic acid on uric acid excretion with a commentary on the renal handling of ascorbic acid. Am J Med 1977;62:71–6.
181. Enomoto A, Kimura H, Chairoungdua A, et al. Molecular identification of a renal urate anion exchanger that regulates blood urate levels. Nature 2002;417:447–52.
182. Pattison DJ, Silman AJ, Goodson NJ, et al. Vitamin C and the risk of developing inflammatory polyarthritis: prospective nested case-control study. Ann Rheum Dis 2004;63:843–7.
183. Knekt P, Ritz J, Pereira MA, et al. Antioxidant vitamins and coronary heart disease risk: a pooled analysis of 9 cohorts. Am J Clin Nutr 2004;80:1508–20.
184. Taylor EN, Stampfer MJ, Curhan GC. Dietary factors and the risk of incident kidney stones in men: new insights after 14 years of follow-up. J Am Soc Nephrol 2004;15:3225–32.
185. Hathcock JN, Azzi A, Blumberg J, et al. Vitamins E and C are safe across a broad range of intakes. Am J Clin Nutr 2005;81:736–45.
186. Emmerson BT. The management of gout. N Engl J Med 1996;334:445–51.
187. Emmerson BT. Alteration of urate metabolism by weight reduction. Aust N Z J Med 1973;3:410–2.
188. Yamashita S, Matsuzawa Y, Tokunaga K, et al. Studies on the impaired metabolism of uric acid in obese subjects: marked reduction of renal urate excretion and its improvement by a low-calorie diet. Int J Obes 1986;10:255–64.
189. Takahashi S, Yamamoto T, Tsutsumi Z, et al. Close correlation between visceral fat accumulation and uric acid metabolism in healthy men. Metabolism 1997;46:1162–5.
190. Bedir A, Topbas M, Tanyeri F, et al. Leptin might be a regulator of serum uric acid concentrations in humans. Jpn Heart J 2003;44:527–36.
191. Fruehwald-Schultes B, Peters A, Kern W, et al. Serum leptin is associated with serum uric acid concentrations in humans. Metabolism 1999;48:677–80.
192. Bakker SJ, Gans RO, ter Maaten JC, et al. The potential role of adenosine in the pathophysiology of the insulin resistance syndrome. Atherosclerosis 2001;155:283–90.
193. Balakrishnan VS, Coles GA, Williams JD. A potential role for endogenous adenosine in control of human glomerular and tubular function. Am J Physiol 1993;265:F504–10.
194. Fransen R, Koomans HA. Adenosine and renal sodium handling: direct natriuresis and renal nerve-mediated antinatriuresis. J Am Soc Nephrol 1995;6:1491–7.
195. Zhu Y, Zhang Y, Choi HK. The serum urate-lowering impact of weight loss among men with a high cardiovascular risk profile: the Multiple Risk Factor Intervention Trial. Rheumatology (Oxford) 2010;49:2391–9.
196. Bhole V, de Vera M, Rahman MM, et al. Epidemiology of gout in women: fifty-two-year followup of a prospective cohort. Arthritis Rheum 2010;62:1069–76.
197. Prevalence of overweight, obesity, and extreme obesity among adults: United States, trends 1976-1980 through 2007-2008. http://www.cdc.gov/nchs/data/hestat/obesity_adult_07_08/obesity_adult_07_08.pdf
198. Sturm R, Wells KB. Does obesity contribute as much to morbidity as poverty or smoking? Public Health 2001;115:229–35.
199. Allison DB, Fontaine KR, Manson JE, et al. Annual deaths attributable to obesity in the United States. JAMA 1999;282:1530–8.
200. Willett WC, Manson JE, Stampfer MJ, et al. Weight, weight change, and coronary heart disease in women. Risk within the 'normal' weight range. JAMA 1995;273:461–5.
201. Rimm EB, Stampfer MJ, Giovannucci E, et al. Body size and fat distribution as predictors of coronary heart disease among middle-aged and older US men. Am J Epidemiol 1995;141:1117–27.
202. Huang Z, Willett WC, Manson JE, et al. Body weight, weight change, and risk for hypertension in women. Ann Intern Med 1998;128:81–8.
203. Colditz GA, Willett WC, Rotnitzky A, et al. Weight gain as a risk factor for clinical diabetes mellitus in women. Ann Intern Med 1995;122:481–6.
204. Taylor EN, Stampfer MJ, Curhan GC. Obesity, weight gain, and the risk of kidney stones. JAMA 2005;293:455–62.
205. Maclure KM, Hayes KC, Colditz GA, et al. Weight, diet, and the risk of symptomatic gallstones in middle-aged women. N Engl J Med 1989;321:563–9.
206. Williams PT. Effects of diet, physical activity and performance, and body weight on incident gout in ostensibly healthy, vigorously active men. Am J Clin Nutr 2008;87:1480–7.
207. Goldberg IJ, Mosca L, Piano MR, et al. AHA Science Advisory: Wine and your heart. Circulation 2001;103:472–5.
208. Choi HK. Diet, alcohol, and gout: how do we advise patients given recent developments? Curr Rheumatol Rep 2005;7:220–6.
209. Mitch WE, Johnson MW, Kirshenbaum JM, et al. Effect of large oral doses of ascorbic acid on uric acid excretion by normal subjects. Clin Pharmacol Ther 1981;29:318–21.

Chapter **12**

Uricosuric Therapy of Hyperuricemia in Gout

Fernando Perez-Ruiz, Ana Maria Herrero-Beites, and Joana Atxotegi Saenz de Buruaga

KEY POINTS

- Inefficient renal excretion of uric acid is the most common cause of hyperuricemia in gout patients.
- Uricosuric drugs tend to normalize renal excretion of uric acid through inhibiting renal tubular reabsorption of uric acid, thus reducing serum urate levels.
- Availability, potency, and safety profile vary greatly among uricosuric drugs, most of them lacking well-designed clinical trials. Some drugs that are not labeled for gout show mild uricosuric effects.
- Patients suitable for uricosuric treatment should be selected based on renal handling of uric acid, preferably with clearance of uric acid.
- The assessment of efficacy and safety can be accomplished with first morning spot blood and urine samples and glomerular filtration rate prediction equations.
- The risk of urolithiasis can be minimized with proper selection of patients and adequate monitoring during follow-up.
- The combination of xanthine oxidase inhibitors and uricosurics is a promising approach in patients failing to reach target serum urate concentration levels with monotherapy with xanthine oxidase inhibitors.

Introduction: Concepts and Historical Background

Uricosuric drugs were the first agents used to control hyperuricemia in patients with gout.[1] Any drug that increases renal excretion of uric acid, independently of the mechanism through which it exerts its effect, may be considered a uricosuric drug. Salicylates were the first drugs to be used to correct hyperuricemia of gout, as they showed a paradoxical effect on renal handling of uric acid: they reduce renal excretion at low doses and increase renal excretion at high doses.[2]

The concept that underlines the term "uricosuric" may be misleading, if one considers that these drugs will exert an effect on the renal handling of urate that will induce what could be considered a hyperuricosuric state. However, it may certainly occur in subjects who show normal renal excretion of uric acid in the hyperuricemic state.

The most actual concept would be to consider uricosuric drugs as drugs to be used to correct hyperuricemia derived from "inefficient renal excretion" (IRE) of uric acid,[3] lately known as "underexcretion," that conceptually means that renal excretion of uric acid is not found to the amount expected based on serum urate concentration (SUR) levels and glomerular filtration, that is to say to the filtered load.[4] Thus, our clinical approach to the use of uricosurics will be to recognize them as means to normalize renal excretion of uric acid in patients with IRE of uric acid.[5]

In this chapter, we will further discuss the concept, targets, and clinical assessment of IRE; drugs that increase renal excretion of uric acid, either approved, not approved, or in development; and clinical management of uricosuric therapy, including combination of xanthine oxidase inhibitors (XOIs) and uricosurics.

Inefficient Renal Excretion of Uric Acid as a Target for Urate-Lowering Therapy

Most patients with gout in the hyperuricemic state will show IRE of uric acid; that is, they show less urinary excretion of uric acid than that expected in relation to the amount of urate that is filtered in the glomerulus. This can be either a primary or secondary (acquired) defect, but overall IRE of uric acid may be present in 90% of the patients with gout and over 80% of patients with primary gout.[6]

In the very early clinical studies of uricosuric drugs, most agents possessing uricosuric properties, such as probenecid, sulfinpyrazone, or salicylates, were found to be organic acids.[1] Investigators empirically proposed that these drugs shared with uric acid a common renal tubular transport system and then would compete with uric acid as substrates for this transporter system, thus inducing renal uric acid leakage through inhibition of tubular reabsorption of uric acid.

Recent investigation has recognized an organic anion transporter (OAT) family mainly located in the proximal renal tubules. Although multiple transporters have been identified, molecular cloning approaches have been used to identify two major tubular transporters of urate: URAT1 and GLUT9 (as reviewed in detail in Chapter 4).

URAT1 (uric acid transporter 1) is the product of the *SCL22A12* gene. URAT1 is expressed only in the kidney and it is located in the epithelium of the proximal, but not of distal renal tubules at the apical membrane (luminal side), with deficient mice and humans showing complete loss of the capacity of reabsorbing uric acid.[7]

Interestingly, most of the drugs well known to exert a uricosuric effect show an inhibitory effect on URAT1, thus enhancing renal excretion of uric acid. On the other hand, diuretics such as furosemide increase uric acid URAT1-mediated transport, favoring the increase in SUR levels.[7] In addition, the most effective uricosuric drug ever tested in clinical practice, benzbromarone,[5] was shown to be the most potent inhibitor of URAT1, completely inhibiting the uric acid uptake in the renal proximal tubule epithelial cell.[7]

A member of the facilitated glucose transporter named GLUT9 has been recently shown to be a uric acid transporter located mainly in the kidney and in the liver. GLUT9 is encoded by the *SCL2A9* gene and is present both in the apical and basolateral membranes of the proximal tubule epithelial cells.[8] It shows different affinities compared to that of URAT1, as it is not influenced by organic anions, suggesting that uric acid may be the only or the primary substrate for GLUT9. Benzbromarone, a strong inhibitor of URAT, only shows a moderate inhibition of uric acid transport through GLUT9. Probenecid and losartan also inhibit GLUT9 moderately.[8] In addition to uric acid, hexoses, such as glucose and fructose, strongly inhibit the uric acid transport via GLUT9.

Assessment of Renal Excretion of Uric Acid in Clinical Practice

A debate has taken place over the past decades regarding whether renal excretion of uric acid assessment should be implemented as a standard in clinical practice.[9] The argument against such procedure is that if patients are to be treated with XOIs estimation of renal excretion of uric acid is less relevant for therapy choice, although still potentially useful to determine the etiology of hyperuricemia.

From a clinical point of view, identifying patients with IRE of uric acid would separate patients with normal excretion and so classify them as showing an overproduction mechanism leading to hyperuricemia and can help in selecting patients suitable for uricosuric therapy. It may also be helpful for differential diagnosis of causes inducing hyperuricemia, with the limitation that the presence of underexcretion in subjects with renal insufficiency cannot exclude the concomitant presence of uric acid overproduction. In addition, identification and correction of the underlying mechanisms leading to hyperuricemia are attractive from a physiopathologic point of view, especially to select patients with IRE of uric acid if they are to be considered candidates for uricosuric therapy.

Several methods have been proposed to be useful to identify subjects with IRE of uric acid, including the 24-hour urinary uric acid (24-UUR) excretion,[10] the clearance (CUR) of uric acid,[6] the urine uric acid–to–creatinine ratio,[11] the uric acid excretion per glomerular filtration volume[12] or Simkin's index (SI), and fractional excretion of uric acid. Some authors even suggested a composite method to "simplify" this assessment.[13] The first two require 24-hour urine collection, while the latter three may be calculated using spot urine and blood samples. Calculations for the different methods and pros and cons for all of them are cited in Table 12-1.

From an academic point of view, clearance of uric acid seems to give a sense of the renal capacity to clear blood of such a substance, and clearance of creatinine (ClCr) is a paradigm of the widespread use of this concept. In addition, CUR shows a good correlation with 24-hour UUR[14]; unlike the other methods, CUR shows no change in patients treated with XOI[6] and may be used to estimate IRE of uric acid in patients taking XOIs; and, finally, high baseline CUR was associated with increased risk for development of renal colic in patients with ongoing uricosuric therapy.[15]

Following a practical clinical approach, SI may be a simple, cheap, and feasible method to estimate the IRE of uric acid. Subjects showing SI less than 0.6 mg/dL will probably suffer from IRE of uric acid. On the other hand, SI greater than 0.6 mg/dL may be associated with normal renal uric acid excretion (overproduction) or with renal function impairment,[14] as the plasma creatinine–to–urinary creatinine (SCR/UCR) ratio will increase in patients with renal dysfunction, leading to high false-positive SI results. If the latter is the case,

Table 12-1 Methods Most Commonly Used in Clinical Practice to Evaluate Real Handling of Urate

Method	Urine Sample	Calculation (UNL)	Pros and Cons
24-hr UUR (mg/day)	24-Hour	UVOL*UUR (880 mg/1.73 m²)	Useful in the hyperuricemic state Good correlation with clearance Not reliable with borderline hyperuricemia or patients treated with XOIs
CLUR (ml/min)	24-Hour	UVOL*UUR/SUR (6 mL/min/1.73 m²)	Conceptually shows renal capacity Useful despite XOIs Associated with risk of urolithiasis
FE_UA (%)	Spot	[UUR*SCR]/[SUR*UCR] (7%)	Dependent on renal function False normal results in patients with chronic kidney disease Useful for follow-up
Simkin's Index (mg/dL glomerular filtration)	Spot	UUR* [UCR/CR] (0.6)	Dependent on renal function False normal results in patients with chronic kidney disease Useful for follow-up

CLUR, Clearance of uric acid; *FE_UA*, fractional excretion of uric acid; *SCR*, serum creatinine concentration; *SUR*, serum urate concentration (mg/dL); *UCR*, urinary creatinine concentration (mg/dL); *UNL*, upper normal limit; *UUR*, urinary uric acid concentration (mg/dL); *24-hr UUR*, 24-hour urinary uric acid; *UVOL*, urinary volume (dL); *XOI*, xanthine oxidase inhibitor.

glomerular filtration (ClCr) should be estimated with any method to ascertain whether patients show normal renal function.

Uricosuric Drugs: Pharmacokinetics, Pharmacodynamics, and Clinical Applicability

Drugs Labeled for the Treatment of Hyperuricemia of Gout

Probenecid

Probenecid, a drug first used to avoid renal excretion of penicillin, was shown to have urate-lowering effects by increasing renal uric acid excretion.[16] Moderate inhibition of both URAT1 and GLUT9 transporter in the renal tubule has been reported, and so probenecid efficacy may be blunted in patients with mild to moderate renal function impairment.[1] However, the GFR level at which probenecid is no longer effective as a uricosuric, although held to be at a GFR less than 50, is not entirely clear from data in the literature.

Probenecid is well absorbed after oral administration, despite being sparingly soluble in water. Peak plasma levels are reached close to 4 hours after oral intake, it is highly bound to proteins, and it has a dose-dependent effect, ranging from 6 to 12 hours,[1] so it is orally administered in a twice-daily prescription but might ideally be suited to three-times-daily dosing.

Dosing is usually started at 500 mg twice daily and increased in a stepwise fashion to reach target SUR levels or up to 2 g/day if tolerated, with an absolute maximum dose of 3 g/day.

Probenecid is mainly metabolized in the liver to glucuronide but it is also hydroxylated and carboxylated derivatives are produced, with all of them excreted renally. Low-dose aspirin seems to not have a significant impact on renal uric acid excretion in patients on probenecid.[17]

The initial reports of the efficacy of probenecid suggested that dosing equal to or greater than 2 g/day in divided doses would not succeed in achieving a reduction over half the baseline levels.[1] Results from a small-population, open-label, randomized, actively controlled 2-month trial in patients failing therapy with allopurinol (85% in first stage of the study) have been reported.[18] Probenecid 2 g/day in divided doses showed a reduction of mean baseline SUR from 9.0 mg/dL to 4.5 mg/dL, with 65% of the patients reaching outcome SUR target of less than 5 mg/dL. Despite adequate efficacy, withdrawals due to intolerance rose up to 15% in this study during the 2-month exposure period.

Severe side effects due to probenecid are not frequent. Cutaneous rash and gastrointestinal complaints are reported in up to 20% of patients, with intolerance being a limitation to this therapy.

Sulfinpyrazone

Sulfinpyrazone was initially used as a uricosuric agent because uricosuric activity was noted during its development as an analog of phenylbutazone.[19]

The tubular target of sulfinpyrazone is URAT1. It is rapidly and well absorbed after oral administration, with its half-life ranging from reaching peak levels and showing a short half-life, close to 3 hours. It is highly bound to plasma proteins. Although sulfinpyrazone is metabolized in the liver, up to one third of the dose is excreted unaltered through the kidneys.[20,21]

It has been withdrawn from most countries due to a bunch of limitations: the loss of its efficacy in the presence of low GFR, its antiaggregating effect on platelets, and poor tolerability.

Benzbromarone

Benzbromarone is to date the most potent uricosuric drug ever tested in clinical practice, being able to totally suppress URAT1-mediated reabsorption of uric acid. Unfortunately, it is not universally available. It is a benzofuran derivative, and after oral intake, it reaches peak plasma concentration in 2 to 4 hours, with its bioavailability being close to 50%.[23] Benzbromarone undergoes liver metabolism and is excreted primarily through the bile, no dose adjustment needed in patients with nonterminal renal dysfunction. Although the half-life of benzbromarone is short, 6-hydroxibenzbromarone is a major metabolite with uricosuric properties and a half-life exceeding 24 hours.[24]

As with other potent urate-lowering drugs, benzbromarone prescription is started at low dose, 50 mg/day, to avoid mobilization flares due to sharp and sudden reduction of SUR levels. Doses may be increased up to the maximum labeled dose of 200 mg/day. The efficacy in reducing SUR levels of benzbromarone 100 mg/day has been shown to be superior to allopurinol 300 mg/day or probenecid 1000 mg/day,[24] its efficacy being close to that of allopurinol 400 mg/day in patients with normal renal function.[5] Recent blinded, randomized, controlled trials have shown that the effectiveness of benzbromarone 200 mg/day to reach target SUR levels lower than 5 mg/dL is superior to allopurinol 2 g/day[18] and that benzbromarone 200 mg/day is comparable to allopurinol 600 mg/day.[25] Limitations inherent to these two recent trials are the short exposure period, limiting any conclusion on safety, and the prescriptions being twice daily for allopurinol but once daily for benzbromarone.

Adding low-dose benzbromarone to standard allopurinol doses has shown an additive effect on SUR level reduction similar to that observed with standard doses of benzbromarone.[26] Contrary to other available uricosuric drugs, which may lose at GFR lower than 50 ml/min, benzbromarone has been shown to maintain its uricosuric properties in patients with mild to moderate reduction of GFR down to 20 mL/min,[27] despite concomitant treatment with drugs that induce hyperuricemia, such as diuretics and cyclosporine, as occurs with renal transplant recipients.[28]

Severe hepatic toxicity has been infrequently reported in patients on benzbromarone. This issue has led the European Medicine Agency to limit the use of benzbromarone.[29]

Drugs With Uricosuric Properties Not Approved for Gout

In addition to the uricosuric drugs labeled for the treatment of hyperuricemia of gout, some other compounds have shown mild uricosuric properties. These drugs could be considered as "adjuvant" urate-lowering treatment that could be useful to control SUR levels in patients not reaching target SUR provided the presence of comorbidities for which their prescription is labeled.[30]

Fenofibrate is a drug labeled for the treatment of type IV hyperlipidemia. At a dose of 200 mg once daily, it was shown to reduce SUR levels by 20% in an open study in patients on stable doses of allopurinol[31] in an open, noncomparative, short-term study. In another short-term open study, fenofibrate 200 mg/day was added to allopurinol 200 mg twice a day, showing a reduction of SUR from 6.2 to 5.2 mg/dL (16% reduction).[32] If added to benzbromarone 50 mg/day, SUR was lowered from 5.9 to 5.1 mg/dL (13% reduction).[32]

Losartan is an antagonist of angiotensin II receptor (ARA-II) labeled for the treatment of hypertension. In a twin study with fenofibrate,[32] patients were to also receive losartan 50 mg once daily. SUR levels were lowered from 6.1 to 5.5 mg/dL (9%) in patients on allopurinol and from 4.8 to 4.4 mg/dL (8%) in patients on benzbromarone.[32] In a small randomized clinical trial in patients with asymptomatic hyperuricemia, losartan 50 mg/day showed a mild uricosuric effect. Interestingly, losartan antagonized the effect of hydrochlorothiazide on SUR levels when given in combination,[33] a clinical applicability that deserves further investigation. In a short-term, small, double-blind, randomized study in patients with gout, losartan 50 mg/day, but not ibesartan 150 mg/day, showed a mild reduction of SUR, from 9.1 to 8.3 mg/dL (9%) but obviously not enough to reduce average SUR to target for urate-lowering therapy.[34]

Atorvastatin, a drug labeled for the treatment of hypercholesterolemia, was shown to mildly reduce SUR levels in patients showing or not showing features of the metabolic syndrome in a post-hoc analysis of the GREACE trial,[35] but the highest benefit was observed in patients with the metabolic syndrome compared with patients without features of the metabolic syndrome. SUR differences between the groups were 1.0 mg/dL versus 0.6 mg/dL, respectively. In a randomized trial comparing atorvastatin 40 mg/day with simvastatin 40 mg/day in patients with primary hyperlipidemia, a significant reduction of SUR from 5.6 to 4.9 mg/dL (12% reduction) was observed in patients treated with atorvastatin, but no change in SUR levels was observed in patients treated with simvastatin.[36] Baseline SUR levels were associated with a greater urate-lowering effect.

Leflunomide is a drug labeled for the treatment of rheumatoid arthritis and psoriatic arthritis with peripheral joint involvement. In patients with rheumatoid arthritis, leflunomide 20 mg/day reduced baseline SUR by 30% and increased fractional excretion of uric acid by 67%. This effect was associated with a decrease of renal tubular reabsorption of phosphate by 5%, suggesting that leflunomide interacts with transporters involved in uric acid and phosphate handling.[37]

Overall, the evaluation of the urate-lowering effect of "adjuvant drugs" is limited by design and external applicability. Data suggest that adding uricosurics to allopurinol is better than adding uricosurics to uricosurics. Despite this, these drugs could be useful in patients with (1) presence of a concomitant disease for which the drug is labeled and (2) borderline SUR levels at baseline or SUR levels close to the target for urate-lowering therapy. In addition, some of these drugs, such as statins or fenofibrate, have drug-drug interaction risks with colchicine that specifically raise the risk for myopathy with or without rhabdomyolysis, which should be taken into consideration for dose prescription and monitoring.[38]

Clinical Management of Hyperuricemia of Gout With Uricosuric Drugs

To properly manage hyperuricemia in patients with gout with uricosuric drugs in daily clinical practice, some issues should be afforded. As any other treatment, the profile of the patient most suitable for this therapy has to be determined and monitoring must be in place to prevent side effects, especially urolithiasis, and document efficacy. This can be accomplished in two different situations: namely uricosuric therapy as monotherapy and the addition of a uricosuric drug to patients on XOIs.

Selection of Patients

Patients with gout showing hyperuricemia and *inefficient renal excretion of uric acid* are, at first sight, the more suitable population to be treated with uricosuric drugs. Selection of patients should be made by assessing the renal handling of uric acid.

Although several methods have been used to classify patients according to renal handling of uric acid, clearance of uric acid at baseline over 6 ml/min/1.73 m^2 of body surface using 24-hour urine collections has been shown to be independently associated in multivariate analysis with increased risk of developing urolithiasis in patients during long-term follow-up[15] but not other indexes such as fractional excretion, SI, or even 24-hour urinary uric acid.

Aging is not by itself a limitation for uricosuric prescription, but renal function impairment independent of age is a limitation. The efficacy of different uricosuric drugs will depend on renal function and their potency, so benzbromarone can be used with GFRs as low as 20 ml/min, while probenecid and sulfinpyrazone seem to lose efficacy with rates lower than 50 ml/min. GFR can be estimated using prediction equations using the MDRD or Cockcroft-Gault formulas.[39]

Patients with a previous history of urolithiasis should not be treated with uricosurics as first-choice drugs, unless no other choice is available. The frequency of urolithiasis (previous renal colic) recalled by history may be increased in 50% if ultrasonographic assessment is used,[40] but the impact of asymptomatic urolithiasis has not yet been evaluated as a risk factor for the development of renal colic during uricosuric therapy.

Patients with tophaceous gout were not at higher risk of developing lithiasis while on uricosurics in a large prospective long-term cohort study.[15] The rationale for this finding is that tophi do not dissolve suddenly or are rapidly reabsorbed during urate-lowering therapy, thus not supplying considerable amounts of uric acid to the kidneys.

It is important to recall that not only patients with previous uric acid lithiasis may be at risk, but also patients with previous urolithiasis due to calcium oxalate stones may be at higher risk of developing urolithiasis due to the increase in urinary uric acid excretion, especially those showing low urinary pH.[41] As the gross amount of clearance of uric acid can change on treatment with XOIs, assessment of renal handling of uric acid can be clinically useful in patients on XOIs, but depends on method employed.[6]

Table 12-2 summarizes laboratory evaluations to properly select and follow patients on uricosuric therapy.

Table 12-2 Laboratory Evaluation for Patients Prior to and During Uricosuric Therapy

	Baseline	Follow-up
Serum urate concentration migration	Evaluation of disease Calculation of clearance	Assessment of efficacy
Glomerular filtration	MDRD or Cockcroft-Gault Low GFR: not suitable for uricosurics	MDRD or Cockcroft-Gault Follow-up of GFR
Clearance of uric acid	Assessment of IRE of uric acid	Not useful
Fractional excretion or Simkin's Index	Assessment of IRE of uric acid Useful if normal GFR	Assessment of response
Spot urine samples • pH • Proteins • Cells • Density	• Assess tubular function • Evaluate for chronic kidney disease • Estimate fluid intake	• Estimate UUur • Altered sediment • Estimate fluid intake

GFR, Glomerular filtration rate; *IRE*, inefficient renal excretion.

Assessment of Efficacy

To evaluate the efficacy of uricosuric therapy, first morning spot blood and urine samples can be used to ascertain that the reduction in SUR is inversely correlated with an increase in fractional excretion of uric acid or SI.[42] In the first days of full-dose uricosuric therapy, a sharp increase of the excretion of uric acid is observed, but it returns to a steady state in 2 weeks.[6] In the face of this fact, progressive steps from low doses are advisable to minimize the risk of early lithiasis.

Monitoring the Risk of Urolithiasis

The risk of urolithiasis during uricosuric therapy can be assessed estimating the concentration of undissociated urinary uric acid (UUur) concentration. For clinical purposes, a nomogram (Fig. 12-1) can be used to estimate UUur basing on urinary uric acid concentration and urinary pH in spot urine samples instead of obtaining 24-hour collections to estimate total daily uric acid urinary excretion. UUur concentration lower than 20 mg/dL has been shown not to be associated with an increased risk of urolithiasis while on uricosuric therapy, compared to patients treated with allopurinol.[15]

The most important factor increasing the UUur concentration is low urinary pH.[43] Low urinary pH is commonly observed in patients with gout, especially in patients with the metabolic syndrome.[44] At this point, patients showing baseline urinary pH equal to or lower than 5.5 should be more closely monitored for UUur concentration during follow-up, and those showing UUur greater than 20 mg/dL should be advised to increase fluid intake in order to augment urinary flow, thus reducing urinary uric acid concentration and then UUur concentration. Spot urine density may be useful to assess adequate fluid intake.[42] In patients unable or not wishing to increase fluid intake, alkali prescription should be considered to increase urinary pH to greater than 5.5.

Combination of Xanthine-Oxidase Inhibitors and Uricosurics

The possibility of combining XOIs and uricosurics opens the possibility of prescription even to patients not showing IRE of uric acid. Patients showing uric acid overproduction who are

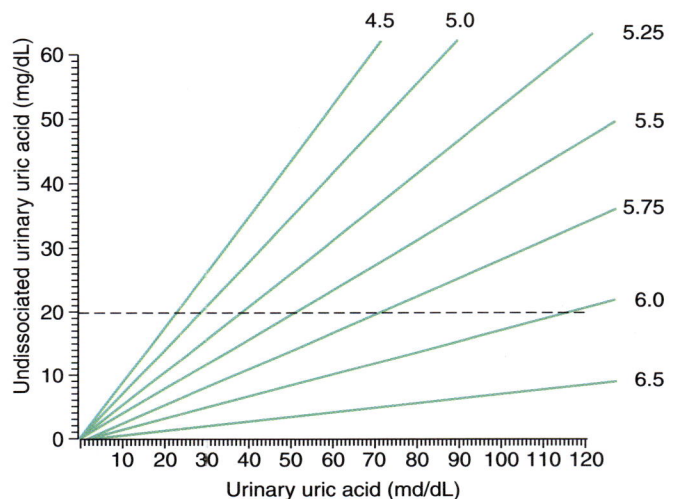

Figure 12-1 Nomogram used to estimate undissociated urinary uric acid (UUur) based on urinary pH and urinary uric acid (UUR) concentration, constructed with data from Maalouf et al.[45] Estimated UUur greater than 20 mg/dL during follow-up is associated with increased risk of urolithiasis. Reduction of UUR (increasing fluid intake should be associated with a decrease increase in urine density) or increasing urinary pH greater than 5.5 (alkali prescription) should be implemented. (© F Perez-Ruiz 2010, used with permission.)

on current treatment with drugs inhibiting XO show a reduction in SUR levels associated with a parallel reduction of the uric acid load filtered to the glomeruli and therefore the urinary uric acid output.[6]

From a practical point of view, patients with efficient renal excretion of uric acid should be first put on XOIs, thus inducing a reduction in urinary uric acid output, and if target SUR levels (at least less than 6 mg/dL) are not achieved, the addition of a uricosuric drug starting at low dose may be considered to achieve target.[22,26]

Combination of XOIs and uricosurics would be a suitable option for patients failing to achieve target SUR levels with monotherapy or in whom target SUR could be settled even lower due to the presence of a great burden of urate crystal deposition. New uricosuric drugs in development for combined therapy with XOIs should afford pharmacodynamic and pharmacokinetic studies to evaluate both efficacy and safety.

References

1. Gutman AB. Uricosuric drugs, with special reference to probenecid and sulfinpyrazone. Adv Pharmacol 1966;4:91–142.
2. Yü TF, Gutman AB. Paradoxical retention of uric acid by uricosuric drugs in low dosage. Proc Soc Exp Biol Med 1955;90:542–7.
3. Simkin PA. New standards for uric acid excretion evidence for an inducible transporter. Arthritis Rheum 2003;49:735–6.
4. Yü TF, Berger L, Gutman AB. Renal function in gout. 2. Effect of uric acid loading on renal excretion of uric acid. Am J Med 1962;33(6):829.
5. Perez-Ruiz F, Alonso-Ruiz A, Calabozo M, et al. Efficacy of allopurinol and benzbromarone for the control of hyperuricaemia. A pathogenic approach to the treatment of primary chronic gout. Ann Rheum Dis 1998;57(9):545–9.
6. Perez-Ruiz F, Calabozo M, Garcia-Erauskin G, et al. Renal underexcretion of uric acid is present in patients with apparent high urinary uric acid output. Arthritis Rheum 2002;47(6):610–3.
7. Enomoto A, Endou H. Roles of organic anion transporters (OATs) and a urate transporter (URAT1) in the pathophysiology of human disease. Clin Exp Nephrol 2005;9:195–205.
8. Anzai N, Ichida K, Jutabha P, et al. Plasma urate level is directly regulated by a voltage-driven urate efflux transporter URATv1 (*SLC2A9*) in humans. J Biol Chem 2008;C800:156–200.
9. Simkin PA. When, why, and how should we quantify the excretion rate of uric acid? J Rheumatol 2001;28:1207–10.
10. Wortmann RL, Fox IH. Limited value of uric acid to creatinine ratios in estimating uric acid excretion. Ann Intern Med 1980;822:825.
11. Moriwaki Y, Yamamoto T, Takahashi S, et al. Spot urine uric acid to creatinine ratio used in the estimation of uric acid excretion in primary gout. J Rheumatol 2001;28:1306–10.
12. Simkin PA. Uric acid excretion: quantitative assessment from spot, midmorning serum and urine samples. Ann Intern Med 1979;91:44–7.
13. Yamamoto T, Moriwaki Y, Takahashi S, et al. A simple method of selecting gout patients for treatment with uricosuric agents, using spot urine and blood samples. J Rheumatol 2002;29:1937–41.
14. Perez-Ruiz F, Herrero-Beites AM. Reply to Dr. Simkin´s letter. Arthritis Rheum 2003;47:736–7.
15. Perez-Ruiz F, Hernandez-Baldizon S, Herrero-Beites AM, et al. Risk factors associated with renal lithiasis during uricosuric treatment of hyperuricemia in patients with gout. Arthritis Care Res (Hoboken) 2010;62(9):1299–305.
16. Bishop C, Rand R, Talbott JR. Effect of Benemid (p-[di-n-propylsufamyl]-benzoic acid) on uric acid metabolism in one normal and one gouty subject. J Clin Invest 1951;30:889–95.
17. Harris M, Bryant LR, Danaher P, et al. Effect of low dose daily aspirin on (SUR) levels and urinary excretion in patients receiving probenecid for gouty arthritis. J Rheumatol 2000;27:1873–6.
18. Reinders MK, van Roon EN, Jansen TL, et al. Efficacy and tolerability of urate-lowering drugs in gout: a randomised controlled trial of benzbromarone versus probenecid after failure of allopurinol. Ann Rheum Dis 2009;68(1):51–6.
19. Yü TF, Paton BC, Chenkin T, et al. Effect of a phenylbutazone analog (4-[phenylthioethyl]-1,2-diphenyl 3,5-pyrazolidinedione) on urate clearance and other discrete renal functions in gouty subjects. Evaluation as uricosuric agent. J Clin Invest 1956;35(4):374–85.
20. Dieterle W, Faigle JW, Mory H. Biotransformation and pharmacokinetics of sulfinpyrazone (Anturan) in man. Eur J Clin Pharmacol 1975;9:135–45.
21. Lecaillon JB, Souppart C, Schiller JP. Sulfinpyrazone kinetics after intravenous and oral administration. Clin Pharmacol Ther 1979;26:611–7.
22. Goldfarb E, Smythe CJ. Effects of allopurinol, a xanthine oxidase inhibitor, and sulfinpyrazone upon the urinary and serum urate concentrations in eight patients with tophaceous gout. Arthritis Rheumatism 1967;9(3):414–23.
23. Heel RC, Brogden RN, Speight TM, et al. Benzbromarone: a review of its pharmacological properties and therapeutic use in gout and hyperuricemia. Drugs 1977;14:349–66.
24. Lee MH, Graham GG, Williams KM, et al. A benefit-risk assessment of benzbromarone in the treatment of gout. Was its withdrawal from the market in the best interest of patients? Drug Saf 2008;31(8):643–65.
25. Reinders MK, Haggsma C, Jansen TL, et al. A randomized-controlled trial on the efficacy and tolerability with dose escalation of allopurinol 300-600 mg/day versus benzbromarone 100-200 mg/day in patients with gout. Ann Rheum Dis 2008. doi:10.1136/ard.2008.091462.
26. Perez-Ruiz F, Calabozo M, Pijoan JI, et al. Effect of urate-lowering therapy on the velocity of size reduction of tophi in chronic gout. Arthritis Rheum 2002;47(4):356–60.
27. Perez-Ruiz F, Calabozo M, Fernandez-Lopez MJ, et al. Treatment of chronic gout in patients with renal function impairment. An open, randomized, actively controlled. J Clin Rheumatol 1999;5:49–55.
28. Perez-Ruiz F, Gomez-Ullate P, Amenabar JJ, et al. Long-term efficacy of hyperuricemia treatment in renal transplant patients. Nephrol Dial Transplant 2003;18:603–6.
29. Jansen TL, Reinders MK, Van Roon EN, et al. Benzbromarone withdrawn from the European market: Another case of "absence of evidence is evidence of absence"? Clin Exp Rheumatol 2004;22:651.
30. Perez-Ruiz F. New treatments for gout. J Bone Joint Spine 2007;74(4):313–5.
31. Feher MD, Hepburn AL, Hogarth MB, et al. Fenofibrate enhances urate reduction in men treated with allopurinol for hyperuricaemia and gout. Rheumatology 2003;42:321–5.
32. Takahashi S, Moriwaki Y, Yamamoto T, et al. Effects of combination treatment using anti-hyperuricaemic agents with fenofibrate and/or losartan on uric acid metabolism. Ann Rheum Dis 2003;62:572–5.
33. Shaninfar SS, Simpson RL, Carides AD, et al. Safety of losartan in hypertensive patients with thiazide-induced hyperuricemia. Kidney Int 1999;56:1879–85.
34. Würzner GC, Gersterb JC, Chiolero A, et al. Comparative effects of losartan and irbesartan on serum uric acid in hypertensive patients with hyperuricaemia and gout. J Hypertens 2001;19(1855):1860.
35. Athyros VG, Elisaf M, Papageorgiou AA, et al. Effect of statins versus untreated dyslipidemia on serum uric acid levels in patients with coronary heart disease: a subgroup analysis of the GREek Atorvastatin and Coronary-heart-disease Evaluation (GREACE) study. Am J Kidney Dis 2004;43(4):589–99.
36. Milionis HJ, Kakafika AI, Tsouli SG, et al. Effects of statin treatment on uric acid homeostasis in patients with primary hyperlipidemia. Am Heart J 2004;148(4):635–40.
37. Perez-Ruiz F, Nolla JM. Influence of leflunomide on renal handling of urate and phosphate in patients with rheumatoid arthritis. J Clin Rheumatol 2003;9:215–8.
38. Colcrys full prescribing information. 2009. www.colcrys.com
39. Levey AS, Coresh J, Balk E, et al. National Kidney Foundation Practice Guidelines for chronic kidney disease: evaluation, classification, and stratification. Ann Intern Med 2003;139:137–47.
40. Alvarez-Nemegyei J, Medina-Escobedo M, Villanueva-Jorge S, et al. Prevalence and risk factors for urolithiasis in primary gout: is a reappraisal needed? J Rheumatol 2005;32(11):2189–91.
41. Pak CY, Poindexter JR, Peterson RD, et al. Biochemical distinction between hyperuricosuric calcium urolithiasis and gouty diathesis. Urology 2002;60:789–94.
42. Perez-Ruiz F, Calabozo Raluy M, Herrero Beites A, et al. Utility of urine spot samples for the follow-up of uricosuric therapy. Rev Esp Reumatol 2001;28:57–61.
43. Khatchdourian J, Preminger GM, Whitson PA, et al. Clinical and biochemical presentation of gout diathesis: comparison of uric acid versus pure calcium stone formation. J Urol 1995;154:1665–9.
44. Maalouf NM, Cameron MA, Moe OW, et al. Low urine pH: a novel feature of the metabolic syndrome. Clin J Am Soc Nephrol 2007;2:883–8.
45. Maalouf NM, Cameron MA, Moe OW, et al. Novel insights into the pathogenesis of uric acid nephrolithiasis. Curr Opin Nephrol Hypertens 2004;13:181–9.

Chapter 13

Xanthine Oxidase Inhibitor Treatment of Hyperuricemia

Nicola Dalbeth and Lisa K. Stamp

KEY POINTS

- Xanthine oxidase is a critical enzyme in the metabolism of purines to uric acid. Both allopurinol and febuxostat reduce serum urate concentration through inhibition of xanthine oxidase.
- The active metabolite of allopurinol, oxypurinol, is largely eliminated unchanged via the kidneys and its half-life is dependent on renal function.
- Risk factors for allopurinol hypersensitivity syndrome (AHS) are impaired renal function, short treatment duration, diuretic use, and *HLA-B*5801*. The role of allopurinol dosing as a risk factor for AHS remains controversial.
- Febuxostat is metabolized by hepatic conjugation and oxidation, and dose adjustment is not required in patients with mild to moderate renal impairment.
- Randomized controlled trials have consistently demonstrated that febuxostat has superior urate-lowering efficacy compared with fixed-dose allopurinol. Further studies are required to determine the comparative efficacy of allopurinol and febuxostat when a treat-to-target serum urate approach is used with allopurinol.
- Effective urate lowering via xanthine oxidase inhibition therapy is associated with a high risk of gout flares at the start of therapy, and intensive gout prophylaxis is required to ensure that adherence to xanthine oxidase inhibitor treatment is maintained in the early phases of treatment.
- In addition to treatment of gout, xanthine oxidase inhibitors have potentially beneficial effects in renal impairment, hypertension, angina, and cardiac failure.

Introduction

Urate-lowering therapy is an essential component in the long-term management of gout. A serum urate (SU) concentration below 6 mg/dL (0.36 mmol/L) is recommended as a treatment target for patients with gout.[1] This is the concentration that corresponds to that required to ultimately, with extended therapy, achieve resolution of monosodium urate (MSU) crystals within synovial fluid, suppression of acute gout attacks, and resolution of gouty tophi.[2-4] Xanthine oxidase (XO) is a critical enzyme in the metabolism of purines to uric acid. It catalyzes the conversion of hypoxanthine to xanthine

and xanthine to uric acid. As such, inhibition of XO has been one of the mainstays of urate-lowering therapy (ULT) in gout since the introduction of allopurinol in 1963. Until the recent development and approval of febuxostat, allopurinol was the only XO inhibitor available for ULT. This chapter will review the XO inhibitors allopurinol and febuxostat and compare the clinical efficacy of these two urate-lowering drugs in controlling the hyperuricemia of gout.

Xanthine Oxidase and Uric Acid Production Pathways

Uric acid is the end product of purine degradation. Purines are obtained either though the diet or from endogenous sources such as cellular turnover. XO is a critical enzyme in the metabolism of purines to uric acid, catalyzing the conversion of hypoxanthine to xanthine and xanthine to uric acid (see Chapter 3).

XO belongs to the family of enzymes known as molybdenum hydroxylases. A common feature of this family of enzymes is the use of water rather than O_2 as the source of the oxygen atoms required for the reaction. Structurally XO consists of flavin molecules (bound as flavin adenine dinucleotide [FAD]), molybdenum, and iron-sulfur clusters. The molybdenum atoms are contained as molybdopterin cofactors and are the active sites of the enzyme. In the reaction with xanthine to form uric acid, an oxygen atom is transferred from molybdenum to xanthine. Active molybdenum is reformed by the addition of water.

In most other mammals, uric acid is broken down by urate oxidase to form allantoin, which is more water soluble and hence more easily excreted. Lack of urate oxidase in humans results in the final product of the purine degradation pathway being uric acid. The critical role of XO in this pathway led to it being a therapeutic target for the management of hyperuricemia.

Allopurinol

Structure and Mechanisms of Action

Allopurinol (4-hydroxypyrazolo[3,4-**d**]pyrimidine) is a structural analog of hypoxanthine, while its active metabolite oxypurinol is a structural analog of xanthine (Fig. 13-1). The mechanisms of action of allopurinol and oxypurinol are summarized in Table 13-1. Both allopurinol and oxypurinol inhibit XO, thereby reducing the production of uric acid. XO exists in both oxidized and reduced forms. Allopurinol weakly inhibits the oxidized form, while oxypurinol binds and inhibits the reduced form of XO. The binding of oxypurinol to the reduced form of XO is strong and renders the binding site inaccessible to reoxidation; thus, dissociation of oxypurinol from XO is slow.[5] Therefore, oxypurinol provides the majority of the inhibition of XO by virtue of its longer half-life and much stronger binding to the reduced form of XO.

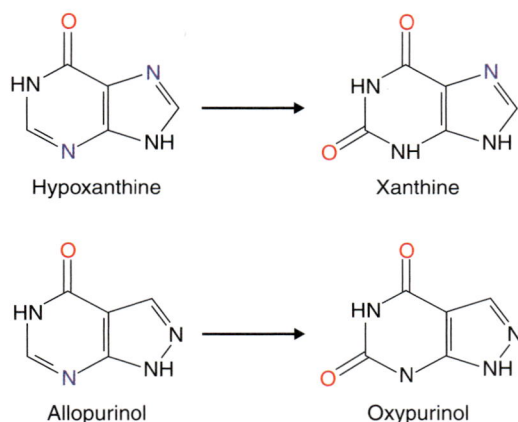

Figure 13-1 Chemical structure of allopurinol and oxypurinol.

Oxypurinol has been described as a mechanism-based inhibitor of XO as it binds to the molybdenum atom of the molybopterin cofactor within XO at sites that are essential for its catalytic reaction.[6]

The importance of oxypurinol in XO inhibition was confirmed by a study comparing the effect of allopurinol and oxypurinol administered at equimolar doses, which reported only a small difference in urate-lowering effect (average reduction in SU from baseline 3.0 mg/dL with allopurinol and 2.6 mg/dL with oxypurinol, $p = .027$).[7]

The structural similarity between allopurinol/oxypurinol and the purines xanthine/hypoxanthine means they may act as a substrate for other metabolic enzymes. Hypoxanthine-guanine phosphoribosyltransferase (HGPRT) and orotate phosphoribosyltransferase (OPRT) can convert allopurinol and oxypurinol to their respective ribonucleotides (allopurinol-1′-ribonucleoside, oxypurinol-1′-ribonucleoside, and oxypurinol-7′-ribonucleoside). Allopurinol, oxypurinol, and allopurinol-1′-ribonucleoside may inhibit other enzymes in the purine and pyrimidine metabolic pathways, including purine nucleoside phosphorylase (PNP) (possibly via accumulation of hypoxanthine and xanthine) and orotidine-5′-monophosphate decarboxylase (OMPDC), respectively.[8]

In addition to its urate-lowering effects through XO inhibition, allopurinol reduces total purine production. Allopurinol utilizes phosphoribosyl pyrophosphate (PRPP), which is required for purine synthesis, in the reaction catalyzed by HGPRT. Increased concentrations of the ribonucleotides also

Table 13-1 Comparison of Febuxostat, Allopurinol, and Oxypurinol Structure and Pharmacokinetics (Febuxostat Data Following Multiple Dosing of Febuxostat 120 mg/day)

	Allopurinol	Oxypurinol	Febuxostat
Structure	Structurally similar to hypoxanthine	Structurally similar to xanthine	No structural resemblance to purines or pyrimidines
Mechanism of XO inhibition	Mechanism-based inhibitor: binds at sites within XO that are critical for enzyme activity		Structure-based inhibitor: binds in a long, narrow channel leading to the molybdenum-pterin active site[96]
Inhibition of XO	Weakly inhibits oxidized form of XO	Inhibits reduced form of XO	Inhibits oxidized and reduced forms of XO[8]
Oral absorption	About 80%[131]	N/A	≥84%[99,100]
Time to maximum plasma drug concentration (t_{max})	1.5 hr[131]	4 hr[131]	1.1 hr[99,100]
Maximum plasma drug concentration (C_{max})	2 mg/L	7 mg/L	5.31 μg/ml[99,100]
Area under the plasma concentration-time curve for the dose administration from 0 to 24 hr (AUC_{24})	4.35 ± 0.67 μg • hr/ml[132]	166 ± 23 μg • h/ml[132]	11.96 μg • hr/ml[99,100]
Metabolism	Metabolized by aldehyde oxidase to oxypurinol	N/A	Hepatic; conjugation by uridine diphosphate-glucuronosyltransferase (UGT) enzymes and oxidation to active metabolites by CYP1A2, CYP2C8, and CYP2C9[102]
Active metabolites	Oxypurinol	N/A	67M-1, 67M-2, and 67M-4
Enterohepatic recirculation	No	No	Yes, above doses of 120 mg/day[99,100]
Volume of distribution at steady state	1.3 L/kg[131]	0.62 L/kg[131]	0.7 L/kg[103]
Plasma protein binding	<1%	No	99.2% (primarily albumin)[102]
Elimination half-life ($t_{½}$)	about 1 hr[131,133]	Depends on renal function, about 23 hr	11.9 hr[99,100]

N/A, Not applicable; *XO,* xanthine oxidase.

cause feedback inhibition of amidophosphoribosyl transferase, a rate-limiting enzyme required for the biosynthesis of purines.

Recent data have shown that allopurinol can also rapidly produce mild inhibition of nociceptive responses induced by injection of capsaicin or glutamate in a dose-dependent manner in a murine model. Furthermore, the effects of allopurinol were reversed by administration of a specific adenosine A_1 receptor antagonist.[9] The exact mechanism by which allopurinol produces such pain-relieving effects remains unclear. To date there are no studies that examine the analgesic effects of allopurinol in gout, other than through its ability to reduce SU, thereby preventing gout flares. Further studies will be required to determine whether allopurinol has a role in acute and/or chronic pain states.

Clinical Pharmacology

The clinical pharmacology of allopurinol and oxypurinol is summarized in Table 13-1. Allopurinol is readily absorbed from the gastrointestinal tract. The major route of elimination of allopurinol is through metabolism to oxypurinol (about 80%), while about 10% is metabolized to allopurinol 1'-riboside. It has been widely assumed that XO is responsible for the conversion of allopurinol to oxypurinol. Given that allopurinol and oxypurinol both inhibit XO, metabolism of allopurinol to oxypurinol should be saturable if XO is also primarily responsible for the metabolism of allopurinol. However, steady-state plasma oxypurinol concentrations increase in a linear fashion as the dose of allopurinol increases, suggesting that the metabolism of allopurinol to oxypurinol is not saturable and that another enzyme must be involved.[10] The closely related enzyme aldehyde oxidase (AO) appears to be more important in the metabolism of allopurinol to oxypurinol. This is supported by the ability of those rare patients who lack XO but who do have AO to metabolize allopurinol to oxypurinol, while those patients who lack both XO and AO cannot convert allopurinol to oxypurinol.[11,12]

In comparison to allopurinol, which has short half-life ($t_{1/2}$ about 1 hour), oxypurinol has a much longer half-life. Oxypurinol is largely eliminated unchanged via the kidneys and thus its half-life is dependent on renal function.

Drug Interactions With Allopurinol
Azathioprine

Gout is common in patients with solid organ transplantation, and azathioprine is a commonly used immunosuppressive agent after transplantation.[13] 6-Mercaptopurine, the active metabolite of azathioprine, is partly inactivated by XO. Inhibition of XO by allopurinol may therefore lead to increased concentrations of 6-mercaptopurine and myelosuppression.[14] It is recommended that the dose of azathioprine be reduced by 50% to 75% before commencing allopurinol and that the starting dose of allopurinol be lower than normal. However, despite dose adjustment patients can become pancytopenic with this combination after months or even years of therapy.[15,16] Thus, the azathioprine-allopurinol combination must be used with great caution and with careful blood monitoring for the duration of combination therapy. While there may be a reluctance to reduce immunosuppression for fear of transplant rejection, there are case reports of successful management of gout by this means.[17]

Furosemide

Furosemide is a powerful loop diuretic that inhibits the absorption of chloride and sodium within the kidney, increasing the rate of urine formation and sodium excretion. Furosemide also decreases urinary excretion of uric acid, which along with the reduction in extracellular fluid results in an increase in SU concentrations. The increase in SU occurs within a few days of commencing diuretics and persists for the duration of therapy.[18] In addition to increasing SU, furosemide has been shown to have effects on plasma oxypurinol concentrations. In a small study of six healthy subjects, a single intravenous dose of 20 mg furosemide reduced urinary oxypurinol excretion by about 40%, although there was no effect on serum oxypurinol concentrations during the study period.[19] However, a significant interaction between furosemide and allopurinol may occur during long-term treatment, and the authors suggest that the hypouricemic effect of allopurinol may become more potent as a result of this interaction.[19] Patients with gout on furosemide require higher doses of allopurinol relative to their renal function to attain SU less than 6 mg/dL (0.36 mml/L) compared to those not on frusemide.[20] Furthermore, concomitant use of furosemide results in a significantly higher plasma oxypurinol concentration for any given allopurinol dose compared to no concomitant furosemide use ($p < .001$) (Lisa Stamp, unpublished data). Combined, these data suggest that allopurinol/oxypurinol is less effective rather than more effective in patients on furosemide. Further studies of this interaction are required.

Thiazide Diuretics

Thiazide diuretics also decrease the renal clearance of uric acid leading to hyperuricemia. Small studies of patients with normal renal function have shown no effect of thiazide diuretics on the renal excretion of oxypurinol or increase in the half-life of oxypurinol.[21-23] However, studies in patients with gout or renal impairment have not been undertaken.

Probenecid and Benzbromarone

Probenecid and benzbromarone are uricosuric agents that may be used in the management of gout. Combination therapy with allopurinol and probenecid may be used in patients who respond poorly to either agent alone, resulting in further reduction in SU.[24,25] Despite this improvement in urate lowering, efficacy studies in healthy volunteers have shown that coadministration of allopurinol and probenecid reduces plasma oxypurinol concentrations with no effect on plasma probenecid concentrations.[25] Thus, the uricosuric effect of probenecid interferes with the reduction in plasma oxypurinol concentrations, resulting in a reduction in SU.

Similar effects are observed when allopurinol and benzbromarone are combined with a reduction in SU concentrations.[26,27] However, the effects of this combination on plasma oxypurinol concentrations are inconsistent with both a reduction in plasma oxypurinol and an increase in the renal elimination rate of oxypurinol,[27,26] and no effect on renal oxypurinol elimination is reported.[28]

Clinical Trials of Allopurinol for the Hyperuricemia of Gout

Key clinical outcomes for patients with gout include number of gout flares, tophus regression, dissolution of crystals, radiographic damage, patient function and quality of life, and cardiovascular outcomes. A recent review has highlighted the role of SU as a biomarker in chronic gout and summarizes the key evidence with respect to the clinical outcomes regardless of the therapy used.[29] Allopurinol has specifically been shown to be effective in reducing SU, resorbing tophi, reducing the number of gout flares, and improving some cardiovascular outcomes (Table 13-2). However, there are no clinical data to date that demonstrate the effect of allopurinol on radiographic joint damage or on patient function or quality of life.

Lowering of Serum Urate Concentration

A number of clinical trials have reported a reduction in SU with allopurinol therapy (see Table 13-2). Compliance with allopurinol therapy is often poor,[30,31] and only one of these studies assessed patient compliance with allopurinol therapy using plasma oxypurinol concentrations.[20] In this study, there was clear evidence of effective SU reduction with allopurinol therapy that was lost when patients became noncompliant.

Tophus Reduction

Allopurinol has been shown to result in a reduction in the size and number of tophi (see Table 13-2). However, the combination of benzbromarone and allopurinol results in a more rapid reduction in tophus size compared to either agent alone.[32]

Flare Rates

A sustained reduction in SU is required for cessation of gout flares. Even after SU reaches the target (less than 6 mg/dL), it may take months for the gouty flares to subside. Furthermore, commencement of allopurinol can precipitate an acute attack of gout. Therefore, careful patient education and use of prophylactic therapy when allopurinol is commenced are required. Studies have confirmed that allopurinol can reduce the number of gout flares (see Table 13-2) and may have an effect even if SU does not reach the target.[33] As expected, patients with gout flares are less likely to be compliant with allopurinol (odds ratio [OR] 0.5; 95% confidence interval [CI] 1.25 to 8.23),[34] highlighting the need for patient education and compliance monitoring.

Other Potential Indications for Allopurinol: Renal Disease, Cardiovascular Disease, and Hypertension
Effects of Allopurinol on Renal Function

Hyperuricemia is an independent risk factor for renal impairment in healthy normotensive individuals,[35] is a predictor of renal progression in IgA nephropathy,[36] and is associated with early glomerular filtration rate (GFR) loss in patients with type 1 diabetes.[37] Furthermore, in a large Japanese cohort study, hyperuricemia was associated with an increased incidence of end-stage renal disease (ESRD) and was an independent predictor of ESRD in women.[38] Allopurinol has been shown to slow the progression of renal disease. In a study of 54 hyperuricemic patients with chronic kidney disease, only 16% of patients receiving allopurinol had a significant deterioration in renal function (serum creatinine increase greater than 40% of baseline) or dialysis dependence after 12 months compared to 46.1% of controls ($p = .015$).[39] In another study of 113 patients with GFR less than 60 ml/min, allopurinol 100 mg/day slowed the progression of renal disease independently of age, gender, C-reactive protein (CRP), diabetes, and use of angiotensin-converting enzyme (ACE) inhibitors.[40]

Effects of Allopurinol on Cardiovascular Disease and Mortality

Hyperuricemia is increasingly recognized as an independent risk factor for a number of vascular disorders including hypertension, cardiovascular disease, and cerebrovascular disease (see review[41]). Hyperuricemia, in the absence of gout, is also associated with poor prognosis in patients with congestive heart failure (CHF).[42,43] More recently, it has been recognized that gout per se is associated with an increase risk of cardiovascular disease and death.[44-46]

Studies in patients with CHF have demonstrated an increase in both the amount and activity of XO, which leads to an increase in production of both SU and reactive oxygen species.[47,48] These data led to the suggestion that XO inhibition may improve long-term cardiovascular outcomes through reduction of both superoxide and SU production.

Recent studies have reported a survival benefit in hyperuricemic patients treated with allopurinol. In a study of 9924 hyperuricemic veterans, therapy with allopurinol was associated with a lower risk of all-cause mortality, even after adjusting for other confounding variables including comorbidities and SU (hazard ratio [HR] 0.77; 95% CI 0.65 to 0.91).[49] In patients with CHF, long-term high-dose allopurinol (300 mg/day or greater) was associated with significantly reduced mortality compared to patients receiving low-dose allopurinol (299 mg/day or less) (risk ratio [RR] 0.59; 95% CI 0.37 to 0.95).[50] More recently, a large retrospective, nested case-control study of 25,090 patients with CHF demonstrated that a history of gout as well as a recent acute episode of gout (within 60 days) were associated with an increased risk of readmission for CHF or death (RR 2.06; 95% CI 1.39 to 3.06; $p < .001$).[51] Allopurinol use was not associated with a reduction in CHF readmission or death in the total population (RR 1.02; 95% CI 0.95 to 1.1; $p = .55$). However, in those patients with gout, allopurinol use was associated with a significant reduction in CHF readmissions or death (RR 0.69; 95% CI 0.60 to 0.79) and reduced all-cause mortality (RR 0.74; 95% CI 0.61 to 0.90).[51] These results are supported by the results of a placebo-controlled trial examining the effect of adding oxypurinol or placebo to standard CHF therapy in 405 patients. Although the addition of oxypurinol (600 mg/day) for 24 weeks did not improve outcomes in the cohort as a whole, there was a trend toward improved outcomes in the subgroup of patients with high baseline SU (9.5 mg/dL or higher) but not those with SU less than 9.5 mg/dL.[52] Furthermore, there was an association between the extent of SU reduction and outcomes, with those patients who had a lesser reduction in

Table 13-2 Summary of Clinical Trials of the Efficacy of Allopurinol

	Reference	Trial Design	Allopurinol Results
SU reduction	134	Allopurinol discontinued in 33 patients with gout and effects observed	Mean serum urate (SU) prior to allopurinol 8.4 ± 1.1 mg/dL, after allopurinol therapy 5.5 ± 1.2 mg/dL, and after withdrawal of allopurinol 8.8 ± 1.2 mg/dL Rise in SU occurred rapidLy with a return to pretreatment SU concentrations within 1 week
	92	Prospective parallel open study of 86 males with gout. Allopurinol 300 mg/day compared to benzbromarone 100 mg/day.	Mean reduction in SU of 2.75 mg/dL in normal urate excretors and 3.34 mg/dL in urate underexcretors. 53% patients on allopurinol 300 mg/day achieved SU <6 mg/dL. Dose of allopurinol increased to 450 mg/day in 21 patients and 600 mg/day in 2 patients to achieve SU <6 mg/dL.
	135	Open randomized study in 36 patients with CrCl 20 to 80 ml/min/1.73 m^2. Allopurinol 100-300 mg/day compared to benzbromarone 100-200 mg/day. Follow-up 9-24 mo	7/19 patients on allopurinol did not achieve SU <6 mg/dL. SU reduced from 8.96 ± 1.84mg/dL to 5.9 ± 0.92 mg/dL.
	2	Prospective study of 57 patients attempting to attain SU <6 mg/dL. All patients received allopurinol. Follow-up 2-10 yr	67% never achieved SU <6 mg/dL—9 patients admitted noncompliance.
	33	Retrospective review of 23 patients with crystal proven gout receiving allopurinol 50-400 mg/d	SU concentrations reduced during a year of allopurinol therapy mean 9.4 mg/dL baseline vs. 7.4 mg/dL in first year of treatment ($p < .0001$). Only 20.4% patients achieved SU <6.4 mg/dL.
	32	Prospective observational study in 63 patients with tophaceous gout. Patients received allopurinol, benzbromarone, or combination. Allopurinol dose adjusted for renal function. Five-year follow-up	Of the 24 patients who received allopurinol mean baseline SU was 8.78 ± 1.34 mg/dL and reduced to a mean SU during follow-up 5.37 ± 0.79 mg/dL ($p < .001$ compared to baseline).
	113	FACT study (n = 762). Patients with gout and SU ≥8.0 mg/dL randomized to febuxostat (80 or 120 mg/day) or allopurinol (300 mg/day) for 52 weeks.	Primary endpoint (SU <6 mg/dL at last 3 monthly visits) achieved by 21% of those on allopurinol
	39	Prospective randomized controlled trial of 54 hyperuricemic patients with chronic kidney disease. Randomized to allopurinol 100 or 300 mg/day or placebo for 12 mo	Allopurinol reduced SU from baseline 9.75 ± 1.18 mg/dL to 5.88 ± 1.01 mg/dL ($p < .0001$) at 12 mo.
	24	Prospective open study in 51 gout patients. Commenced allopurinol 200-300 mg/day. Probenecid added if SU >5.0 mg/dL at 2 mo.	After 2 mo 8/32 (25%) SU <5.0 mg/dL and 53% ≤6 mg/dL SU reduced by 36 ± 11% from baseline
	114	APEX study (n = 1072). Patients with gout and SU ≥8.0 mg/dL and serum creatinine ≤2.0 mg/dL randomized to febuxostat (80, 120, or 240 mg/day), allopurinol (100 or 300 mg/day depending on renal function) or placebo for 28 weeks.	Last 3 monthly SU <6 mg/dL achieved in 22%
	136	Prospective open-label study of 12 patients with-stage renal disease undergoing hemodialysis. All patients received allopurinol 300 mg/day for 3 mo	Allopurinol resulted in a reduction in SU from baseline median of 10.13 mg/dL to a median of 6.6 mg/dL at 3 mo ($p < .01$). The mean reduction in SU was −3.53 ± 2.4 mg/dL.
	137	Randomized open labeled trial in gout patients (n = 65) with CrCl ≥50 ml/min. Patients randomized to allopurinol 300 mg/day, which was increased to 600 mg/day if SU not ≤5 mg/dL after 2 mo OR benzbromarone 100 mg/day increased to 200 mg/day at 2 mo	8/31 (26%) patients achieved SU ≤5.0 mg/dL on allopurinol 300 mg/day. 21/27 (78%) patients achieved SU ≤5.0 mg/dL on allopurinol 300 or 600 mg/day. Mean SU reduction from baseline −33 ± 13% for allopurinol 300 mg/day and −49 ± 14% for allopurinol 600 mg/day

Table 13-2 Summary of Clinical Trials of the Efficacy of Allopurinol—cont'd

	Reference	Trial Design	Allopurinol Results
	4	EXCEL study (n = 1086) 3-yr open-label extension study febuxostat 80 or 120 mg/day vs. allopurinol 300 mg/day. Primary endpoint SU <6 mg/dL.	46% achieved SU <6 mg/dL after 1 mo. 56.6% allopurinol-treated patients reassigned to febuxostat to attain target SU. Between 12 and 36 mo 75% to 100% maintained target SU
	20	Open labeled 12-mo dose escalation study of 45 patients on allopurinol. Dose of allopurinol increased by 50-100 mg/mo to attain target SU <6 mg/dL	88% patients achieved target SU at 12 mo. Mean % reduction in SU from baseline ranged from 10% to 37% depending on the dose of allopurinol in mg/day above the CrCl-based dose. Increase in SU associated with noncompliance with therapy as assessed by plasma oxypurinol concentration
	115	CONFIRMS study (n = 2269). Patients with gout and SU ≥8.0 mg/dL and CrCl ≥30 ml/min randomized to febuxostat (40 or 80 mg/day), allopurinol (200 or 300 mg/day depending on renal function) for 28 weeks. Primary endpoint SU <6 mg/dL at the final visit.	Primary endpoint achieved by 42% of all patients on allopurinol. In those with renal impairment (CrCl 30-89 ml/min), primary endpoint achieved by 42% of patients on allopurinol.
Gout flare rates	135	Open randomized study in 36 patients with CrCl 20-80 ml/min/1.73 m². Allopurinol 100-300 mg/day compared to benzbromarone 100-200 mg/day. Follow-up 9-24 mo	Number of flares reduced: 3.4 ± 1.62/yr before ULT to 0.93 ± 1.16 in first year of follow-up and 0.06 ± 0.25/yr during second year of follow-up. No difference between allopurinol and benzbromarone groups
	2	Prospective study of 57 patients attempting to attain SU <6 mg/dL. All patients received allopurinol. Follow-up 2-10 yr	Of the 33% patients who achieved SU ≤6 mg/dL for at least a year the mean number of attacks in the last year was 1 (range 0-3) compared to a mean of 6 (range 4-12) in those patients with SU >6 mg/dL.
	33	Retrospective review of 23 patients with crystal proven gout receiving allopurinol 50-400 mg/day	Mean dose of allopurinol was 211 mg/day. There was a significant reduction in the number of gout flares during a year of allopurinol therapy. Mean flares in year prior to allopurinol 2.69/yr compared to 0.3/yr during the first year of treatment ($p < .0001$)
	4	EXCEL study (n = 1086) 3-yr open-label extension study febuxostat 80 or 120 mg/day vs. allopurinol 300 mg/day. Primary endpoint SU <6 mg/dL.	Maintenance of SU <6 mg/dL resulted in progressive reduction in flare rates such that flares occurred in <4% patients after 18 mo of ULT
	32	Prospective observational study in 63 patients with tophaceous gout. Patients received allopurinol, benzbromarone or combination. Allopurinol dose adjusted for renal function. Five-year follow-up	Of the 24 patients who received allopurinol mean diameter of target tophus at baseline was 16.2 ± 6.1mm. The time until tophus resolution was 29.1 ± 8.3 mo with a velocity of tophus reduction of 0.57 ± 0.18 mm/mo.
Tophus resorption	2	Prospective study of 57 patients attempting to attain SU <6 mg/dL. All patients received allopurinol. Follow-up 2-10 yr	Mean of 3 tophi in patients with SU ≤6 mg/dL compared to 14 tophi in patients with SU >6 mg/dL.
	113	FACT study (n = 762). Patients with gout and SU ≥8.0 mg/dL randomized to febuxostat (80 or 120 mg/day) or allopurinol (300 mg/day) for 52 wk.	Median reduction in tophus area was 50%
	4	EXCEL study (n = 1086) open label extension study febuxostat 80 or 120 mg/day vs. allopurinol 300 mg/day.	Tophus resolution achieved by 29%

SU having worse outcomes. Taken together, these data suggest that in the subgroup of patients with gout or hyperuricemia (9.5 mg/dL or higher), XO inhibition improves long-term outcomes.

Allopurinol, through its ability to reduce myocardial oxygen demand, may also be beneficial in patients with ischemic heart disease. In patients with chronic stable angina, allopurinol 600 mg/day for 6 weeks increased the median time to ST-segment depression on exercise testing, increased median total exercise time, and increased the time to chest pain compared to placebo.[53] In another placebo-controlled study of 40 patients with ST-segment elevation myocardial

Table 13-3 Effects of Allopurinol on the Cardiovascular System

Effect	References
Improves myocardial contractility by restoring myocardial calcium sensitivity and β-adrenergic responsiveness in heart failure	138
Decreases oxidative stress leading to improved endothelial function	139
Decreases myocardial oxygen consumption for a particular stroke volume	47, 140
May reduce plasma renin leading to reduced blood pressure	141

infarction who underwent primary coronary intervention, the addition of allopurinol 400 mg stat followed by 100 mg/day for 1 month resulted in lower peak troponin I ($p = .04$) and creatinine kinase (CK) ($p = .01$) concentrations and more effective ST-elevation recovery ($p < .05$). In addition, at 1 month, those patients who received allopurinol had a 13% lower incidence of major adverse cardiac events compared to placebo ($p < .002$).[54]

While further larger studies are required, these data give further weight to the need for ULT in patients with gout who are at high risk of cardiovascular disease. Whether the current target SU of less than 6 mg/dL is appropriate for preventing cardiovascular events remains to be determined. Finally, further studies will be required to determine the role of allopurinol in patients with asymptomatic hyperuricemia with cardiovascular disease. The effects of allopurinol on the cardiovascular system are summarized in Table 13-3.

Serum Urate, Allopurinol, and Blood Pressure

Hypertension and hyperuricemia are commonly associated; 25% of patients with untreated hypertension, 50% of patients on diuretics, and more than 75% of patients with malignant hypertension have hyperuricemia.[55] In patients with gout, up to about 40% have hypertension.[56,57] While hyperuricemia may have a pathogenic role in hypertension (see review[58]), medications frequently used in the management of hypertension also contribute. Loop and thiazide diuretics both increase SU. In comparison, the angiotensin II receptor antagonist losartan[59] and the calcium channel blocker amlodipine significantly increase uric acid clearance, thereby reducing SU.[60,61] Thus, clinicians need to consider the underlying reasons for the use of loop or thiazide diuretics and whether alternative agents, which do not result in retention of uric acid, could be used in patients with gout.

Allopurinol may also contribute to a reduction in blood pressure. In a small study of 48 patients with hyperuricemia, allopurinol 300 mg/day for 3 months resulted in a significant reduction in both systolic and diastolic blood pressures.[62] In another study of 30 adolescents (aged 11 to 17 years) with newly diagnosed essential hypertension, allopurinol 200 mg twice daily for 4 weeks resulted in a significant reduction in blood pressure.[63] Similar studies have not been undertaken in patients with gout.

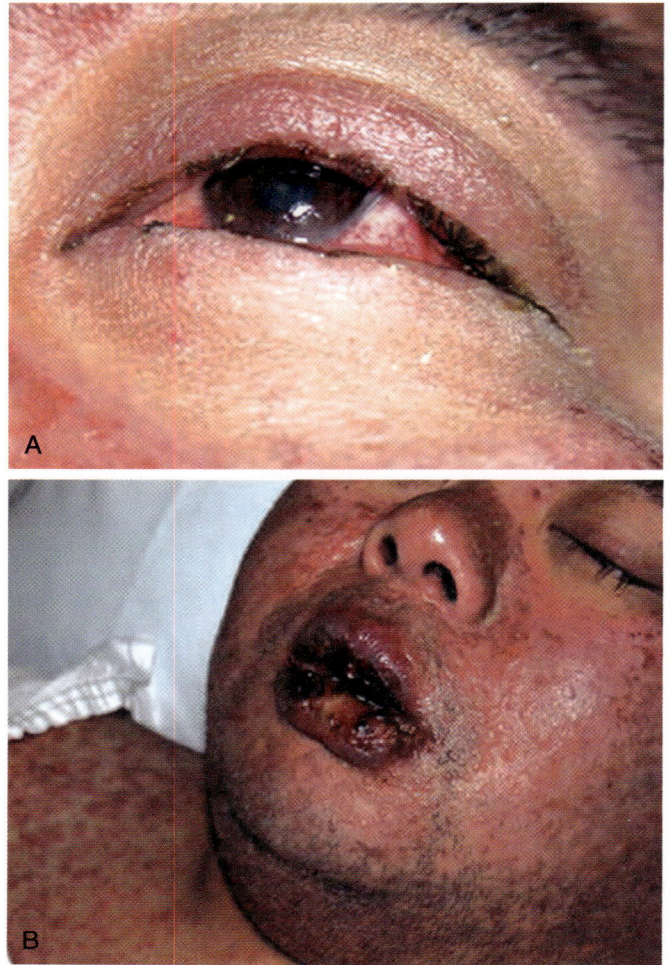

Figure 13-2 Ocular, mucosal and cutaneous involvement in allopurinol hypersensitivity syndrome. *(From Fernando SL, Broadfoot AJ. Prevention of severe cutaneous adverse drug reactions: the emerging value of pharmacogenetic screening. CMAJ 2010;182(5):476-80.)*

Allopurinol Hypersensitivity Syndrome

Allopurinol is generally well tolerated. Approximately 2% of patients develop a mild rash[64] and up to 5% of patients stop allopurinol due to adverse events. The most devastating adverse effect is the potentially life-threatening allopurinol hypersensitivity syndrome (AHS). AHS is characterized by rash (e.g., Stevens-Johnson syndrome [SJS], toxic epidermal necrolysis [TEN], exfoliative dermatitis) (Fig. 13-2), eosinophilia, leukocytosis, fever, hepatitis, and progressive renal failure. Criteria for the diagnosis of AHS that incorporate the clinical features after exposure to allopurinol have been published (Table 13-4).[65] Although SJS is not included in these criteria, it is common in AHS and should be included as one of the forms of rash in the major criteria.

The incidence of AHS is estimated to be about 0.1%. In the hospital-based Boston Collaborative Drug Surveillance Program, 7 of 1835 (0.38%) patients treated with allopurinol had a life-threatening reaction, although not all of these were AHS.[64] A more recent European study of patients with SJS or TEN reported that allopurinol was the most common causative drug and that the incidence of allopurinol-associated SJS or TEN had increased in the past 15 years.[66]

Table 13-4 Diagnostic Criteria for Allopurinol Hypersensitivity Syndrome

Diagnostic Criteria for Allopurinol Hypersensitivity Syndrome

Clear history of exposure to allopurinol

Lack of exposure to another drug that may have caused the same clinical picture

Clinical picture including:
    At least two of the following major criteria
    Worsening renal function
    Acute hepatocellular injury
    Rash, including toxic epidermal necrolysis, erythema multi-forme, or a diffuse maculopapular or exfoliative dermatitis

OR

One of the major criteria and at least one of the following minor criteria
    Fever
    Eosinophilia
    Leukocytosis

From Gutierrez-Macias A, Lizarralde-Palacios E, Martinez-Odriozola P, et al. Fatal allopurinol hypersensitivity syndrome after treatment of asymptomatic hyperuricemia. Br Med J 2005;331:623-4.

Table 13-5 Risk Factors for Allopurinol Hypersensitivity Reactions[142]

Risk Factor	References
Recent onset of allopurinol treatment	67, 71-73
Renal impairment	67, 71, 72, 74, 75, 143, 144
Diuretic therapy	71, 72, 74, 75, 143
Presence of *HLA-B*5801* allele	67-70
? Allopurinol dose	Positive association: 71, 72, 74, 145 Negative association: 67, 88, 89

Risk Factors for AHS

Risk factors for the development of AHS include renal impairment, diuretic use, and recent commencement of allopurinol therapy (Table 13-5). More recently, *HLA-B*5801* has been identified as a significant risk factor for AHS and allopurinol-associated SJS and TEN. In Han Chinese, the *HLA-B*5801* allele was found in 100% of AHS cases and 15% of allopurinol-tolerant controls (OR 580.3; 95% CI 34.4 to 9780.9).[67] A similar association has been observed in several ethnic populations including Thai, Japanese, and a mixed population of Europeans.[68-70] Whether HLA profiling can help prevent these life-threatening reactions remains to be determined and will likely require large international trials within different ethnic groups. Many cases of AHS have been reported in patients receiving allopurinol for asymptomatic hyperuricemia.[71-74] It remains unclear whether asymptomatic hyperuricemia is a specific risk factor for AHS, although a recent case-control study of AHS did report lower rates of gout in AHS cases than in allopurinol-tolerant controls.[67]

Outcome and Treatment of AHS

AHS is a life-threatening condition with mortality associated reported to be as high as 27%.[74,75] There is no cure for AHS, and early recognition and drug withdrawal are critical. Supportive care is the mainstay of treatment. Corticosteroids have been used; however, their role is controversial.[72,74] Whether increased excretion of oxypurinol through uricosuric drugs (such as probenecid[76]) or hemodialysis has a role in the management of AHS is unknown.

Mechanism of AHS

The exact mechanism of AHS is unclear. Some cases of AHS occur as a result of T-cell–mediated immune reactions to oxypurinol.[77] Although it has been suggested that AHS may be due to an accumulation of oxypurinol, AHS can occur even with low oxypurinol concentrations.[78]

Other Adverse Effects of Allopurinol

Allopurinol has been reported to be the most common cause of drug reaction with eosinophilia and systemic symptoms (DRESS).[79] DRESS is characterized by fever, rash, eosinophilia, multiorgan involvement, and lymphocyte activation. There is some debate as to whether DRESS is a separate clinical entity from other drug-induced reactions such as AHS.[80] While there may be some pathologic differences between AHS and DRESS, the clinical picture can be very similar. Whether *HLA-B*5801* is also a risk factor for DRESS is unclear.

Allopurinol has also been associated with hypersensitivity vasculitis with a variety of clinical manifestations, including rash, cerebral vasculitis, eosinophilia, glomerulonephritis, and liver disease.[81,82] Less commonly, allopurinol has been associated with drug-induced antineutrophil cytoplasmic antibody (ANCA)-associated vasculitis.[83]

Some allopurinol adverse effects may be related to effects on pyrimidine metabolism. Murine studies have shown that high-dose allopurinol results in abnormal pyrimidine metabolism and nephrotoxicity, an effect that was limited by provision of uridine.[84]

Allopurinol, through its ability to increase purines, including adenosine, may have effects on the central nervous system (CNS). Adenosine has a number of inhibitory effects within the CNS including anticonvulsant, sedative, antipsychotic, and antiaggression effects. Such effects may be of benefit in the treatment of conditions such as schizophrenia.[85] However, these effects, particularly the sedating effects, can be considered unwanted adverse effects in patients receiving allopurinol for the treatment of hyperuricemia.

Allopurinol Dosing

There is currently no clear evidence base or consensus regarding allopurinol dosing, especially in patients with renal impairment. The U.S. Food and Drug Administration (FDA) has approved allopurinol in doses up to 800 mg/day in patients with gout,[86] while the British Society of Rheumatology (BSR) recommends a maximum dose of 900 mg/day.[87] The FDA, BSR, and European League Against Rheumatism (EULAR) all recommend that allopurinol is commenced at a

Table 13-6 Allopurinol Dose Based on Creatinine Clearance

Creatinine Clearance (ml/min)	Maintenance Dose Allopurinol
0	100 mg every 3 days
10	100 mg every 2 days
20	100 mg/day
40	150 mg/day
60	200 mg/day
80	250 mg/day
100	300 mg/day
120	350 mg/day
140	400 mg/day

Data from Hande K, Noone R, Stone W. Severe allopurinol toxicity. Description and guidelines for prevention in patients with renal insufficiency. Am J Med 1984;76:47-56.

low dose (50 to 100 mg/day) and increased in 50- to 100-mg increments until the target SU is achieved,[1,86,87] a measure that could reduce development of gout attacks when commencing urate-lowering therapy. However, all acknowledge that the maximum dose of allopurinol should be reduced in patients with renal impairment.

Dose reduction in renal impairment is based on reports of a relationship between full-dose allopurinol (300 mg/day or greater) in patients with renal impairment and development of AHS.[71] This observation, along with the recognition that oxypurinol excretion was significantly reduced in patients with impaired renal function, led to the suggestion that allopurinol should be dosed according to creatinine clearance (CrCl) (Table 13-6).

While CrCl-based allopurinol dosing has been widely accepted, it has had two important consequences. First, many patients fail to achieve the target SU of 6 mg/dL or less on the CrCl-based dose. For example, in a study of 250 patients with gout, target SU concentrations were only achieved in 28% of non-Polynesian patients receiving CrCl-based allopurinol doses, compared with 60% of those on higher-than-CrCl–based doses ($p < .05$).[88] Thus, many patients remain undertreated with CrCl-based allopurinol dosing.

Second, there is no clear evidence that CrCl-based dosing reduces serious allopurinol-related adverse events—in particular, AHS. In a recent large case-control study of severe AHS, there was a trend to lower allopurinol doses in the AHS group compared to allopurinol-tolerant controls.[67] In another case-control study of allopurinol dosing, AHS did not occur more frequently in those taking higher-than-CrCl–based doses, compared with those receiving the CrCl-based dose.[89] Furthermore, in a case-control study, AHS cases were more likely in patients taking the CrCl-based dose of allopurinol.[90] Thus, the net result of CrCl-based allopurinol dosing may be undertreatment of a potential treatable condition with no obvious improvement in safety.

Recent data suggest that allopurinol can be used safely in higher-than-CrCl–based doses even in patients with renal impairment. In a prospective study of 45 gouty patients with

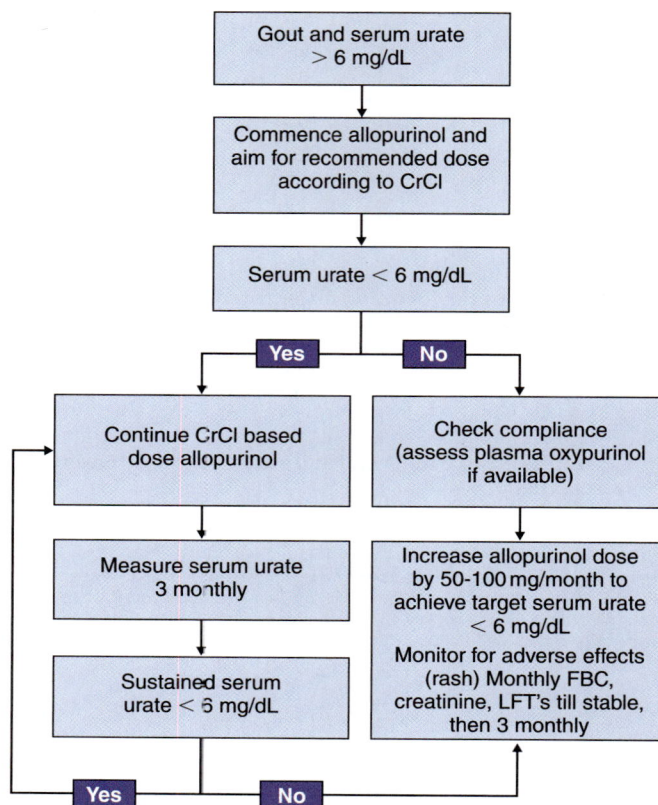

Figure 13-3 Dosing of allopurinol to achieve target SU concentrations.

SU of 6 mg/dL or greater despite receiving allopurinol at the CrCl-based dose, the dose was systematically increased until the target SU was achieved. Of 35 patients who completed the study, 31 (88%) achieved the target SU (less than 6 mg/dL) at 12 months. Two of five patients who had SU of 6 mg/dL or greater had undetectable plasma oxypurinol, indicating noncompliance. There was a significant reduction in SU at all allopurinol doses above CrCl-based doses ($p < .001$). The highest dose of allopurinol required to achieve the target was 400 mg/day *above* the CrCl-based dose.[91] While three patients developed rashes, these responded to dose reduction or cessation of allopurinol. There were no serious adverse events or cases of AHS. Perez-Ruiz et al.[92] have also shown that higher doses of allopurinol are more effective in lowering SU. Of the 49 patients with gout and CrCl greater than 60 ml/min enrolled in that study, 23 (47%) failed to achieve SU less than 6 mg/dL on allopurinol 300 mg/day. The target SU less than 6 mg/dL was achieved in 21 patients (55%) when the allopurinol dose was increased to 450 mg/day and in 2 patients when allopurinol was increased to 600 mg/day.[92] These data, along with results from the study by Stamp et al.,[91] suggest that a gradual increase in allopurinol dose, especially in patients with more significant renal impairment, is appropriate and effective. A revised strategy for allopurinol dosing aiming for the target SU is outlined in Figure 13-3.

When doses of allopurinol greater than 300 mg/day are used, there may be some advantages of twice-daily divided dosing. Such an approach may help reduce CNS and gastrointestinal adverse effects.

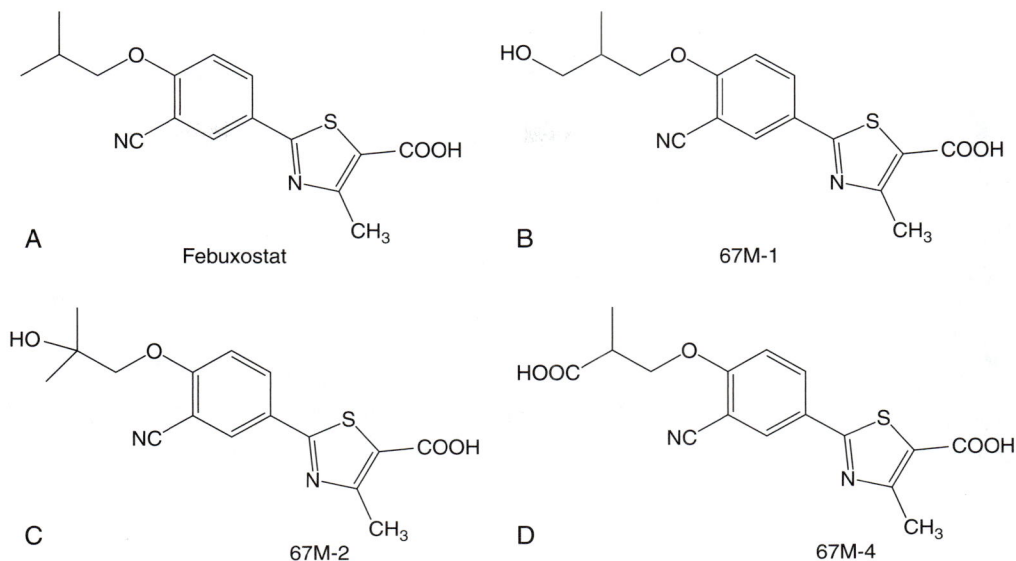

Figure 13-4 Chemical structure of febuxostat and active metabolites 67M-1, 67M-2, and 67M-4. (*From Khosravan R, Grabowski BA, Mayer MD, et al. The effect of mild and moderate hepatic impairment on pharmacokinetics, pharmacodynamics, and safety of febuxostat, a novel nonpurine selective inhibitor of xanthine oxidase. J Clin Pharmacol 2006;46(1):88-102. Reprinted by permission of SAGE Publications.*)

Role of Oxypurinol in Monitoring Allopurinol Therapy

The current role of plasma oxypurinol is in assessing patient compliance with allopurinol therapy. In patients who fail to achieve an SU less than 6 mg/dL, measurement of plasma oxypurinol should be undertaken to assess compliance with therapy. Measurement of plasma oxypurinol has been suggested as a means of monitoring allopurinol therapy. However, there is scant clinical trial data on which to base a plasma oxypurinol therapeutic range. A plasma oxypurinol concentration of 100 μmol/L (15 mg/L) at 6 to 9 hours post allopurinol has been suggested as the upper limit of the therapeutic range.[93,94] However, in these early studies, the target SU was 7.1 mg/dL (0.42 mmol/L), which is substantially higher than the current target SU of 6 mg/dL (less than 0.36 mmol/L). We have recently shown that the majority of patients require a plasma oxypurinol greater than 100 μmol/L to achieve the target SU (less than 6 mg/dL) (Lisa Stamp, unpublished data). This is substantially higher than previously suggested oxypurinol target concentrations. However, there is wide variability in range above plasma oxypurinol 100 μmol/L to achieve the target SU for a particular individual, so how high above 100 μmol/L the plasma oxypurinol needs to be remains uncertain. Furthermore, patients with renal impairment (CrCl 60 ml/min or less) may require higher plasma oxypurinol concentrations to achieve the target SU than will patients with "normal" renal function. There are no convincing data supporting an association between adverse events and plasma oxypurinol concentrations.

Febuxostat

Febuxostat is a recently developed XO inhibitor that was approved by the European Medicines Agency in 2008 and the FDA in 2009 for management of hyperuricemia in patients with gout.

Structure and Mechanisms of Action

Febuxostat [TEI-6720, TMX-67, chemical name (2-(3-cyano-4-isobutoxyphenyl)-4-methyl-5-thiazolecarboxylic acid, empiric formula $C_{16}H_{16}N_2O_3S$, molecular weight 316.38] is a potent nonpurine inhibitor of the oxidized and reduced forms of XO with an in vitro inhibition (K_i) value of less than 1 nM.[8,95,96] The mechanisms of action of febuxostat are summarized in Table 13-1. The molecular structure and mechanism of XO inhibition of febuxostat are quite different from those of allopurinol or oxypurinol (Fig. 13-4). Febuxostat has at least three pharmacologically active metabolites: 67M-1, 67M-2, and 67M-4 (see Fig. 13-4). Analysis of the crystal structure of the enzyme–drug interaction showed that febuxostat binds in a long, narrow channel leading to the molybdenum-pterin active site of XO, preventing substrate binding and activity of the enzyme[96] (Fig. 13-5). The enzyme–inhibitor complex is very stable and specific.[8,96] Unlike allopurinol, febuxostat does not alter the activity of other enzymes in the purine or pyrimidine pathways, such as guanine deaminase, hypoxanthine-guanine phosphoribosyltransferase, purine nucleoside phosphorylase, orotate phosphoribosyltransferase, and orotidine-5′-monophosphate decarboxylase.[8,97]

Preclinical Studies

In vitro studies of bovine milk XO have shown that febuxostat showed potent mixed-type inhibition of both the oxidized and reduced forms of XO.[8] Oral administration of febuxostat had a marked urate-lowering effect in both normal rodents and rats with oxonate-induced hyperuricemia and was more potent than allopurinol. ED$_{50}$ values (the dose causing a 50% reduction in SU) were 1.5 mg/kg for febuxostat and 5 mg/kg for allopurinol in oxonate-treated hyperuricemic rats.[95] The potent urate-lowering effect was confirmed in chimpanzees; after 3 days of treatment (5 mg/kg/day), febuxostat reduced SU by 74%, compared with 45% in the allopurinol-treated group.[98]

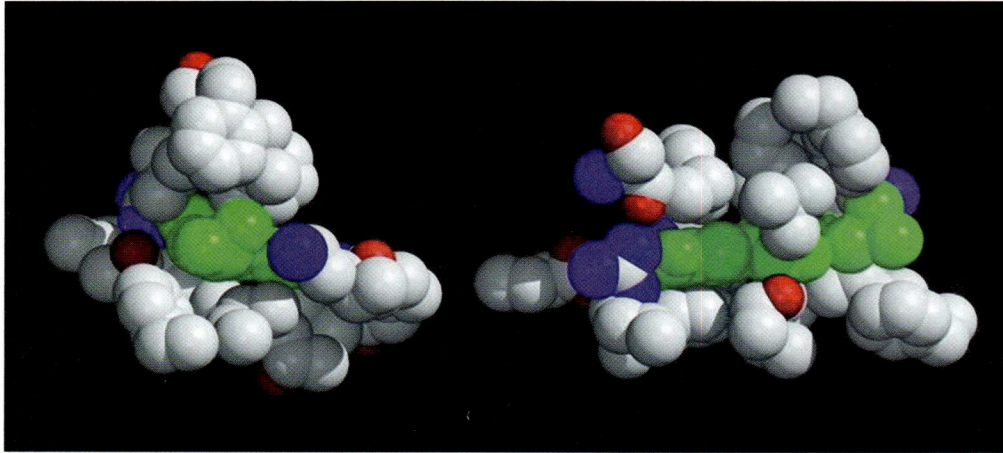

Figure 13-5 Febuxostat in access channel to molybdenum-pterin active site of xanthine oxidase. *Green,* Febuxostat. *(From Okamoto K, Eger BT, Nishino T, et al. An extremely potent inhibitor of xanthine oxidoreductase: crystal structure of the enzyme-inhibitor complex and mechanism of inhibition. J Biol Chem 2003;278:1848-55, Fig. 8B.)*

Clinical Pharmacology

The clinical pharmacology of febuxostat is summarized in Table 13-1.

Healthy Volunteers

A phase 1, 2-week, multiple-dose, placebo-controlled, dose-escalation study of febuxostat in 154 healthy adults confirmed that this agent is a potent urate-lowering agent.[99,100] Progressive reductions in SU were observed in a linear relationship with febuxostat doses in the range of 10 to 120 mg/day (25% to 70% reduction in SU respectively). Corresponding increase in serum xanthine concentration, reduction in urinary uric acid excretion, and increases in hypoxanthine and xanthine excretion were observed. All of these effects reached a plateau at doses above 120 mg/day. Adverse events were mild and self-limited (most commonly headache, nausea, flushing, and vasodilatation) and no serious adverse events were observed.

Studies of healthy volunteers also showed that the dose-adjusted pharmacokinetics were neither time- nor dose-dependent in the 10 to 120 mg/day range.[99,100] Febuxostat was readily absorbed (approximately 85%) after oral dosing,[101] and time to maximum concentration (t_{max}) was constant at approximately 1 hour, indicating rapid gastrointestinal absorption. Multiple oral dosing of febuxostat at the 120 mg/day dose resulted in the following values: area under the plasma concentration-time curve for the dose administration from 0 to 24 hours (AUC_{24}) 11.96 μg • hr/ml, maximum plasma drug concentration (C_{max}) 5.31 μg/ml, t_{max} 1.1 hours, elimination half-life ($t_{1/2}$) 11.9 hours. At doses above 120 mg/day, greater than dose proportional increases in AUC were observed, consistent with enterohepatic recirculation. The volume of distribution at steady state was 0.7 L/kg and drug was highly bound to plasma proteins, primarily albumin.[102] Febuxostat was metabolized in the liver mainly by conjugation via uridine diphosphate-glucuronosyltransferase (UGT) enzymes (UGT1A1,UGT1A3, UGT1A7, UGT1A9, UGT1A10, and UGT2B7), with a small portion oxidized into the active metabolites (67M-1, 67M-2, and 67M-4) by cytochrome P450 enzymes (CYP1A2, CYP2C8, and CYP2C9).[101,102] Febuxostat

and its metabolites were eliminated in the urine. Multiple oral administration of febuxostat led to urinary excretion of 25% to 45% of drug dose as either intact febuxostat or its conjugate (1% to 6% as unchanged drug) and 2% to 8% as oxidative metabolites.[99]

Effects of Renal Impairment

In a 7-day multiple-dosing study (febuxostat 80 mg/day) of participants with normal renal function (CrCl greater than 80 ml/min/1.73 m², n = 11) or mild (CrCl 50 to 80 ml/min/1.73 m², n = 6), moderate (CrCl 30 to 49 ml/min/1.73 m², n = 7), or severe (CrCl 10 to 29 ml/min/1.73 m², n = 7) renal impairment, the percentages of decrease in SU were comparable regardless of the renal function group.[103] Regardless of the renal function group, the mean SU concentrations decreased by 55% to 64% by day 7. Febuxostat was well tolerated in all groups. The t_{max} and C_{max} values of unbound febuxostat were not affected by CrCl. However, a relationship was observed between CrCl and the $t_{1/2}$, steady state clearance, and AUC_{24} of unbound febuxostat. A linear relationship was also observed between C_{max} for 67M-2 and 67M-4 and AUC_{24} for all three metabolites (67M-1, 67M-2, and 67M-4) and CrCl. Overall, these increases were not considered to be clinically important, and dose adjustment of febuxostat is not considered necessary in patients with mild to moderate renal impairment.

Effects of Hepatic Impairment

In a 7-day multiple-dosing study (febuxostat 80 mg/day) of participants with normal hepatic function (n = 12) or mild (Child-Pugh class A, n = 8) or moderate (Child-Pugh class B, n = 8) hepatic impairment, a significant reduction in SU was observed in those with mild and moderate hepatic impairment (49% reduction and 48% reduction, respectively).[104] However, this reduction in SU was lower than that observed for the participants with normal hepatic function (63% reduction, $p \le .005$ for both comparisons). Febuxostat was well tolerated in all groups. No significant differences were observed between those with hepatic impairment and those with normal liver function in the plasma pharmacokinetic parameters (including t_{max}, C_{max}, AUC_{24}, and $t_{1/2}$) for unbound febuxostat or its active metabolites. Thus, dose adjustment of febuxostat in patients with mild or moderate hepatic impairment is not considered necessary. No data are available for use in patients with severe hepatic impairment.

Effects of Age and Gender

In a 7-day multiple-dosing study of healthy participants (n = 48), designed to examine the effects of gender and age on the pharmacodynamics, pharmacokinetics, and safety of febuxostat 80 mg/day, a significant reduction in SU was observed in all groups.[105] Similar reductions in SU were observed in the younger participants (18 to 40 years) and the elderly participants (≥65 years). However, the percentage reduction in SU was significantly less in male participants compared with female participants (52% versus 59%, $p \leq .01$). No significant differences were observed between the two age groups in the plasma pharmacokinetic parameters (including t_{max}, C_{max}, AUC_{24}, and $t_{1/2}$). Although C_{max} and AUC_{24} for unbound febuxostat were higher in women as compared with men, the differences were not considered clinically significant and could be largely accounted for by weight differences between male and female participants. Accordingly, dose adjustment of febuxostat based on age or gender is not considered necessary.

Effects of Food

Following multiple 80 mg/day doses with a high-fat meal, there was a 49% decrease in C_{max} and an 18% decrease in AUC.[106] However, no clinically significant change in the reduction in SU was observed following multiple 80 mg doses. Therefore, febuxostat can be taken without regard to food intake.

Drug Interactions With Febuxostat

Drug-drug interaction studies have not identified clinically significant interactions between febuxostat and a number of other coadministered drugs, including ibuprofen, verapamil, nitrendipine, captopril, bezafibrate, warfarin, digoxin, colchicine, naproxen, indomethacin, hydrochlorothiazide, antacid, and theophylline.[102,106-109] Although febuxostat is a mild inhibitor of the CYP2D6 enzyme, studies with desipramine (a CYP2D6 substrate) did not show any clinically significant interactions.[110] Drug interaction studies with furosemide have not been reported. An important potential interaction that has not been tested in clinical studies is the interaction of febuxostat with azathioprine or 6-mercaptopurine; as outlined earlier, metabolism of these drugs is dependent on XO, and bone marrow toxicity can occur when allopurinol is coadministered with azathioprine or 6-mercaptopurine. The combination of febuxostat with azathioprine or 6-mercaptopurine should be avoided because of the risk of significant toxicity.

Clinical Trials of Febuxostat for the Hyperuricemia of Gout

In addition to the clinical pharmacology studies outlined earlier, one phase 2 controlled double-blind study, three phase 3 controlled double-blind studies, and two open-label long-term extension studies of febuxostat in patients with gout and hyperuricemia have been published. These studies have established the dose range, clinical efficacy, and safety of febuxostat for management of hyperuricemia of gout and are summarized here. In all of these clinical trials except the phase 2 study, allopurinol was used as an active comparator (results comparing febuxostat and allopurinol are summarized in Table 13-7). In all of these studies, patients had hyperuricemia (SU 8 mg/dL or greater) and a history of gout as defined by the American College of Rheumatology preliminary criteria for acute gout.[111] Typical exclusion criteria included severe renal impairment (CrCl less than 30 ml/min), pregnancy or lactation, use of azathioprine or 6-mercaptopurine, severe obesity (body mass index greater than 50 kg/m^2), hepatic impairment, history of alcohol abuse, or alcohol intake of greater than 14 drinks per week. The majority of participants were middle-aged Caucasian men. Comorbidities such as obesity, hypertension, and dyslipidemia were frequently present in participants at baseline. The primary endpoint was the proportion of patients achieving an SU concentration of less than 6 mg/dL at various time points.

Phase 2 Dose-Ranging Study

In a 28-day, randomized, double-blind, placebo-controlled trial, 153 patients were randomized to febuxostat (40 mg, 80 mg, or 120 mg/day) or placebo, with colchicine prophylaxis.[112] Exclusion criteria included serum creatinine greater than 1.5 mg/dL (CrCl less than 50 ml/min). The primary endpoint was the proportion of patients achieving SU less than 6 mg/dL on day 28. The primary endpoint was achieved in 0% of those taking placebo, 56% of those taking 40 mg, 76% taking 80 mg, and 94% taking 120 mg/day of febuxostat. Mean SU reduction from baseline was 2% in the placebo group and 37% in the 40 mg, 44% in the 80 mg, and 59% in the 120 mg febuxostat groups. Despite colchicine prophylaxis, gout flares were more frequently observed in those patients taking higher doses of febuxostat (37% in the placebo group and 35% in the 40 mg, 43% in the 80 mg, and 55% in the 120 mg febuxostat groups). Incidences of treatment-related adverse events were similar in the febuxostat and placebo groups. The most frequent adverse events were abdominal pain, diarrhea, and abnormal liver function tests.

The Febuxostat versus Allopurinol Controlled Trial (FACT)

A phase 3 randomized, double-blind, 52-week trial compared the safety and efficacy of febuxostat (80 mg or 120 mg/day) with allopurinol (300 mg/day) in 762 patients.[113] Prophylaxis against gout flares with colchicine or naproxen was given for the first 8 weeks of treatment. Exclusion criteria included serum creatinine greater than 1.5 mg/dL (CrCl less than 50 ml/min). The primary endpoint was the proportion of patients achieving SU less than 6 mg/dL at the last three monthly measurements. Clinical secondary endpoints were percentage change in index tophus area from baseline, change in the number of tophi at each visit, and proportion of patients requiring treatment for gout flares from weeks 9 to 52. The primary endpoint was achieved in 21% of those on allopurinol, 53% of those on 80 mg febuxostat, and 62% of those on 120 mg febuxostat ($p < .001$ for each febuxostat group

Table 13-7 Summary of Clinical Trials of the Efficacy of Allopurinol and Febuxostat

	Reference	Trial Design	Allopurinol	Febuxostat
SU reduction	113	FACT study (n = 762). Patients with gout and SU ≥8.0 mg/dL randomized to febuxostat (80 or 120 mg/day) or allopurinol (300 mg/day) for 52 wk. Primary endpoint SU <6 mg/dL at last 3 monthly visits.	Primary endpoint achieved by 21% of those on allopurinol	Primary endpoint achieved by 53% of those on febuxostat 80 mg/day and 62% on those on 120 mg/day
	114	APEX study (n = 1072). Patients with gout and SU ≥8.0 mg/dL and serum creatinine ≤2.0 mg/dL randomized to febuxostat (80, 120, or 240 mg/day), allopurinol (100 or 300 mg/day depending on renal function) or placebo for 28 wk. Primary endpoint SU <6 mg/dL at last 3 monthly visits.	Primary endpoint achieved by 22% of those on allopurinol	Primary endpoint achieved by 48% on febuxostat 80 mg/day, 65% on febuxostat 120 mg/day, and 69% febuxostat on 240 mg/day
	115	CONFIRMS study (n = 2269). Patients with gout and SU ≥8.0 mg/dL and CrCl ≥30 ml/min randomized to febuxostat (40 or 80 mg/day), allopurinol (200 or 300 mg/day depending on renal function) for 28 wk. Primary endpoint SU <6 mg/dL at the final visit.	Primary endpoint achieved by 42% of all patients on allopurinol. In those with renal impairment (CrCl 30-89 ml/min), primary endpoint achieved by 42% of patients on allopurinol.	Primary endpoint achieved by 45% of all patients on febuxostat 40 mg/day, 67% on febuxostat 80 mg/day. In those with renal impairment (CrCl 30-89 ml/min), primary endpoint achieved by 50% of patients on febuxostat 40 mg/day, 72% on febuxostat 80 mg/day.
	4	EXCEL study (n = 1086) 3-yr open label extension study febuxostat 80 or 120 mg/day vs. allopurinol 300 mg/day. Primary endpoint SU <6 mg/dL at each visit.	46% achieved SU<6 mg/dL after 1 mo. 56.6% allopurinol treated patients reassigned to febuxostat to attain target SU. Between 12 and 36 mo, 75%-100% maintained target SU irrespective of treatment	After 1 mo, SU <6 mg/dL in 81% (80 mg/day) and 87% (120 mg/day).
Gout flare rates	113	FACT study (n = 762). Patients with gout and SU ≥8.0 mg/dL randomized to febuxostat (80 or 120 mg/day) or allopurinol (300 mg/day) for 52 wk.	Between wk 9 and 52, 64% of patients on allopurinol had flares. Between wk 49-52, only 11% patients flared.	Between wk 9 and 52, 64% of patients on febuxostat 80 mg/day and 70% patients on febuxostat 120 mg/day had flares Between wk 49 and 52, only 8% of patients on febuxostat 80 mg/day and 6% patients on febuxostat 120 mg/day flared
	4	EXCEL study (n = 1086) 3-yr open label extension study febuxostat 80 or 120 mg/day vs. allopurinol 300 mg/day.	Maintenance of SU <6 mg/dL resulted in progressive reduction in flare rates such that flares occurred in <4% patients after 18 mo of ULT irrespective of treatment arm.	
Tophus resorption	113	FACT study (n = 762). Patients with gout and SU ≥8.0 mg/dL randomized to febuxostat (80 or 120 mg/day) or allopurinol (300 mg/day) for 52 wk.	Median reduction in tophus area was 50%	Median reduction in tophus area was 83% in febuxostat 80 mg/day and 66% in febuxostat 120 mg/day
	4	EXCEL study (n = 1086) open label extension study febuxostat 80 or 120 mg/day vs. allopurinol 300 mg/day.	Baseline tophus resolution achieved by 29%	Baseline tophus resolution achieved by 46% (80 mg/day) and 36%(120 mg/day)

Table 13-7 Summary of Clinical Trials of the Efficacy of Allopurinol and Febuxostat—cont'd

	Reference	Trial Design	Allopurinol	Febuxostat
Adverse event rates	113	FACT study (n = 762). Patients with gout and SU ≥8.0 mg/dL randomized to febuxostat (80 or 120 mg/day) or allopurinol (300 mg/day) for 52 wk.	Adverse event and serious adverse event rates similar between allopurinol and febuxostat.	
	114	APEX study (n = 1072). Patients with gout and SU ≥8.0 mg/dL and serum creatinine ≤2.0 mg/dL randomized to febuxostat (80, 120 or 240 mg/day), allopurinol (100 or 300 mg/day depending on renal function) or placebo for 28 wk.	Adverse event and serious adverse event rates similar between allopurinol and febuxostat.	
	115	CONFIRMS study (n = 2269). Patients with gout and SU ≥8.0 mg/dL and CrCl ≥30 ml/min randomized to febuxostat (40 or 80 mg/day), allopurinol (200 or 300 mg/day depending on renal function) for 28 wk.	Adverse event and serious adverse event rates similar between allopurinol and febuxostat	
	4	EXCEL study (n = 1086) open label extension study febuxostat 80 or 120 mg/day vs. allopurinol 300 mg/day.	Adverse event and serious adverse event rates similar between allopurinol and febuxostat	

compared with allopurinol) (Fig. 13-6). No difference in the frequency of gout flares was observed between weeks 9 and 52, but gout flares were significantly more common in the 120 mg febuxostat group in the first 8 weeks of treatment (21% in those on allopurinol, 22% in those on 80 mg febuxostat, and 36% in those on 120 mg febuxostat). No significant difference in sentinel tophus reduction was observed between treatment groups. Apart from gout flares, the incidence of adverse events and serious adverse events was similar in the three treatment groups; any treatment-emergent event was observed in 85% of patients in the allopurinol group, 80% in the 80 mg febuxostat group, and 75% in the 120 mg febuxostat group, and any serious adverse event was observed in 8% of patients in the allopurinol group, 4% in the 80 mg febuxostat group, and 8% in the 120 mg febuxostat group. The most common treatment-related adverse events for all groups were liver function test abnormalities, diarrhea, headache, and musculoskeletal signs and symptoms. More patients in the 120 mg febuxostat group discontinued from the study (39.0% compared with 26.0% in the allopurinol group and 34.2% in the 80 mg febuxostat group), due to higher rates of gout flares in the 120 mg febuxostat group. There was no significant difference in the number of deaths between the treatment groups (0% in those on allopurinol and 0.8% in those on febuxostat).

Allopurinol and Placebo-Controlled Efficacy Study of Febuxostat (APEX)

A phase 3 randomized, double-blind, 28-week trial compared the safety and efficacy of febuxostat (80 mg, 120 mg, or 240 mg/day) with allopurinol (300 mg or 100 mg/day, based on renal function) or placebo in 1072 patients.[114] This study included patients with normal renal function (serum

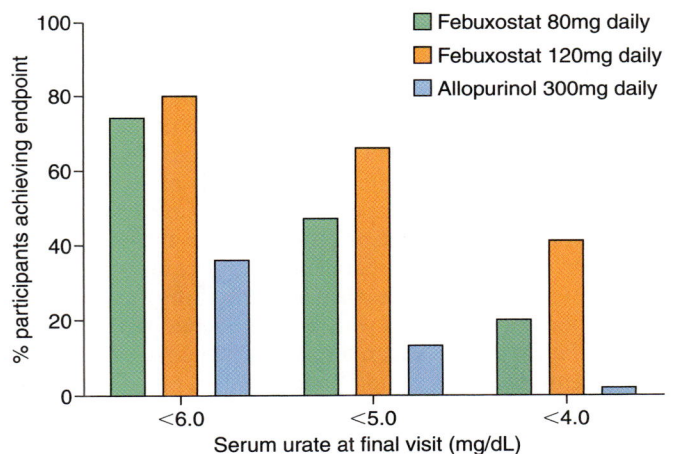

Figure 13-6 Serum urate concentrations in a 52-week randomized controlled trial of urate lowering therapy. *(From Becker MA, Schumacher HR Jr, Wortmann RL, et al. Febuxostat compared with allopurinol in patients with hyperuricemia and gout. N Engl J Med 2005;353(23):2450-61.)*

creatinine concentration 1.5 mg/dL or less, n = 1032) and impaired renal function (serum creatinine concentration greater than 1.5 to 2.0 mg/dL or less, n = 40). Prophylaxis against gout flares with colchicine or naproxen was given for the first 8 weeks of treatment. The primary endpoint was the proportion of patients achieving SU less than 6 mg/dL at the last three monthly measurements. The primary endpoint was achieved in 48% of patients treated with febuxostat 80 mg, 65% of those on 120 mg febuxostat, 69% of those on 240 mg febuxostat, 22% of those on allopurinol, and 0% of those on placebo ($p < .05$ for each febuxostat group compared with both allopurinol and placebo groups). In patients with impaired renal function, the primary endpoint was achieved in 44% of those treated with febuxostat 80 mg, 45% with febuxostat 120 mg, 60% with febuxostat 240 mg, and 0% with allopurinol ($p < .05$ for each febuxostat group compared with allopurinol). Premature withdrawal rates were higher in the febuxostat 80 mg and 240 mg groups (35% and 36%, respectively) than in the febuxostat 120 mg (26%) or allopurinol (21%) groups. The primary reasons for withdrawal were similar across all treatment groups except for gout flares, which were more frequently reported in the 120 mg and 240 mg febuxostat groups in the first 8 weeks compared with the other groups. After week 8 there was no difference between groups in the frequency of gout flares. No significant difference in tophus size reduction was observed between treatment groups. Generally, adverse events occurred with similar frequency across treatment groups and were mild or moderate in severity. A significantly higher incidence of diarrhea and dizziness was observed in the febuxostat 240 mg group compared with each of the other active treatment groups. Serious adverse events were reported with similar frequencies in all groups, the most common of which were cardiovascular disorders. No deaths were reported.

Phase 3, Double-Blind Randomized Controlled Trial Further Examining the Comparative Urate-Lowering Efficacy and Safety of Febuxostat and Allopurinol (the CONFIRMS Trial)

A further phase 3 randomized, double-blind, 28-week trial compared the safety and efficacy of febuxostat (40 mg or 80 mg/day) with allopurinol (300 mg or 200 mg/day, based on renal function) in 2269 patients.[115] At least 35% of patients enrolled were to have mild or moderate renal impairment, defined as baseline estimated CrCl (eCrCl) of 60 to 89 ml/min or 30 to 59 ml/min, respectively. Prophylaxis against gout flares with colchicine or naproxen was given throughout the treatment period. The primary endpoint was the proportion of patients achieving SU less than 6 mg/dL at the final visit and the proportion of patients with mild/moderate renal impairment achieving SU less than 6 mg/dL at the final visit. Safety assessments included blinded adjudication of each cardiovascular adverse event and death. The primary endpoint was achieved in 45% of patients treated with febuxostat 40 mg, 67% of those on 80 mg febuxostat, and 42% of those on allopurinol ($p < .001$ for the 80 mg febuxostat group compared with both 40 mg febuxostat and allopurinol, $p > .05$ for 40 mg febuxostat compared with allopurinol). In the 1483 patients with mild/moderate renal impairment, SU less than 6 mg/dL was achieved in 50% of patients treated with febuxostat 40 mg, 72% of those on 80 mg febuxostat, and 42% of those on allopurinol ($p \leq .001$ for the 80 mg febuxostat group compared with both 40 mg febuxostat and allopurinol, $p = .02$ for 40 mg febuxostat compared with allopurinol). Rates of adverse events and serious adverse events did not differ across treatment groups. Adjudicated cardiovascular event rates were 0% for febuxostat 40 mg and 0.4% for both febuxostat 80 mg and allopurinol. One death occurred in each febuxostat group and three occurred in the allopurinol group.

Further analysis of the CONFIRMS trial showed that a number of baseline clinical factors predicted higher urate-lowering

response rates to febuxostat; these factors included the presence of moderate renal impairment, older age, female sex, high adherence, nonsmoking, lower baseline SU, lower body mass index, and absence of tophi.[116]

Phase 2 Open-Label Extension Study (FOCUS)

Patients who completed the previous 28-day phase 2 study were entered into a 5-year open-label extension study.[117] Patients initially received febuxostat 80 mg/day, and dosing could be adjusted to febuxostat 40 or 120 mg between weeks 4 and 24. All patients received gout flare prophylaxis during the first 4 weeks. The primary efficacy endpoint was the proportion of patients who achieved and maintained SU less than 6 mg/dL. Additional efficacy endpoints included the proportion of patients requiring treatment for gout flare and the resolution of palpable tophi. Among 116 patients initially enrolled, dose adjustments were made for 44 (38%) patients. At 5 years, 93% (54 of 58) of the remaining patients had SU less than 6 mg/dL. Fifty-eight patients (50%) discontinued prematurely; 38 did so in the first year. Thirteen patients withdrew due to an adverse event, most commonly abnormal liver function test results (n = 3), cancer (n = 3), and increased serum creatinine (n = 2). Sustained reduction of SU was associated with nearly complete elimination of gout flares. In the 26 patients with a tophus at baseline, resolution of the index tophus was achieved in 69% (18 of 26) on study drug. There were no deaths reported during the study.

Febuxostat vs. Allopurinol Comparative Extension Long-term Study (EXCEL)

To evaluate long-term clinical efficacy and safety of febuxostat, an open-label extension of the FACT and APEX trials was undertaken[4] in which 1086 patients were assigned to fixed-dose daily ULT with febuxostat (80 mg or 120 mg/day) or allopurinol (300 mg/day). Treatment reassignment was permitted during months 1 to 6 to achieve SU concentrations between 3.0 and less than 6 mg/dL. Flares requiring treatment, tophus size, safety, and SU levels were monitored during up to 40 months of maintenance treatment. After 1 month of initial treatment, greater than 80% of patients receiving either febuxostat dose, but only 46% of subjects receiving allopurinol achieved SU less than 6 mg/dL. After treatment reassignment, 606 patients were on febuxostat 80 mg/day, 388 were on febuxostat 120 mg/day, and 92 were on allopurinol. After treatment reassignment, greater than 80% of all remaining patients maintained the primary efficacy endpoint of SU less than 6 mg/dL at each visit. Sustained reduction of SU was associated with nearly complete elimination of gout flares. Resolution of the index tophus was achieved by 46%, 36%, and 29% of subjects maintained on febuxostat 80 mg, febuxostat 120 mg, and allopurinol, respectively. Overall adverse event rates (including cardiovascular adverse event rates) did not differ significantly among treatment groups.

Special Populations/Subgroups

The majority of patients in the clinical trials just described were middle-aged Caucasian men. Subgroup analysis of other groups in these trials has been reported. In the

CONFIRMS study, the 374 patients aged 65 years or older had a similar clinical response to the entire CONFIRMS population with no increased rate of adverse events.[118] Post-hoc analysis of the 182 African American patients in the APEX and FACT studies showed a similar number of participants achieved sustained normouricemia with febuxostat as the entire study population and had similar rates of adverse events.[119] Similarly, analysis of the 226 women in the CONFIRMS, APEX, and FACT studies showed that febuxostat was effective in reducing the SU to less than 6 mg/dL, independent of renal function, and was well tolerated in female patients.[120]

Because allopurinol was used as an active comparator in the phase 3 trials of febuxostat, patients with intolerance or hypersensitivity to allopurinol were excluded from these studies. The safety of febuxostat was reported in a case series of 13 patients with previous severe AHS and renal impairment.[121] Febuxostat treatment was initiated at 40 mg/day in 12 patients and 20 mg/day in 1 patient. Febuxostat was well tolerated in 12 patients. One patient (an 85-year-old woman), previously hospitalized with documented exfoliative erythroderma during allopurinol treatment, developed biopsy-confirmed cutaneous leukocytoclastic vasculitis after 4-day exposure to febuxostat 40 mg/day. No evidence for other organ system involvement was detected, and the rash resolved promptly after febuxostat withdrawal. This patient had also received seasonal influenza vaccination on day 1 of febuxostat treatment. Ten of the 12 patients remaining on febuxostat maintained the SU less than 6 mg/dL. Thus, febuxostat appears to be a therapeutic option for those patients who were intolerant of allopurinol. However, the report of a hypersensitivity-type cutaneous vasculitis (likely but not definitively febuxostat-related) early in treatment emphasizes the need for careful dosing and close monitoring when febuxostat is considered in such patients.

Summary of Clinical Trial Data

Together, these trials have demonstrated the efficacy of febuxostat as a urate-lowering agent. A dose of 40 mg/day may be effective in achieving a target SU of less than 6 mg/dL and is the recommended starting dose.[122] However, a higher dose of 80 mg or 120 mg/day may be required to achieve this target. Febuxostat appears to be well tolerated and does not require dose adjustment in patients with mild to moderate renal or hepatic impairment. Liver function tests should be monitored while patients are taking febuxostat. Intensive prophylaxis against gout flares using colchicine or nonsteroidal antiinflammatory drugs should be prescribed for up to 6 months when commencing febuxostat. While febuxostat has been shown to be more effective than allopurinol at standard doses for reduction of SU, it is not yet known whether this drug is also superior with respect to other patient outcomes such as musculoskeletal function, joint damage, and tophus regression. Use of this drug in patients with severe renal impairment or dialysis, severe liver disease, tumor lysis syndrome, Lesch-Nyhan syndrome, and organ transplantation has not been evaluated. Similarly, use of febuxostat in children younger than 18 years has not been reported. Long-term safety data beyond 5.5 years are awaited.

Other Potential Indications for Febuxostat: Preclinical Studies of Renal Disease, Metabolic Syndrome, and Heart Failure

A number of studies in rodents have suggested a beneficial role for febuxostat in hypertension, renal disease, and metabolic syndrome. In the oxonic acid–induced rat model of hyperuricemia, febuxostat lowered SU, systolic blood pressure, and glomerular pressure.[123] Morphologic changes in the glomerulus were also observed with febuxostat treatment in this model, including reduction in afferent arteriole medial area, media-to-lumen ratio, glomerular cellularity, and mesangial matrix fraction. In normal rats, no effects on blood pressure or renal hemodynamics were observed with febuxostat, despite SU reduction. In rats with fructose-induced metabolic syndrome, treatment with febuxostat significantly lowered SU, blood pressure, triglycerides, and insulin.[124] Febuxostat treatment was also associated with reduced glomerular pressure, renal vasoconstriction, and afferent arteriolar area in this model. No significant effects were observed in rats on a normal diet treated with febuxostat. In 5/6 nephrectomized rats with and without oxonic acid–induced hyperuricemia, febuxostat reduced proteinuria, preserved renal function, and prevented glomerular hypertension.[125] These functional improvements were accompanied by preservation of afferent arteriolar morphology and reduced tubulointerstitial fibrosis.

In the clinical trials of febuxostat for treatment of hyperuricemia in patients with gout, changes in blood pressure or lipids have not been reported. However, post-hoc analysis of the FOCUS study has shown that intensive urate lowering with febuxostat was associated with improved renal function, as measured by the eGFR.[126] Human studies specifically designed to assess the effects of febuxostat on blood pressure, renal function, and parameters of metabolic syndrome have not yet been published.

As inhibition of XO with allopurinol and oxypurinol has been reported to have benefits on cardiac function in CHF in animal models and also in human disease, preclinical studies have been conducted to determine whether selective XO inhibition using febuxostat can improve cardiac hemodynamics in models of CHF. In the transverse aortic constriction (TAC) rodent model of left ventricular (LV) hypertrophy and dysfunction, daily administration of febuxostat commencing 60 minutes after TAC attenuated LV hypertrophy, dysfunction, and fibrosis and reduced measures of myocardial oxidative stress.[127] However, delayed treatment with febuxostat did not reverse the established changes of TAC-induced LV hypertrophy.[128] Similarly, in a rabbit model of CHF induced by coronary artery ligation, early treatment with febuxostat significantly lessened the reduction of LV function and attenuated the changes in LV dimensional parameters.[129] In contrast, when treatment with febuxostat was started after the establishment of CHF, no significant improvements in cardiac functional or dimensional parameters were observed. In dogs with pacing-induced CHF, febuxostat improved LV function with no change of myocardial oxygen consumption.[130] The role of febuxostat in human CHF has not been reported.

Role of Allopurinol and Febuxostat in Patients With Gout

Allopurinol has been the mainstay of ULT in patients with gout for more than 40 years. This agent is inexpensive and is effective for many patients, particularly when the dose is

Table 13-8 Comparison of the Advantages and Disadvantages of Allopurinol and Febuxostat

	Allopurinol	Febuxostat
Advantages	Single daily dose	Single daily dose
	Low drug cost	More effective urate-lowering than allopurinol when allopurinol dose limited by CrCl
	>40 yr clinical experience and safety data	Dose adjustment not required in mild-moderate renal impairment.
		Limited data on efficacy and safety in severe renal impairment
Disadvantages	Severe cutaneous reactions and potentially fatal AHS and DRESS	More expensive than allopurinol
	Drug interactions—azathioprine, 6-MP, theophylline, furosemide, ampicillins, warfarin	Drug interactions—azathioprine, 6-MP
	Limited safety data for doses above 300 mg daily, particularly in chronic kidney disease	Limited safety data beyond 5.5 yr
	Often ineffective in urate lowering at CrCl-based dose	
Dose	50-900 mg/day (maximum of 800 mg/day FDA-approved in USA)—can be titrated to achieve target SU	40-120 mg/day (maximum of 80 mg/day FDA-approved in USA)—can be titrated to achieve target SU

adjusted according to target SU concentrations rather than CrCl. There is extensive clinical experience of allopurinol in most relevant patient groups. However, dosing is controversial and severe life-threatening toxicity may occur, particularly in patients with renal impairment (Table 13-8).

As outlined earlier and summarized in Table 13-7, the clinical trials of febuxostat have consistently demonstrated that febuxostat has superior urate-lowering efficacy compared with allopurinol. However, in these studies, the dose of allopurinol was fixed and limited to a maximum of 300 mg/day. Furthermore, in those trials that included patients with even mild to moderate renal impairment, the allopurinol dose was further restricted (100 or 200 mg/day). Further studies are required to determine the comparative efficacy of allopurinol and febuxostat when a treat-to-target SU approach is used with allopurinol.

Febuxostat should be considered for those patients with gout who are intolerant to allopurinol or who have failed to achieve a target SU of less than 6 mg/dL on an adequate dose of allopurinol. Febuxostat may be particularly useful in the context of renal impairment, where allopurinol dosing is most complicated and carries the greatest risk of toxicity. However, clinical experience of febuxostat in patients with severe renal impairment, severe liver disease, and transplantation is very limited, and the safety of febuxostat in these situations is unknown. Importantly, the frequency of gout flares was consistently higher when commencing febuxostat compared with allopurinol in the FACT trial, a finding linked in post-hoc analysis to more extensive early serum urate lowering, and intensive gout prophylaxis is required to ensure that adherence to XO inhibitor treatment is maintained in the early phases of treatment.

Authors' Note

Since this book went into production, new studies of importance have been reported. A study of Korean patients with chronic renal impairment commencing allopurinol examined the role of HLA-B*5801 in development of severe cutaneous adverse reactions (SCARs).[147] One hundred percent of patients with allopurinol-SCAR were HLA-B*5801 positive compared to 9.5% allopurinol-tolerant patients (OR 179, p < 0.001). The frequency of HLA-B*5801 is high in certain populations (up to 20% in Han Chinese living in Taiwa1[148]) compared with other populations (1% to 3% in most European populations[149]). The role of routine HLA testing before commencing allopurinol in high-risk patients remains uncertain at present, noting that allopurinol-SCAR is a rare adverse event.

A study of allopurinol hypersensitivity syndrome (AHS) was reported at the European League Against Rheumatism meeting in 2011.[150] This case-controlled study examined the role of allopurinol starting dose as a risk factor for AHS, after carefully controlling for other known risk factors including renal function and diuretic use. Allopurinol starting doses were assessed using the Hande allopurinol dosing guidelines, based on creatinine clearance.

Patients with AHS were more likely to be commenced on a higher-than-recommended dose compared to controls (OR 16.7, p < 0.001). A clear relationship was observed between starting dose of allopurinol and risk of AHS. However, AHS also occurred in patients starting allopurinol at recommended doses. These data suggest that allopurinol should be commenced at low doses and that vigilance regarding AHS is important for all patients starting allopurinol.

References

1. Zhang W, Doherty M, Bardin T, et al. EULAR evidence based recommendations for gout. Part II: Management. Report of a task force of the EULAR Standing Committee for International Clinical Studies Including Therapeutics (ESCISIT). Ann Rheum Dis 2006;65(10):1312–24.
2. Li-Yu J, Clayburne G, Sieck M, et al. Treatment of chronic gout. Can we determine when urate stores are depleted enough to prevent attacks of gout? J Rheumatol 2001;28(3):577–80.
3. Shoji A, Yamanaka H, Kamatani N. A retrospective study of the relationship between serum urate level and recurrent attacks of gouty arthritis: evidence for reduction of recurrent gouty arthritis with antihyperuricemic therapy. Arthritis Rheum 2004;51(3):321–5.

4. Becker MA, Schumacher HR, MacDonald PA, et al. Clinical efficacy and safety of successful longterm urate lowering with febuxostat or allopurinol in subjects with gout. J Rheumatol 2009;36(6):1273–82.

5. Spector T. Inhibition of urate production by allopurinol. Biochem Pharmacol 1977;26(5):355–8.

6. Okamoto K, Eger BT, Nishino T, et al. Mechanism of inhibition of xanthine oxidoreductase by allopurinol: crystal structure of reduced bovine milk xanthine oxidoreductase bound with oxipurinol. Nucleosides Nucleotides Nucl Acids 2008;27(6):888–93.

7. Walter-Sack I, de Vries JX, Ernst B, et al. Uric acid lowering effect of oxipurinol sodium in hyperuricemic patients: therapeutic equivalence to allopurinol. J Rheumatol 1996;23(3):498–501.

8. Takano Y, Hase-Aoki K, Horiuchi H, et al. Selectivity of febuxostat, a novel non-purine inhibitor of xanthine oxidase/xanthine dehydrogenase. Life Sci 2005;76(16):1835–47.

9. Schmidt AP, Bohmer AE, Antunes C, et al. Anti-nociceptive properties of the xanthine oxidase inhibitor allopurinol in mice: role of A1 adenosine receptors. Br J Pharmacol 2009;156(1):163–72.

10. Graham S, Day R, Wong H, et al. Pharmacodynamics of oxypurinol after administration of allopurinol to healthy subjects. Br J Clin Pharmacol 1996;41:299–304.

11. Reiter S, Simmonds HA, Zollner N, et al. Demonstration of a combined deficiency of xanthine oxidase and aldehyde oxidase in xanthinuric patients not forming oxipurinol. Clin Chim Acta 1990;187(3):221–34.

12. Shibutani Y, Ueo T, Yamamoto T, et al. A case of classical xanthinuria (type 1) with diabetes mellitus and Hashimoto's thyroiditis. Clin Chim Acta 1999;285(1-2):183–9.

13. Stamp L, Ha L, Searle M, et al. Gout in renal transplant recipients. Nephrology 2006;11:367–71.

14. Venkat Raman G, Sharman V, Lee H. Azathioprine and allopurinol: a potentially dangerous combination. J Int Med 1990;228:69–71.

15. Cummins D, Sekar M, Halil O, et al. Myelosuppression associated with azathioprine-allopurinol interaction after heart and lung transplantation. Transplantation 1996;61(11):1661–2.

16. Wluka A, Ryan P, Miller A, et al. Post-cardiac transplantation gout: incidence and therapeutic complications. J Heart Lung Transplant 2000;19:951–6.

17. Bryne P, Fraser A, Pritchard M. Treatment of gout following cardiac transplantation. Rheumatology 1996;35(12):1329.

18. Reyes A. Cardiovascular drugs and serum uric acid. Cardiovasc Drug Ther 2003;17(5/6):397–414.

19. Yamamoto T, Moriwaki Y, Takahashi S, et al. Effect of frusemide on renal excretion of oxypurinol and purine bases. Metabolism 2001;50(2):241–5.

20. Stamp L, O'Donnell J, Zhang M, et al. Using allopurinol above the dose based on creatinine clearance is effective and safe in chronic gout, including in those with renal impairment. Arthritis Rheum 2010.

21. Hande KR. Evaluation of a thiazide-allopurinol drug interaction. Am J Med Sci 1986;292(4):213–6.

22. de Vries JX, Voss A, Ittensohn A, et al. Interaction of allopurinol and hydrochlorothiazide during prolonged oral administration of both drugs in normal subjects. II. Kinetics of allopurinol, oxipurinol, and hydrochlorothiazide. Clin Investig 1994;72(12):1076–81.

23. Loffler W, Landthaler R, de Vries JX, et al. Interaction of allopurinol and hydrochlorothiazide during prolonged oral administration of both drugs in normal subjects. I. Uric acid kinetics. Clin Investig 1994;72(12):1071–5.

24. Reinders M, Van Roon E, Houtmann P, et al. Biochemical effectiveness of allopurinol and allopurinol-probenecid in previously benzbromarone-treated gout patients. Clin Rheumatol 2007;26:1459–65.

25. Stocker S, Williams K, McLachlan A, et al. Pharmacokinetic and pharmacodynamic interaction between allopurinol and probenecid in healthy subjects. Clin Pharmacokinet 2008;47(2):111–8.

26. Muller F, Schall R, Groenewound G, et al. The effect of benzbromarone on allopurinol/oxypurinol kinetics in patients with gout. Eur J Clin Pharmacol 1993;44:69–72.

27. Colin J, Farinotti R, Fredj G, et al. Kinetics of allopurinol and oxipurinol after chronic oral administration. Interaction with benzbromarone. Eur J Clin Pharmacol 1986;31:53–8.

28. Mertz D, Eichhorn R. Does benzbromarone in therapeutic doses raise renal excretion of oxipurinol? Klin Wochenschr 1984;62(24):1170–2.

29. Stamp L, Xiaoyu Z, Dalbeth N, et al. Serum urate as a soluble biomarker in chronic gout: evidence that serum urate fulfils the OMERACT validation criteria for soluble biomarkers. Semin Arthritis Rheum 2010.

30. Riedel A, Nelson M, Joseph-Ridge N, et al. Compliance with allopurinol therapy among managed care enrollees with gout: a retrospective analysis of administrative claims. J Rheumatol 2004;31(8):1575–81.

31. Harrold L, Andrade S, Briesacher B, et al. Adherence with urate-lowering therapies for the treatment of gout. Arthritis Res Ther 2009;11:R46.

32. Perez-Ruiz F, Calabozo M, Pijoan J, et al. Effect of urate-lowering therapy on the velocity of size reduction of tophi in chronic gout. Arthritis Care Res 2002;47(4):356–60.

33. Beutler A, Rull M, Schlesinger N, et al. Treatment with allopurinol decreases the number of acute gout attacks despite persistently elevated serum uric acid levels. Clin Exp Rheumatol 2001;19(5):595.

34. Sarawate CA, Brewer KK, Yang W, et al. Gout medication treatment patterns and adherence to standards of care from a managed care perspective. Mayo Clin Proc 2006;81(7):925–34.

35. Bellomo G, Venanzi S, Verdura C, et al. Association of uric acid with change in kidney function in healthy normotensive individuals. Am J Kidney Dis 2010;56:264–73.

36. Ohno I, Hsoya T, Gomi H, et al. Serum uric acid and renal prognosis in patients with IgA nephropathy. Nephron 2001;87(4):333–9.

37. Ficociello L, Rosolowsky E, Niswczas M, et al. High-normal serum uric acid increases risk of early progressive renal function loss in type 1 diabetes. Diabetes Care 2010;33(6):1337–43.

38. Iseki K, Ikemiya Y, Inoue T, et al. Significant hyperuricemia as a risk factor for developing ESRD in a screened cohort. Am J Kidney Dis 2004;44(4):642–50.

39. Siu Y-P, Leung K-T, Tong M, et al. Use of allopurinol in slowing the progression of renal disease through its ability to lower serum uric acid level. Am J Kidney Dis 2006;47(1):51–9.

40. Goicoechea M, de Vinuesa S, Verdalles U, et al. Effect of allopurinol in chronic kidney disease progression and cardiovascular risk. Clin J Am Soc Nephrol 2010:5.

41. Edwards N. The role of hyperuricemia in vascular disorders. Curr Opin Rheumatol 2009;21:132–7.

42. Jankowska E, Ponikowska B, Majda J, et al. Hyperuricemia predicts poor outcome in patients with mild to moderate chronic heart failure. Int J Cardiol 2007;115(2):151–5.

43. Anker S, Doehner W, Rauchhaus M, et al. Uric acid and survival in chronic heart failure. Validation and application in metabolic, functional and hemodynamic staging. Circulation 2003;107(15):1991–7.

44. Krishnan E, Baker J, Furst D, et al. Gout and the risk of acute myocardial infarction. Arthritis Rheum 2006;54(8):2688–96.

45. Krishnan E, Svendsen K, Neaton J. Long-term cardiovascular mortality among middle-aged men with gout. Arch Int Med 2008;168(10):1104–10.

46. Choi H, Curhan G. Independent impact of gout on mortality and risk for coronary heart disease. Circulation 2007;116:894–900.

47. Cappola TP, Kass DA, Nelson GS, et al. Allopurinol improves myocardial efficiency in patients with idiopathic dilated cardiomyopathy. Circulation 2001;104(20):2407–11.

48. Spiekermann S, Landmesser U, Dikalov S, et al. Electron spin resonance characterization of vascular xanthine and NAD(P)H oxidase activity in patients with coronary artery disease. Circulation 2003;107:1383–9.

49. Luk AJ, Levin GP, Moore EE, et al. Allopurinol and hyperuricaemic patients. Rheumatology (Oxford) 2009;48(7):804–6.

50. Struthers A, Donnan P, Lindsay P, et al. Effect of allopurinol on mortality and hospitalisations in chronic heart failure; a retrospective cohort study. Heart 2002;87(3):229–34.

51. Thanassoulis G, Brophy J, Richard H, et al. Gout, allopurinol use and heart failure outcomes. Arch Intern Med 2010;170(15):1358–64.

52. Hare JM, Mangal B, Brown J, et al. Impact of oxypurinol in patients with symptomatic heart failure. J Am Coll Cardiol 2008;51(24):2301–9.

53. Norman A, Ang D, Ogston S, et al. Effect of high dose allopurinol on exercise in patients with chronic stable angina: a randomised, placebo controlled crossover trial. Lancet 2010;375:2161–7.

54. Rentoukas E, Tasarouhas K, Tsitsimpikou C, et al. The prognostic impact of allopurinol in patients with acute myocardial infarction undergoing primary percutaneous coronary intervention. Int J Cardiol 2009.doi:10.1016/j.ijcard.2009.08.037.

55. Cannon P, Stason W, Demartini F, et al. Hyperuricemia in primary and renal hypertension. N Engl J Med 1966;275:457–64.

56. Annemans L, Spaepen E, Gaskin M, et al. Gout in the UK and Germany: prevalence, comorbidities and management in general practice 2000-2005. Ann Rheum Dis 2008;67(7):960–6.

57. Chen S-Y, Chen C-L, Shen M- L. Manifestations of metabolic syndrome associated with male gout in different age strata. Clin Rheumatol 2007;26:1453–7.

58. Johnson R, Kang D-H, Feig D, et al. Is there a pathogenic role for uric acid in hypertension and cardiovascular renal disease? Hypertension 2003;41:1183–90.

59. Burnier M, Rutschmann B, Nussberger J, et al. Salt-dependent renal effects of an angiotensin II antagonist in healthy subjects. Hypertension 1993;22:339–47.

60. Chanard J, Toupance O, Lavaud S, et al. Amlodipine reduces cyclosporin-induced hyperuricemia in hypertensive renal transplant recipients. Nephrol Dial Transplant 2003;18:2147–53.

61. Sennesael J, Lamote J, Violet I, et al. Divergent effects of calcium channel and angiotensin converting enzyme blockade on glomerulotubular function in cyclosporin-treated renal allograft recipients. Am J Kidney Dis 1996;27(5):701–8.

62. Kanbay M, Ozkara A, Selcoki Y, et al. Effect of treatment of hyperuricemia with allopurinol on blood pressure, creatinine clearance, and proteinuria in patients with normal renal functions. Int Urol Nephrol 2007;39(4):1227–33.

63. Feig D, Soletsky B, Johnson R. Effect of allopurinol on blood pressure of adolescents with newly diagnosed essential hypertension. JAMA 2010;300(8):924–32.

64. McInnes G, Lawson D, Jick H. Acute adverse reactions attributed to allopurinol in hospitalised patients. Ann Rheum Dis 1981;40:245–9.

65. Gutierrez-Macias A, Lizarralde-Palacios E, Martinez-Odriozola P, et al. Fatal allopurinol hypersensitivity syndrome after treatment of asymptomatic hyperuricemia. Br Med J 2005;331:623–4.

66. Halevy S, Ghislain PD, Mockenhaupt M, et al. Allopurinol is the most common cause of Stevens-Johnson syndrome and toxic epidermal necrolysis in Europe and Israel. J Am Acad Dermatol 2008;58(1):25–32.

67. Hung S, Chung W, Liou L, et al. HLA-B*5801 allele as a genetic marker for severe cutaneous adverse reactions caused by allopurinol. Proc Natl Acad Sci USA 2005;102(11):4134–9.

68. Kaniwa N, Saito Y, Aihara M, et al. HLA-B locus in Japanese patients with anti-epileptics and allopurinol-related Stevens-Johnson syndrome and toxic epidermal necrolysis. Pharmacogenomics 2008;9(11):1617–22.

69. Tassaneeyakul W, Jantararoungtont T, Chen P, et al. Strong association between HLA-B*5801 and allopurinol-induced Stevens-Johnson syndrome and toxic epidermal necrolysis in a Thai population. Pharmacogenet Genom 2009;19(9):704–9.

70. Lonjou C, Borot N, Sekula P, et al. A European study of HLA-B in Stevens-Johnson syndrome and toxic epidermal necrolysis related to five high risk drugs. Pharmacogenet Genom 2008;18(2):99–107.

71. Hande K, Noone R, Stone W. Severe allopurinol toxicity. Description and guidelines for prevention in patients with renal insufficiency. Am J Med 1984;76:47–56.

72. Lupton G, Odom R. Severe allopurinol hypersensitivity syndrome. J Am Acad Dermatol 1979;72:1361–8.

73. Singer J, Wallace S. The allopurinol hypersensitivity syndrome. Unnecessary morbidity and mortality. Arthritis Rheum 1986;29:82–7.

74. Arellano F, Sacristan J. Allopurinol hypersensitivity syndrome: a review. Ann Pharmacother 1993;27:337–43.

75. Lang P. Severe hypersensitivity reactions to allopurinol. South Med J 1979;72(11):1361–8.

76. Elion G, Yu T-F, Gutman A, et al. Renal clearance of oxipurinol, the chief metabolite of allopurinol. Am J Med 1968;45:69–77.

77. Emmerson BT, Hazelton RA, Frazer IH. Some adverse reactions to allopurinol may be mediated by lymphocyte reactivity to oxypurinol. Arthritis Rheum 1988;31(3):436–40.

78. Puig J, Casas E, Ramos T, et al. Plasma oxypurinol concentration in a patient with allopurinol hypersensitivity. J Rheumatol 1989;16(6):842–4.

79. Chen YC, Chiu HC, Chu CY. Drug reaction with eosinophilia and systemic symptoms: a retrospective study of 60 cases. Arch Dermatol 2010.

80. Peyriere H, Dereure O, Breton H, et al. Variability in the clinical pattern of cutaneous side-effects of drugs with systemic symptoms: does a DRESS syndrome really exist? Br J Dermatol 2006;155(2):422–8.

81. Rothwell PM, Grant R. Cerebral vasculitis following allopurinol treatment. Postgrad Med J 1996;72(844):119–20.

82. Boyer TD, Sun N, Reynolds TB. Allopurinol-hypersensitivity vasculitis and liver damage. West J Med 1977;126(2):143–7.

83. Choi HK, Merkel PA, Walker AM, et al. Drug-associated antineutrophil cytoplasmic antibody-positive vasculitis: prevalence among patients with high titers of antimyeloperoxidase antibodies. Arthritis Rheum 2000;43(2):405–13.

84. Horiuchi H, Ota M, Kaneko H, et al. Nephrotoxic effects of allopurinol in dinitrofluorobenzene-sensitized mice: comparative studies on TEI-6720. Res Commun Mol Pathol Pharmacol 1999;104(3):293–305.

85. Brunstein MG, Ghisolfi ES, Ramos FL, et al. A clinical trial of adjuvant allopurinol therapy for moderately refractory schizophrenia. J Clin Psychiatry 2005;66(2):213–9.

86. Medicine UNLoMD. FDA information: allopurinol tablet.

87. Jordan KM, Cameron JS, Snaith M, et al. British Society for Rheumatology and British Health Professionals in Rheumatology guideline for the management of gout. Rheumatology 2007;46(8):1372–4.

88. Dalbeth N, Kumar S, Stamp LK, et al. Dose adjustment of allopurinol according to creatinine clearance does not provide adequate control of hyperuricemia in patients with gout. J Rheumatol 2006;33(8):1646–50.

89. Vazquez-Mellado J, Meono Morales E, Pacheco-Tena C, et al. Relationship between adverse events associated with allopurinol and renal function in patients with gout. Ann Rheum Dis 2001;60:981–3.

90. Silverberg M, Mallela R, Lesse A, et al. Allopurinol hypersensitivity reactions: a case-control study of the role of renal dosing. Arthritis Rheum 2009;60(Suppl. 10):S414.

91. Stamp L, O'Donnell J, Zhang M, et al. Increasing allopurinol dose above the recommended range is effective and safe in chronic gout, including in those with renal impairment. Arthritis Rheum 2009;60(suppl. 10):S729.

92. Perez-Ruiz F, Alonso-Ruiz A, Calabozo M, et al. Efficacy of allopurinol and benzbromarone for the control of hyperuricemia. A pathogenic approach to the treatment of primary chronic gout. Ann Rheum Dis 1998;57:545–9.

93. Emmerson B, Gordon R, Cross M, et al. Plasma oxypurinol concentrations during allopurinol therapy. Br J Rheumatol 1987;26:445–9.

94. Peterson G, Boyle R, Francis H, et al. Dosage prescribing and plasma oxypurinol levels in patients receiving allopurinol therapy. Eur J Clin Pharmacol 1990;39:419–21.

95. Osada Y, Tsuchimoto M, Fukushima H, et al. Hypouricemic effect of the novel xanthine oxidase inhibitor, TEI-6720, in rodents. Eur J Pharmacol 1993;241(2-3):183–8.

96. Okamoto K, Eger BT, Nishino T, et al. An extremely potent inhibitor of xanthine oxidoreductase. Crystal structure of the enzyme-inhibitor complex and mechanism of inhibition. J Biol Chem 2003;278(3):1848–55.

97. Yamamoto T, Moriwaki Y, Fujimura Y, et al. Effect of TEI-6720, a xanthine oxidase inhibitor, on the nucleoside transport in the lung cancer cell line A549. Pharmacology 2000;60(1):34–40.

98. Komoriya K, Osada Y, Hasegawa M, et al. Hypouricemic effect of allopurinol and the novel xanthine oxidase inhibitor TEI-6720 in chimpanzees. Eur J Pharmacol 1993;250(3):455–60.

99. Becker MA, Kisicki J, Khosravan R, et al. Febuxostat (TMX-67), a novel, non-purine, selective inhibitor of xanthine oxidase, is safe and decreases serum urate in healthy volunteers. Nucleosides Nucleotides Nucleic Acids 2004;23(8-9):1111–6.

100. Khosravan R, Grabowski BA, Wu JT, et al. Pharmacokinetics, pharmacodynamics and safety of febuxostat, a non-purine selective inhibitor of xanthine oxidase, in a dose escalation study in healthy subjects. Clin Pharmacokinet 2006;45(8):821–41.

101. Grabowski BA, Khosravan R, Vernillet L, et al. Metabolism and excretion of [14C] febuxostat, a novel nonpurine selective inhibitor of xanthine oxidase, in healthy male subjects. J Clin Pharmacol 2010.

102. Mukoyoshi M, Nishimura S, Hoshide S, et al. In vitro drug-drug interaction studies with febuxostat, a novel non-purine selective inhibitor of xanthine oxidase: plasma protein binding, identification of metabolic enzymes and cytochrome P450 inhibition. Xenobiotica 2008;38(5):496–510.

103. Mayer MD, Khosravan R, Vernillet L, et al. Pharmacokinetics and pharmacodynamics of febuxostat, a new non-purine selective inhibitor of xanthine oxidase in subjects with renal impairment. Am J Ther 2005;12(1):22–34.

104. Khosravan R, Grabowski BA, Mayer MD, et al. The effect of mild and moderate hepatic impairment on pharmacokinetics, pharmacodynamics, and safety of febuxostat, a novel nonpurine selective inhibitor of xanthine oxidase. J Clin Pharmacol 2006;46(1):88–102.

105. Khosravan R, Kukulka MJ, Wu JT, et al. The effect of age and gender on pharmacokinetics, pharmacodynamics, and safety of febuxostat, a novel nonpurine selective inhibitor of xanthine oxidase. J Clin Pharmacol 2008;48(9):1014–24.

106. Khosravan R, Grabowski B, Wu JT, et al. Effect of food or antacid on pharmacokinetics and pharmacodynamics of febuxostat in healthy subjects. Br J Clin Pharmacol 2008;65(3):355–63.

107. Khosravan R, Wu T, Joseph-Ridge N, et al. Pharmacokinetic interactions of concomitant administration of febuxostat and NSAIDs. J Clin Pharmacol 2006;46(8):855–66.

108. Grabowski B, Khosravan R, Wu JT, et al. Effect of hydrochlorothiazide on the pharmacokinetics and pharmacodynamics of febuxostat, a non-purine selective inhibitor of xanthine oxidase. Br J Clin Pharmacol 2010;70(1):57–64.

109. Tsai M, Wu J, Gunawardhana L, et al. Effect of multiple doses of febuxostat on the pharmacokinetics of a single dose of theophylline. Presented at the American College of Rheumatology Annual Scientific Meeting, Atlanta, GA, 2010, abstract 149.

110. Khosravan R, Erdman K, Vernillet L, et al. Effect of febuxostat on pharmacokinetics of desipramine, a CYP2D6 substrate, in healthy subjects. Clin Pharmacol Ther 2005;77:43.

111. Wallace SL, Robinson H, Masi AT, et al. Preliminary criteria for the classification of the acute arthritis of primary gout. Arthritis Rheum 1977;20(3):895–900.

112. Becker MA, Schumacher Jr HR, Wortmann RL, et al. Febuxostat, a novel nonpurine selective inhibitor of xanthine oxidase: a twenty-eight-day, multicenter, phase II, randomized, double-blind, placebo-controlled, dose-response clinical trial examining safety and efficacy in patients with gout. Arthritis Rheum 2005;52(3):916–23.

113. Becker MA, Schumacher Jr HR, Wortmann RL, et al. Febuxostat compared with allopurinol in patients with hyperuricemia and gout. N Engl J Med 2005;353(23):2450–61.

114. Schumacher Jr HR, Becker MA, Wortmann RL, et al. Effects of febuxostat versus allopurinol and placebo in reducing serum urate in subjects with hyperuricemia and gout: a 28-week, phase III, randomized, double-blind, parallel-group trial. Arthritis Rheum 2008;59(11):1540–8.

115. Becker MA, Schumacher HR, Espinoza LR, et al. The urate-lowering efficacy and safety of febuxostat in the treatment of the hyperuricemia of gout: the CONFIRMS trial. Arthritis Res Ther 2010;12(2):R63.

116. Becker MA, MacDonald P, Chefo S, et al. Baseline (BL) characteristics of gout subjects influence urate-lowering (UL) efficacy during febuxostat and allopurinol treatment. Presented at the American College of Rheumatology Annual Scientific Meeting, Philadelphia, PA, 2009, abstract 704.

117. Schumacher Jr HR, Becker MA, Lloyd E, et al. Febuxostat in the treatment of gout: 5-yr findings of the FOCUS efficacy and safety study. Rheumatology (Oxford) 2009;48(2):188–94.

118. Krishnan E, MacDonald PA, Hunt B, et al. Febuxostat versus allopurinol in the treatment of gout in subjects ≥65 years of age: a subgroup analysis of the CONFIRMS trial. Presented at the American College of Rheumatology Annual Scientific Meeting, Atlanta, GA, 2010, abstract 154.

119. Becker MA, MacDonald PA, Lloyd EJ, et al. Urate-lowering pharmacotherapy with febuxostat (FEB) or allopurinol (ALLO) in African-American subjects with gout. Presented at the American College of Rheumatology Annual Scientific Meeting, Atlanta, GA, 2010, abstract 1622.

120. Chohan S, Becker MA, MacDonald PA, et al. Urate-lowering (UL) efficacy and safety of febuxostat (FEB) and allopurinol (ALLO) in women with gout, an older subset of gout subjects with increased comorbidity. Presented at the American College of Rheumatology Annual Scientific Meeting, Atlanta, GA, 2010, abstract 165.

121. Chohan S, Becker MA. Safety and efficacy of febuxostat (FEB) treatment in subjects with gout and severe allopurinol (ALLO) adverse reactions. Presented at the American College of Rheumatology Annual Scientific Meeting, Atlanta, GA, 2010, abstract 158.

122. Takeda Pharmaceuticals. Febuxostat prescribing information. http://www.uloric.com/hcp/.

123. Sanchez-Lozada LG, Tapia E, Soto V, et al. Treatment with the xanthine oxidase inhibitor febuxostat lowers uric acid and alleviates systemic and glomerular hypertension in experimental hyperuricemia. Nephrol Dial Transplant 2008;23(4):1179–85.

124. Sanchez-Lozada LG, Tapia E, Bautista-Garcia P, et al. Effects of febuxostat on metabolic and renal alterations in rats with fructose-induced metabolic syndrome. Am J Physiol Renal Physiol 2008;294(4):F710–8.

125. Sanchez-Lozada LG, Tapia E, Soto V, et al. Effect of febuxostat on the progression of renal disease in 5/6 nephrectomy rats with and without hyperuricemia. Nephron Physiol 2008;108(4):69–78.

126. Whelton A, MacDonald P, Lloyd E, et al. Beneficial relationship of serum urate (sUA) reduction and estimated glomerular filtration rate (eGFR) improvement/maintenance in hyperuricemic gout subjects treated for up to 5.5 years with febuxostat (FEB). Presented at the American College of Rheumatology Annual Scientific Meeting, San Francisco, CA, 2008, abstract L7.

127. Xu X, Hu X, Lu Z, et al. Xanthine oxidase inhibition with febuxostat attenuates systolic overload-induced left ventricular hypertrophy and dysfunction in mice. J Card Fail 2008;14(9):746–53.

128. Xu X, Zhao L, Hu X, et al. Delayed treatment effects of xanthine oxidase inhibition on systolic overload-induced left ventricular hypertrophy and dysfunction. Nucleosides Nucleotides Nucl Acids 2010;29(4-6):306–13.

129. Zhao L, Roche BM, Wessale JL, et al. Chronic xanthine oxidase inhibition following myocardial infarction in rabbits: effects of early versus delayed treatment. Life Sci 2008;82(9-10):495–502.

130. Hou M, Hu Q, Chen Y, et al. Acute effects of febuxostat, a nonpurine selective inhibitor of xanthine oxidase, in pacing induced heart failure. J Cardiovasc Pharmacol 2006;48(5):255–63.

131. Day R, Graham G, Hicks M, et al. Clinical pharmacokinetics and pharmacodynamics of allopurinol and oxypurinol. Clin Pharmacokinet 2007;46(8):623–44.

132. Turnheim K, Krivanek P, Oberbauer R. Pharmacokinetics and pharmacodynamics of allopurinol in elderly and young subjects. Br J Clin Pharmacol 1999;48:501–9.

133. Hande K, Reed E, Chabner B. Allopurinol kinetics. Clin Pharmacol Ther 1978;23(5):598–605.

134. Loebl WY, Scott JT. Withdrawal of allopurinol in patients with gout. Ann Rheum Dis 1974;33(4):304–7.

135. Perez-Ruiz F, Calaabozo M, Fernardez-Lopez J, et al. Treatment of chronic gout in patients with renal function impairment: an open, randomised, actively controlled study. J Clin Rheumatol 1999;5(2):49–55.

136. Shelmadine B, Bowden R, Wilson R, et al. The effects of lowering uric acid levels using allopurinol on markers of metabolic syndrome in end-stage renal disease patients: a pilot study. Anadolu Kardiyol Derg 2009;9:385–9.

137. Reinders M, Haagsma C, Jansen T, et al. A randomised controlled trial on the efficacy and tolerability with dose escalation of allopurinol 300-600 mg/day versus benzbromarone 100-200 mg/day in patients with gout. Ann Rheum Dis 2009;68:892–7.

138. Saliaris AP, Amado LC, Minhas KM, et al. Chronic allopurinol administration ameliorates maladaptive alterations in Ca2+ cycling proteins and beta-adrenergic hyporesponsiveness in heart failure. Am J Physiol Heart Circ Physiol 2007;292(3):H1328–35.

139. George J, Carr E, Davies J, et al. High-dose allopurinol improves endothelial function by profoundly reducing vascular oxidative stress and not by lowering uric acid. Circulation 2006;114(23):2508–16.

140. Perez N, Gao W, Marban E. Novel myofilament Ca^{2+}-sensitizing property of xanthine oxidase inhibitors. Circ Res 1998;83(4):423–30.

141. Mazzali M, Hughes J, Kim YG, et al. Elevated uric acid increases blood pressure in the rat by a novel crystal-independent mechanism. Hypertension 2001;38(5):1101–6.

142. Dalbeth N, Stamp L. Allopurinol dosing in renal impairment: walking the tightrope between adequate urate lowering and adverse events. Semin Dialysis 2007;20(5):391–5.

143. Young J, Boswell R, Nies A. Severe allopurinol hypersensitivity. Arch Int Med 1974;134:553–8.

144. Khanna D, Pandya B, D'Souza A, et al. Incidence of allopurinol hypersensitivity syndrome (AHS) among renally impaired patients. Arthritis Rheum 2009;60(suppl. 10):S761.

145. Perez-Ruiz F, Hernando I, Villar I, et al. Correction of allopurinol dosing should be based on clearance of creatinine, but not plasma creatinine levels: another insight into allopurinol related toxicity. J Clin Rheumatol 2005;11:129–33.

146. Fernando SL, Broadfoot AJ. Prevention of severe cutaneous adverse drug reactions: the emerging value of pharmacogenetic screening. CMAJ 2010;182(5):476–480.

147. Jung JW, Song WJ, Kim YS, et al. HLA-B58 can help the clinical decision on starting allopurinol in patients with chronic renal insufficiency. Nephrol Dial Transplant 2011.

148. Hung SI, Chung WH, Liou LB, et al. HLA-B*5801 allele as a genetic marker for severe cutaneous adverse reactions caused by allopurinol. Proc Natl Acad Sci USA 2005;102(11):4134–4139.

149. Middleton D, Menchaca L, Rood H, Komerofsky R. New allele frequency database. http://www.allelefrequencies.net. Tissue Antigens 2003;61(5):403–407.

150. Stamp LK, Dockerty J, Frampton C, et al. Allopurinol starting dose as a risk factor for allopurinol hypersensitivity syndrome in patients with gout. EULAR Annual Scientific Meeting 2011; London.

Chapter 14

Uricase Therapy of Gout

George Nuki

KEY POINTS

- Uricolytic therapy with uricase (urate oxidase) degrades uric acid, ultimately resulting in the production of allantoin, which is much more soluble and readily excreted in the urine than is uric acid.
- As a result of loss of expression of uricase during hominid evolution and a delicate balance of uric acid production and elimination in man, humans are unusually predisposed to develop gout because tissue levels of urate are close to its solubility threshold.
- As all uricases are highly immunogenic in humans, PEGylated enzymes with reduced antigenicity and prolonged duration of action have been developed for therapeutic use in patients with severe, refractory gout who cannot tolerate, or do not respond to, available uricostatic or uricosuric drugs.
- Pegloticase is a recombinant PEG modified mammalian uricase that is effective in about half of patients with severe gout refractory to other urate-lowering drugs.
- Gout patients who are persistent responders to pegloticase demonstrate marked serum urate lowering and a remarkable, rapid decrease (over months) in the size of tophi.
- Treatment-emergent antibodies limit the therapeutic efficacy of pegloticase and are associated with infusion reactions in a sizeable subset of patients.
- Plasma urate should be measured before each infusion of pegloticase and treatment discontinued if the PUA is repeatedly ≥6 mg/dL (0.36 mmol/L).

Introduction

Uricase or urate oxidase (EC 1.7.3.3) is a copper-binding enzyme that catalyses the oxidation of uric acid to 5-hydroxy-isourate and hydrogen peroxide (H_2O_2) (Fig. 14-1). Subsequent hydrolysis and decarboxylation leads to the formation of allantoin as the end product of purine metabolism in most prokaryotic and eukaryotic organisms[1] (see Fig. 14-1).

As a consequence of two independent mutations in the urate oxidase gene during hominoid evolution,[2,3] humans and some primates are unusual, among mammals, in lacking active uricase and in having uric acid as the end product of purine catabolism. Allantoin is 5 to 10 times more water-soluble than uric acid and readily excreted in the urine. Plasma and tissue urate concentrations in humans are 5- to 10-fold higher than those in mammals that express uricase and, even in the absence of genetic, dietary, and other environmental risk factors for hyperuricemia, are close to the solubility threshold of urate. This renders humans intrinsically prone to urate crystal deposition and gout.

Development of Uricolytic Drug Therapy

The possibility of developing uricolytic therapy with uricase for gout, and the hyperuricemia associated with tumour lysis in patients with malignant disease, has been considered for more than 50 years. In an elegant *proof of principle* study, published in *Science* in 1957, London and Hudson were able to demonstrate transient reduction of serum urate in a patient with gout, and in a nongouty subject, following intravenous administration of small quantities of a purified porcine liver uricase[4] (Fig. 14-2). This followed earlier studies in chickens and a single patient by Oppenheimer and Kunkel in the 1940s.[5,6] Over the years, a number of urate oxidase preparations from a variety of sources have been developed and investigated (Table 14-1). One of these, pegloticase (Krystexxa, Puricase), a recombinant, mammalian, uricase conjugated to methoxypolyethylene glycol (mPEG), received marketing authorization in the United States in September 2010 as an orphan drug for the treatment of adults with chronic gout refractory to conventional therapy. Another PEGylated recombinant uricase, pegadricase (formerly pegsiticase), is currently in early clinical trials, as this is written in 2011.

Nonrecombinant Uricase From *Aspergillus flavus*

Nonrecombinant fungal uricase from *A. flavus* (Uricozyme) was developed in France in the 1960s.[7] After an early phase I/II study in 61 adults demonstrated reduction in serum urate levels and urinary excretion of allantoin following intravenous administration of 800 units/day,[8] it was used widely for the prevention and treatment of tumor lysis in Europe in the 1970s and 1980s.[9,10] A review of children in France with advanced Burkitt lymphoma and mature B-cell acute lymphoblastic leukemia treated with nonrecombinant uricase showed that only 1.7% required dialysis for acute renal failure during induction chemotherapy.[11] This compared very favorably with a report of U.S. experience using standard prophylaxis with allopurinol, hydration, and alkalinization of the urine, in which there were six deaths from renal and metabolic complications and 21% of children with comparable malignancies required hemodialysis following chemotherapy.[12]

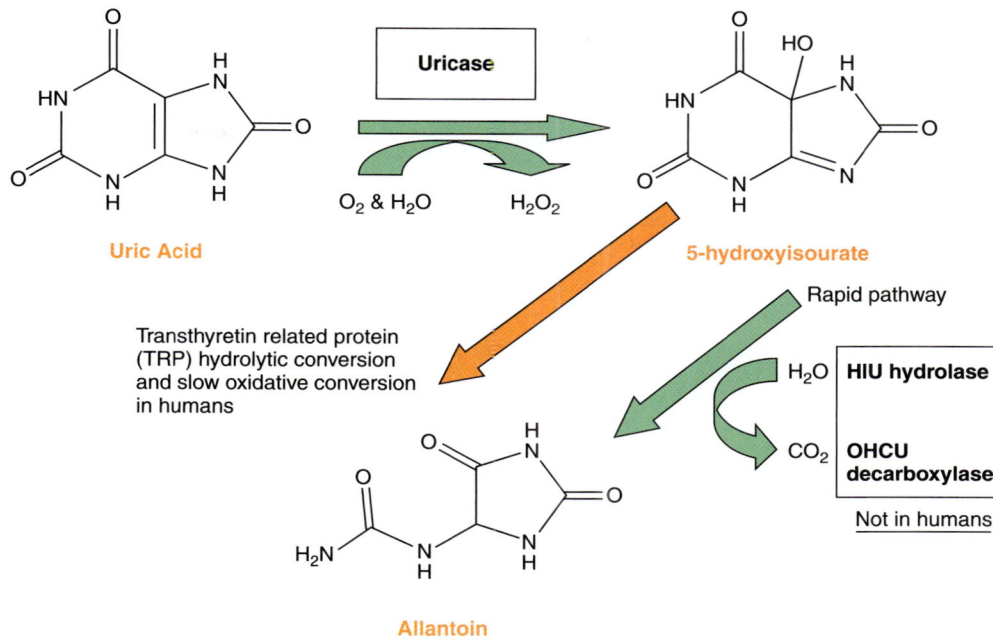

Figure 14-1 Pathway for the degradation by uricase of urate to allantoin in most mammals and other organisms. Uricase (urate oxidase) catalyses the oxidation of urate to 5-hydroxyisourate. Allantoin is rapidly generated after enzymatic hydrolysis and decarboxylation in lower species. In humans, in addition to the loss of uricase, enzymes that specifically degrade 5-hydroxyisourate to allantoin were lost in evolution, and slower alternative hydrolysis (by transthyretin-related protein) and/or oxidative degradation (over hours) occurs to generate allantoin. Not depicted here is oxidative degradation, in humans and other species, of uric acid to 5-hydroxyisourate via myeloperoxidase and peroxide. This can occur in human inflammatory loci and on the endothelial surface, and neutrophils have been observed to generate allantoin from uric acid.

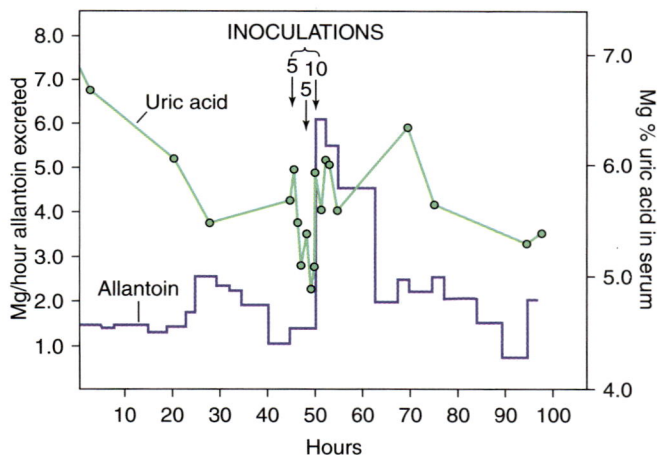

Figure 14-2 Serum uric acid and urine allantoin in a patient with gout before and after intravenous administration of purified porcine uricase in 1957. *(From London M, Hudson PB. Uricolytic activity of purified uricase in two human beings. Science 1957;125:937-8.)*

In a subsequent review of 134 children with acute leukemia and Burkitt lymphoma treated with chemotherapy in the United States, prophylaxis with nonrecombinant uricase was found to be associated with lower mortality and morbidity from tumor lysis, as well as lower levels of serum urate, than historical controls managed with allopurinol.[13] However, serious allergic reactions including urticaria, bronchospasm with hypoxia, and anaphylaxis occurred in 4.5%; and methemoglobinemia developed in one patient.[13]

There were a few case reports of the use of Uricozyme for the management of hyperuricemia in patients with gout

following organ transplants in the 1990s,[14,15] but more widespread use in patients with treatment-resistant gout was limited by the short half-life, low enzyme yields, and difficulties in purification during the manufacturing process, as well as by the significant risk of severe allergic reactions.

Production of Uricozyme was discontinued following the development and availability of recombinant *A. flavus* enzyme.

Recombinant *Aspergillus flavus* Uricase (Rasburicase)

The gene encoding *A. flavus* urate oxidase was first cloned and expressed in *Escherichia coli* in 1992.[16] Rasburicase (Elitek, Fasturtek) is a purified, recombinant *A. flavus* uricase expressed in a genetically modified strain of *Saccharomyces cerevisiae*. In the United States, rasburicase has had U.S. Food and Drug Administration (FDA) approval since 2002 for short-term, initial control of hyperuricemia in children with leukemia, lymphoma, and solid tumor malignancies who are receiving anticancer therapies expected to result in tumor lysis. In Europe, rasburicase has EMA approval for the prevention and treatment of hyperuricemia associated with tumor lysis in adults, as well as in children, but it is not currently licensed for the treatment of hyperuricemia in patients with gout.

Pharmacokinetics and Pharmacodynamics

Rasburicase is tetramer composed of four monomeric subunits, each with a molecular mass of 34 kDa. It has a half-life of 16 to 21 hours following intravenous administration at doses of 0.15 mg/kg and 0.2 mg/kg. There is no evidence of drug

Table 14-1 Uricases Developed for Clinical Studies/Therapy

Name	Method Production	Species of Origin	Current Status	References
Hog liver uricase	Purified from liver	Pig	Not in clinical development	4, 61
Uricozyme	Nonrecombinant, purified from fungal cultures	*Aspergillus flavus*	No longer manufactured	7–15
Rasburicase Fasturtec Elitek	Non-PEGylated, recombinant protein produced in strain of *Saccharomyces cerevisiae*	Uricase cDNA from *A. flavus*	Approved for prevention/treatment tumor lysis in children in United States (FDA) Adults and children in Europe (EMA)	16–26
Uricase-PEG5	Nonrecombinant, purified from fungal cultures and PEGylated (5-kDa PEG strands)	*Candida utilis*	No longer in clinical development	61
Uricase-PEG5	Nonrecombinant, bacterial protein, PEGylated (5-kDa PEG strands)	*Arthrobacter protophormiae*	Not in clinical development	62
Uricase-PEG 20 Pegadricase (formerly known as pegsiticase)	Recombinant, PEGylated (20-kDa PEG strands linked via succinimidyl succinimide)	Uricase cDNA from *Candida utilis*	Phase II studies	30, 63, 64
Pegloticase Krystexxa Puricase	Recombinant, PEGylated (9 strands 10-kDa PEG covalently attached to each subunit)	Mammalian cDNA (mainly porcine, with baboon C-terminal sequence)	FDA approval Sept 2010 for treatment of adults with chronic gout refractory to conventional therapy.	30, 36-54, 65

Adapted from Terkeltaub R. Learning how and when to employ uricase as bridge therapy in refractory gout. J Rheumatol 2007;34:1955-8.

accumulation in children after steady-state levels are achieved at 48 to 72 hours, but there are few data on the pharmacokinetics of rasburicase in adults and the elderly.[17] Clearance of enzyme, by peptide hydrolysis, is not, however, influenced by renal or hepatic function and rasburicase has no effect on cytochrome P450 activity. The licensed recommendation for dosing for the prevention or treatment of tumor lysis is 0.15 to 0.2 mg/kg once daily in 50 ml of normal saline as an intravenous infusion over 30 minutes for 5 days, but there is much data to suggest that lower doses, and single doses, can be used to control hyperuricemia in adults as well as children following tumor lysis.[18]

Efficacy of Rasburicase in Preventing and Treating Tumor Lysis Syndrome

In an open-label phase I/II study of the efficacy and safety of rasburicase in 131 patients, 20 years old or younger, receiving chemotherapy for acute lymphoblastic leukemia or advanced non-Hodgkin lymphoma, treatment with rasburicase 0.2 mg/kg every 12 hours for 48 hours was followed by reduction of plasma urate levels from 9.7 mg/dL to 1.0 mg/dL in 65 children who were hyperuricemic and from 4.3 mg/dL to 0.5 mg/dL in 66 children who did not have raised plasma urate levels before therapy (p = .0001).[19] None of the patients required dialysis and none developed tumor lysis syndrome. In a single nonblinded randomized controlled comparison of treatment with rasburicase or allopurinol in 52 pediatric patients with lymphoma or leukemia receiving chemotherapy,[20] the frequency of normalization of serum urate was significantly greater in hyperuricemic patients receiving rasburicase (risk ratio [RR] 19.09, 95% confidence interval [CI] 1.28 to 285.41) and the area under the curve of serum urate at 96 hours was significantly lower in the rasburicase group (MD-201, 95% CI −258.05 to −143.95).[20,21] However, a recent Cochrane

systematic review of trials of nonrecombinant and recombinant urate oxidase for the treatment and prevention of tumor lysis syndrome in children with cancer concluded that while it was effective in reducing the serum urate, there was currently no conclusive evidence that it was effective in reducing renal failure or mortality from tumor lysis syndrome in children with malignancies.[21]

Efficacy of Rasburicase in Primary Purine Overproducers

There is a single case report recording the safety and efficacy of intravenous rasburicase (0.2 mg/kg/day for 3 days) in preserving renal function in a 26-day-old boy with Lesch-Nyhan syndrome presenting with renal insufficiency, metabolic acidosis, hyperuricemia, and hyperuricosuria associated with overproduction of uric acid and severe deficiency of hypoxanthine-guanine phosphoribosyl transferase.[22]

Use of Rasburicase for the Treatment of Gout

Although no controlled trials of rasburicase for the treatment of gout have been undertaken, and rasburicase is not licensed or approved for treating gout anywhere in the world, it has been used to treat a small number of difficult cases, where other approaches to lowering urate levels had failed or were inappropriate.

In 2000, Phillips et al. reported regression of tophi following treatment with rasburicase in a patient with end-stage renal disease and severe tophaceous gout that was resistant to allopurinol.[23]

In 2005, Vogt documented successful treatment of a 33-year-old woman with severe progressive tophaceous gout, allopurinol

A Before rasburicase

B After 1 year of rasburicase

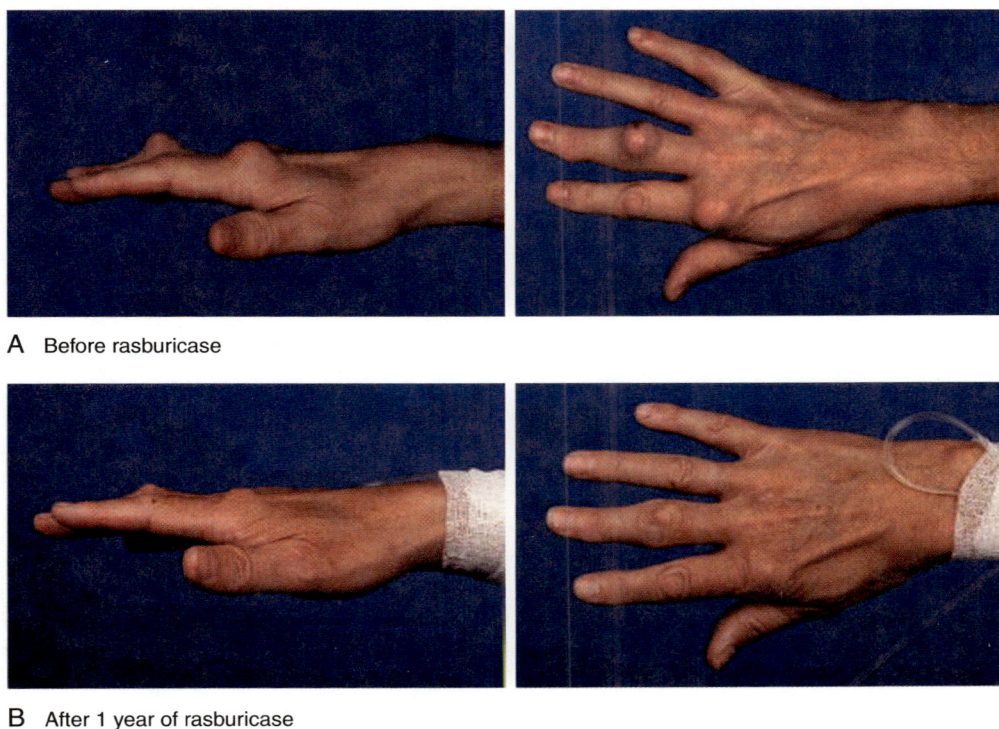

Figure 14-3 Reduction in the size of tophi in a patient with gout following 12 months treatment with rasburicase (0.2 mg/kg weekly). *(From Moolenburgh JD, Reinders MK, Jansen TLThA. Rasburicase treatment in severe tophaceous gout: a novel therapeutic option. Clin Rheumatol 2006;25:749-52.)*

hypersensitivity, and chronic renal insufficiency following transplantation for end-stage renal failure.[24] Serum urate decreased from baseline levels of about 850 µmol/L to less than 50 µmol/L a few days after commencing rasburicase 0.15 mg/kg IV but then returned to baseline despite continuing therapy with infusions every second week for 6 months. However, gout flares gradually ceased, tophi diminished in size, and the recombinant uricase was well tolerated with continuing infusions of rasburicase fortnightly, and subsequently monthly, over 3 years.[24] The prolonged efficacy and tolerance of repeated infusions of rasburicase over such a long period in this patient may have been in part attributable to the co-administration of immunosuppressive treatment with cyclosporine A and prednisolone.

Moolenburgh et al.[25] reported on a 57-year-old man with primary gout who had progressive tophaceous disease, recurrent flares, and persistent hyperuricemia despite combination therapy with allopurinol 900 mg and benzbromarone 200 mg/day. Hyperuricemia persisted in the range 0.45 to 0.55 mmol/L even after further escalation of the allopurinol dose to 1800 mg/day. Treatment with rasburicase 0.2 mg/kg IV over 60 minutes daily for 1 week resulted in an immediate fall in serum urate to less than 0.01 mmol/L. Continuing treatment with weekly infusions of rasburicase was initially associated with serum urate levels that sometimes rose again to more than 0.6 mmol/L immediately before the next infusion, as well as with regular postinfusion flares of gout requiring intravenous dexamethasone for symptom control. These ceased, however, after 3 months of therapy when serum urate levels were consistently in the normal range. Decreasing the frequency of the rasburicase infusions from 1 to 2 weeks was followed by a rise in serum urate to greater than 0.6 mmol/L and a recurrence of gout attacks, but subsequent maintenance treatment with weekly infusions of rasburicase (0.2 mg/kg)

was followed by gradual cessation of gout flares, stabilization of the serum urate in the range 0.25 to 0.27 mmol/L and measurable decrease in the size of tophi[25] (Fig. 14-3).

One small retrospective study[26] in 10 patients with tophaceous gout, that could not be treated with allopurinol, compared outcomes and short-term safety in five patients who had received IV infusions of rasburicase 0.2 mg/kg daily for 5 days with five patients treated with 6 consecutive monthly infusions of raburicase. Patients in both groups were given 60 mg dexamethasone to prevent gout flares. In the first group a rapid and profound fall in the serum urate immediately following infusion was not sustained at 1 month (511.5 ± 128.4 µmol/L) or 2 months (572 ± 96.2 µmol/L) compared with the baseline serum urate of 573.6 ± 48.2 µmol/L. Infusions were followed by gout flares and there was no noticeable change in the size of tophi. In those given monthly treatment, the serum urate fell significantly from 612.6 ± 162.4 µmol/L at baseline to 341.2 ±91.8 µmol/L ($p = .001$) after six infusions, and reduction in the size of tophi was observed in two patients. However, one patient developed bronchospasm and one developed urticaria during the sixth infusion. Two others from this group, who continued with monthly injections of rasburicase, had to discontinue therapy after 8 months because of cutaneous allergic reactions, and one patient developed a new tophus, as well as hyperuricemia that was refractory to further rasburicase after 14 monthly infusions; presumably because of the development of neutralizing antibodies.

Wider use of rasburicase as a debulking agent in patients with tophaceous gout or for the long-term management of patients with gout that cannot be treated with other urate-lowering drugs is limited by its short half-life,[19] the development of neutralizing antibodies,[18] significant risk of immune-mediated serious side effects,[27] and with loss of efficacy after 6 to 15 months of therapy.[26]

Immunogenicity and Adverse Effects Associated With Non-PEGylated Uricases

Most of the information about the immunogenicity and adverse effects associated with the administration of non-PEGylated, nonrecombinant, and recombinant A. *flavus* urate oxidase comes from trials and clinical experience in children and young adults with malignancy-associated hyperuricemia.

Rasburicase was remarkably well tolerated in both children and adults in the North American multicenter, compassionate use trial with a low (6%) incidence of adverse events. Only 10 of 1069 patients (less than 1%) were withdrawn as a result of events that might be drug related.[27] During the first course of treatment, 12 patients (1.1%) had hypersensitivity reactions (pruritis, urticaria, bronchospasm, or edema) and one had an anaphylactic reaction. Antibodies to rasburicase were detected in 13% of patients after a single infusion.[19] However, the incidence of hypersensitivity reactions in patients treated with rasburicase is much lower after both single and repeated infusions[20,27,28] than in patients treated with nonrecombinant uricase,[10,13] presumably because of greater purity of the recombinant protein and possibly because of increased immunogenicity associated with modification of an active cysteine during the extraction and purification of Uricozyme.[29]

Side Effects Associated With the Generation of Hydrogen Peroxide

Among the more serious adverse events that followed treatment with rasburicase that were not attributable to hypersensitivity were four cases of hemolytic anemia and three patients with methemoglobinemia.[27] In one of the patients who developed hemolysis, glucose-6-phosphate dehydrogenase (G6PD) deficiency was subsequently diagnosed. Hydrogen peroxide (H_2O_2) is generated during uricolysis with uricase (see Fig. 14-1). Treatment with all urate oxidase preparations, including rasburicase, is contraindicated in patients with G6PD deficiency because of markedly increased risks of inducing hemolysis and/or methemoglobinemia. Guidelines for the management of tumor lysis syndrome in adults and children[18] recommend screening for G6PD deficiency before treatment with rasburicase in patients with a previous history of drug-induced hemolytic anemia and in patients from certain ethnic groups in which G6PD deficiency occurs more frequently (African, Mediterranean, and Southeast Asian ancestry). Patients should be monitored for evidence of cyanosis during uricase infusions and full blood counts should be undertaken during and after treatment.

It is also important to monitor plasma urate levels regularly. Blood should be collected in prechilled heparinized tubes and plasma urate assayed at 4°C within 4 hours of collection, to avoid spuriously low measurements of serum urate, as a result of urate degradation in vitro by uricase activity in serum at room temperature.

PEGylated Recombinant Uricases

To prolong the duration of uricase activity and reduce antigenicity, efforts in recent years have focused on the development of polyethylene glycol (PEG)–modified forms of recombinant uricase. Some that are, or have been, in development are included in Table 14-1. One form of PEG-uricase, pegloticase (Krystexxa, Puricase) was given FDA approval for the treatment of adults with chronic gout refractory to conventional therapy in the United States in 2010. It is a recombinant, porcine-like uricase produced in *Escherichia coli* that is covalently conjugated to methoxypolyethylene glycol (mPEG).

Pegloticase (PEG-uricase, Krystexxa, Puricase)

The preclinical development of pegloticase and some other PEG-uricases is well described in a recent review by Sherman et al.[30] The earliest U.S. patent for "water-soluble non-immunogenic polypeptide compositions" filed by Davis et al. in 1979 included a description of a synthesis of a PEGylated uricase.[31] The development of the PEG-uricase that is pegloticase resulted from collaborative experimental work undertaken by scientists at Duke University and Mountain View Pharmaceuticals between 1995 and 1999.[30] A predominantly porcine-like recombinant uricase containing a few residues from the baboon sequence was chosen from a number of recombinant uricases for coupling to a variable number of strands of methoxy-PEG with differing molecular weights, using *p*-nitrophenolcarbonate to form stable, covalent urethane bonds between the polymers and the solvent-accessible amino groups on the protein.[30] As had previously been demonstrated,[32] it was found that the number of strands of 5-kDa PEG that inactivated the enzyme by greater than 50% was smaller than the number needed to confer a longer half-life in rodents or to suppress the binding of antiuricase antibodies in vitro. Experiments showed that conjugates with six strands of 10-kDA PEG per subunit had a significantly longer half-life in mice than conjugates with smaller numbers of strands of 20- or 30-kDa PEG, while retaining approximately 90% of the uricolytic activity of the unmodified enzyme. Conjugates with 9 ± 1 strands of 10-kDa PEG per subunit were, however, 10-fold less antigenic than conjugates with six strands.

Previous work had demonstrated that the immunogenicity of of PEGylated porcine-like uricase conjugates could be reduced below the level conferred by the PEGylation alone if the conjugates were prepared from uricase from which all traces of aggregated protein, detectable by light scattering measurements, had been removed.[33] However, even extensive PEGylation with 24 strands of 10-kDa PEG per tetramer could not completely block the immunogenicity in mice of a porcine-like uricase that contained traces of large aggregates.[30] Conjugates with nine strands of 10-kDa PEG per subunit were taken forward for clinical development as they came closest to fulfilling the requirements proposed for the clinical usefulness of a PEGylated drug[30] (Table 14-2). Figure 14-4 shows a molecular model of this conjugate in which 36 strands of 10-kDa PEG are coupled to the most accessible lysine residues of the uricase tetramer using a program adapted from the *Add ..PEG program* described by Lee et al.[34]

Phase I Clinical Studies: Pharmacokinetics and Pharmacodynamics

In the first open-label phase I trial, PEG-uricase (Puricase) was administered by subcutaneous (SC) injection.[35] Thirteen patients with treatment-failure gout received single SC injections of 4, 8, 12, or 24 mg of protein. The mean plasma urate

From Sherman MR, Saifer MGP, Perez-Ruiz F. PEG-uricase in the management of treatment–resistant gout and hyperuricemia. Adv Drug Deliv Rev 2008;60(1):60.

Table 14-2 Requirements for a Clinically Useful PEG-Uricase[30]

1. Sufficient reduction of immunogenicity of nonhuman enzyme to permit repeated dosing.
2. Retention of sufficient enzymatic activity to be effective at a reasonable dose, e.g., retention of at least 75% of the intrinsic activity of the conjugate.
3. Sufficient solubility under physiologic conditions to enable reasonable bioavailability.
4. Reproducible and cost-effective synthesis of a conjugate with adequate stability during storage, during shipping, and in vivo.
5. A sufficiently long half-life in patients to permit a convenient schedule of administration, e.g., once or twice a month.

was reduced from 11 mg/dL to 3 mg/dL after 7 days and six patients had the anticipated gout flares that frequently accompany all forms of urate-lowering drug therapy. However, three patients had injection site reactions, and while the circulating half–life of the enzyme was unexpectedly prolonged in eight patients, with activity detectable after 21 days, there was also evidence of accelerated clearance in the other five patients with no detectable enzyme activity after 10 days,[35] possibly associated with the development of antidrug antibodies.

A second phase I study was then undertaken to examine the efficacy, immunogenicity, tolerability, pharmacokinetics, and pharmacodynamics of pegloticase following intravenous administration.[36] Six groups of four patients received single intravenous doses of 0.5, 1, 2, 4, 8, or 12 mg of protein. Following doses of 4 to 12 mg, the plasma urate fell within 24 to 72 hours from a mean ± SEM of 11.1 ± 0.6 mg/dL to 1.0 ± 0.5 mg/dL. The plasma half-life of uricase activity ranged from 6 to 14 days but area under the curve measurements

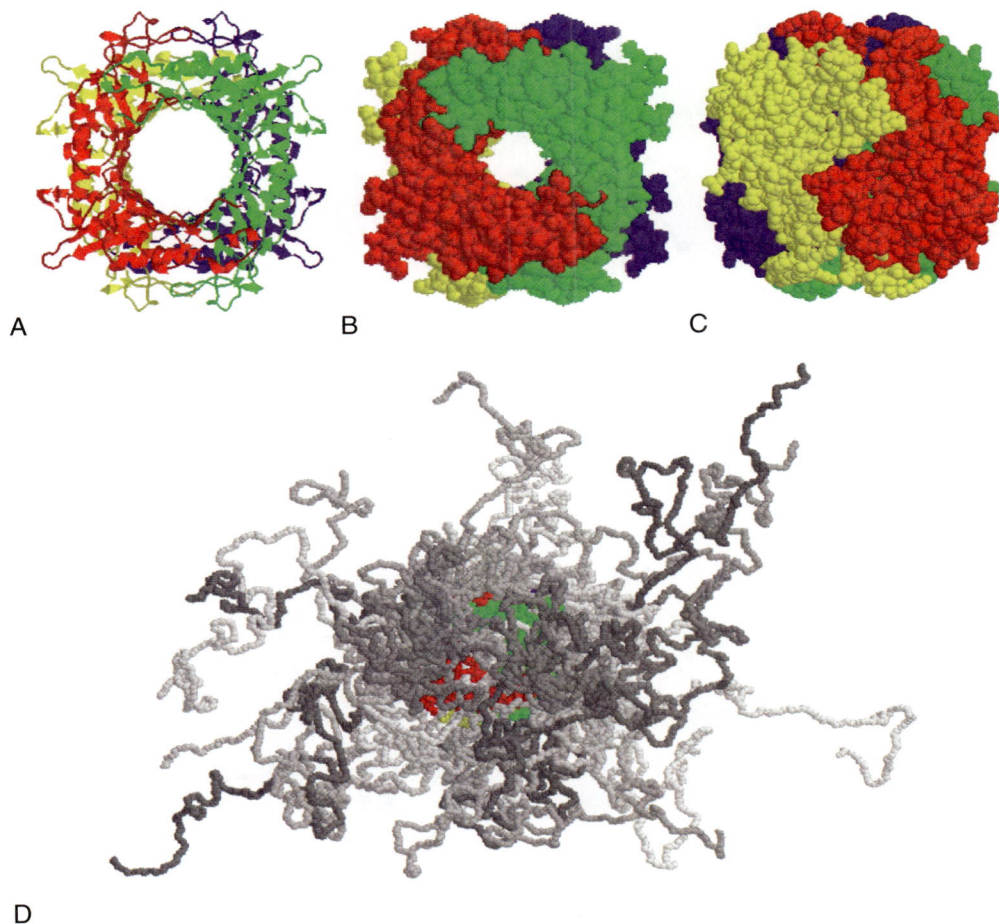

Figure 14-4 Molecular models of uricase tetramer (**A–C**) and of pegloticase (Puricase, Krystexxa) containing 36 strands of 10-kDa PEG per uricase tetramer. **A,** Cartoon model of uricase tetramer based on crystal structure of *Aspergillus flavus*. Each subunit is shown in a different color (*red, blue, green,* or *yellow*). **B,** Space-filling model of *A. flavus* uricase tetramer showing the central tunnel. **C,** Space-filling model of *A. flavus* uricase rotated around the vertical axis so that tunnel is not visible. **D,** Space-filling model of uricase tetramer, in the same orientation as in **B,** to which nine strands of 10-kDa PEG are attached to each uricase subunit. The structures of the PEG strands, shown in various shades of gray, were generated using a program adapted from that of Lee.[34] The scale of **D** is about half that of **A–C**. *(From Sherman MR, Saifer MGP, Perez-Ruiz F. PEG-uricase in the management of treatment-resistant gout and hyperuricemia. Adv Drug Deliv Rev 2008;60(1):59-68, Fig 1, p 63.)*

of the plasma urate suggested that plasma urate levels were maintained in the range 1.2 to 4.7 mg/dL for 21 days following infusion of these doses. Anti-PEG IgG_2 antibodies developed in nine patients who had more rapid clearance of enzyme but there were no associated allergic reactions.[36]

Phase II Clinical Studies

An open-label, multicenter, parallel-group study of a number of differing doses and dose regimens of intravenous pegloticase was undertaken to assess the efficacy and safety of multiple doses of pegloticase over 12 to 14 weeks in 41 patients with hyperuricemia associated with treatment-failure gout,[37] and this was also the subject of a Cochrane systematic review.[38] Patients were randomized to receive six infusions of 4 mg or 8 mg every 2 weeks or three infusions of 8 mg or 12 mg every

4 weeks. The primary efficacy endpoint was the percentage of patients achieving a plasma urate level of 6 mg/dL or less for at least 80% of the study period in each treatment group. Efficacy analyses were undertaken on the intention-to-treat (ITT) population, which received at least one dose of pegloticase, and on the population that completed the study. The mean plasma urate level fell to 6 mg/dL or less within 6 hours in all groups, and this was sustained through week 10 in all groups except the group treated with 4 mg every 2 weeks (Fig. 14-5, A). The mean plasma urate (area under the curve) over the whole study period up to 28 days after the last administered dose remained below 6 mg/dL in all the treatment groups with mean ± SD plasma urate levels of 4.12 ± 2.02 mg/dL (4 mg every 2 weeks), 1.42 ± 2.06 mg/dL (8 mg every 2 weeks), 3.21 ± 2.26 mg/dL (8 mg every 4 weeks), and 3.09 ± 2.46 mg/dL (12 mg every 4 weeks). Mean plasma urate levels rose between each infusion

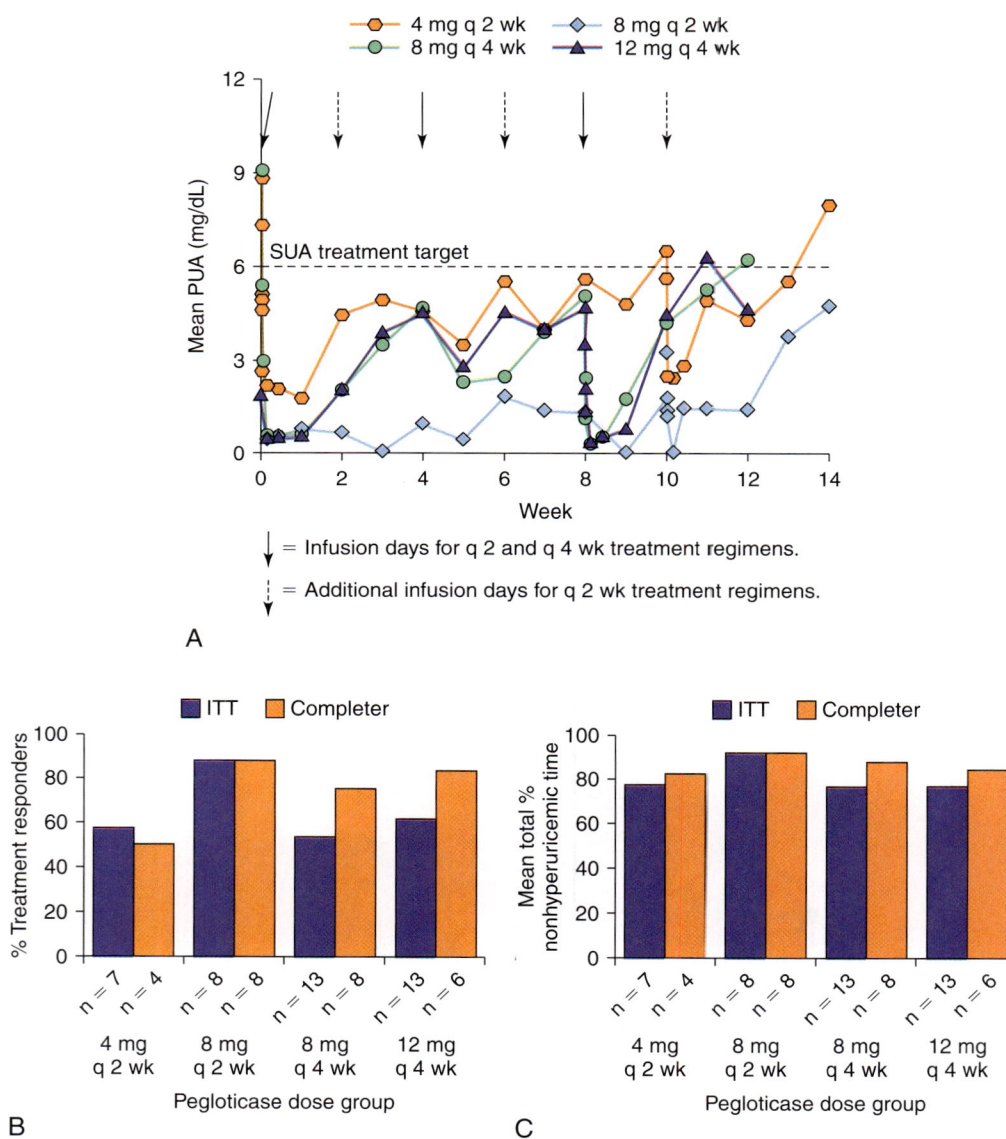

Figure 14-5 Phase II study of pegloticase to establish optimum dosing regimen. **A,** Weekly plasma urates in the four treatment groups. **B,** Proportion of treatment responders in intent-to-treat (ITT) and completer populations. **C,** Percentage of time without hyperuricemia in the ITT and completer populations. (*From Sundy JS, Becker MA, Baraf HSB, et al. Pegloticase Phase 2 Study Investigators. Reduction of plasma urate levels following treatment with multiple doses of pegloticase (polyethylene glycol-conjugated uricase) in patients with treatment-failure gout: results of a phase II randomized study. Arthritis Rheum 2008;58(9):2882-91.*)

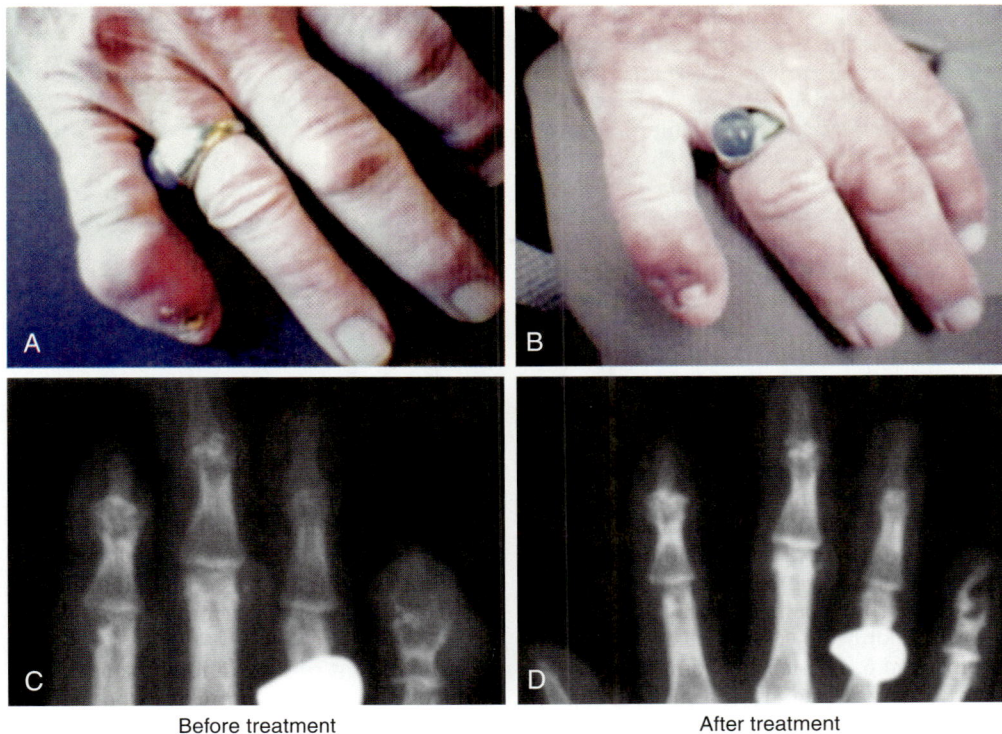

Before treatment   After treatment

Figure 14-6 Photograph of hand of patient with chronic gouty arthritis (**A**) demonstrating resolution of tophus (**B**) following 12 weeks' treatment with pegloticase. Corresponding radiographs (**C**) and (**D**) taken before, and 15 months after termination of treatment show resolution of soft tissue swelling and some healing of erosive changes in the DIP joint of the fifth finger. *(From Baraf HS, Matsumoto AK, Maroli AN, et al. Resolution of gouty tophi after twelve weeks of pegloticase treatment. Arthritis Rheum 2008;58(11):3632-4.)*

but remained below the target level of 6 mg/dL throughout, except in the group treated with 4 mg every 2 weeks (Fig. 14-5, *A*). The proportion of patients who were treatment responders and the percentage of time without hyperuricemia can be seen in Figure 14-5, *B* and *C*. Transient responsiveness, associated with development of antibodies, was seen in 20% to 25% of patients and was apparently unrelated to the dosing regimen.

Pharmacokinetics

Measurements of serum pegloticase showed very variable pharmacokinetics. The mean serum half-life after the first infusion ranged from 181 to 403 hours (mean 289 hours) and from 93 to 940 hours (mean 268 hours) after the last infusion, with some evidence of accumulation of pegloticase in patients receiving infusions every 2 weeks. The incidence of adverse events was, however, similar across all treatment groups. Gout flares occurred in 88% of patients. Infusion reactions developed in 18 patients and were the most frequent reason for study withdrawal (12 of 15 withdrawals). Antipegloticase antibodies were detected in 31 of 41 patients and were associated with reduced serum half-life of the pegloticase in some patients.

Overall, fortnightly injections of 4 mg of pegloticase were less effective than was 8 mg every 2 or 4 weeks, while the higher-dose regimen of 12 mg monthly did not appear to be associated with greater efficacy. Withdrawals due to adverse events did not differ significantly between groups. Additional pharmacokinetic and pharmacodynamic analyses suggested that intravenous infusions of 8 mg pegloticase every 2 to 4 weeks would maintain plasma urate levels well below

the recommended target of 6 mg/dL.[39] These dosing regimens were therefore taken forward for study in randomized controlled trials (RCTs).

Early Evidence of Rapid Resolution of Tophi

During the course of the 3-month phase II open-label study, visible reduction in tophus size was observed in a number of patients. The cases of two such patients were reported.[40] Figure 14-6 shows the photographic evidence of tophus resolution and associated radiographic changes in one of these patients following 6 infusions of 8mg of pegloticase at intervals of 2 weeks.[40]

Phase III Clinical Trials

Two replicate, multicenter, pivotal, phase III placebo-controlled RCTs, the Gout Outcome and Urate Therapy trials (GOUT 1 and 2), were undertaken in 212 patients with treatment-failure gout in the United States, Canada, and Mexico.[41-43] Patients who completed the 6-month placebo-controlled trial were eligible to enroll in a 2-year open-label extension study (GOUT 3).

Patients *included* in GOUT 1 and 2 either had a history of allopurinol hypersensitivity, intolerance, or toxicity or were deemed to have failed treatment with allopurinol. Treatment failure was defined as failure to normalize the plasma urate with 3 months' or more treatment with allopurinol at the maximum labeled dose (800 mg/day in the United States) or at a medically appropriate lower dose based on toxicity or dose-limiting comorbidity. *Exclusions* were patients with cardiovascular pathology (unstable angina, uncontrolled arrhythmia, uncompensated congestive heart failure, uncontrolled hypertension greater than 150/90 mm Hg), patients with organ transplants, and patients on renal dialysis. Pregnancy and G6PD deficiency were additional exclusions.

Subjects were randomized (2:2:1), after stratification for the presence or absence of tophi, to receive pegloticase 8 mg every 2 weeks (n = 85) or 8 mg every 4 weeks (n = 84) or placebo (n = 43) in 250 ml saline by intravenous infusion over 2 to 4 hours every 2 weeks for 6 months. All urate-lowering therapy was withdrawn 1 week or more prior to randomization, and subjects not already receiving colchicine 0.6 mg daily or twice daily or a labeled analgesic dose of a nonsteroidal antiinflammatory drug were started on gout flare prophylaxis. Patients were also given prophylaxis against infusion reactions comprising: oral fexofenadine (60 mg evening before and immediately before each infusion), oral acetaminophen 1000 mg, and intravenous hydrocortisone 200 mg prior to each infusion.

The primary efficacy endpoint was reduction of the plasma urate to less than 6 mg/dL for 80% of the time or more during treatment months 3 and 6. Secondary efficacy endpoints included measured reduction of tophi using digital photography, the incidence and frequency of gout flares during months 4 to 6, the number of tender and/or swollen joints, and the clinician's global assessment of disease activity. Patient-reported secondary outcomes were patient global assessment of disease activity, pain (using a visual analogue scale), physical function (using the Health Assessment Questionnaire Disability Index [HAQDI]), and health-related quality of life (HRQOL) (using the SF-36 physical component score).

The patients participating in these studies were predominantly male (82%) with a mean age of 55 years. They had severe gout with about 10 acute flares in the 18 months prior to study entry, 73% had tophi, and 58% suffered chronic pain associated with synovitis/arthritis. They were also characterized by a very high prevalence of comorbidities, with cardiovascular disease or cardiovascular risk factors in 84%. Sixty-one percent were obese (body mass index ≥ 30 kg/m^2), 32% had osteoarthritis, and 28% had renal insufficiency (creatinine clearance less than 60 ml/min).

In both the GOUT 1 and GOUT 2 trials, the primary endpoint was achieved following pegloticase 8 mg every 2 weeks (47% and 38%) and pegloticase 8 mg every 4 weeks (20% and 49%), with no responses in the placebo-treated patients. The pooled results from the replicate studies showed that 42% of patients given pegloticase 8 mg every 2 weeks and 35% receiving pegloticase 8 mg every 4 weeks were persistent responders (Fig. 14-7), who maintained the plasma urate at less than 6 mg/dL for 80% of the 6-month study period. All patients who received pegloticase responded with a fall in plasma urate within 24 hours, but 58% of those given pegloticase 8 mg every 2 weeks and 65% of those given pegloticase every 4 weeks were transient responders who did not sustain the response (Fig. 14-8). The loss of plasma urate response typically occurred within 3 months and was associated with the presence of antibodies engaging the drug and accelerated drug clearance.

There was complete resolution of one tophus or more in at least 40% of patients on pegloticase every 2 weeks (*p* = .002), in 21% of those on pegloticase every 4 weeks, and in 7% of the

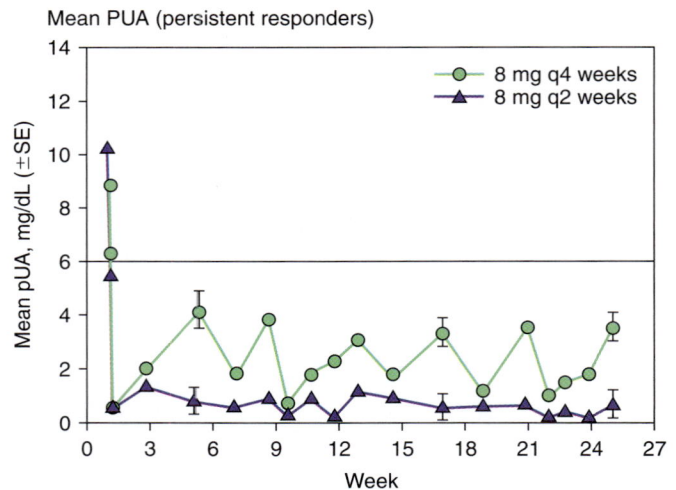

Figure 14-7 Mean plasma urate (PUA) levels in persistent pegloticase responders in phase III RCT. *(Data from Food and Drug Administration, Center for Drug Evaluation and Research, Division of Anesthesia, Analgesia and Rheumatology Products. AAC briefing document Krystexxa (Pegloticase), June 16, 2009. http://www.fda.gov/downloads/AdvisoryCommittees/CommitteesMeetingMaterials/Drugs/ArthritisDrugsAdvisory Committee/UCM1657 14.pdf)*

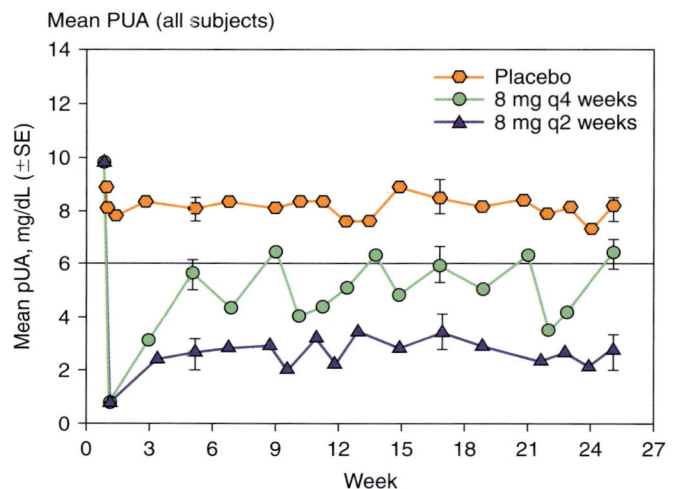

Figure 14-8 Mean plasma urate (PUA) levels in all subjects in the phase III placebo-controlled RCT. Includes transient and persistent responders to pegloticase receiving 8 mg every 2 weeks or 8 mg monthly. *(Data from Food and Drug Administration, Center for Drug Evaluation and Research, Division of Anesthesia, Analgesia and Rheumatology Products. AAC briefing document Krystexxa (Pegloticase), June 16, 2009. http://www.fda.gov/downloads/AdvisoryCommittees/CommitteesMeetingMaterials/Drugs/ArthritisDrugsAdvisory Committee/UCM1657 14.pdf)*

placebo-treated patients. Tophus resolution occurred within 13 weeks in 22%.[44,45]

Despite prophylactic drug therapy, there was an increase in the number of flares during the first 3 months of therapy (77% in pegloticase every 2 weeks, 83% in pegloticase every 4 weeks, and 81% in the placebo group). These were followed, however, by a statistically significant decrease in the incidence and frequency of flares during months 4 to 6 in patients receiving pegloticase 8 mg every 2 weeks, compared with placebo-treated patients (41% versus 67%, *p* = .007), or

Table 14-3 Summary of Treatment-Emergent Adverse Effects (AEs) Including Infusion Reactions and Gout Flares Reported[48,65]

	GOUT 1 and 2 RCTs (pooled)			GOUT 3 (open extension)	
	Placebo (n = 43)	Pegloticase q2wk (n = 85)	Pegloticase q4wk (n = 84)	Pegloticase q2wk (n = 85)	Pegloticase q4wk (n = 84)
AEs	370	693	870	1044	1411
Subjects with AEs	41 (95%)	80 (94%)	84 (100%)	83 (98%)	84 (100%)
Subjects with serious AEs	5 (12%)	20 (24%)	19 (23%)	24 (28%)	27 (32%)
Subjects with infections	22 (51%)	30 (35%)	40 (48%)	41 (48%)	54 (64%)
Subjects with serious infections	4 (9%)	3 (4%)	5 (6%)	3 (4%)	7 (8%)
Subjects with malignancy	1 (2%)	0 (0%)	1 (1%)	0 (0%)	1 (1%)
Subjects with infusion reactions	2 (5%)	22 (26%)	34 (41%)	26 (31%)	38 (45%)
Subjects who discontinued due to AEs	1 (2%)	16 (19%)	17 (20%)	18 (21%)	21 (25%)
Deaths	1 (2%)	3 (4%)	1 (1%)	0 (0%)	2 (2%)

Data from Food and Drug Administration, Center for Drug Evaluation and Research, Division of Anesthesia, Analgesia and Rheumatology Products. AAC briefing document Krystexxa (Pegloticase), June 16, 2009. http://www.fda.gov/downloads/AdvisoryCommittees/CommitteesMeetingMaterials/Drugs/ArthritisDrugsAdvisory Committee/UCM1657 14.pdf; Reinders MK, Jansen TLTHa. New advances in the treatment of gout: review of pegloticase. Ther Clin Risk Manage 2010;6:543-50.

with the incidence and frequency of flares during the first 3 months of treatment.

Treatment with 8 mg pegloticase every 2 weeks resulted in a significant reduction in the number of tender joints and in improved physicians' global assessments compared with placebo-treated patients. Patient-reported outcomes (global assessment of disease activity and pain) were also significantly improved in the patients receiving pegloticase 8 mg every 2 weeks. Physical disability (HAQDI) and HRQOL (SF-36 physical component scores) improved significantly in both pegloticase-treated groups compared with the placebo-treated patients.[46]

Adverse Events

Gout flares were the most frequent adverse events and occurred in 77% of the patients treated with pegloticase 8 mg every 2 weeks, 83% of those having pegloticase every 4 weeks, and 81% of the placebo-treated group (Table 14-3). Infusion reactions were the most frequent reason for discontinuing treatment (19 of 34) and occurred in 26% of those treated with pegloticase every 2 weeks, 41% of those having pegloticase every 4 weeks and in 5% of the placebo-treated group. Adverse events classified as serious adverse events (SAEs) were also predominantly gout flares and infusion reactions (pegloticase every 2 weeks [26%], pegloticase every 4 weeks [23%], placebo [12%]). In a post-hoc analysis, 5% of the patients who had received pegloticase were considered to have suffered anaphylactic reactions, although only one required treatment with epinephrine.[47]

Five patients died during the course of the trials—three in the group receiving pegloticase every 2 weeks, two in the group receiving pegloticase monthly, and one in the placebo-treated group. None of the deaths were judged to be related to the treatment with pegloticase.

More serious adverse cardiovascular events (arrhythmias, ischemic events, and congestive heart failure) were recorded in the groups of patients treated with pegloticase than in the placebo-treated patients, but the difference was not statistically significant and there was no relationship to dose. The FDA concluded that the number and distribution of cardiovascular deaths and SAEs were not unexpected, considering the high prevalence of cardiovascular disease and cardiovascular risk factors in the patients being studied, as well as the smaller number of patients randomized to the placebo group.[48] Nevertheless, exacerbation of congestive heart failure was observed in two patients who had received pegloticase every 2 weeks in the RCTs and in four patients during the open-label extension.[47] There was a history of cardiac failure in 12% of patients participating in the phase III trials, and it should be noted that the label advises that pegloticase should be used with caution in patients with congestive heart failure.

Antipegloticase antibodies engaging the PEG were detected in 89% of patients who received pegloticase. They were associated with increased clearance of pegloticase and loss of treatment response, as well as with increased risk of infusion reactions in some patients.[49] Analysis of the results indicated that monitoring the serum urate can predict antibody-mediated loss of response and infusion reaction risk during therapy with pegloticase.[50] This has led to the recommendation that pegloticase treatment should be discontinued in patients whose serum urate levels (typically measured ~14 days after the most recent infusion) rise above 6 mg/dL as well as in patients who have moderate or severe infusion reactions.[43,47,51] Since the majority of pegloticase infusion reactions in the phase 3 trial studies occurred in those who lost the urate-lowering response, it is important to adhere to the recommendation to discontinue the course of pegloticase after one (or at most two consecutive) reading(s) of serum urate greater than 6 mg/dL are obtained during the every 2 week regimen of infusions.

Antioxidant and Pro-oxidant Effects of Urate Metabolism Potentially Pertinent to Uricase Therapy

Thirty years ago, Ames et al.[52] advanced the hypothesis that the mutational loss of uricase, which led to humans having uric acid as the end product of purine metabolism, was associated with evolutionary advantage through protection from cancers and other life-shortening disorders as a result of the properties of uric acid as a free radical scavenger. In the range of concentrations that occur in humans, urate is widely believed to be the most important soluble antioxidant in plasma,[53] although cellular enzymes such as superoxide dismutase, catalase, and glutathione peroxidase have much greater antioxidant capacity.[54] Nevertheless, there has been a theoretical concern that treatment with uricase will both increase oxidative stress through the generation of H_2O_2 (see Fig. 14-1) and reduce antioxidant capacity by lowering the concentration of urate in the plasma and tissues. Hershfield et al. have recently examined this hypothesis in patients with refractory gout undergoing treatment with pegloticase in the phase II studies.[55] Following infusions of pegloticase, there was no accumulation of disulfide-linked peroxiredoxin-2 dimer in erythrocytes, suggesting that their peroxidase capacity was not exceeded by the H_2O_2 generated during treatment with pegloticase. Plasma levels of F2-isoprostanes, which are markers of oxidative stress and which were elevated in the hyperuricemic gout patients before therapy, did not increase further during treatment with pegloticase despite profound and prolonged hypouricemia.[55] These studies suggest that plasma urate is probably not the major circulating antioxidant in vivo in humans and that, except in patients with G6PD deficiency, or possibly with catalase deficiency (in which erythrocyte antioxidant defences are globally impaired),[56] the H_2O_2 generated during treatment with pegloticase does not exceed the antioxidant capacity of erythrocytes.

Pro-oxidant effects resulting from hyperuricemia and uric acid metabolism, on the other hand, are likely significant and are not simply due to superoxide generation by xanthine oxidase (a topic partly discussed in Chapter 19). Specifically, myeloperoxidase, with peroxide present, oxidizes uric acid to 5-hydroxyisourate (5-HIU),[57] and activated human neutrophils can generate allantoin. Moreover, 5-HIU is generated by uricase oxidation of uric acid (see Fig. 14-1). Humans lost expression, in evolution, of the key enzyme (5-HIU hydrolase) that rapidly catabolizes 5-HIU.[58] In humans, 5-HIU and the 5-HIU derivative 2-oxo-4-hydroxy-4-carboxy-5-ureidoimidazoline (OHCU) can undergo hydrolysis (by transthyretin-related protein) or alternatively, slow (i.e., in hours) oxidative (nonenzymatic) degradation to allantoin.[58] Biologic effects of the oxidative intermediates are not clear. It was observed that 5-HIU hydrolase knockout mice develop hepatomegaly and liver carcinogenesis,[59] which suggests oxidant effects of 5-HIU and its metabolism in hepatic cells, since uricase is expressed only in hepatic cell peroxisomes in mice. However, PEGylated forms of uricase given therapeutically to humans would only generate extrahepatic 5-HIU. It is not clear what effects, if any, plasma 5-HIU and its metabolites would have during the course of intravenous uricase treatment in humans.

Summary of Indications, Precautions, and Conclusions

Expert recommendations for the use of uricases in treating patients with severe refractory gout have evolved over a number of years as new and safer products have become available or are undergoing refinement in development[41,47,60,63,64].

Table 14-4 Key Points for the Use of Pegloticase in Clinical Practice

- Pegloticase is a recombinant PEG modified mammalian uricase that offers a new option for the effective treatment of about half of a small subgroup of patients with severe, refractory gout who cannot tolerate, or do not respond to available uricostatic or uricosuric drugs.
- Pegloticase (Krystexxa) has FDA approval for the treatment of chronic gout in adult patients who are refractory to conventional therapy.
- Patients with recurring gout, with or without overt tophi or structural joint damage, associated with persistent hyperuricemia should only be considered for uricolytic treatment with pegloticase after it has been established that they cannot tolerate, or do not respond to, allopurinol or febuxostat at optimum doses.
- Pegloticase 8 mg in 250 ml of normal saline should be administered by IV infusion over 2 hours by physicians with experience and facilities for dealing with infusion reactions. The treatment can be repeated every 2 weeks.
- Patients receiving infusions of pegloticase should be pretreated with antihistamines and steroids to reduce the risk of infusion reactions, in addition to low-dose colchicine or NSAIDs for flare prophylaxis for at least 3 months.
- Pegloticase is contraindicated in patients with G6PD deficiency because of the risk of hemolysis and methemoglobinemia and screening should be considered in patients from ethnic groups in which G6PD deficiency is more frequent.
- Pegloticase should be used with particular caution in patients with congestive heart failure.
- Plasma urate should be measured before each infusion and treatment with pegloticase discontinued if the plasma urate level is repeatedly ≥6 mg/dL (0.36 mmol/L) as such transient responders may be at increased risk for infusion reactions and anaphylaxis.

Table 14-5 Uricolytic Therapy for Gout: Unanswered Questions and Future Prospects

- Optimal duration of treatment with pegloticase has yet to be determined.
- The costs and cost-effectiveness of therapy with pegloticase need to be established.
- The safety, efficacy, and cost-effectiveness of repeated courses of pegloticase need to be investigated.
- Trials are required to investigate the possibility of using pegloticase as a more rapid "debulking" or "bridging" therapy followed by maintenance treatment with other uric acid–lowering drugs.
- In view of the frequency and severity of the gout flares that occur in the first few weeks of uricolytic therapy despite conventional prophylaxis with colchicine, NSAIDs, or corticosteroids, trials of prophylaxis with interleukin-1β antibodies or inhibitors should be considered.
- Postmarketing information on long-term safety and cardiovascular events need to be accumulated.
- Registers of patients receiving uricolytic therapy should be established, as they have for other biological agents used to treat chronic rheumatic diseases.

Table 14-4 summarizes some clinical points to consider when using pegloticase, and Table 14-5 lists some unresolved questions and future prospects. Preliminary data have suggested that successful retreatment with pegloticase is feasible, with a substantial response rate (in initial responders). However, the database of patients treated with pegloticase and other uri-colytic agents in clinical trials and open studies remains very small at this time, and evidence-based, expert consensus practice guidelines have yet to be developed.

References

1. Kahn K, Serfozo P, Tipton PA. Identification of the true product of the urate oxidase reaction. J Am Chem Soc 1997;274:5435–42.
2. Wu XW, Muzny DM, Lee CC, et al. Two independent mutational events in the loss of urate oxidase during hominoid evolution. J Mol Evol 1992;34:74–82.
3. Oda M, Satta Y, Takenaka O, et al. Loss of urate oxidase activity in hominoids and its evolutionary implications. Mol Biol Evol 2002;19:640–53.
4. London M, Hudson PB. Uricolytic activity of purified uricase in two human beings. Science 1957;125:937–8.
5. Oppenheimer EH. The lowering of blood uric acid by uricase injections. Bull Johns Hopkins Hosp 1941;68:190–5.
6. Oppenheimer EH, Kunkel HG. Further observations on the lowering of blood uric acid by uricase injections. Bull Johns Hopkins Hosp 1943;73:40–53.
7. Laboureur P, Langlois C. Urate-oxydase d'Aspergillus flavus: I. Obtention, purification, proprietes. Bull Soc Chim Biol 1968;50:811–25.
8. Kissel P, Lamarche M, Royer R. Modification of uricaemia and the excretion of uric acid nitrogen by an enzyme of fungal origin. Nature 1968;217:72–4.
9. Masera G, Jankovic M, Zurlo MG, et al. Urate-oxidase prophylaxis of uric acid-induced renal damage in childhood leukemia. J Pediatr 1982;100:152–5.
10. Patte C, Sakiroglu O, Sommelet D. European experience in the treatment of hyperuricemia. Semin Hematol 2001;38(Suppl. 10):9–12.
11. Patte C, Michon J, Bouffet E, et al. High survival rate of childhood B-cell lymphoma and leukemia (ALL) as a result of LMB 89 protocol of the SFOP (French Pediatric Oncology Society) [abstract]. Proc Am Soc Clin Oncol 1992:11.
12. Bowman WP, Shuster JJ, Cook B, et al. Improved survival for children with B-cell acute lymphoblastic leukaemia and stage IV noncleaved-cell lymphoma: a Pediatric Oncology Group study. J Clin Oncol 1996;14:1252–61.
13. Pui CH, Relling MV, Lascombes F, et al. Urate oxidase in prevention and treatment of hyperuricemia associated with lymphoid malignancies. Leukemia 1997;11:1813–6.
14. Rozenberg S, Roche B, Dorent R, et al. Urate-oxidase for the treatment of tophaceous gout in heart transplant recipients. A report of three cases. Rev Rhum Engl Ed 1995;62:392–4.
15. Ippoliti G, Negri M, Campana C, et al. Urate oxidase in hyperuricemic heart transplant recipients treated with azathioprine. Transplantation 1997;63:1370–1.
16. Legoux R, Delpech B, Dumont X, et al. Cloning and expression in Escherichia coli of the gene encoding Aspergillus flavus urate oxidase. J Biol Chem 1992;267:8565–70.
17. Ueng S. Rasburicase. (Elitek): a novel agent for tumor lysis syndrome. Proc (Bayl Univ Med Cent) 2005;18:275–9.
18. Coiffier B, Altman A, Pui C-H, et al. Guidelines for the management of pediatric and adult tumor lysis syndrome: an evidence-based review. J Clin Oncol 2008;26:2767–8.
19. Pui CH, Mahmoud HH, Wiley JM, et al. Recombinant urate oxidase for the prophylaxis or treatment of hyperuricemia associated with leukemia or lymphoma. J Clin Oncol 2001;19:697–704.
20. Goldman SC, Holcenberg JS, Finkelstein JZ, et al. A randomized comparison between rasburicase and allopurinol in chidren with lymphoma or leukaemia at high risk for tumor lysis. Blood 2001;97:2998–3003.
21. Cheuk DKL, Chiang AKS, Chan GCF, et al. Urate oxidase for the prevention and treatment of tumor lysis syndrome in children with cancer. Cochrane Database Syst Rev 2010:CD006945. doi:10.1002/14651858.CD006945.pub2.
22. Roche A, Perez-Duenas B, Camacho JA, et al. Efficacy of rasburicase in hyperuricemia secondary to Lesch-Nyhan syndrome. Am J Kidney Dis 2009;53:677–80.
23. Phillips M, Hunt RE, Shergy WJ, et al. Urate-oxidase in the treatment of severe tophaceous gout resistant to high-dose allopurinol: case report and review. Arthritis Rheum 2000;43:S401:[abstract].
24. Vogt B. Urate oxidase (rasburicase) for treatment of severe tophaceous gout. Nephrol Dial Transplant 2005;20:431–3.
25. Moolenburgh JD, Reinders MK. Jansen TLThA. Rasburicase treatment in severe tophaceous gout: a novel therapeutic option. Clin Rheumatol 2006;25:749–52.
26. Richette P, Briere C, Hoenen-Claverrt V, et al. Rasburicase for tophaceous gout not treatable with allopurinol: an exploratory study. J Rheumatol 2007;34:2093–8.
27. Jeha S, Kantarjian H, Irwin D, et al. Efficacy and safety of rasburicase, a recombinanant urate oxidase (Elitek™), in the management of malignancy associated hyperuricemia in pediatric and adult patients: final results of a multicenter compassionate use trial. Leukemia 2005;19:34–8.
28. Bosly A, Sonnet A, Pinkerton CR, et al. Rasburicase (recombinant urate oxidase) for the management of hyperuricemia in patients with cancer: report of an International Compassionate Use Study. Cancer 2003;98:1045–54.
29. Bayol A, Capdevielle J, Malazzi P, et al. Modification of a reactive cysteine explains differences between rasburicase and Uricozyme, a natural Aspergillus flavus uricase. Biotechnol Appl Biochem 2002;36:12–31.
30. Sherman MR, Saifer MGP, Perez-Ruiz F. PEG-uricase in the management of treatment–resistant gout and hyperuricemia. Adv Drug Deliv Rev 2008;60:59–68.
31. Davis FF, Van Es T, Paczuk NC. Non-immunogenic polypeptides 1979; US patent 4,179,337, Enzon, Inc.
32. Nishimura H, Asihara Y, Matsushima A, et al. Modification of yeast uricase with polyethylene glycol: disappearance of binding ability towards anti-uricase serum. Enzyme 1979;24:261–4.
33. Sherman MR, Saifer MGP, Williams LD, et al. Aggregate-free urate oxidase for preparation of non-immunogenic polymer conjugates 2004; US patent 6,783,965 B1, Mountain View Pharmaceuticals Inc. and Duke University.
34. Lee LS, Conover C, Shi C, et al. Prolonged circulating lives of single-chain Fv proteins conjugated with polyethylene glycol: a comparison of conjugation chemistries and compounds. Bioconjug Chem 1999;10:973–81.
35. Ganson NJ, Kelly SJ, Scarlett E, et al. Control of hyperuricemia in subjects with refractory gout and induction of antibody against poly(ethylene glycol) PEG, in a phase I trial of subcutaneous PEGylated urate oxidase. Arthritis Res Ther 2006;8:R12.
36. Sundy JS, Ganson NJ, Kelly SJ, et al. Pharmacokinetics and pharmacodynamics of intravenous PEGylated recombinant mammalian urate oxidase in patients with refractory gout. Arthritis Rheum 2007;56:1021–8.
37. Sundy JS, Becker MA, Baraf HSB, et al. Reduction of plasma urate levels following treatment with multiple doses of pegloticase (polyethylene glycol-conjugated uricase) in patients with treatment failure gout. Results of a phase II randomized study. Arthritis Rheum 2008;58:2882–91.
38. Anderson A, Singh JA. Pegloticase for chronic gout. Cochrane Database Syst Rev 2010(3):CD0083335. doi:10.1002/14651858.CDCD008335.pub2.
39. Yue CS, Huang W, Alton M, et al. Population pharmacokinetic and pharmacodynamic analysis of pegloticase in subjects with hyperuricaemia and treatment-failure gout. J Clin Pharmacol 2008;48:708–18.
40. Baraf HS, Matsumoto AK, Maroli AN, et al. Resolution of gouty tophi after twelve weeks of pegloticase treatment. Arthritis Rheum 2008;58:3632–4.
41. Sundy JS, Baraf HS, Becker MA, et al. Efficacy and safety of intravenous (IV) pegloticase (PGL) in subjects with treatment: failure gout (TFG): phase 3 results from GOUT 1 and GOUT 2 [abstract]. Arthritis Rheum 2008;58(Suppl. 9):S635.
42. Sundy JS, Baraf HS, Becker MA, et al. Efficacy and safety of intravenous (IV) pegloticase (PGL) in treatment failure gout (TFG): results from GOUT 1 and GOUT 2 [abstract]. Ann Rheum Dis 2009;68(Suppl. 3):S318.
43. US Food and Drug Administration. FDA labeling information: Krystexxa (pegloticase). FDA website 2010. http://www.accessdata.fda.gov/drugsatfdad ocs/label/2010/125293s0000lbl.pdf.
44. Baraf HS, Becker MA, Edwards NL, et al. Tophus response to pegloticase (PGL) therapy: pooled results from the GOUT 1 and GOUT 2, PGL phase 3 randomized, double blind, placebo-controlled trials [abstract]. Arthritis Rheum 2008;58(Suppl. 9):S22.
45. Baraf HS, Becker MA, Edwards NL, et al. Reduction of tophus size with pegloticase (PGL) in treatment failure gout (TFG): results from GOUT 1 and GOUT 2 [abstract]. Ann Rheum Dis 2008;68(Suppl. 3):S84.
46. Edwards NL, Baraf HS, Becker MA, et al. Improvement in health-related quality of life (HRQOL) and disability index in treatment failure gout (TFG) after pegloticase (PGL) therapy: pooled results from GOUT 1 and GOUT 2, phase 3, randomized, double-blind, placebo (PBO)-controlled trials [abstract]. Arthritis Rheum 2008;58(Suppl. 9):S27.
47. Sundy JS. American College of Rheumatology Hotline: pegloticase for the treatment of gout. http://www.rheumatology.org/publications/hotline/2010_11_01_pegloticase.asp.
48. Food and Drug Administration, Center for Drug Evaluation and Research, Division of Anesthesia, Analgesia and Rheumatology Products. AAC briefing document Krystexxa (Pegloticase). June 16, 2009. http://www.fda.gov/d ownloads/AdvisoryCommittees/CommitteesMeetingMaterials/Drugs/Arthri tisDrugsAdvisory Committee/UCM1657 14.pdf.

49. Becker MA, Treadwell EL, Baraf HS, et al. Immunoreactivity and clinical response to pegloticase (PGL): pooled data from GOUT 1 and GOUT 2 PGL phase 3, randomized, double-blind, placebo-controlled trials [abstract]. Arthritis Rheum 2008;58(Suppl. 9):S1945.

50. Wright D, Sundy JS, Rosario-Jansen T. Routine serum uric acid (SUA) monitoring predicts antibody-mediated loss of response and infusion reaction risk during pegloticase therapy [abstract]. Arthritis Rheum 2009;60(Suppl. 10):S413.

51. Schlesinger N, Yasothan U, Kirkpatrick P. Pegloticase. Nat Rev 2011;10: 17–8.

52. Ames BN, Cathcart R, Schwiers E, et al. Uric acid provides an antioxidant defense in humans against oxidant- and radical-caused aging and cancer: a hypothesis. Proc Natl Acad Sci USA 1981;78:6858–62.

53. Ghiselli A, Serafini M, Natella F, et al. Total antioxidant capacity as a tool to assess redox status: critical view and experimental data. Free Radic Biol Med 2000;29:1106–14.

54. Mates JM, Perez-Gomez C, De Castro IN. Antioxidant enzymes and human diseases. Clin Biochem 1999;32:595–603.

55. Hershfield MS, Jackson Roberts II L, Ganson NJ, et al. Treating gout with pegloticase, a PEGylated urate oxidase, provides insight into the importance of uric acid as an antioxidant in-vivo. Proc Natl Acad Sci USA 2010;107:14351–6.

56. Goth L, Bigler NW. Catalase deficiency may complicate urate oxidase (rasburicase) administration. Free Radic Res 2007;41:953–5.

57. Meotti FC, Jameson GN, Turner R, et al. Urate as a physiological substrate for myeloperoxidase: implications for hyperuricemia and inflammation. J Biol Chem 2011 Jan 25. [Epub ahead of print].

58. Ramazzina I, Folli C, Secchi A, et al. Completing the uric acid degradation pathway through phylogenetic comparison of whole genomes. Nat Chem Biol 2006;2(3):144–8.

59. Stevenson WS, Hyland CD, Zhang JG, et al. Deficiency of 5-hydroxyisourate hydrolase causes hepatomegaly and hepatocellular carcinoma in mice. Proc Natl Acad Sci USA 2010;107(38):16625–30.

60. Terkeltaub R. Learning how and when to employ uricase as bridge therapy in refractory gout. J Rheumatol 2007;34:1955–8.

61. Chen RH-L, Abuchowski A, Van Es T, et al. Properties of two urate oxidases that have been modified by the covalent attachment of polyethylene glycol. Biochim Biophys Acta 1981;660:293–8.

62. Chua CC, Greenberg ML, Viau AT, et al. Use of polyethylene glycol-modified uricase (PEG-uricase) in a patient with non-Hodgkin lymphoma. Ann Intern Med 1988;109:114–7.

63. Bomalski JS, Clark MA. Serum uric acid lowering therapies: where are we heading in management of hyperuricemia and the potential role of uricase? Curr Rheumatol Rep 2004;6:240–7.

64. Bomalski JS, Holtsberg FW, Ensor CM, et al. Uricase formulated with polyethylene glycol (uricase-PEG 20): biochemical rationale and preclinical studies. J Rheumatol 2002;29(9):1942–9.

65. Reinders MK. Jansen TLThA. New advances in the treatment of gout: review of pegloticase. Ther Clin Risk Manage 2010;6:543–50.

Prophylaxis of Attacks of Acute Gouty Arthritis

Robert Terkeltaub

KEY POINTS

- Gout attacks (also called "flares") are commonly precipitated by factors that induce rapid rise (e.g., diet and alcohol excess, intensive diuresis for congestive heart failure) or decline of serum urate (e.g., initiation of urate-lowering therapy [ULT]).

- Acute gout attacks that occur early in ULT are likely due to proinflammatory effects in joint tissue via remodeling and altered stability of tophi in the joint, particularly in response to rapid, extensive lowering of serum urate.

- All forms of alcohol, ingested in a concentrated time period (e.g., more than three servings in a 24-hour period), promote gout flares.

- Dehydration appears central to promotion of many gout attacks, can be promoted by "binges" of alcohol or caffeine consumption, and may help account for seasonal increases in rates of acute gout attacks in spring and summer. Conversely, consumption of five to eight 250-ml servings of water daily (unless medically contraindicated) may help suppress gout flares.

- In clinical practice, gout flare prophylaxis should be combined with the initiation of the pharmacologic ULT program in all patients. Oral ULT should start a submaximal dose, and then build up to the dose of ULT that achieves the serum urate target. Gout attacks contribute to decreased adherence in the first months after initiation of ULT, and patient education on the likelihood of gout flares is essential.

- Low-dose colchicine therapy is effective for prophylaxis of acute gout, and low-dose oral nonsteroidal antiinflammatory drug therapy (e.g., naproxen 250 mg twice daily) is an alternative. Colchicine prophylaxis should be started 1 to 2 weeks before initiation of ULT and continued for at least 6 months, and longer if visible tophi remain or ULT has not achieved the target level (typically less than 6 mg/dl).

- Even low doses of daily prophylactic colchicine treatment can be associated with toxicities. Colchicine dose should be reduced, or the drug should be avoided where drug-drug interactions are likely (e.g., clarithromycin, erythromycin, disulfiram), in chronic kidney disease, and in those over age 70.

- Use of low-dose corticosteroids for gout attack prophylaxis is not evidence based and should generally be avoided, or used as a last resort; we do not know what the minimum doses of corticosteroids are for efficacy in gout flare prophylaxis.

- Therapy with interleukin-1 antagonists is an emerging approach for prophylaxis of gout attacks that has been successful in phase II and III clinical trials, although this is not Food and Drug Administration approved at the time in 2011 that this is written.

Introduction

A key therapeutic objective in gout is to prevent the acute, painful, and debilitating attacks (also called "flares") that make such an impact on quality of life in the disease. Understanding therapeutic strategies to prevent gout attacks, beyond pharmacologic and nonpharmacologic measures for lowering of serum urate to ultimately dissolve tissue urate crystal deposits, requires appreciation of the most common precipitating factors of acute gout flares, which are listed in Table 15-1.

Factors That Precipitate Gout Attacks
Urate-Lowering Therapy

Accelerated rises or declines of serum urate, due to altered purine intake, hydration, and urate-lowering drugs, are the most common fundamental factors driving flares of acute gout. Gout flares driven by urate-lowering therapy (ULT) are most likely mediated by inflammatory effects in joint tissue brought about by remodeling and altered stability of tophi in the joint, and release of naked urate crystals (i.e., lacking protein coat) from tophi may be responsible.[1] The more rapid and extensive the lowering of serum urate, by any pharmacologic means, the more likely it is that attacks will develop in the first 3 to 6 months of ULT.[2] As such, the most recent U.S. Food and Drug Administration (FDA)–approved advanced therapeutics for urate lowering (febuxostat and pegloticase) have produced substantially high rates of gout flares in the first few months

Supported by the VA Research Service.

Table 15-1 Major Factors That Precipitate Attacks of Gout

Initial phase (first 3-6 months in particular) of urate-lowering therapy

Dehydration

Joint trauma or abnormal biomechanical loading: e.g., at first metatarsophalangeal joint

Intercurrent medical or surgical illness: e.g., pneumonia, deep venous thrombosis, congestive heart failure, exacerbation, general surgery (especially in first 48 hours of postoperative state)

Excess consumption, in a period of hours to 1 to 2 days, of:

    Alcohol (beer, wine, or spirits)

    Caffeine (4 or more servings of caffeinated beverages in a 24-hour period)

Sudden extreme nutrient deprivation (e.g., "crash diets", or initial post–bariatric surgery period)

of therapy in clinical trials, particularly when adequate gout flare prophylaxis is not used or prematurely discontinued.[2] For example, the early flare rate in phase II studies of pegloticase (in which patients were not premedicated with corticosteroids) approached 80%.[3] In the Febuxostat Versus Allopurinol Control Trial in Subjects With Gout (FACT trial), acute gout attacks were reported in about 30% to 45% of subjects between weeks 8 and 16.[2] This time frame was in conjunction with the discontinuation, by trial design, of pharmacologic gout attack prophylaxis with low-dose colchicine (or low-dose nonsteroidal antiinflammatory drugs [NSAIDs]).[2]

Dehydration, Concomitant Illness, and Trauma

Dehydration, with associated elevation in serum urate, appears to promote gout flares in instances such as intensive diuresis with intravascular volume depletion in congestive heart failure and may, with increased activity, account for seasonal increases in gout-flare rates in spring and summer.[4] In an Internet-based case-crossover study, water consumption was associated with decreased risk of gout flares.[5] Ingestion in a 24-hour period of five to eight servings of water (250 ml per serving, which is the volume of the standard drinking glass) was associated with decreased odds ratio (OR) of gout flare of 0.6 (95% confidence interval [CI] 0.4 to 0.9). Moreover, drinking more than eight servings per day was associated with adjusted OR 0.54 (95% CI 0.32 to 0.9) ($p = .02$)[5]; adjustments in this study were for diuretic use and for purine and alcohol.[5] Extreme nutrient deprivation (e.g., via "crash diets" or in the initial postoperative period of bariatric surgery) also has the potential to induce gout flares by promoting fluctuations in serum urate.

Gout attacks commonly occur in the first 1 to 2 days postoperatively in the setting of major surgery and general anesthesia. Maintenance of adequate hydration would likely be a factor in preventing postoperative gout attacks, although gout attacks in this clinical scenario also likely are provoked by tissue trauma with consequent systemic cytokine release. In fact, gout flares can be triggered by systemic and regional medical illnesses as well, including pneumonia and deep venous

thrombosis. Trauma to joints, exemplified by subtle excesses in biomechanical forces on the first metatarsophalangeal joint mediated both by ambulation and poor-fitting footwear, also can promote gout attacks, likely by effects on tophus stability, inflammation, and fluid and solute shifts in the joint space.

Excesses in Diet, Alcohol, and Caffeine

It has long been recognized by medical and lay public alike that precipitating factors for gout attacks include excesses in dietary purine and alcohol intake, which induce fluctuation (typically rapid rise and fall) of serum urate that could modify tophus structure. In addition, dietary excesses also have been suggested to have a priming effect on urate crystal–induced inflammation by increasing free fatty acid–driven TLR2-mediated activation of cells in the joint including mononuclear phagocytes.[6]

Although middle-aged male wine drinkers without gout do not, unlike beer and spirit drinkers, have an increased risk of developing gout, all forms of alcohol, when ingested in a condensed period of time, appear to be associated with an increased risk of gout attacks.[7] Specifically, in an Internet-based case-crossover study, five or more standard servings of alcohol (beer, wine, or spirits) in a 24- or 48-hour period at least doubled the risk of gout attack.[7] A dose response for alcohol was more clear for consumption patterns in a 24-hour period, and three or more servings of alcohol in 1 day appears to be a critical number linked with the onset of gout attacks.[7] One suspects that the effects of intense alcohol consumption to promote gout attacks may relate not simply to acute elevation in serum urate but also to decreased hydration. In this context, "binges" of caffeine-containing beverage consumption (four or more servings per 24-hour period prior to the gout attack) also were suggested to be associated with gout attacks in an Internet-based case-crossover study.[8]

Therapeutic Options for Gout Attack Prophylaxis

Nonpharmacologic Strategies of Attack Prevention

Table 15-2 summarizes approaches to gout attack prophylaxis. Some patients who decline, do not adhere to, or are not prescribed pharmacologic ULT, attempt, on their own, or are advised to manage their gout indefinitely by prophylaxis of attacks by itself. "Moderation" of diet and alcohol serving sizes and frequency is the most common first step, and it clearly has benefits to overall health. Each portion size (appetizer, main course, dessert) needs to be moderated in size with such a strategy. A useful concept for the main course is to have the patient conceptualize a dinner portion for a 9-inch diameter plate size (about 800 to 900 food calories on average) rather than the current U.S. standard of 12 inches for a dinner plate (about 1800 food calories on average). Maintenance of oral hydration with repeated servings of water (five to eight per day) and avoidance of "binges" of caffeine-containing beverages (four or more servings per day) are best advised.[8] Other dietary excesses that are advisable to avoid include "crash weight-loss diets" (due to dehydration and lactic acidosis that can raise serum urate) and "yeast-based diets" (due to their high purine content). The role of the folk remedy of cherries (or commercially available

Table 15-2 Nonpharmacologic and Pharmacologic Gout Attack Prophylaxis Regimens

Nonpharmacologic

Employ well-fitted footwear

Maintain hydration daily (e.g., 5-8 servings of water daily)

Avoid so-called "crash diets" built on a foundation of extreme nutrient deprivation for days to weeks

Avoid concentrated excesses of:

Purine-rich food (e.g., meat, shellfish, seafood)

Any form of alcohol

Caffeine

Yeast

Pharmacologic

For ULT initiation:

Oral colchicine 0.6 mg once or twice daily for at least 6 months; start colchicine prophylaxis 1 week before starting ULT.

Continue colchicine prophylaxis longer than 6 months in patients with visible tophi, continuing gout flares, or for at least 3 months after serum urate is normalized to <6.0 mg/dl in those with refractory hyperuricemia

Reduce colchicine dose in those:

In stage 3 or worse chronic kidney disease (i.e., CrCl <60 ml/min adjusted for ideal body weight)

With potential drug-drug interactions

Patients >70 years of age (extent of dose reduction is not yet evidence based)

Alternative Regimen

Low-dose NSAID prophylaxis for same duration as for colchicine, (e.g., naproxen 250 mg twice daily, or indomethacin 25 mg PO twice daily)

Caveat: The evidence basis for NSAID-based gout attack prophylaxis regimens is less established than for colchicine

Avoid use of low-dose corticosteroids as prophylaxis for gout flares:

The dose level of corticosteroids adequate to prevent gout attacks is not known, and it is difficult to wean gout patients from low-dose prednisone due to rebound flares

Experimental

Interleukin-1 inhibition; this strategy has given positive results compared to both placebo and the active comparator colchicine 0.5 mg daily in advanced clinical trials

cherry juice extract), which theoretically provides urate-lowering activity of ascorbate and antiinflammatory effects of the anthocyanins particularly enriched in sour or tart cherries,[9] has not yet been subjected to adequate study.

Pharmacologic Strategies of Attack Prevention

Since the vast majority of gout patients with a history of at least one acute attack will have additional gout flares in future years, pharmacologic therapy with colchicine or NSAID alone (without ULT) is not recommended in clinical practice.[10,11] The general principles when initiating ULT with allopurinol,

febuxostat, and uricosurics include starting at a submaximal dose and gradually titrating upward, over a period of weeks to months, to achieve the target serum urate level. This strategy of upward dose adjustments is held to reduce the incidence of early acute gout attacks in ULT and is the FDA-recommended and European League Against Rheumatism (EULAR)–recommended strategy for allopurinol, for example.[12]

For prophylaxis of acute gout attacks, low-dose colchicine therapy is the first choice and, as an alternative, low-dose NSAID therapy is commenced when colchicine is not well tolerated or is contraindicated. It should be noted that colchicine intolerance may be overstated by some patients, based on previous, non–FDA-approved regimens of acute gout in which colchicine was administered hourly over an extended period until diarrhea, pain relief, or a maximum of dose of about 5 to 7 mg was achieved.

In clinical practice, colchicine for gout attack prophylaxis is commenced 1 to 2 weeks before initiation of serum ULT and continued for at least 6 months (if successful serum urate lowering less than 6 mg/dl is achieved and no tophi are visibly detectable).[10-13] It is noteworthy that in the FACT trial, prophylactic low-dose colchicine or low-dose NSAID therapy was discontinued 8 weeks into ULT with allopurinol or febuxostat, and gout attacks markedly increased between 8 and 12 weeks into ULT.[2] In contrast, there was continual gout attack prophylaxis therapy through 6 months in the CONFIRMS trial of the same ULT drugs and, under these conditions, a flatter incidence of acute gout attacks.[14]

Early gout flares contribute to decreased adherence with ULT, a major problem in clinical practice for gout care. Since gout patients appear to be much less adherent overall than patients with many other medical disorders,[15] patient expectations must be adequately addressed when starting ULT.

Evidence basis for low-dose colchicine prophylaxis of acute gout flares after starting ULT becomes clear from comparison of the FACT and CONFIRMS trial data.[2,14] It is buttressed by a small (N = 43), randomized, placebo-controlled study of patients starting allopurinol as ULT[13] (Fig. 15-1). In this study by Borstad et al., colchicine was continued for at least 3 months beyond the point at which the serum urate target level was reached, and subjects who remained on colchicine for 6 months retained significant clinical benefit.[13] Acute gout attacks developed in 33% on colchicine 0.6 mg twice daily and 77% taking placebo (p = .008). Gout attacks were less severe with colchicine than placebo (p = .018).[13]

In the average-sized patient with intact renal and hepatobiliary function and no predicted drug-drug interactions, colchicine 0.5 or 0.6 mg twice daily for at least 6 months is the recommended dosage/duration regimen.[10,16] That said, colchicine at such doses can induce gastrointestinal tract symptoms such as loose stools. The minimum effective dose of colchicine for prophylaxis of gout attacks is not yet established,[16] and in clinical practice and some key ULT clinical trials, colchicine 0.5 or 0.6 mg daily has been the dose used. Even such low colchicine doses used in daily prophylactic treatment may be associated with side effects and substantial toxicities. Gastrointestinal side effects and alopecia can occur,[16] and colchicine rarely induces reversible oligospermia/azoospermia.[17] Effects have not been clarified for colchicine on chromosomal integrity of sperm or potential effects of colchicine, taken during pregnancy, on chromosomal integrity, birth defects, or pregnancy complications. Effects of colchicine on breastfed infants are not clear.

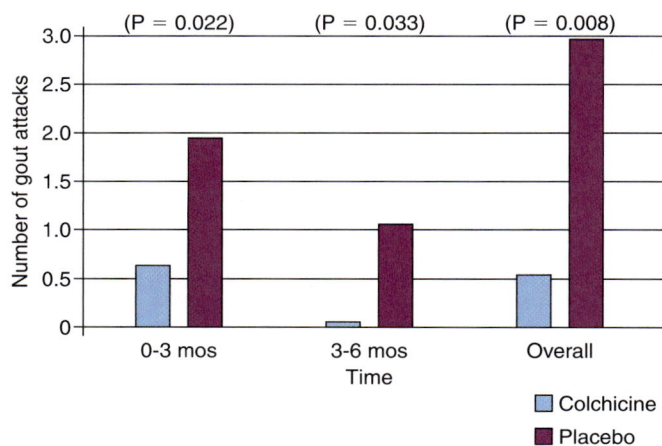

Figure 15-1 Summarized results of placebo-controlled trial (N = 43) of colchicine 0.6 mg orally twice daily (starting dose) in subjects with preserved renal function, with primary outcome being gout attacks after allopurinol initiation. The study results of Borstad et al.[13] showed significant benefit of colchicine prophylaxis for ULT-induced gout attacks. *[Data from Borstad GC, Bryant LR, Abel MP. Colchicine for prophylaxis of acute flares when initiating allopurinol for chronic gouty arthritis. J Rheumatol 2004;31(12):2429-32.]*

Bone marrow suppression and a combined myopathy and neuropathy characteristically associated with weakness and creatine kinase elevation can develop on colchicine,[16] with development of the latter syndrome accelerated by cyclosporine. Statins and colchicine appear to accentuate each other's potential to promote myopathy.[16] Routine surveillance of the hemogram and creatine kinase is recommended during sustained colchicine prophylaxis therapy.

Colchicine Mechanism of Action and Clinical Pharmacology
Mechanism of Action

Colchicine binds to soluble nonpolymerized tubulin with high activation energy in an equimolar and not readily reversible manner.[18-20] Colchicine thereby forms a tubulin-colchicine complex (TC-complex).[18-20] This action is central to colchicine mechanism of action,[16] since heterodimers of α- and β-tubulin form dynamic polymers (microtubules) that elongate and contract as filaments, thereby regulating structure and function of the cytoskeleton.[18-20] The TC-complex bound to the ends of microtubules physically prevents elongation of the microtubule polymer, although at high concentrations colchicine promotes depolymerization of the microtubules.[18] In this context, microtubules are involved in mitosis, signal transduction, gene expression, migration, and secretion.[16,18,19] Studies of certain colchicine analog have revealed partial dissociation of antiinflammatory effects from tubulin binding.[16] In this light, colchicine binds not only tubulin but also certain leukocyte membrane proteins that might provide sites for attachment of microtubules and consequent cytoskeletal reorganization.[12] Nevertheless, the primary antiinflammatory actions of colchicine appear mediated by disruption of microtubule function.[21] With respect to colchicine toxicity, cells with high proliferative rates are disproportionately affected by the drug (e.g., gastrointestinal tract–lining cells and bone marrow precursors).[21,22]

Low-dose prophylactic colchicine treatment decreases total leukocyte and absolute neutrophil counts in asymptomatic gouty knee joints,[23] arguing that colchicine acts by suppressing baseline subclinical joint inflammation and holding back augmentation of urate crystal–induced inflammation.[24-26] Important in the context of crystal-induced inflammation, colchicine concentrates in leukocytes, and this effect persists even after a single dose.[16,25] Colchicine used at low prophylaxis regimen doses achieves steady-state nanomolar serum concentrations that suppress redistribution of the endothelial cell adhesion molecule E-selectin, a key mediator of neutrophil adhesion,[26] and colchicine at low concentrations also potently suppresses superoxide production by neutrophils.[27] At higher doses, colchicine achieves a circulating C_{max} of about 6 ng/ml that is associated with more generalized suppression of neutrophil functions (phagocytosis, mobility, secretion).[28] The capacity of colchicine to suppress NLRP3 inflammasome activation emerges only at elevated concentrations (10^{-5} mol/L) in vitro that are not achieved with conventional, FDA-approved low-dose regimens of colchicine therapy.

Colchicine also modulates of expression of pyrin and cytosolic colchicine-pyrin contributes to colchicine efficacy in Familial Mediterranean Fever,[16] but colchicine effects via pyrin in crystal arthropathy are not clear. At high concentrations, colchicine also regulates expression of multiple genes in cultured endothelial cells, but it is not clear what contribution such effects make to colchicine action in gout attack prophylaxis.[16]

Clinical Pharmacology of Colchicine

After oral administration, colchicine is readily bioavailable via uptake in the jejunum and ileum, although absolute colchicine bioavailability is less than 50%.[29,30] The lipophilic nature of colchicine allows for absorption by multiple cell types and for binding to its primary target tubulin, which serves as a reservoir of the drug.[16]

Colchicine bioavailability is similar in young and aged subjects, but colchicine pharmacokinetics differ. Specifically, in elderly subjects, the volume of colchicine distribution at steady state (V_{ss}) and total body clearance are significantly reduced; this makes the plasma C_{max} significantly higher in older than younger subjects at comparable colchicine doses.[16] As such, the dose of prophylactic colchicine is routinely lowered in the elderly,[16] although detailed, evidence-based dosing regimens are not available for the elderly.

Colchicine Metabolism: P-glycoprotein, CYP3A4, and Potential for Drug-Drug Interactions

Elimination of colchicine is predominantly driven by the multidrug resistance transporter P-glycoprotein (P-gp) (also known as ABCB1). This occurs in the feces and by biliary excretion[16] (Fig. 15-2). Extrusion of colchicine from cells (including intestinal lining cells), enterohepatic recirculation, and marked drug enrichment in bile are central to elimination of colchicine.[16] In the plasma membrane, P-gp extrudes a multiplicity of compounds in an adenosine triphosphate (ATP)–driven manner; as such, P-gp mediates clinically significant drug-drug interactions[16] (Fig. 15-3); but it should be noted that most drugs that inhibit P-gp also inhibit

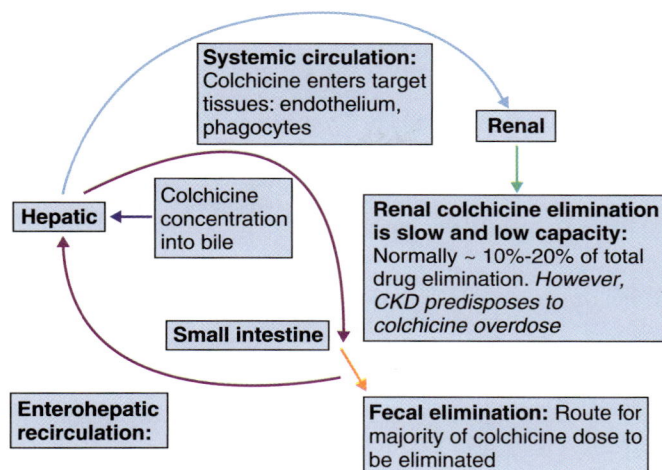

Figure 15-2 Principal sites involved in colchicine pharmacology and elimination. This paradigm summarizes key points of colchicine pharmacology reviewed in the text. Colchicine is readily bioavailable after oral administration via uptake in the jejunum and ileum, and the lipophilic nature of colchicine allows it to be absorbed readily by multiple cell types and to bind to its primary target tubulin, which serves as a reservoir of the drug. Colchicine is predominantly eliminated by biliary excretion and through the stool, and a major role for colchicine elimination by the gut is via the multidrug resistance transporter molecule P-glycoprotein (P-gp) (also known as ABCB1). P-gp extrudes colchicine from cells. Colchicine undergoes hepatobiliary excretion (and marked concentration in bile) against the bile-to-blood concentration gradient, mediated in part by P-gp. Colchicine elimination driven by hepatic metabolism and intestinal excretion follows a first-order process, and enterohepatic circulation plays a significant role. In addition, enteric and hepatic cytochrome P450 3E4 (CYP3A4) catalyzes demethylation of colchicine to inactive metabolites. Renal elimination also plays a role in colchicine metabolism. CYP3A4 and renal disposition of colchicine become more critical with certain drug-drug interactions that affect P-gp and the scenarios of aging and hepatobiliary dysfunction. Unresolved questions in colchicine pharmacology include the net roles in colchicine disposition of transporters other than P-gp.

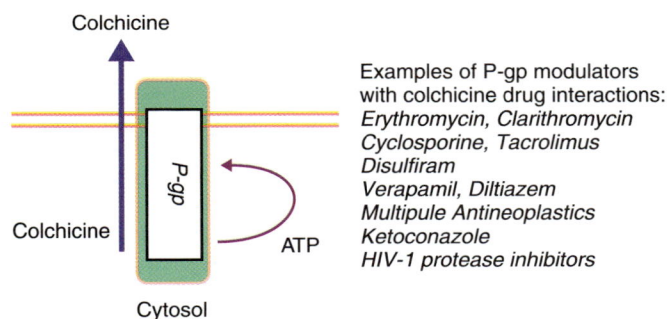

Figure 15-3 Colchicine extrusion from cells actively driven by P-gp: Potential effects of different drugs on colchicine metabolism by modulation of P-gp. This figure summarizes effects of the plasma membrane-localized multidrug transporter P-gp, which actively extrudes multiple classes of substrates from cells in an ATP-driven manner. Changes in intestinal P-gp expression and activity alter absorption of drugs transported by P-gp and can thereby critically regulate bioavailability and plasma concentrations, leading to suboptimal therapeutic effects or alternatively, to drug toxicity. P-gp also clearly participates in removal of drug metabolites into bile, the intestinal lumen, and urine. The diagram lists several drugs or drug classes that modulate P-gp activity, thereby contributing to the potential adverse drug-drug interactions with colchicine.

cytochrome P-450 3E4 (CYP3A4). The CYP3A4 enzyme demethylates colchicine to inactive metabolites in the liver, an event that precedes hepatobiliary elimination of colchicine.[16]

The clearest examples of adverse colchicine drug interactions are with cyclosporine and clarithromycin.[16,31] Colchicine neuromyopathy can develop weeks after starting cyclosporine,[16] and the fact that cyclosporine and certain other drugs can delay or obscure colchicine-induced diarrhea can render screening of colchicine intolerance more difficult. Importantly, the calcineurin inhibitors cyclosporine and tacrolimus are commonly associated with accelerated development of chronic, tophaceous gout in the setting of major organ transplantation. Colchicine is useful in gout attack prophylaxis in many such patients. Hence, attention to dosing and monitoring for clinical weakness and of the creatine kinase and hemogram are critical in this situation, especially with any renal or hepatobiliary disease.

More than one macrolide antibiotic (clarithromycin, erythromycin) has been reported to promote severe colchicine toxicity. This includes multiple reports of death due to clarithromycin-colchicine drug-drug interaction.[16,31] As a general rule, use of clarithromycin, erythromycin, and disulfiram (the latter putatively working by modulating P-gp)[16,31,32] should be avoided with colchicine. In contrast, azithromycin, which only weakly inhibits P-gp and CYP3A4, appears safe to use with colchicine, since azithromycin did not significantly increase plasma concentration of colchicine in healthy volunteers.[16]

Prophylactic Colchicine Dosing Models Regarding Concurrent Drugs and Chronic Kidney Disease

A sample dosing model for maintenance low-dose colchicine in gout attack prophylaxis is shown in Table 15-3, with the caveat that paradigms such as this are flawed. In this context, colchicine demethylation plays a minor role relative to P-gp in colchicine disposition, but CYP3A4 becomes a greater factor in elimination of colchicine in aging (due to decreased P-gp expression), and also with hepatobiliary dysfunction.[16] It is critical to note that drugs that interfere with both P-gp and CYP3A4 (e.g., erythromycin, clarithromycin, cyclosporine, and certain statins) potentiate colchicine toxicity in renal impairment.[16]

Gout is common in aged patients with renal impairment, and the risk of NSAID toxicity is increased by this clinical scenario. Therefore, colchicine remains particularly useful in gout attack prophylaxis in the elderly, and especially with chronic kidney disease (or congestive heart failure, or other contraindications to NSAIDs), Table 15-4 presents a model low-dose prophylactic colchicine dosing schedule, albeit non–evidence-based, that is calibrated to renal function and geared for maximum drug safety.[16]

Use of NSAIDs for Gout Attack Prophylaxis

Low-dose NSAID therapy is not fully evidence based for gout attack prophylaxis at the time this is written. Low-dose NSAID gout attack prophylaxis regimens commonly used in clinical practice include naproxen 250 mg twice daily, indomethacin 25 mg twice daily, and ibuprofen 600 mg twice daily,[2,10] although other NSAIDs and selective cyclooxygenase

Table 15-3 Examples of Dose Adjustments of Chronic Low-Dose Colchicine Prophylaxis to Avoid Significant Drug-Drug Interactions*

FDA Drug Classification		Drug	Prophylaxis of Gout Flares Adjusted Colchicine Dose (per 24 hours) Recommendations
Strong P-gp inhibitors		Cyclosporine[3]	Decrease dose by three-fourths and monitor CK and hemogram regularly.
	Other examples include:	Ranolazine. (potentially tacrolimus)	
Strong CYP3A4 inhibitors		Clarithromycin, ketoconazole, ritonavir	Avoid clarithromycin use entirely. Decrease dose by three-fourths for the other agents, and monitor CK and hemogram regularly.
	Other examples include:	Atazanavir, itraconazole, saquinavir telithromycin,	
Moderate CYP3A4 inhibitors		Diltiazem, verapamil	Decrease dose by one-half and monitor CK and hemogram regularly.
	Other examples include:	Erythromycin, fluconazole,	
—		Azithromycin	No dose reduction required.

*Other parameters, such as renal or hepatic function, and advanced age, may necessitate further colchicine dose reduction.
This table is adapted from: Terkeltaub RA, Furst DE, Digiacinto JL, Kook KA, Davis MW. Evidence basis of a novel colchicine dose reduction algorithm to predict & prevent colchicine toxicity in the presence of P-gp/CYP P450 3A4 inhibitors. Arthritis Rheum. 2011 Apr 7. doi: 10.1002/art.30389. [Epub ahead of print]

Table 15-4 Dosing Guidelines for Oral Low-Dose Colchicine Prophylaxis of Gout Flares in Subjects With Chronic Kidney Disease*

Colchicine 0.6 mg PO twice daily with CrCl >60 ml/min

Colchicine 0.6 mg PO once daily with CrCl 49-59 ml/min

Colchicine 0.6 mg once every 2 days with CrCl 30-39 ml/min

Colchicine 0.6 mg once every 2 to 3 days with CrCl 11-29 ml/min

Avoid colchicine or limit the dose to 0.6 mg once or twice a week with CrCl <10 ml/min, in patients on hemodialysis and those with severe hepatobiliary dysfunction

Patients with combined significant hepatic and renal disease appear to be at particular risk for colchicine toxicity.

*This table is not evidence-based and does not take into account drug-drug interactions of colchicine that necessitate further dose adjustments.

(COX)-2 inhibitors can be used. Proton pump inhibitor therapy may be indicated for cytoprotection when chronic NSAIDs are used, a determination made after considering risk factors (including past peptic ulcer disease, current gastrointestinal symptoms, and age). NSAIDs and COX-2 inhibitors can induce fluid retention and a decline in renal function, and can complicate management of hypertension and congestive heart failure, and these are substantial considerations in many gout patients.

Corticosteroids in Gout Attack Prophylaxis

Low-dose prednisone or prednisolone (i.e., up to 10 mg daily) is sometimes used as a measure of last resort for gout attack prophylaxis. This practice should be avoided unless absolutely necessary, since it is not evidence-based and effective minimum doses of corticosteroids for gout attack prophylaxis have not been established. It is illuminating that chronic low-dose prednisone often fails to prevent gout flares in major organ transplant recipients. Moreover, prednisone can be difficult to taper in gout, since gout attacks can rebound when corticosteroids are tapered or discontinued.[10]

Interleukin-1 Inhibition in Gout Attack Prophylaxis

Interleukin (IL)-1 inhibition therapy at the time this is written in 2011, is a strategy presently in advanced clinical trials for prophylaxis and treatment of gouty arthritis. As such, gout is not, in 2011, an FDA-approved indication for IL-1 inhibition treatment. Strikingly similar results for effectiveness in gout attack prophylaxis of distinct IL-1 have been observed in recent clinical trials, using the IL-1α and IL-1β inhibitor rilonacept (as a soluble receptor form of IL-1 inhibition therapy), and the humanized monoclonal antibody to IL-1β canakinumab. Specifically, weekly subcutaneous injection of rilonacept (80 to 160 mg), in both phase II and III trials, gave a marked, significant reduction of ULT-induced early gout attack frequency of approximately 80% (over several months) compared with placebo in randomized, double-blind studies.[33,34] Rilonacept had an acceptable safety and tolerability profile in these studies. Single-dose canakinumab provided a relative risk reduction to single-dose intramuscular riamcinolone acetate (40 mg) of 94% for recurrent gout flare at 8 weeks after treatment of acute gout attack.[35] In this study, canakinumab also was superior to triamcinolone for acute gout attack, as assessed by endpoints including pain relief within 72 hours.[35]

Canakinumab was further analyzed, using as an active comparator colchicine 0.5 mg daily, in large, 24-week, double-blind study of gout attack prevention in 432 randomized patients starting allopurinol therapy and followed for 16 weeks.[36] In this study, gout patients between 20 and 79 years of age were randomized (1:1:1:1:1:1:2) to canakinumab (subcutaneous single doses of 25, 50, 100, 200, or 300 mg or 150 mg divided into doses every 4 weeks [as a regimen of 50, 50, 25, 25 mg (given every 4 weeks)]) compared to colchicine. Each of the canakinumab doses except for the 25 mg colchicine single dose was associated with statistically significant reductions in gout attacks compared to colchicine.[36] Specific breakdown of percentage of patients with gout attacks was lower for all canakinumab groups given different doses (25 mg [27.3%], 50 mg [16.7%], 100 mg [14.8%], 200 mg [18.5%], 300 mg [15.1%], and for 150 mg [divided into doses given every 4 weeks; 16.7%]) than for the colchicine group (44.4%). In addition, canakinumab, which was well tolerated overall, also significantly reduced C-reactive protein from baseline levels.[36]

Collectively, the data for IL-1 inhibition in gout attack prophylaxis suggest that the role of IL-1 inhibition will be particularly valuable for both patients prone to breakthrough gout flares on ULT and those intolerant of colchicine and NSAIDs. Those patients with more intensive urate lowering indicated for more severe disease, such as chronic tophaceous gouty arthropathy, could particularly benefit from advanced biologic gout attack prophylaxis using IL-1 inhibition.

References

1. Liu-Bryan R, Terkeltaub R. Evil humors take their toll as innate immunity makes gouty joints TREM-ble. Arthritis Rheum 2006;54(2):383–6.
2. Becker MA, Schumacher Jr HR, Wortmann RL, et al. Febuxostat compared with allopurinol in patients with hyperuricemia and gout. N Engl J Med 2005;353(23):2450–61.
3. Sundy JS, Becker MA, Baraf HS, et al. Pegloticase Phase 2 Study Investigators. Reduction of plasma urate levels following treatment with multiple doses of pegloticase (polyethylene glycol-conjugated uricase) in patients with treatment-failure gout: results of a phase II randomized study. Arthritis Rheum 2008;58(9):2882–91.
4. Schlesinger N. Acute gouty arthritis is seasonal: possible clues to understanding the pathogenesis of gouty arthritis. J Clin Rheumatol 2005;11(4):240–2.
5. Neogi T, Chen C, Chiasson C, et al. Drinking water can reduce the risk of recurrent gout attacks. Arthritis Rheum 2009;60(Suppl):S762.
6. Joosten LA, Netea MG, Mylona E, et al. Engagement of fatty acids with Toll-like receptor2 drives interleukin-1β production via the ASC/caspase 1 pathway in monosodium urate monohydrate crystal-induced gouty arthritis. Arthritis Rheum 2010;62(11):3237–48.
7. Zhang Y, Woods R, Chaisson CE, et al. Alcohol consumption as a trigger of recurrent gout attacks. Am J Med 2006;119(9):800.e13-8.
8. Neogi T, Chen C, Chiasson C, et al. Short-term effects of caffeinated beverage intake on risk of recurrent gout attacks. Arthritis Rheum 2010 [Abstract 1362], in Programs and Abstracts of the 74th Annual Scientific Meeting of the American College of Rheumatology Meeting, Atlanta, GA, 2010. p. S565.
9. Zhang Y, Chen C, Hunter DJ, et al. Cherry consumption and risk of recurrent gout attacks. Arthritis Rheum 2010 [Abstract 1366], in Programs and Abstracts of the 74th Annual Scientific Meeting of the American College of Rheumatology Meeting, Atlanta, GA, 2010. p. S567.
10. Terkeltaub RA. Clinical practice. Gout. N Engl J Med 2003;349(17):1647–55.
11. Terkeltaub R. Update on gout: new therapeutic strategies and options. Nat Rev Rheumatol 2010;6(1):30–8.
12. Zhang W, Doherty M, Bardin T, et al. EULAR Standing Committee for International Clinical Studies Including Therapeutics. EULAR evidence based recommendations for gout. Part II: Management. Report of a task force of the EULAR Standing Committee for International Clinical Studies Including Therapeutics (ESCISIT). Ann Rheum Dis 2006;65(10):1312–24.
13. Borstad GC, Bryant LR, Abel MP. Colchicine for prophylaxis of acute flares when initiating allopurinol for chronic gouty arthritis. J Rheumatol 2004;31(12):2429–32.
14. Becker MA, Schumacher Jr HR, Espinoza L, et al. The urate-lowering efficacy and safety of febuxostat in the treatment of the hyperuricemia of gout: the CONFIRMS trial. Arthritis Res Ther 2010;12(2):R63.
15. Harrold LR, Andrade SE, Briesacher BA. Adherence with urate-lowering therapies for the treatment of gout. Arthritis Res Ther 2009;11(2):R46.
16. Terkeltaub RA. Colchicine update: 2008. Semin Arthritis Rheum 2009;38(6):411–9.
17. Haimov-Kochman R, Ben-Chetrit E. The effect of colchicine treatment on sperm production and function: a review. Hum Reprod 1998;13(2):360–2.
18. Bhattacharyya B, Panda D, Gupta S, et al. Anti-mitotic activity of colchicine and the structural basis for its interaction with tubulin. Med Res Rev 2008;28:155–83.
19. Wilson L, Panda D, Jordan MA. Modulation of microtubule dynamics by drugs: a paradigm for the actions of cellular regulators. Cell Struct Funct 1999;24(5):329–35.
20. Ravelli RB, Gigant B, Curmi PA, et al. Insight into tubulin regulation from a complex with colchicine and a stathmin-like domain. Nature 2004;428:198–202.
21. Niel E, Scherrmann JM. Colchicine today. Joint Bone Spine 2006;73(6):672–8.
22. Bibas R, Gaspar NK, Ramos-e-Silva M. Colchicine for dermatologic diseases. J Drugs Dermatol 2005;4(2):196–204.
23. Pascual E, Castellano JA. Treatment with colchicine decreases white cell counts in synovial fluid of asymptomatic knees that contain monosodium urate crystals. J Rheumatol 1992;19(4):600–3.
24. Cronstein BN, Terkeltaub R. The inflammatory process of gout and its treatment. Arthritis Res Ther 2006;8(Suppl. 1):S3.
25. Nuki G. Colchicine: its mechanism of action and efficacy in crystal-induced inflammation. Curr Rheumatol Rep 2008;10(3):218–27.
26. Cronstein BN, Molad Y, Reibman J, et al. Colchicine alters the quantitative and qualitative display of selectins on endothelial cells and neutrophils. J Clin Invest 1995;96(2):994–1002.
27. Chia EW, Grainger R, Harper JL. Colchicine suppresses neutrophil superoxide production in a murine model of gouty arthritis: a rationale for use of low-dose colchicine. Br J Pharmacol 2008;153(6):1288–95.
28. Terkeltaub RA, Furst DE, Bennett K, et al. High versus low dosing of oral colchicine for early acute gout flare: twenty-four-hour outcome of the first multicenter, randomized, double-blind, placebo-controlled, parallel-group, dose-comparison colchicine study. Arthritis Rheum 2010;62(4):1060–8.
29. Ferron GM, Rochdi M, Jusko WJ, et al. Oral absorption characteristics and pharmacokinetics of colchicine in healthy volunteers after single and multiple doses. J Clin Pharmacol 1996;36(10):874–83.
30. Rochdi M, Sabouraud A, Girre C, et al. Pharmacokinetics and absolute bioavailability of colchicine after i.v. and oral administration in healthy human volunteers and elderly subjects. Eur J Clin Pharmacol 1994;46(4):351–4.
31. Hung IF, Wu AK, Cheng VC, et al. Fatal interaction between clarithromycin and colchicine in patients with renal insufficiency: a retrospective study. Clin Infect Dis 2005;41(3):291–300.
32. Chen SC, Huang MC, Fan CC. Potentially fatal interaction between colchicines and disulfiram. Prog Neuropsychopharmacol Biol Psychiatry 2009;33(7):1281.
33. Sundy JS, Terkeltaub R, Knapp HR, et al. Placebo-controlled study of rilonacept for gout flare prophylaxis during initiation of urate-lowering therapy. Arthritis Rheum 2009;60(Suppl):S410.
34. Terkeltaub R, Schumacher HR, Saag KG, et al. Evaluation of rilonacept for prevention of gout flares during initiation of urate-lowering therapy: results of a phase 3, randomized, double-blind, placebo-controlled trial. Arthritis Rheum 2010 [Abstract 152], in Programs and Abstracts of the 74th Annual Scientific Meeting of the American College of Rheumatology Meeting, Atlanta, GA, 2010. p. S64.
35. So A, De Meulemeester M, Pikhlak A, et al. Canakinumab for the treatment of acute flares in difficult-to-treat gouty arthritis: results of a multicenter, phase II, dose-ranging study. Arthritis Rheum 2010;62(10):3064–76.
36. Schlesinger N, Lin H-Y, De Meulemeester M, et al. Efficacy of Canakinumab (ACZ885), a fully human anti-interleukin (IL)-1beta monoclonal antibody, in the prevention of flares in gout patients initiating allopurinol therapy. Arthritis Rheum 2010 [Abstract 2087], in Programs and Abstracts of the 74th Annual Scientific Meeting of the American College of Rheumatology Meeting, Atlanta, GA, 2010. p. S872.

Overview of Gout Therapy Strategy and Targets, and the Management of Refractory Disease

Frédéric Lioté and Robert Terkeltaub

KEY POINTS

- Comprehensive management of gout involves identifying and addressing comorbid cause(s) of the hyperuricemia, treating and preventing attacks of gouty inflammation, and lowering serum urate to an appropriate target level indefinitely.

- The ideal serum urate target is, at a minimum, less than 6 mg/dL (360 µmol/L). The serum urate target should remain at less than 6 mg/dL indefinitely in all gout patients and should initially be well under that in patients with extensive tophaceous disease until tophi have resolved.

- Patient education and adherence are enormous and often-neglected aspects of the optimal management of gout. Adherence can be monitored in part by continuing, regular assessment of the serum urate level.

- Difficult-to-treat gout often warrants combination drug therapy strategies for both refractory hyperuricemia and chronic tophaceous polyarthritis. Chronic tophaceous gouty arthropathy inadequately responsive to optimized oral antihyperuricemic therapy warrants consideration of the use of pegloticase.

Introduction

Gout has grown more prevalent (see Chapter 6), especially in the United States, and we have accumulated many more cases with difficult management problems.[1] The long-term management goals of gout are closely linked, with each step promoting the effectiveness of the other steps in a "therapeutic wheel" (Fig. 16-1).

Disclosures: Frederic Lioté is consultant or has contributed to CME sessions for Novartis France, Novartis global, Mayoly-Spindler, LGV, Ipsen, and Ménarini.
Robert Terkeltaub has recently served as, or is, a consultant for URL, Regeneron, Novartis, ARDEA, BioCryst, Pfizer, Takeda, and Savient.
Dr. Terkeltaub's research is supported by the VA Research Service.

Effective Communication to Address the Problem of Poor Patient Adherence in Gout

Achieving patient adherence and "buy in" to the program is critical but is markedly underachieved in gout patients (Table 16-1), especially those who are younger and reported fewer office visits and comorbidities.[2-6]

Gout requires patient education via effective communication, as discussed in part in Chapter 28. In short, explaining gout and treatment objectives to patients in terms they can readily comprehend (at a basic level of education), and clarifying the important, modifiable comorbidities with which gout and hyperuricemia are associated, must be part of a systematic program approach. This promotes optimum quality of care and outcomes, each aspect of which is covered in chapters elsewhere in this book.

A variety of reliable Internet-based sites exist for practical approaches to physician-patient communication for gout. Handbooks, leaflets, memos, and websites have been implemented in some countries [USA: www.update.com/patient; http://www.mayoclinic.com/health/gout; France and French-speaking countries: www.crisedegoutte.fr) (HON); UK: http://www.ukgoutsociety.org]. One terse, current monograph for patients available on this subject is cited in Doghramji et al.[7] One approach we have found useful is the analogy of gout being like deposits of matches in and around the joints[8] (Table 16-2).

Monitoring for Outcome and Quality of Care

The comprehensive gout management plan is consistently monitored for outcome, in part by regular assessment of serum urate level (SUA), and quality of care and quality of life hinge on decreasing acute and chronic arthritis, which should always include appropriate use of antiinflammatory prophylaxis to suppress arthritis attacks in early urate-lowering therapy (ULT).

Unlike most other rheumatic disorders, gout can be quite readily placed into permanent remission and, in some cases,

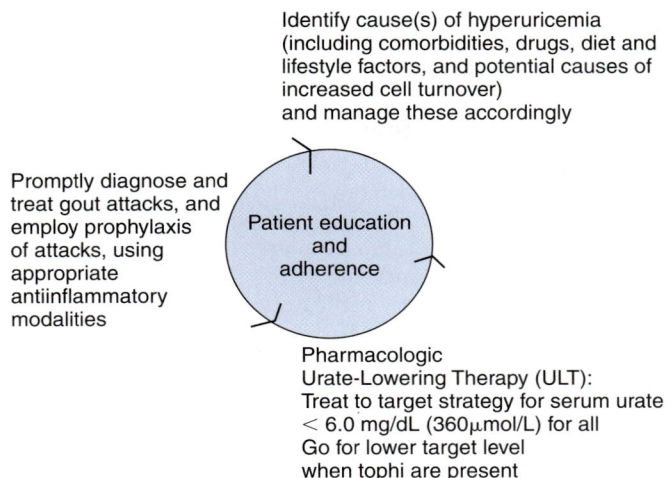

Figure 16-1 General principles for gout management emphasizing patient education and related issue of adherence to treatment and lifestyle changes.

Table 16-1 Nonadherence to Medical Therapy Is Disproportionately High in Gout Patients

	Adherence Rates of ≥80%
Hypertension	72.3%
Hypothyroidism	68.4%
Type 2 diabetes	65.4%
Seizure disorders	60.8%
Hypercholesterolemia	54.6%
Osteoporosis	51.2%
Gout	*36.8%*

Health care claims data 706,032 adults over 18 years old.
Data from Briesacher BA, et al. Pharmacotherapy 2008;28:437-43.

Table 16-2 Use of the Analogy "Gout Is Like Deposits of Matches in and Around the Joints" as a Tool to Concisely and Effectively Communicate Both Disease Pathogenesis and Treatment Options and Objectives in Gout

What to say to the patients with gout in readily comprehensible terms
- Uric acid is a normal breakdown product of genetic material, termed "purines," which are naturally present in your body, and also rich in certain foods and beverages.
- In gout, uric acid has accumulated in the body, most often because the kidneys cannot clear the uric acid quickly enough every day.
- In gout, crystals formed of a salt of uric acid deposit in and around the joints, like "matches."
- Gout attacks come on when the "matches" are lit and catch fire.
- A brief course of drugs that fight inflammation, such as naproxen, prednisone or prednisolone, or colchicine, puts out such "fires."
- Low, regular doses of some medications such as colchicine keep the "matches" moist so that they do not light on fire.
- Urate-lowering therapies, such as allopurinol and febuxostat, reduce the size of the "matches."
- With successful, long-term urate-lowering therapy, which is typically needed for the rest of one's life, the "matches" eventually disappear and gout is no longer a problem.

Adapted from Wortmann RL. Am J Med 1998;105:513-4.

Table 16-3 Checklist of Major Co-morbidities and Factors Clinicians should Consider when Assessing Each Gout Patient

- Age
- Comorbidities
  - Obesity
  - Metabolic syndrome or diabetes mellitus
  - Hypertension
  - Chronic kidney disease, end-stage renal disease, hemodialysis
  - Alcohol abuse
  - Congestive heart failure
  - Coronary heart disease
  - Upper (gastric or duodenal ulcer, bleeding) gastrointestinal conditions
  - Lower (sigmoid diverticular disease) gastrointestinal conditions
- Major organ transplantation
- Drug-drug interactions or predisposition to drug toxicity

truly cured. Despite that consideration, gout is often mismanaged, with adequately effective ULT either not achieved or not sustained indefinitely as the typical, appropriate measure. With the development of new drug options and treatment guidelines, a better outcome for gout patients is expected. Indeed in 2005, the European League Against Rheumatism (EULAR) reported and then published the first international recommendations for the diagnosis and treatment of gout.[9,10] The development of EULAR and British Society for Rheumatology (BSR) guidelines,[11] as well as the development of new drugs, stimulated the need for better care and for quality indicators. Deliberation on the American College of Rheumatology guidelines is ongoing at the time this is being written, and will address new epidemiological data and recently approved therapeutics (febuxostat, pegloticase).

Gout Treatment Strategy

Once gout is definitively diagnosed, treatment is dependent on a global strategy that includes five clinical aims, each of which is discussed in detail elsewhere in this book:

1. Evaluation of hyperuricemia and its causes via disorders of renal urate disposition and/or uric acid production (see Chapters 3 and 4)
2. Treatment of acute gout attacks (see Chapter 10), as an urgent patient need
3. Gout attack prophylaxis implementation (see Chapter 15) followed by ULT (see Chapters 12 through 14)
4. Identification and management of associated comorbidities, such as the metabolic syndrome, and diet and lifestyle factors (see Chapters 11 and 19)
5. Patient (and other health professional) education in order to emphasize adherence to treatment and quality of care and quality of life (see Chapters 17, 18, and 27)

Evaluation of comorbidities (Table 16-3) and disease severity are parts of any "case-by-case" discussion. These five clinical aims of the strategy have to be systematically considered in every patient presenting with gout, and overall management has to take into account the balance between risks and benefits of drugs at any part of the management. Treatment should be tailored to the individual, but general principles and strategies should be borne in mind.

Pathophysiology is also a key point to consider when treating gout and guides us in providing key information to the patient. Indeed, gout is a metabolic storage and deposition disease, with gradual accumulation of urate as monosodium urate (MSU) crystals in bone and joints, soft tissues, and sometimes the renal medulla, or precipitation of uric acid uroliths. Urate crystal masses can degrade tissues in bone, joints, bursae, and skin. Reducing body urate burden and MSU crystal mass using efficient ULT can be followed by imaging and clinical means, but relationship to the SUA is very valuable, since the SUA level should be substantially lower than the MSU crystallization threshold (urate solubility limit) of above 6.8 to 7.0 mg/dl for urate in physiologic buffers. This is done by aiming for an SUA target below 6.0 mg/dl, less than 360 μmol/L, in all patients with gout.

Striking differences exist between undertreated and nonadherent gout patients, and "refractory gout," which is related to patients not able to achieve the target for SUA lowering,[12] and "difficult-to-treat" (DTT) gout, which includes patients with uncontrolled gout attacks. For treatment-refractory disease,[13] DTT patients, or specific settings (e.g., major organ transplantation), referral to a rheumatologist is strongly considered.[14]

This chapter will consider general approaches and drug choices in management and discuss DTT gout with respect to aging, renal dysfunction, patients with uncontrolled recurrent attacks and chronic tophaceous gout arthropathy, and gout in major organ transplant recipients. We also cite differences that exist with respect to drug availability in the United States and other countries,[15] to proper label use according to each drug, and to national (BSR) or transnational recommendations (EULAR).

General Therapeutic Strategy

The strategy schematized in Figure 16-1 should be implemented in all patients with gout with or without comorbidities.

Specific Education on Diet and Lifestyle Factors Pertinent to Gout

Immediately after the first gout attack or the firm diagnosis of gout, the patient should be educated about the disease, with respect to precipitating factors for attacks, the destructive potential of excess urate due to tophi, cardiovascular disease risks, and how lifestyle modifications can lessen the risk for recurrent bouts and other medical complications. A discussion with the patient about diet (given in detail in Chapter 11) is vital. In brief, many different diets have been advocated to avoid gout; indeed, diet should be thought of as "nutritional behavior": restriction of calories and animal protein intake (seafood, shellfish, and meat [especially organ meats]) along with the "portion size" of meals in countries such as the United States, alcohol moderation (especially marked limits or abstinence with respect to beer and prohibition of binges of alcohol consumption), and limitation of intake of table sugar and high fructose corn syrup–sweetened beverages and foods (particularly carbonated beverages ["sodas"] and energy drinks). A shift to diet beverages and

maintenance of hydration are core aspects of dietary advice. "Heart-healthy" foods in moderation such as seafood, vegetables, nuts, and low-fat dairy products are encouraged.[15] Physical exercise (30-minute walk per day) is also important in order to consume calories and to help achieve ideal body weight. These measures will contribute also to better control of hypertension, the metabolic syndrome, diabetes mellitus, and dyslipidemia. These lifestyle adjustments should be encouraged and monitored regularly by physicians, other health professionals, and key family members. Diet and physical fitness measures, as illustrated in the Multiple Risk Factor Intervention Trial (MRFIT),[16] can drop serum urate by at least 10% to 15%, but most patients with gout do not achieve a serum urate target of through 6 mg/dL by diet and lifestyle measures alone.

Exclusion of Secondary Hyperuricemia and Gout

As discussed extensively in this book, primary hyperuricemia is related to a combination of genetics, including reduced urinary uric acid clearance, and environmental overload of purines and fructose, and overall calories, with obesity and insulin resistance that largely raise serum urate by inhibiting renal uric acid excretion (see Chapters 4, 5, and 12). At time of diagnosis, secondary causes of hyperuricemia should also be considered and can be related to various conditions. Chapter 12 reviews the value of 24-hour and spot urine–based methods to screen and assess for uric acid overproduction relative to the more common condition of uric acid underexcretion. A complete hemogram, liver function tests, urinalysis, and chemistry panel are essential baseline studies in all gout patients, and psoriasis should be ruled out. In those with moderate to severely impaired renal function, spot collection becomes a valuable approach. The 24-hour urine uric acid measurement is used as a more definitive analysis, including after screening of spot urine, in those with preserved renal function.

Commonly, in clinical practice, it is not necessary to screen urine for uric acid excretion values, since the cause of the hyperuricemia is evident (e.g., diuretic or cyclosporine use, advanced renal impairment). Furthermore, the urine testing may not need to be done if the most appropriate first-line ULT option is xanthine oxidase inhibition.

Elimination of Nonessential Drugs That Promote Hyperuricemia

Physicians should systematically consider discontinuing nonessential use of drugs that promote hyperuricemia. Thiazide diuretics are commonly used in patients with hypertension, since they positively impact on hypertension outcomes and are inexpensive. However, diuretics can be switched to other antihypertensive drugs, such as losartan (see Chapter 12) and amlodipine, which also has been associated with serum urate–lowering effects in some studies. Chronic heart failure and renal insufficiency may require substantial dosages of loop diuretics such as furosemide, but we know this to be a major contributor to hyperuricemia. Nonessential use of niacin should be discontinued. In contrast, low-dose aspirin (acetylsalicylic acid) should not be discontinued in gout patients requiring cardiovascular event prophylaxis.

Therapy Choices in Acute Gout Management

As reviewed in Chapter 10, a patient presenting with an acute gout attack is typically in excruciating pain. At this stage, the specific treatment goals for acute attacks of gouty arthritis are rapid analgesia and inhibition of inflammation, such that a swift return of pain-free function can be restored for the involved joint(s) in a safe, highly effective, and cost-efficient manner.[17]

The antiinflammatory therapies used to treat acute gout do reduce pain as well as inflammation in this condition, but analgesics (typically opiates and acetaminophen-paracetamol) and local measures (e.g., rest, elevation, upper limb splint, and topical ice packs) can be used as adjunctive therapies. We do not yet know if topical nonsteroidal antiinflammatory drug (NSAID) gels add significantly to the armamentarium in acute gout.

This crucial part of management, at least for the patient, can be addressed with a variety of antiinflammatory medications (Table 16-4). If therapy with any one of these is initiated promptly after the onset of symptoms, much relief should occur quickly, with unbearable pain becoming bearable as the inflammation resolves. In most drug trials for therapy of acute gout, there is an approximately 50% decrease in pain within 2 to 3 days. The earlier acute gout is treated, the better the clinical response, but this is particularly so when using colchicine (which is most effective if started within the first day of the gouty attack). Duration of gout attack treatment should be long enough (7 to 15 days, optimally with treatment stopped 1 to 2 days after complete resolution of symptoms) to avoid early relapse.[17]

It should be recalled that septic arthritis should have been ruled out since fever, acute phase reagents, and leukocytosis can accompany acute attacks; synovial fluid analysis should be done where appropriate, and in particular if one contemplates using systemic or intraarticular steroids.

Choices of treatment for acute gout (Fig. 16-2) are dictated by the patient's comorbidities rather than by any evidence-based medicine survey. However, recent antiinflammatory agents such as interleukin (IL)-1 inhibitors have been investigated using "state-of-the-art" protocols (canakinumab, rilonacept),[18,19] as well as classic medications such as colchicine.[20] New, "lower-dose" colchicine regimens have been implemented in the United States and in Europe.

Choices of NSAIDs and Cyclooxygenase (COX)-2 Selective Inhibition as an Alternative Strategy in Gout

Any NSAID can be considered in acute gout, despite the traditional preference for indomethacin, naproxen, or sulindac, each of which is U.S. Food and Drug Administration (FDA) approved for gout in the United States. Alternatives include other short half-life NSAIDs, such as diclofenac. Full doses should be prescribed for the first 2 to 3 days and then tapered off in most cases. NSAIDs with more favorable gastrointestinal side effect profiles than indomethacin, with naproxen being a prime example, should be used more widely, in our opinion.*

Use of high doses of aspirin (acetylsalicylic acid) or of nonacetylated salicylates has not been formally evaluated for

Table 16-4 Treatment for Acute Gouty Attacks: Current Dosing Recommendations

A. Oral NSAIDs and selective COX-2 inhibitors: Therapeutic regimens are discussed in extensive detail in Chapter 10 for this category, which remains the most frequently prescribed group of drugs for acute gouty arthritis
B. Colchicine regimen in acute gouty attacks. Early treatment of acute gout attack is essential.
For attack within 12 hours of onset (U.S.)
- Use 1.2 mg, with 0.6 mg 1 hour later (FDA-approved regimen); gout flare prophylaxis can be started on day 2
- Previous, extended higher-dose regimens are no longer recommended
- Caution is required to avoid adding oral colchicine for acute gout attacks in patients already loaded in low-dose colchicine for gout attack prophylaxis
For other gout attacks (U.S., Europe)
- 0.6 mg or 0.5 mg tid for a few days (2005–2006 EULAR and BSR recommendations)
- 3 mg (maximal dosage per day) on day 1, then decrease to 1 mg after few days (France)
C. Corticosteroid regimen in acute gouty attacks.
- 30 to 50 mg/day for 3 days, then tapering and discontinuation by day 7
- Oral prednisone 30 mg/day × 5 days (as effective as naproxen 500 mg bid 3 days)
- Oral prednisolone 35 mg/day × 5 days (as effective as and better tolerated than indomethacin 150 mg/day × 2 days then 75 mg/day for 3 days)*
D. Intramuscular corticosteroid regimen: no adequate studies are available
- Triamcinolone acetate 60 mg IM for acute gout attack, followed by oral prednisone 20 to 30 mg maximum for 5 days

*Has been studied in clinical trial setting where subjects also received acetaminophen and, at onset, IM diclofenac 75 mg, before such regimens were started.

urate handling could substantially alter serum urate during the acute gout attack and thereby theoretically worsen acute gout. Also an issue is the time needed for acetylsalicylic acid to reach therapeutic serum levels for adequate analgesia to control the severe pain of gout.

Comparisons of NSAIDs and Corticosteroids

Collectively, the choice of NSAIDs can be decided based on availability, past tolerance, age, risk of cardiovascular* and gastrointestinal adverse events, cost and reimbursement, and personal prescriber choice. Indomethacin has been considered a "gold standard" in the past, but gastrointestinal and central nervous side effects are substantial with this agent, including in aged patients. High-dose prednisone or prednisolone appears at least as effective as indomethacin (or naproxen) and relatively well tolerated, and it is more cost-effective in most patients.[21-24]

*Harmful effects of NSAIDs should be recognized. Bavry et al have shown that there is an increased cardiovascular (CV) risk (CV death, nonfatal myocardial infarction [MI], nonfatal stroke) in patients with hypertension and coronary heart disease[20a]; based upon a nationwide cohort of patients over 30 years old with prior MI, even short-term treatment (less than 7 days) with most NSAIDs, except naproxen, was associated with increased risk of death and recurrent MI in patients with prior MI. As such, alternatives to short- and long-term treatment with NSAIDs should be considered in this population, NSAIFs used with caution in this population, and any NSAID use strictly limited from a CV safety point of view.[20b]

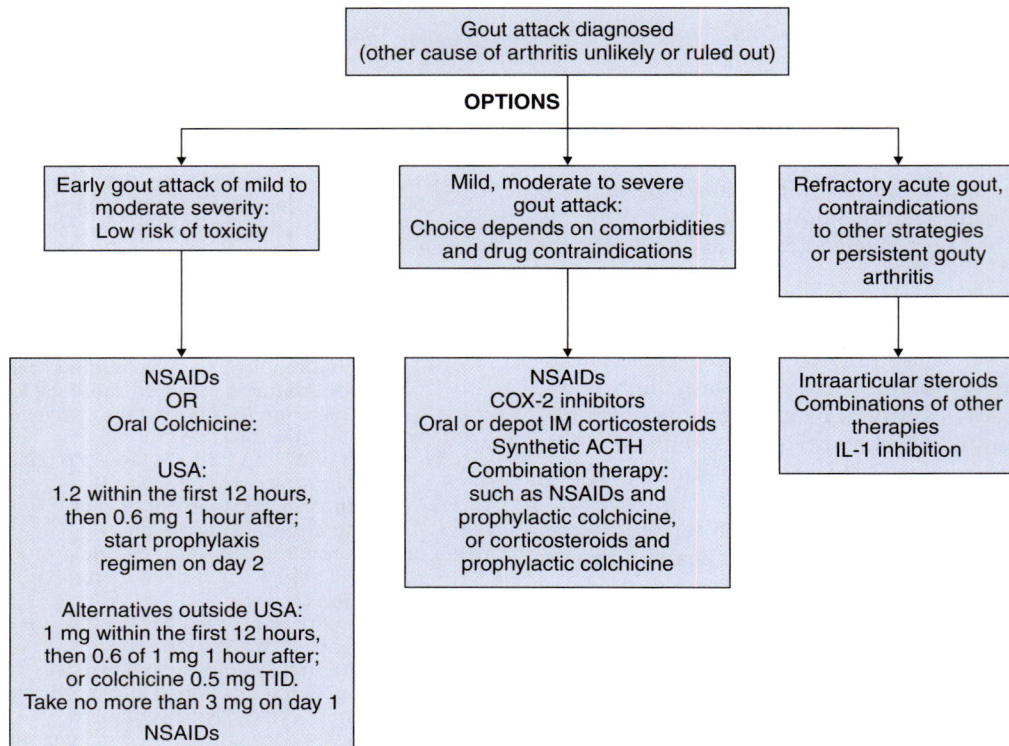

Figure 16-2 Proposed algorithm for pharmacological treatment of acute gout attack. Note that general measures also are adapted for each patient: rest, immobilization, elevation, ice pack, and analgesics.

Use of COX-2 Selective Inhibition

Some comparative studies have shown comparable effects with selective COX-2 inhibitors (coxibs) to ketoprofen and indomethacin; indeed, there is noninferiority between lumiracoxib and etoricoxib, and naproxen or indomethacin at full dosage. It should be mentioned that etoricoxib at the dosage used in gout trials (120 mg) has not been approved in Europe. Cardiovascular safety of all COX-2 selective agents clearly remains under review. In addition, the European Committee recommended that the existing contraindication on the use of etoricoxib in patients with high blood pressure that is not adequately controlled should be amended to state that patients whose blood pressure is persistently above 140/90 mm Hg and has not been adequately controlled must not take the medicine. Warnings on the risk of heart-related side effects should also be added, stating that (1) high blood pressure should be controlled before treatment is begun and (2) blood pressure should be monitored for 2 weeks after the start of treatment and regularly thereafter. In gout, cardiovascular safety questions still exist regarding the use of coxibs.

Use of celecoxib is not universally accepted for treatment of acute gout. Importantly, it appears that use of celecoxib to treat acute gout requires substantial doses. Schumacher and colleagues have reported preliminary results in which celecoxib to be as effective as indomethacin in acute gout, and better tolerated.[25] However, substantial doses of celecoxib appeared necessary in a randomized, double-blind, double-dummy, active-controlled trial of acute gout, with onset of pain up to 48 hours prior to enrollment. The study was randomized 1:1:1:1 for celecoxib 50 mg twice daily, celecoxib 400 mg followed by 200 mg on day 1 and then 200 mg twice daily for 7 days, celecoxib 800 mg

followed by 400 mg on day 1 and then 400 mg twice daily for 7 days, or indomethacin 50 mg three times daily. The high-dose celecoxib (800/400 mg) regimen was associated with greater pain reduction on day 2 compared to low-dose celecoxib (50 mg twice daily; $p = .0014$), and it also was superior to the middle-dose celecoxib regimen. The high-dose celecoxib 800/400 mg regimen gave results for pain relief from baseline to day 2 comparable to indomethacin 50 mg three times daily but was better tolerated.

Colchicine

The EULAR and BSR recommendations have mainly focused on NSAIDs as a first-line choice for acute gout, since colchicine was not widely used in North European countries.[10,11] By contrast, in southern European countries such as Spain, Portugal, France, Italy, and even Switzerland, colchicine is long used as a therapeutic but also as a "diagnostic" compound in gout, but that practice is unreliable.

In the United States, a recent randomized, placebo-controlled trial (AGREE) has shown that low-dose oral colchicine 1.8 mg self-administered by the patient over 2 hours, and given within the first 12 hours after acute attack began, was as effective as high-dose 4.8 mg colchicine (given in divided doses over 7 hours) on day 1.[20] With this regimen, 38% of patients are expected to be responders, meaning that additional therapy should be necessary in other patients. EULAR recommendations, based on expert opinions, suggested that a low colchicine dose of up to 1.5 mg (0.5 mg twice daily) daily will be effective in some patients.[10]

Therefore, a low-dose colchicine regimen is now advocated for early gout and is a regimen the patient can quickly

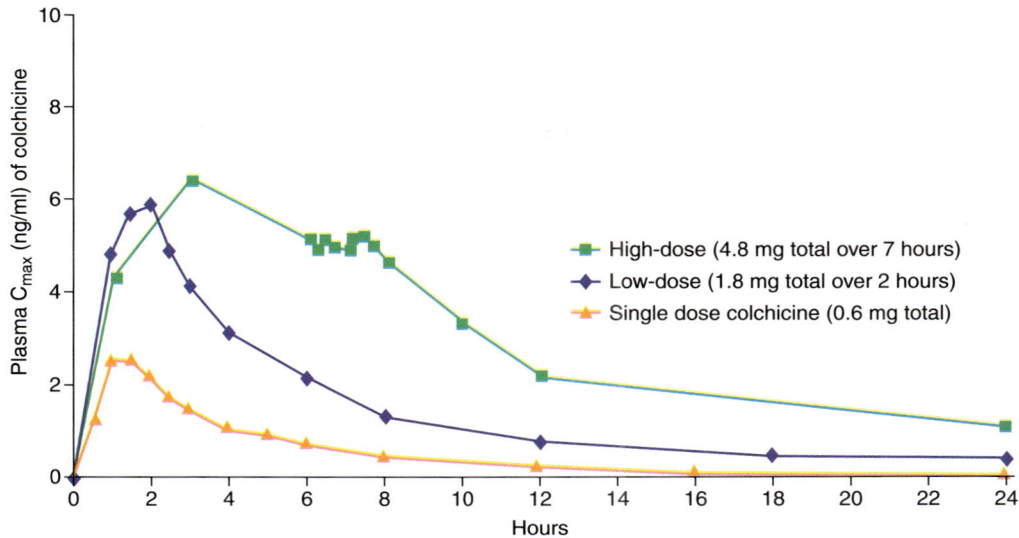

Figure 16-3 Low-dose and high-dose colchicine pharmacokinetics in acute gout treatment regimens. Identical plasma C_{max} of about 6 ng/ml is achieved by high-dose and low-dose colchicine, likely accounting for the major therapeutic effects. Total drug exposure is proportional to dose and likely accounts for the majority of side effects. *(From Terkeltaub RA, et al. High versus low dosing of oral colchicine for early acute gout flare: twenty-four-hour outcome of the first multicenter, randomized, double-blind, placebo-controlled, parallel-group, dose-comparison colchicine study. Arthritis Rheum 2010;62(4):1060-8.)*

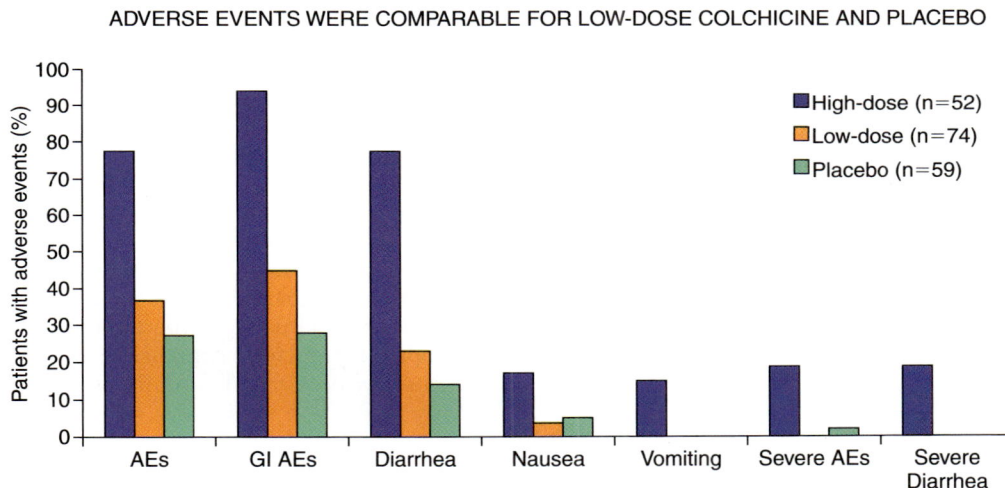

Figure 16-4 Comparison of side effects of low-dose and high-dose colchicine pharmacokinetics in acute gout treatment regimens. "Low-dose" oral colchicine: 1.2 mg, then 0.6 mg 1 hour later; "high-dose" oral colchicine: 1.2 mg, then 0.6 mg every hour afterward for 6 more hours (4.8 mg total). *(From Terkeltaub RA, et al. High versus low dosing of oral colchicine for early acute gout flare: twenty-four-hour outcome of the first multicenter, randomized, double-blind, placebo-controlled, parallel-group, dose-comparison colchicine study. Arthritis Rheum 2010;62(4):1060-8.)*

self-administer to limit acute gout attacks. Gout patients can also test their sensitivity to such a colchicine regimen at the inception of gout attacks, early in the course of their disease. There is absolutely no evidence basis to support "inundating" the patient with early gout attack with repeated doses of colchicine clustered over several hours. This opinion is buttressed by key pharmacokinetics and side effects results of the AGREE trial (Figs. 16-3 and 16-4). In particular, both low- and high-dose colchicine attained circulating C_{max} of approximately 6 ng/ml in the AGREE trial (see Fig. 16-3) under conditions where their efficacy was comparable but total drug exposure was proportional to dose and, under these conditions, toxicity was remarkably high in the high-dose colchicine group, but

no significant difference was seen between placebo and low-dose colchicine (see Fig. 16-4).

When colchicine is started later than 12 hours after flare onset, 1.5 or 1.8 mg might be inefficient.[26,27] One option is to increase colchicine dosage up to the maximum daily dose allowed by each current national formulary. In France, the current updated maximal colchicine dosage is 3 mg/day, but, in our opinion, a superior option is to add another therapeutic to the low-dose colchicine, such as an NSAID or corticosteroid, for refractory acute gout.

It is not advised in the U.S. to use extra colchicine for an acute gout attack that occurs despite 1 mg or 1.2 mg/day colchicine prophylaxis. Higher colchicine doses, and more extended early-dosing regimens over multiple hours, do not clearly add efficacy and they increase toxicity in early gout attack treatment.

Differences in Colchicine Formulations Internationally

Each country has its own labeled colchicines with different unitary dosages (0.5, 0.6, or 1 mg, scored tablet or not, with anticholinergic compound), giving the opportunity to precisely adjust the dosage. Combination of colchicine with intestinal "protector" (dicycloverine [anticholinergic], tiemonium [antispasmodic]) should not be used since this can mask diarrhea as a sign of colchicine toxicity. Examples are 1 mg Colchicine (colchicine) or 1 mg Colchimax (colchicine + opium + tiemonium methylsulfate) in France, 0.6 mg Colchrys (colchine) in the United States, and 1 mg Colchicina (colchicine) and 0.5 mg Colchimax (colchicine + dicycloverine) in Spain.

Intravenous (IV) colchicine is no longer approved in the United States and is not available in Europe. Inappropriate use and the life-threatening side effects of overdosage of IV colchicine (including deaths) were behind the FDA edict for withdrawal from the U.S. market.

Factor in Choosing Corticosteroids or ACTH (Corticotrophin) for Acute Gout

Corticosteroids have justifiably become much more popular for acute gout because of efficacy and safety in patients with contraindications to colchicine and NSAIDs, let alone low cost. Oral or parenteral steroids and intraarticular steroid injections are the most common modes of prescription.[28] In some countries, corticotropin (ACTH) is also used and appears to be effective in many cases, with rapidity of therapeutic action seen in a matter of hours. Cost is inexpensive for ACTH in many European countries, but in the United States, it can be significant for the synthetic ACTH (which is the preferred form). Adequate, comparative controlled trials of ACTH in gout are still lacking.

Oral Therapy

Prednisone or prednisolone is a valuable frontline treatment for acute gout, with best practice guidelines to use a starting dose of at least 0.5 mg/kg prednisone on the first day. Indeed, the fact that attacks of acute gout develop in many major-organ transplant patients maintained on daily prednisone (in the range of 7.5 to 10 mg/day) is a good illustration of the need for relatively high initial doses of systemic corticosteroids to effectively treat acute gouty arthritis. Sample regimens include 30 to 60 mg prednisone daily for 3 days (depending on severity of the flare, then decreasing by 10 to 15 mg/day every 3 days until discontinuation). Alternatively, for relatively mild attacks of acute gout, a methylprednisolone single dose is sometimes used in clinical practice, but this is not an evidence-based regimen.

Two randomized, controlled, clinical trials have shown equivalence between prednisolone 30 to 35 mg/day for 5 days and full-dose NSAIDs. Prednisolone 35 mg/day for 5 days and naproxen 500 mg twice daily for 5 days were similar in efficacy and tolerance for acute gout,[13] and prednisolone (6 doses of 30 mg over 5 days) was similar in efficacy to indomethacin (150 mg/day for 2 days followed by 75 mg/day for 3 other days) and was superior in tolerance.[14]

Parenteral Systemic Corticosteroid Therapy

In severe cases of acute polyarticular gout or when the patient is unable to ingest oral medication, a short course of intravenous methylprednisolone appears to be an appropriate strategy. Using 100 to 150 mg IV methylprednisolone as an initial dose, followed by 50 to 75 mg twice daily for a few days, is considered to be a reasonable starting point for acute gout. A single dose of 60 mg IM triamcinolone acetonide (a potent antiinflammatory with a relatively long half-life) has been suggested to be effective for acute gout. Single intramuscular corticosteroid dose administration allows controlling drug intake, avoiding some side effects due to repeated oral steroid dosing.[29] However, continuation with oral prednisone for several additional days after the IM triamcinolone is better clinical practice for most patients. Duration of oral corticosteroid treatment is not defined but should be limited to 5 to 14 days in order to limit side effects.[24]

Rebound Attacks of Gout After Discontinuation of Systemic Corticosteroids

The use of corticosteroids and ACTH for treatment of acute gout attack is associated with the potential for rebound attacks when the short courses of corticosteroids are stopped. The best practice is to initiate or continue low-dose colchicine for gout-flare prophylaxis as an adjunct to therapy when systemic glucocorticoids are used to treat acute gout, particularly in the setting of recent initiation of ULT. This practice is much preferable to having to administer sustained or multiple courses of systemic corticosteroids, even at low doses, in patients with gout. Chronic steroid side effects should be monitored, including diabetes mellitus and hypertension. Concerns regarding development or increase of tophi size in corticosteroid-treated patients have been raised,[30] but this is not yet substantiated.

Anti–Interleukin-1 Agents

Because IL-1β is the pivotal cytokine in MSU crystal–induced inflammation, development of anti–IL-1 agents, already approved in orphan autoinflammatory conditions, in the treatment and prophylaxis of acute gout will allow for addressing unmet needs. Off-label use of anakinra, a soluble IL-1 receptor antagonist, typically administered at 100 mg subcutaneously for 3 consecutive days, was linked with rapid control of pain and local symptoms within 48 hours in the majority of patients with sustained gouty arthritis in two small open reports.[31,32] Moreover, rilonacept, another soluble IL-1 inhibitor, was associated with significant decrease in symptoms and decreased C-reactive protein, in a small controlled crossover study of patients with chronic gouty arthritis.[19] This far, in clinical trials, as discussed elsewhere in this book, canakinumab was superior to 40 mg IM single-dose triamcinolone for acute gout, whereas rilonacept was not significantly superior to rilonacept and indomethacin for acute gout. In patients with comorbidities, namely chronic kidney disease (CKD) and congestive heart failure (CHF), which limit or forbid the use or the dosage of NSAIDs, anti–IL-1β agents can be helpful, under strict supervision.[31]

Urate-Lowering Therapy and Management
Objectives

The roles of ULT are to suppress the formation and deposition of MSU crystals and to promote tophus dissolution.[1,10,11,15] The main SUA targets are regularly less than 6.0 mg/dL (360 μmol/L) or less than 5.0 mg/dL (300 μmol/L).[26] Achieving these targets is effective in controlling and remitting the disease as long as this level of urate-lowering is maintained. In cases of tophaceous gout, levels less than 250 or 300 μmol/L may be required for resolution of tophi[12]; the velocity of tophus size reduction appears to be linked to the lowest attained SUA levels. A mean of 20 or 29 months is required to achieve complete resolution of tophi, according to SUA of 4.0 mg/dl and 5.4 mg/dl, respectively, achieved using combined allopurinol-benzbromarone and allopurinol alone.

Ultimately, adjusted ULT prescription will prevent disease progression by reducing the body urate burden. Any patient presenting with advanced gout or demonstrating clinical tophi or recurrent attacks (two or more per year) should be treated. In Europe, it is recommended to start ULT after the first two attacks. In uncomplicated gout, ULT should be started if a second attack or further attacks occur within 1 year.[1,11,15] Indications for ULT drug therapy are summarized in Table 16-5, and sites of ULT action are schematized in Figure 16-5.

Hyperuricemia alone is NOT currently an indication to use ULT but rather to control comorbid, dietary, and iatrogenic factors that promote hyperuricemia. Recent, preliminary ultrasound studies suggest that subclinical tophi or the "double contour" sign might be detected in up to a third of patients with chronic asymptomatic hyperuricemia.[33]

Studies will be needed to provide insights on potential utility of early ULT in such a subset of patients.

Choice of Drugs in ULT

As first-line drugs in the average patient (Fig. 16-6), both allopurinol and febuxostat, xanthine oxidase inhibitors (XOIs), or uricostatics, are effective in treating gout patients, regardless of the mechanism of hyperuricemia.[34] Uricosurics are mainly used as second-line drugs after XOI failure: they include probenecid and, outside the United States, benzbromarone and sulfinpyrazone, with availability varying according to country.[35] Fenofibrate is less potent than these primary uricosurics, and losartan is even less potent and often only temporarily effective in urate lowering. Both potent uricosuric drug therapy and XOI therapy have comparable efficacy in normalizing SUA and ultimately in decreasing and abolishing gout attacks and shrinking tophi (see Fig. 16-6). Uricosurics should generally be avoided as primary therapy for serum urate–lowering if the 24-hour urine uric acid excretion is greater than 700 mg/day. Since XOI therapy decreases urine uric acid excretion, it

Table 16-5 Indications for Pharmacologic Urate-Lowering Therapy (ULT)

Recurrent gout attacks (at a frequency of two or more per year)
OR clinical tophi or tophi seen on imaging (it is not resolved if "double contour" sign on high-resolution ultrasound, by itself, is an absolute indication for ULT)
OR chronic tophaceous gouty arthropathy
OR severe, polyarticular, or difficult to treat gout attacks (e.g., in advanced chronic kidney disease, congestive heart failure, or major organ transplant recipient)
OR documented state of uric acid overproduction
OR history of urolithiasis

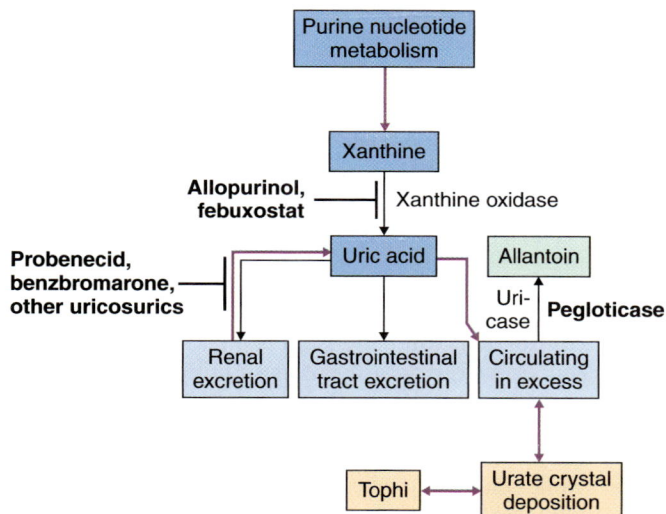

Figure 16-5 Schematic pathways of urate and tophi formation and targets for urate-lowering therapy. (Adapted from Schlesinger N, Yasothan U, Kirkpatrick P. Pegloticase. Nat Rev Drug Discov 2011;10(1):17-8.)

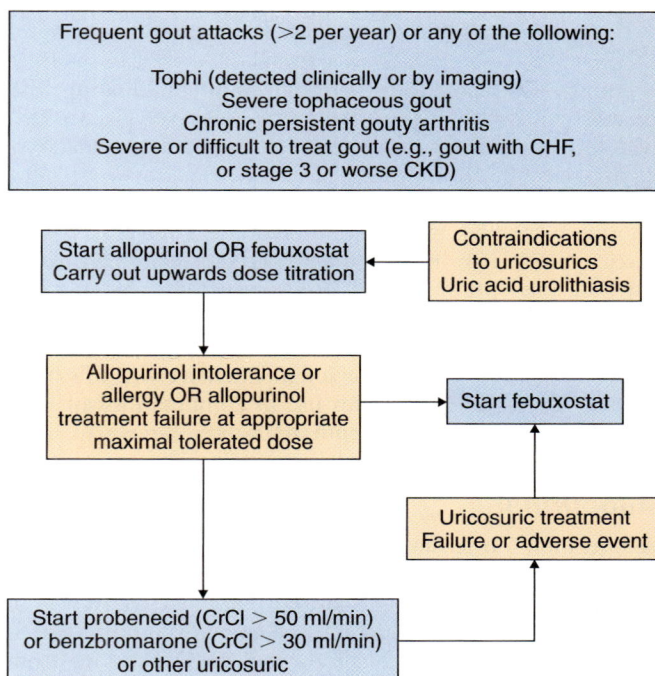

Figure 16-6 Proposed "single-agent" therapeutic algorithm for serum urate lowering in the average case of gout. This algorithm shows the authors' recommended strategy for therapeutic SUA lowering in patients with gout, taking onto account alternative approaches in the event of therapeutic failures of specific treatment choices (allopurinol). Not shown in the figure is the strategy (discussed in the text) of using uricosuric therapy to provide additive effects with xanthine oxidase inhibition, since xanthine oxidase inhibitors decrease urinary uric acid excretion. Also not shown is pegloticase therapy for severe cases.

Refractory gout
Defined primarily by failure to adequately lower serum urate (SUA)
Examples of settings: Severe and frequent gout attacks and/or polyarticular tophaceous gout
Limitations in treatment options due to comorbidities such as CKD or CHF, or due to hypersensitivity or intolerance with urate-lowering drug(s)

↓

Difficult to lower SUA to target (e.g., < 6.0 mg/gL in the average case) with allopurinol, febuxostat, or uricosuric alone

↓

Titrate single urate-lowering agent to maximum appropriate dose AND/OR consider combination of appropriately dosed xanthine oxidase inhibitor and uricosuric

↓

Failure to lower SUA to target after optimally dosed oral therapy, or drug intolerance, AND patient has active symptoms from arthritis and tophi and/or connective tissue destruction from tophaceous disease

↓

Consider pegloticase, especially as limited-term ≪tophus debulking≫ therapy

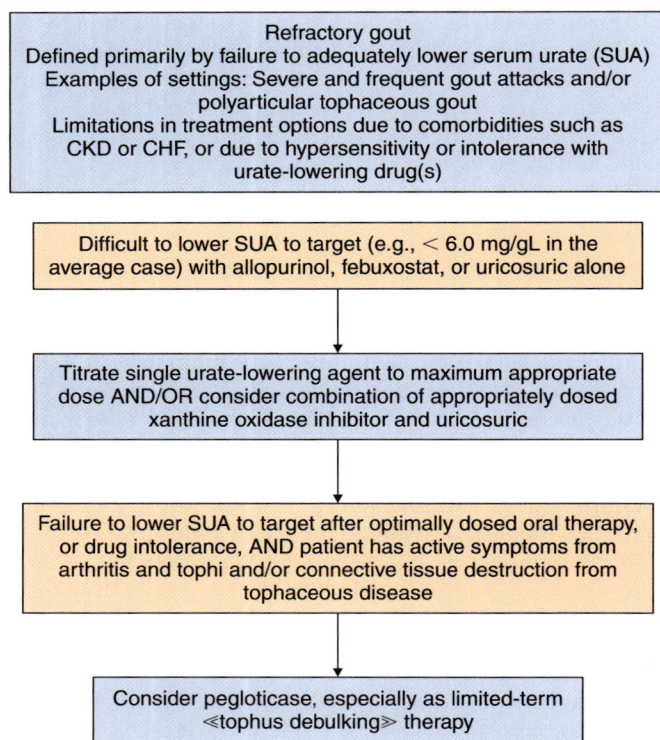

Figure 16-7 Proposed algorithm for urate-lowering therapy in refractory gout. This model is related to failure to properly lower chronic hyperuricemia to a serum urate target of less than 6.0 mg/dl; 360 μmol/L, or lower in tophaceous gout (at least below 5.0 mg/dl [300 μmol/L]).

is entirely acceptable to use uricosurics in combination with established XOI therapy in refractory cases (see Fig. 16-7),[36] with one caveat being that probenecid can increase renal oxypurinol clearance.[37]

Recently pegloticase, a recombinant uricase, has been approved for the most severe, treatment-refractory gout cases, particularly in chronic tophaceous gouty arthropathy that fails optimized oral antihyperuricemic therapy (see Fig. 16-7).[13] Pegloticase can achieve rapid tophus resolution (in months) in responders (see Chapter 14). Uses of each of these classes of agents are reviewed extensively in this book (see Chapters 12 to 14), with use of combinations of ULT drugs discussed in further depth in Chapter 27.

Allopurinol

Allopurinol, a uricostatic drug, is currently the most widely used ULT, and most often the first-line ULT, because of its ease of use (once daily) and low cost and its effectiveness in both uric acid overproduction and underexcretion.[1,34] It is standard practice to titrate allopurinol dosage, starting from 100 mg/day, increasing by 100 mg (or 50 mg with advanced renal impairment) every 15 to 30 days to an appropriate maximum dose in order to achieve the serum urate target.

Chi va piano va sano, or "the slower the safer," since slow adjustment of allopurinol will reduce gout attacks and improve compliance. Indeed, there is no rush to lower SUA to target or below this threshold. However, a "standard," but relatively ineffective dose, is 300 mg/day. A slight increase to 400 mg/day can be sufficient.[38] In patients with normal renal function, maximal allopurinol dosage is 800 to 900 mg/day according to differing national formulary standards. In CKD, lowered maximum dosages of allopurinol will be relatively ineffective in adequately controlling hyperuricemia and do not avoid severe allopurinol hypersensitivity.[39]

Febuxostat

Febuxostat[40,41] is structurally different from allopurinol, and it is standard practice to turn to febuxostat in those with prior allergy or intolerance to allopurinol, or ineffectiveness of allopurinol at maximum appropriate dose (see Chapter 13). It is taken orally in doses of 40 mg initially, with escalation to 80 mg after 2 to 3 weeks if the target serum urate of less than 6.0 mg/dl is not achieved on the lower dose. In Europe, the two available dosages are 80- and 120-mg tablets. There are inadequate safety data to this point for assessing risks of increasing febuxostat above 120 mg/day over the long term.[42] Unlike allopurinol, there is no recommended need for reduction of the maximum dose in mild-to-moderate renal impairment (stage 2 and stage 3 CKD). Relative performance of febuxostat and allopurinol in clinical trials was reviewed in Chapter 13. In renally impaired subjects, febuxostat is a particularly valuable option, although there are not yet safety data for febuxostat in stage 4 CKD.

Ultimately, the choice between the first-line XOI agents, allopurinol or febuxostat, largely depends on factors including cost and third party payer approval, history of drug allergy, renal and liver function, and prior success in achieving the serum urate target on appropriate maximum doses of XOI therapy. Clearly, dose maximums for allopurinol should not be calculated according to the non–evidence-based Hande et al. criteria of the 1980s. Instead, one approach is to carefully titrate allopurinol upward (e.g., increase by 50 to 100 mg/day every 4 weeks, between the 200 to 600 mg/day range, in those with no worse than stage 2 CKD, with a lower dose maximum of allopurinol applied to those with stage 3 or worse CKD).[43] No matter which XOI agent is chosen, liver function studies should be monitored prior to and during therapy.

Practical Management, Including Gout Attack Prophylaxis

Gout attack triggers and prophylaxis (pharmacologic and nonpharmacologic approaches) were reviewed in (see Chapter 15). In brief, in patients requiring pharmacologic ULT (Table 16-6), the following approach should be applied:

1. Initiate antiinflammatory prophylaxis with low-dose daily colchicine (0.5 or 0.6 mg once or twice a day or 1 mg/day) or a low-dose NSAID, at least 1 to 2 weeks prior to starting ULT and continue prophylaxis for 6 months or longer (see Table 16-6).
2. ULT should not be started at time of attacks but after control of inflammation and pain.
3. Initiate a uricostatic agent at an initial low dose (100 mg/day for allopurinol or 40 mg/day for febuxostat in the United States, or a higher febuxostat dose outside the United States), monitor SUA every 2 to 3 weeks while increasing allopurinol or febuxostat. In the United States, gradual increase in febuxostat dosage is achieved, while in Europe an initial dose of 80 mg febuxostat might more sharply reduce hyperuricemia, triggering more early gout attacks; 40 mg febuxostat

Table 16-6 Gout Attack Prophylaxis Regimens: Start Prophylaxis 1 to 2 Weeks Before Starting Urate-Lowering Therapy

Preferred regimen
- Oral colchicine 0.6 mg once or twice daily (U.S.) or 1.0 mg (0.5 mg twice daily or 1.0 mg daily (Europe) for at least 6 months (minimal mandatory duration with febuxostat in Europe)
- Continue longer than 6 months in patients with visible tophi, continuing gout attacks, or for at least 3 months after serum urate is normalized to <6.0 mg/dL in those with refractory hyperuricemia
- Reduce daily colchicine dose in those:
  - With stage 3 or worse chronic kidney disease (i.e., creatinine clearance <60 mL/min adjusted for ideal body weight)
  - With potential drug-drug interactions (e.g., 50% colchicine dose reduction with verapamil or diltiazem)
  - Possibly aged >70 years

Alternative regimen
- Low-dose NSAID prophylaxis for same time-frame as described for colchicine (e.g., naproxen 250 mg PO twice daily, or indomethacin 25 mg PO twice daily, or diclofenac 25 mg twice daily)
- The evidence basis for NSAID-based prophylaxis regimens is less established than for colchicine, and cardiovascular/gastrointestinal safety issues are unknown. Consider proton pump inhibitor where appropriate.

Avoid use of low-dose prednisone or prednisolone as prophylaxis for gout attacks
- Low-dose prednisone often fails to prevent gout attacks and it is difficult to wean gout patients from low-dose prednisone due to rebound attacks

Experimental, in advanced clinical trials: Interleukin-1 inhibitors

Table 16-7 Strategies That Use Adjunctive Drugs or Compounds With Urate-Lowering Effects

- Antihypertensive drugs: Discontinue diuretics, in particular thiazides and loop diuretics, and replace by other antihypertensive agents (e.g., losartan, which is uricosuric, and amlodipine in patients with CKD).
- Lipid-lowering drugs: Fenofibrate,* atorvastatin†
- Diet and vitamins†: Low-fat or nonfat dairy products, vitamin C (500-1000 mg/day): caution is needed, because this may increase the risk of urolithiasis
- Hormones: Estrogens*

*Can reduce serum urate by more than 0.6 mg/dL (36 µmol/L); uricosuric effect of estrogens contributes to the low risk of gout before menopause.
†Can reduce serum urate by 0.4–0.6 mg/dl (24–36 µmol/L) due to uricosuric effects.

can be considered everywhere as an initiation therapy, in part to reduce gout attacks in early ULT. Due to half-life issues, febuxostat should always be used as an everyday medication, and the drug should not be used as an alternate day treatment (in order to avoid day-to-day swings in serum urate).

4. If gout attack occurs, patients should be aware that they should NOT stop uricostatic agent but should maintain the dosage and treat by adding or optimizing NSAIDs or colchicine prophylaxis.
5. Prophylaxis should be reinforced (see later).

Prophylaxis of Gout Attacks

Nonpharmacologic and pharmacologic gout attack prophylaxis (see Table 16-6) was reviewed in depth in Chapter 15. Unfortunately, this arm of therapy is frequently neglected in clinical practice. Patients also need to appreciate that early gout attacks do not represent failure of ULT or adverse events of ULT but rather evidence for reduction in SUA level and are the "price you have to pay for cure."[15] Patients should be warned that attacks can occur for months with decreased frequency as a first outcome. Efficacy of colchicine is evidence based (see Chapter 15), and the drug dose can be titrated in renal impairment.

In patients who cannot tolerate colchicine, an NSAID or coxib can be substituted provided that there are no contraindications, but the duration of NSAID or coxib prophylactic use should be limited to weeks to months.[11] Indomethacin 25 mg twice daily appears to be effective, as are other NSAIDs such as diclofenac 25 mg twice daily or naproxen 250 mg

twice daily. Combination of 0.6 or 0.5 mg colchicine and low-dose NSAIDs is another possibility but there are no evidence-based data.

Duration of Prophylaxis

Because of potential toxicity, the continued use of colchicine or NSAID is not recommended after achieving stable normalization of serum urate, unless tophi remain detectable on physical examination. Duration of prophylaxis is related to clinical settings and regulatory facts. Colchicine (as low-dose prophylaxis) should be continued for at least 6 months (6 months is mandatory in Europe for febuxostat use) when there is no clinical detection of tophi. A 12-month course of prophylaxis is not unusual, because gout attacks can continue over this period of time, and potential drug interactions should be monitored. The optimal duration of prophylaxis when tophi are present is debated: most experts recommend continuing gout attack prophylaxis as long as tophi are clinically detectable. Duration of prophylaxis with NSAIDs has been recommended, by the BSR, to be only 6 weeks; this is not a viable duration of prophylaxis in most patients.[11]

Management of comorbidities to help reduce serum urate

Besides obesity, primary caregivers and treating specialists should pay attention to comorbidities, since specific management could be needed. Nonpharmacologic measures aimed at reducing uric acid (Table 16-7) will also contribute by reducing blood pressure, blood sugar level, and insulin resistance and will improve general health. Drugs that are hypouricemic agents via uricosuric effects, such as losartan for hypertension and atorvastatin or fenofibrate for dyslipidemia, can also have a salutary effect in management of patients with gout (see Table 16-7).

Targets and Management of Refractory Disease

Particularly to avoid treatment failure, quality of care should also be proposed to physicians.[44-46] Quality indicators can be suggested to improve the treat to target process (Table 16-8). Special situations include the following.

Table 16-8 Quality Indicators Proposed in the Management of Gout

1. Urate-lowering therapy (ULT) should be offered to patients with gouty arthritis with recurrent attacks, radiographic changes, tophaceous deposits, or history of urolithiasis or to difficult-to-treat patients.
2. No pharmacologic treatment of asymptomatic hyperuricemia with ULT in absence of related symptoms or complications or with malignancy under chemotherapy*
3. Measure creatinine clearance (using the MDRD formula) before allopurinol or febuxostat prescription.
4. Initial allopurinol dosage: 100 mg/day, or initial febuxostat dose 40 mg/day (U.S.) or 80 mg/day (Europe)
5. Maximal allopurinol dosage defined according to national formularies
6. Mandatory prophylaxis of ULT-triggered gout attacks before initiating ULT†
7. Once SUA target achieved (<6.0 mg/dl [360 μmol/L] in all), monitor SUA level regularly every 6 months to ensure drug maintenance and target.
8. Avoid severe drug interactions with colchicine (e.g., clarithromycin) during prophylaxis of gout attacks.
9. Limit diuretic use strictly to CHF or CKD, with consideration of discontinuation of nonessential diuretics and switching to other antihypertensive agents in hypertension.
10. Educate patients and monitor regularly for diet modifications and lifestyle changes; education should include avoidance of dehydration in order to reduce gout attack frequency; warning on the possibility of frequent gout attacks early after initiation of ULT; stress importance of adherence to treatment.

*Hyperuricemia without gouty arthritis attacks but with the "double contour" sign or a subclinical tophi detected by ultrasonography alone is not yet an unequivocal indication for ULT.
†Duration of prophylaxis is at least 6 months.
Adapted from Zhang W, et al. Ann Rheum Dis 2006;65:1312-24 and from Jordan KM, et al. Rheumatology (Oxford) 2007;46:1372-4.

Management of Patients With Allopurinol Allergy or Failure

Allopurinol side effects occur in 6% to 10% of patients.[47] The most difficult issue is related to drug discontinuation when allergic reaction occurs, ranging from skin "rash" to DRESS (drug reaction with eosinophilia and systemic symptoms) or even Lyell syndrome. The DRESS syndrome usually commences symptomatically 1 to 8 weeks after exposure to the responsible drug. The classic combination is rash, fever, and major internal organ involvement (most commonly hepatitis but can include nephritis and pneumonitis). Eosinophilia is often present. Allopurinol should not be continued or reintroduced, since there is a high risk for more severe adverse reaction, including fatal outcome.

Febuxostat

Skin reactions have been reported in RCT comparing febuxostat to allopurinol; a similar prevalence of skin reactions (about 2% overall) has been reported. Severe cutaneous hypersensitivity appears rare with febuxostat, and febuxostat use is appropriate in those with a history of prior hypersensitivity reaction to allopurinol. It is not yet known whether those with past severe hypersensitivity reaction to allopurinol are also at increased risk for

hypersensitivity to febuxostat[41]; hence, caution is needed in this setting.

Uricosurics

Urinary pH should be checked before starting urocosurics, since urine pH < 6 is a risk factor for precipitating uric acid lithiasis in urine when urinary uric acid excretion is increased by drugs. Sodium or potassium citrate or fresh lemon juice every day can provide an inexpensive and safe way to reduce frequency of urinary tract uric acid stones. Patients should ensure adequate hydration (1500 to 2000 ml of water intake daily) in order to dilute the urine. Overall, these measures will reduce the risk of urolithiasis (see Chapter 12).

Probenecid

Renal function should be adequate (as discussed in Chapter 12; probenecid does lose effectiveness with stage 3 CKD, but the evidence basis is not fully established as to what degree of GFR is associated with marked loss of probenecid effect). Drug dosage is started at 250 mg twice a day because of its short half-life, and the dose should be gradually increased up to 1000 mg twice daily as a typical maximum (with 3000 mg/day an absolute maximum). However, probenecid can be effective at submaximal doses. Probenecid exerts drug-drug interactions that should be avoided. Efficacy has been observed in monotherapy or in association with allopurinol (see Chapter 12),[48] and probenecid can be added to febuxostat. However, probenecid side effects are potentially substantial.[48]

Benzbromarone

Benzbromarone is available only outside the United States and is still available in Europe and other countries, on a regular prescription form or on a restricted basis after failure, contraindication, or side effects of probenecid.[35] Standard dosages of benzbromarone (100 mg/day) tend to produce greater hypouricemic effects than the most frequently prescribed doses of allopurinol (300 mg/day) or probenecid 1000 mg/day.[48,49] Adverse effects associated with benzbromarone are relatively infrequent but potentially severe. Four cases of benzbromarone-induced hepatotoxicity were identified from the literature with debatable causality.[35] Benefit-risk assessment based on total exposure to the drug does not support the decision by the drug company (Sanofi-Synthélabo) to withdraw benzbromarone from the market, given the paucity of alternative options at that time. It is likely that risks of hepatotoxicity could be ameliorated by using a graded dosage increase, together with regular (monthly) monitoring of liver function.

Sulfinpyrazone

This uricosuric is available in a few European countries but is no longer available in the United States. Sulfinpyrazone (200 to 800 mg/day) can be used only in patients with adequate renal function, as discussed in Chapter 12. Initial dosage is 50 mg twice daily, with increase to the usual dosage of 200 mg (BSR recommendations). The drug, which is related to phenylbutazone, has antiplatelet activity and other potential toxicities that can be severe.

Refractory Gout or Treatment-Failure Gout

There are no universally accepted definitions of refractory or treatment-failure gout (TFG) (see Fig. 16-7). This uncommon clinical presentation should be distinguished from DTT gout, in which optimal ULT treatment or attack management cannot be achieved because of intolerance, contraindications, or allergy. DTT gout therefore encompasses gout with uncontrolled gout attacks because of contraindications, adverse events including intolerance and allergy, or drug interaction. These cases are clearly related to aging, CKD, CHF, and other cardiovascular events.

Among patients diagnosed with gout, only 60% will be treated with ULT and only 25% of them will remain on treatment for longer than 1 month. Thereafter, only 25% will adhere to treatment but only 40% will reach target. Then, a genuine treatment failure, defined as reaching target despite appropriate management, is limited to these adherent treat-to-target failure patients. Since failure-to-treat gout is not synonymous with treat-to-target failure, namely below an SUA level of 6.0 mg/dl (60 mg/L), it is essential to identify patients who do not adhere to their ULT. With allopurinol treatment, a serum trough oxypurinol level may be helpful, especially if it is subtherapeutic, and many patients on allopurinol, especially those with CKD, require supratherapeutic oxypurinol levels to achieve the serum urate target,[43,51,52] but long-term safety issues above the baseline therapeutic levels of oxypurinol are not yet clear.

Ultimately, DTT gout patients, or nonadherent patients, can evolve to TFG. TFG affects approximately 40,000 to 100,000 patients, or about 1% or slightly more of the overall population of patients with gout in the United States.[13] The severity of TFG is manifested by frequent gout attacks, chronic deforming arthropathy, destructive tophi on bones and joints, progressive physical disability, and poor health-related quality of life. Notably, some patients with hands and feet involved by tophi[53] can have severely impaired function and major complications such as superinfection or joint and soft tissue destruction leading to amputation. Pegloticase responders clearly can have improved quality of life in this clinical scenario, as discussed later and in Chapter 14.

Interleukin-1 Antagonist

When TFG is related to poor control of gout attacks or failure to achieve proper prophylaxis, the use of anti–IL-1 agents can be helpful, as discussed here earlier and in other chapters, although this is not yet FDA or EMEA approved at the time of writing.

Uncontrolled Serum Urate Level and Marked Tophaceous Disease

When TFG is related to uncontrolled hyperuricemia due to ineffective ULT, several strategies can be proposed (see Fig. 16-7), as follows.

Combination Therapy

In some patients with advanced disease and multiple tophaceous deposits, lowering the serum urate level to well below 6.0 mg/dL, such as less than 5.0 or even 4.0 mg/day, appears to help optimize therapy. The velocity of size reduction of tophi is greater when SUA is lower.[54] Add-on of uricosuric agent to allopurinol has been proved to be effective to lower SUA below 5.0 mg/dL (300 μmol/L) or even 4.0 mg/dL (240 μmol/L).[36] Probenecid and benzbromarone have been evaluated in small but randomized controlled trials[36,48,49] with this low SUA target. However, uricosurics have specific contraindications (see Chapter 12).

Uricases are reviewed in Chapter 14. Rasburicase[55] is non-PEGylated and use is limited by immunogenicity. In September 2010, pegloticase (Krystexxa; Savient Pharmaceuticals), a recombinant urate oxidase conjugated to polyethylene glycol (PEG) to increase half-life, was approved by the FDA for the treatment of chronic gout in adult patients refractory to conventional therapy.[63] Pegloticase is intended for use in TFG at a dose of 8 mg (of uricase protein) by IV infusion every 2 weeks. The active substance is a genetically engineered, recombinant, PEG-conjugated mammalian (porcine-baboon) uricase enzyme. In a 6-month, placebo-controlled clinical trial, 8 mg of pegloticase for every 2 weeks induced a striking decrease of SUA concentrations, leading to dissolution of tophi in 40% of patients at final visit, and further responses in some patients in open-label extension, with retreatment tolerated in many responders. However, 58% were nonresponders to the defined target SUA of 6.0 mg/dl (360 μmol/L), associated with treatment-emergent antibodies. Moreover, 26% to 31% experienced infusion reactions and 77% suffered from gout attacks. Since infusion reactions occurred in line with antibodies raised against the product, infusion reaction prophylaxis consisted of oral anti-H1 and paracetamol-acetaminophen and a corticosteroid such as hydrocortisone 200 mg IV before pegloticase infusion.

The majority of infusion reactions in the clinical trials of pegloticase occurred at a point in time where serum urate–lowering effect was lost due to treatment-emergent antibodies. Hence, it is very important to check the serum urate level just prior to each pegloticase infusion once treatment is started and to stop pegloticase infusion if one or more serum urate levels rise to 6 mg/dl or more occurs.

According to current FDA approval, pegloticase might have an important role as bridging treatment, e.g., for 6 months in SUA-responsive patients for rapid urate debulking in severe (treatment refractory) gout.[15,57] Interestingly, the uricolytic effect of pegloticase is independent of kidney function. After a successful extent of dissolution of clinically detected tophi, another ULT regimen with oral agents would likely be sufficient in most patients for maintaining normalized total body urate burden.

Chronic Kidney Disease and Renal Insufficiency

At present it is recognized as good clinical practice to use the *Modification of Diet in Renal Disease* (MDRD) study equation to define estimated GFR. This equation is more accurate in the elderly, in patients with large weight scale including high muscle mass, and in African Americans or Africans. At least 40% of gout patients have at least stage 2 CKD (estimated GFR, creatinine clearance between 60 and 89 ml/min). Electronic devices or software available on the Internet will allow easy MDRD calculation. Indeed, the DTT patients are related to patients with stage 3 CKD (defined as GFR between 30 and 59 ml/min). Defining GFR and CKD at baseline (see Table 16-8) is a key quality indicator for management, including dosing of many of the medications used to treat gout attacks and hyperuricemia.

Therapy Choices in Management of Gout Attacks

NSAIDs (and coxibs) should be avoided (or used with great caution) in patients with GFR less than 60 ml/min and limited to well-hydrated patients. Co-prescriptions with angiotensin-converting enzyme inhibitors or angiotensin II receptor blockers should be avoided. Some clinical settings put patients at high risk of renal dysfunction: dehydration, uncontrolled hypertension, hepatic cirrhosis, ascites. Corticosteroids are difficult-to-use drugs in treating attacks in these patients. Colchicine becomes a central tool for prophylaxis and treatment of acute attacks. Dosing should be adapted to CKD (see Chapter 15). In some CKD patients, IL-1 inhibitors present a valuable option for prophylaxis and management of gouty inflammation.

ULT in Renal Disease and Renal Failure

The FDA, EULAR, and national (United Kingdom, France) recommendations are to reduce the maximum allopurinol dosage in CKD.[10,15,47] However, such renal dose adjustment, if set at 100 to 300 mg/day, clearly fails to normalize SUA in most patients with CKD. Upward dose titration above "renally adjusted" doses of allopurinol is always an option, but alternatives are available, such as febuxostat and some uricosurics.

In stage 2 and 3 CKD, 40 and 80 febuxostat daily is superior to renally adjusted dosages (200 to 300 mg/day) of allopurinol, without safety issues.[40] To date, the effect and safety of febuxostat in stage 4 CKD and above have not been yet evaluated.

The potent uricosuric probenecid is not effective when GFR is below 50 ml/min. Benzbromarone, a major uricosuric agent available as mentioned earlier, can be used with lower GFR (greater than 25 to 30 ml/min). New uricosuric drugs are currently under investigation but have not yet been evaluated and reported in stage 3 CKD; they will add to the armamentarium in these DTT patients.

Gout in Major Organ Transplant Recipients

Gout in solid organ transplantation is an increasing and challenging clinical problem; it impacts adversely on quality of life.[58] These patients should be managed by rheumatologists. Gout markedly increases after kidney and cardiac transplantation,[59] due in large part to the drug regimens used. Nephropathy-induced calcineurin inhibitor regimens and, in particular, the marked rise of serum urate promoted by cyclosporine (see Chapter 4) are enormous factors in driving rapid development of tophi) within a few years, rather than a decade, and gout that can rapidly affect atypical joints such as the hip. Hypertensive nephropathy and hyperuricemia occurring well before heart or kidney transplantation are other factors, but cases occurring before adulthood are well described.

Organ transplant patients will develop acute gout attacks while being already treated with low-dose corticosteroids as part of the immunosuppressive regimen. NSAIDs are generally contraindicated, especially heart and kidney transplantation, since they can trigger acute renal failure and related complications such as pulmonary edema. ACTH may be ineffective due to adrenal atrophy while on long-term corticosteroids, and there is a major drug-drug interaction of colchicine with cyclosporine (see Chapter 15). With respect to XOI therapy, drug interactions with 6-mercaptopurine or azathioprine can trigger severe toxicity.

Acute Attacks

There is no clinical trial in this specific setting. In clinical practice, treatment regimens include (1) increased prednisone dosage for few days as previously discussed and (2) a short course of low-dose colchicine in combination with steroids added for 1 or 2 weeks. Colchicine neuromyotoxicity,[60] although reversible, is of particular concern in transplant recipients with renal impairment or when used in combination with cyclosporine. Off-label anakinra 100 mg SC daily, according to the So et al. regimen,[31] could be suggested, but safety data are particularly lacking, and formal drug trials are needed.

Urate-Lowering Therapy

There are no specific trials using ULT in these transplant patients. Sirolimus use in place of a calcineurin inhibitor should be considered, and mycophenolate mophetil also is a useful immunosuppression alternative. Marked asymptomatic hyperuricemia in a major organ transplant patient who truly requires long-term calcineurin inhibitor treatment warrants XOI ULT treatment, in our opinion. Allopurinol dosage can be adjusted to target SUA level or to maximal dosage.[34,39] The risk of side effects, including major hypersensitivity syndrome, has not been studied in organ transplant recipients. Uricase treatment has been used in some major transplant recipients with gout. However, the safety and efficacy of pegloticase have not yet been assessed in this patient population. While loop and thiazide diuretics increase SUA, amlodipine and losartan have the same antihypertensive effect with the additional benefit of lowering SUA level. Atorvastatin, but not simvastatin, may lower SUA, and while fenofibrate may reduce serum urate, caution is needed in stage 3 or worse CKD.

Gout in Hemodialysis Patients

Because urate is dialyzable, hemodialysis diminishes total body urate burden, and this assists in urate-lowering and often stabilizes the clinical course of gout. Serum urate levels should always be measured prior to dialysis rather than during or immediately after dialysis. Importantly, gout attacks most commonly, but do not always, lessen in frequency after hemodialysis is started. In this context, end-stage renal disease and hemodialysis do modulate inflammatory responses. In clinical trials, the phosphate-reducing agent sevelamer moderately decreased serum urate in dialysis patients, and the drug absorbs urate and likely lessens the effects of secondary hyperparathyroidism on serum urate. For prophylaxis of gout attacks, if absolutely necessary, colchicine can be used but should be dosed with great caution, since it is not dialyzable. Pseudogout also occurs in dialysis patients (see Chapter 23), promoted in part by secondary hyperparathyroidism. Therefore, differential diagnosis of gout and pseudogout mandate careful consideration in dialysis patients (see Chapter 23).

Surgery in Gout

Surgical procedures in the management of gout are limited to complications of tophaceous disease and should generally be avoided due to poor vascularization and healing of some tophi. Infections and neurologic compression (spinal cord or cauda equina compression, nerve root compressions, carpal tunnel syndrome) should be performed as an emergency procedure. Other clinical settings are joint deformity, distal joint destruction, and olecranon bursitis with skin lesions at risk of infection. It is possible that pegloticase will be able to reduce severe tophaceous masses, leading to fewer surgeries. In rare cases, tophus fractures can occur in particular at the patella,[61] and resection, reconstruction, or fixation can be needed.

References

1. Terkeltaub RA. Clinical practice. Gout. N Engl J Med 2003;349:1647–55.
2. Silva L, Miguel ED, Peiteado D, et al. Compliance in gout patients. Acta Reumatol Port 2010;35(5):466–74.
3. Harrold LR, Mazor KM, Velten S, et al. Patients and providers view gout differently: a qualitative study. Chron Ill 2010;6(4):263–71.
4. Wall GC, Koenigsfeld CF, Hegge KA, et al. Adherence to treatment guidelines in two primary care populations with gout. Rheumatol Int 2010;30(6):749–53.
5. Harrold LR, Andrade SE, Briesacher BA, et al. Adherence with urate-lowering therapies for the treatment of gout. Arthritis Res Ther 2009;11(2):R46.
6. Briesacher BA, Andrade SE, Fouayzi H, et al. Comparison of drug adherence rates among patients with seven different medical conditions. Pharmacotherapy 2008;28(4):437–43.
7. Doghramji PP, Edwards NL, McTigue J. Managing gout in the primary care setting: what you and your patients need to know. Am J Med 2010;123(8):S2.
8. Wortmann RL. Effective management of gout: an analogy. Am J Med 1998;105(6):513–4.
9. Zhang W, Doherty M, Pascual E, et al. EULAR Standing Committee for International Clinical Studies Including Therapeutics. EULAR evidence based recommendations for gout. Part I: Diagnosis. Report of a task force of the Standing Committee for International Clinical Studies Including Therapeutics (ESCISIT). Ann Rheum Dis 2006;65:1301–11.
10. Zhang W, Doherty M, Bardin T, et al. EULAR Standing Committee for International Clinical Studies Including Therapeutics. EULAR evidence based recommendations for gout. Part II: Management. Report of a task force of the EULAR Standing Committee for International Clinical Studies Including Therapeutics (ESCISIT). Ann Rheum Dis 2006;65:1312–24.
11. Jordan KM, Cameron JS, Snaith M, et al. British Society for Rheumatology and British Health Professionals in Rheumatology Standards, Guidelines and Audit Working Group (SGAWG). British Society for Rheumatology and British Health Professionals in Rheumatology guideline for the management of gout. Rheumatology (Oxford) 2007;46:1372–4.
12. Perez-Ruiz F, Lioté F. Lowering serum uric acid levels: what is the optimal target for improving clinical outcomes in gout? Arthritis Rheum 2007;57:1324–8.
13. Edwards NL. Treatment-failure gout: a moving target. Arthritis Rheum 2008;58:2587–90.
14. Barber C, Thompson K, Hanly JG. Impact of a rheumatology consultation service on the diagnostic accuracy and management of gout in hospitalized patients. J Rheumatol 2009;36:1699–704.
15. Terkeltaub R, Zelman D, Scavulli J, et al. Gout Study Group: update on hyperuricemia and gout. Joint Bone Spine 2009;76:444–6.
16. Choi HK. A prescription for lifestyle change in patients with hyperuricemia and gout. Curr Opin Rheumatol 2010;22(2):165–72.
17. Terkeltaub RA. Colchicine update: 2008. Semin Arthritis Rheum 2009;38:411–9.
18. So A, De Meulemeester M, Pikhlak A, et al. Canakinumab for the treatment of acute flares in difficult-to-treat gouty arthritis: results of a multicenter, phase II, dose-ranging study. Arthritis Rheum 2010;62:3064–76.
19. Terkeltaub R, Sundy JS, Schumacher HR, et al. The interleukin 1 inhibitor rilonacept in treatment of chronic gouty arthritis: results of a placebo-controlled, monosequence crossover, non-randomised, single-blind pilot study. Ann Rheum Dis 2009;68:1613–7.
20. Terkeltaub RA, Furst DE, Bennett K, et al. High versus low dosing of oral colchicine for early acute gout flare: twenty-four-hour outcome of the first multicenter, randomized, double-blind, placebo-controlled, parallel-group, dose-comparison colchicine study. Arthritis Rheum 2010;62:1060–8.
20a. Bavry AA, Khaliq A, Gong A, et al. Harmful effects of nonsteroidal anti-inflammatory drugs among patients with hypertension and coronary artery disease. Am J Med 2011:doi:10.1016/j.amjmed.2011.02.025.
20b. Schjerning Olsen AM, Fosbøl EL, Lindhardsen J, et al. Duration of treatment with nonsteroidal anti-inflammatory drugs and impact on risk of death and recurrent myocardial infarction in patients with prior myocardial infarction: a nationwide cohort study.. Circulation 2011;123:2226–35.
21. Cattermole GN, Man CY, Cheng CH, et al. Oral prednisolone is more cost-effective than oral indomethacin for treating patients with acute gout-like arthritis. Eur J Emerg Med 2009;16(5):261–6.
22. Man CY, Cheung IT, Cameron PA, et al. Comparison of oral prednisolone/paracetamol and oral indomethacin/paracetamol combination therapy in the treatment of acute goutlike arthritis: a double-blind, randomized, controlled trial. Ann Emerg Med 2007;49(5):670–7.
23. Janssens HJ, Janssen M, van de Lisdonk EH, et al. Use of oral prednisolone or naproxen for the treatment of gout arthritis: a double-blind, randomised equivalence trial. Lancet 2008;371(9627):1854–60.
24. Janssens HJ, Lucassen PL, Van de Laar FA, et al. Corticosteroids for acute gout. Cochrane Database Syst Rev 2008;(2):CD005521.
25. Schumacher HR, Berger M, Li-Yu J, et al. Efficacy and tolerability of celecoxib in the treatment of moderate to extreme pain associated with acute gouty arthritis: a randomized controlled trial. Atlanta, GA: Presented at the American College of Rheumatology Annual Scientific Meeting; November 7-11, 2010, Abstract 151.
26. Lioté F. Advances in the proper use of colchicine and adapting dosages in other countries: comment on the article by Terkeltaub et al. Arthritis Rheum 2010;62:3126–7.
27. Richette P, Bardin T. Colchicine for the treatment of gout. Exp Opin Pharmacother 2010;11:2933–8.
28. Janssens HJ, Lucassen PL, Van de Laar FA, et al. Systemic corticosteroids for acute gout. Cochrane Database Syst Rev 2008; (2):CD005521.
29. Werlen D, Gabay C, Vischer TL. Corticosteroid therapy for the treatment of acute attacks of crystal-induced arthritis: an effective alternative to nonsteroidal antiinflammatory drugs. Rev Rhum Engl Ed 1996;63:248–54.
30. Raso AA, Sto Niño OV, Li-Yu J. Does prolonged systemic glucocorticoid use increase risk of tophus formation among gouty arthritis patients? Int J Rheum Dis 2009;12:243–9.
31. So A, De Smedt T, Revaz S, et al. Pilot study of IL-1 inhibition by anakinra in acute gout. Arthritis Res Ther 2007;9:R28.
32. Chen K, Fields T, Mancuso CA, et al. Anakinra's efficacy is variable in refractory gout: report of ten cases. Semin Arthritis Rheum 2010;40:210–4.
33. Pineda C, Amezcua-Guerra LM, Solano C, et al. Joint and tendon subclinical involvement suggestive of gouty arthritis in asymptomatic hyperuricemia: an ultrasound controlled study. Arthritis Res Ther 2011;13(1):R4.
34. Chao J, Terkeltaub R. A critical reappraisal of allopurinol dosing, safety, and efficacy for hyperuricemia in gout. Curr Rheumatol Rep 2009;11:135–40.
35. Lee MH, Graham GG, Williams KM, et al. A benefit-risk assessment of benzbromarone in the treatment of gout: was its withdrawal from the market in the best interest of patients? Drug Saf 2008;31:643–65.
36. Reinders MK, van Roon EN, Houtman PM, et al. Biochemical effectiveness of allopurinol and allopurinol-probenecid in previously benzbromarone-treated gout patients. Clin Rheumatol 2007;26:1459–65.
37. Stocker SL, Graham GG, McLachlan AJ, et al. Pharmacokinetic and pharmacodynamic interaction between allopurinol and probenecid in patients with gout. J Rheumatol 2011;38:306–10.
38. Mikuls TR, Farrar JT, Bilker WB, et al. Suboptimal physician adherence to quality indicators for the management of gout and asymptomatic hyperuricaemia: results from the UK General Practice Research Database (GPRD). Rheumatology (Oxford) 2005;44:1038–42.
39. Dalbeth N, Kumar S, Stamp L, et al. Dose adjustment of allopurinol according to creatinine clearance does not provide adequate control of hyperuricemia in patients with gout. J Rheumatol 2006;33:1646–50.
40. Becker MA, Schumacher HR, Espinoza LR, et al. The urate-lowering efficacy and safety of febuxostat in the treatment of the hyperuricemia of gout: the CONFIRMS trial. Arthritis Res Ther 2010;12:R63.
41. Jansen TL, Richette P, Perez-Ruiz F, et al. International position paper on febuxostat. Clin Rheumatol 2010;29:835–40.

42. Khosravan R, Grabowski BA, Wu JT, et al. Pharmacokinetics, pharmacodynamics and safety of febuxostat, a non-purine selective inhibitor of xanthine oxidase, in a dose escalation study in healthy subjects. Clin Pharmacokinet 2006;45(8):821–41.

43. Stamp LK, O'Donnell JL, Zhang M, et al. Using allopurinol above the dose based on creatinine clearance is effective and safe in patients with chronic gout, including those with renal impairment. Arthritis Rheum 2011;63(2):412–21.

44. Mikuls TR, MacLean CH, Olivieri J, et al. Quality of care indicators for gout management. Arthritis Rheum 2004;50:937–43.

45. Sarawate CA, Brewer KK, Yang W, et al. Gout medication treatment patterns and adherence to standards of care from a managed care perspective. Mayo Clin Proc 2006;81:925–34.

46. Singh JA, Hodges JS, Toscano JP, et al. Quality of care for gout in the US needs improvement. Arthritis Rheum 2007;57:822–9.

47. Bardin T. Current management of gout in patients unresponsive or allergic to allopurinol. Joint Bone Spine 2004;71:481–5.

48. Reinders MK, van Roon EN, Jansen TL, et al. Efficacy and tolerability of urate-lowering drugs in gout: a randomised controlled trial of benzbromarone versus probenecid after failure of allopurinol. Ann Rheum Dis 2009;68:51–6.

49. Reinders MK, Haagsma C, Jansen TL, et al. A randomised controlled trial on the efficacy and tolerability with dose escalation of allopurinol 300-600 mg/day versus benzbromarone 100-200 mg/day in patients with gout. Ann Rheum Dis 2009;68:892–7.

50. Stamp LK, O'Donnell JL, Zhang M, et al. Using allopurinol above the dose based on creatinine clearance is effective and safe in chronic gout, including in those with renal impairment. Arthritis Rheum 2011;63:412–21.

51. Panomvana D, Sripradit S, Angthararak S. Higher therapeutic plasma oxypurinol concentrations might be required for gouty patients with chronic kidney disease. J Clin Rheumatol 2008;14(1):6–11.

52. Takada M, Okada H, Kotake T, et al. Appropriate dosing regimen of allopurinol in Japanese patients. J Clin Pharm Ther 2005;30(4):407–12.

53. Andracco R, Zampogna G, Parodi M, et al. Risk factors for gouty dactylitis. Clin Exp Rheumatol 2009;27:993–5.

54. Perez-Ruiz F, Calabozo M, Pijoan JI, et al. Effect of urate-lowering therapy on the velocity of size reduction of tophi in chronic gout. Arthritis Rheum 2002;47:356–60.

55. Richette P, Brière C, Hoenen-Clavert V, et al. Rasburicase for tophaceous gout not treatable with allopurinol: an exploratory study. J Rheumatol 2007;34:2093–8.

56. Reinders MK, Jansen TL. New advances in the treatment of gout: review of pegloticase. Ther Clin Risk Manag 2010;6:543–50.

57. Becker MA, Schumacher HR, Espinoza LR, et al. The urate-lowering efficacy and safety of febuxostat in the treatment of the hyperuricemia of gout: the CONFIRMS trial. Arthritis Res Ther 2010;12(2):R63.

58. Stamp L, Searle M, O'Donnell J, et al. Gout in solid organ transplantation: a challenging clinical problem. Drugs 2005;65:2593–611.

59. Schwab P, Lipton S, Kerr GS. Rheumatologic sequelae and challenges in organ transplantation. Best Pract Res Clin Rheumatol 2010;24(3):329–40.

60. Guis S, Mattéi JP, Lioté F. Drug-induced and toxic myopathies. Best Pract Res Clin Rheumatol 2003;17:877–907.

61. Nguyen C, Ea HK, Palazzo E, et al. Tophaceous gout: an unusual cause of multiple fractures. Scand J Rheumatol 2010;39:93–6.

62. Anderson A, Singh JA. Pegloticase for chronic gout. Cochrane Database Syst Rev 2010; (3):CD008335.

63. US Food and Drug Administration. FDA labeling information: Krystexxa (pegloticase). 2010.

64. Schlesinger N, Yasothan U, Kirkpatrick P. Pegloticase. Nat Rev Drug Discov 2011;10:17–8.

65. Dalbeth N, Schauer C, Macdonald P, et al. Methods of tophus assessment in clinical trials of chronic gout: a systematic literature review and pictorial reference guide. Ann Rheum Dis 2011;70:597–604.

Quality of Care in Gout

Jasvinder A. Singh and Supriya G. Reddy

KEY POINTS

- Surprisingly, instances of suboptimal treatment of gout remain frequent, even in this era of expanded and well-understood treatment options. These include errors in medication use and dosages and inadequate use of the laboratory and diagnostic approaches.
- Common diagnostic and therapeutic errors include infrequent use of diagnostic joint aspiration and crystal analysis, infrequent monitoring of serum urate, and failure to achieve an adequate target level for serum urate.
- Inappropriate dosings of allopurinol and colchicine, particularly in those with renal dysfunction, are the most common medication errors.
- Higher number of outpatient visit days, more primary care or rheumatology visits, and lower comorbidities are associated with better gout care patterns.
- Efforts aimed at improving quality of care should first focus on high-risk patients such as elderly patients and those with higher comorbidity load, most severe forms of gout, and polypharmacy. Multimodal low-cost interventions are most likely to be associated with improvements that are sustainable and can be implemented in multiple health care systems.
- Data from several studies confirmed gaps in quality of care, pertaining to both treatment and laboratory monitoring and for both effectiveness and safety.
- Most significant gaps were evident in lack of monitoring of serum urate levels after starting urate-lowering therapy, failure to achieve target serum urate, use of inappropriate doses of allopurinol, and lack of use of colchicine or NSAID prophylaxis when starting allopurinol.
- These quality care gaps can be overcome by systems-based interventions, although patient- and physician-based interventions may also help.
- The quality gaps present opportunity for improvement in quality of gout care.

Introduction

Gout, characterized by acute and chronic inflammatory arthritis, affects up to 3% to 4% of the adult population in the United States (see Chapter 6), with a similar prevalence in most Western countries. Furthermore, the prevalence of gout in the United States may have approximately doubled in the

past 20 years[1] with the greatest increase occurring in males that are 65 or older.[1] Gout accounts for significant health care burden and costs. A diagnosis of gout was associated with 1.4 million outpatient visits in the United States in 2002.[2] A recent study estimated that $27 million is spent annually for care of new acute gout cases in the United States.[3] Thus, gout is a significant problem with public health implications.

Effective treatment options for acute and chronic gout have been available for more than half a century, yet instances of suboptimal treatment of gout remain frequent.[4-6] A simulation study found that urate-lowering therapy is cost-effective in most scenarios and cost-saving in the patients with two or more acute gout attacks per year.[7] Although new approaches are currently being developed for the treatment of gout, treating symptomatic gout with available therapies is still a major concern. Available treatment options for gout include non-steroidal antiinflammatory drugs (NSAIDs), corticosteroids (oral, parenteral, and intraarticular), colchicine, urate-lowering medications such as allopurinol, febuxostat, and pegloticase, and uricosurics such as probenecid. With currently available therapies being effective in a majority of the patients, efficacy needs to be balanced against safety in a given patient, especially in the elderly patients with bone marrow, liver, or kidney problems. Many patients with gout continue to experience recurrent gouty attacks,[8] which has a negative impact on health-related quality of life, function, mobility, and social roles.[8] Thus, there is an urgent need for improving the quality of care (QOC) for patients with gout.

In this chapter, we describe the results of a systematic review of the published literature regarding compliance with evidence-based QOC indicators for gout[9] and errors in medication use and laboratory monitoring in gout. Using the search terms "gout," "quality of care," "treatment guidelines," "recommendations," "medical errors," and similar terms, an experienced librarian from the Cochrane musculoskeletal group (L.F.) performed a systematic search in the following databases in July 2010: (1) Ovid MEDLINE 1950 to June week 1 2010; (2) EMBASE 1980 to 2010 week 23; and

Grant support: This material is the result of work supported by the resources and the use of facilities at the VA Medical Center, Birmingham, Alabama, USA.

Financial conflict: There are no financial conflicts related to this work. J.A.S. has received speaker honoraria from Abbott; research and travel grants from Allergan, Takeda, Savient, Wyeth, and Amgen; and consultant fees from Savient, URL Pharmaceuticals, and Novartis.

The views expressed in this article are those of the authors and do not necessarily reflect the position or policy of the Department of Veterans Affairs or the United States government.

(3) The Cochrane Library (including Cochrane database of systematic reviews, DARE, CENTRAL, HTA database, and NHS EED), second quarter 2010. We previously published a review of studies on QOC in gout,[12] and several studies included in this chapter were also included in the previous review. This chapter provides an updated systematic review of studies of QOC in gout.

Definition and Measurement of Quality of Care

The Agency for Health Care Research (AHRQ) defines *quality of care* as the "degree to which health care services for individuals and populations increase the likelihood of desired health outcomes and are consistent with current professional knowledge." QOC for gout has been frequently measured using quality indicators (QIs) since the description of 10 gout QIs by Mikuls et al. in 2004.[9] These QIs for gout related to medication prescription, laboratory monitoring, and behavioral modifications were derived using evidence-based UCLA appropriateness method using a panel of rheumatologists and internists.[9] QIs are process measures of health care quality. QIs are easily measurable since they have well-defined numerator and denominator, easily extractable from readily available health care data. Prior to description of QIs for gout, QOC was measured based on what was accepted as appropriate treatment regimens and laboratory monitoring in patients with gout. The gout QIs cover the spectrum of gout management, including both effectiveness/efficacy and safety/adverse events. Efficacy QIs consist of treatment of acute gouty arthritis, urate-lowering therapies to prevent gouty arthritis flares and damage from tophaceous deposits, behavioral modification to prevent gout and gouty flares, antiinflammatory prophylaxis during the initiation of urate-lowering therapy for the prevention of acute gouty flares, and serum urate monitoring. Safety QIs address the areas of safety related to adverse events related to use of colchicine, NSAIDs, and urate-lowering therapy.

Gout QIs are in the IF-THEN-BECAUSE format. An example of a gout QI as described by Mikuls et al.[9] is, "**IF** a gout patient is given a prescription for a xanthine oxidase inhibitor, **THEN** a serum urate level should be checked at *least once* during the first 6 months of continued use, **BECAUSE** periodic serum urate measurements are required for appropriate dose adjustments of xanthine oxidase inhibitors (escalations or reductions)."

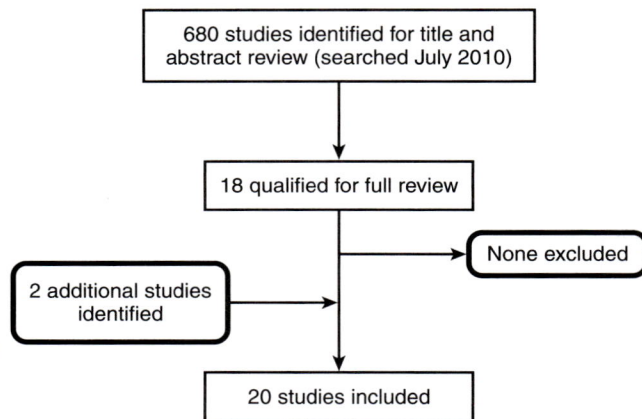

Figure 17-1

Table 17-1 Overview of Studies of Quality of Care

	Type of Study	No. of Patients	Follow-up Duration
Petersel and Schlesinger, 2007[11]	Retrospective cohort	184	Not provided
Neogi et al., 2006[12]	Prospective case crossover Internet study	232	268 days (SD, 178)
Dalbeth et al., 2006[13]	Retrospective	250	Not reported
Annemans et al., 2007, United Kingdom[14]	Retrospective	7443	Not reported
Annemans et al., 2007, Germany[14]	Retrospective	4006	Not reported
Ly, Gow, and Dalbeth, 2007[15]	Retrospective	100	Not reported
Mikuls et al., 2005[16]	Retrospective	63,105	3.8 y (SD, 2.8)
Mikuls et al., 2006[17]	Retrospective	Not reported, number of medication errors 582,397	5-y study
Sarawate, 2006[17,19]	Retrospective	5942	1 y
Singh, 2007[18]	Retrospective	3658	2 y
Singh, 2009[29]	Retrospective	643 with new allopurinol	2 y
Pal, 2000[20]	Retrospective	429	Not reported
Smith, 2000[21]	Retrospective	73	Not reported
Evans, 1996[22]	Retrospective	19	Inpatient stay
Ho, 1993[23]	Retrospective	67	Inpatient stay
Stamp, 2000[24]	Prospective, cross-sectional	31	Cross-sectional

SD, standard deviation.

Search Results

The search identified 680 articles related to the QOC in gout. Eighteen articles qualified for full text review and all were included in the summary synthesis, since there were no exclusions[11-28] (Fig. 17-1). Two additional articles were identified as pertinent literature not captured in the search.[29-30] In this chapter, we summarize all the available data in Tables 17-1 and 17-2 and highlight key studies and findings in the narrative.

Key Studies of Quality of Care and Findings

Petersel et al.[11] performed a retrospective chart review at their medical center to assess the practice patterns of treatment of acute gout in hospitalized patients. Patients were identified using *International Classification of Disease (ICD)* codes of 274.0 or 274.9 for gout in a 2-year period. Of the 79 diagnosed with acute gout during hospitalization, consultations from rheumatology, orthopedic surgery, or podiatry were obtained

Table 17-2 Detailed Characteristics of Patients Included in Quality of Care Studies of Gout

	No. of Patients	Age, y, Mean (SD or Range)	Male, %	Body Mass Index, kg/m², mean (SD or range)	Tophaceous Gout, %	Comorbidities
Petersel and Schlesinger, 2007[11]	184	71 (range 40–96 y)	100%	NR	NR	Heart disease: 15 (19%) Renal insufficiency: 149 (80.9%)
Neogi et al., 2006[12]	232	53 (range 23–85)	81%	30.8 (17.8–53.5)	35%	16% peptic ulcer disease, renal disease, or congestive heart failure
Dalbeth et al., 2006[13]	250	56 (range 26–86)	82%	NR	134 (53.6%)	8 patients with end-stage renal failure were excluded; n was originally 258
Annemans et al., 2007, United Kingdom[14]	7443	65.6 (SD, 13.8)	81.6%	NR	NR	Heart disease: 14.5% Renal failure: 9.5%
Annemans et al., 2007, Germany[14]	4006	58.6 (SD, 13.1)	80.4%	NR	16.6%	Heart disease: 16.6% Diabetes: 25.9% Renal failure: 4.8%
Ly et al., 2007[15]	100	NR	82%	NR	56 (56%)	Renal impairment: 44% of acute gout; 100% of chronic gout*
Mikuls et al., 2005[16]	63,105	61 (SD,15 y)	78%	NR	NR	Heart disease: 26% Diabetes: 7% Renal failure: 1%
Mikuls et al., 2006[17]	Number of medication errors: 582,397	NR	NR	NR	NR	NR
Sarawate, 2006[17,19]	5942	57.4 (SD, 14.1)	76%	NR	9.1%	Hypertension: 39.8% Coronary artery disease: 24.7% Diabetes: 18.3% Renal impairment: 13%
Singh, 2007[18]	643	67.9 (SD, 9.7)	99%	NR	NR	Mean Charlson score, 2.5
Singh, 2009[29]	643	67.9 (SD, 9.7)	99%	NR	NR	Mean Charlson score, 2.5
Pal, 2000[20]	429	64.5 y	80%	NR	NR	NR
Smith, 2000[21]	73	77 y	55%	NR	NR	NR
Evans, 1996[22]	19	59 y	80%	NR	NR	Multiple comorbidities including renal and hepatic disease
Ho, 1993[23]	67	72 y	83%	NR	NR	Hypertension: 59% Congestive heart failure: 34% Peptic ulcer disease: 32%
Stamp, 2000[24]	31	58 y	81%	NR; weight 92 kg	55%	Renal insufficiency: 55%

*Cohort was chosen by presence of chronic renal failure with Creatinine clearance ≤50 ml/minute or creatinine ≥2 mg/dL.
SD, standard deviation; *NR,* not reported.

in 66%. Only 25% of study patients diagnosed with acute gout underwent joint aspiration, despite the fact that joint aspiration is considered the gold standard for the diagnosis of gout. Combination antiinflammatory agents (prednisone, NSAIDs, colchicine) were used in 50% of the patients despite the lack of evidence supporting the use of combination therapies to treat gout. Only 27% of all patients with gouty arthritis had been receiving allopurinol prior to admission, and serum urate levels were checked in only 27%. Serum urate was greater than 6 mg/dl in 60% of patients receiving allopurinol. Renal failure was present in 73% of patients with gout: 86% of patients treated with colchicine and 80% treated with NSAID had renal failure.[11]

In an Internet-based case-crossover study, Neogi et al.[12] found that approximately one fourth of their sample size (n = 232) had inappropriate management for some or all of their recurrent gout attacks. Among inappropriate therapy, most common was no medication in 60%, analgesics in 22%, and alternative remedies in 2%. In 13%, allopurinol was prescribed during an acute attack. A majority (53%) always consulted their physicians for each of their recurrent attacks and 24% did it sometimes.

In a retrospective study, Dalbeth et al.[13] examined whether the allopurinol dosing in 227 patients attending a rheumatology clinic was adjusted to creatinine clearance, with the maximum allowed dose of allopurinol being 400 mg/day. Twenty-two of the patients (10%) were taking less than the recommended dosage, 161 (71%) patients were given the recommended dose of allopurinol, and 44 patients (14%) were given more than the recommended dosage. Serum urate levels were lower in those patients receiving higher doses of allopurinol compared to the other two groups of patients.[13] There were significant differences between the groups that received higher doses of allopurinol compared to those that received the recommended dose ($p < .01$).[13] Serum urate lower than 0.36 mmol/L (equivalent to 6 mg/dl) were achieved in 22.4% of patients treated with allopurinol: 19% of those taking recommended allopurinol doses versus 15% taking lower-than-recommended doses versus 38% taking higher-than-recommended doses of allopurinol.

Annemans et al.[14] conducted a retrospective cohort study using the IMS Disease Analyzer, a longitudinal database containing anonymous patient records maintained by 650 general practitioners in both the United Kingdom and Germany. They included patients with an ICD code for gout and at least one additional recording of gout in their history (consultation with diagnosis of gout or prescription for gout treatment). Only 2.1% in the United Kingdom and 3.4% in Germany were prescribed allopurinol doses greater than 300 mg/day.[14] Persistence with allopurinol treatment at 1 year was 61.2% in the United Kingdom and 96% in Germany. The number of comorbidities increased with an increase in serum urate levels. Serum urate was tested in 14% of patients in the United Kingdom and 9% in Germany during an observation period and in less than 1% annually in both countries. In unadjusted analyses, the study found a positive association between serum urate levels above 7 mg/dl and the number of gout flares, in both U.K. and German cohorts.[13]

Ly et al.[15] conducted a study to assess current colchicine prescribing and safety monitoring in 50 patients each with acute gout or chronic gout with renal impairment receiving long-term colchicine therapy. All 50 patients with acute gout received colchicine for treatment of acute gout and 96% of the patients received colchicine doses at less than 2.5 mg in a 24-hour period, according to the New Zealand Rheumatology Association guidelines. However, 60% had at least one risk factor and 32% had more than one risk factor for colchicine toxicity; no patient developed severe toxicity. In the 50 patients with chronic gout with renal failure (creatinine of 2 mg/dl or greater or creatinine clearance of 50 mL/min or less) who were taking long-term prophylactic colchicine, 76% had a full blood count as well as monitoring of their creatine kinase (CK) levels, in compliance with a QI described by Mikuls et al.,[9] which identified one patient with colchicine myopathy. However, other risk factors for colchicine toxicity were present in 58% of the patients.[15]

Mikuls et al. used the General Practice Research Database (GPRD), which collects data from participating general practices in the United Kingdom.[16] The database was used to examine adherence to QIs such as dosing in renal impairment, concomitant use of azathioprine or 6-mercaptopurine, and use in the treatment of asymptomatic hyperuricemia. They examined compliance with three QIs: 26% received an incorrect initial allopurinol dose in the presence of renal failure, 25% received an inadequate dose adjustment while receiving allopurinol and azathioprine or 6-mercaptopurine, and 57% were inappropriately treated with urate-lowering therapy for asymptomatic hyperuricemia.

Mikuls et al.[17] also conducted another study in which the MEDMARX database was used to examine medication errors related to the treatment of gout. The database is an Internet-accessible error-reporting system specially designed for use by health care systems and hospitals in the United States. Errors involving allopurinol, colchicine, probenecid, and sulfinpyrazone were all examined from 1999 to 2003. Of the 582,397 medication errors found, 891 errors (0.15%) were specifically related to errors with gout-related medications. The most frequent error occurred with allopurinol (524 of 891), followed by colchicines (315 of 891).[17] The most frequent errors associated with colchicine and allopurinol involved illegible or incomplete orders followed by excessive dosing in several patients with renal failure. In comparison to errors involving other musculoskeletal treatments, errors were more often attributed to physician prescribing (7% for other therapies versus 23% to 39%, $p < .0001$) and less often due to drug administration of nursing error (50% versus 23% to 27%, $p < .0001$).[17]

In a retrospective database study of a large southeastern U.S. health care plan, Sarawate et al.[19] analyzed claims of 5942 gout patients from January 1, 2000, to December 31, 2002, of whom 1,077 were newly diagnosed gout patients allopurinol during follow-up. Among gout patients taking allopurinol, 64.9% received 300 mg/day. Only 3% received more than 300 mg/day of allopurinol. The mean duration of continuous allopurinol therapy was 8.5 months (SD 11 months; median 3 months), with frequent interruptions in 88% of patients. However, suggested QOC indicators for gout had low performance: 53% of gout patients with renal impairment were receiving a daily allopurinol dose of 300 mg or higher and 83% of patients who had started taking allopurinol did not have their serum urate levels checked within 180 days of starting treatment.[19]

Singh et al.[18] examined evidence-based QIs in a cohort of 663 veterans at Minneapolis Veterans Affairs Medical Center with a diagnosis of gout who qualified for one or more QIs among a cohort of 3658 gout patients. Three QIs were examined: initial allopurinol dose of less than 300 mg for those individuals with renal insufficiency, uric acid monitoring within 6 months of starting a new allopurinol prescription, and complete blood count and creatine kinase monitoring for patients receiving prolonged prophylactic colchicine therapy. There were 663 patients who qualified for one or more QI. Of these 663 patients, therapy in 144 patients (22%) adhered to all applicable QIs. Also, 59 of 76 (78%) adhered to the QI involving initial allopurinol dosage, 155 of 643 (24%) adhered to obtaining uric acid checks within 6 months of allopurinol initiation, and 18 of 52 (35%) adhered to monitoring of creatine kinase and complete blood count during prolonged colchicine therapy.[18]

In another study using the same cohort as just described, Singh et al.[29] studied the compliance with urate-lowering therapy, use of antiinflammatory prophylaxis before starting allopurinol, and success of achieving target serum urate of less than 6 mg/dl. Only 46% of patients prescribed allopurinol took it without significant gaps in prescription. Only 26% received NSAID or colchicine prophylaxis at least 2 weeks before starting allopurinol. Only 20% of those receiving allopurinol reached a target serum urate level of less than 6 mg/dl.

Pal et al.[20] conducted a study of 429 patients with a diagnosis of gout or taking known treatment for gout (e.g., allopurinol). A sample was chosen among 74,111 patients from 12 general practices in the United Kingdom. The mean age of gout patients was 64.5, and 80% were men; 6% of patients had received NSAIDs for more than 2 years after the start of allopurinol.[20] In the majority of patients, allopurinol was administered prior to the resolution of acute gout. Study findings illustrate that 61% of patients had no laboratory tests performed while on medication for the treatment of gout. Inadequate doses of allopurinol were given in a significant proportion (19%) of gout patients. Counseling on reducing alcohol intake was given to only 42% of patients.[20]

Smith et al.[21] conducted a retrospective study to determine whether the dose of allopurinol was in accordance with the patients' estimated creatinine clearance. The study was conducted at an Australian hospital among 73 patients, who were identified using pharmacy records. Mean age of the patients was 77.7 years. Serum urate was measured in only a total of 12 patients (16.4%), even though all of these patients were taking allopurinol. Allopurinol dosage was higher than recommended (for creatinine clearance) in 34 patients (47%) and lower in 17 patients (40%).[21]

Predictor of Poor-Quality Care in Patients With Gout: Evidence From Published Studies

Table 17-3 summarizes the key findings of correlates of poor QOC from each study that described these care patterns.

Sarawate et al.[19] examined the predictors of high medication:prescription ratio (MPR) and serum urate testing after initiation of a new allopurinol prescription in a large claims database. Previously diagnosed gout (versus new diagnosis) and presence of hypertension were associated with an MPR of 80% or higher for allopurinol, while occurrence of gout flare was associated with a lower MPR (see Table 17-3). Factors associated with odds of serum urate testing after

allopurinol initiation were renal impairment (odds ratio 3.2), colchicine use (0.55), number of medications (1.53 per medication), and baseline serum urate level (1.14/1 mg/dl uric acid level).

Neogi et al.[12] described factors associated with inappropriate therapy during an acute gout attack. The authors reported that risk of inappropriate therapy was significantly higher in patients who consulted with a physician during acute attack (odds ratio 2.5, 95% confidence interval 1.3–4.7) and lower in patients with a higher number of gout attacks (odds ratio 0.8, 95% confidence interval 0.7–0.9).[12] Body mass index, age, sex, race, education, and self-reported comorbidities were not associated with risk of inappropriate therapy.

Singh et al.[18] examined physician, patient, and systems factors associated with overall physician adherence with three QIs in their study of 663 veterans with gout. The authors reported that older age and more inpatient visits per year were associated with lower adherence to all applicable QIs. In contrast, patients with higher number of outpatient visits or with greater number of health care providers had higher adherence with all applicable QIs.

Mikuls et al.,[16] in their study of QIs in GPRD patients, found that male gender, older age, chronic renal failure, and a greater number of concomitant medications were significantly associated with inappropriate treatment for asymptomatic hyperuricemia. Hypertension and use of diuretics were associated with lower odds of the treatment of asymptomatic hyperuricemia.[16]

Singh et al.[29] examined the predictors of continuous allopurinol, of use of colchicine or NSAID prophylaxis, and of achieving target serum uric acid in veterans with gout receiving a new allopurinol prescription, the same cohort as described in their first study. Higher number of outpatient visit days, more primary care or rheumatology visits, and lower comorbidities were associated with better care patterns.

As described earlier, we found that patient-, physician-, and systems-level factors are associated with poor QOC in patients with gout. Thus, several potential targets exist for improving the QOC. We believe that efforts aimed at improving QOC should first focus on high-risk patients such as elderly patients and those with higher comorbidity load, most severe forms of gout, and polypharmacy. Multimodal low-cost interventions are most likely to be associated with improvements that are sustainable and can be implemented in multiple health care systems.

Physician Surveys: Potential Reasons for Noncompliance With Gout Quality Indicators

The evidence summarized earlier highlights variables associated with poor QOC. Although these studies provide some insight into the correlates of poor QOC, it is important to survey physicians to identify what they perceive as barriers to good-quality gout care. Therefore, we searched for additional surveys of physicians and practitioners related to gout care. The few published surveys of practitioners that have examined the reasons for physician noncompliance with QIs and physician opinions regarding gout QIs are summarized next. Most patients with gout receive gout-related care from nonrheumatologists, primarily general practitioners, family practitioners,

Table 17-3 Significant Predictors of Quality of Care in Patients With Gout

Study	Outcome	Potential Predictors	Significant Predictors	Odds/Risk Ratio (95% Confidence Interval)	p Value
Sarawate et al., 2006[19]	MPR ≥80% for allopurinol (n = 2318)	Age, sex, preindex comorbidities, newly or previously diagnosed gout, and gout flare before postindex serum urate testing	Previously diagnosed gout vs. newly diagnosed gout	2.95 (2.45–3.55)	<.001
			Preindex hypertension vs. postindex hypertension	1.44 (1.20–1.73)	<.001
			Gout flare before postindex serum urate test vs. no gout flare before postindex serum urate test	0.50 (0.40–0.63)	<.001
			Age	1.01	…
	Getting serum urate test after initiation of allopurinol (n = 337)	Age, sex, preindex comorbidities, all postindex concomitant medications, gout-specific drugs, and mean baseline serum urate level	Baseline renal impairment vs. postindex renal impairment	3.20 (1.25–8.23)	.003
			Increasing number of medications (per medication increase)	1.53 (1.21–1.94)	<.05
			Increasing baseline serum urate level (per mg/dl increase)	1.14 (1.02–1.29)	<.05
			Colchicine use vs. allopurinol use (related to getting a postindex serum urate test)	0.55 (0.35–0.89)	<.05
Neogi et al., 2006[12]	Definitely or possibly inappropriate drug therapy during acute gouty arthritis (n = 202)	Age, sex, race, highest education level attained, self-reported comorbidities, body mass index, duration of gout, consulting a physician, and the total number of recurrent attacks	Increasing number of gout attacks in patients with documented gout (risk per attack increase per y)	0.8 (0.7–0.9)	<.01
			Consultation with physician during acute attack vs. no consultation	2.5 (1.3–4.7)	.006
Mikuls et al., 2005[16]	Inappropriate treatment of asymptomatic hyperuricemia with allopurinol	Age, gender, comorbidity, concomitant medication use, follow-up duration	Male sex vs. female	1.82 (1.10–2.99)	<.05
			Chronic renal failure that was definite or probable vs. no renal failure	4.89 (1.58–15.11)	<.05
			Diuretic use vs. no diuretic use	0.46 (0.27–0.77)	<.05
			Total medications or concomitant drug use (diuretics and cyclosporine or FK-506) vs. no concomitant drug use	1.25 (1.12–1.40)	<.05
Singh et al., 2007[18]	Overall physician-adherence with three quality indicators: initial allopurinol dose <300 mg in renal insufficiency, uric acid check within 6 months of starting a new allopurinol prescription, and complete blood count and creatine kinase check every 6 months when receiving prolonged colchicine therapy (n = 643)	Race; age; inpatient stays per year; inpatient stays per year with gout as the primary diagnosis; primary care, rheumatology, and other outpatient visits per year; percent service connection and Charlson Comorbidity Index; and number of health care providers.	Age	0.78 (0.64–0.96)	.02
			Race other vs. white	1.41 (0.52–3.84)	.035
			Inpatient stays per year with gout as primary diagnosis	0.71 (0.52–0.97)	.015
			Inpatient stays per year	0.57 (0.40–0.81)	<.001
			Primary care visits per year	1.28 (1.02–1.62)	.037
			Number of health care providers	1.69 (1.32–2.15)	<.001

Table 17-3 Significant Predictors of Quality of Care in Patients With Gout—Cont'd

Study	Outcome	Potential Predictors	Significant Predictors	Odds/Risk Ratio (95% Confidence Interval)	p Value
Singh et al., 2009[29]	Allopurinol discontinuations (n = 643)	Same variables as in study above	Visits per year to rheumatology or primary care		
	Colchicine prophylaxis with new allopurinol prescriptions (n = 643)	Same variables as above	Days per year with any outpatient visits	2.08 (1.54–2.80)	<.0001
			Most frequent clinic (ref: rheumatology) Primary care Specialty medicine Surgery Other	0.16 (0.07–0.36) 0.12 (0.02–0.58) 0.12 (0.01–1.22) 0.13 (0.03–0.53)	.0006
	Getting serum urate test within 6 months after initiation of allopurinol (n = 643)	Same variables as above	Days per year with any outpatient visits	1.60 (1.15–2.22)	.0034
			Charlson Comorbidity Index	0.61 (0.44–0.83)	.0012
Annemans et al., 2007, UK and Germany,[14]	Number of gout flares	Serum urate levels	UK (unadjusted analyses) 6–7 mg/dl >7–8 mg/dl >8–9 mg/dl ≥9 mg/dl Germany (unadjusted analyses) 6–7 mg/dl >7–8 mg/dl >8–9 mg/dl ≥ 9 mg/dl	1.33 (0.92–1.94) 1.49 (1.21–2.42) 1.71 (1.04–2.13) 2.15 (1.53–3.01) 1.37 (0.91–2.05) 1.65 (1.17–2.33) 2.37 (1.67–3.36) 2.48 (1.77–3.49)	NS <.01 <.01 <.01 NS <.01 <.01 <.01
Mikuls et al., 2006[17]	Risk factors for drug-related toxicity	Error related to gout medication versus other musculoskeletal medications	Physician error in prescribing allopurinol	7% error for other therapies vs. 23%–39% for allopurinol and colchicine	<.0001
			Drug administration or nursing error	50% for other therapies vs. 23%–27% for allopurinol and colchicine	<.0001

Studies that did not describe risk factors for noncompliance with treatment recommendations or QIs: Ly et al., 2007[15]; Petersel and Schlesinger, 2007[11]; Dalbeth et al., 2006[13]; Smith et al., 2000[21]; and Pal, 2000.[20]

and internists. Rheumatologists provide gout care to a smaller proportion of gout patients, usually those with the most severe disease. Surveys of general practitioners in Europe[25,26] and China[27] have assessed reasons for lack of adherence to good-quality gout care and published recommendations.

Owens et al.[25] surveyed 170 general practitioners (82 responded; 47% response rate) with questions regarding gout diagnosis and management. Of the respondents, 89% usually made the diagnosis of gout on the basis of tenderness and erythema (with or without tophi) and initiated treatment on this basis. In addition, 77% usually measured serum urate in suspected gout, and 3% aspirated joint in suspected gout. Reasons for not aspirating the joint were lack of experience (78%), lack of time (47%), uncertainty regarding analysis (51%), and uncertainty regarding management of results (32%). Of the 82 general practitioners, 93% used NSAIDs or colchicine for acute gout, 73% did not start urate-lowering therapy during an acute attack, and only 26% rechecked urate levels after an acute attack; and 32% routinely monitored levels in those receiving long-term therapy.

Roberts et al.[26] surveyed 446 general practitioners in England and 240 general practitioners responded (54%); 87% of the general practitioners were confident to manage gout with their own skills and knowledge, and 32% of gout cases were referred to rheumatologists by primary care physicians. Reasons for not aspirating joints were little opportunity to learn (64%), not enough opportunity for regular practice to keep up the skills (61%), medicolegal worries (45%), and lack of time (42%).

In a survey of practicing physicians and those in training at a tertiary care center in China, composed of generalists, rheumatologists, and other specialists (one third in each group), 70% responded to the survey.[27] Among the 82 eligible responders/surveys, 78% indicated that synovial fluid examination for crystals should be done when acute gouty arthritis is suspected, but only 4% actually reported performing the procedure in this scenario. In contrast, 84% examined the serum urate in patients with diagnosed gout more than 75% of the time. Factors associated with agreement with synovial fluid examination included being a resident (versus a professor), less than 5 years in practice, training in health ministry–affiliated medical school, and having received a CME in gout. For acute gout, 77% preferred oral colchicine and 17% preferred NSAIDs. In patients with creatinine of 2.2 mg/dl, 48% preferred corticosteroids, 17% preferred NSAIDs, and 26% preferred oral colchicine. Of the respondents, 54% said they would start treatment with urate-lowering drugs within 1 week of acute gout, 32% said they would start in the second week, and only 11% would start after 2 weeks.

Schlesinger et al.[28] surveyed 2500 rheumatologists and 2500 internists: 21% of rheumatologists (n = 518) and 0.9% of internists (n = 22) responded. Analyses were restricted to rheumatologists, due to the small number of internists responding to the survey. Rheumatologists reported performing crystal analyses 80% of the time for new suspected gout; 64% used combination therapy for acute gout, with the most common combination being NSAIDs and intraarticular corticosteroids, followed by NSAIDs with oral corticosteroids. Antiinflammatory prophylaxis is used by 90% of the respondents when initiating urate-lowering therapy. Rheumatologists prescribed lifelong urate-lowering therapy in 91% of cases.

In a national survey of 99 rheumatologists at Veterans Affairs medical centers, relevance of gout QIs to U.S. veterans with gout was assessed.[30] Initiation of urate-lowering therapy and monitoring of serum urate after initiation of urate lowering therapy were ranked as the highest 2 indicators among 10 QIs for both relevance to veterans with gout and likelihood to improve gout care. All 10 QIs were ranked higher than 8 on a 0 to 10 scale. This study implied that rheumatologists view the current gout QIs to be appropriate for measuring and improving the care of gout.

More studies are needed to examine underlying reasons for physician noncompliance to better inform future interventions so they can be designed to improve gout care. While the focus of quality research is on the physician noncompliance, further research is needed to define issues regarding patients and lack of access to health care, which may contribute to suboptimal care.

In conclusion, there are several gaps in the quality of gout care. Patient-, physician-, and systems-level factors are associated with deficits in gout care. Therefore, interventions targeting QOC have the potential to not only improve standard of care but also perhaps improve the quality of life in patients with gout.

References

1. Arromdee E, Michet CJ, Crowson CS, et al. Epidemiology of gout: is the incidence rising? J Rheumatol 2002;29(11):2403–6.
2. Krishnan E, Griffith C, Kwoh K. Burden of illness from gout in ambulatory care in the United States. Arthritis Rheum 2005;52(Suppl. 9):S656.
3. Kim KY, Ralph Schumacher H, Hunsche E, et al. A literature review of the epidemiology and treatment of acute gout. Clin Ther 2003;25(6):1593–617.
4. McClintock AD, Egan AJ, Woods DJ, et al. A survey of allopurinol dosage prescribing. N Z Med J 1995;108(1006):346–7.
5. Smith P, Karlson N, Nair BR. Quality use of allopurinol in the elderly. J Qual Clin Pract 2000;20(1):42–3.
6. Stamp L, Gow P, Sharples K, et al. The optimal use of allopurinol: an audit of allopurinol use in South Auckland. Aust N Z J Med 2000;30(5):567–72.
7. Ferraz MB, O'Brien B. A cost effectiveness analysis of urate lowering drugs in nontophaceous recurrent gouty arthritis. J Rheumatol 1995;22(5):908–14.
8. Lee SJ, Hirsch JD, Terkeltaub R, et al. Perceptions of disease and health-related quality of life among patients with gout. Rheumatology (Oxford) 2009;48(5):582–6.
9. Mikuls TR, MacLean CH, Olivieri J, et al. Quality of care indicators for gout management. Arthritis Rheum 2004;50(3):937–43.
10. Singh JA. Quality of life and quality of care for patients with gout. Curr Rheumatol Rep 2009;11(2):154–60.
11. Petersel D, Schlesinger N. Treatment of acute gout in hospitalized patients. J Rheumatol 2007;34(7):1566–8.
12. Neogi T, Hunter DJ, Chaisson CE, et al. Frequency and predictors of inappropriate management of recurrent gout attacks in a longitudinal study. J Rheumatol 2006;33(1):104–9.
13. Dalbeth N, Kumar S, Stamp L, et al. Dose adjustment of allopurinol according to creatinine clearance does not provide adequate control of hyperuricemia in patients with gout. J Rheumatol 2006;33(8):1646–50.
14. Annemans L, Spaepen E, Gaskin M, et al. Gout in the UK and Germany: prevalence, comorbidities and management in general practice 2000-2005. Ann Rheum Dis 2008;67(7):960–6.
15. Ly J, Gow P, Dalbeth N. Colchicine prescribing and safety monitoring in patients with gout. N Z Med J 2007;120(1265):U2808.
16. Mikuls TR, Farrar JT, Bilker WB, et al. Suboptimal physician adherence to quality indicators for the management of gout and asymptomatic hyperuricaemia: results from the UK General Practice Research Database (GPRD). Rheumatology (Oxford) 2005;44(8):1038–42.
17. Mikuls TR, Curtis JR, Allison JJ, et al. Medication errors with the use of allopurinol and colchicine: a retrospective study of a national, anonymous Internet-accessible error reporting system. J Rheumatol 2006;33(3):562–6.
18. Singh JA, Hodges JS, Toscano JP, et al. Quality of care for gout in the US needs improvement. Arthritis Rheum 2007;57(5):822–9.
19. Sarawate CA, Brewer KK, Yang W, et al. Gout medication treatment patterns and adherence to standards of care from a managed care perspective. Mayo Clin Proc 2006;81(7):925–34.
20. Pal B, Foxall M, Dysart T, et al. How is gout managed in primary care? A review of current practice and proposed guidelines. Clin Rheumatol 2000;19(1):21–5.
21. Smith P, Karlson N, Nair BR. Quality use of allopurinol in the elderly. J Qual Clin Pract 2000;20(1):42–3.
22. Evans TI, Wheeler MT, Small RE, et al. A comprehensive investigation of inpatient intravenous colchicine use shows more education is needed. J Rheumatol 1996;23(1):143–8.
23. Ho Jr G, DeNuccio M. Gout and pseudogout in hospitalized patients. Arch Intern Med 1993;153(24):2787–90.
24. Stamp L, Gow P, Sharples K, et al. The optimal use of allopurinol: an audit of allopurinol use in South Auckland. Aust N Z J Med 2000;30(5):567–72.
25. Owens D, Whelan B, McCarthy G. A survey of the management of gout in primary care. Ir Med J 2008;101(5):147–9.
26. Roberts C, Adebajo AO, Long S. Improving the quality of care of musculoskeletal conditions in primary care. Rheumatology (Oxford) 2002;41(5):503–8.
27. Fang W, Zeng X, Li M, et al. The management of gout at an academic healthcare center in Beijing: a physician survey. J Rheumatol 2006;33(10):2041–9.
28. Schlesinger N, Moore DF, Sun JD, et al. A survey of current evaluation and treatment of gout. J Rheumatol 2006;33(10):2050–2.
29. Singh JA, Hodges JS, Asch SM. Opportunities for improving medication use and monitoring in gout. Ann Rheum Dis 2009;68(8):1265–70.
30. Singh JA, Alpert MD, Kerr G. A national survey of Veterans Affairs Rheumatologists for relevance of quality of care indicators for gout management. Arthritis Care Res (Hoboken) 2010;62(9):1306–11.
31. Wallace SL, Singer JZ. Review: Systemic toxicity associated with the intravenous administration of colchicine—guidelines for use. J Rheumatol 1988;15(3):496–9.
32. Roberts WN, Liang MH, Stern SH. Colchicine in acute gout. Reassessment of risks and benefits. JAMA 1987;257(14):1920–2.

Health-Related Quality of Life and Outcome Measures in Gout

Puja P. Khanna and Dinesh Khanna

KEY POINTS

- Despite the growing prevalence of gout, only a few studies have examined the overall impact of gout on patient's health-related quality of life (HRQOL). HRQOL refers to the physical, mental, and social well-being and is shaped by a person's perception and expectations of their health.
- Studies in chronic gout have documented decrements in HRQOL using Short Form (SF)-36, with the number of joints involved during a typical and worst gout attack having the greatest impact on patient's SF-36 scores. Patients with chronic gout generally have marked decrements in their SF-36 physical domain scores.
- Gout confers substantial economic impact on the patient, employer, and society with loss of productivity at work and home and increased health care utilization.
- Feasible, reliable, and valid outcome measures have been developed in gout for clinical trials.
- For clinical trials in acute gout, patient-reported pain is usually the primary outcome measure.
- For trials in chronic gout, serum urate is used as the primary outcome measure.
- Other outcome measures in acute and chronic gout are discussed in detail.

Introduction

Gout is known to have a wide spectrum of presentation that ranges from infrequent acute painful attacks to chronic persistent swelling and pain, and once it becomes tophaceous due to the deposition of urate crystals in joints and soft tissues results in significant disability. Despite the growing prevalence of gout, only a few studies have examined the overall impact of gout on patient's health-related quality of life (HRQOL).[1-4] HRQOL refers to the physical, psychosocial, and social domains of health and is shaped by a person's perception and expectations

Grant support: Dr. P. Khanna was supported by American College of Rheumatology Research and Education Foundation Clinical Investigator Fellowship Award 2009-2011. Dr. D. Khanna was supported by a National Institutes of Health Award (NIAMS K23 AR053858-04). In addition, Drs. Khanna are supported by a National Institutes of Health Award (NIH/NIAMS U01 AR057936A) and the National Institutes of Health through the NIH Roadmap for Medical Research Grant (AR052177).

of their health. Work in HRQOL has originated from two fundamentally different approaches: health status and health value/preference/utility assessment[5] (Figures 18-1 and 18-2).

Health Status

In general, health status measures describe a person's functioning in one or more domains (e.g., physical functioning or mental well-being).

Medical Outcomes Short Form-36 (SF-36)

Currently, one of the most commonly used generic health status instruments (i.e., the concepts are not specific for any age, disease, or treatment group) is the Medical Outcomes Short Form-36 (SF-36), a 36-item measure encompassing eight domains—physical functioning, social functioning, mental health, role limitations due to physical problems, role limitations due to emotional problems, vitality (energy and fatigue), bodily pain, and general health perceptions—with higher scores denoting better HRQOL. The SF-36 domains can be summarized into physical component summary (PCS) and mental component summary (MCS) scores. Studies in chronic gout have documented decrements in HRQOL using SF-36 compared with the general population.[1-4,6] The impact of HRQOL, especially physical domains, was significant in unadjusted analysis from a large observational U.S. study.[2] After adjusting for sociodemographics and coexisting comorbidities, only bodily pain was significantly worse ($p < .01$).[2] In another observational study, Lee et al. assessed SF-36 in patients with gout in three U.S. cities.[7] The SF-36 PCS and MCS were significantly lower for gout patients ($p < .05$). In patients, the mean SF-36 PCS and MCS were lower for those with more frequent gout attacks and greater number of affected joints ($p < .005$ and $p < .001$, respectively). After adjusting for age, gender, and comorbidities, the number of joints involved during a typical and the worst gout attack had the greatest impact on patients' SF-36 PCS and MCS. In general, patients with chronic gout had marked decrements in their SF-36 PCS scores (ranged from 32.2 to 40.3), which translates into 1.0 to 1.8 standard deviations below the general U.S. population. Using another HRQOL instrument,

HEALTH-RELATED QUALITY OF LIFE

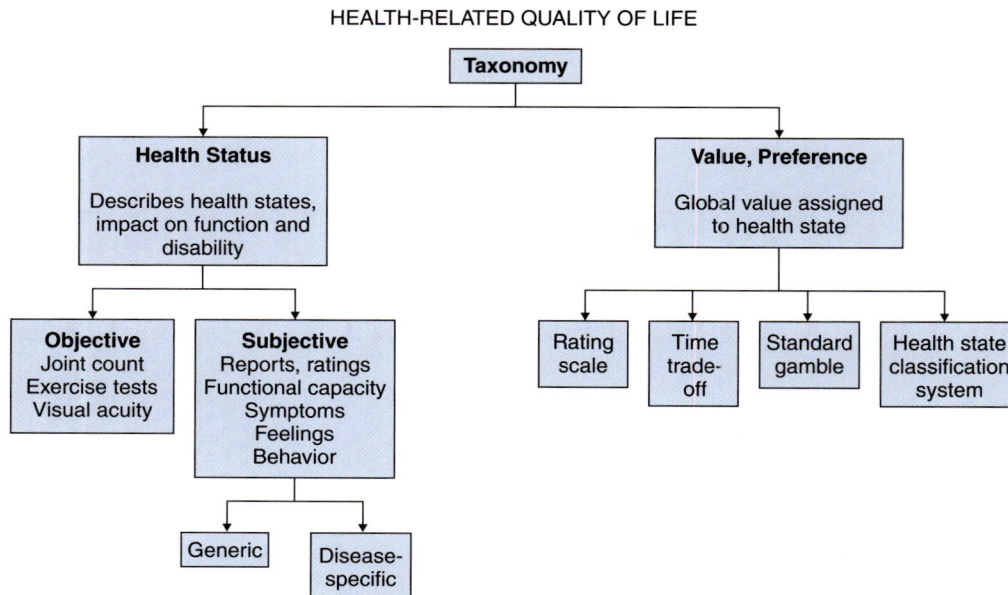

Figure 18-1 Work in health-related quality of life (HRQOL) has originated from two fundamentally different approaches: health status and health value/preference/utility assessment. In general, health status measures describe a person's functioning in one or more domains (e.g., physical functioning or mental well-being). As an example, reports of pain, fatigue, etc. are health status measures. Generic and disease-specific instruments are schematized in this figure and in Figure 18-2. Health value/preference/utility measures, in contrast, assess the *value* or *desirability* of a state of health against an external metric, are generic HRQOL measures, and summarize HRQOL as a single number. There are two major families of utility measures: direct and indirect (also known as *multiattribute utilities* or *health state classification systems*). *(From Khanna D, Tsevat J. Health-related quality of life: an introduction. Am J Manag Care 2007;13(suppl 9):S218-23.)*

HEALTH STATUS

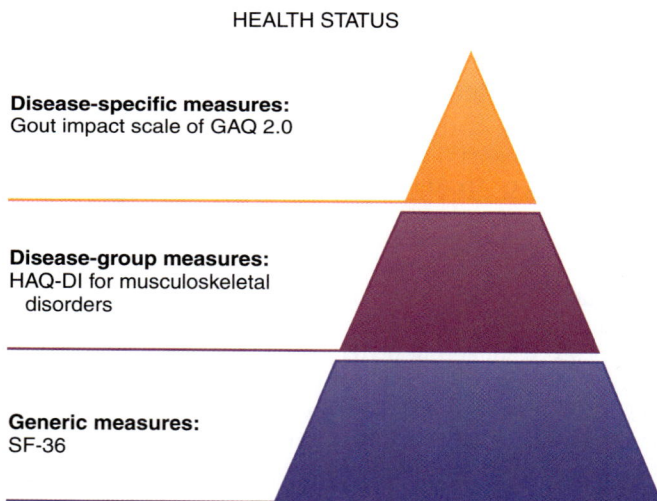

Disease-specific measures:
Gout impact scale of GAQ 2.0

Disease-group measures:
HAQ-DI for musculoskeletal disorders

Generic measures:
SF-36

Figure 18-2 Distinct types of health status measures applied to gout. Disease-targeted measures complement generic instruments. Short Form 36 (SF-36) is a generic health-related quality of life measure and can be used across disease and populations. Health Assessment Questionnaire–Disability index (HAQ-DI) is a musculoskeletal-targeted measure that can be used across different musculoskeletal disorders. Gout Impact Scale (GIS) of Gout Assessment Questionnaire 2.0 (GAQ2.0) is a gout-specific instrument. Advantages of HAQ-DI and GIS include their relevance to gout, clinical sensibility (face validity), and more sensitive to smaller differences and smaller changes over time.

the World Health Organization's WHOQOL-BREF instrument, Roddy et al. showed that patients with gout have poor HRQOL compared to control patients.[6] Although the association between overall HRQOL and gout lessened when adjusted for comorbidities, it remained significant between gout and the physical domain of HRQOL even after adjusting for several medical comorbidities.

SF-36 domain scores can be presented as Spydergrams that offer a simplified means to visualize results across all domains of SF-36 in a single figure: depicting disease- and population-specific patterns of decrements in HRQOL compared with age- and gender-matched normative data, as well as providing a tool for interpreting treatment-associated changes or longitudinal changes.[8] In addition, follow-up scores of the SF-36 domains and summary measures can be interpreted to see if the changed scores are clinically meaningful to the patients. Minimal clinically important differences (MCID) represent the smallest improvement in score of an HRQOL instrument that patients perceive as beneficial and that may lead to a change in the patient's management.[9] The MCID can help clinicians understand whether score differences between two treatment groups are considered clinically meaningful and if the changes within one group over time are clinically meaningful and relevant. MCID for the SF-36 domains and summary scores are defined as an improvement of 5 to 10 points and 2.5 to 5 points, respectively[4,10,11] (Table 18-1). In a recent observational study, treatment of patients with long-term urate-lowering therapy and daily colchicine was associated with 38% (for SF-36 MCS) to 79% (for bodily pain domain) patients achieving the MCID threshold at 12 months.[4]

Health Assessment Questionnaire–Disability Index (HAQ-DI)

The HAQ-DI is a self-administered 20-question instrument that assesses a patient's level of functional ability and includes questions on fine movements of the upper extremities, locomotor activities of the lower extremities, and activities that involve both the upper and lower extremities. The HAQ-DI

Table 18-1 Minimal Clinically Important Differences for Patient-Reported Outcome Measures

Scale	MCID Estimates
SF-36 domains (0–100)[†]	5–10 points
SF-36 summary scores (PCS and MCS)*[†]	2.5–5.0 points
Health Assessment Questionnaire-Disability Index (0–3)[†]	0.22 point
Gout Impact Scales (0–100)[‡]	5–8 points
Pain visual analog scale (0–100)[†]	10 points
Patient Global Assessment (0–100)[†]	10 points
Physician Global Assessment (0–100)[†]	10 points

*Adjusted for U.S. general population.
[†]Estimated in other arthritides.
[‡]Estimated in gout population.

score is determined by summing the highest item score in each of the eight domains and dividing the sum by 8, yielding a score ranging from 0 (no disability) to 3 (severe disability). HAQ-DI has been used in different observational studies in gout.[3,12-14] Studies have shown that patients with chronic gout (without recent history of acute attacks) have mild disability—the HAQ-DI scores range from 0.54 to 0.61[3,12-14] where scores of less than 1.0 are indicative of mild functional disability. In pegloticase randomized controlled trials (RCTs), the patients with chronic moderate-to-severe gout had moderate disability (1.10 to 1.24).[15] In contrast, patients with other rheumatic diseases (rheumatoid arthritis and scleroderma) have moderate-to-severe disability[16,17] and are predictive of poor outcomes and survival. Patients in gout observational cohorts had a high ceiling effect (percentages of respondents scoring at the highest possible scale level) ranging from 28% to 34%, signifying no functional disability. This may limit its applicability in longitudinal clinical care. Utility of HAQ-DI in gout clinical care (especially in patients with acute gout) needs to be determined.

Gout Impact Scale (GIS)

To capture the impact of gout per se, a gout-specific HRQOL instrument, called the Gout Impact Scale (GIS), has been developed.[18] This scale was originally the Gout Impact Section of the Gout Assessment Questionnaire 2.0 ($GAQ_{2.0}$).[7,19] The GIS allows patients to describe the impact of gout on their HRQOL, while the remaining $GAQ_{2.0}$ questions allow patients to describe their gout overall (e.g., recent gout attacks, treatment, gout history, demographics). The GIS contains five scales—three assess the impact of gout overall (Gout Concern Overall, Gout Medication Side Effects, and Unmet Gout Treatment Need) and two assess the impact of gout during an attack (Gout Well-being during Attack and Gout Concern during Attack). Response options for GIS items are on a 5-point ordinal scale (e.g., strongly agree to strongly disagree or all of the time to none of the time). Each GIS scale is scored from 0 to 100, with higher scores on each scale indicating "worse condition" or "greater gout impact." The scale was developed in a large observational cohort[19] and its use in real life needs to be determined.

Patient-Reported Outcomes Measurement Information System (PROMIS)

The National Institutes of Health (NIH) Patient-Reported Outcomes Measurement Information System (PROMIS) Roadmap initiative (www.nihpromis.org) is a cooperative research program designed to develop, evaluate, and standardize item banks to measure patient-reported outcomes (PROs) across common medical conditions.[20] The goal of PROMIS is to develop reliable and valid item banks using item response theory (IRT) that can be administered as computerized adaptive tests (CATs).[20-22] A CAT selects the most informative questions from an item bank on the basis of a person's previous responses; this process determines an individualized score using a minimum number of questions while preserving precision. Eleven adult domains have been developed to date as short forms and CATs in physical, mental, and social health and are available free to researchers at www.nihpromis.org.[20] These CATs include anger, anxiety, depression, fatigue, pain behavior, pain impact, physical function, sleep disturbance, wake disturbance, satisfaction with participation in social roles, and satisfaction with participation in discretionary social activities (available at www.nihpromis.org). NIH PROMIS scales have been successfully used in other chronic diseases including different arthritides.[23]

Bottom Line

Both SF-36 and HAQ-DI have robust data to support their use in clinical care. However, SF-36 requires computer software to calculate scores limiting its applicability in clinical care. HAQ-DI has advantages in that it takes 3 to 5 minutes to complete and less than 1 minute to score. However, in a real-life cohort of patients with no recent acute flares, there is a high ceiling effect that may limit its usefulness in longitudinal follow-up. Although NIH PROMIS scales have not been tested in gout, they have been successfully tested in other chronic diseases including different arthritides.[23] PROMIS provides validated item banks that are easy to administer, and the computer automatically calculates an individualized score using a minimum number of questions while preserving precision and provides a comparison with the general U.S. population.

Health Value/Preference/Utility Measures

Health values assess the *value* or *desirability* of a state of health against an external metric, are generic HRQOL measures, and summarize HRQOL as a single number.[5] There are two major families of utility measures: direct and indirect (also known as multiattribute utilities or health state classification systems). These values can be used for decision analysis and cost-effectiveness analysis. On an individual level, one's own health utilities may be used to help make decisions regarding testing and treatment. Khanna et al.[3] interviewed 80 subjects with gout and assessed direct preference based measures including a health rating scale, the time tradeoff, and standard gamble for one's current health state with gout and current health state without gout; indirect preference-based measures including the SF-6D and the EQ-5D. Disutilities for chronic stable gout were small compared to other chronic conditions. However, the patients who rank their gout as their top health concern tended to assign greater disutility to gout than did other patients. In another ongoing study presented as an abstract, patients with tophaceous gout assigned a higher disutility to their health compared to patients without it.[24] Further research is important in this area as new drugs are being developed for acute and chronic gout.

There is increasing evidence showing that inadequate control of gout results in continued suffering in a significant number of patients thus not only has detrimental effects on patient-reported outcomes but also confers substantial economic impact on the patient, employer, and society.[2,25] The next section discusses the data on work productivity and health care utilization in gout.

Work Productivity

Kleinman et al.[26] evaluated the impact of gout (defined by *International Classification of Diseases [ICD]-9* code) on an employed population's health-related work absence and objectively measured productivity output in a retrospective study. They used two comparison cohorts selected from the Human Capital Management Services Research Reference Database: a cohort of 300,000 employees with gout and without gout. Sick leave, short- and long-term disability, and workers' compensation data were collected from employers during 2001 to 2004. Data on employee-specific at-work productivity that can be measured in units of work processed per hour for a subset of the overall population were analyzed for hourly productivity and a 12-month period (total annual productivity). Employees with gout had 4.6 more annual absence days for all categories of health-related work absence than did those without gout. Objective productivity (units of work processed) was available in 86 employees with gout. It showed that these patients processed 3.51% fewer units per hour worked and 2.38% fewer units per year than did employees without gout.

Edwards et al.[27] recently assessed patient work productivity and social participation in chronic gout refractory to conventional therapy in a 1-year prospective observational study (N = 81). For patients who were less than 65 years of age, an average of 25.1 work days were lost annually. At least one flare per year was reported in 54% patients with a mean of 17.1 social days lost.

Work productivity using the Work Productivity Survey was assessed in an ongoing Veterans Administration cohort of tophaceous and nontophaceous gout patients to evaluate the impact of gout on productivity at home and in the workplace.[28] The authors found that patients missed 3.7 days during the past month and had an additional 3 days with impaired productivity at work. Tophaceous gout was associated with greater loss of productivity at home and in the workplace compared to nontophaceous gout. The patients with tophi reported 4.5 days of work lost compared to 3.2 days per month in the non-tophaceous group and an additional 4.2 days of reduced productivity at home compared to 2.4 in the nontophaceous group. Thus, the literature conclusively suggests that gout negatively impacts workplace and home productivity.

Health Care Utilization

Patterns of health care utilization have been examined by Singh et al. across a variety of settings such as primary care, rheumatology, and emergency/urgent health care utilization in patients with gout in patients recruited from three large U.S. cities.[25] The most utilized gout-related health care resource in the past year was primary care physicians, used by 60% of patients with a mean annual utilization of 3.1 visits, followed by visits to rheumatologists (51% of patients utilized with a mean annual number of visits of 3.7). Other providers such as nurse practitioners, physician assistants, urgent care, and emergency department resources were each used by about one-fourth of patients, averaging approximately two visits each in the past year. Overnight hospitalization for gout was reported by less than 10% of patients. Overall gout severity (physician defined), recent gout attack, elevated serum urate, and history of heart disease were significantly associated with whether patients utilized each resource category, with the exception of rheumatologist utilization. In another population of veterans in the United States, Singh and Strand[25] showed that gout patients had significantly more annual primary care visits (3.5 versus 2.7) and hospitalizations (18% versus 15%) and fewer mental health visits (10% versus 14%, $p < .01$) compared to patients without gout.

Measurement Properties of an Instrument—Feasibility, Reliability, and Validity

An outcome measure should be feasible, reliable, and valid.[29,30] A feasible measure is accessible, easily interpretable, and associated with low cost. Reliability (precision) is extent to which a measure yields the same score each time it is administered if the underlying health condition has not changed. A reliability coefficient of 0.90 or higher (means that 90% of the score is accurate while the remaining 10% denotes error) is considered satisfactory for individual comparisons and 0.70 or higher is considered satisfactory for group comparisons.[5] Reliability can be assessed by conducting test-retest (where scores are assessed at two different time points) and assessing internal consistency (assesses correlation between items within each scale). Validity is the extent to which the score a health measure yields accurately reflects the health concept and includes face (sensible), content (comprehensive), construct (measures or correlates with a theorized health construct), and criterion validity (predicts or correlates with gold standard). Sensitivity to change (also known as responsiveness to change), an aspect of construct validity, assesses whether an instrument score changes in the right direction when underlying health construct changes; the ability of an instrument to detect clinically important change is crucial to its usefulness as an outcome measure in a clinical trial. Magnitude of the change can be assessed using effect size. Effect size is the ratio of observed change to a measure of variance (also known as signal-to-noise ratio). An effect size of 0.20 to 0.49 represents a small change; 0.50 to 0.79, a medium change; and 0.80 or greater, a large change.[31]

Table 18-2 presents the instruments that are ready for RCTs and clinical care in patients with gout. Most of these instruments have been included in different RCTs of acute and chronic gout and endorsed by OMERACT.[32-34]

Table 18-2 Proposed Outcome Measures for Clinical Trials and Clinical Practice for Acute and Chronic Gout

Instruments	Ready for RCT	Can be used in clinical practice
Health-Related Quality of Life		
Short Form-36[¶]	Yes[†]	No
Health Assessment Questionnaire-Disability Index[¶]	Yes[†]	Yes
Gout Impact Scale (GAQ 2.0)[¶]	Yes[†]	No
PROMIS item banks[¶]	No	Yes
Global Assessment		
Patient global assessment using visual analog scale (VAS), numeric rating scale, or Likert scale[¶]	Yes[*†]	Yes
Investigator global assessment using visual analog scale (VAS), numeric rating scale, or Likert scale[§]	Yes[*†]	Yes
Patient global assessment of response to treatment[¶]	Yes[*]	Yes
Investigator global assessment of response to treatment[§]	Yes[*]	Yes
Patient assessment of pain using Visual Analog Scale (VAS), Numeric Rating Scale, or Likert scale[¶]	Yes[*†]	Yes
Patient-reported acute flare[¶]	Yes[*†]	Yes
Laboratory tests		
Serum urate <6 mg/dL	Yes[†]	Yes
Musculoskeletal		
Tender joint count[§]	Yes[*†]	Yes
Swollen joint count[§]	Yes[*†]	Yes
Tophus Measurement	Yes[†]	Yes
Vernier Calipers[§]	Yes[†]	Yes
Digital photography[‡]	Yes[†]	No
Tape measure[§]	No	Yes

*For acute gout studies.
[†]For chronic gout studies.
[‡]Standardized central reading strongly encouraged in multicenter randomized controlled trial.
[§]Assessed by the same investigator.
[¶]Completed by the patient.

Acute Gout

Pain

Pain is a cardinal symptom of acute gout that is used as the primary outcome in all RCTs for acute gout. It has face and content validity in acute gout. Pain has been captured as a Likert scale (0 = none, 1 = mild, 2 = moderate, 3 = severe, and 4 = extreme), 11-point numeric rating scale (0 to 10), or visual analog scale ranging from 0 ("no pain") to 100 ("severe or intolerable pain"). Construct validity has been published as an abstract using two large RCTs comparing etoricoxib versus

indomethacin (N = 339)[35,36]; there were moderate to strong cross-sectional and longitudinal correlations with other outcome measures.[37] Discriminant validity was supported by statistical significant differences in pain scores between patients categorized into "none/fair" versus "good/excellent" based on responses to patient and physician global assessments. Sensitivity to change has been demonstrated in multiple clinical trials of acute gout.[35,38-40]

Patient Global Assessment

Patient global assessment evaluates the patient's overall global assessment of the disease. In acute gout trials, researchers have used patient global assessment of response to treatment (PGART) as a secondary outcome measure. This asks the patient at every visit (or using daily diary) his or her response to the therapy on a 5-point ordinal scale (4 = poor, 3 = fair, 2 = good, 1 = very good, 0 = excellent).[41] Construct validity has been published as an abstract from two large RCTs comparing etoricoxib versus indomethacin (N = 339).[42] PGART had a high correlation with investigator assessment of response to treatment (r = 0.59). PGART also had significant correlations with pain, joint tenderness, and swelling but no association with laboratory tests.

Investigator Global Assessment

Investigators in the RCTs are asked to provide an overall rating of the patient's disease activity or severity as a result of gout. In acute gout trials, researchers have used investigator global assessment of response to treatment (IGART rather than global assessment) as a secondary outcome measure. As an example, in the etoricoxib versus indomethacin RCTs, investigators were asked to rate the response on a 5-point Likert scale[41,42] (4 = none—no response, absence of drug effect; 3 = poor—minimal response, unacceptable; 2 = definite response, but could be better; 1 = good—good response, but less than best possible anticipated result; 0 = excellent—best possible anticipated response, considering severity of gout attack). Similar to PGART, IGART had a significant correlation with pain, joint swelling, and tenderness. There was no significant correlation between IGART and laboratory data.

BOTTOM LINE

Both global assessment (patient and investigator) and assessment of response to treatment (PGART and IGART) should be included in acute gout trials. Both provide complementary information— global assessment provides baseline severity of gout and a changed score that can be assessed for statistical significance and clinically important improvements. PGART and IGART are Likert scales and provide a treatment response.

Joint Swelling and Joint Tenderness

Joint swelling, tenderness, and redness are integral parts of an acute attack of gout (supporting its face and content validity). There is a lack of published data on the construct validity of joint swelling and tenderness during an acute attack, although data are available from multiple RCTs. Reliability (interreader and intrareader) has also not been reported. Sensitivity to change has been shown in multiple trials for treatment of acute gout.[35,43] Studies have used a 4-point scale for joint swelling

(0 = no swelling, 1 = palpable, 2 = visible, 3 = distended joint) and tenderness (0 = no tenderness, 1 = responds that tender, 2 = winces, 3 = withdraws). We also suggest including redness of index joint on a 0-to-4 Likert scale (0 = no redness, 1 = subtle, 2 = moderate, 3 = dramatic). OMERACT-9 has proposed that when more than one joint is involved, an index joint must be selected.[34] The method of index joint selection is not defined, but patient nomination of most severe joint is considered a practical solution. It may be necessary for investigators to exclude certain joints where other factors, like overlying tophi, ulceration, or concomitant degenerative joint disease, may preclude assessment or influence response. In addition, the same investigator should assess joint swelling and tenderness to decrease variability among investigators. The inclusion of joint swelling and tenderness in chronic gout is also discussed in the next section, Chronic Gout.

There is a lack of data on assessment of HRQOL (SF-36 using 1-week recall, GIS, and HAQ-DI) in acute gout. Future studies should incorporate these outcome measures to assess them.

Chronic Gout
Gout Flare

Gout flare is a significant concern for individuals with gout and thus has face and content validity. Chronic prophylaxis for gout includes acute flares and gout flare was chosen as a mandatory item by gout experts for chronic gout trials.[33] Construct validity was demonstrated in a large observational study where patients with recent gout flares had poor HRQOL (SF-36 summary scores) compared to those who didn't have a flare.[7] Traditionally, the gout flare has been patient-reported and usually includes an acute onset of joint swelling, tenderness, and redness associated with pain. Also, there is lack of data on agreement between physician-defined gout flare (gold standard) versus patient-defined flare. Different clinical trials have used different definitions.[44-47] A uniform definition to define flare is urgently needed. Potential items for an operational definition of gout flare have been identified by consensus and were validated against physician-diagnosed flare. It includes patient self-report flare, overall pain at rest, warm joints, and swollen joints.[48]

Serum Urate Level

Serum urate (SUA) is a key outcome measure for chronic gout trials and is accepted by regulatory agencies as the primary outcome measure for chronic gout therapy. SUA is a feasible measure of hyperuricemia in gout. SUA as a biomarker for chronic gout was recently reviewed in detail by Stamp et al.[49] It is widely available and internationally standardized and remains stable after repeat freeze-and-thaw cycles as frozen specimens in long-term storage. The assay is reproducible and generally reliable with between-laboratory and between-method coefficient of variation of less than 5%. The factors that have been known to cause variability in SUA concentrations include age, sex, ethnicity, circadian rhythms, body mass index, renal/hepatic function, and fasting/nonfasting status (reviewed in detail[49]).

The relationship between SUA and gout makes inherent sense (face and content validity). The risk of gout increases with increasing SUA with a 5-year cumulative incidence of gout of 22% for those with SUA of 9.0 mg/dL or greater compared to only 3% for those with SUA of 7.0 to 8.9 mg/dL.[50] SUA is a surrogate biomarker for clinical and patient-reported endpoints/outcomes in gout, including number of gout flares, reduction in tophus size, dissolution of monosodium urate crystals within joints, radiological progression, and HRQOL.

Construct validity of SUA is demonstrated in different studies. Higher SUA is associated with increased risk of having gouty flares over 12 months (SUA 9 mg/dL or greater versus SUA less than 6 mg/dL [odds ratio 3.4]). The average number of flares also increase with increasing SUA (1.5 for SUA less than 6 mg/dL, 1.6 for SUA between 6 and 8.99 mg/dL, and 1.7 for SUA of 9 mg/dL or greater). The average number of gout flares increased by 11.9% with each unit increased when SUA was 6 mg/dL or greater.[51] The presence of tophi in patients with gout is associated with higher SUA concentrations. SUA was significantly higher in patients with clinically evident tophi compared to those without tophi (9.2 mg/dL versus 7.3 mg/dL; $p < .006$).[52]

Association between HRQOL and SUA was recently demonstrated by Hirsch et al.[19] during the development of GIS. Mean scores for the "gout concern overall" and "unmet gout treatment need" scales were lower for subjects with lower versus higher SUA levels ($p = .001$ and $p = .012$). In another observational study, Khanna et al. divided baseline SUA at median value (8.7 or less versus greater than 8.7 mg/dL). The mean (SD) bodily pain domain of the SF-36 was lower (worse HRQOL) in patients with SUA greater than 8.7 (37.02 [10.97] versus 42.47 [10.92], $p < .02$ [unpublished data]). There were no statistical differences in other SF-36 domains and summary scores.

Reduction in SUA is associated with disappearance of monosodium urate crystals from synovial fluid,[53] decrease in gout flares, and tophi resolution.[15,54] In pegloticase trials, responders were defined as the percentage of patients achieving plasma uric acid concentrations less than 6 mg/dL for at least 80% of the time during months 3 and 6. The data from these two RCTs have been combined, because the trials had the same methodology, design, duration (6 months), interventions (pegloticase every 2 weeks versus every 4 weeks versus placebo), and outcomes. In responders for the U.S. Food and Drug Administration (FDA)-approved dose (8 mg every 2 weeks, 38% to 47%), patients had statistically significant improvements in the tender joint count, swollen joint count, and patient-reported outcome measures (SF-36 and HAQ-DI).[15] In addition, a higher proportion of patients had complete resolution of tophi (prescribing information).

Improvement in SUA is also associated with an improvement in HRQOL. Khanna et al.[4] showed that when chronic gout patients with a baseline serum urate level of 8.9 mg/dL and mean number of flares 4.7 over last year were treated with daily urate-lowering therapy and colchicine, there was a reduction in SUA (mean 5.46 mg/dL) and number of flares ($p < .001$ for both) over 12 months.

Tophus Measurement

Tophus formation is a result of untreated and uncontrolled chronic gout and is a surrogate for more severe gout and poor HRQOL.[1,4] Tophi measurement in clinical studies range from simple physical measurement techniques such as counting the total number of visible subcutaneous tophi, tape measurement of the tophus, and the diameter measurement of the tophus using Vernier calipers, to the more complex advanced imaging methods such as computed tomography (CT) and magnetic resonance imaging (MRI).[55] Among these methods, Vernier calipers involve identification and serial measurement of the longest diameter of an index tophus in an observational study and was shown to have acceptable reliability (interobserver and intraobserver) and construct validity with a very high correlation coefficient between CT and Vernier caliper measurement (coefficient 0.91).[56] In another longitudinal study, caliper measurement of tophi was found to be sensitive to change when all index tophi completely resolved with urate-lowering therapy after 21 months.[55,57] It was also able to discriminate between types of urate-lowering therapy. Tape measurement of the index tophus was used in febuxostat studies. This measure is feasible, reliable, and sensitive to change over time. However, data on construct validity are lacking at this time.[55] Digital photography of the tophus that uses standardized digital photography was performed in clinical trials of pegloticase.[15] Electronic calipers were placed along the longest dimension with distinguishable borders and margins were identified of the longest perpendicular diameter; the computer measured the length of the two diameters and calculated the area. Response was graded as an ordinal response from progressive disease to complete resolution. Sensitivity to change and between-group discrimination (active drug versus placebo) were demonstrated, but reliability and validity data are not yet available. Future analysis should assess interreader and intrareader agreement, and the digital pictures from longitudinal data should be read in random order (as done for the radiographic assessment in rheumatoid arthritis clinical trials) to prevent bias for an improvement. Also, further validation studies are needed that compare it with the simple physical methods.

Another potential inexpensive and relative easy to perform imaging technique for measurement of tophus diameter and volume is ultrasonography, which has been assessed in a longitudinal observational study of patients on urate-lowering therapy.[58] It correlates highly with MRI measurements, and intraobserver and interobserver reliability is acceptable. Sensitivity to change has been demonstrated, but this method was not able to discriminate between different urate-lowering therapies.[58,59] Although ultrasonography is quickly becoming a popular noninvasive imaging modality in rheumatology clinics, operator variability remains a potential problem in large multicenter studies.

Other advanced imaging methods of tophus assessment such as CT, MRI, and dual-energy computed tomography (DECT) are potentially useful methods of tophus size measurement as they can measure both subcutaneous and intraarticular tophi.[58-60] Data from these modalities are easy to store and centrally read; however, costs can be expensive and nonavailability of these modalities (DECT). The other major drawback is the cumulative life dose of radiation received on CT; the time required to complete the volume assessments limits the feasibility of this imaging technique. DECT can differentiate between healthy volunteers and in patients with tophaceous gout.[61] DECT was recently evaluated in 12 patients with tophaceous gout.[62] In patients who responded to urate-lowering therapy (n = 10), an improvement in the articular region corresponded to a decrease in total tophus volume by DECT. In contrast, in two nonresponders, there was an increase in total tophus volume. DECT is still in the investigational phase and its feasibility and reliability are yet to be reported.

Health-Related Quality of Life

SF-36 and HAQ-DI have been included in chronic gout clinical trials.[15] Both instruments have face and content validity as they measure constructs that are important to patients with gout, and both measures are easy to administer. The test-retest and Cronbach's alpha reliability for SF-36 and HAQ-DI are acceptable in chronic gout.[1,12,13] Construct validity for SF-36 was recently demonstrated in a large observational trial where SF-36 physical and bodily pain domains and PCS scores were able to discriminate patients with versus those without palpable tophi, presence versus absence of comorbidities, monoarticular/oligoarticular versus polyarticular joint involvement, and absence versus presence of radiographic damage.[4] In another observational study, HAQ-DI was able to differentiate between the presence and absence of tophi, swollen joints, tender joints, and limited joint mobility.[12] In the pegloticase clinical trials, both HAQ-DI and SF-36 (especially the physical domains and PCS) showed sensitivity to change with statistically significant and clinical important improvements.[15] Another observational study also showed that SF-36 (especially the physical domains and PCS) was sensitive to change with chronic urate-lowering therapy.[4]

The GIS of the $GAQ_{2.0}$ is a 24-item instrument that has acceptable feasibility, reliability (test-retest and Cronbach alpha), and validity in a large observational trial.[19] GIS scales were recently administered in an RCT assessing rilonacept versus placebo for the prevention of gout flares during the initiation of allopurinol therapy[63] and showed feasibility of the GIS scales. The Cronbach alpha coefficients were calculated for four scales (not for Gout Medication Side Effects due to lack of an appropriate anchor) and ranged from 0.59 for Unmet Gout Treatment Need to 0.94 for Gout Well-being during Attack. The study also provided estimates for minimally important differences for future interpretation of GIS scales in RCTs that range from 5 to 8 points (on a 0-to-100 scale). The instrument, however, lacks a conceptual model on what it intends to measure—it has questions that ask about impact of gout on social and emotional well-being; impact of gout on activities of daily living, vocational and avocational activities; and side effects and perceptions of medication. In addition, it lacks a recall period. Further studies will clarify its utility in clinical studies.

Pain

Pain assessment is the primary outcome measure in acute gout RCTs. However, pain is also a common symptom of chronic moderate-to-severe gout. Pain was assessed on a 0-to-100 visual analog scale in the pegloticase RCTs.[15] In these studies, treatment with pegloticase was associated with statistical improvement in pain scores compared to the placebo group. In addition, SF-36 bodily pain scale has been assessed recently in an observational study.[4] SF-36 bodily pain scale was able to discriminate patients with versus without palpable tophi, monoarticular/oligoarticular versus polyarticular joint involvement, and absence versus presence of radiographic damage. In addition, chronic treatment with urate-lowering therapy and colchicine was associated with significant improvement in bodily pain at 1 year with large effect sizes (1.09).

Patient and Investigator Global Assessments

Patient and investigator global assessments in the pegloti-case RCTs were assessed on a 0-to-100 visual analog scale.[15] Construct validity has yet to be assessed in chronic gout, but treatment with pegloticase was associated with statistically significant improvements in patient and investigator global scores compared to the placebo group.

Joint Inflammation

Joint inflammation has been assessed in chronic arthritides using joint count. Joint involvement is associated with poor HRQOL in patients with chronic gout.[4] Investigator assessment of joint tenderness and swelling was found to be feasible, reliable, and valid (including sensitive to change) in rheumatoid arthritis and psoriatic arthritis RCTs. Joint count can be assessed by examining either 28 joints or 66 of 68 joints of the upper and lower extremities. In patients with chronic severe gout, baseline data from RCTs showed a high prevalence of SJC and TJC, supporting its face and content validity.[15] Although its construct validity needs to be determined in this population and may be confounded by associated tophi, the RCTs supported its sensitivity to change. Future studies should incorporate 66 of 68 joint count as it involves feet and lower extremities (an area of high prevalence in gout) and should be evaluated by the same investigator to decrease interreader variability (as done in rheumatoid arthritis and psoriatic arthritis trials).

Conclusion

Gout has a detrimental impact on HRQOL and productivity at work and home. We present outcome measures that are ready to use for answering research questions asked in RCTs and those who will use the end results (e.g., patients , physicians, providers, and other stakeholders such as policymakers). These can be used easily in the day-to-day management of patients to measure attributes or specific symptoms, such as an individual's pain, stiffness, and specific disability, or as a broader global measure of health.

Author's Note

Schlesinger et al. recently studied the effect of canakinumab, a fully human anti-interleukin-1β monoclonal antibody on HRQOL. In an 8-week, single-blind, double-dummy, dose-ranging study in patients with acute gout flares who were unresponsive or intolerant to or had contraindications for nonsteroidal antiinflammatory drugs and/or colchicine, improvements were noted in physical health at 7 days in all treatment groups. In the 150-mg group, the mean SF-36 PCS increased by 12.0 points from baseline to 48.3 at 7 days. SF-36 scores for physical functioning and bodily pain for the canakinumab 150-mg group approached those for the US general population by 7 days and reached norm values by 8 weeks.[64]

References

1. Becker MA, Schumacher HR, Benjamin KL, et al. Quality of life and disability in patients with treatment-failure gout. J Rheumatol 2009;36(5):1041–8.
2. Singh JA, Strand V. Gout is associated with more comorbidities, poorer health related quality of life and higher health care utilization in US veterans. Ann Rheum Dis 2008.
3. Khanna D, Ahmed M, Yontz D, et al. The disutility of chronic gout. Qual Life Res 2008.
4. Khanna PP, Perez-Ruiz F, Maranian P, et al. Long-term therapy for chronic gout results in clinically important improvements in the Health-Related Quality of Life: Short Form-36 is responsive to change in chronic gout. Oxford: Rheumatology; 2010.
5. Khanna D, Tsevat J. Health-related quality of life: an introduction. Am J Manag Care 2007;13(Suppl. 9):S218–23.
6. Roddy E, Zhang W, Doherty M. Is gout associated with reduced quality of life? A case-control study. Rheumatology (Oxford) 2007;46(9):1441–4.
7. Lee SJ, Hirsch JD, Terkeltaub R, et al. Perceptions of disease and health-related quality of life among patients with gout. Rheumatology (Oxford) 2009;48(5):582–6.
8. Strand V, Crawford B, Singh J, et al. Use of "spydergrams" to present and interpret SF-36 health-related quality of life data across rheumatic diseases. Ann Rheum Dis 2009;68(12):1800–4.
9. Jaeschke R, Singer J, Guyatt GH. Measurement of health status. Ascertaining the minimal clinically important difference. Control Clin Trials 1989;10(4):407–15.
10. Khanna D, Yan X, Tashkin DP, et al. Impact of oral cyclophosphamide on health-related quality of life in patients with active scleroderma lung disease: results from the Scleroderma Lung Study. Arthritis Rheum 2007;56(5):1676–84.
11. Kosinski M, Zhao SZ, Dedhiya S, et al. Determining minimally important changes in generic and disease-specific health-related quality of life questionnaires in clinical trials of rheumatoid arthritis. Arthritis Rheum 2000;43(7):1478–87.
12. Alvarez-Hernandez E, Pelaez-Ballestas I, Vazquez-Mellado J, et al. Validation of the Health Assessment Questionnaire disability index in patients with gout. Arthritis Rheum 2008;59(5):665–9.
13. Ten Klooster PM, Oude Voshaar MA, Taal E, et al. Comparison of measures of functional disability in patients with gout. Oxford: Rheumatology; 2010.
14. van Groen MM, Ten Klooster PM, Taal E, et al. Application of the Health Assessment Questionnaire Disability Index to various rheumatic diseases. Qual Life Res 2010;19(9):1255–63.
15. KRYSTEXXA™ (pegloticase) for intravenous infusion. Briefing document for Arthritis Advisory Committee Division of Anesthesia, Analgesia, and Rheumatology Products FDA Arthritis Advisory Committee Meeting. Accessed January 1, 2011. http://www.fda.gov/downloads/AdvisoryCommittees/CommitteesMeetingMaterials/Drugs/ArthritisDrugsAdvisoryCommittee/UCM165814.pdf.
16. Cole JC, Motivala SJ, Khanna D, et al. Validation of single-factor structure and scoring protocol for the Health Assessment Questionnaire-Disability Index. Arthritis Rheum 2005;53(4):536–42.
17. Cole JC, Khanna D, Clements PJ, et al. Single-factor scoring validation for the Health Assessment Questionnaire-Disability Index (HAQ-DI) in patients with systemic sclerosis and comparison with early rheumatoid arthritis patients. Qual Life Res 2006;15(8):1383–94.
18. Hirsch J, Lee S, Terkeltaub R, et al. Evaluation of the psychometric properties of a gout-specific patient reported outcomes (PRO) instrument. Arthritis Rheum 2006;54(9):S102.
19. Hirsch JD, Lee SJ, Terkeltaub R, et al. Evaluation of an instrument assessing influence of Gout on health-related quality of life. J Rheumatol 2008;35(12):2406–14.
20. Cella D, Yount S, Rothrock N, et al. The Patient-Reported Outcomes Measurement Information System (PROMIS): progress of an NIH Roadmap cooperative group during its first two years. Med Care 2007;45(5 Suppl. 1):S3–11.
21. Reeve BB, Hays RD, Bjorner JB, et al. Psychometric evaluation and calibration of health-related quality of life item banks: plans for the Patient-Reported Outcomes Measurement Information System (PROMIS). Med Care 2007;45(5 Suppl. 1):S22–31.
22. Hays RD, Liu H, Spritzer K, et al. Item response theory analyses of physical functioning items in the medical outcomes study. Med Care 2007;45(5 Suppl. 1):S32–8.
23. Fries JF, Bruce B, Cella D. The promise of PROMIS: using item response theory to improve assessment of patient-reported outcomes. Clin Exp Rheumatol 2005;23(5 Suppl. 39):S53–7.

24. Khanna P, Persselin J, Hays RD, et al. Health related quality of life (HRQOL) in tophaceous versus non-tophaceous gout. Arthritis Rheum 2010.

25. Singh JA, Sarkin A, Shieh M, et al. Health care utilization in patients with gout. Semin Arthritis Rheum 2010.

26. Kleinman NL, Brook RA, Patel PA JE, et al. The impact of gout on work absence and productivity. Value Health 2007;10(4):231–7.

27. Edwards NL, Sundy JS, Forsythe A, et al. Work productivity loss due to flares in patients with chronic gout refractory to conventional therapy. J Med Econ 2010.

28. Khanna P, Persselin J, Hays RD, et al. Healthcare utilization and productivity at home and work place in tophaceous versus non-tophaceous gout. Arthritis Rheum 2010.

29. Hays RD. Reliability and validity (including responsiveness). In: Fayers P, Hays RD, editors. Assessing Quality of Life in Clinical Trials. 2nd ed. New York: Oxford; 2005:25–39.

30. Khanna D. Assessing disease activity and outcomes in scleroderma. In: Hochberg M, Silman A, Smolen J, editors. Rheumatology. 5th ed. St Louis: Mosby; 2010:1367–71.

31. Cohen J. A power primer. Psychol Bull 1992;112:155–9.

32. Brooks P, Boers M, Simon LS, et al. Outcome measures in rheumatoid arthritis: the OMERACT process. Exp Rev Clin Immunol 2007;3(3):271–5.

33. Taylor WJ, Schumacher Jr HR, Baraf HS, et al. A modified Delphi exercise to determine the extent of consensus with OMERACT outcome domains for studies of acute and chronic gout. Ann Rheum Dis 2008;67(6):888–91.

34. Grainger R, Taylor WJ, Dalbeth N, et al. Progress in measurement instruments for acute and chronic gout studies. J Rheumatol 2009;36(10):2346–55.

35. Rubin BR, Burton R, Navarra S, et al. Efficacy and safety profile of treatment with etoricoxib 120 mg once daily compared with indomethacin 50 mg three times daily in acute gout: a randomized controlled trial. Arthritis Rheum 2004;50(2):598–606.

36. Schumacher Jr HR, Boice JA, Daikh DI, et al. Randomised double blind trial of etoricoxib and indomethacin in treatment of acute gouty arthritis. BMJ 2002;324(7352):1488–92.

37. Schlesinger N, Norquist J, Holmes R, et al. Validation of a patient-reported assessment of pain in acute gouty arthritis. Ann Rheum Dis 2011;66:234.

38. Cheng TT, Lai HM, Chiu CK, et al. A single-blind, randomized, controlled trial to assess the efficacy and tolerability of rofecoxib, diclofenac sodium, and meloxicam in patients with acute gouty arthritis. Clin Ther 2004;26(3):399–406.

39. Man CY, Cheung IT, Cameron PA, et al. Comparison of oral prednisolone/paracetamol and oral indomethacin/paracetamol combination therapy in the treatment of acute goutlike arthritis: a double-blind, randomized, controlled trial. Ann Emerg Med 2007;49(5):670–7.

40. Terkeltaub RA, Furst DE, Bennett K, et al. High versus low dosing of oral colchicine for early acute gout flare: twenty-four-hour outcome of the first multicenter, randomized, double-blind, placebo-controlled, parallel-group, dose-comparison colchicine study. Arthritis Rheum 2010;62(4):1060–8.

41. Schumacher Jr HR, Boice JA, Daikh DI, et al. Randomised double blind trial of etoricoxib and indomethacin in treatment of acute gouty arthritis. BMJ 2002;324(7352):1488–92.

42. Norquist J, Levine K, Schlesinger N, et al. Critical evaluation of recommended outcome assessments in acute gouty arthritis. Ann Rheum Dis 2008;67(Suppl. II):247.

43. Schumacher Jr HR, Boice JA, Daikh DI, et al. Randomised double blind trial of etoricoxib and indometacin in treatment of acute gouty arthritis. BMJ 2002;324(7352):1488–92.

44. Becker MA, Schumacher Jr HR, Wortmann RL, et al. Febuxostat compared with allopurinol in patients with hyperuricemia and gout. N Engl J Med 2005;353(23):2450–61.

45. Sundy JS, Becker MA, Baraf HS, et al. Reduction of plasma urate levels following treatment with multiple doses of pegloticase (polyethylene glycol-conjugated uricase) in patients with treatment-failure gout: results of a phase II randomized study. Arthritis Rheum 2008;58(9):2882–91.

46. Becker MA, Schumacher HR, Espinoza LR, et al. The urate-lowering efficacy and safety of febuxostat in the treatment of the hyperuricemia of gout: the CONFIRMS trial. Arthritis Res Ther 2010;12(2):R63.

47. Terkeltaub RA, Furst DE, Bennett K, et al. High- vs low-dosing of oral colchicine for early acute gout flare: twenty-four hour outcome results of the first randomized, placebo-controlled, dose comparison colchicine trial. Arthritis Rheum 2010.

48. Gaffo A, Schumacher HR, Saag K, et al. Developing American College of Rheumatology and European League against Rheumatism criteria for definition of a flare in patients with gout. Arthritis Rheum 2010.

49. Stamp LK, Zhu X, Dalbeth N, et al. Serum urate as a soluble biomarker in chronic gout-evidence that serum urate fulfills the OMERACT validation criteria for soluble biomarkers. Semin Arthritis Rheum 2010.

50. Campion EW, Glynn RJ, DeLabry LO. Asymptomatic hyperuricemia. Risks and consequences in the Normative Aging Study. Am J Med 1987;82(3):421–6.

51. Wu EQ, Patel PA, Mody RR, et al. Frequency, risk, and cost of gout-related episodes among the elderly: does serum uric acid level matter? J Rheumatol 2009;36(5):1032–40.

52. Nakayama DA, Barthelemy C, Carrera G, et al. Tophaceous gout: a clinical and radiographic assessment. Arthritis Rheum 1984;27(4):468–71.

53. Pascual E, Sivera F. Time required for disappearance of urate crystals from synovial fluid after successful hypouricaemic treatment relates to the duration of gout. Ann Rheum Dis 2007;66(8):1056–8.

54. Schumacher Jr HR, Becker MA, Lloyd E, et al. Febuxostat in the treatment of gout: 5-yr findings of the FOCUS efficacy and safety study. Rheumatology (Oxford) 2009;48(2):188–94.

55. Dalbeth N, McQueen F, Singh J, et al. Tophus measurement as an outcome measure for clinical trials of chronic gout: progress and research priorities. J Rheumatol 2011:In press.

56. Dalbeth N, Clark B, Gregory K, et al. Computed tomography measurement of tophus volume: comparison with physical measurement. Arthritis Rheum 2007;57(3):461–5.

57. Perez-Ruiz F, Calabozo M, Pijoan JI, et al. Effect of urate-lowering therapy on the velocity of size reduction of tophi in chronic gout. Arthritis Rheum 2002;47(4):356–60.

58. Perez-Ruiz F, Martin I, Canteli B. Ultrasonographic measurement of tophi as an outcome measure for chronic gout. J Rheumatol 2007;34(9):1888–93.

59. Perez-Ruiz F, Dalbeth N, Urresola A, et al. Imaging of gout: findings and utility. Arthritis Res Ther 2009;11(3):232.

60. Schumacher Jr HR, Becker MA, Edwards NL, et al. Magnetic resonance imaging in the quantitative assessment of gouty tophi. Int J Clin Pract 2006;60(4):408–14.

61. Choi HK, Al-Arfaj AM, Eftekhari A, et al. Dual energy computed tomography in tophaceous gout. Ann Rheum Dis 2009;68(10):1609–12.

62. Abufayyah M, Nicolaou S, Eftekhari A, et al. quantitative documentation of tophus volume change using dual energy computed tomography scans. Arthritis Rheum 2010;62(Suppl. 10).

63. Khanna D, Sarkin A, Khanna PP, et al. Minimally important differences of the gout impact scale in a randomized controlled trial. Rheumatology (Oxford) 2011:In press.

64. Schlesinger N, De Meulemeester M, Pikhlak A, et al. Canakinumab relieves symptoms of acute flares and improves health-related quality of life in patients with difficult-to-treat gouty arthritis by suppressing inflammation: results of a randomized, dose-ranging study. *Arthritis Res Ther* 2011;13(2):R53. [Epub ahead of print].

Asymptomatic Hyperuricemia: Cardiovascular and Renal Implications

Tuhina Neogi

KEY POINTS

- There are a number of in vitro and in vivo models supporting a complex potential relation of hyperuricemia to both cardiovascular and renal outcomes.
- Definitive evidence of clinical benefits of urate reduction for cardiovascular endpoints is lacking from randomized controlled trials, although preliminary evidence from trials suggests potential efficacy for hypertension in adolescents and for renal disease.
- Whether any potential clinical effects are mediated by urate-lowering versus xanthine oxidase inhibition itself is unclear.
- Clinical trials of urate-lowering, including agents that act via mechanisms other than xanthine oxidase inhibition, specifically designed to assess cardiovascular endpoints are needed to address potential clinical benefits of such a strategy.
- There are insufficient data at the present time to recommend treatment of asymptomatic hyperuricemia in the absence of clinical gout.

Hyperuricemia: Definition

Uric acid, a product of purine metabolism, is degraded in most mammals by the hepatic enzyme urate oxidase (uricase) to more highly soluble allantoin, which is freely excreted in the urine. During the Miocene epoch (24 to 6 million years ago), mutations occurred in early hominids that rendered the uricase gene nonfunctional.[1] As a consequence, humans and the great apes have higher urate levels than do most other mammals, resulting in an inability of the liver to convert uric acid to the more soluble compound allantoin as the end product of purine metabolism. Hyperuricemia is best defined by serum urate concentrations in excess of 6.8 mg/dL, the limit of urate solubility in vitro at physiologic temperature, and pH.[2] Hyperuricemia, due to uric acid overproduction or, more commonly, renal uric acid underexcretion, is necessary but not sufficient to cause clinical gout; only 22% of individuals with urate levels of 9.0 mg/dL or higher developed gout over 5 years in one cohort study.[3] Hyperuricemia in the absence of clinical gout, tophi, or urolithiasis is considered "asymptomatic" and currently is not itself an indication for urate-lowering therapy.

Hypothetical Evolutionary Advantages of Hyperuricemia

It has been hypothesized that, because independent functional mutations in different evolutionary lineages are unlikely to occur due to chance, the loss of uricase may have had evolutionary advantages, particularly since 90% of urate filtered by the kidneys is reabsorbed rather than being eliminated.

One hypothesis is that the advantage conferred was related to uric acid functioning as an antioxidant.[4] The loss of uricase was preceded by the loss of ability to synthesize ascorbic acid (vitamin C), another antioxidant, during a period in which primates consumed large quantities of fruits containing vitamin C.[5,6] In later epochs, when diets contained lower levels of vitamin C, the higher serum urate levels related to the loss of uricase could have become an important source of antioxidant activity necessary for the prevention and repair of oxidative damage. For example, some have postulated that the relative "hyperuricemia" of higher primates and humans may have promoted the evolution of higher intelligence through antioxidant, neuroprotective effects of extracellular soluble urate.

Another hypothesis is related to salt sensitivity. The low-salt intakes of early hominids, combined with a shift toward more arid conditions occurring in the middle to late time periods of this epoch, could have led to selection pressure on early hominids toward a genotype that would enhance sodium retention to maintain blood pressure. This hypothesis has been supported by the observation of maintenance or a rise in blood pressure among rats in which hyperuricemia was induced while being maintained on a low-salt dietary condition.[7]

The latest hypothesis for the evolutionary benefit of uricase loss appears more sound than the blood pressure hypothesis and is related to complex effects of uric acid on fructose disposition, with hyperuricemia promoting increased fat stores in part by effects on hepatic fructose metabolism.[8]

The potentially important linkages between hyperuricemia and fructose intake and metabolism (and consequent metabolic effects on liver and adiposity, and potentially vascular disease)[8] are partially reviewed later, but a full discussion is beyond the scope of the summary provided here.

Potential Adverse Effects of Hyperuricemia in the Modern Era: Cardiovascular and Renal Consequences

In modern times, there has been a change to a higher salt diet in combination with food abundance throughout the seasons, eliminating the need to undergo physiologic adaptation for periods of hibernation or fasting. Further, average serum urate concentrations have been increasing over the past several decades,[9] likely contributed to by increased consumption of purine-rich foods and fructose intake. Thus, while there may have been potential evolutionary advantages for elevated serum urate concentrations in early hominids, some of those very same benefits are now potentially harmful to humans in the modern era, particularly with changes that have led to even higher urate levels.

Clarifying the relation of uric acid to cardiovascular and renal disease risk has clinical implications and public health importance. First, there is an ongoing secular increase in the incidence and prevalence of gout and hyperuricemia in recent years.[10-12] Second, asymptomatic hyperuricemia is presently not an indication for urate-lowering therapy. If hyperuricemia is indeed an independent risk factor for cardiovascular or renal disease, it might motivate a change in traditional treatment recommendations.

Link Between Uric Acid and Hypertension

Hypertension is a well-known strong risk factor for cardiovascular disease. A potential mechanistic link between uric acid and hypertension has been postulated. In vitro studies have pointed toward potential vascular effects of soluble urate. In the presence of urate concentrations seen in vivo in human plasma, levels of vasodilatory nitric oxide are suppressed,[13] and vascular smooth muscle cells proliferate, migrate, and express inflammatory mediators, as do cultured endothelial cells.[9,14-16] The soluble urate–induced vascular smooth muscle cell proliferation has been linked to suggested urate-related increased platelet-derived growth factor expression, local thromboxane production, cyclooxygenase-2 stimulation, and activation of the renin-angiotensin system in these cells.[16-18] Additionally, results of in vitro studies have suggested that soluble urate could modulate intravascular C-reactive protein (CRP) production, endothelial cell function, inflammation, and platelet adhesiveness.[14,18-21] Intracellular pro-oxidant effects of soluble uric acid have been proposed to be responsible for many of these changes, but conclusive proof is lacking. Also, one caveat to interpretation of soluble exogenous uric acid effects in some in vitro studies is a concern that contamination of the uric acid with endotoxin has not been adequately addressed in all studies.

In vivo evidence of a relation between uric acid and hypertension also exists. A rat model of mild hyperuricemia without crystalline disease affecting the renal parenchyma has been developed by use of oxonic acid, a uricase inhibitor. In this rat model, salt-sensitive hypertension and vascular remodeling were induced by hyperuricemia and prevented by treatment with a urate-lowering drug but not by treatment of the hypertension alone with hydrochlorothiazide.[18] Further, both a xanthine oxidase inhibitor and a uricosuric agent prevented the rise in blood pressure and arteriolar thickening, supporting a specific role for uric acid in the vascular remodeling and resultant hypertension. In another model of spontaneously hypertensive rats, uric acid was associated with vascular smooth muscle cell proliferation, while allopurinol suppressed neointimal formation in the carotid artery.[22] The hypertension related to elevated urate in rats in vivo appears to occur, at least partly, via effects on the renin-angiotensin system and afferent glomerular arteriolopathy.[9,17,23] Additionally, after removing oxonic acid, which was used to induce hyperuricemia, maintenance of the rats on a low-salt diet still resulted in blood pressure elevations and arteriolar thickening, despite no longer being hyperuricemic. It is not known, however, whether oxonic acid has nonspecific effects at work in vivo other than uricase inhibition. Nonetheless, the hyperuricemia itself can lead to decreased renal plasma flow and glomerular filtration rate, as well as interstitial renal parenchymal changes without any urate crystal deposition, contributing to renal disease that can itself contribute to hypertension.[21,24,25]

These findings have led to the development of a two-stage hypertension model with respect to serum urate effects: early hypertension being dependent on the renin-angiotensin system and nitric oxide pathways,[7] while at later stages, when preglomerular vascular disease develops, hypertension is driven by the kidney and arteriosclerosis, at which time lowering serum urate levels is no longer protective[26] (Figure 19-1). To test this hypothesis, the response of pediatric/adolescent "essential" hypertension (i.e., in the absence of a secondary cause) to urate-lowering therapy with allopurinol has been studied in a randomized, double-blind, placebo-controlled crossover trial.[27] In this study, the mean change in systolic blood pressure for allopurinol was −6.3 mm Hg

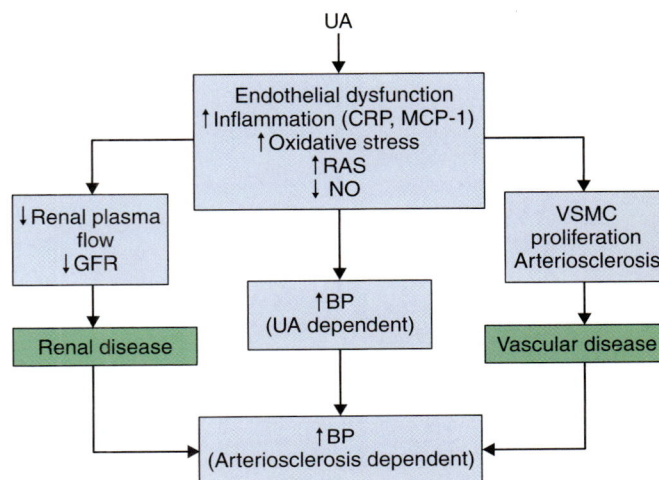

Figure 19-1 Potential conceptual model for the two-stage model of hypertension: one is urate dependent and the other is urate independent. *BP,* Blood pressure; *CRP,* C-reactive protein; *GFR,* glomerular filtration rate; *MCP-1,* monocyte chemotactic protein-1; *NO,* nitric oxide; *RAS,* renin angiotensin system; *VSMC,* vascular smooth muscle cell.

(95% confidence interval [CI] 3.8 to 8.9 mm Hg) compared with 0.8 mm Hg for placebo (95% CI −2.9 to 3.4 mm Hg), and two thirds of participants achieved a normal blood pressure while taking allopurinol compared with only one participant while taking placebo ($p < .001$).[27] Interpretation of these results as attributable to urate lowering is of course limited by the antioxidant effects of xanthine oxidase (the primary target of allopurinol and an enzyme that is active in the vasculature[28-30]), let alone the lack of specificity of allopurinol, which affects pyrimidine metabolism and acts at several points in purine metabolism (see Chapter 13).

Given the postulated model of later stages of hypertension being independent of prior hyperuricemia that could have driven the earlier stages, one may expect the relationship between serum urate and hypertension in adults to be less clear cut. In the largest meta-analysis to date, representing data from over 55,000 participants in 18 prospective cohorts, hyperuricemia was associated with a 41% increased risk of incident hypertension (95% CI for risk ratio (RR) 1.23 to 1.58).[31] However, the possibility of reverse causation cannot be excluded since preclinical hypertension can potentially drive renal changes leading to hyperuricemia itself. Further, the randomized clinical trials of febuxostat, a xanthine oxidase inhibitor that results in substantial urate lowering, did not report beneficial blood pressure lowering effects despite having substantial proportions of hypertensive participants included in the trials.[32-35] In one study, the incidence of hypertension was higher in the febuxostat 80 mg/day arm compared with allopurinol but was no different than placebo, and allopurinol had a lower incidence of hypertension than placebo, while the other doses of febuxostat did not differ from placebo or allopurinol with regard to incidence of hypertension.[33] Thus, the specific role of uric acid in adult hypertension requires further clarification.

It may well be that antihyperuricemic therapy is only beneficial at the earliest stages of the onset of hypertension. This is somewhat supported by the finding that the risk ratios for incident hypertension are higher among those of a younger age[36] (Figure 19-2), although this may represent the phenomenon of being able to demonstrate larger relative risks among lower risk populations. That is, it is easier to demonstrate larger risk ratios in a population whose baseline risk is low. Nonetheless, there are likely numerous pathways that can lead to hypertension, and therefore better mechanistic phenotyping will be needed to identify those in whom hyperuricemia may be playing a role and to identify the particular stage at which hyperuricemia may be important.

Link Between Uric Acid and Metabolic Syndrome and Diabetes

Persons with metabolic syndrome and diabetes are also at increased risk for cardiovascular disease. Elevated serum urate in the metabolic syndrome has historically been attributed to hyperinsulinemia given that insulin decreases renal excretion of uric acid. However, hyperuricemia may predate hyperinsulinemia, obesity, and diabetes. For example, using data from two cohorts of the Framingham Study (Original and Offspring), the Finnish Diabetes Prevention Study, the Rancho Bernardo Study, and the Rotterdam Study, serum urate levels were associated with an increased risk of developing type 2 diabetes.[37-40] Although only a cross-sectional association, persons with higher serum urate levels have a substantially higher prevalence of the metabolic syndrome, even among those without hypertension, those without diabetes, and those who are not overweight.[41] At the very least, such an association should encourage physicians to evaluate hyperuricemic (gout) patients for the presence of the metabolic syndrome.

Interestingly, fructose may be a potential link between uric acid and the metabolic syndrome. Fructose intake in the forms of table sugar (sucrose, which is a crystalline disaccharide of glucose and fructose) and the widely used beverage and food sweetening additive high-fructose corn syrup (which is enriched in monosaccharide fructose) has increased dramatically over the past two to three decades and is associated with increased incidence of obesity and diabetes as well as with hyperuricemia and incident gout.[42-47] Hepatic adenosine triphosphate (ATP) depletion via fructose metabolism could be a component in nonalcoholic steatotic hepatic disease (NASH). In an animal study, fructose-fed rats, but not those that were dextrose-fed, developed the metabolic syndrome.[48] Further, use of either allopurinol or benzbromarone (a uricosuric agent) in the fructose-fed rats prevented or reversed features of the metabolic syndrome. The effects of fructose in this animal model were seen even with caloric restriction. The fructose transporter SLC2A9 (also known as GLUT9) was recently noted to also be a urate transporter (and more potent as a urate than a hexose transporter), and genetic studies have demonstrated an association of single nucleotide polymorphisms of the gene with gout and urate levels.[49] In sum, these studies provide a potential link between fructose, hyperuricemia, and the metabolic syndrome.

Link Between Uric Acid and Cardiovascular Disease (Coronary Heart Disease)

There are many potential mechanisms linking uric acid to cardiovascular disease. While not all individuals with hyperuricemia have clinical gout despite urate's ability to promote inflammation, a proinflammatory state is likely associated with hyperuricemia.[15,50] The insulin resistance so often associated with hyperuricemia can also contribute to both a low-grade

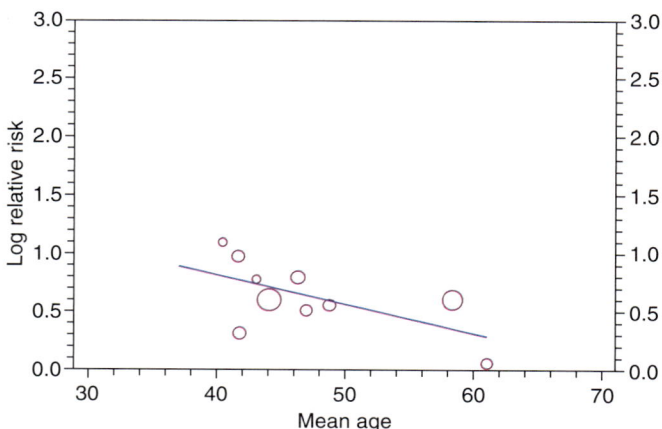

Figure 19-2 Unadjusted risk ratios for association of hyperuricemia with risk of incident hypertension versus mean study age in 11 cohort studies from meta-analysis. Bubble size represents sample size of study. *(From Grayson PC, et al. Hyperuricemia and incident hypertension: a systematic review and meta-analysis. Arthritis Care Res 2011;63:102-10. doi:10.1002/acr.20344.)*

inflammatory state and cardiovascular risk.[51] Further, in addition to its elevated levels in atherosclerotic plaques,[52] soluble urate has been reported by approximately half a dozen different research groups to promote proliferative and pro-inflammatory responses in cultured vascular smooth muscle cells[14,53] and a variety of inflammatory responses in cultured endothelial cells.[15,21] As outlined earlier, there is in vivo evidence from rat models that hyperuricemia may have a pathogenic role through vascular effects, partly via effects on nitric oxide metabolism and on the renin-angiotensin system.[9] On the other hand, direct effects of soluble urate on the vasculature have not been conclusively established. For example, urate infusion into the human circulation in vivo failed to demonstrate impairment of cardiovascular function,[54] possibly related to antioxidant effects of soluble extracellular urate. However, urate may also be pro-oxidative under certain conditions, particularly when inside the cell, and when other antioxidants are at low levels, which could potentially contribute to promotion of cardiovascular abnormalities through oxidative stress.[20] The net effects of these complex and, in some cases, competing functions of soluble urate are unknown, although they provide considerable support for the possibility that uric acid may have direct biological effects on the vasculature.

The difficulty with such indirect evidence is that hyperuricemia is also associated with a number of comorbidities that could contribute to cardiovascular disease risk. Persons with gout and underlying hyperuricemia have an increased risk for cardiovascular disease and increased prevalence of associated cardiovascular comorbidities than expected.[55-57] These comorbidities include obesity, diabetes, dyslipidemia, and hypertension.[57-61] Thus, it is unclear as to whether the increased association between hyperuricemia and cardiovascular disease is due to the associated cardiovascular comorbidities or the demographic characteristics of persons who are typically hyperuricemic (males who are often older and overweight) or whether uric acid itself plays a role in the development of cardiovascular disease. Epidemiologic studies have been conflicting with respect to whether hyperuricemia is independently associated with cardiovascular disease, with some showing a positive independent association[56,62-67] and others demonstrating no independent association.[68-70]

Approximately two thirds of more than 30 observational cohort studies over the years have demonstrated an association of uric acid and cardiovascular disease. Contradictory results can be due to differences in adjustment for certain covariates and definitions used for such covariates, resulting in residual confounding. Some prior studies, with both negative and positive associations reported, have either failed to adjust for low-dose aspirin use or for renal insufficiency (both of which can increase serum urate levels and risk for cardiovascular disease[71,72]), have not used current standard definitions for hypertension, and/or have adjusted for the presence of hypertension and use of antihypertensive agents, which may cause problems of collinearity.[62-64,66,68,70,73-75] Additionally, the definition for hyperuricemia can vary from study to study, and most studies have only assessed urate levels at a single time point, whereas it is possible that a cumulative effect of serum urate could be important in conferring risk of cardiovascular events.

Another problem is in the statistical modeling of the potential effects of serum urate on cardiovascular disease in such observational studies. Most analyses aim to determine whether serum urate has a *direct* effect on cardiovascular disease, independent of other risk factors. Such an approach does not allow for consideration of the possibility that uric acid may exert its effects *indirectly* through other risk factors, such as hypertension or renal disease (Figure 19-3). For example, assume that hyperuricemia is causally related to hypertension, which in turn is itself a strong risk factor for cardiovascular disease, and that uric acid has no other direct effects on cardiovascular disease. In this example, hypertension is on the causal pathway between uric acid and cardiovascular disease (i.e., an intermediate). In the typical approach to statistical modeling, hypertension would be adjusted for to discern the independent effects of uric acid. However, by doing so, no effect of uric acid would be seen if uric acid has no other effects on cardiovascular disease except through hypertension. With such a modeling approach, one would correctly conclude that uric acid has no association with cardiovascular disease independent of hypertension but will have importantly missed identifying hyperuricemia as an important modifiable risk factor for hypertension, which in turn is a risk factor for cardiovascular disease.

Thus understanding the potential biologic mechanisms is crucial to appropriate statistical modeling. Indeed, if the question is about the sum total effect of uric acid on cardiovascular disease, both those that are *direct* and those that are *indirect*, then special analytic methods[76] need to be used as one should not simply adjust for risk factors that are intermediates along the pathway from uric acid to cardiovascular disease (see Figure 19-3) since such an approach can introduce bias. This is a particularly difficult and prevalent problem since many factors, such as hypertension, can be considered to be both a confounder and an intermediate, and therefore the standard approach of simply adjusting for such factors results in biased effect estimates.

Finally, as any effect of serum urate is likely to be small given the multifactorial nature of cardiovascular disease, studies with relatively small numbers of events may not be able to demonstrate an association, particularly when populations studied are at low risk for the outcome under study.[68-70] Thus, individual studies may be underpowered to detect a small effect. An approach to dealing with potential lack of power in individual studies is to perform a meta-analysis. One of the first such meta-analyses to evaluate the relationship between serum urate and coronary heart disease

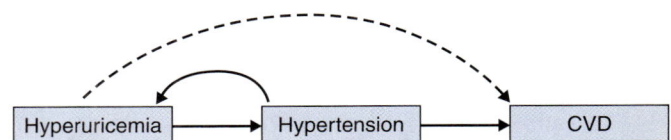

Figure 19-3 A key issue in analysis of observational data is the bias introduced by adjusting for potential intermediate factors (e.g., hypertension) in the causal pathway from the exposure of interest (here, hyperuricemia) to the outcome (here, cardiovascular disease [CVD]), particularly when that intermediate factor can also act as a confounder. In the example illustrated here, hypertension is acting as both an intermediate in the pathway from hyperuricemia to cardiovascular disease, as well as a confounder since it can potentially also contribute to hyperuricemia (e.g., through effects on the kidneys). Special analytic techniques are needed to address such complex relationships to avoid biased effect estimates obtained from standard analytic approaches.

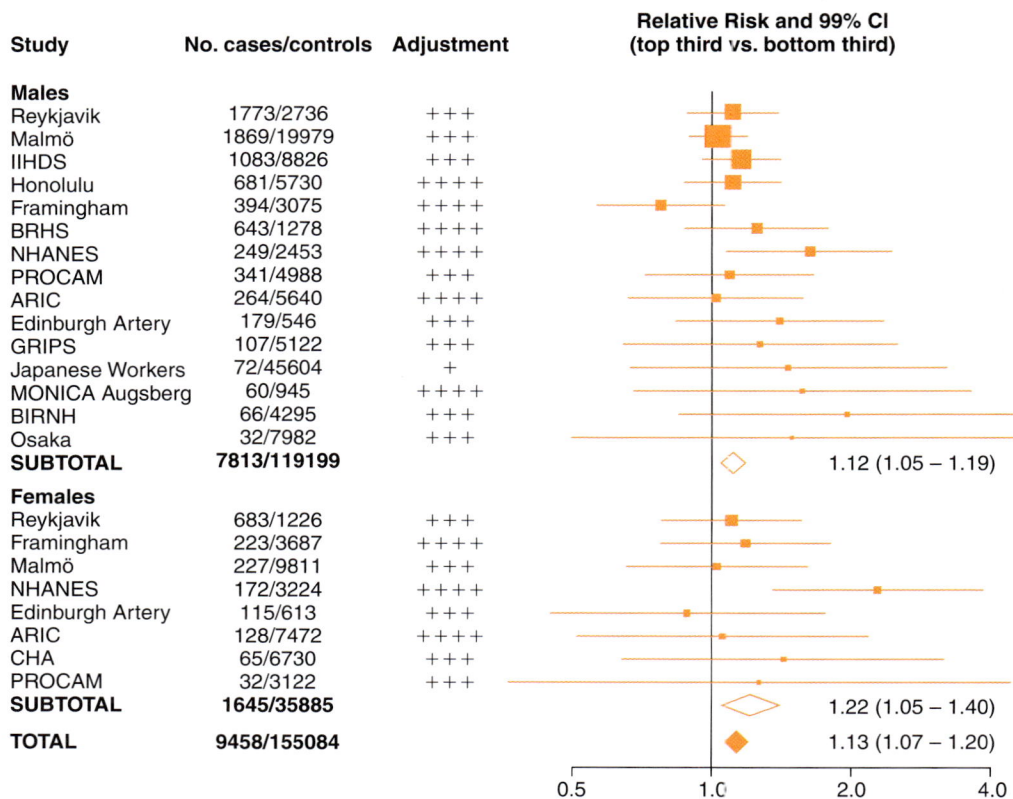

Figure 19-4 Meta-analysis results of prospective observational general population studies of serum urate and coronary heart disease, subdivided by sex. (*Data from Wheeler JG, et al. Serum uric acid and coronary heart disease in 9,458 incident cases and 155,084 controls: prospective study and meta-analysis. PLoS Med 2005;2:e76, Figure 2. doi:10.1371/journal.pmed.0020076.g002.*)

included close to 9,500 cases from 16 studies and found a 13% increased risk (RR = 1.13, 95% CI 1.07 to 1.20) of coronary heart disease among those in the top tertile of serum urate levels compared with the lowest tertile[77] (Figure 19-4). The authors of this report downplay their main results and state that their results indicate that serum urate does not appear to be an important predictor of coronary heart disease when taking into account other potential risk factors, and in fact, conclude no association despite a statistically significant result. However, most cardiac risk factors have small effects. Further, a modifiable risk factor that has a high prevalence in the population can have a substantial public health impact if intervened upon, even if the noted effect estimate appears to be small.

A more recently updated meta-analysis that included 26 studies (only 8 of which were included in the previous meta-analysis) with data from over 400,000 participants reported similar results, with 9% (RR = 1.09, 95% CI 1.03 to 1.16) and 16% (RR = 1.16, 95% CI 1.01 to 1.30) increased risk of coronary heart disease incidence and mortality, respectively, among those who were hyperuricemic compared with those who were normouricemic[78] (Figure 19-5). This largest meta-analysis to date supports a significant but modest association between hyperuricemia and cardiovascular events, independent of traditional cardiovascular risk factors.

In addition to attempting to discern whether hyperuricemia is associated with adverse cardiovascular outcomes, many investigators have focused on potential differential risk by sex. Such differences reflect effect measure modification, which is

typically formally assessed by a statistical test for interaction to discern whether the differences in effect estimates between the groups being compared are truly statistically significantly different from one another. However, not all studies addressing this question support their conclusions by such formal statistical evaluations. Another difficulty in interpretation of differences in effect estimates is that, as discussed above, a higher relative risk may be a reflection of a lower baseline risk rather than a true difference in absolute risk difference. In a study using data from the National Health and Nutrition Examination Survey (NHANES) I, the authors concluded that although higher urate levels were associated with cardiovascular outcomes for both men and women, the risk was higher among women.[64] The highest quartile of serum urate was associated with 1.77 times higher risk of ischemic heart disease mortality among men, and a 3.00 times higher risk among women than the lowest quartiles, respectively. However, in terms of absolute rate differences, the highest quartile of serum urate was associated with 3.55 more deaths per 1000 person-years among men, and 4.03 more deaths per 1000 person-years among women than the lowest quartiles, respectively. This example illustrates that the absolute risk differences were similar between the sexes, despite the seemingly large disparities in the relative measures of effect. Further, the cut-points for the quartiles were different between men and women, making direct comparison difficult. This is one reason that biologically meaningful cut-points are potentially better than sample-specific quartiles to aid in interpretation of the data.

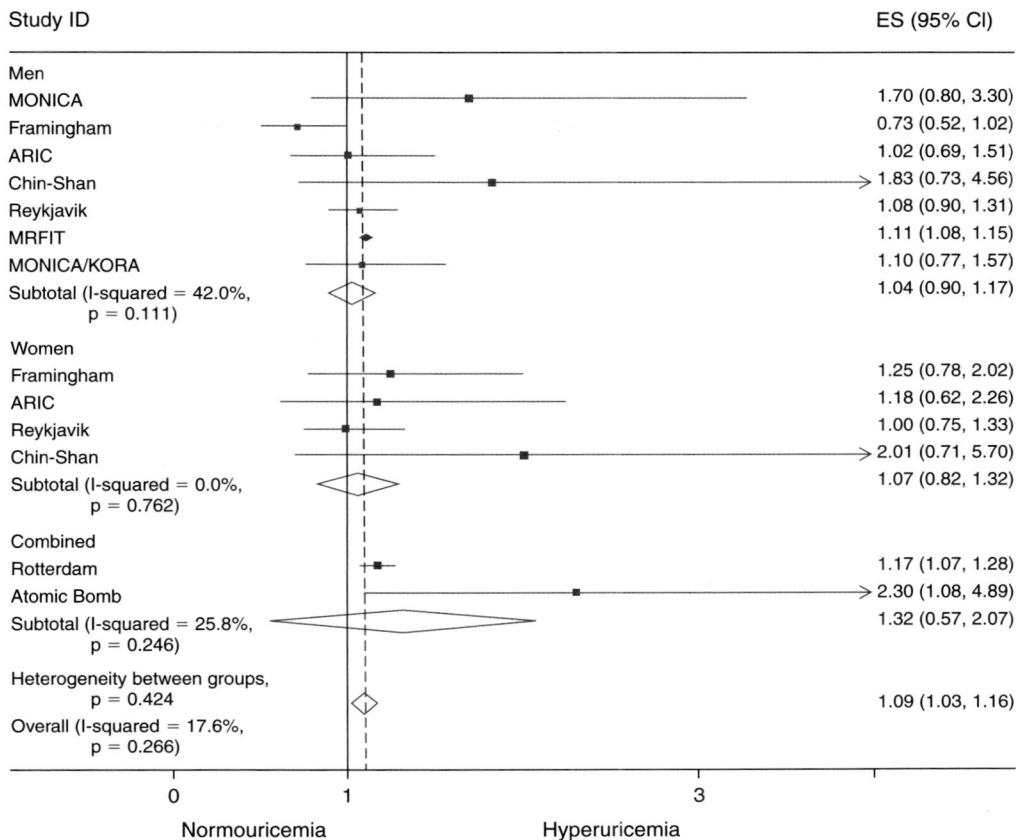

A

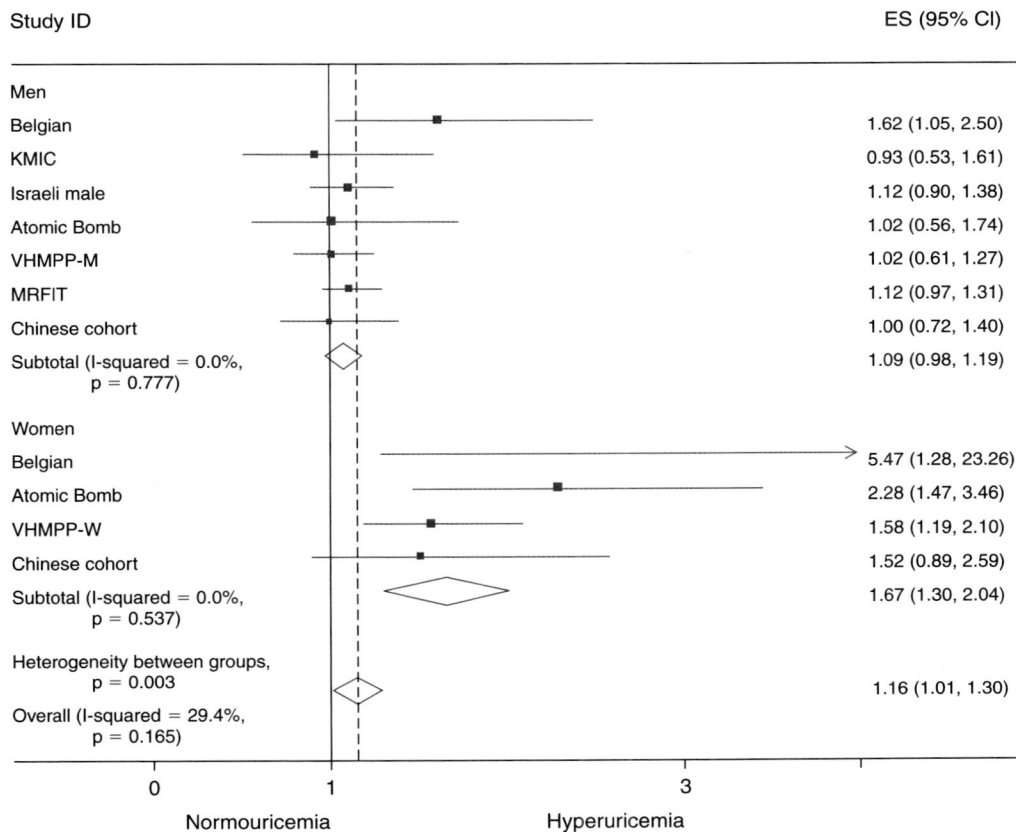

B

Figure 19-5 Meta-analysis results of prospective observational studies of association of hyperuricemia with coronary heart disease incidence (**A**) and mortality (**B**). *(Data from Kim SY, et al. Hyperuricemia and coronary heart disease: a systematic review and meta-analysis. Arthritis Care Res 2010;62:170-80, Figure 2. doi:10.1002/acr.20065.)*

In the Wheeler et al. meta-analysis, the top tertile of serum urate was associated with higher risk of coronary heart disease to a similar extent with overlapping confidence intervals in both men (RR = 1.12, 95% CI 1.05 to 1.19) and women (RR = 1.22, 95% CI 1.05 to 1.40), compared with the lowest tertile[77] (see Figure 19-4). In the Kim et al. meta-analysis, the association of hyperuricemia with incident coronary heart disease was not significant for men (RR = 1.04, 95% CI 0.90 to 1.17) or for women (RR = 1.32, 95% CI 0.57 to 2.07), even though the pooled effect of both sexes combined was significant (see Figure 19-5, A).[78] For coronary heart disease mortality, hyperuricemia among men was associated with a nonsignificant 1.09 times higher risk (95% CI 0.98 to 1.19), while among women hyperuricemia was associated with a 1.67 times higher risk (95% CI 1.30 to 2.04) (see Figure 19-5, B).[78] Thus the results are conflicting regarding effect measure modification by sex in these two meta-analyses, highlighting the difficulty in definitively answering this question even with the large amounts of data available in these meta-analyses.

Another way to address the question of whether uric acid is harmful is to evaluate whether reducing urate levels improves outcomes. This is best accomplished in a randomized trial (discussed later). Observational studies can also attempt to address such a question by evaluating whether individuals on urate-lowering therapy have better outcomes than those who are not on such therapies. The difficulty in interpreting such observational studies, though, is that people on urate-lowering therapy are systematically different than those who are not, and without taking into account those differences, such studies are prone to substantial bias. In particular, confounding by indication is a common problem in pharmaco-epidemiologic studies.

Confounding by indication refers to a type of bias that occurs when one cannot account for factors that influence why individuals receive or do not receive a certain exposure (in this case, urate-lowering therapy). For example, an individual with more comorbidities may be less likely to receive allopurinol than a relatively healthier individual with fewer medical contraindications to allopurinol; individuals who have better medical management of their comorbidities, and are therefore at lower risk of adverse outcomes, may be more likely to have medications such as allopurinol prescribed to them. A recent study concluded that use of urate-lowering therapy was associated with substantially lower risk of cardiovascular mortality and stroke-related mortality based on a clinical database linked to prescription records.[79] However, whether confounding by indication was appropriately accounted for is not clear, and could importantly bias their results to show a protective effect when there may not be one, or at least a much smaller effect. A further caveat is that the event rate was quite low, at 1% or substantially lower for the various outcomes assessed.

Link Between Uric Acid and Associated Cardiovascular Disorders: Congestive Heart Failure and Stroke

Another approach that may mitigate against potential for low event rates is to study related outcomes of potentially higher prevalence. One potential phenotype related to cardiovascular disease is congestive heart failure. Serum urate has been associated with increased risk for incident congestive heart failure,[80,81] and changes in serum urate have been associated with flares of congestive heart failure.[82] Potentially complementing this latter finding, a study that used data from a universal health care coverage program that included clinical and prescription data found use of allopurinol to be associated with lower risk of heart failure readmission or death among persons with gout, but not among their whole study population.[83] It is possible that by reducing urate levels and the attendant risk for gout flares, that heart failure outcomes could improve. However, it's not clear as to why a large proportion of individuals would be on allopurinol in the absence of a gout diagnosis, or why that should make a difference for heart failure outcomes. Further, and importantly, a concern about confounding by indication exists in this study since, compared with the cases, a larger proportion of controls were on various cardiovascular medications, potentially suggesting they were more likely to be appropriately medically managed, and by extension, more likely to be prescribed allopurinol.

In terms of urate as a risk factor for another related phenotype, stroke, a meta-analysis demonstrated hyperuricemia to be associated with a 47% increased risk of stroke (95% CI 1.19 to 1.76) after adjusting for known risk factors, and a 26% increased risk for stroke mortality (95% CI 1.12 to 1.39), compared with those who were normouricemic.[84]

Link Between Uric Acid and Preclinical Atherosclerotic Disease

Noninvasive assessment of preclinical lesions may provide another strategy for avoiding low power resulting from studies using clinical endpoints that suffer from low event rates. Further, as opposed to adverse clinical events such as myocardial infarction or stroke, such studies of preclinical lesions may provide insight into potential pathophysiologic mechanisms of risk factors. Advances in imaging technology have enabled the evaluation of markers of preclinical atherosclerotic disease, such as carotid plaques, which have been associated with prevalent and incident cardiovascular disease and strokes.[85-88] Carotid plaques as measured by ultrasound may be a result of atherosclerosis causing intimal expansion and/or a result of vascular hypertrophy and remodeling causing an increased thickness in the media.[89] Unfortunately, the association between hyperuricemia and preclinical carotid atherosclerosis has been conflicting, although the majority of studies have supported an association.[73-75,90-96]

Coronary artery calcification is another such preclinical marker of cardiovascular disease.[97] The extent of intimal artery calcification correlates with the extent of atherosclerosis.[98,99] Coronary artery calcification has been associated with death from coronary disease and all-cause mortality,[100-102] which may be mediated by the capacity of hydroxyapatite crystals deposited in the calcified intima to promote low-grade inflammation in the artery wall.[103] With regard to atherosclerosis, soluble urate is held to play a pathogenic role in the vascular remodeling of cardiovascular disease by biologic mechanisms detailed above, including low level uptake by endothelial and vascular smooth muscle cells, induction of oxidative stress and inflammatory cytokine expression, and modulation of the renin-angiotensin system.[9,14,15,17,53,104] Thus, there may be different atherosclerotic phenotypes reflected by coronary artery calcification versus carotid plaques. While there are many potential mechanisms linking serum urate levels to cardiovascular disease through vascular remodeling and other risk factors, soluble urate has not been investigated as a potential direct inducer of arterial calcification. In observational studies to date, the association of serum urate with coronary artery calcification has been conflicting.[105-107] In this light, not all vascular calcification is related to atherosclerosis. For example, aging, end-stage renal disease, and diabetes mellitus can cause nonatherosclerotic artery tunica media calcification. Soluble urate potentially decreases nitric oxide bioavailability through suppression of its production, promotion of its inactivation, and stimulation of its degradation.[9] Thus, with respect to reported vascular effects of soluble urate, by suppressing nitric oxide levels in the artery, urate theoretically has the potential to suppress ectopic osteoblastic differentiation of vascular smooth muscle cells,[108] which in theory could result in less vascular calcification than otherwise predicted in a disease such as atherosclerosis.

Again, many of the same potential explanations as have been explored for the contradictory results of the numerous studies of clinical coronary heart disease just presented also apply here, including methodologic and definitional issues.

Lessons Learned From Randomized Clinical Trials of Urate-Lowering Therapies Regarding Potential Cardiovascular Effects

Well-conducted randomized clinical trials avoid many (but not all) of the pitfalls faced by observational studies. If uric acid is truly a causal factor in cardiovascular disease, one should expect that lower serum urate levels would be associated with lower risk for cardiovascular endpoints. Indeed, in the Losartan Intervention For Endpoint reduction in hypertension (LIFE) study, approximately a third of the improved cardiovascular mortality was attributed to an independent effect on serum urate levels in those who received losartan, a drug with uricosuric effects, compared with those who received atenolol, a beta-blocker with no such effects.[109] However, such interpretations should be viewed with caution. It is possible that losartan has effects beyond lowering of blood pressure that beta-blockers do not have that mediated such effects and that serum urate is simply a biomarker or epiphenomenon of such an effect. On the other hand, in the Systolic Hypertension in the Elderly (SHEP) trial, the authors found that those who had their hypertension appropriately controlled with a thiazide diuretic but who concomitantly also had an increase in their serum urate levels failed to demonstrate a cardiovascular benefit compared with placebo.[63] A similar mitigation of beneficial effect was not seen for stroke or "any cardiovascular event." It is not clear as to why this would be the case, and it raises a concern about a false-positive result. Three secondary coronary heart disease studies using sulfinpyrazone, which has both antiplatelet and uricosuric effects, demonstrated reduced risk of sudden cardiac death[110,111] and fatal and nonfatal myocardial infarction,[112] while another demonstrated no benefit of sulfinpyrazone on risk of cardiac death or nonfatal myocardial infarction among persons with unstable angina.[113] In the Heart and Estrogen/progestin Replacement Study (HERS) trial, the active treatment arm had significantly lower serum urate levels compared with placebo, but this was not associated with lower overall risk for cardiovascular events.[114] These latter two studies provide examples of urate lowering in the context of a trial that was not associated with improved outcomes.

Urate-lowering effects on surrogate endpoints have also been studied. Although oxypurinol improved left ventricular ejection fraction in a post-hoc analysis of a select subset whose baseline ejection fractions were less than 40% in a small trial,[115] another trial for moderate-to-severe congestive heart failure did not demonstrate a beneficial effect except for persons with serum urate levels above 9.5 mg/dL in post-hoc analyses.[116] Another surrogate endpoint that has been examined is exercise capacity. In one study, conducted among persons with unstable angina, exercise capacity increased with use of high-dose (600 mg/day) allopurinol compared with placebo. In another study conducted among persons with chronic heart failure,[117] allopurinol at 300 mg/day did not improve exercise capacity.[118] Whether these discrepancies are related to dose, a difference in underlying pathophysiology of the two conditions or other factors is not clear.

If more effective urate-lowering may be needed to demonstrate a beneficial cardiac effect, as may have been achieved with higher doses of allopurinol in the unstable angina study described earlier, one may expect that randomized clinical trials of febuxostat should demonstrate positive effects. However, such trials have not demonstrated a cardiovascular benefit. In fact, there has even been some concern that there may be a nonsignificant increase in cardiovascular events in those who took febuxostat compared with allopurinol in the initial trial, which necessitated further study into the cardiovascular safety of febuxostat.[32-35] If urate contributed to cardiovascular disease, drugs with substantial urate-lowering effects in such trials should have been able to demonstrate positive effects. It is possible that such studies were too short in duration, enrolled patients with a high risk of cardiovascular disease, and were not powered for cardiovascular outcomes, all of which could affect one's ability to detect a small positive effect. Moreover, increased flares of gout, which are well documented to occur with more intense serum urate-lowering regimens, can induce systemic inflammation, with release of cytokines (e.g., interleukin [IL]-1β, tumor necrosis factor [TNF]α, IL-6, IL-8) and other mediators such as CRP, which in turn have the potential to promote a variety of adverse cardiovascular events, including arrhythmia mediated by IL-6. Nonetheless, with the best evidence available to date based on these randomized trials, urate-lowering does not appear to have a substantial cardiovascular benefit. A potentially smaller beneficial effect cannot be ruled out as appropriately designed studies to address cardiovascular outcomes using specifically urate-lowering drugs have not been carried out to date. Ideally, one would need to evaluate a uricosuric agent as well as a xanthine oxidase inhibitor and uricase to demonstrate that the effect is truly due to urate lowering rather than another drug-related mechanism.

Potential Role for Xanthine Oxidase in Cardiovascular Disease

Some investigators have argued that rather than uric acid itself being harmful, it is xanthine oxidase and its capacity for oxidative damage that are the culprits in cardiovascular disease. As such, the potential positive effects of xanthine oxidase

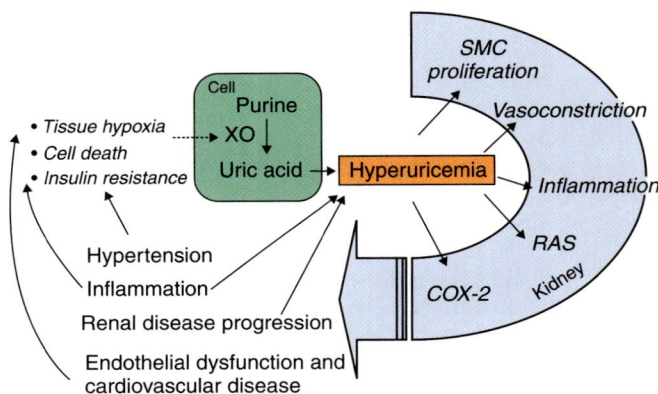

Figure 19-6 The potential interrelationships of uric acid, xanthine oxidase activity, and clinical endpoints of cardiovascular and renal disease. *(From Kang DH, Nakagawa T. Uric acid and chronic renal disease: possible implication of hyperuricemia on progression of renal disease. Semin Nephrol 2005;25:43-9.)*

inhibition, as would be obtained with allopurinol or febuxostat, are argued to not be related to urate-lowering effects but rather to their effects on suppressing xanthine oxidase activity. Xanthine oxidase itself has been demonstrated in vitro to become activated in mononuclear phagocytes and to contribute to the inflammatory state of the mononuclear phagocyte, the major cell type that drives atherogenesis.[119] The role of xanthine oxidase on the human cardiovascular system has been studied primarily in the setting of congestive heart failure, where it is thought that xanthine oxidase contributes to abnormal excitation-contraction coupling and cardiac remodeling in heart failure. Such features have been altered by use of the xanthine oxidase inhibitor, allopurinol.[120] Treatment in another study with allopurinol improved endothelial function among subjects with heart failure, whereas comparable uric acid reduction with probenecid, a uricosuric agent, did not.[121] These studies suggest that the potential association between hyperuricemia and cardiovascular disease may be due to free-radical generation by xanthine oxidase and that the hyperuricemia–cardiovascular disease link may just be an epiphenomenon (Figure 19-6).

Link Between Uric Acid and Renal Disease

In vivo rat models have demonstrated hyperuricemia to not only affect renal plasma blood flow but also cause interstitial changes.[21,24,25] In a cross-sectional study using data from the Normative Aging Study, no association was noted between serum urate and renal failure as defined by an elevated serum creatinine level.[3] However, this was a cross-sectional study without appropriate adjustment for important potential confounders. In contrast, two Japanese observational studies, both using the same data source (Okinawa General Health Maintenance Association Study) with some overlapping follow-up time, noted an association between serum urate and development of end-stage renal disease.[122,123] In two observational studies of IgA nephropathy, which has a substantial risk of end-stage renal disease, uric acid was found to be a predictor of renal progression.[124,125] One of the largest epidemiologic studies on renal progression to date, including over 177,000 patients in the U.S. Renal Data System followed over 25 years, found serum urate to be associated with an increased

risk for end-stage renal disease.[126] However, as discussed earlier, it is difficult to make definitive causal inferences from observational studies alone.

Testing the effects of lowering serum urate on renal disease has some practical considerations. Uricosuric drugs cannot be used in the setting of advanced renal impairment, leaving only xanthine oxidase as a therapeutic option for testing. There is concern, though, about using allopurinol in the setting of renal insufficiency due to increased potential for hypersensitivity. However, more recent studies have not confirmed a dose-response relationship between allopurinol and the hypersensitivity reaction.[127] Likely as a consequence of these issues, there have been only few trials of urate-lowering in renal disease to date. In a small nonrandomized study of 59 patients, hyperuricemic patients given allopurinol for 3 months experienced an improvement in glomerular filtration rate, while there were no changes in the normouricemic control group who did not receive any change to therapy.[128] Only one patient in the allopurinol arm developed an urticarial rash. In the first randomized trial of urate-lowering therapy for renal progression, which enrolled 54 participants, those in the allopurinol arm had 65% lower risk of experiencing significant deterioration in renal function and dialysis dependence compared with usual therapy after 12 months (16% versus 46.1%, RR = 0.35).[129] Similar to the nonrandomized trial, only one participant developed an urticarial rash in the allopurinol treatment arm. In another small randomized trial, this time double-blinded but with unclear allocation concealment, 40 subjects with type 2 diabetes and nephropathy received either allopurinol 100 mg/day or placebo for 4 months.[130] Along with a documented reduction in serum urate levels, the allopurinol arm had significantly lower 24-hour urinary protein than the placebo group. No participants experienced any adverse events.

A recent larger randomized trial, comprising 113 participants randomized to allopurinol (100 mg/day) versus usual therapy, found estimated glomerular filtration rate to have increased slightly after 24 months for the allopurinol group (1.3 ± 1.3 ml/min/1.73 m^2), while it decreased in the comparator group (3.3 ± 1.2 ml/min/1.73 m^2). In an adjusted model, treatment with allopurinol was associated with a 47% lower risk of renal progression compared with the usual treatment arm (hazard ratio = 0.43, 95% CI 0.28 to 0.99).[131] Interestingly, none of the allopurinol-treated participants developed a hypersensitivity reaction in this study either. Thus, despite these studies enrolling participants with renal insufficiency, there did not appear to be an elevated risk of hypersensitivity among their participants. None of the randomized clinical trials of febuxostat reported renal endpoints, positive or negative, but a post-hoc analysis of the Febuxostat Open-label Clinical trial of Urate-lowering efficacy and Safety (FOCUS) study, during which 116 hyperuricemic gout subjects received daily doses of febuxostat (40, 80, or 120 mg) for up to 5 years, suggested that decreases in serum urate are associated with maintenance or improvement in estimated glomerular filtration rate.[132]

In terms of the effects being mediated through urate-lowering versus xanthine oxidase inhibition, it has been argued that human kidneys do not have substantial xanthine oxidase activity, and therefore the effects are likely mediated through reduction of urate.

Link Between Uric Acid and Neurologic Disorders

There has been a growing literature regarding the potential adverse neurologic effects of having serum urate levels that are too low.[133] A concern regarding an observed association between low urate levels and progressive neurologic conditions, such as Parkinson disease, or impaired stroke recovery, is the possibility of reverse causation. That is, mental and/or physical impairment as a consequence of those underlying neurologic conditions can lead to poor nutritional status, and serum urate may merely be a reflection of that status. However, more recently, studies have demonstrated an association between lower serum or dietary urate with onset of Parkinson disease,[134,135] which limits the likelihood of reverse causation. Given that uric acid suppresses neuronal damage by the potent oxidant peroxynitrite, the consideration that having serum urate levels that are too low could potentially contribute to adverse neurologic issues later in life certainly merits further investigation. In addition, increasing serum urate has been investigated as a measure to reduce nervous system damage in experimental multiple sclerosis.[136]

The role of uric acid in poststroke recovery has been controversial, with one study demonstrating better outcomes among those with higher urate levels,[137] while others demonstrated better outcomes with lower urate levels,[138,139] and another demonstrating a U-shaped relationship, suggesting that levels that are low and high are problematic.[140] Such observational studies are difficult to interpret because serum urate levels are typically assessed at the time of stroke diagnosis (i.e., the exposure [urate level] is assessed after the outcome [stroke] has occurred), and therefore the possibility of reverse causation exists. In contrast to the theory that higher levels of uric acid may be neuroprotective, a small randomized, double-blind placebo-controlled trial tested efficacy of allopurinol poststroke.[141] This trial did not demonstrate improvement in cerebrovascular reactivity compared with placebo despite lowering urate levels, although the study was likely underpowered. Further, there is a lack of evidence of a predilection to neurologic disease in individuals with inherited hypouricemic conditions. Thus, clinically significant neuroprotective effects of higher serum urate remain speculative at this point in human beings.

Conclusions

There are a number of in vitro and in vivo models to support a complex interrelationship between uric acid and clinical outcomes of cardiovascular and renal disease (see Figure 19-6). Nonetheless, despite numerous observational data supporting a link between hyperuricemia and cardiovascular disease, definitive evidence from trial data has been lacking as to the benefits of urate reduction. However, no study to date has been ideally designed to specifically address this question. Further, whether any potential effects are mediated by the specific urate-lowering properties of the drugs used versus xanthine oxidase inhibition itself is not clear. Preliminary data support the possibility that urate-lowering may benefit early stages of hypertension in adolescents, but larger trials, and study of other mechanisms of urate-lowering (e.g., uricosuric or uricase agents), will be required before specific recommendations can be made. In contrast, there appear to be more supportive data for the utility of urate-lowering in suppressing progression of renal disease, although more and larger randomized trials will be required for a more definitive answer and a more comprehensive evaluation of potential risks to such a management strategy. Importantly, urate-lowering therapy is not without risk, including hypersensitivity reaction with allopurinol, which can be severe and life-threatening in a fraction of patients, and the possibility has been raised, without conclusive evidence, of potential neurologic effects later in life.

In summary, current clinical treatment guidelines do not recommend treatment of asymptomatic hyperuricemia. Should serum urate be confirmed as a risk factor for cardiovascular or renal disease, this may provide another indication for urate-lowering therapy irrespective of the presence of clinical gout, but such recommendations are premature at the present time.

References

1. Wu XW, Muzny DM, Lee CC, et al. Two independent mutational events in the loss of urate oxidase during hominoid evolution. J Mol Evol 1992;34:78–84.
2. Loeb JN. The influence of temperature on the solubility of monosodium urate. Arthritis Rheum 1972;15:189–92.
3. Campion EW, Glynn RJ, DeLabry LO. Asymptomatic hyperuricemia. Risks and consequences in the Normative Aging Study. Am J Med 1987;82:421–6.
4. Ames BN, Cathcart R, Schwiers E, et al. Uric acid provides an antioxidant defense in humans against oxidant- and radical-caused aging and cancer: a hypothesis. Proc Natl Acad Sci U S A 1981;78:6858–62.
5. Johnson RJ, Titte S, Cade JR, et al. Uric acid, evolution and primitive cultures. Semin Nephrol 2005;25:3–8.
6. Spitsin SV, Scott GS, Mikheeva T, et al. Comparison of uric acid and ascorbic acid in protection against EAE. Free Radic Biol Med 2002;33:1363–71.
7. Mazzali M, Hughes J, Kim YG, et al. Elevated uric acid increases blood pressure in the rat by a novel crystal-independent mechanism. Hypertension 2001;38:1101–6.
8. Johnson RJ, Andrews P, Benner SA, et al. Woodward award. The evolution of obesity: insights from the mid-Miocene. Trans Am Clin Climatol Assoc 2010;121:295–305:discussion 308.
9. Feig DI, Kang DH, Johnson RJ. Uric acid and cardiovascular risk. N Engl J Med 2008;359:1811–21.
10. Wallace KL, Riedel AA, Joseph-Ridge N, et al. Increasing prevalence of gout and hyperuricemia over 10 years among older adults in a managed care population. J Rheumatol 2004;31:1582–7.
11. Zhu Y, Pandya B, Choi H. Increasing gout prevalence in the US over the last two decades: the National Health and Nutrition Examination Survey (NHANES). Arthritis Rheum 2010;62:S901.
12. Arromdee E, Michet CJ, Crowson CS, et al. Epidemiology of gout: is the incidence rising? J Rheumatol 2002;29:2403–6.
13. Zharikov S, Krotova K, Hu H, et al. Uric acid decreases NO production and increases arginase activity in cultured pulmonary artery endothelial cells. Am J Physiol Cell Physiol 2008;295:C1183–90.
14. Kanellis J, Watanabe S, Li JH, et al. Uric acid stimulates monocyte chemoattractant protein-1 production in vascular smooth muscle cells via mitogen-activated protein kinase and cyclooxygenase-2. Hypertension 2003;41:1287–93.
15. Kang DH, Park SK, Lee IK, et al. Uric acid-induced C-reactive protein expression: implication on cell proliferation and nitric oxide production of human vascular cells. J Am Soc Nephrol 2005;16:3553–62.
16. Rao GN, Corson MA, Berk BC. Uric acid stimulates vascular smooth muscle cell proliferation by increasing platelet-derived growth factor A-chain expression. J Biol Chem 1991;266:8604–8.
17. Corry DB, Eslami P, Yamamoto K, et al. Uric acid stimulates vascular smooth muscle cell proliferation and oxidative stress via the vascular renin-angiotensin system. J Hypertens 2008;26:269–75.
18. Mazzali M, Kanellis J, Han L, et al. Hyperuricemia induces a primary renal arteriolopathy in rats by a blood pressure-independent mechanism. Am J Physiol Renal Physiol 2002;282:F991–7.
19. Alderman MH. Uric acid and cardiovascular risk. Curr Opin Pharmacol 2002;2:126–30.

20. Johnson RJ, Kang DH, Feig D, et al. Is there a pathogenetic role for uric acid in hypertension and cardiovascular and renal disease? Hypertension 2003;41:1183–90.

21. Khosla UM, Zharikov S, Finch JL, et al. Hyperuricemia induces endothelial dysfunction. Kidney Int 2005;67:1739–42.

22. Yamamoto Y, Ogino K, Igawa G, et al. Allopurinol reduces neointimal hyperplasia in the carotid artery ligation model in spontaneously hypertensive rats. Hypertens Res 2006;29:915–21.

23. Mazzali M, Kanbay M, Segal MS, et al. Uric acid and hypertension: cause or effect? Curr Rheumatol Rep 2010;12:108–17.

24. Kang DH, Nakagawa T, Feng L, et al. A role for uric acid in the progression of renal disease. J Am Soc Nephrol 2002;13:2888–97.

25. Sanchez-Lozada LG, Tapia E, Avila-Casado C, et al. Mild hyperuricemia induces glomerular hypertension in normal rats. Am J Physiol Renal Physiol 2002;283:F1105–10.

26. Watanabe S, Kang DH, Feng L, et al. Uric acid, hominoid evolution, and the pathogenesis of salt-sensitivity. Hypertension 2002;40:355–60.

27. Feig DI, Soletsky B, Johnson RJ. Effect of allopurinol on blood pressure of adolescents with newly diagnosed essential hypertension: a randomized trial. JAMA 2008;300:924–32.

28. George J, Struthers AD. Role of urate, xanthine oxidase and the effects of allopurinol in vascular oxidative stress. Vasc Health Risk Manage 2009;5:265–72.

29. Li JM, Shah AM. Endothelial cell superoxide generation: regulation and relevance for cardiovascular pathophysiology. Am J Physiol Regul Integr Comp Physiol 2004;287:R1014–30.

30. Meneshian A, Bulkley GB. The physiology of endothelial xanthine oxidase: from urate catabolism to reperfusion injury to inflammatory signal transduction. Microcirculation 2002;9:161–75.

31. Grayson PC, Kim SY, Lavalley M, et al. Hyperuricemia and incident hypertension: a systematic review and meta-analysis. Arthritis Care Res (Hoboken) 2011;63:102–10.

32. Becker MA, Schumacher HR, Espinoza LR, et al. The urate-lowering efficacy and safety of febuxostat in the treatment of the hyperuricemia of gout: the CONFIRMS trial. Arthritis Res Ther 2010;12:R63.

33. Schumacher Jr HR, Becker MA, Wortmann RL, et al. Effects of febuxostat versus allopurinol and placebo in reducing serum urate in subjects with hyperuricemia and gout: a 28-week, phase III, randomized, double-blind, parallel-group trial. Arthritis Rheum 2008;59:1540–8.

34. Becker MA, Schumacher Jr HR, Wortmann RL, et al. Febuxostat compared with allopurinol in patients with hyperuricemia and gout. N Engl J Med 2005;353:2450–61.

35. Schumacher Jr HR, Becker MA, Lloyd E, et al. C. Febuxostat in the treatment of gout: 5-yr findings of the FOCUS efficacy and safety study. Rheumatology (Oxford) 2009;48:188–94.

36. Grayson PC, Kim SY, Lavalley M, et al. Hyperuricemia and incident hypertension: a systematic review and meta-analysis. Arthritis Care Res (Hoboken) 2010.

37. Bhole V, Choi JW, Kim SW, et al. Serum uric acid levels and the risk of type 2 diabetes: a prospective study. Am J Med 2010;123:957–61.

38. Dehghan A, van Hoek M, Sijbrands EJ, et al. High serum uric acid as a novel risk factor for type 2 diabetes. Diabetes Care 2008;31:361–2.

39. Kramer CK, von Muhlen D, Jassal SK, et al. Serum uric acid levels improve prediction of incident type 2 diabetes in individuals with impaired fasting glucose: the Rancho Bernardo Study. Diabetes Care 2009;32:1272–3.

40. Niskanen L, Laaksonen DE, Lindstrom J, et al. Serum uric acid as a harbinger of metabolic outcome in subjects with impaired glucose tolerance: the Finnish Diabetes Prevention Study. Diabetes Care 2006;29:709–11.

41. Choi HK, Ford ES. Prevalence of the metabolic syndrome in individuals with hyperuricemia. Am J Med 2007;120:442–7.

42. Ludwig DS, Peterson KE, Gortmaker SL. Relation between consumption of sugar-sweetened drinks and childhood obesity: a prospective, observational analysis. Lancet 2001;357:505–8.

43. Bray GA, Nielsen SJ, Popkin BM. Consumption of high-fructose corn syrup in beverages may play a role in the epidemic of obesity. Am J Clin Nutr 2004;79:537–43.

44. Choi HK, Curhan G. Soft drinks, fructose consumption, and the risk of gout in men: prospective cohort study. BMJ 2008;336:309–12.

45. Choi HK, Willett W, Curhan G. Fructose-rich beverages and risk of gout in women. JAMA 2010.

46. Choi JW, Ford ES, Gao X, et al. Sugar-sweetened soft drinks, diet soft drinks, and serum uric acid level: the Third National Health and Nutrition Examination Survey. Arthritis Rheum 2008;59:109–16.

47. Schulze MB, Manson JE, Ludwig DS, et al. Sugar-sweetened beverages, weight gain, and incidence of type 2 diabetes in young and middle-aged women. JAMA 2004;292:927–34.

48. Nakagawa T, Hu H, Zharikov S, et al. A causal role for uric acid in fructose-induced metabolic syndrome. Am J Physiol Renal Physiol 2006;290:F625–31.

49. Le MT, Shafiu M, Mu W, et al. SLC2A9–a fructose transporter identified as a novel uric acid transporter. Nephrol Dial Transplant 2008;23:2746–9.

50. Shi Y, Evans JE, Rock KL. Molecular identification of a danger signal that alerts the immune system to dying cells. Nature 2003;425:516–21.

51. Dessein PH, Shipton EA, Stanwix AE, et al. Beneficial effects of weight loss associated with moderate calorie/carbohydrate restriction, and increased proportional intake of protein and unsaturated fat on serum urate and lipoprotein levels in gout: a pilot study. Ann Rheum Dis 2000;59:539–43.

52. Patetsios P, Rodino W, Wisselink W, et al. Identification of uric acid in aortic aneurysms and atherosclerotic artery. Ann N Y Acad Sci 1996;800:243–5.

53. Kang DH, Han L, Ouyang X, et al. Uric acid causes vascular smooth muscle cell proliferation by entering cells via a functional urate transporter. Am J Nephrol 2005;25:425–33.

54. Waring WS, Adwani SH, Breukels O, et al. Hyperuricaemia does not impair cardiovascular function in healthy adults. Heart 2004;90:155–9.

55. Chen SY, Chen CL, Shen ML, et al. Trends in the manifestations of gout in Taiwan. Rheumatology (Oxford) 2003;42:1529–33.

56. Krishnan E, Baker JF, Furst DE, et al. Gout and the risk of acute myocardial infarction. Arthritis Rheum 2006;54:2688–96.

57. Rott KT, Agudelo CA. Gout. JAMA 2003;289:2857–60.

58. Emmerson B. Hyperlipidaemia in hyperuricaemia and gout. Ann Rheum Dis 1998;57:509–10.

59. Mikuls TR, Farrar JT, Bilker WB, et al. Gout epidemiology: results from the UK General Practice Research Database, 1990-1999. Ann Rheum Dis 2005;64:267–72.

60. Moriwaki Y, Yamamoto T, Takahashi S, et al. Apolipoprotein E phenotypes in patients with gout: relation with hypertriglyceridaemia. Ann Rheum Dis 1995;54:351–4.

61. Takahashi S, Yamamoto T, Moriwaki Y, et al. Impaired lipoprotein metabolism in patients with primary gout–influence of alcohol intake and body weight. Br J Rheumatol 1994;33:731–4.

62. Bos MJ, Koudstaal PJ, Hofman A, et al. Uric acid is a risk factor for myocardial infarction and stroke: the Rotterdam study. Stroke 2006;37:1503–7.

63. Franse LV, Pahor M, Di Bari M, et al. Serum uric acid, diuretic treatment and risk of cardiovascular events in the Systolic Hypertension in the Elderly Program (SHEP). J Hypertens 2000;18:1149–54.

64. Fang J, Alderman MH. Serum uric acid and cardiovascular mortality the NHANES I epidemiologic follow-up study, 1971-1992. National Health and Nutrition Examination Survey. JAMA 2000;283:2404–10.

65. Madsen TE, Muhlestein JB, Carlquist JF, et al. Serum uric acid independently predicts mortality in patients with significant, angiographically defined coronary disease. Am J Nephrol 2005;25:45–9.

66. Freedman DS, Williamson DF, Gunter EW, et al. Relation of serum uric acid to mortality and ischemic heart disease. The NHANES I Epidemiologic Follow-up Study. Am J Epidemiol 1995;141:637–44.

67. Verdecchia P, Schillaci G, Reboldi G, et al. Relation between serum uric acid and risk of cardiovascular disease in essential hypertension. The PIUMA study. Hypertension 2000;36:1072–8.

68. Culleton BF, Larson MG, Kannel WB, et al. Serum uric acid and risk for cardiovascular disease and death: the Framingham Heart Study. Ann Intern Med 1999;131:7–13.

69. Brand FN, McGee DL, Kannel WB, et al. Hyperuricemia as a risk factor of coronary heart disease: the Framingham Study. Am J Epidemiol 1985;121:11–8.

70. Moriarity JT, Folsom AR, Iribarren C, et al. Serum uric acid and risk of coronary heart disease: Atherosclerosis Risk in Communities (ARIC) Study. Ann Epidemiol 2000;10:136–43.

71. Go AS, Chertow GM, Fan D, et al. Chronic kidney disease and the risks of death, cardiovascular events, and hospitalization. N Engl J Med 2004;351:1296–305.

72. Segal R, Lubart E, Leibovitz A, et al. Early and late effects of low-dose aspirin on renal function in elderly patients. Am J Med 2003;115:462–6.

73. Crouse JR, Toole JF, McKinney WM, et al. Risk factors for extracranial carotid artery atherosclerosis. Stroke 1987;18:990–6.

74. Cuspidi C, Valerio C, Sala C, et al. Lack of association between serum uric acid and organ damage in a never-treated essential hypertensive population at low prevalence of hyperuricemia. Am J Hypertens 2007;20:678–85.

75. Kawamoto R, Tomita H, Oka Y, et al. Association between uric acid and carotid atherosclerosis in elderly persons. Intern Med 2005;44:787–93.

76. Robins JM, Greenland S. Identifiability and exchangeability for direct and indirect effects. Epidemiology 1992;3:143–55.

77. Wheeler JG, Juzwishin KD, Eiriksdottir G, et al. Serum uric acid and coronary heart disease in 9,458 incident cases and 155,084 controls: prospective study and meta-analysis. PLoS Med 2005;2:e76.

78. Kim SY, Guevara JP, Kim KM, et al. Hyperuricemia and coronary heart disease: a systematic review and meta-analysis. Arthritis Care Res (Hoboken) 2010;62:170–80.

79. Chen JH, Pan WH. Effects of urate lowering therapy on cardiovascular mortality: a Taiwanese cohort study. Arthritis Rheum 2010;62:S872.

80. Ekundayo OJ, Dell'Italia LJ, Sanders PW, et al. Association between hyperuricemia and incident heart failure among older adults: a propensity-matched study. Int J Cardiol 2010;142:279–87.

81. Krishnan E. Hyperuricemia and incident heart failure. Circ Heart Fail 2009;2:556–62.

82. Misra D, Zhu Y, Zhang Y, et al. The independent impact of congestive heart failure status and diuretic use on serum uric acid among men with a high cardiovascular risk profile: a prospective longitudinal study. Semin Arthritis Rheum 2011, published online 24 March 2011. doi:10.1016/j.semarthrit.2011.02.002.

83. Thanassoulis G, Brophy JM, Richard H, et al. Gout, allopurinol use, and heart failure outcomes. Arch Intern Med 2010;170:1358–64.

84. Kim SY, Guevara JP, Kim KM, et al. Hyperuricemia and risk of stroke: a systematic review and meta-analysis. Arthritis Rheum 2009;61:885–92.

85. Chambless LE, Heiss G, Folsom AR, et al. Association of coronary heart disease incidence with carotid arterial wall thickness and major risk factors: the Atherosclerosis Risk in Communities (ARIC) Study, 1987-1993. Am J Epidemiol 1997;146:483–94.

86. O'Leary DH, Polak JF, Kronmal RA, et al. Carotid-artery intima and media thickness as a risk factor for myocardial infarction and stroke in older adults. Cardiovascular Health Study Collaborative Research Group. N Engl J Med 1999;340:14–22.

87. Bots ML, Hoes AW, Koudstaal PJ, et al. Common carotid intima-media thickness and risk of stroke and myocardial infarction: the Rotterdam Study. Circulation 1997;96:1432–7.

88. Salonen JT, Salonen R. Ultrasound B-mode imaging in observational studies of atherosclerotic progression. Circulation 1993;87:1156–65.

89. Devine PJ, Carlson DW, Taylor AJ. Clinical value of carotid intima-media thickness testing. J Nucl Cardiol 2006;13:710–8.

90. Ishizaka N, Ishizaka Y, Toda E, et al. Association between serum uric acid, metabolic syndrome, and carotid atherosclerosis in Japanese individuals. Arterioscler Thromb Vasc Biol 2005;25:1038–44.

91. Montalcini T, Gorgone G, Gazzaruso C, et al. Relation between serum uric acid and carotid intima-media thickness in healthy postmenopausal women. Intern Emerg Med 2007;2:19–23.

92. Pacifico L, Cantisani V, Anania C, et al. Serum uric acid and its association with metabolic syndrome and carotid atherosclerosis in obese children. Eur J Endocrinol 2009;160:45–52.

93. Neogi T, Ellison RC, Hunt S, et al. Serum uric acid is associated with carotid plaques: the National Heart, Lung, and Blood Institute Family Heart Study. J Rheumatol 2009;36:378–84.

94. Tavil Y, Kaya MG, Oktar SO, et al. Uric acid level and its association with carotid intima-media thickness in patients with hypertension. Atherosclerosis 2008;197:159–63.

95. Iribarren C, Folsom AR, Eckfeldt JH, et al. Correlates of uric acid and its association with asymptomatic carotid atherosclerosis: the ARIC Study. Atherosclerosis Risk in Communities. Ann Epidemiol 1996;6:331–40.

96. Kawamoto R, Tomita H, Oka Y, et al. Relationship between serum uric acid concentration, metabolic syndrome and carotid atherosclerosis. Intern Med 2006;45:605–14.

97. Demer LL, Tintut Y. Mineral exploration: search for the mechanism of vascular calcification and beyond: the 2003 Jeffrey M. Hoeg Award lecture. Arterioscler Thromb Vasc Biol 2003;23:1739–43.

98. Frink RJ, Achor RW, Brown Jr AL, et al. Significance of calcification of the coronary arteries. Am J Cardiol 1970;26:241–7.

99. LaMonte MJ, FitzGerald SJ, Church TS, et al. Coronary artery calcium score and coronary heart disease events in a large cohort of asymptomatic men and women. Am J Epidemiol 2005;162:421–9.

100. Greenland P, LaBree L, Azen SP, et al. Coronary artery calcium score combined with Framingham score for risk prediction in asymptomatic individuals. JAMA 2004;291:210–5.

101. Kondos GT, Hoff JA, Sevrukov A, et al. Electron-beam tomography coronary artery calcium and cardiac events: a 37-month follow-up of 5635 initially asymptomatic low- to intermediate-risk adults. Circulation 2003;107:2571–6.

102. Shaw LJ, Raggi P, Schisterman E, et al. Prognostic value of cardiac risk factors and coronary artery calcium screening for all-cause mortality. Radiology 2003;228:826–33.

103. Nadra I, Boccaccini AR, Philippidis P, et al. Effect of particle size on hydroxyapatite crystal-induced tumor necrosis factor alpha secretion by macrophages. Atherosclerosis 2008;196:98–105.

104. Robinson KM, Morre JT, Beckman JS. Triuret: a novel product of peroxynitrite-mediated oxidation of urate. Arch Biochem Biophys 2004;423:213–7.

105. Coutinho Tde A, Turner ST, Peyser PA, et al. Associations of serum uric acid with markers of inflammation, metabolic syndrome, and subclinical coronary atherosclerosis. Am J Hypertens 2007;20:83–9.

106. Neogi T, Terkeltaub R, Ellison RC, et al. Serum urate is not associated with coronary artery calcification: the NHLBI Family Heart Study. J Rheumatol 2011;38:111–7.

107. Santos RD, Nasir K, Orakzai R, et al. Relation of uric acid levels to presence of coronary artery calcium detected by electron beam tomography in men free of symptomatic myocardial ischemia with versus without the metabolic syndrome. Am J Cardiol 2007;99:42–5.

108. Kanno Y, Into T, Lowenstein CJ, et al. Nitric oxide regulates vascular calcification by interfering with TGF-signalling. Cardiovasc Res 2008;77:221–30.

109. Hoieggen A, Alderman MH, Kjeldsen SE, et al. The impact of serum uric acid on cardiovascular outcomes in the LIFE study. Kidney Int 2004;65:1041–9.

110. Sulfinpyrazone in the prevention of cardiac death after myocardial infarction. The Anturane Reinfarction Trial. N Engl J Med 1978;298:289–95.

111. The Anturane Reinfarction Trial Research Group. Sulfinpyrazone in the prevention of sudden death after myocardial infarction. N Engl J Med 1980;302:250–6.

112. Sulphinpyrazone in post-myocardial infarction. Report from the Anturan Reinfarction Italian Study. Lancet 1982;1:237–42.

113. Cairns JA, Gent M, Singer J, et al. Aspirin, sulfinpyrazone, or both in unstable angina. Results of a Canadian multicenter trial. N Engl J Med 1985;313:1369–75.

114. Simon JA, Lin F, Vittinghoff E, et al. The relation of postmenopausal hormone therapy to serum uric acid and the risk of coronary heart disease events: the Heart and Estrogen-Progestin Replacement Study (HERS). Ann Epidemiol 2006;16:138–45.

115. Cingolani HE, Plastino JA, Escudero EM, et al. The effect of xanthine oxidase inhibition upon ejection fraction in heart failure patients: La Plata Study. J Card Fail 2006;12:491–8.

116. Hare JM, Mangal B, Brown J, et al. Impact of oxypurinol in patients with symptomatic heart failure. Results of the OPT-CHF study. J Am Coll Cardiol 2008;51:2301–9.

117. Noman A, Ang DS, Ogston S, et al. Effect of high-dose allopurinol on exercise in patients with chronic stable angina: a randomised, placebo controlled crossover trial. Lancet; 375:2161–7.

118. Gavin AD, Struthers AD. Allopurinol reduces B-type natriuretic peptide concentrations and haemoglobin but does not alter exercise capacity in chronic heart failure. Heart 2005;91:749–53.

119. Gibbings S, Elkins ND, Fitzgerald H, et al. Xanthine oxidoreductase promotes the inflammatory state of mononuclear phagocytes through effects on chemokine expression, peroxisome proliferator-activated receptor-γ sumoylation, and HIF-1α. J Biol Chem 2011;286:961–75.

120. Saliaris AP, Amado LC, Minhas KM, et al. Chronic allopurinol administration ameliorates maladaptive alterations in Ca2+ cycling proteins and beta-adrenergic hyporesponsiveness in heart failure. Am J Physiol Heart Circ Physiol 2007;292:H1328–35.

121. George J, Carr E, Davies J, et al. High-dose allopurinol improves endothelial function by profoundly reducing vascular oxidative stress and not by lowering uric acid. Circulation 2006;114:2508–16.

122. Iseki K, Ikemiya Y, Inoue T, et al. Significance of hyperuricemia as a risk factor for developing ESRD in a screened cohort. Am J Kidney Dis 2004;44:642–50.

123. Iseki K, Oshiro S, Tozawa M, et al. Significance of hyperuricemia on the early detection of renal failure in a cohort of screened subjects. Hypertens Res 2001;24:691–7.

124. Ohno I, Hosoya T, Gomi H, et al. Serum uric acid and renal prognosis in patients with IgA nephropathy. Nephron 2001;87:333–9.

125. Syrjanen J, Mustonen J, Pasternack A. Hypertriglyceridaemia and hyperuricaemia are risk factors for progression of IgA nephropathy. Nephrol Dial Transplant 2000;15:34–42.

126. Hsu CY, Iribarren C, McCulloch CE, et al. Risk factors for end-stage renal disease: 25-year follow-up. Arch Intern Med 2009;169:342–50.

127. Dalbeth N, Kumar S, Stamp L, et al. Dose adjustment of allopurinol according to creatinine clearance does not provide adequate control of hyperuricemia in patients with gout. J Rheumatol 2006;33:1646–50.

128. Kanbay M, Ozkara A, Selcoki Y, et al. Effect of treatment of hyperuricemia with allopurinol on blood pressure, creatinine clearance, and proteinuria in patients with normal renal functions. Int Urol Nephrol 2007;39:1227–33.

129. Siu YP, Leung KT, Tong MK, et al. Use of allopurinol in slowing the progression of renal disease through its ability to lower serum uric acid level. Am J Kidney Dis 2006;47:51–9.

130. Momeni A, Shahidi S, Seirafian S, et al. Effect of allopurinol in decreasing proteinuria in type 2 diabetic patients. Iran J Kidney Dis 2010;4:128–32.

131. Goicoechea M, de Vinuesa SG, Verdalles U, et al. Effect of allopurinol in chronic kidney disease progression and cardiovascular risk. Clin J Am Soc Nephrol 2010;5:1388–93.

132. Whelton A, MacDonald PA, Zhao L, et al. Renal function in gout: long-term treatment effects of febuxostat. J Clin Rheumatol 2011;17(1):7–13.

133. Kutzing MK, Firestein BL. Altered uric acid levels and disease states. J Pharmacol Exp Ther 2008;324:1–7.

134. Chen H, Mosley TH, Alonso A, et al. Plasma urate and Parkinson's disease in the Atherosclerosis Risk in Communities (ARIC) study. Am J Epidemiol 2009;169:1064–9.

135. Gao X, Chen H, Choi HK, et al. Diet, urate, and Parkinson's disease risk in men. Am J Epidemiol 2008;167:831–8.

136. Hooper DC, Spitsin S, Kean RB, et al. Uric acid, a natural scavenger of peroxynitrite, in experimental allergic encephalomyelitis and multiple sclerosis. Proc Natl Acad Sci U S A 1998;95:675–80.

137. Chamorro A, Obach V, Cervera A, et al. Prognostic significance of uric acid serum concentration in patients with acute ischemic stroke. Stroke 2002;33:1048–52.

138. Cherubini A, Polidori MC, Bregnocchi M, et al. Antioxidant profile and early outcome in stroke patients. Stroke 2000;31:2295–300.

139. Weir CJ, Muir SW, Walters MR, et al. Serum urate as an independent predictor of poor outcome and future vascular events after acute stroke. Stroke 2003;34:1951–6.

140. Seet RC, Kasiman K, Gruber J, et al. Is uric acid protective or deleterious in acute ischemic stroke? A prospective cohort study. Atherosclerosis 2010;209:215–9.

141. Dawson J, Quinn TJ, Harrow C, et al. The effect of allopurinol on the cerebral vasculature of patients with subcortical stroke; a randomized trial. Br J Clin Pharmacol 2009;68:662–8.

Section III

Calcific Crystal Arthropathies

Chapter 20

Pathogenesis and Molecular Genetics of Calcium Pyrophosphate Dihydrate Crystal Deposition Disease

Robert Terkeltaub and Kenneth P.H. Pritzker

KEY POINTS

- By far the majority of calcium pyrophosphate dihydrate (CPPD) crystal deposition disease is an idiopathic/sporadic disease with onset in later life, but early-onset familial disease also occurs.

- Familial CPPD crystal deposition disease is primarily an autosomal dominant disorder linked to a variety of mutations in *ANKH*, a chromosome 5 gene that encodes an inorganic pyrophosphate (PP_i) transporter.

- Disordered PP_i metabolism is central to the pathogenesis of CPPD crystal deposition disease, but dysregulated chondrocyte growth factor responsiveness and differentiation are also involved, as is the biology of aging.

- The connective tissue matrix of fibrocartilaginous menisci, of articular hyaline cartilage, and of some ligaments and tendons are susceptible to pathologic calcification with CPPD crystals. Dehydration of the fibrocartilaginous menisci in aging may be a factor in particularly promoting PP_i excess there.

- Activation of the NLRP3 (cryopyrin) inflammasome, and consequent maturation and release of interleukin-1β, mediate CPPD crystal–induced inflammation.

Genetics of Calcium Pyrophosphate Dihydrate Crystal Deposition Disease

The vast majority of calcium pyrophosphate dihydrate (CPPD) crystal deposition disease is an idiopathic/sporadic disorder related to aging, and some cases are related to joint trauma or certain metabolic diseases. However, some CPPD crystal deposition disease is familial, and typically these cases

have early onset (defined as onset before age 55).[1] Familial chondrocalcinosis is heterogeneous. For example, osteoarthritis (OA) with prominent CPPD and hydroxyapatite (HA) crystal deposits and cartilage and periarticular calcification were described in a kindred that has not yet been linked to a specific chromosomal locus.[2] One chromosomal linkage of familial CPPD crystal deposition disease (with early-onset OA) is with 8q, and this was previously designated CCAL1.[1] Chromosome 5p–linked chondrocalcinosis (termed CCAL2) is more common and is mediated by mutants of the gene *ANKH* (which encodes a transmembrane protein with PP_i transport and other apparent functions discussed later); has been established in these studies.[1,3,4] ANKH structure-function is reviewed in detail later and in a recent review.[5]

A syndrome of spondyloepiphyseal dysplasia tarda, brachydactyly, precocious OA, and intraarticular calcifications with CPPD and/or HA crystals, as well as periarticular calcifications, was linked to mutation of the procollagen type II gene in indigenous natives of the Chiloe Island region of Chile.[6] This population has a high prevalence of familial CPPD deposition disease. Families affected with diffuse idiopathic skeletal hyperostosis (DISH) and/or chondrocalcinosis have been identified in the Azores Islands, and this may reflect a shared pathogenesis, although the specific mechanism is not clear.[7]

Pathogenesis of CPPD Crystal Deposition Disease

This discussion supplements and complements the review of this topic, with emphasis on pathology, by Kenneth P.H. Pritzker in Chapter 1. The connective tissue matrix of fibrocartilaginous menisci, of articular hyaline cartilage, and of certain ligaments and tendons is particularly susceptible to calcification with CPPD[8] (chemical formula $Ca_2P_2O_7 \cdot H_2O$, calcium:phosphate ratio 1.0). In addition, basic calcium phosphate (BCP) crystals can be deposited in articular cartilage, most commonly in OA. Unlike growth plate cartilage, joint

This work was supported by the VA Research Service.

cartilages are specialized to avoid developing matrix calcification, with lack of vascularity and abundant, intact proteoglycans among factors that limit access to phosphatases that liberate inorganic phosphate (P_i). However, altered matrix composition and hydration in aging and OA compromise these defense mechanisms.[9,10]

CPPD crystals will precipitate where PP_i concentration is highest. This is usually where matrix is most efficient at sequestering PP_i and the furthest from pyrophosphatase activities.[11] Phosphatases have broad substrate specificity, as exemplified by extracellular alkaline phosphatase, which has phosphatase, pyrophosphatase, and CPPD crystal dissolution activity, as discussed below. Classically, the locations for CPPD crystal deposition are in meniscal fibrocartilage and in middle zones of hyaline cartilage in synovial and symphyseal sites. However, CPPD sometimes forms in reparative fibrocartilage on the articular cartilage surface. Dehydration of the fibrocartilaginous menisci in aging may be a factor in particularly promoting PP_i excess there.

It is rare for CPPD and BCP crystals to coexist at a single finite locus, since the physical formation conditions are mutually exclusive. However, this does occur at some sites, and, at these sites, the crystals likely have formed at different times; for example, HA might form when CPPD deposits dissolve. Usually, BCP in human cartilage forms near the surface of the articular cartilage. At times, driven by intraarticular steroids, BCP crystals form around the chondrons. Also, in advanced OA, BCP can form in the advancing calcification front of cartilage. Many, if not most cases, however, represent BCP debris from exposed or dislodged bone.

Major factors in the deposition of CPPD in joint cartilages are schematized in Figure 20-1. Alterations in many of the same factors alternatively can promote BCP crystal deposition; for example, decreased and increased PP_i can promote BCP crystal deposition, with increased tissue nonspecific alkaline phosphatase (TNAP) activity a cofactor. CPPD deposition reflects a breakdown of checks and balances imposed heterogeneously by genetics, inflammation, dysregulated chondrocyte growth factor responsiveness and differentiation, ATP and PP_i transport and metabolism, and extracellular matrix environment, especially with aging. Increase in the concentrations of PP_i, and the solubility product of PP_i and ionic calcium clearly are factors in promoting CPPD crystal formation.[12] However, concentration of magnesium, P_i, iron, and cartilage extracellular matrix content (including high density of negative charges in intact proteoglycans) regulates the dynamics of CPPD crystal formation and helps to determine whether monoclinic and/or triclinic CPPD crystals are formed.[13-16] In this context, monoclinic CPPD crystals appear more inflammatory than triclinic CPPD crystals.[17]

The influence of the extracellular matrix on CPPD crystal formation (reviewed in part in Chapter 1) has typically been analyzed in model gel systems.[13,18-21] Such studies, in particular using type I collagen as a variable in the gel system to promote CPPD deposition, have revealed stimulation of CPPD formation by ATP, osteopontin (a sialoprotein increased with chondrocyte hypertrophic differentiation and in OA cartilage), and addition of corticosteroids; in contrast, type II collagen and intact proteoglycans can suppress ATP-induced CPPD crystal formation in vitro.[13,14,22,23]

Some experimental systems to analyze CPPD (and BCP) crystal deposition also have used matrix vesicles isolated from

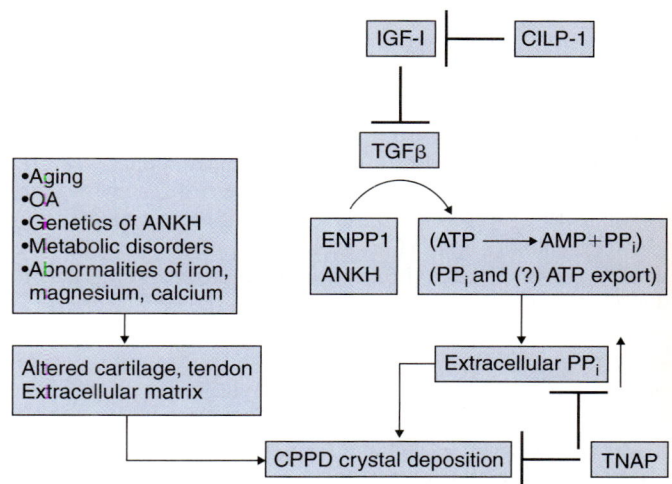

Figure 20-1 Proposed inorganic pyrophosphate (PP_i)–dependent mechanisms stimulating CPPD crystal deposition. This model accounts for the association of elevated extracellular PP_i concentration with CPPD crystal deposition, a scenario that in the aged cartilage in idiopathic CPPD deposition disease, and in osteoarthritis (OA) cartilages, is mediated in part by increased nucleotide pyrophosphatase phosphodiesterase 1 (ENPP1). Other factors promoting CPPD crystal deposition in joint cartilages include genetic factors particularly via the multiple-pass transmembrane protein ANKH, metabolic disorders that affect both chondrocyte differentiation and levels of solutes such as iron, calcium, and magnesium, or tissue-nonspecific alkaline phosphatase (TNAP). Alterations in cartilage matrix composition in OA and aging also appear to favor CPPD crystal deposition. The enzyme activity of ENPP1 acts in part to hydrolyze adenosine triphosphate (ATP) and other nucleoside triphosphates to generate PP_i and adenosine monophosphate. ANKH and ENPP1 expression, and ENPP1 movement to the plasma membrane are stimulated by transforming growth factor (TGF)β, and TGFβ also stimulates release of PP_i and ATP. The multiple-pass transmembrane protein ANKH drives transport to the cell exterior of PP_i and also may mediate ATP release. Insulin-like growth factor (IGF-I) inhibits extracellular PP_i levels, in part by suppressing responses to TGFβ, but the IGF-I effect is inhibited by the matrix protein cartilage intermediate layer protein-1 (CILP-1), whose expression rises in aging and osteoarthritic cartilages. TNAP is normally sparse in articular chondrocytes. TNAP hydrolyzes PP_i to P_i, and also induces CPPD crystal dissolution, mediated by binding to the crystal surface. A central point of the model is that excess extracellular PP_i is promoted by heightened "leakiness" of intracellular PP_i by increased ANKH expression in OA or abnormal function of mutant ANKH in familial chondrocalcinosis. Alterations in many of the same factors illustrated here alternatively can promote basic calcium phosphate (BCP) crystal deposition; for example, either increased or decreased PP_i promotes BCP crystal deposition, with increased TNAP activity a cofactor.

chondrocytes. Matrix vesicles are small, membrane-limited bodies released from chondrocytes (and other calcifying cells such as osteoblasts) that are enriched in constituents that regulate and can promote calcification.[13] Matrix vesicles initially have intracellular $[Mg^{2+}]$, $[Ca^{2+}]$, and pro-calcifying protein molecules in their interior and TNAP on outside.[24] As the vesicle "deflates," Ca^{2+} diffuses in and $[Mg^{2+}]$ diffuses out. Toward the end of this process, the vesicle has an extracellular ion environment, but the remnant has protein and, in particular, lipids that bind calcium and promote calcification of the BCP crystal type, which may be an amorphous calcium phosphate before it becomes BCP crystals.

Matrix vesicles are clearly involved in cartilage growth plate calcification with BCP. However, it is not yet clear whether

BCP crystal formation in articular cartilages is initiated more by matrix vesicles or by nucleation of crystals in the extracellular matrix. Moreover, areas in which CPPD crystals are deposited clearly include areas removed from collagen and matrix vesicles (and from pyrophosphatases) in cartilages affected by CPPD deposition disease (see Chapter 1). Matrix vesicles can provide phospholipids, proteinases, enzymes that regulate PP_i metabolism, and other regulators of articular cartilage calcification.[24] However, CPPD crystal deposition is likely to be initiated in the extracellular matrix and unlikely to be initiated within matrix vesicles, due to the very large size of CPPD (micron size, unlike submicroscopic BCP) crystals relative to matrix vesicles, and the substantial content of TNAP on the exterior of the vesicles, and magnesium and P_i[24] in the interior of matrix vesicles.

Loci of pericellular concentration of PP_i may be needed to drive CPPD crystal formation at low micromolar PP_i concentrations developing in cartilages with chondrocalcinosis. Moreover, it is not clear what the effects on CPPD deposition are of apoptotic bodies, which have an inside-out vesicle orientation (i.e., where calcification-regulating mediators, such as the PP_i-generating enzyme ENPP1, may be functionally misplaced on the surface of the structure).[25]

There are unequivocal physical effects of calcium, P_i, and PP_i on crystal nucleation and propagation.[14,26,27,27a] These solutes also regulate mineralization by effects on gene expression, differentiation, and viability in chondrocytes, mediated partly by calcium-sensing receptors and sodium-dependent P_i cotransport in chondrocytes.[27-29] Excess PP_i on chondrocytes also appears to be sensed (by unclear mechanisms) in chondrocytes, as evidenced by deleterious induction of matrix metalloproteinase-13 (MMP-13) expression,[30] suppression of chondrogenesis,[31] and promotion of apoptosis.[32] These observations support the long-used clinical term "pyrophosphate arthropathy" as an umbrella term for the phenotype of chronic cartilage degeneration seen in CPPD crystal deposition disease.

Altered PP_i Metabolism in CPPD Deposition Disease

PP_i is a potent, physiologic inhibitor of the nucleation and propagation of BCP crystals,[11] and this has been well illuminated in mouse models of pathologic soft tissue calcification linked with deficient PP_i generation and transport.[27,27a,33] Chondrocytes and osteoblasts are unique in robustly producing extracellular PP_i. Depending on the ambient levels of cartilage ATP and PP_i and the level of activity of P_i-generating ATPases and TNAP, and the PP_i-degrading effects of TNAP, formation of CPPD and HA crystals may be promoted in the same cartilages, an event that can occur in OA. However, the physical-chemical conditions favoring CPPD and BCP crystal formation are largely mutually exclusive.[14,34] Where CPPD and BCP are found in adjacent domains, such as occasionally seen in OA, the crystal types formed at different times; in some cases secondary to partial dissolution of preexisting CPPD crystals.

Role of ENPP1 in PP_i Metabolism in Chondrocalcinosis

Sporadic/idiopathic CPPD crystal deposition disease associated with aging is consistently linked with an excess chondrocyte PP_i-generating nucleotide pyrophosphatase phosphodiesterase (NPP) activity and increased PP_i generation by chondrocytes.[11,35,36] The NPP family isoenzymes ENPP1 (formerly known as NPP1 and plasma cell membrane glycoprotein-1 [PC-1]) and ENPP3 (formerly known as B10) actively generate PP_i via hydrolysis of nucleoside triphosphates, principally ATP.[11,35,36] Notably, some of the ATP used by chondrocytes to generate extracellular PP_i is extracellular, and some is generated by the mitochondria.[11]

ENPP1 plays a core role in driving extracellular PP_i in chondrocytes (see Figure 20-1), and in some other cell types. Increased ENPP1 also is associated with apoptosis in vitro and in degenerative human cartilages.[32,35] ENPP1 deficiency states in vivo and in vitro are linked with up to a 50% decrease in plasma and extracellular PP_i.[26,33] Contrastingly, in sporadic/idiopathic chondrocalcinosis of aging, cartilage NPP activity and PP_i levels have been reported to average approximately double those of normal subjects.[37,38] This PP_i concentration is insufficient to cause CPPD deposition. Therefore, sequestration of PP_i in pericellular matrix is thought to be necessary to raise PP_i levels sufficiently to achieve CPPD crystal deposition).[11]

ANKH in the Molecular Genetics and Pathogenesis of CPPD Crystal Deposition Disease

ANKH encodes a multiple-pass transmembrane protein that functions in PP_i channelling[39-42] (Figure 20-2) and also appears to directly or indirectly promote ATP release.[42] ANKH also appears to regulate P_i metabolism and uptake of P_i by the type III sodium-dependent P_i cotransporter Pit-1.[43] ANKH also promotes bidirectional movement of PP_i at the plasma membrane,[32] but the gradient for ANKH-stimulated PP_i movement in chondrocytes is from cytosol to the extracellular space.[11] Chondrocytes produce abundant PP_i in the cell both by ENPP1 and as a byproduct of matrix biosynthesis and other biochemical (e.g., intramitochondrial) reactions, and ANKH transport of PP_i that is generated intracellularly by ENPP1,[30] is likely the fundamental means by which chondrocytes regulate extracellular PP_i concentrations.[11] Molecular models of ANKH have limitations, but the PP_i channelling function of ANKH may be via 10 or 12 membrane-spanning domains in the molecule that have an alternating inside-out orientation and provide a central channel for movement of PP_i[32,39] (see Figure 20-2).

ANKH is unequivocally involved in pathogeneses of both familial and idiopathic/sporadic chondrocalcinosis.[1,44] Importantly, ANKH expression is regulated, and ANKH is increased in OA and chondrocalcinotic cartilages,[30] and increased chondrocyte ANKH expression may drive secondary chondrocalcinosis in OA.[30] Hypoxia inhibits ANKH expression,[45] via the transcription factor hypoxia inducible actor-1α; it is possible that that increased permeability to oxygen via fissures and fibrillation in OA cartilage promotes increased ANKH expression. Conjoint effects of ANKH and signaling by extracellular P_i promote chondrocyte maturation to the hypertrophic differentiation state that promotes calcification.[46]

Figure 20-1 summarized a paradigm in which alterations in chondrocyte expression of both ANKH and ENPP1 drive PP_i supersaturation in cartilage in idiopathic/sporadic and

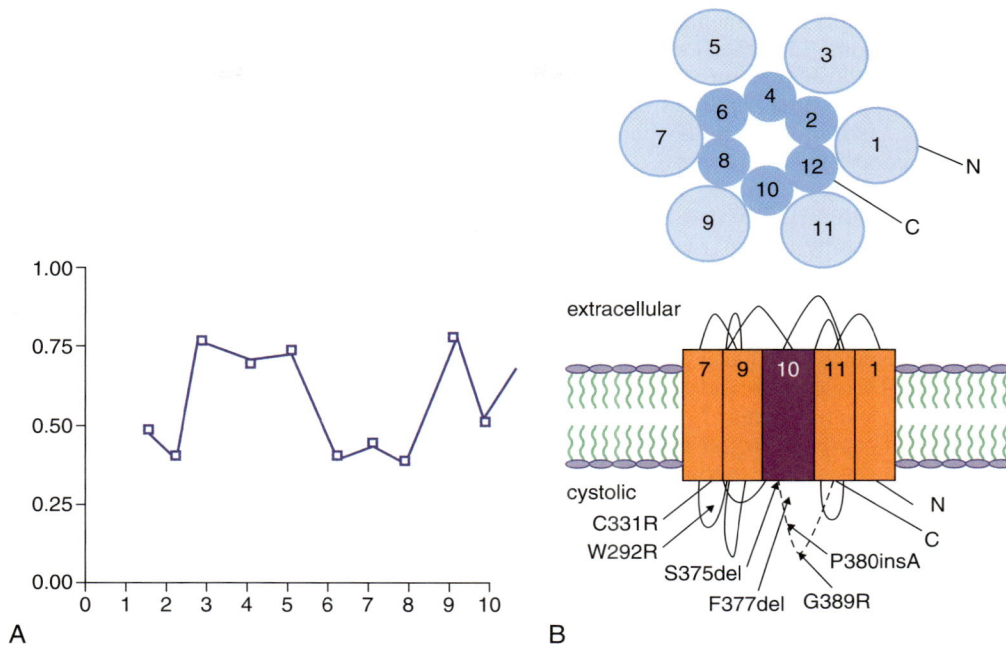

Figure 20-2 Channel model of ANKH structure, and predicted cytosolic location of most mutants of ANKH linked to craniometaphyseal dysplasia. **A,** Overall hydrophobicity plot of the transmembrane helical segments. Note the alternating hydrophobicity of the predicted 12 consecutive helices. **B,** Schematic representation of ANKH transmembrane helix assembly with sites of mutation indicated (*arrows*). Views from above and from the side are shown. Only even-numbered helices (*black*) are predicted to contribute directly to the channel. The six-membered helical assembly results in a central channel wide enough to permit the passage of an inorganic pyrophosphate (PP$_i$) molecule, whereas the channel of a five-membered ring would be too narrow (for instance, the five-helix channel of phospholamban [PDB code 1PLN] has an inner diameter of about 4 Å, but the lowest diameter for PP$_i$ is 5.3 Å, even without Mg^{2+} or water ligands), and that of a circular 12- (or 10-) membered helix assembly would be far too wide to be selective for PP$_i$. Note that nearly all mutations occurred at the cytosolic side. Loops in *black* are in the background and connect helices not visible in the side view. The fact that most ANKH mutations found here affect only one of the five intracellular loops (*hatched*) indicates that this loop may have a critical role in control of ANK function. *(Adapted by permission from Macmillan Publishers Ltd: Nürnberg P, Thiele H, Chandler D, et al. Heterozygous mutations in ANKH, the human ortholog of the mouse progressive ankylosis gene, result in craniometaphyseal dysplasia. Nat Genet 2001;28:37-41.)*

Table 20-1 *ANKH* Mutations Associated With CPPD Deposition Disease

Location (cDNA Position*)	Nucleotide Variation (Amino Acid Change)	Role in Sporadic CPPD Deposition	Change in *ANKH* Expression
5'-UTR (−11 bp)	C>T (+4 amino acids†)	No role	Unknown
5'-UTR‡ (−4 bp)	G>A (NA)	Yes	↑
Exon 1 (+13 bp)	C>A (Pro→Thr)	Unknown	↔
Exon 1 (+14 bp)	C>T (Pro→Leu)	No role	↑ or ↔
Exon 2 (+143 bp)	T>C (Met→Thr)	No role	↔
Exon 12§ (+490 bp)	GAGdel (Glu deletion)	No role	↑

With the exceptions of mutants designated by ‡ and §, each mutant ANKH cited has been linked to autosomal dominant familial CPPD deposition disease.
*Relative to the ATG initiation codon.
†Generates an alternative ATG codon adding four amino acids to the N-terminus.
§This mutant in exon 12 was found only in a single case of sporadic CPPD deposition disease.
Adapted by permission from Macmillan Publishers Ltd: Abhishek A, Doherty M. Pathophysiology of articular chondrocalcinosis-role of ANKH. Nat Rev Rheumatol 2010 Nov 23. Epub ahead of print.

OA-associated CPPD crystal deposition arthropathy. Alternatively, mutations at different locations in *ANKH* can affect postnatal skeletal development, inducing autosomal dominant chondrocalcinosis[1,38-41] (Table 20-1) or a variety of other phenotypes, such as murine progressive ankylosis (*ank/ank* mouse). In humans, craniometaphyseal dysplasia (CMD) is another phenotype of multiple mutations of *ANKH* (nine to date), most of which are in predicted cytosolic regions of central exons in the molecule. This phenotype has been linked with decreased transport of PP$_i$ within bone, which modulates bone resorption and remodeling likely directly and indirectly on the function of osteoclasts, as elucidated in *Ank*-deficient mice,[38,41,47] and by a knock-in mouse model homozygous for the phenylalanine 377 deletion.[48]

Recently, a consanguineous family was defined in which homozygous ANK missense mutation L244S was detected in all those with a novel phenotype of mental retardation, in addition to deafness (a finding in some CMD kindreds), and joint ankylosis, and with skeletal features such as painful small joint soft tissue calcifications, progressive spondyloarthropathy, osteopenia, and mild hypophosphatemia.[49] In this kindred, the mutant ANKH was transcribed and synthesized and moved into the plasma membrane. However, fibrosis and mineralization of the articular soft tissues developed in homozygotes. Significantly, heterozygous carriers of this L244S mutation developed mild osteoarthritis, without altered serum phosphate or the bone changes of the homozygotes.[49] Such findings suggest a fundamental homeostatic role of PP$_i$ metabolism in maintenance of articular cartilage, likely through maintenance of physiologic articular chondrocyte differentiation, but other mechanisms may be at play, since ANKH affects bone geometry at the joint,[50-52] and affects differentiation of bone marrow cells (of the erythroid lineage).[53]

Chondrocalcinosis associated with ANKH mutations demonstrates clinical and mechanistic heterogeneity (see Table 20-1).[1] This is consistent with the concept of differing functional effects of ANKH mediated by specific regions of the molecule that cause either chondrocalcinosis (largely the N-terminal ANKH domain) or CMD (certain cytosolic regions). Most N-terminal ANKH mutations identified, to date, in association with familial chondrocalcinosis (see Table 20-1) appear to elevate PP$_i$ transport,[40] but some of ANKH mutations have differing effects on chondrocyte differentiation.[44] Moreover, the M48T ANKH mutant, originally characterized in a French kindred, appears to have unique effects; first, it is linked with increased intracellular PP$_i$,[54] and, second, it interrupts ANKH interaction of with the sodium-dependent P$_i$ cotransporter Pit-1.[43] The significance of such an effect may be because elevated P$_i$ increases both ANKH and Pit-1 expression; in addition, ANKH and Pit-1 colocalize in the plasma membrane in chondroctyres.[43] Moreover, P$_i$ and P$_i$ uptake modulate chondrocyte differentiation and promote chondrocyte hypertrophy.[55,56] The findings of a single case with sporadic CPPD deposition disease also are instructive, via linkage with the ANKH mutation ΔE590[3]; ANKHΔE590 appears to indirectly suppress PP$_i$ catabolism by association with impairment of TNAP expression.[57] This suggests an alternative mechanism of disrupting PP$_i$ metabolism by mutant ANKH.

Collectively, the capacity of ANKH to promote chronic, low-grade chondrocyte "PP$_i$ leakiness" clearly can promote CPPD crystal deposition via extracellular matrix supersaturation with PP$_i$.[1,39,58] In this context, homozygosity for a single nucleotide substitution (−4 G to A) in the ANKH 5′-untranslated region (see Figure 20-2) that promotes increased ANKH mRNA expression was present in about 4% of British subjects identified as having idiopathic/sporadic chondrocalcinosis of aging.[44] These findings indicate that a small but significant subset of CPPD deposition disease in late middle to later life likely has a slow onset familial component.

TNAP and CPPD Crystal Dissolution and CPPD Deposition Disease, Including in Hypophosphatasia

TNAP is a major physiologic antagonist of ENPP1-mediated elevation of extracellular PP$_i$.[27a] Conversely, physiologic ENPP1-induced PP$_i$ generation antagonizes the essential pro-mineralizing effects of TNAP mediated by P$_i$ generation,[27a] and presumed PP$_i$ excess in the joint space promotes a scenario to drive chondrocalcinosis in young adults in hypophosphatasia. The rate-limiting factor for PP$_i$ concentration in extracellular fluid is TNAP activity. TNAP hydrolyzes PP$_i$ to more soluble P$_i$. TNAP chondrocyte alkaline phosphatase has been shown to dissolve the normally very insoluble CPPD crystals at physiologic pH.[59-61] To do so, TNAP must be attached to the surface of the CPPD crystal,[62] indicating that that TNAP must act on soluble PP$_i$ that is in equilibrium with solid state PP$_i$ on the crystal surface. This provides a formidable challenge to crystal dissolution strategies that are less efficient than TNAP. Further, TNAP inhibition, by decreasing PP$_i$ hydrolysis, inhibits CPPD crystal dissolution. Endogenous small molecules such as cysteine[63] and mercaptopyruvate[64] can inhibit TNAP and CPPD crystal dissolution in vitro. Interestingly, relative elevation of cysteine and mercaptopyruvate substances may occur in vivo in hypoxic states.

Hypophosphatasia is due to deficient activity of TNAP, consequently with effects including limitation of hydrolysis PP$_i$ to generate P$_i$.[27a, 65-67] Generalized PP$_i$ excess in hypophosphatasia is evidenced by increased PP$_i$ excretion in urine. Enpp1 knockout mice and mice homozygous for the ENPP1 truncation mutant ttw demonstrate marked articular cartilage calcification with HA and OA, as well as ankylosing spinal ligament hyperostosis and synovial joint ossific fusion; extracellular PP$_i$ levels and mineralization disturbances in soft tissues (but not long bones) of Enpp1 knockout and TNAP-deficient mice are mutually corrected by crossbreeding.[26]

Imbalance of Chondrocyte Growth Factor Responses on PP$_i$ Metabolism in CPPD Deposition Disease

Insulin-like growth factor (IGF)-I and transforming growth actor (TGFβ) are major chondrocyte anabolic growth factors, but they have antagonistic effects on chondrocyte PPi metabolism. Specifically, TGFβ stimulates ENPP1 expression and ENPP1 movement to the plasma membrane, and ATP release by chondrocytes,[42] which stimulate increased extracellular PP$_i$.[36,65] TGFβ also stimulates ANKH expression, mediated in part by calcium entry into the cell through voltage-operated channels, and associated calcium-mediated signal transduction. The capacity of TGFβ to raise chondrocyte PP$_i$ rises with aging in humans, and TGFβ-stimulated NPP activity also does so.[69] Growth-promoting effects in articular chondrocytes of TGFβ, on the other hand, decrease with aging.[70] Moreover, TGFβ suppresses TNAP in chondrocytes, an effect mediated by P$_i$.[71]

In contrast to TGFβ, IGF-I physiologically suppresses extracellular PP$_i$ (as well as ATP release),[42] in chondrocytes[72] (see Figure 20-1). Importantly, chondrocyte IGF-I resistance develops in aging and osteoarthritic cartilages[73] (see Figure 20-1). Significantly, IGF-I induces expression of cartilage intermediate layer protein (CILP) (see Figure 20-1), and this large cartilage interterritorial matrix protein rises in expression in cartilage in aging and OA. CILP is most prevalent in the middle zone of articular cartilage, and it is this cartilage zone where CPPD crystal deposition is most abundant. The CILP-1 isoform, but not CILP-2, promotes increased extracellular PP$_i$

CHONDROCYTE HYPERTROPHY:
CHANGES PERTINENT TO
PATHOLOGIC CALCIFICATION AND OSTEOARTHRITIS

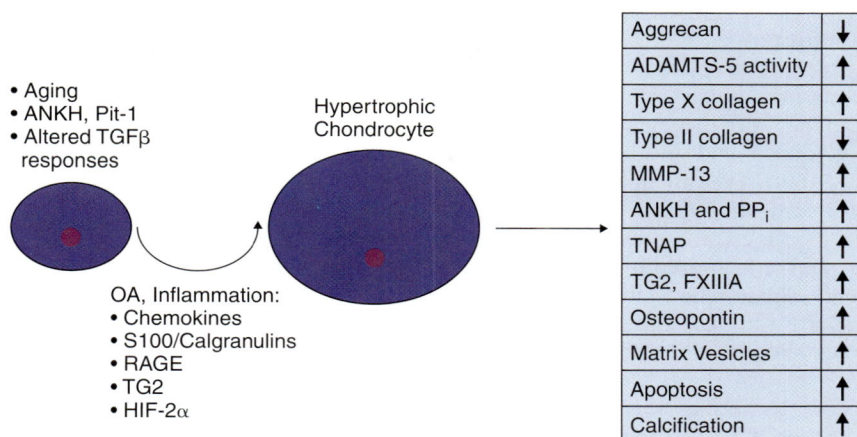

Figure 20-3 Factors that promote chondrocyte hypertrophy in articular cartilage and the effects of chondrocyte on articular cartilage germane to CPPD deposition disease. Since hypertrophic (and apoptotic) chondrocytes are observed adjacent to calcifications in joint cartilages, this figure provides a partial listing of major forces that promote chondrocyte maturation to hypertrophy held to be operative in osteoarthritis. Chondrocyte hypertrophy clearly is a differentiation state specialized for calcification via the characteristics listed in the schematic, which are discussed in detail in the text. Enhanced release of matrix vesicles and the increased susceptibility of hypertrophic chondrocytes to apoptotic death are among the factors that promote pathologic calcification. It should be noted that chondrocyte hypertrophy as a driving force for CPPD crystal deposition is neither universally accepted nor adequately established, as reviewed and discussed in detail in Chapter 1.

in chondrocytes in an indirect manner by inhibiting IGF-I signaling at the receptor level.[73]

It should be noted that the inflammatory cytokine IL-1β, whose expression rises in OA, and which promotes OA progression, also suppresses both ENPP1 expression and extracellular PP_i in chondrocytes. IL-1β also inhibits the effects of TGFβ on PP_i.[36,68]

Inflammation, Hypertrophic Chondrocyte Differentiation, and Transglutaminase 2 in Joint Cartilage Calcification

Changes in chondrocyte differentiation and viability appear to promote joint cartilage calcification, not simply OA.[74] Multifocal development of chondrocyte maturation to hypertrophy[74] is found in OA, and also chondrocyte hypertrophy is seen adjacent to CPPD crystal deposits.[75,76] Chapter 1 presents several arguments against chondrocyte hypertrophy being central in CPPD crystal deposition disease, including the fact that TNAP, which promotes PP_i hydrolysis and dissolution of CPPD crystals, is actually upregulated in hypertrophic chondrocytes. On the other hand, articular chondrocyte hypertrophy[74] (Figure 20-3) is associated with ANKH expression as a marker (at least in growth plate cartilage), increased PP_i elaboration, and increased release of matrix vesicles,[77] and certain other calcification-promoting changes such as increased expression of certain transglutaminases (transglutaminase 2 [TG2] and FXIIIA) and of osteopontin (which promote CPPD crystal formation) and loss of physiologic extracellular matrix composition that suppresses calcification.[78] Significantly, changes in TGFβ signal transduction in aging (and OA) likely are involved in promoting chondrocyte maturation to hypertrophy.[79] One can strongly argue that the

key studies linking chondrocyte hypertrophy to CPPD deposition have not yet been done, since the classic hypertrophy marker type X collagen has not been analyzed in situ. Moreover, it is possible that CPPD crystals deposited in chondrons of hypertrophic chondrocytes eventually kill such chondrocytes, making the chondrocyte characterization problematic.

Other changes that can promote chondrocyte hypertrophy and apoptosis include P_i taken up by Pit-1 sodium-dependent cotransport, calcium sensing by the calcium sensing receptor, and responses to TGFβ that regulate PP_i.[11,35,55,80-82] Increased PTHrP expression in cartilage also could turn on endochondral-type differentiation changes in articular chondrocytes that promote calcification.[19] Chondrocyte apoptosis also promotes calcification, and this is in part due to the release of apoptotic bodies that function as calcifying "inside-out" matrix vesicles.[82-84]

Inflammation-associated chondrocyte hypertrophy is driven by a variety of inflammation-modulated pathways, such as through hypoxia inducible factor-2α and Indian hedgehog,[74] and the effects of multiple cytokines and calgranulins, oxidative stress, P_i transport, RAGE signaling, and release of TG2. Moreover, IL-1β stimulates articular chondrocytes to calcify extracellular matrix,[69,78] an effect mediated through induction of nitric oxide (NO),[83] alterations in extracellular matrix, and induction of increased chondrocyte TG activity mediated dually via the TG family enzymes factor XIIIA and TG2.[69,78] TG2 and factor XIIIA function in part to cross-link proteins by transamidation. Both transglutaminases are markers of chondrocyte hypertrophy,[69,78] and there is upregulated TG2 and factor XIIIA in hypertrophic chondrocytes in OA cartilage.[69] Increased factor XIIIA and TG2 stimulate calcification by chondrocytes,[69] and OA severity-linked and age-dependent IL-1–induced increases in TG activity occur in chondrocytes from human knee menisci.[69] TG2 drives the capacity of IL-1β to stimulate articular chondrocytes to calcify in vitro.[78] TG2-independent and TG2-dependent mechanisms promote articular chondrocyte hypertrophy and calcification in vitro, and increased TG2 release is sufficient to promote chondrocyte hypertrophy.[78,85,86]

Other inflammatory pathways that promote chondrocyte hypertrophy include effects of S100/calgranulins, a class of small, calcium-binding polypeptides through the multiligand receptor for advanced glycation end products (RAGE).[87] CXCL8 and TNFα induce S100A11 release in chondrocytes,[87] and S100A11 induces chondrocyte hypertrophy in vitro,[88] dependent on S100A11 homodimerization catalyzed by TG2-mediated transamidation, and antagonized by the alternative S100A11 receptor CD36.[88,89] Chemokine-induced and TNFα-induced chondrocyte hypertrophy also have been demonstrated to require RAGE signaling.[87]

Pathogenic Features of CPPD Deposition Disease in Primary Metabolic Disorders: Relationship to PP$_i$ Metabolism and Chondrocyte Differentiation

Not only hypophosphatasia, but also hypomagnesemic conditions (such as Gitelman's variant of Bartter syndrome), and also apparently thiazide diuretic use, are associated with CPPD deposition disease.[90] Hemochromatosis and hyperparathyroidism are characterized primary metabolic disorders linked with secondary CPPD crystal deposition disease.[91] Increased joint fluid PP$_i$ levels, as has been described in each of these conditions, suggests at least one shared mechanism in the pathogenesis of chondrocalcinosis via cartilage PP$_I$ excess.[92] Magnesium is a cofactor in pyrophosphatase activity. Conversely, iron excess can suppress pyrophosphatase activity. Hypercalcemia likely promotes CPPD crystal deposition in hyperparathyroidism (and in familial hypocalciuric hypercalcemia),[93] by effects beyond those on cartilage matrix supersaturation with ionized calcium. These include calcium service as a cofactor in ENPP1 catalytic activity; in addition, chondrocyte-activating effects mediated by the calcium-sensing receptor may be at play.[29] Pertinent to hyperparathyroidism, articular chondrocytes express parathyroid hormone/parathyroid hormone–related protein (PTH/PTHrP) receptors, Last, the functional PTH responses of chondrocytes of proliferation, altered matrix synthesis, and calcification[94,95] likely promote CPPD deposition disease in hyperparathyroidism.

CPPD Crystal–Induced Inflammation

CPPD crystals primarily deposited in joint cartilages can traffic to synovial fluid and synovium, and CPPD crystals can directly stimulate chondrocytes, synovial lining cells, and intraarticular phagocytes.[96-102] CPPD crystals unequivocally stimulate inflammation that can promote cartilage matrix degradation and thereby contribute to the progression of OA.[96-102] Many of the inflammatory mechanisms active in gout (see Chapter 5) also appear to be involved in synovitis and cartilage degeneration associated with CPPD crystal deposition disease.[96-102] For example, CPPD crystals activate cells in part via innate immune mechanisms through complement activation and Toll-like receptor 2 (TLR2) activation.[103] CPPD-triggered signal transduction pathways include mitogen-activated protein kinases, activation of cyclooxygenase-derived and lipooxygenase-derived metabolites of arachidonic acid, and induction of cytokines (e.g., TNFα, IL-1, and CXCL8).[96-102] Importantly, CPPD crystal–induced activation of the cytosolic NLRP3 (cryopyrin) inflammasome stimulates caspase-1 activation and IL-1β processing and release, a central mechanism that drives cellular responses to CPPD crystals in vitro and CPPD crystal–induced inflammation in vivo.[104] As in gout, CPPD crystal–induced neutrophil ingress into the joint space is at the core of the execution phase of acute crystal-induced synovitis. In this context, IL-8/CXCL8 and related chemokines that bind the receptor CXCR2 appear to be central to neutrophil ingress in acute CPPD crystal–induced inflammation.[105] Likewise, as in gout, colchicine effects on neutrophil–endothelial adhesion likely are a primary locus for prophylactic effects of low concentrations of colchicine for acute pseudogout.[106]

References

1. Zaka R, Williams CJ. Genetics of chondrocalcinosis. Osteoarthritis Cartilage 2005;13(9):745–50.
2. Pons-Estel BA, Gimenez C, Sacnun M, et al. Familial osteoarthritis and Milwaukee shoulder associated with calcium pyrophosphate and apatite crystal deposition. J Rheumatol 2000;27(2):471–80.
3. Pendleton A, Johnson MD, Hughes A, et al. Mutations in ANKH cause chondrocalcinosis. Am J Hum Genet 2002;71(4):933–40.
4. Williams JC, Zhang Y, Timms A, et al. Autosomal dominant familial calcium pyrophosphate dihydrate deposition disease is caused by mutation in the transmembrane protein ANKH. Am J Hum Genet 2002;71(4):985–91.
5. Abhishek A, Doherty M. Pathophysiology of articular chondrocalcinosis: role of ANKH. Nat Rev Rheumatol 2010 Nov 23:[Epub ahead of print].
6. Reginato AJ, Passano GM, Neumann G, et al. Familial spondyloepiphyseal dysplasia tarda, brachydactyly, and precocious osteoarthritis associated with an arginine 75→cysteine mutation in the procollagen type II gene in a kindred of Chiloe Islanders. I. Clinical, radiographic, and pathologic findings. Arthritis Rheum 1994;37(7):1078–86.
7. Bruges-Armas J. Couto AR, Timms A, et al. Ectopic calcification among families in the Azores: clinical and radiologic manifestations in families with diffuse idiopathic skeletal hyperostosis and chondrocalcinosis. Arthritis Rheum 2006;54(4):1340–9.
8. Mandel N, Mandel G. Calcium pyrophosphate crystal deposition in model systems. Rheum Dis Clin North Am 1988;14(2):321–40.
9. Hunter GK, Grynpas MD, Cheng PT, et al. Effect of glycosaminoglycans on calcium pyrophosphate crystal formation in collagen gels. Calcif Tissue Int 1987;41(3):164–70.
10. Cheng PT, Pritzker KP. Inhibition of calcium pyrophosphate dihydrate crystal formation: effects of carboxylate ions. Calcif Tissue Int 1988;42(1):46–52.
11. Pritzker KP. Calcium pyrophosphate crystal arthropathy: a biomineralization disorder. Hum Pathol 1986;17(6):543–5.
12. Terkeltaub R. Inorganic pyrophosphate (PP$_i$) generation and disposition in pathophysiology. Am J Physiol Cell Physiol 2001;281(7):C1–11.
13. Jubeck B, Gohr C, Fahey M, et al. Promotion of articular cartilage matrix vesicle mineralization by type I collagen. Arthritis Rheum 2008;58(9):2809–17.
14. Pritzker KP, Cheng PT, Omar SA, Nyburg SC. Calcium pyrophosphate crystal formation in model hydrogels. II. Hyaline articular cartilage as a gel. J Rheumatol 1981;8(3):451–5.
15. Pritzker KP, Cheng PT, Adams ME, Nyburg SC. Calcium pyrophosphate dihydrate crystal formation in model hydrogels. J Rheumatol 1978;5(4):469–73.
16. Cheng PT, Pritzker KP. Pyrophosphate, phosphate ion interaction: effects on calcium pyrophosphate and calcium hydroxyapatite crystal formation in aqueous solutions. J Rheumatol 1983;10(5):769–77.
17. Cheng PT, Pritzker KP. Ferrous [Fe2=] but not ferric [Fe] ions inhibit de novo formation of calcium pyrophosphate dihydrate crystals: possible relationships to chondrocalcinosis and hemochromatosis. J Rheumatol 1988;15(2):321–4.
18. Cheng PT, Pritzker KP. The effect of calcium and magnesium ions on calcium pyrophosphate crystal formation in aqueous solutions. J Rheumatol 1981;8(5):772–82.

19. Swan A, Heywood B, Chapman B, et al. Evidence for a causal relationship between the structure, size, and load of calcium pyrophosphate dihydrate crystals, and attacks of pseudogout. Ann Rheum Dis 1995;54(10):825–30.

20. Mandel GS, Halverson PB, Rathburn M, et al. Calcium pyrophosphate crystal deposition: a kinetic study using a type I collagen gel model. Scanning Microsc 1990;4(1):175–80.

21. Mandel N, Mandel G. Calcium pyrophosphate crystal deposition in model systems. Rheum Dis Clin North Am 1988;14(2):321–40.

22. Fahey M, Mitton E, Muth E, et al. Dexamethasone promotes calcium pyrophosphate dihydrate crystal formation by articular chondrocytes. J Rheumatol 2009;36(1):163–9.

23. Rosenthal AK, Gohr CM, Uzuki M, et al. Osteopontin promotes pathologic mineralization in articular cartilage. Matrix Biol 2007;26(2):96–105.

24. Anderson HC, Mulhall D, Garimella R. Role of extra cellular membrane vesicles in the pathogenesis of various diseases, including cancer, renal diseases, atherosclerosis, and arthritis. Lab Invest 2010;90(11):1549-47.

25. Kirsch T, Wang W, Pfander D. Functional differences between growth plate apoptotic bodies and matrix vesicles. J Bone Miner Res 2003;18(10):1872–81.

26. Thouverey C, Bechkoff G, Pikula S, et al. Inorganic pyrophosphate as a regulator of hydroxyapatite or calcium pyrophosphate dihydrate mineral deposition by matrix vesicles. Osteoarthritis Cartilage 2009;17(1):64–72.

27. Johnson K, Goding J, van Etten D, et al. Linked deficiencies in extracellular inorganic pyrophosphate and osteopontin expression mediate pathologic calcification in PC-1 null mice. Am J Bone Miner Res 2003;18(6):994–1004.

27a. Hessle L, Johnson KA, Anderson HC, et al. Tissue-nonspecific alkaline phosphatase and plasma cell membrane glycoprotein-1 are central antagonistic regulators of bone mineralization. Proc Natl Acad Sci U S A 2002;99(14):9445–9.

28. Wang D, Canaff L, Davidson D, et al. Alterations in the sensing and transport of phosphate and calcium by differentiating chondrocytes. J Biol Chem 2001;276(36):33995–4005.

29. Burton DW, Foster M, Johnson KA, et al. Chondrocyte calcium-sensing receptor expression is up-regulated in early guinea pig knee osteoarthritis and modulates PTHrP, MMP-13, and TIMP-3 expression. Osteoarthritis Cartilage 2005;13(5):395–404.

30. Johnson K, Terkeltaub R. Upregulated ank expression in osteoarthritis can promote both chondrocyte MMP-13 expression and calcification via chondrocyte extracellular PPi excess. Osteoarthritis Cartilage 2004;12(4):321–35.

31. Johnson K, Polewski M, van Etten D, et al. Chondrogenesis mediated by PPi depletion promotes spontaneous aortic calcification in NPP1-/- mice. Arterioscler Thromb Vasc Biol 2005;25(4):686–91.

32. Johnson K, Pritzker K, Goding J, et al. The nucleoside triphosphate pyrophosphohydrolase (NTPPPH) isozyme PC-1 directly promotes cartilage calcification through chondrocyte apoptosis and increased calcium precipitation by mineralizing vesicles. J Rheumatol 2001;28(12):2681–91.

33. Rutsch F, Ruf N, Vaingankar S, et al. Mutations in ENPP1 are associated with 'idiopathic' infantile arterial calcification. Nat Genet 2003;34(4):379–81.

34. Pritzker KP, Cheng PT, Renlund RC. Calcium pyrophosphate crystal deposition in hyaline cartilage. Ultrastructural analysis and implications for pathogenesis. J Rheumatol 1988;15(5):828–35.

35. Johnson K, Hashimoto S, Lotz M, et al. Up-regulated expression of the phosphodiesterase nucleotide pyrophosphatase family member PC-1 is a marker and pathogenic factor for knee meniscal cartilage matrix calcification. Arthritis Rheum 2001;44(5):1071–81.

36. Johnson K, Vaingankar S, Chen Y, et al. Differential mechanisms of inorganic pyrophosphate production by plasma cell membrane glycoprotein-1 and B10 in chondrocytes. Arthritis Rheum 1999;42(1):1986–97.

37. Pattrick M, Hamilton E, Hornby J, et al. Synovial fluid pyrophosphate and nucleoside triphosphate pyrophosphatase: comparison between normal and diseased and between inflamed and non-inflamed joints. Ann Rheum Dis 1991;50(4):214–8.

38. Ho A, Johnson M, Kingsley DM. Role of the mouse ank gene in tissue calcification and arthritis. Science 2000;289(5477):265–70.

39. Zaka R, Stokes D, Dion AS, et al. P5L mutation in Ank results in an increase in extracellular PPi during proliferation and non-mineralizing hypertrophy in stably transduced ATDC5 cells. Arthritis Res Ther 2006;8:R164.

40. Williams CJ, Pendleton A, Bonavita G, et al. Mutations in the amino terminus of ANKH in two US families with calcium pyrophosphate dihydrate crystal deposition disease. Arthritis Rheum 2003;48(4):2627–31.

41. Gurley KA, Reimer RJ, Kingsley DM. Biochemical and genetic analysis of ANK in arthritis and bone disease. Am J Hum Genet 2006;79(6):1017–29.

42. Costello JC, Rosenthal AK, Kurup IV, et al. Parallel regulation of extracellular ATP and inorganic pyrophosphate: roles of growth factors, transduction modulators, and ANK. Connect Tiss Res 2010; Jul 6:[Epub ahead of print].

43. Wang J, Tsui HW, Beier F, et al. The CPPDD-associated ANKH M48T mutation interrupts the interaction of ANKH with the sodium/phosphate cotransporter PiT-1. J Rheumatol 2009;36(6):1265–72.

44. Zhang Y, Johnson K, Russell RG, et al. Association of sporadic chondrocalcinosis with a -4-basepair G-to-A transition in the 5'-untranslated region of ANKH that promotes enhanced expression of ANKH protein and excess generation of extracellular inorganic pyrophosphate. Arthritis Rheum 2005;52(4):1110–7.

45. Zaka R, Dion AS, Kusnierz A, et al. Oxygen tension regulates the expression of ANK (progressive ankylosis) in an HIF-1-dependent manner in growth plate chondrocytes. J Bone Miner Res 2009;24(11):1869–78.

46. Wang W, Xu J, Du B, et al. Role of the progressive ankylosis gene (ank) in cartilage mineralization. Mol Cell Biol 2005;25(1):312–23.

47. Nürnberg P, Thiele H, Chandler D, et al. Heterozygous mutations in ANKH, the human ortholog of the mouse progressive ankylosis gene, result in craniometaphyseal dysplasia. Nat Genet 2001;28(1):37–41.

48. Chen IP, Wang CJ, Strecker S. Introduction of a Phe377del mutation in ANK creates a mouse model for craniometaphyseal dysplasia. J Bone Miner Res 2009;24(7):1206–15.

49. Morava E, Kohnisch J, Drijvers JM, et al. Autosomal recessive mental retardation, deafness, ankylosis, and mild hypophosphatemia associated with a novel ANKH mutation in a consanguineous family. J Clin Endocrinol Metab 2010; Oct 13:[Epub ahead of print].

50. Cheung CL, Livshits G, Zhou Y. Hip geometry variation is associated with bone mineralization pathway gene variants: the Framingham Study. J Bone Miner Res 2009 Nov 5:[Epub ahead of print].

51. Kiel DP, Demissie S, Dupuis J. Genome-wide association with bone mass and geometry in the Framingham Heart Study. BMC Med Genet 2007;8(Suppl. 1):S14.

52. Malkin I, Ermakov S, Kobyliansky E. Strong association between polymorphisms in ANKH locus and skeletal size traits. Hum Genet 2006;120(1):42–51.

53. Wang J, Wang C, Tsui HW. Microcytosis in ank/ank mice and the role of ANKH in promoting erythroid differentiation. Exp Cell Res 2007;313(20):4120–9.

54. Lust G, Faure G, Netter P, et al. Increased pyrophosphate in fibroblasts and lymphoblasts from patients with hereditary diffuse articular chondrocalcinosis. Science 1981;214(4522):809–10.

55. Cecil DL, Rose DM, Terkeltaub R, et al. Role of interleukin-8 in PiT-1 expression and CXCR1-mediated inorganic phosphate uptake in chondrocytes [Erratum in: Arthritis Rheum 2006;54:2320]. Arthritis Rheum 2005;52(1):144–54.

56. Alini M, Carey D, Hirata S. Cellular and matrix changes before and at the time of calcification in the growth plate studied in vitro: arrest of type X collagen synthesis and net loss of collagen when calcification is initiated. J Bone Miner Res 1994;9(7):1077–87.

57. Wang J, Tsui HW, Beier F, et al. The ANKH deltaE490 mutation in calcium pyrophosphate dihydrate crystal deposition disease (CPPDD) affects tissue non-specific alkaline phosphatase (TNAP) activities. Open Rheumatol J 2008;2:23–30:Epub 2008 Apr 10.

58. Williams CJ, Pendleton A, Bonavita G, et al. Mutations in the amino terminus of ANKH in two US families with calcium pyrophosphate dihydrate crystal deposition disease. Arthritis Rheum 2003;48(9):2627–31.

59. Xu Y, Cruz TF, Pritzker KP. Alkaline phosphatase dissolves calcium pyrophosphate dihydrate crystals. J Rheumatol 1991;18(10):1606–10.

60. Shinozaki T, Pritzker KP. Regulation of alkaline phosphatase: implications for calcium pyrophosphate dihydrate crystal dissolution and other alkaline phosphatase functions. J Rheumatol 1996;23(4):677–83.

61. Xu Y, Pritzker KP, Cruz TF. Characterization of chondrocyte alkaline phosphatase as a potential mediator in the dissolution of calcium pyrophosphate dihydrate crystals. J Rheumatol 1994;21(5):912–9.

62. Shinozaki T, Xu Y, Cruz TF, et al. Calcium pyrophosphate dihydrate (CPPD) crystal dissolution by alkaline phosphatase: interaction of alkaline phosphatase on CPPD crystals. J Rheumatol 1995;22(1):117–23.

63. So PP, Tsui FW, Vieth R, et al. Inhibition of alkaline phosphatase by cysteine: implications for calcium pyrophosphate dihydrate crystal deposition disease. J Rheumatol 2007;34(6):1313–22.

64. Kannampuzha JV, Tupy JH, Pritzker KP. Mercaptopyruvate inhibits tissue-specific alkaline phosphatase and calcium pyrophosphate dihydrate crystal dissolution. J Rheumatol 2009;36(12):2758–65.

65. Chuck AJ, Pattrick MG, Hamilton E, et al. Crystal deposition in hypophosphatasia: a reappraisal. Ann Rheum Dis 1989;48(7):571–6.

66. Eade AW, Swannell AJ, Williamson N. Pyrophosphate arthropathy in hypophosphatasia. Ann Rheum Dis 1981;40:164–70.

67. O'Duffy JD. Hypophosphatasia associated with calcium pyrophosphate dihydrate deposits in cartilage. Report of a case. Arthritis Rheum 1970;13(4):381–8.
68. Lotz M, Rosen F, McCabe G, et al. Interleukin 1 beta suppresses transforming growth factor-induced inorganic pyrophosphate [PP_i] production and expression of the PP_i-generating enzyme PC-1 in human chondrocytes. Proc Natl Acad Sci U S A 1995;92(22):10364–8.
69. Johnson K, Hashimoto S, Lotz M, et al. IL-1 induces pro-mineralizing activity of cartilage tissue transglutaminase and factor XIIIa. Am J Pathol 2001;159(1):149–63.
70. Rosen F, McCabe G, Quach J, et al. Differential effects of aging on human chondrocyte responses to transforming growth factor beta: increased pyrophosphate production and decreased cell proliferation. Arthritis Rheum 1997;40(7):1275–81.
71. Hamade T, Bianchi A, Sebillaud S, et al. Inorganic phosphate (Pi) modulates the expression of key regulatory proteins of the inorganic pyrophosphate (PPi) metabolism in TGFβ1-stimulated chondrocytes. Biomed Mater Eng 2010;20(3-4):209–15.
72. Olmez U, Ryan LM, Kurup IV, et al. Insulin-like growth factor-1 suppresses pyrophosphate elaboration by transforming growth factor beta1-stimulated chondrocytes and cartilage. Osteoarthritis Cartilage 1994;2(3):149–54.
73. Johnson K, Farley D, Hu S-I, et al. One of two chondrocyte-expressed isoforms of cartilage intermediate layer protein functions as an IGF-I antagonist. Arthritis Rheum 2003;48(5):1302–14.
74. Husa M, Liu-Bryan R, Terkeltaub R. Shifting HIFs in osteoarthritis [Erratum in: Nat Med 2010;16(6):828]. Nat Med 2010;16:641–4.
75. Kirsch T, Swoboda B, Nah H. Activation of annexin II and V expression, terminal differentiation, mineralization and apoptosis in human osteoarthritic cartilage. Osteoarthritis Cartilage 2000;8(4):294–302.
76. Masuda I, Ishikawa K, Usuku G. A histologic and immunohistochemical study of calcium pyrophosphate dihydrate crystal deposition disease. Clin Orthop 1991;263:272–87.
77. Kirsch T, Nah HD, Shapiro IM, et al. Regulated production of mineralization competent matrix vesicles in hypertrophic chondrocytes. J Cell Biol 1997;137(5):1149–60.
78. Johnson K, Van Etten D, Nanda N, et al. Distinct transglutaminase II/TG2-independent and TG2-dependent pathways mediate articular chondrocyte hypertrophy. J Biol Chem 2003;278(21):18824–32.
79. Serra R, Johnson M, Filvaroff EH, et al. Expression of a truncated, kinase-defective TGF-beta type II receptor in mouse skeletal tissue promotes terminal chondrocyte differentiation and osteoarthritis. J Cell Biol 1997;139(2):541–52.
80. Adams CS, Shapiro IM. The fate of the terminally differentiated chondrocyte: evidence for microenvironmental regulation of chondrocyte apoptosis. Crit Rev Oral Biol Med 2002;13(6):465–73.
81. Adams CS, Mansfield K, Perlot RL, et al. Matrix regulation of skeletal cell apoptosis. Role of calcium and phosphate ions. J Biol Chem 2001;276(23):20316–22.
82. Hashimoto S, Ochs RL, Rosen F, et al. Chondrocyte-derived apoptotic bodies and calcification of articular cartilage. Proc Natl Acad Sci U S A 1998;95(6):3094–9.
83. Cheung HS, Ryan LM. Phosphocitrate blocks nitric oxide-induced calcification of cartilage and chondrocyte-derived apoptotic bodies. Osteoarthritis Cartilage 1999;7(4):409–12.
84. Kirsch T, Wang W, Pfander D. Functional differences between growth plate apoptotic bodies and matrix vesicles. J Bone Miner Res 2003;18(10):1872–81.
85. Merz D, Liu R, Johnson K, et al. IL-8/CXCL8 and growth-related oncogene alpha/CXCL1 induce chondrocyte hypertrophic differentiation. J Immunol 2003;171(8):4406–15.
86. Johnson KA, Terkeltaub RA. External GTP-bound transglutaminase 2 is a molecular switch for chondrocyte hypertrophic differentiation and calcification. J Biol Chem 2005;280(15):15004–12.
87. Cecil DL, Johnson K, Rediske J, et al. Inflammation-induced chondrocyte hypertrophy is driven by receptor for advanced glycation end products. J Immunol 2005;175(12):8296–302.
88. Cecil DL, Appleton CT, Polewski MD, et al. The pattern recognition receptor CD36 is a chondrocyte hypertrophy marker associated with suppression of catabolic responses and promotion of repair responses to inflammatory stimuli. J Immunol 2009;182(8):5024–31.
89. Cecil DL, Terkeltaub R. Transamidation by transglutaminase 2 transforms S100A11 calgranulin into a procatabolic cytokine for chondrocytes. J Immunol 2008;180(12):8378–85.
90. Richette P, Bardin T, Doherty M. An update on the epidemiology of calcium pyrophosphate dihydrate crystal deposition disease. Rheumatology (Oxford) 2009;48(7):711–5.
91. Jones AC, Chuck AJ, Arie EA, et al. Diseases associated with calcium pyrophosphate deposition disease. Semin Arthritis Rheum 1992;22(3):188–202.
92. Doherty M, Belcher C, Regan M, et al. Association between synovial fluid levels of inorganic pyrophosphate and short term radiographic outcome of knee osteoarthritis. Ann Rheum Dis 1996;55(7):432–6.
93. Volpe A, Guerriero A, Marchetta A, et al. Familial hypocalciuric hypercalcemia revealed by chondrocalcinosis. Joint Bone Spine 2009;76(6):708–10.
94. Terkeltaub R, Lotz M, Johnson K, et al. Parathyroid hormone related protein (PTHrP) expression is abundant in osteoarthritic cartilage, and the PTHrP 1-173 isoform is selectively induced by TGFβ in articular chondrocytes, and suppresses extracellular inorganic pyrophosphate generation. Arthritis Rheum 1998;41(12):2152–64.
95. Goomer R, Johnson K, Burton D, et al. A tetrabasic C-terminal motif determines intracrine regulatory effects of PTHrP 1-173 on PP_i metabolism and collagen synthesis in chondrocytes. Endocrinology 2000;141:4613–22.
96. Liu R, O'Connell M, Johnson K, et al. Extracellular signal-regulated kinase 1/extracellular signal-regulated kinase 2 mitogen-activated protein kinase signaling and activation of activator protein 1 and nuclear factor kappaB transcription factors play central roles in interleukin-8 expression stimulated by monosodium urate monohydrate and calcium pyrophosphate crystals in monocytic cells. Arthritis Rheum 2000;43(5):1145–55.
97. Morgan MP, McCarthy GM. Signaling mechanisms involved in crystal-induced tissue damage. Curr Opin Rheumatol 2002;14(3):292–7.
98. Sun Y, Wenger L, Brinckerhoff CE, et al. Basic calcium phosphate crystals induce matrix metalloproteinase-1 through the Ras/mitogen-activated protein kinase/c-Fos/AP-1/metalloproteinase 1 pathway. Involvement of transcription factor binding sites AP-1 and PEA-3. J Biol Chem 2002;277(2):1544–52.
99. Molloy ES, Morgan MP, Doherty GA, et al. Microsomal prostaglandin E2 synthase 1 expression in basic calcium phosphate crystal-stimulated fibroblasts: role of prostaglandin E2 and the EP4 receptor. Osteoarthritis Cartilage 2009;17(5):686–92.
100. Molloy ES, Morgan MP, Doherty GA, et al. Mechanism of basic calcium phosphate crystal-stimulated cyclo-oxygenase-1 up-regulation in osteoarthritic synovial fibroblasts. Rheumatology (Oxford) 2008;47(7):965–71.
101. Molloy ES, Morgan MP, Doherty GA, et al. Mechanism of basic calcium phosphate crystal-stimulated matrix metalloproteinase-13 expression by osteoarthritic synovial fibroblasts: inhibition by prostaglandin E2. Ann Rheum Dis 2008;67(12):1773–9.
102. Molloy ES, Morgan MP, McDonnell B, et al. BCP crystals increase prostacyclin production and upregulate the prostacyclin receptor in OA synovial fibroblasts: potential effects on mPGES1 and MMP-13. Osteoarthritis Cartilage 2007;15(4):414–20.
103. Liu-Bryan R, Pritzker K, Firestein GS, et al. TLR2 signaling in chondrocytes drives calcium pyrophosphate dihydrate and monosodium urate crystal-induced nitric oxide generation. J Immunol 2005;174(8):5016–23.
104. Martinon F, Petrilli V, Mayor A, et al. Gout-associated uric acid crystals activate the NALP3 inflammasome. Nature 2006;440:237–41.
105. Terkeltaub R, Baird S, Sears P, et al. The murine homolog of the interleukin-8 receptor CXCR-2 is essential for the occurrence of neutrophilic inflammation in the air pouch model of acute urate crystal-induced gouty synovitis. Arthritis Rheum 1998;41(5):900–9.
106. Cronstein BN, Molad Y, Reibman J, et al. Colchicine alters the quantitative and qualitative display of selectins on endothelial cells and neutrophils. J Clin Invest 1995;96(2):994–1002.

Calcium Pyrophosphate Dihydrate Crystal Deposition: Epidemiology, Clinical Features, Diagnosis, and Treatment

Pierre-André Guerne and Robert Terkeltaub

KEY POINTS

- Calcium pyrophosphate dihydrate (CPPD) crystal deposition is a metabolic disorder that manifests substantially more often as joint pathology than it does as a symptomatic arthropathy.

- The vast majority of CPPD crystal deposition is idiopathic/sporadic and is a disorder linked to aging, but other factors that promote CPPD deposition include prior joint trauma, osteoarthritis (OA), and possibly hypomagnesemia associated with diuretic use.

- Diagnosis of CPPD deposition prior to age 50 to 55, particularly if CPPD deposition is widespread, should prompt differential diagnostic consideration of a primary metabolic disease (e.g., hemochromatosis, hyperparathyroidism, hypomagnesemia) or a familial disorder.

- CPPD crystal deposition disease is a tremendous mimic and can clinically resemble (or coexist with) gout, septic arthritis, primary OA, and rheumatoid arthritis.

- Chronic degenerative arthropathy in CPPD deposition commonly affects certain joints that are typically spared in primary OA, such as the metacarpophalangeal, wrist, and elbow joints.

- Pseudogout is a major cause of acute monoarticular or oligoarticular arthritis in the elderly. The attacks typically involve a large joint, most often the knee, and less often the wrist or ankle; unlike gout, pseudogout rarely involves the first metatarsophalangeal joint.

- Definitive diagnosis of CPPD crystal deposition requires demonstration of CPPD crystals (in synovial fluid or biopsy), typical calcifications on plain radiographs, and/or typical findings for CPPD crystal deposition in articular hyaline cartilage or fibrocartilage by high-resolution ultrasound. However, ultrasound is incompletely sensitive, diagnostic criteria are not fully validated, and false-positive and -negative results occur with ultrasound.

- The guidelines for treatment of attacks of acute pseudogout in CPPD crystal deposition disease are predominantly expert opinion–based rather than evidence-based and have been modeled on treatment of acute gout.

- Pseudogout can respond to nonsteroidal antiinflammatory drugs (NSAIDs) (or selective cyclooxygenase-2 inhibitors) and to colchicine but sometimes more slowly and, overall, less consistently than for acute gout treatment. Since comorbidities in the elderly often limit the aforementioned modalities, systemic glucocorticosteroids or intraarticular steroids, typically given as described for acute gout attack, are useful and broadly effective primary treatment choices in acute pseudogout and valuable in refractory cases.

- Low-dose daily colchicine or NSAID prophylaxis, prescribed as is done to prevent gout attacks, is a useful treatment modality.

- Hydroxychloroquine, methotrexate, and interleukin-1 antagonism have been suggested, without definitive proof, to be of some benefit to patients with refractory chronic polyarticular CPPD deposition disease. Moreover, these approaches also can have prophylactic efficacy for attacks of pseudogout.

- There remains a lack of proven therapies to both inhibit CPPD crystal deposition and to effectively preserve articular cartilage already affected by the disorder. However, the clinical course and outcomes of CPPD deposition disease are variable, and the primary idiopathic disorder is not always anatomically progressive.

Introduction

The molecular genetics, molecular epidemiology, and pathogenesis of calcium pyrophosphate dihydrate (CPPD) deposition disease are reviewed in Chapter 20, with this review focusing on clinical aspects of the condition.

The terminology, diagnostic criteria for CPPD deposition disease, and treatment strategies have recently undergone

Dr. Terkeltaub's work is supported by the VA Research Service.

Table 21-1 EULAR Consensus Propositions and Strength of Recommendation (SOR), Ordered According to Topic (Clinical Features, Synovial Fluid Testing, Imaging, Comorbidities, and Risk Factors)

No.	Proposition	LoE	SOR (95% CI)
1	Although often asymptomatic, CPPD can present variable clinical phenotypes, most commonly OA with CPPD, acute CPP crystal arthritis and chronic inflammatory arthritis.	IIb	90 (86 to 94)
2	The rapid development of severe joint pain, swelling and tenderness that reaches its maximum within 6 to 24 hours, especially with overlying erythema, is highly suggestive of acute crystal inflammation though not specific for acute CPP crystal arthritis.	IV	88 (84 to 93)
3	Presentation with features suggesting crystal inflammation involving the knee, wrist or shoulder of a patient over age 65 years is likely to be acute CPP crystal arthritis. The presence of radiographic CC and advanced age increases this likelihood, but definitive diagnosis needs to be crystal proven.	IIb	81 (74 to 89)
4	OA with CPPD particularly targets knees with chronic symptoms and/or acute attacks of crystal-induced inflammation. Compared to OA without CPPD, it may associate with more inflammatory symptoms and signs, an atypical distribution (e.g., radiocarpal or midcarpal, glenohumeral, hindfoot or midfoot involvement) and prominent cyst and osteophyte formation on radiographs.	Ib/IIb	53 (38 to 68)
5	Chronic CPP crystal inflammatory arthritis presents as chronic oligoarthritis or polyarthritis with inflammatory symptoms and signs and occasional systemic upset (with elevation of CRP and ESR); superimposed flares with characteristics of crystal inflammation support this diagnosis. It should be considered in the differential diagnosis of rheumatoid arthritis and other chronic inflammatory joint diseases in older adults. Radiographs may assist diagnosis, but the diagnosis should be crystal proven.	IIb	83 (72 to 93)
6	Definitive diagnosis of CPPD is by identification of characteristic CPP crystals (parallelepipedic, predominantly intracellular crystals with absent or weak positive birefringence) in synovial fluid, or occasionally biopsied tissue.	Ib	94 (90 to 97)
7	A routine search for CPP (and urate) crystals is recommended in all synovial fluid samples obtained from undiagnosed inflamed joints, especially from knees or wrists of older patients.	IV	99 (97 to 100)
8	Radiographic CC supports the diagnosis of CPPD, but its absence does not exclude it.	IIb	97 (92 to 102)
9	Ultrasonography can demonstrate CPPD in peripheral joints, appearing typically as thin hyperechoic bands within hyaline cartilage and hyperechoic sparkling spots in fibrocartilage. Sensitivity and specificity appear excellent and possibly better than those of conventional x-rays.	IIb	78 (70 to 87)
10	Acute CPP crystal arthritis and sepsis may coexist, so when infection is suspected microbiological investigation should be performed even if CPP crystals and/or CC are identified.	III	96 (93 to 100)
11	In patients with CPPD, risk factors and associated comorbidities should be assessed, including OA, prior joint injury, predisposing metabolic disease (including hemochromatosis, primary hyperparathyroidism, hypomagnesaemia) and rare familial predisposition. Metabolic or familial predisposition should particularly be considered in younger patients (<55) and if there is florid polyarticular CC.	Ib/IIb	94 (89 to 99)

CC, Chondrocalcinosis; CPP, calcium pyrophosphate; CPPD, calcium pyrophosphate disease; ESR, erythrocyte sedimentation rate; LoE, level of evidence (Ia = meta-analysis of cohort studies, Ib = meta-analysis of case control or cross sectional studies, IIa = cohort study, IIb = case control or cross-sectional studies, III = noncomparative descriptive studies, IV = expert opinion); OA, osteoarthritis; SOR, strength of recommendation on visual analog scale (0 to 100 mm, 0 = not recommended at all, 100 = fully recommended).
From Zhang W, Doherty M, Bardin T, et al. European League Against Rheumatism recommendations for calcium pyrophosphate deposition. Part I: terminology and diagnosis. Ann Rheum Dis 2011 Jan 7 [Epub ahead of print], Table 1.

a timely, systematic examination by the European League Against Rheumatoid Arthritis (EULAR)[1,2] (Table 21-1). Several changes in terminology have been proposed,[1] but the authors' choice, in this chapter, was to use the more precise biochemical terminology for CPPD crystals, rather than the calcium pyrophosphate (CPP) terminology proposed by EULAR. In addition, this chapter uses the original, broadly employed and clinically attractive terminology for acute arthritis linked with CPPD crystals (i.e., "pseudogout"). This chapter also liberally applies the conventionally used term "chondrocalcinosis" to the major aspect of CPPD crystal deposition, with the caveat that CPPD crystallization is not the only type of pathologic calcification of articular cartilage. One difference between this chapter's viewpoint and the EULAR guidelines is that this chapter views CPPD crystal deposition as a distinct primary cause of chronic degenerative arthropathy in a distinct subset of patients beyond those with familial CPPD deposition disease. EULAR has predominantly emphasized linkages between osteoarthritis (OA) and secondary CPPD deposition as drivers of chronic joint degeneration.[1]

Epidemiology and Clinical Aspects of the Genetics of the Disorder

The vast majority of CPPD crystal deposition disease is idiopathic/sporadic and with onset in later life,[3] but heritable early-onset disease does occur, and there are genetic influences on development of late-onset disease. These issues are discussed, in Chapter 20, particularly with respect to ANKH

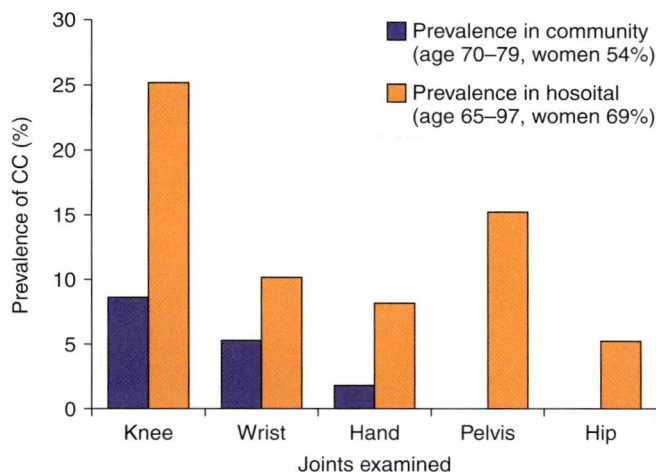

Figure 21-1 Prevalence of chondrocalcinosis in different joints. *(Reprinted from Zhang W, Doherty M, Bardin T, et al. European League Against Rheumatism recommendations for calcium pyrophosphate deposition. Part I: terminology and diagnosis. Ann Rheum Dis 2011 Jan 7 [Epub ahead of print], Fig. 1; data from Bergström G, Bjelle A, Sundh V, et al. Br J Rheumatol 1986;25:333-41, and from Wilkins E, Dieppe P, Maddison P, et al. Ann Rheum Dis 1983;42:280-4.)*

Table 21-2 Conditions and Factors Promoting or Associated With CPPD Deposition

High prevalence—strong association:
- Aging (idiopathic chondrocalcinosis, most frequent)
- Osteoarthritis (relationship with CPPD deposition probably bidirectional; see text)
- Joint trauma or knee meniscectomy

Moderate prevalence—strong association:
- Familial-genetic
- Hemochromatosis
- Primary hyperparathyroidism
- Hypomagnesemia from:
  - Gitelman syndrome (hypomagnesemia—tubular hypokalemia with hypocalciuria)
  - Malabsorption
    - Extensive small bowel resection (short bowel syndrome)
  - Certain drugs
    - Thiazidic and loop diuretics
    - Potentially also from proton pump inhibitors, tacrolimus, cyclosporine
- Hypophosphatasia

Low prevalence—questionable association (essentially based on case reports):
- X-linked hypophosphatemic rickets
- Familial hypocalciuric hypercalcemia
- Ochronosis
- Articular amyloidosis
- Myxedematous hypothyroidism
- Osteochondrodysplasias and spondyloepiphyseal dysplasias
- Wilson disease

Modified from Terkeltaub R. Diseases associated with articular deposition of calcium pyrophosphate dihydrate and basic calcium phosphate crystals. In Firestein GS et al., eds. Kelley's Textbook of Rheumatology. 8th ed. Philadelphia: Elsevier Saunders; 2009:1507-24; 1513, Table 88-2, with data from Zhang W, Doherty M, Bardin T, et al. European League Against Rheumatism recommendations for calcium pyrophosphate deposition. Part I: terminology and diagnosis. Ann Rheum Dis 2011 Jan 7 [Epub ahead of print].

in the molecular genetics of CPPD crystal deposition disease, and the low disease prevalence in Chinese in Beijing is cited later.

Most of what we know about the epidemiology of CPPD crystal deposition disease is the product of inexact science. Prior analyses of prevalence of CPPD deposition disease[4-7] were principally built on plain radiographic features characteristic of the disease, with assessments confined to only a few joints. The limits in sensitivity and specificity of this approach are profound.[4] Studies of CPPD deposition epidemiology via synovial fluid analyses (see Chapter 2) are also inherently limited. There is a need for definitive epidemiologic studies based on pathology of articular cartilages and other tissues and on imaging approaches more sensitive than plain radiography, such as high-resolution ultrasound. However, high-resolution ultrasound also has limits in sensitivity and specificity, as discussed later.

What we do know with certainty is that the prevalence of CPPD crystal deposition disease, including clinically silent disease, increases progressively with aging[4-7] (Figure 21-1, Tables 21-2 and 21-3). The idiopathic/sporadic form of CPPD crystal deposition disease uncommonly presents before age 55, except with monoarticular disease following a history of joint trauma or knee meniscectomy. Studies of prevalence of CPPD crystal deposition disease, using plain radiographs as the screening tool, have estimated higher prevalence when the hands, wrists, pelvis, and knees have been the joints surveyed. Importantly, the majority of aged patients with CPPD crystal deposition disease of the knee also have chondrocalcinosis detected by plain radiography in other joints. Involvement of the meniscal fibrocartilage of the knee was detected in 16% of women aged 80 to 89 and in 30% of women older than 89,[8] and this has been reproduced in other studies.[9] In one plain x-ray survey study of hands, wrists, pelvis, and knees of patients admitted to a geriatrics ward, chondrocalcinosis was detected in 44% of patients older than 84 and in 36% of 75- to 84-year-olds, with a prevalence of 15% in 65- to

74-year-olds.[10] Other studies of cohorts in the United Kingdom and Italy were limited to fewer joint regions (the knee, or knee and pelvis, respectively) and, predictably, gave lesser numbers for prevalence.[4-7]

In a unique, and sizeable U.K. community study, adults over age 40 had an age-, sex-, and knee pain–adjusted prevalence of knee chondrocalcinosis of 4.5%.[5] In this study, as in a meta-analysis by EULAR,[1] there was no sex predisposition (unlike in some past studies that suggested a slight female predominance). However, a strong association between OA and chondrocalcinosis was present,[5] which appeared linked more to presence of osteophytes than joint space narrowing with OA. The association between CPPD deposition disease and diuretic use in the U.K. community is potentially due to diuretic-induced hypomagnesemia.[5]

Lack of uniformity of CPPD crystal deposition disease prevalence between populations has been illuminated by a comparison of a random sample of Beijing residents aged more than 60 years old with whites in the U.S. Framingham OA Study.[10] The Chinese participants had a much lower prevalence of knee chondrocalcinosis, and wrist chondrocalcinosis was quite uncommon in the aged Chinese cohort.[10] These findings were unexpected, because there is an excess of knee OA in Beijing and because of the common association between OA and secondary chondrocalcinosis, particularly in

Table 21-3 Risk Factors and Comorbidities Associated With Calcium Pyrophosphate Dihydrate Deposition

	No. of Studies	No. of Subjects	OR (95% CI)*	References
Age (every 10 years from 40 to 90)	1	1851	2.25 (1.79 to 2.82)	91
Female gender	8	5042	0.89 (0.58 to 1.38)	3, 5, 92-97
BMI (WHO grade)	1	1851	0.90 (0.70 to 1.14)	91
Familial aggregation	2	2000	1.10 (0.58 to 2.08)	91, 98
OA	9	4517	2.66 (2.00 to 3.54)	3, 5, 92, 94, 97, 99-102
OST	3	1906	1.26 (0.76 to 2.09)	5, 103-104
JSN	4	2043	1.24 (0.91 to 1.69)	5, 99, 103, 105
Cysts	3	367	2.94 (0.92 to 4.96)	103-104, 106
Trauma/injury	1	100	5.00 (1.77 to 14.11)	107
RA	2	818	0.18 (0.08 to 0.41)	94, 108
Hyperparathyroidism	5	976	3.03 (1.15 to 8.02)	109-113
Hypomagnesemia	1	144	13.5 (2.76 to 127.3)	114
Diuretics	1	1727	2.17 (1.02 to 4.19)	5

*Meta-analysis was undertaken to pool results from multiple studies.
BMI, Body mass index; *CPPD; JSN,* joint space narrowing; *OA,* osteoarthritis; *OST,* osteophyte; *RA,* rheumatoid arthritis.

the knee joint. Whether the low prevalence of CPPD deposition in the Chinese in Beijing reflects a racial disparity, environmental influences, or both is not yet clear but is discussed further later, with respect to the relatively high levels of calcium in drinking water in Beijing.

Clinical Genetic Aspects of Epidemiology of CPPD Deposition Disease

Early-onset CPPD crystal deposition disease is variably defined as onset before age 50 or 55. Familial disease with such early onset is well recognized,[11] and sporadic early-onset disease also occurs. In such cases, exclusion of metabolic diseases as primary etiology must be done. Major chromosomal linkages with 8q and 5p are established in studies of familial CPPD crystal deposition disease. Linkage to chromosome 8q of both early-onset OA and chondrocalcinosis has been designated CCAL1, but chromosome 5p–linked chondrocalcinosis (CCAL2) appears more common and has been better characterized,[11-13] via linkage to *ANKH* on chromosome 5p studies.[11-13] Biology and molecular genetics and structure-function of ANKH, a transmembrane protein with functions in inorganic pyrophosphate (PP$_i$) transport and other cell functions, is addressed in detail in Chapter 20. Importantly, homozygosity for a single nucleotide substitution (−4 G to A) in the *ANKH* 5′-untranslated region promotes increased ANKH mRNA expression and was detected in about 4% of subjects in the United Kingdom previously identified as having "idiopathic" CPPD crystal deposition disease related to aging.[14] There are likely other, unrecognized genetic factors in late onset "sporadic" chondrocalcinosis.

The clinical heterogeneity of familial chondrocalcinosis, and associations with mixed forms of pathologic calcification, are noteworthy. For example, CPPD and basic calcium phosphate crystal (BCP), and cartilage and periarticular calcifications, in association with OA were described in one kindred, without a specific chromosomal linkage established.[15]

A syndrome of spondyloepiphyseal dysplasia tarda, brachydactyly, precocious OA, and intraarticular calcifications with CPPD and/or BCP crystals, in addition to periarticular calcifications, has been linked to mutation of the procollagen type II gene in indigenous natives of the Chiloe Islands in Chile.[16] Importantly, this population has a high prevalence of familial CPPD deposition disease, for reasons that are not clear. Last, in the Azores Islands, families affected with diffuse idiopathic skeletal hyperostosis (DISH) and/or chondrocalcinosis have been described, posing as yet-unanswered questions on a potential, shared pathogenic mechanism.[17]

CPPD Deposition Disease Secondary to Primary Metabolic Disorders

Hemochromatosis, hyperparathyroidism, hypophosphatasia, and hypomagnesemic conditions (including the Gitelman's variant of Bartter syndrome) are the best-characterized primary metabolic disorders linked to secondary CPPD crystal deposition disease.[18] A complete listing of such conditions, and EULAR weighting of risk factors, is provided in Tables 21-2 and 21-3. The relationships of many of these disorders to disordered PP$_i$ metabolism and chondrocyte differentiation are discussed in Chapter 20. CPPD crystal deposition disease linked to primary metabolic conditions (such as hemochromatosis, hyperparathyroidism, dialysis-dependent renal failure[18]) can present earlier than age 55. We do not understand the basis for the heterogeneous presentation of hemochromatosis either as premature degenerative joint disease, or with prominent CPPD crystal deposition. We now increasingly recognize that hypomagnesia can be caused by diuretic therapy, short bowel syndrome and malabsorption, and treatment with proton pump inhibitors, cyclosporine, and tacrolimus).[19-22] Diagnostic approaches to these conditions are discussed in this chapter.

Development of CPPD crystal deposition disease in end-stage renal disease and hemodialysis, linked to secondary hyperparathyroidism, is a common problem and is reviewed

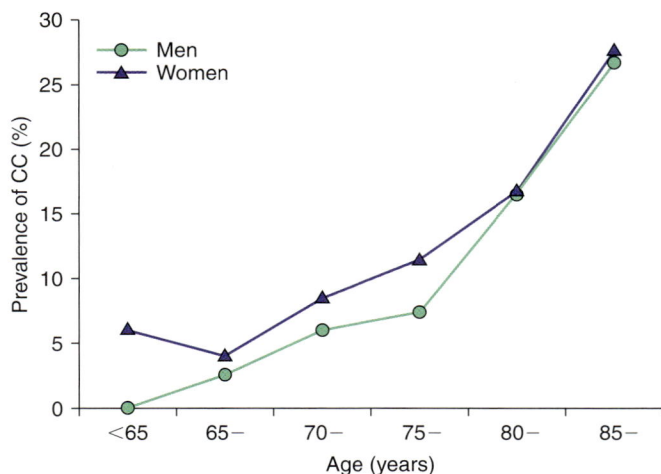

Figure 21-2 Prevalence of knee chondrocalcinosis by age and gender. *(Reprinted from Zhang W, Doherty M, Bardin T, et al. European League Against Rheumatism recommendations for calcium pyrophosphate deposition. Part I: terminology and diagnosis. Ann Rheum Dis 2011 Jan 7 [Epub ahead of print], Fig. 2; data from Felson DT, Anderson JJ, Naimark A, et al. J Rheumatol 1989;16:1241-5.)*

Table 21-4 EULAR Proposed Classification of the Main Clinical Phenotypes of CPPD Crystal Deposition

Clinical Phenotype	Characteristics—Comments
1. Asymptomatic	Fortuitous radiographic or ultrasound finding
2. Acute CPP crystal arthritis	Generally called pseudogout; the rapid development of severe joint pain, swelling and tenderness that reaches its maximum within 6 to 24 hours, especially with overlying erythema, is highly suggestive of acute crystal inflammation though not specific for acute CPP crystal arthritis
3. Chronic CPP crystal inflammatory arthritis	Presents as chronic oligoarthritis or polyarthritis with inflammatory symptoms and signs, and occasional systemic upset (with elevation of CRP and ESR); superimposed flares with characteristics of crystal inflammation support this diagnosis. It should be considered in the differential diagnosis of rheumatoid arthritis and other chronic inflammatory joint diseases in older adults. Radiographs may assist diagnosis, but the diagnosis should be crystal proven.
4. Osteoarthritis with CPP deposition	Particularly targets knees with chronic symptoms and/or acute attacks of crystal-induced inflammation. Compared to OA without CPPD, it may associate with more inflammatory symptoms and signs, an atypical distribution (see Table 21-2). Some causal responsibility of CPP crystals is very likely but not well established, and the relationship is most probably in two directions (see text).

CPPD; CRP, C-reactive protein; ESR, erythrocyte sedimentation rate; OA, osteoarthritis.
Classification types from Zhang W, Doherty M, Bardin T, et al. European League Against Rheumatism recommendations for calcium pyrophosphate deposition. Part I: terminology and diagnosis. Ann Rheum Dis 2011 Jan 7 [Epub ahead of print].

in detail in Chapter 23. Association of CPPD crystal deposition with gout is not rare in the clinic, particularly in elderly patients. It is likely that cartilage abnormalities and intraarticular inflammation from preexisting CPPD crystal deposition disease can promote urate crystal deposition in the joint, and possibly vice versa for CPPD deposition superimposed on gout. However, CPPD deposition disease and gout are both quite common conditions, and it is not surprising that they coexist in some patients, particularly among the elderly.

Clinical Features

Although CPPD deposition is prevalent and a substantial public health problem in the elderly, the "disease and health-related quality of life impact" and the long-term course of various forms of CPPD-associated arthropathies have not been adequately evaluated. Furthermore, we do not yet understand the relative contributions, to each clinical phenotype of arthritis, of the forms of CPPD crystals deposited (i.e., monoclinic versus triclinic crystals), and the influences of host factors are poorly understood.

Clinical Presentations of CPPD Deposition Disease

Most aged individuals with CPPD deposition disease have a primary idiopathic/sporadic form of the disorder (see Table 21-1), which most often appears only after age 50 or 55, and favors large joints[3,23-24] (Figure 21-2). Those with antecedent repetitive joint trauma or knee meniscectomy can clinically present with nonsystemic (monoarticular) CPPD deposition disease before age 55, often first recognized on plain radiographs (see Tables 21-2 and 21-3).

The heterogeneous clinical presentations of familial CPPD crystal deposition disease are discussed next[25] (Tables 21-4 and 21-5, Figures 21-3 and 21-4) Commonly, this is an asymptomatic disorder rather than a disease or a disorder that coexists with symptomatic OA and could contribute to

baseline symptoms and/or flares of OA. Alternatively, CPPD crystal deposition disease is a versatile mimic. The disease can resemble primary OA ("pseudo-osteoarthritis"), gout ("pseudogout") (see Figure 21-4), "pseudo-septic arthritis," acute-onset or insidious RA ("pseudo rheumatoid arthritis") (see Figures 21-3 and 21-4), or "pseudo-polymyalgia rheumatica" or present as a fever of unknown origin or "pseudo-neuropathic" arthropathy. Patients with CPPD crystal deposition disease also can present with episodic hemarthrosis, often post-traumatic and in the knee. In some patients, CPPD deposition disease and rheumatoid arthritis (RA) coexist, but this is likely by chance association in elderly subjects.

Acute Synovitis of Pseudogout

Pseudogout, a common etiology of acute, inflammatory monoarticular or oligoarticular arthritis in the aged, presents as attacks typically involving a large joint. This is most often the knee, and less often the wrist or ankle and, rarely, the first metatarsophalangeal joint, unlike the case for gout. Acute

Table 21-5 Common Clinical Presentations and Diseases Mimicked by CPPD Deposition Disease

Clinical Presentations	Mimicked conditions	Peculiarities—Differences*
Chronic degenerative arthritis	Osteoarthritis	Unusual locations (radiocarpal, mediocarpal, mediotarsal, hindfoot-tarsal, MCPs, elbows, glenohumeral. Prominent cysts and osteophytes.
Recurrent acute inflammatory monoarticular or oligoarticular arthritis ("pseudogout")	Gout	MTPs less often involved. Lower or absent effectiveness of colchicine
"Pseudoseptic Arthritis"	Septic arthritis	Clinically indistinguishable apart from the response to NSAIDs (that one cannot afford to wait; in principle, puncture always needed)
Chronic symmetric inflammatory polyarthritis ("pseudo rheumatoid arthritis")	Rheumatoid arthritis	Rare rheumatoid factor and absent ACPAs. Mild or no local osteopenia but sclerosis and osteophytes on radiography notably on MCPs
Systemic illness with proximal limb pain and stiffness	Polymyalgia rheumatica	Frequent involvement of wrists, ankles, MCPs, PIPs, DIPs, knees, and MTPs. Common tendinous calcifications
Ligamentum flavum or transverse ligament of atlas involvement	Spondylodiscitis, cervical canal stenosis, cervical myelopathy, meningismus, foramen magnum syndrome, odontoid fracture	Cervical spine: calcification of the transverse ligament of atlas (crowned dens) most visible on CT scan. Dorsolumbar spine: possible discal thinning and erosions but no abscess. Response to NSAIDs
Rapidly destructive arthritis (frequently in dialysis-dependent renal failure)	Neuropathic arthropathy	Extensive and progressive joint destruction, but without neurologic signs. Responsibility of CPPD crystals in the destruction is likely but poorly demonstrated
Wrist pain and median nerve compression signs	Carpal tunnel syndrome	Improvement with NSAIDs and/or GC
Tumoral and pseudotophaceous CPPD crystal deposits	Gouty tophus, tumor	Generally painless. Histiocytes, giant cells and characteristic rhomboid shaped crystals with basophilic calcified material on microscopic examination

ACPAs, Anti-CCP antibodies; *CPPD,* calcium pyrophosphate dihydrate; *CT,* computed tomography; *DIP,* distal interphalangeal; and *GC,* glucocorticosteroids; *MCP,* metacarpophalangeal; *MTP,* metatarsophalangeal; *NSAID,* nonsteroidal antiinflammatory drug; *PIP,* proximal interphalangeal.
*In addition to the presence of CPPD crystals in synovial fluid and visible chondrocalcinosis on radiography.

attacks of pseudogout usually are sudden in onset and often excruciatingly painful and can be accompanied by periarticular erythema, warmth, and swelling, similar to gout attacks. In some patients, pseudogout can manifest as migratory, additive, polyarticular, and bilateral arthritis. For example, familial chondrocalcinosis and hyperparathyroidism can present with polyarticular pseudogout.

Factors that promote acute pseudogout include not only minor trauma but also illnesses that require hospitalization, such as intercurrent medical or surgical problems (e.g., pneumonia, myocardial infarction, cerebrovascular accident, and, in occasional cases, pregnancy). Parathyroid surgery for hyperparathyroidism commonly triggers acute pseudogout. Moreover, pseudogout of the knee can be precipitated by arthroscopy or by intraarticular hyaluronan injection,[26] the latter possibly reflecting innate immune inflammation through Toll-like receptors, or triggering of CPPD crystal shedding from cartilage. Granulocyte colony-stimulating factor (G-CSF)[27] and bisphosphonates[28] also can trigger pseudogout attacks, the former likely by fueling an increase in smoldering, subclinical joint inflammation, and the latter possibly via pyrophosphatase inhibition, since bisphosphonates are nonhydrolyzable PP_i analogues.

It has been suggested that initiation of thyroid hormone replacement can precipitate acute attacks of pseudogout.[29] On the other hand, hypothyroidism (with the probable exception of myxedematous hypothyroidism) has not been tied to increased prevalence of CPPD crystal deposition disease in

controlled studies, and both disorders are quite prevalent in the aged.[18,30,31]

Acute and subacute cases of pseudogout, like gout, can be associated with fever, chills, elevated sedimentation rate and acute phase reactants, and systemic leukocytosis, particularly in those with polyarticular arthritis and in the aged.[32] Synovial fluid leukocytosis (with a markedly elevated percentage of neutrophils) is present, and, on occasion, the joint fluid leukocyte count in pseudogout can exceed 50,000 per mm^3 with predominant neutrophilia ("pseudoseptic arthritis"). CPPD crystals (within and outside of phagocytes) are most often (but not universally) detectable by compensated polarized light microscopy in the acute phase of pseudogout (see Chapter 2). Although pseudogout attacks usually flare for 7 to 10 days, they also can be clustered and last for weeks to months, even with NSAID therapy. There has been reported to be a favorable prognosis for initial CPPD deposition disease in the knee presenting as acute pseudogout attacks alone.[33]

CPPD Crystal Deposition in OA

Articular cartilage and synovial fluid CPPD crystals, frequently in association with BCP crystals, are commonly detectable (about 60%) in knee OA at the advanced stage of total joint arthroplasty.[34,35] Higher mean radiographic scores correlated with the presence of these types of crystals.[34] In a recent study, patients with primary OA and detectable CPPD crystals in joint fluids required knee arthroplasty more than those with

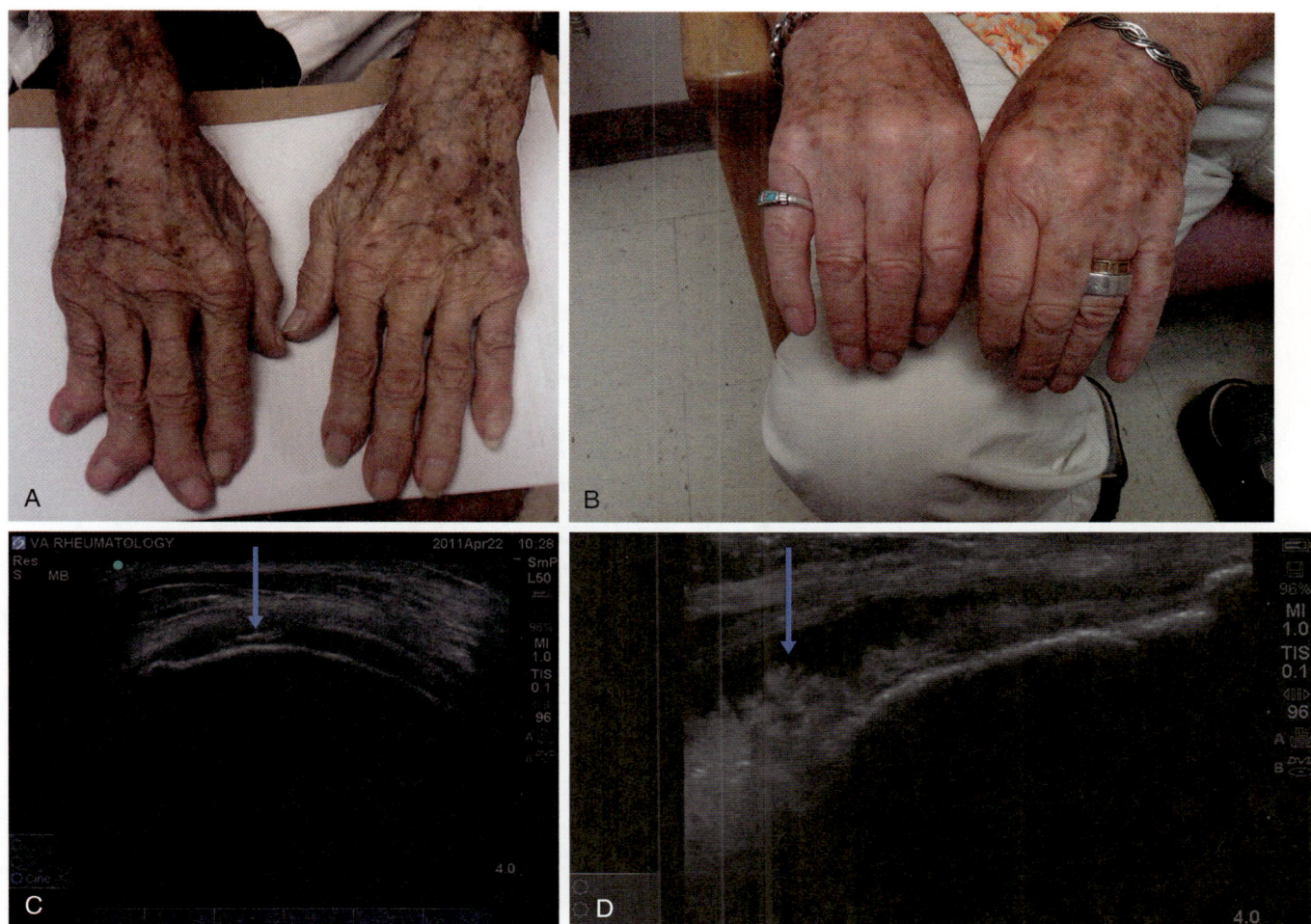

Figure 21-3 Panel A: Idiopathic symmetric pseudorheumatoid calcium pyrophosphate dihydrate (CPPD) deposition arthropathy in an elderly man. This 78-year-old patient presented with a history of bilateral knee and wrist symmetric proliferative synovitis, complicated by a *Staphylococcus aureus* septic arthritis of his left knee. Physical findings included synovial and dorsal extensor tenosynovial swelling of both wrists and the right second metacarpophalangeal joint. Distal hand joint osteoarthritis also was present in this patient, and was severe. Changes on knee, hand, and wrist plain radiographs were consistent with the diagnosis of CPPD deposition disease (not shown). (Source: Robert Terkeltaub, MD) Figure 21.3B. Low grade symmetric, diffuse synovitis of the metacarpophalangeal joint row (pseudo rheumatoid arthritis picture) in another 78-year-old male with CPPD deposition disease, established by plain radiography and exclusion of RA by serologic testing and radiography. (Source: Robert Terkeltaub, MD) Figure 21-3, Panels C and D. High resolution ultrasound images from the knee of the 78-year-old male patient with CPPD crystal deposition associated "pseudo rheumatoid arthritis" shown in Figure 21-3A. **C.** Knee hyaline articular cartilage demonstrating large linear "chunk" of CPPD crystal deposition *(arrow)* in the middle zone of the cartilage. **D.** Large synovial fronds *(arrow)* protruding into sizeable knee joint effusion consistent with the "pseudo rheumatoid arthritis" picture of CPPD crystal deposition disease. These ultrasound images from the collection of Dr. Robert Terkeltaub were taken at the San Diego VA Medical Center using a Sonosite M-Turbo apparatus equipped with high resolution transducer. The ultrasound diagnostic approach to CPPD deposition disease is reviewed in detail by Dr. Ralf Thiele in Chapter 26 in this book.

OA without crystals.[35] The clinical significance of BCP crystals is reviewed in Chapter 22. The presence of CPPD crystals in joints with primary OA can contribute to OA symptoms (partially from synovitis) and flares, and potentially OA progression, since CPPD crystals induce synovial proliferation, and can cause chondrocyte cytotoxicity, and synovial and chondrocyte metalloproteinase expression.[35-37]

Chronic Degenerative and Inflammatory Arthropathies Driven by CPPD Crystals

A small subset of subjects with CPPD deposition develop prolonged, recurring polyarticular inflammation. Progressive degenerative arthropathy is more common.

It has been suggested that acute flares of pseudogout become less common in those with established chronic degenerative CPPD deposition arthropathy,[38] but acute pseudogout episodes still do occur in those with chronic arthropathy in CPPD crystal deposition disease. The chronic form of CPPD deposition disease often involves certain joints characteristically spared in primary OA (e.g., metacarpophalangeal joints, wrists, elbows, glenohumeral joints). The development of cartilage degenerative changes in CPPD deposition disease in typical as well as atypical joints for primary OA is consistent with CPPD deposition disease being a systemic disorder.

Not just familial CPPD crystal deposition disease, but also idiopathic/sporadic CPPD crystal deposition disease, can

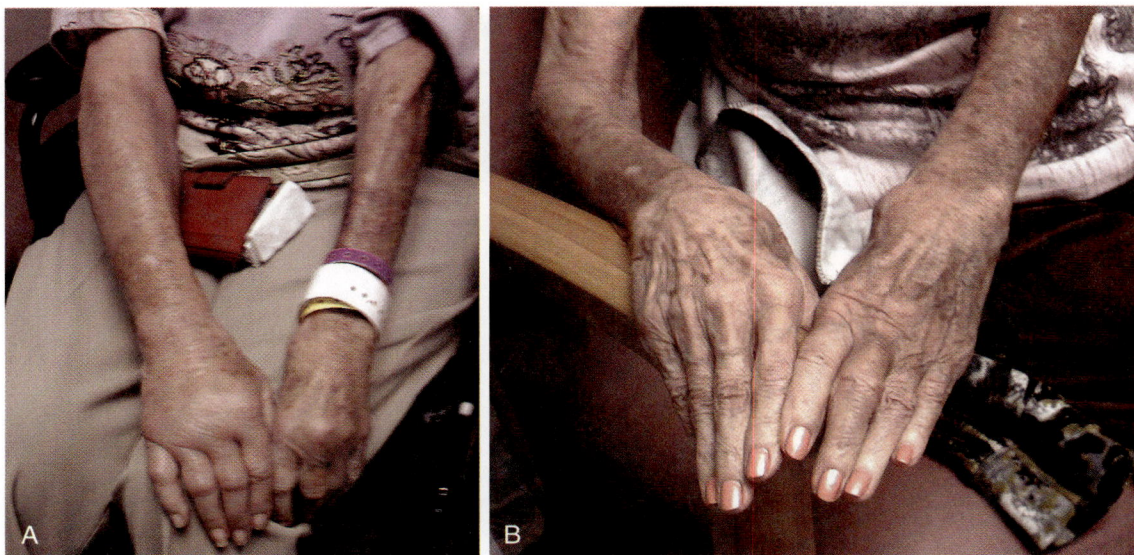

Figure 21-4 Acute polyarticular pseudogout and chronic pseudo rheumatoid calcium pyrophosphate dihydrate (CPPD) deposition arthropathy. This 85-year-old woman had chronic pseudo rheumatoid CPPD deposition disease of both wrists, and following admission for an upper gastrointestinal bleed, the patient developed an acute polyarthritis. **A,** Marked swelling of the right elbow, and bilateral hand and wrist swelling, with marked synovitis and swelling of both proximal interphalangeal and metacarpophalangeal joint rows. **B,** Marked improvement in all findings, though persistent bilateral, chronic wrist proliferative synovitis, 3 weeks after treatment with systemic corticosteroids and daily low-dose prophylactic colchicine.

cause destructive arthropathy, but the aggressiveness of CPPD crystal arthropathy-associated degenerative disease is highly variable. Prospective analysis of CPPD deposition disease predominantly of the knee suggested relatively slow radiographic worsening of degenerative arthropathy, and a nonprogressive course in some patients.[33] Although the majority of affected subjects develop changes in radiographic chondrocalcinosis with time, there is no clear correlation between the extent of calcification and progression of disease with CPPD deposition arthropathy.

Pseudo Rheumatoid Arthritis in CPPD Deposition Disease

Pseudo rheumatoid arthritis occurs in a small but significant fraction of patients with CPPD deposition disease. It presents as a chronic, bilateral, symmetric, inflammatory polyarthropathy (see Figures 21-3 and 21-4), and loss of joint motion and rheumatoid arthritis–like deformities may develop in the wrists and hands. Bilateral wrist and metacarpophalangeal joint involvement is a classic presentation, and wrist extensor tenosynovitis and tendon rupture and carpal tunnel syndrome may occur. Elbow cubital tunnel syndrome also may develop. Radiographic changes of CPPD deposition are characteristically present at the stage of pseudo rheumatoid disease associated with CPPD deposition disease.

Mechanisms driving synovial and tenosynovial proliferation, and synovitis, in response to CPPD crystal deposition, likely include uptake of CPPD crystals by synovial lining cells, and synovial proliferation, partly via solubilization of the crystalline calcium.[39] Other mechanisms, including the role of the NLRP3 inflammasome and interleukin (IL)-1β release, are discussed in Chapter 20.

Other Clinical Presentations of Idiopathic CPPD Crystal Deposition

Concentrated (tumoral or pseudotophaceous) CPPD crystal deposition can develop in bone and in periarticular structures such as tendons, ligaments, and bursae.[25,40] CPPD deposits in tendons (e.g., Achilles, triceps, obturator tendons) are usually fine and linear on plain radiography and readily detected on high-resolution ultrasound. Plantar fascial involvement also occurs. Pseudotophaceous CPPD crystal deposition has also been reported in the temporal bone, the knee and hip regions, and in the acromioclavicular, temporomandibular, elbow, and small hand joints.[40] Tumoral CPPD crystal deposits can present with acute attacks of arthritis and, in the knee region, can clinically mimic osteonecrosis.[41] Tumoral deposits of CPPD crystals are characteristically associated with chondroid metaplasia and clinical behavior equivalent to a locally aggressive but benign chondroid tumor. CPPD crystal–induced metalloproteinase expression and other inflammatory responses likely drive the connective tissue invasion and destruction in this condition.

CPPD crystal deposition in the axial skeleton occasionally involves the intervertebral disc and the sacroiliac or lumbar facet joints, and spinal ankylosis may develop.[42] Among the clinical syndromes reported are meningismus and clinical manifestations that mimic intervertebral disc herniation and ankylosing spondylitis; acute pseudogout of lumbar facet joints has been reported.[42,43]

Notably, CPPD deposition disease can present as neurologic disturbance and painful cervical mass, especially in the aged. Specifically, CPPD crystal deposition in the ligamentum flavum or the transverse ligament of atlas can be quite robust and may progress to cause symptomatic cervical spinal canal stenosis, cervical myelopathy, and foramen magnum syndrome.[43-45] Odontoid fracture due to the calcification of the atlantoaxial joint also has been reported.[43-46]

Familial CPPD Crystal Deposition Disease

Familial CPPD crystal deposition disease often declares itself clinically in the third or fourth decades of life but is sometimes detected, or clinically present, later than that or before age 20. Familial CPPD deposition disease has been reported in numerous countries and ethnic groups. This includes kindreds from Czechoslovakia, Holland, France, England, Germany, Sweden, Israel, the United States, Canada, and Japan, and the familial disease may be most prevalent in Chile and Spain. Multiple members of a British kindred with CPPD deposition disease linked to *ANKH* mutation manifested recurrent childhood seizures strongly associated with later development of CPPD deposition disease.[47] Kindreds with *ANKH* linkage have had heterogeneous phenotypes. Early-onset polyarthritis, including ankylosing intervertebral and sacroiliac joint disease, has been seen in some, whereas others have presented with late-onset CPPD crystal deposition disease. In some kindreds, mild oligoarticular disease resembling idiopathic CPPD deposition disease has been observed.[14,48,49] Argentinian and Alsatian French *ANKH* mutant–linked kindreds had similar phenotypic features of CPPD crystal deposition, including early onset (third decade of life), premature OA in many, and some with pseudo rheumatoid arthritis peripheral joint disease. Commonly affected joints and regions in these kindreds were knees, wrists, symphysis pubis, and intervertebral discs.

Diagnosis and Diagnostic Tests

The original diagnostic criteria for CPPD crystal deposition disease were proposed by Daniel J McCarty and colleagues and are adapted here principally to include diagnostic use of ultrasound (Table 21-6). EULAR expert- and evidence-based diagnostic propositions and weighing of diagnostic measures also are very helpful to consider[1] (Tables 21-1 and 21-7, respectively). Diagnosis is based on a foundation of the detection of CPPD crystals by at least one method. The diagnostic tools include plain radiography and high-resolution ultrasound, which detect hyaline articular cartilage and/or fibrocartilage calcifications characteristic of CPPD crystal deposition. The gold standard for diagnosis of CPPD crystal deposition disease, particularly for acute pseudogout, is identification of CPPD crystals by compensated polarized light microscopic analysis of synovial fluid in the absence of joint infection or other cause of arthritis. Detection of CPPD crystals in tissue sections (see Chapter 1) also is useful and is possible whether specimens are fixed in formaldehyde or ethanol, unlike the case for monosodium urate crystals (which are dissolved by formaldehyde fixation). Usually, specialized crystal analytic approaches (see Chapter 22) such as atomic force microscopy, Fourier transform infrared spectroscopy (FTIR), x-ray energy spectroscopy, and powder diffraction analysis are not required to establish or confirm CPPD crystal deposition. Spacing of x-ray powder diffraction lines and determination of the calcium/phosphate ratios provide the most specific information when specialized analyses are needed to assess deposited crystals in calcifications.

Table 21-6 Proposed Diagnostic Criteria for CPPD Crystal Deposition Disease

Criteria:

I. Demonstration of CPPD crystals, obtained by biopsy or aspirated synovial fluid, by definitive means (such as characteristic x-ray diffraction powder pattern).

II. A. Identification of monoclinic or triclinic crystals showing a weak positive birefringence (or no birefringence) by compensated polarized light microscopy.
   B. Presence of typical calcifications on radiographs (as discussed in text): heavy punctate and linear calcifications in fibrocartilages, articular (hyaline) cartilages, and joint capsules, especially if bilaterally symmetric.
   C. Presence of typical findings for CPPD crystal deposition in articular hyaline cartilage or fibrocartilage by high-resolution ultrasound.

III. A. Acute arthritis, especially of knees, wrists, or other large joints.
   B. Chronic arthritis, especially of knee, hip, wrist, carpus, elbow shoulder, and metacarpophalangeal joints, particularly if accompanied by acute exacerbations.

Diagnostic Categories:

A. Definite: criteria I or IIA must be fulfilled.
B. Probable: criteria IIA or IIB or IIC must be fulfilled.
C. Possible: criteria IIIA or IIIB suggests possible underlying CPPD deposition disease

Adapted from McCarty DJ: Crystals and arthritis. Dis Month 6:255, 1994; reprinted from Terkeltaub R. Diseases associated with articular deposition of calcium pyrophosphate dihydrate and basic calcium phosphate crystals. In: Firestein GS et al., eds. Kelley's Textbook of Rheumatology. 8th ed. Philadelphia: Elsevier Saunders; 2009:1507-24, 1508, Table 88-1.

Differential Diagnosis

Clinical syndromes of CPPD crystal deposition disease, as cited earlier, can resemble multiple conditions and vice versa (see Table 21-5). This warrants careful attention to the diagnostic criteria for CPPD deposition disease (see Tables 21-1, 21-6, and 21-7). A diagnostic algorithm is presented here (Figure 21-5). It is important to remember that radiographic chondrocalcinosis is a common finding in the elderly and does not necessarily indicate that the patient's symptomatic arthritis is due to CPPD deposition disease, and this is of particular importance when septic arthritis or concomitant gout must be ruled out.

The ability of pseudogout to resemble septic arthritis and vice versa highlights the diagnostic value of arthrocentesis with synovial fluid crystal analysis and, in appropriate instances, concurrent exclusion of joint infection. In this context, crystal deposits can be "enzymatically strip-mined" by inflammation primarily driven by infection of the joint. As such, CPPD and urate crystals can be detected in synovial fluids in some infected joints.

Certain clinical and imaging features help distinguish chronic degenerative arthritis in CPPD crystal deposition disease from OA. These include involvement of joints not typically affected by primary OA, such as the wrist, metacarpophalangeal joints, elbow, or shoulder. The presence on plain radiographs of heavy punctate and linear calcifications in fibrocartilages, articular (hyaline) cartilages, and joint capsules, especially if bilaterally symmetric, points to CPPD deposition (see Chapter 25), although faint or atypical calcifications may be due to BCP-related vascular calcifications.

Table 21-7 Validity of Diagnostic Tests for Calcium Pyrophosphate Deposition

Test	Target Joints	No. of Studies (subjects)	Age Range, (yr)	Reference Standard	Sensitivity (95% CI)	Specificity (95% CI)	Positive LR (95% CI)	References
Clinical								
Acute CPP crystal arthritis								
Acute attacks	Knee	1 (100)	36 to 80	Radiographic CC	(0.28 to 0.72)	0.90 (83 to 0.97)	5.00 (27 to 11.02)	107
Chronic CPP crystal inflammatory arthritis								
Pain	Knee, wrist, elbow, shoulder and hip	4 (429)	36 to 97	SF crystals and/or radiographic CC	0.21 (12 to 0.30)	0.80 (72 to 0.89)	1.18 (82 to 1.71)	24, 92, 95, 107
Stiffness	Knee	2 (227)	36 to 80	Radiographic CC	0.35 (19 to 0.50)	0.81 (74 to 0.88)	1.96 (12 to 3.44)	92, 107
Swelling/ effusion	Knee, wrist, elbow, shoulder and hand	5 (432)	36 to 97	Radiographic CC	0.40 (23 to 0.56)	0.77 (68 to 0.87)	1.56 (16 to 2.11)	24, 92, 104, 107, 115
Tenderness	Knee	2 (227)	36 to 80	Radiographic CC	0.13 (02 to 0.24)	0.85 (79 to 0.91)	0.91 (37 to 2.24)	92, 107
Instability	Knee	2 (227)	36 to 80	Radiographic CC	0.18 (06 to 0.31)	0.82 (51 to 1.14)	0.95 (44 to 2.04)	92, 107
Synovial fluid								
CPP crystals	Not specified	194		Expert diagnosis	0.95 (92 to 1.00)	0.86 (80 to 0.93)	7.09 (27 to 11.76)	116
Radiograph								
CC	Wrist	18	71 (41 to 95)	CPP crystals	0.29 (−0.05 to 0.62)	0.20 (−0.15 to 0.55)	0.36 (10 to 1.25)	115
Ultrasound								
cartilage calcification	Knee	43	68 (40 to 92)	CPP crystals	0.87 (69 to 1.04)	0.96 (90 to 1.03)	24.2 (51 to 168.01)	117
Achilles tendon calcification	Heel	107	65 (42 to 92)	Radiographic CC plus CPP crystals	0.56 (0.45 to 0.71)	0.98 (0.94 to 1.02)	29 (4.11 to 204.05)	65
Plantar fascia calcification	Heel	107	65 (42 to 92)	Radiographic CC plus CPP crystals	0.16 (0.06 to 0.25)	0.98 (0.94 to 1.02)	7.89 (1.04 to 60.16)	65

CC, Chondrocalcinosis; CPP, calcium pyrophosphate; LR, likelihood ratio.
Table reprinted from Zhang W, Doherty M, Bardin T, et al. European League Against Rheumatism recommendations for calcium pyrophosphate deposition. Part I: terminology and diagnosis. Ann Rheum Dis 2011 Jan 7 [Epub ahead of print], Table 2. Data from references as cited.

Nonpathologic dicalcium phosphate dihydrate (DCPD) ($CaHPO_4 \cdot 2H_2O$, calcium:phosphate ratio 1.0) ("brushite") crystals can cause some atypical calcifications. Brushite crystals can develop as an artefact of acid preparation of calcified tissue for pathologic analyses.[50]

As reinforced by EULAR,[1] the diagnosis of CPPD deposition disease prior to age 55, particularly when CPP deposition is widespread (polyarticular), should prompt consideration of a primary metabolic or familial disorder in the differential diagnosis (see Table 21-1). In the elderly, CPPD deposition disease can present as diffuse pain and/or fever of unknown origin,[52] thereby mimicking infection, polymyalgia rheumatica and RA. Furthermore, a false-positive rheumatoid factor (RF) test is common (about one-third positive) in the elderly, and patients with pseudo rheumatoid CPPD crystal deposition disease can be positive for RF.

Use of Synovial Fluid Crystal Analysis and Other Laboratory Tests in Diagnosis

The finding of CPPD crystals in synovial fluid or in tissues, via compensated polarized light microscopy, is definite evidence for CPPD deposition disease only if the observers are reliable (see Chapter 2). Some CPPD crystals can be rod-shaped and

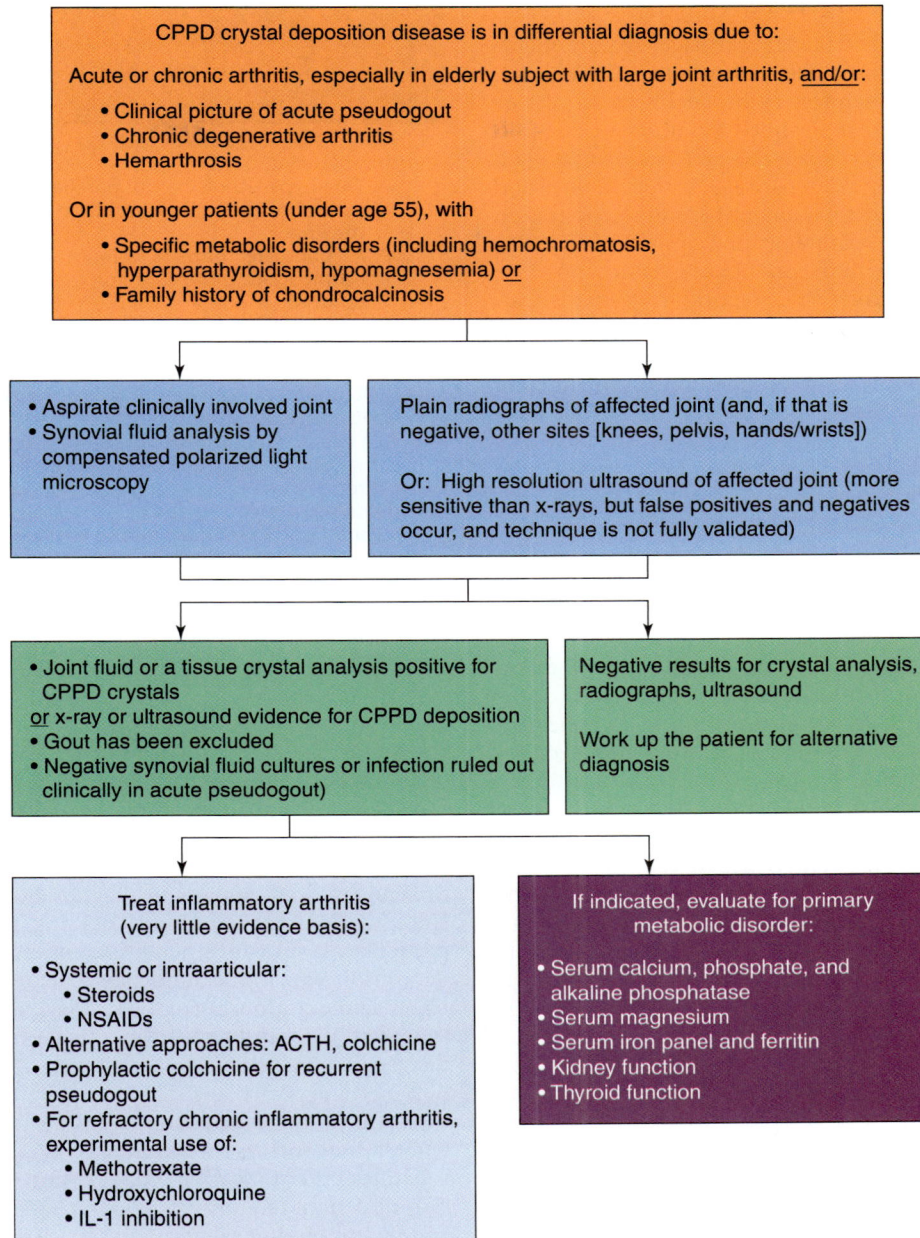

Figure 21-5 Algorithm for diagnosis, evaluation, and treatment of calcium pyrophosphate dihydrate deposition disease. The algorithm is discussed in detail in the text.

intracellular and resemble urate crystals, and some CPPD crystals are nonbirefringent[51]; and the appearance and number of CPPD crystals can change with storage (as reviewed in Chapter 2). Relatively fresh specimens are desirable and should be collected in vials free of calcium-chelating anticoagulants such as EDTA. Cytocentrifugation increases sensitivity of detection of CPPD crystals. One study, using cytocentrifugation, demonstrated both urate and CPPD crystals in 7% to 8% of synovial fluid samples (of subjects with gout and OA).[52]

When synovial fluid specimens are not fresh, Gram stain and Diff Quick staining have been suggested to provide information beyond that obtained from compensated polarized light microscopy.[53-55] The demonstration of CPPD crystals in

tissues can be challenging in specimens stained with hematoxylin-eosin, since the acidity of hematoxylin solutions promotes decalcification. Fortunately, the decalcifying effect of hematoxylin can be lessened by curtailing to 3 minutes the staining period with Mayer's hematoxylin.[56]

Conventional radiography or ultrasound is usually the first method to evaluate patients with suspected CPPD deposition disease. Nevertheless, laboratory evaluation of the newly diagnosed patient with CPPD deposition disease should include, as appropriate, serum calcium, phosphate, magnesium, alkaline phosphatase, ferritin, and iron and total iron binding capacity, and a thyroid function evaluation is useful (see Figure 21-5).

Use of Imaging in Diagnosis

BCP crystal deposits in articular cartilage require high-resolution radiography to be detected, whereas CPPD crystal deposits frequently manifest as broad linear streaks or linear "chunks" in articular hyaline and fibrocartilages on plain radiographs. However, it is important to note that plain radiographic findings may fail to correlate with pathology and clinical features of CPPD deposition. For example, correlation between radiographic and pathology findings was only 39.2% in one study of patients with the use of knee arthroscopy.[57]

A radiographic screen for CPPD deposition disease is usually not necessary in differential diagnosis, but can be done by obtaining an anteroposterior (AP) view of each knee, an AP view of the pelvis (to detect symphysis pubis involvement), and Posterior-anterior (PA) views of both hands that include visualization of both wrists (see Chapter 25). Calcific deposits may or may not be detectable by plain radiographic screening of an affected area in CPPD deposition disease, and radiographic evidence other than chondrocalcinosis may point to the correct diagnosis[58] (see Chapter 25). Such radiographic findings suggesting CPPD deposition disease, as opposed to primary OA, include radiocarpal or marked patellofemoral joint space narrowing, especially if isolated (such as the patella "wrapped around" the femur). Scaphoid-lunate widening and femoral cortical erosion superior to the patella also suggest CPPD deposition (see Chapter 25). "Pseudo-neuropathic" CPPD deposition disease can manifest as severe progressive degeneration in the knee, with subchondral bony collapse (microfractures), and fragmentation, with formation of intraarticular radiodense bodies. CPPD deposition disease involving the metacarpophalangeal joints radiographically can manifest as metacarpal squaring associated with "beaklike" osteophytes and subchondral cyst formation. Tendon calcifications (e.g., Achilles, triceps, and obturator tendons) are a valuable characteristic of CPPD deposition, in differential diagnosis. Osteophyte formation is variable with CPPD deposition disease, more so than with OA.

High-Resolution Ultrasound in Diagnosis of CPPD Crystal Deposition

Ultrasound has many advantages for imaging CPPD deposition, starting with convenience, low cost, lack of radiation, ability to detect effusion and to help with joint aspiration, and ability to detect the presence or absence of active inflammation with power Doppler technique as an adjunct.[59] Ultrasound can recognize a greater number of inflamed knee joints than does clinical assessment.[60]

Preliminary criteria proposed for CPPD calcifications by ultrasound are summarized in Table 21-8, and Chapter 26 reviews and illustrates characteristic ultrasound features of CPPD deposits. In small studies to date, this approach has correlated quite well with positive results for CPPD crystals in synovial fluid analysis and has detected CPPD deposition in some patients in whom plain radiographs were negative in affected joints[60-65] (see Chapter 26). However, further validation is needed for reliance on high-resolution ultrasound in CPPD deposition diagnosis, since false-positive results occur (possibly due to fibrotic changes), and false-negative results also occur due to limits in sensitivity. Current generation high-resolution equipment and operator expertise are essential elements to the approach. Limitations of ultrasound also include difficulty in visualizing crystal deposits in deep recesses of the joint space, whereas the approach is likely most

Table 21-8 Preliminary Criteria for Diagnosis of CPPD Crystal Deposition by High Resolution Ultrasound*

1. All CPPD deposits are hyperechoic and present as one of the following patterns:
   - Thin hyperechoic bands, parallel to (but below) the surface of the hyaline cartilage (frequently observed in the knee)
   - A "punctate" pattern, composed of several thin hyperechoic spots, more common in fibrous cartilage and in tendons
   - Homogeneous hyperechoic nodular or oval deposits localized in bursae and articular recesses (frequently mobile)
2. CPPD crystal deposit calcifications always have a sparkling appearance and create posterior shadowing only when they reach dimensions of greater than 10 mm. In contrast, calcifications that present a hypoechoic appearance with posterior shadowing even at an early stage (2 to 3 mm in diameter) are considered as crystalline deposits of another nature, most commonly due to basic calcium phosphate crystal deposition disease.

*These criteria are not validated by pathology examination and are incompletely sensitive and incompletely specific.
Adapted from Frediani B, Filippou G, Falsetti P, et al. Diagnosis of calcium pyrophosphate dihydrate crystal deposition disease: ultrasonographic criteria proposed. Ann Rheum Dis 2005;64:638-40.

specific for detection of CPPD crystal deposition in fibrocartilages (e.g., triangular fibrocartilage of the wrist, knee menisci) and in the middle zones of articular hyaline cartilages.

Ultrasound should complement, not totally replace, the use of synovial fluid analysis in diagnosis of acute pseudogout, since one does not want to risk missing infectious arthritis, in particular. Gout can generally be differentiated from CPPD deposition with ultrasound (see Chapter 26). For example, hyperechoic contouring of the cartilage surface ("double contour sign") is seen in gout, whereas CPPD crystal deposition disease is characteristically visualized within the middle zone of the articular cartilage. The diagnostic value for CPPD disease of ultrasound detection of calcification in plantar fascia and tendons such as the Achilles[65] is not entirely clear; enthesopathies other than CPPD disease also give rise to calcification of certain tendons and plantar fascia, although Achilles and triceps tendon calcification, for example, are highly suggestive of CPPD deposition.

Dual-energy computed tomography (DECT) has not been specifically studied for CPPD detection but is useful for specific discrimination of urate from BCP deposits[66] (see Chapter 25). Magnetic resonance imaging (MRI) is not yet a reliable approach for detecting CPPD crystal deposition disease due to a lack of mobile protons in CPPD crystals. Nonenhanced MRI is less sensitive in detecting knee meniscal fibrocartilage calcification than it is for hyaline cartilage calcification.[67]

Treatment

Primary Approaches to Management and Prophylaxis of Acute, CPPD Crystal–Associated Inflammation

A treatment algorithm is presented at the bottom of Figure 21-5 that is in line with recent EULAR expert opinion–based guidelines.[2] As in gout, therapeutic approaches to patients

Table 21-9 Current and Potential Therapies for CPPD Crystal Deposition Disease

Accepted Benefits Based Mainly on Expert Opinion and Some Clinical Study:
  NSAIDs or COX-2 inhibitors
  Intraarticular corticosteroids
  Systemic corticosteroids
  ACTH
  Prophylactic low-dose colchicine
Possible Benefits Observed Clinically:
  Methotrexate for refractory chronic inflammation and recurrent pseudogout
  Hydroxychloroquine for refractory chronic inflammation
  IL-1 antagonism for CPPD crystal–induced inflammation
  Oral magnesium (for patients with hypomagnesemia); typically magnesium oxide in divided doses titrated to tolerability and therapeutic effect on serum magnesium
Theoretical Benefits:
  Caspase-1 antagonism for CPPD crystal–induced inflammation
  (?) Oral calcium supplementation to suppress PTH levels
  Inhibition of ANKH anion channel-mediated PP$_i$ transport (e.g., Probenecid)
  Polyphosphates
Promotion of Crystal Dissolution by Alkaline Phosphatase or Polyamines

ACTH, Adrenocorticotropic hormone; *COX,* cyclooxygenase; *IL,* interleukin; *NSAID,* nonsteroidal antiinflammatory drug; *PP$_i$,* inorganic pyrophosphate; *PTH,* parathyroid hormone.
Modified from Terkeltaub R. Diseases associated with articular deposition of calcium pyrophosphate dihydrate and basic calcium phosphate crystals. In: Firestein GS et al., eds. Kelley's Textbook of Rheumatology. 8th ed. Philadelphia: Elsevier Saunders; 2009:1507-24, 1519, Table 88-4.

with CPPD deposition disease involve treatment and prophylaxis of acute attacks of arthritis (Tables 21-9 and 21-10). In contrast, therapies to lessen crystal deposition, as well as chronic and anatomically progressive sequelae of crystal deposition, are not adequately developed for CPPD deposition (Tables 21-9 and 21-10).

All guidelines for treatment of attacks of acute pseudogout in CPPD crystal deposition disease (e.g., EULAR guidelines in Table 21-10) are predominantly expert opinion–based rather than evidence-based and have been modeled on treatment of acute gout.[2] This is an unsatisfactory state of affairs, but the fact that pseudogout has not been subjected to adequate clinical trials presents substantial opportunities.

Pseudogout can respond to NSAIDs (or selective cyclooxygenase-2 inhibitors) and to colchicine[2,68] but sometimes more slowly and, overall, less consistently than for acute gout treatment. Some of the evaluations of colchicine for pseudogout employed intravenous therapy, which is no longer marketed in the United States, and even so, responses were less consistent than for acute gout. Since comorbidities in the elderly often limit the use of NSAIDs, COX-2 inhibitors, and colchicine, a very useful approach is to use, as primary treatment, systemic glucocorticosteroids or intraarticular steroids (particularly so because pseudogout typically affects large joints).[2] Systemic or intraarticular glucocorticosteroids can be essentially given as described for acute gout attacks (see Chapters 10 and 16; also see Table 21-10). Glucocorticosteroids are not only broadly effective primary treatment choices in acute pseudogout but also valuable in refractory cases. ACTH,[69] generally given as described for acute gout, also can be effective in many cases of acute pseudogout.

The self-limited nature of most acute pseudogout attacks in the knee can be enhanced by simple arthrocentesis and thorough drainage of the joint effusion.[2] However, there are no data for tidal irrigation in the acute arthritis of CPPD deposition disease, unlike the case for chronic Milwaukee shoulder syndrome linked to BCP crystal deposition.[70,71]

Low-dose daily colchicine prophylaxis of pseudogout attacks, prescribed as is done to prevent gout attacks, is a useful treatment modality, as first established for low-dose colchicine prophylaxis by Alvarellos and Spilberg.[72] Low-dose NSAID prophylaxis has not been formally studied for pseudogout, and extra caution is needed when using NSAIDs in elderly patients.

Approaches to CPPD Deposition and Chronic Sequelae of CPPD Deposition Disease

Administration of oral magnesium (with magnesium oxide as a practical method) has appeared to reduce meniscal fibrocartilage calcification over a long period in association in secondary CPPD deposition disease due to hypomagnesemia.[73] Otherwise, there is no specific treatment validated to prevent or lessen CPPD crystal deposition in idiopathic disease. Even with proven primary metabolic disorders that cause secondary CPPD crystal deposition, which obviously mandate treatment, the potential benefits of such treatment for prevention of cartilage degeneration (and pseudogout attacks) remain unclear. This may be the case because detection of chondrocalcinosis on plain radiographs indicates an already advanced state of CPPD crystal deposition.

Hydroxychloroquine[74] may provide some benefit in refractory chronic polyarticular CPPD deposition disease and may reduce flares of pseudogout. The theoretical mechanism of action of hydroxychloroquine in these settings would be via stabilization of phagolysosomes in macrophage lineage cells, thereby suppressing NLRP3 inflammasome activation triggered by CPPD crystal uptake (see Chapter 5). Methotrexate appeared beneficial in a small open study of five consecutive patients with refractory chronic polyarticular CPPD deposition disease, with reduction of pseudogout attacks.[75] In this study, the status of patients prior to methotrexate served as the internal control. IL-1 antagonism (such as off-label use of anakinra as in gout; see Chapter 16) has had anecdotal success.[76,77] In contrast, breakthrough pseudogout was recently reported during TNF antagonism therapy.[78] Collectively, at this point, a sufficient evidence basis is lacking for hydroxychloroquine, methotrexate, and IL-1 antagonism as standard therapies for refractory inflammation in CPPD crystal deposition disease. However, these approaches appear reasonable to clinically explore in refractory disease (see Tables 21-9 and 21-10) and merit well-controlled clinical trials.

There is no known, effective cartilage preservation therapy for idiopathic CPPD deposition disease. There is no evidence to support arthroscopic debridement. Limited evidence suggested that OA patients with cartilage calcification respond distinctly to arthroscopic irrigation[79] and low dose colchicine,[80-81] but substantial clinical trials would be required to support this approach. Since intraarticular hyaluronan therapy can precipitate pseudogout in those with CPPD deposition in the knee, this approach to degenerative arthropathy should be avoided in the presence of CPPD deposition.

Table 21-10 EULAR Expert Guidelines for Management of Clinical Manifestations of CPPD Crystal Deposition

No.	Proposition	LoE	SOR (95% CI)
1	Optimal treatment of CPPD requires both nonpharmacologic and pharmacologic modalities and should be tailored according to clinical features (isolated CC, acute, chronic CPP crystal inflammatory arthritis, OA with CPPD) and general risk factors (age, comorbidities).	IV	93 (85 to 100)
2	For acute CPP crystal arthritis, optimal and safe treatment comprises application of ice or cool packs, temporary rest, joint aspiration, and intraarticular injection of long-acting GCS. For many patients these approaches alone may be sufficient.	IIa-IV	95 (92 to 98)
3	Both oral NSAID (with gastroprotective treatment if indicated) and low-dose oral colchicine (e.g., 0.5 mg up to 3 or 4 times a day with or without an initial dose of 1 mg) are effective systemic treatments for acute CPP crystal arthritis, although their use is often limited by toxicity and comorbidity, especially in the older patient.	Ib-IIb	79 (66 to 91)
4	A short tapering course of oral GCS, or parenteral GCS or ACTH, may be effective for acute CPP crystal arthritis that is not amenable to intraarticular GCS injection and is an alternative to colchicine and/or NSAID.	IIb-III	87 (76 to 97)
5	Prophylaxis against frequent recurrent acute CPP crystal arthritis can be achieved with low-dose oral colchicine (eg, 0.5-1 mg daily) or low-dose oral NSAID (with gastroprotective treatment if indicated).	IIb-IV	81 (70 to 92)
6	The management objectives and treatment options for patients with OA and CPPD are the same as those for OA without CPPD.	Ia	84 (74 to 94)
7	For chronic CPP crystal inflammatory arthritis, pharmacologic options in order of preference are oral NSAID (plus gastroprotective treatment if indicated) and/or colchicine (0.5-1.0 mg daily), low-dose corticosteroid, methotrexate and hydroxychloroquine.	Ib-IV	79 (67 to 91)
8	If detected, associated conditions such as hyperparathyroidism, haemochromatosis or hypomagnesaemia should be treated.	Ib	89 (81 to 98)
9	Currently, no treatment modifies CPP crystal formation or dissolution and no treatment is required for asymptomatic CC.	IV	90 (83 to 97)

LoE and SOR: order according to topic (general, acute attacks, prophylaxis and chronic CPPD management).
ACTH, Adrenocorticotropic hormone; *CC*, chondrocalcinosis; *CPP*, calcium pyrophosphate; *CPPD*, calcium pyrophosphate deposition; *GCS*, glucocorticosteroids; *LoE*, level of evidence (see Table 1 for further details); *NSAID*, nonsteroidal antiinflammatory drug; *OA*, osteoarthritis; *SOR*, strength of recommendation on visual analog scale (0-100 mm, 0 = not recommended at all, 100 = fully recommended).
Level of Evidence Key:
Ia —Meta-analysis of randomized controlled trials
Ib—Randomized controlled trial
IIa —Controlled study without randomization
IIb—Quasi-experimental study
III—Nonexperimental descriptive studies, such as comparative, correlation, and case-control studies
IV—Expert committee reports or opinion or clinical experience of respected authorities, or all
From Zhang W, Doherty M, Pascual E, et al. EULAR recommendations for calcium pyrophosphate deposition. Part II: Management. Ann Rheum Dis 2011 Jan 20 [Epub ahead of print].

Outcome and Prognosis of CPPD Crystal Deposition Disease

Detection of CPPD deposition had been proposed to be a predictive factor for more frequent knee replacement surgery in primary knee OA.[37] In addition, mean radiographic scores directly correlated with detection of calcium-containing crystals in OA at time of total joint arthroplasty in one study.[35] On the other hand, there is evidence that degenerative arthropathy associated with idiopathic/sporadic CPPD crystal deposition disease is less destructive than in primary OA. In one prospective study, degenerative arthritis was slow to progress (as assessed by radiography) in CPPD deposition disease of the knee.[33] Moreover, bidirectional changes in radiographic extent of chondrocalcinosis are observed over time with CPPD deposition,[33] and there is no clear, direct correlation between the extent of joint cartilage calcification and the progression of arthropathy linked with CPPD deposition.

The Boston OA Knee Study (BOKS) and the Health, Aging and Body Composition (Health ABC) Study[82] prospectively evaluated the relationship between chondrocalcinosis and progression of knee OA in a longitudinal manner, using MRI. Knees with chondrocalcinosis had a lower risk of cartilage loss than without chondrocalcinosis. A study from Thailand, in which CPPD deposition was identified by radiographs and/or by synovial fluid analysis in 52.9% of 102 patients undergoing total knee arthroplasty, revealed that those with and without chondrocalcinosis did not differ in activities of daily living or in age at time of total knee arthroplasty.[83] Such studies paint a different picture of the impact of CPPD deposition in OA than that previously hypothesized. Specifically, dysregulated cartilage matrix homeostasis and repair that produces CPPD deposition may be at least as effective at delaying cartilage tissue degradation as other phenotypes of cartilage repair in OA.

Potential Future Developments in Treatment of CPPD Deposition Disease

The low prevalence of CPPD deposition in Beijing is noteworthy, since high oral calcium intake can limit parathyroid hormone production, and calcium levels in tap water in Beijing are very high.[10] Deficient calcium intake, including in the elderly, is a major public health problem in Western countries. CPPD deposition may be more influenced by dietary and environmental factors than previously appreciated, with variability in calcium intake, parathyroid function, and possible vitamin D metabolism all warranting further investigation.

Probenecid, an anion transport inhibitor, suppresses ANKH-induced and TGFβ-induced increases in extracellular PP_i in vitro.[84,85] The potential to develop therapies for both CPPD crystal–associated arthropathies based on new molecular targets has been further illuminated by molecular structure, regulation, and function studies on ANKH, ENPP1, and TG2 (see Chapter 20). Prevention of CPPD deposition by polyphosphates or stimulation of CPPD crystal degradation by alkaline phosphatase and by polyamines (via pyrophosphatase activation) could provide alternative therapeutic modalities.[86-88] One caveat is that accelerated but incomplete CPPD crystal dissolution by intraarticular knee lavage with disodium EDTA and magnesium ions was a therapeutic failure, due to postlavage attacks of pseudogout mediated by crystal shedding and removal of only small amounts of CPPD crystals.[89] Slower, intraarticular "depot"-based or systemic means of modulation of CPPD crystals might be more successful due to fewer "crystal mobilization" flares of pseudogout. Last, the roles of the NLRP3 inflammasome, caspase-1 activation, and IL-1β processing in CPPD crystal–induced inflammation[90] collectively point to novel potential therapeutic targets for CPPD crystal–associated inflammation and cartilage degradation.

CPPD Deposition Disease–Related Internet Sites of Interest

Familial Chondrocalcinosis Recruitment Page for Wellcome Trust Centre for Human Genetics. http://www.well.ox.ac.uk/brown/chondro.shtml.
Teaching resource page for radiographic images of CPPD arthropathy. http://www.orthopaedicweblinks.com/Teaching_Resources/Radiology/more3.html.

References

1. Zhang W, Doherty M, Bardin T, et al. European League Against Rheumatism recommendations for calcium pyrophosphate deposition. Part I: terminology and diagnosis. Ann Rheum Dis 2011 Jan 7:[Epub ahead of print].
2. Zhang W, Doherty M, Pascual E, et al. EULAR recommendations for calcium pyrophosphate deposition. Part II: Management. Ann Rheum Dis 2011 Jan 20:[Epub ahead of print].
3. Felson DT, Anderson JJ, Naimark A, et al. The prevalence of chondrocalcinosis in the elderly and its association with knee osteoarthritis: the Framingham Study. J Rheumatol 1989;16(9):1241–5.
4. Richette P, Bardin T, Doherty M. An update on the epidemiology of calcium pyrophosphate dihydrate crystal deposition disease. Rheumatology (Oxford) 2009;48(7):711–5.
5. Neame RL, Carr AJ, Muir K, et al. UK community prevalence of knee chondrocalcinosis: evidence that correlation with osteoarthritis is through a shared association with osteophyte. Ann Rheum Dis 2003;62(6):513–8.
6. Ramonda R, Musacchio E, Perissinotto E, et al. Prevalence of chondrocalcinosis in Italian subjects from northeastern Italy. The Pro.V.A. (PROgetto Veneto Anziani) study. Clin Exp Rheumatol 2009;27(6):981–4.
7. Salaffi F, De Angelis R, Grassi W, et al. INvestigation Group (MAPPING) study. Prevalence of musculoskeletal conditions in an Italian population sample: results of a regional community-based study. I. The MAPPING study. Clin Exp Rheumatol 2005;23(6):819–28.
8. Ellman MH, Levin B. Chondrocalcinosis in elderly persons. Arthritis Rheum 1975;18(1):43–7.
9. Mitrovic DR, Stankovic A, Iriarte-Borda O, et al. The prevalence of chondrocalcinosis in the human knee joint. An autopsy survey. J Rheumatol 1988;15(4):633–41.
10. Zhang Y, Terkeltaub R, Nevitt M, et al. Lower prevalence of chondrocalcinosis in Chinese subjects in Beijing than in white subjects in the United States: The Beijing Osteoarthritis Study. Arthritis Rheum 2006;54(11):3508–12.
11. Zaka R, Williams CJ. Genetics of chondrocalcinosis. Osteoarthritis Cartilage 2005;13(9):745–50.
12. Pendleton A, Johnson MD, Hughes A, et al. Mutations in ANKH cause chondrocalcinosis. Am J Hum Genet 2002;71(4):933–40.
13. Williams JC, Zhang Y, Timms A, et al. Autosomal dominant familial calcium pyrophosphate dihydrate deposition disease is caused by mutation in the transmembrane protein ANKH. Am J Hum Genet 2002;71(4):985–91.
14. Zhang Y, Johnson K, Russell RG, et al. Association of sporadic chondrocalcinosis with a -4-basepair G-to-A transition in the 5'-untranslated region of ANKH that promotes enhanced expression of ANKH protein and excess generation of extracellular inorganic pyrophosphate. Arthritis Rheum 2005;52(4):1110–7.
15. Pons-Estel BA, Gimenez C, Sacnun M, et al. Familial osteoarthritis and Milwaukee shoulder associated with calcium pyrophosphate and apatite crystal deposition. J Rheumatol 2000;27(2):471–80.
16. Reginato AJ, Passano GM, Neumann G, et al. Familial spondyloepiphyseal dysplasia tarda, brachydactyly, and precocious osteoarthritis associated with an arginine 75→cysteine mutation in the procollagen type II gene in a kindred of Chiloe Islanders. I. Clinical, radiographic, and pathologic findings. Arthritis Rheum 1994;37(7):1078–86.
17. Bruges-Armas J, Couto AR, Timms A, et al. Ectopic calcification among families in the Azores: clinical and radiologic manifestations in families with diffuse idiopathic skeletal hyperostosis and chondrocalcinosis. Arthritis Rheum 2006;54(4):1340–9.
18. Jones AC, Chuck AJ, Arie EA, et al. Diseases associated with calcium pyrophosphate deposition disease. Semin Arthritis Rheum 1992;22(3):188–202.
19. Richette P, Ayoub G, Bardin T, et al. Hypomagnesemia and chondrocalcinosis in short bowel syndrome. J Rheumatol 2005;32(12):2434–6.
20. Hoorn EJ, van der Hoek J, de Man RA, et al. A case series of proton pump inhibitor-induced hypomagnesemia. Am J Kidney Dis 2010;56(1):112–6.
21. Van Laecke S, Desideri F, Geerts A, et al. Hypomagnesemia and the risk of new-onset diabetes after liver transplantation. Liver Transpl 2010;16(11):1278–87.
22. Sabbagh F, El Tawil Z, Lecerf F, et al. Impact of cyclosporine A on magnesium homeostasis: clinical observation in lung transplant recipients and experimental study in mice. Transplantation 2008;86(3):436–44.
23. Bergström G, Bjelle A, Sundh V, et al. Joint disorders at ages 70, 75 and 79 years—a cross-sectional comparison. Br J Rheumatol 1986;25(4):333–41.
24. Wilkins E, Dieppe P, Maddison P, et al. Osteoarthritis and articular chondrocalcinosis in the elderly. Ann Rheum Dis 1983;42(3):280–4.
25. Canhao H, Fonseca JE, Leandro MJ, et al. Cross-sectional study of 50 patients with calcium pyrophosphate dihydrate crystal arthropathy. Clin Rheumatol 2001;20(2):119–22.
26. Bernardeau C, Bucki B, Lioté F. Acute arthritis after intra-articular hyaluronate injection: onset of effusions without crystals. Ann Rheum Dis 2000;60(5):518–20.
27. Sandor V, Hassan R, Kohn E. Exacerbation of pseudogout by granulocyte colony-stimulating factor. Ann Intern Med 1996;125(9):781.
28. Wendling D, Tisserand G, Griffond V, et al. Acute pseudogout after pamidronate infusion. Clin Rheumatol 2008;27(9):1205–6.
29. Benito-Lopez P, Ramos-Rolon G, Ysamat-Marfa R, et al. Pseudogout caused by thyroid hormone replacement therapy. Rev Clin Esp 1981;163(5):349–50.
30. Chaisson CE, McAlindon TE, Felson DT, et al. Lack of association between thyroid status and chondrocalcinosis or osteoarthritis: the Framingham Osteoarthritis Study. J Rheumatol 1996;23(4):711–5.
31. Job-Deslandre C, Menkes CJ, Guinot M, et al. Does hypothyroidism increase the prevalence of chondrocalcinosis? Br J Rheumatol 1993;32(3):197–8.
32. Mavrikakis ME, Antoniades LG, Kontoyannis SA, et al. CPPD crystal deposition disease as a cause of unrecognised pyrexia. Clin Exp Rheumatol 1994;12(4):419–21.
33. Doherty M, Dieppe P, Watt I. Pyrophosphate arthropathy: a prospective study. Br J Rheumatol 1993;32(3):189–96.
34. Derfus BA, Kurian JB, Butler JJ, et al. The high prevalence of pathologic calcium crystals in pre-operative knees. J Rheumatol 2002;29(3):570–4.
35. McCarthy GM, Cheung HS. Point: hydroxyapatite crystal deposition is intimately involved in the pathogenesis and progression of human osteoarthritis. Curr Rheumatol Rep 2009;11(2):141–7.

36. Reuge L, Lindhoudt DV, Geerster J. Local deposition of calcium pyrophosphate crystals in evolution of knee osteoarthritis. Clin Rheumatol 2001;20(6):428–31.
37. van Linthoudt D, Beutler A, Clayburne G, et al. Morphometric studies on synovium in advanced osteoarthritis: is there an association between apatite-like material and collagen deposits? Clin Exp Rheumatol 1997;15(5):493–7.
38. Schlesinger N, Hassett AL, Neustadter L, et al. Does acute synovitis (pseudogout) occur in patients with chronic pyrophosphate arthropathy (pseudo-osteoarthritis)? Clin Exp Rheumatol 2009;27(6):940–4.
39. Nakase T, Takeuchi E, Sugamoto K, et al. Involvement of multinucleated giant cells synthesizing cathepsin K in calcified tendinitis of the rotator cuff tendons. Rheumatology (Oxford) 2000;39(10):1074–7.
40. Yamakawa K, Iwasaki H, Ohjimi Y, et al. Tumoral calcium pyrophosphate dihydrate crystal deposition disease. Pathology 2001;197(7):499–506.
41. Kwak SM, Resnick D, Haghighi P. Calcium pyrophosphate dihydrate crystal deposition disease of the knee simulating spontaneous osteonecrosis. Clin Rheumatol 1999;18(5):390–3.
42. el Maghraoui A, Lecoules S, Lechavalier D, et al. Acute sacroiliitis as a manifestation of calcium pyrophosphate dihydrate crystal deposition disease. Clin Exp Rheumatol 1999;17(4):477–8.
43. Fujishiro T, Nabeshima Y, Yasui S, et al. Pseudogout attack of the lumbar facet joint: a case report. Spine 2002;27(17):396–8.
44. Cabre P, Pascal-Moussellard H, Kaidomar S, et al. Six cases of ligamentum cervical flavum calcification in blacks in the French West Indies. Joint Bone Spine 2001;68(2):158–65.
45. Assaker R, Louis E, Boutry N, et al. Foramen magnum syndrome secondary to calcium pyrophosphate crystal deposition in the transverse ligament of atlas. Spine 2001;26(12):1396–400.
46. Kakitsubata Y, Boutin RD, Theodorou DJ, et al. Calcium pyrophosphate dihydrate crystal deposition in and around the atlantoaxial joints: association with type 2 odontoid fractures in nine patients. Radiology 2000;216:213–9.
47. Doherty M, Hamilton E, Henderson J, et al. Familial chondrocalcinosis due to calcium pyrophosphate dihydrate crystal deposition in English families. Br J Rheumatol 1991;30(1):10–5.
48. Williams CJ, Pendleton A, Bonavita G, et al. Mutations in the amino terminus of ANKH in two US families with calcium pyrophosphate dihydrate crystal deposition disease. Arthritis Rheum 2003;48(9):2627–31.
49. Andrew LJ, Brancolini V, Serrano de la Pena L, et al. Refinement of the chromosome 5p locus for familial calcium pyrophosphate dihydrate deposition disease. Am J Human Genet 1999;64(1):136–45.
50. Keen CE, Crocker PR, Brady K, et al. Intraosseous secondary calcium salt crystal deposition: an artefact of acid decalcification. Histopathology 1995;27(2):181–5.
51. Ivorra J, Rosas J, Pascual E. Most calcium pyrophosphate crystals appear as non-birefringent. Ann Rheum Dis 1999;58(9):582–4.
52. Robier C, Neubauer M, Quehenberger F, et al. Coincidence of calcium pyrophosphate and monosodium urate crystals in the synovial fluid of patients with gout determined by the cytocentrifugation technique. Ann Rheum Dis 2010 Oct 21:[Epub ahead of print].
53. Galvez J, Saiz E, Linares LF, et al. Delayed examination of synovial fluid by ordinary and polarized light microscopy to detect and identify crystals. Ann Rheum Dis 2002;61(5):444–7.
54. Petrocelli A, Wong AL, Sweezy RL. Identification of pathologic synovial fluid crystals on Gram stains. J Clin Rheumatol 1998;4(2):103–5.
55. Selvi E, Manganelli S, Catenaccio M, et al. Diff Quik staining method for detection and identification of monosodium urate and calcium pyrophosphate crystals in synovial fluids. Ann Rheum Dis 2001;60(3):194–8.
56. Ohira T, Ishikawa K. Preservation of calcium pyrophosphate dihydrate crystals: effect of Mayer's haematoxylin staining period. Ann Rheum Dis 2001;60(1):80–2.
57. Fisseler-Eckhoff A, Muller KM. Arthroscopy and chondrocalcinosis. Arthroscopy 1992;8(1):98–104.
58. Steinbach LS, Resnick D. Calcium pyrophosphate dihydrate crystal deposition disease: imaging perspective. Curr Probl Diagn Radiol 2000;29(6):209–29.
59. Filippucci E, Scire CA, Delle Sedie A, et al. Ultrasound imaging for the rheumatologist. XXV. Sonographic assessment of the knee in patients with gout and calcium pyrophosphate deposition disease. Clin Exp Rheumatol 2010;28(1):2–5.
60. Grassi W, Meenagh G, Pascual E, et al. "Crystal clear"-sonographic assessment of gout and calcium pyrophosphate deposition disease. Semin Arthritis Rheum 2006;36(3):197–202.
61. Frediani B, Filippou G, Falsetti P, et al. Diagnosis of calcium pyrophosphate dihydrate crystal deposition disease: ultrasonographic criteria proposed. Ann Rheum Dis 2005;64(4):638–40.
62. Foldes K. Knee chondrocalcinosis: an ultrasonographic study of the hyalin cartilage. Clin Imaging 2002;26(3):194–6.
63. Sofka CM, Adler RS, Cordasco FA. Ultrasound diagnosis of chondrocalcinosis in the knee. Skeletal Radiol 2002;31(1):43–5.
64. Monteforte P, Brignone A, Rovetta G. Tissue changes detectable by sonography before radiological evidence of elbow chondrocalcinosis. Int J Tissue React 2000;22(1):23–5.
65. Falsetti P, Frediani B, Acciai C, et al. Ultrasonographic study of Achilles tendon and plantar fascia in chondrocalcinosis. J Rheumatol 2004;31(11):2242–50.
66. Choi HK, Al-Arfaj AM, Eftekhari A, et al. Dual energy computed tomography in tophaceous gout. Ann Rheum Dis 2009;68(10):1609–12.
67. Abreu M, Johnson K, Chung CB, et al. Calcification in calcium pyrophosphate dihydrate (CPPD) crystalline deposits in the knee: anatomic, radiographic, MR imaging, and histologic study in cadavers. Skeletal Radiol 2004;33(7):392–8.
68. Meed SD, Spilberg I. Successful use of colchicine in acute polyarticular pseudogout. J Rheumatol 1981;8(4):689–91.
69. Ritter J, Kerr LD, Valeriano-Marcet J, et al. ACTH revisited: effective treatment for acute crystal induced synovitis in patients with multiple medical problems. J Rheumatol 1994;21(4):696–9.
70. Halverson PB, Ryan LM. Tidal lavage in Milwaukee shoulder syndrome: do crystals make the difference? J Rheumatol 2007;34(7):1446–7.
71. Epis O, Caporali R, Scire CA, et al. Efficacy of tidal irrigation in Milwaukee shoulder syndrome. J Rheumatol 2007;34(7):1545–50.
72. Alvarellos A, Spilberg I. Colchicine prophylaxis in pseudogout. J Rheumatol 1986;13(4):804–5.
73. Smilde TJ, Haverman JF, Schipper P, et al. Familial hypokalemia/hypomagnesemia and chondrocalcinosis. J Rheumatol 1994;21(8):1515–9.
74. Rothschild B, Yakubov LE. Prospective 6-month, double-blind trial of hydroxychloroquine treatment of CPPD. Compr Ther 1997;23(5):327–31.
75. Chollet-Janin A, Finckh A, Dudler J, et al. Methotrexate as an alternative therapy for chronic calcium pyrophosphate deposition disease: an exploratory analysis. Arthritis Rheum 2007;56(2):688–92.
76. Announ N, Palmer G, Guerne PA, et al. Anakinra is a possible alternative in the treatment and prevention of acute attacks of pseudogout in end-stage renal failure. Joint Bone Spine 2009;76(4):424–6.
77. McGonagle D, Tan AL, Madden J, et al. Successful treatment of resistant pseudogout with anakinra. Arthritis Rheum 2008;58(2):631–3.
78. Josefina M, Ana CJ, Ariel V, et al. Development of pseudogout during etanercept treatment. J Clin Rheumatol 2007;13(3):177.
79. Kalunian KC, Ike RW, Seeger LL, et al. Visually-guided irrigation in patients with early knee osteoarthritis: a multicenter randomized, controlled trial. Osteoarthritis Cartilage 2000;8(6):412–8.
80. Das SK, Mishra K, Ramakrishnan S, et al. A randomized controlled trial to evaluate the slow-acting symptom modifying effects of a regimen containing colchicine in a subset of patients with osteoarthritis of the knee. Osteoarthritis Cartilage 2002;10(4):247–52.
81. Das SK, Ramakrishnan S, Mishra K, et al. A randomized controlled trial to evaluate the slow-acting symptom modifying effects of colchicine in osteoarthritis of the knee: a preliminary report. Arthritis Care Res 2002;47(3):280–4.
82. Neogi T, Nevitt M, Niu J, et al. Lack of association between chondrocalcinosis and increased risk of cartilage loss in knees with osteoarthritis: results of two prospective longitudinal magnetic resonance imaging studies. Arthritis Rheum 2006;54(6):1822–8.
83. Viriyavejkul P, Wilairatana V, Tanavalee A, et al. Comparison of characteristics of patients with and without calcium pyrophosphate dihydrate crystal deposition disease who underwent total knee replacement surgery for osteoarthritis. Osteoarthritis Cartilage 2007;15(2):232–5.
84. Ho A, Johnson M, Kingsley DM. Role of the mouse ank gene in tissue calcification and arthritis. Science 2000;14;289(5477):265–70.
85. Rosenthal AK, Ryan LM. Probenecid inhibits transforming growth factor-beta 1 induced pyrophosphate elaboration by chondrocytes. J Rheumatol 1994;21(5):896–900.
86. Kannampuzha JV, Tupy JH, Pritzker KP. Mercaptopyruvate inhibits tissue-nonspecific alkaline phosphatase and calcium pyrophosphate dihydrate crystal dissolution. J Rheumatol 2009;36(12):2758–65.
87. Cini R, Chindamo D, Catenaccio M, et al. Dissolution of calcium pyrophosphate crystals by polyphosphates: an in vitro and ex vivo study. Ann Rheum Dis 2001;60(10):962–7.

88. Shinozaki T, Pritzker KP. Polyamines enhance calcium pyrophosphate dihydrate crystal dissolution. J Rheumatol 1995;22(10):1907–12.

89. Bennett RM, Lehr JR, McCarty DJ. Crystal shedding and acute pseudogout. An hypothesis based on a therapeutic failure. Arthritis Rheum 1976;19(1):93–7.

90. Martinon F, Petrilli V, Mayor A, et al. Gout-associated uric acid crystals activate the NALP3 inflammasome. Nature 2006;440:237–41.

91. Zhang W, Neame R, Doherty S, et al. Relative risk of knee chondrocalcinosis in siblings of index cases with pyrophosphate arthropathy. Ann Rheum Dis 2004;63(8):969–73.

92. Gordon TP, Smith M, Ebert B, et al. Articular chondrocalcinosis in a hospital population: an Australian experience. Aust N Z J Med 1984;14(5):655–9.

93. Cruz J, Aviña-Zubieta A, Martínez de la Escalera G, et al. Molecular heterogeneity of prolactin in the plasma of patients with systemic lupus erythematosus. Arthritis Rheum 2001;44(6):1331–5.

94. Doherty M, Dieppe P, Watt I. Low incidence of calcium pyrophosphate dihydrate crystal deposition in rheumatoid arthritis, with modification of radiographic features in coexistent disease. Arthritis Rheum 1984;27(9):1002–9.

95. Viriyavejkul P, Wilairatana V, Tanavalee A, et al. Comparison of characteristics of patients with and without calcium pyrophosphate dihydrate crystal deposition disease who underwent total knee replacement surgery for osteoarthritis. Osteoarthr Cartil 2007;15(2):232–5.

96. Ellman MH, Brown NL, Levin B. Prevalence of knee chondrocalcinosis in hospital and clinic patients aged 50 or older. J Am Geriatr Soc 1981; 29(4):189–92.

97. Sanmartí R, Serrarols M, Galinsoga A, et al. Diseases associated with articular chondrocalcinosis: an analysis of a series of 95 cases. Med Clin (Barc) 1993;101(8):294–7.

98. Fernandez Dapica MP, Gómez-Reino JJ. Familial chondrocalcinosis in the Spanish population. J Rheumatol 1986;13(3):631–3.

99. Riestra JL, Sánchez A, Rodríques-Valverde V, et al. Roentgenographic features of the arthropathy associated with CPPD crystal deposition disease. A comparative study with primary osteoarthritis. J Rheumatol 1985;12(6):1154–8.

100. Al-Arfaj AS. The relationship between chondrocalcinosis and osteoarthritis in Saudi Arabia. Clin Rheumatol 2002;21(6):493–6.

101. Menkes CJ, Decraemere W, Postel M, et al. Chondrocalcinosis and rapid destruction of the hip. J Rheumatol 1985;12(1):130–3.

102. Stucki G, Hardegger D, Böhni U, et al. Degeneration of the scaphoid-trapezium joint: a useful finding to differentiate calcium pyrophosphate deposition disease from osteoarthritis. Clin Rheumatol 1999;18(3):232–7.

103. Bourqui M, Vischer TL, Stasse P, et al. Pyrophosphate arthropathy in the carpal and metacarpophalangeal joints. Ann Rheum Dis 1983;42(6):626–30.

104. Hansen SE, Herning M. A comparative study of radiographic changes in knee joints in chondrocalcinosis, osteoarthrosis and rheumatoid arthritis. Scand J Rheumatol 1984;13(1):85–92.

105. Schouten JS, van den Ouweland FA, Valkenburg HA. A 12 year follow up study in the general population on prognostic factors of cartilage loss in osteoarthritis of the knee. Ann Rheum Dis 1992;51(8):932–7.

106. Ledingham J, Regan M, Jones A, et al. Factors affecting radiographic progression of knee osteoarthritis. Ann Rheum Dis 1995;54(1):53–8.

107. Doherty M, Dieppe P, Watt I. Low incidence of calcium pyrophosphate dihydrate crystal deposition in rheumatoid arthritis, with modification of radiographic features in coexistent disease. Arthritis Rheum 1984;27(9):1002–9.

108. Brasseur JP, Huaux JP, Devogelaer JP, et al. Articular chondrocalcinosis in seropositive rheumatoid arthritis. Comparison with a control group. J Rheumatol 1987;14(1):40–1.

109. Yashiro T, Okamoto T, Tanaka R, et al. Prevalence of chondrocalcinosis in patients with primary hyperparathyroidism in Japan. Endocrinol Jpn 1991;38(5):457–64.

110. Alexander GM, Dieppe PA, Doherty M, et al. Pyrophosphate arthropathy: a study of metabolic associations and laboratory data. Ann Rheum Dis 1982;41:377–81.

111. Huaux JP, Geubel A, Koch MC, et al. The arthritis of hemochromatosis. A review of 25 cases with special reference to chondrocalcinosis, and a comparison with patients with primary hyperparathyroidism and controls. Clin Rheumatol 1986;5(3):317–24.

112. Pritchard MH, Jessop JD. Chondrocalcinosis in primary hyperparathyroidism. Influence of age, metabolic bone disease, and parathyroidectomy. Ann Rheum Dis 1977;36:146–51.

113. Rynes RI, Merzig EG. Calcium pyrophosphate crystal deposition disease and hyperparathyroidism: a controlled, prospective study. J Rheumatol 1978;5(4):460–8.

114. Richette P, Ayoub G, Lahalle S, et al. Hypomagnesemia associated with chondrocalcinosis: a cross-sectional study. Arthritis Rheum 2007;57(8):1496–501.

115. Utsinger PD, Resnick D, Zvaifler NJ. Wrist arthropathy in calcium pyrophosphate dihydrate deposition disease. Arthritis Rheum 1975;18(5): 485–91.

116. Lumbreras B, Pascual E, Frasquet J, et al. Analysis for crystals in synovial fluid: training of the analysts results in high consistency. Ann Rheum Dis 2005;64(4):612–5.

117. Filippou G, Frediani B, Gallo A, et al. A "new" technique for the diagnosis of chondrocalcinosis of the knee: sensitivity and specificity of high-frequency ultrasonography. Ann Rheum Dis 2007;66(8):1126–8.

Chapter 22

Basic Calcium Phosphate Crystal Arthropathy

Paul MacMullan, Gillian McMahon and Geraldine M. McCarthy

KEY POINTS

- Basic calcium phosphate (BCP) crystals are a group of ultramicroscopic crystals that are mainly composed of hydroxyapatite and are frequently deposited in articular tissues.
- BCP crystal deposition gives rise to a number of specific clinical syndromes, affecting both periarticular (e.g., calcific periarthritis) and intraarticular joint structures (e.g., Milwaukee shoulder syndrome).
- An emerging body of evidence indicates a significant pathogenic role for BCP crystals in osteoarthritis (OA). These crystals are produced by diseased articular cartilage and contribute directly to the synovium-derived joint inflammation often seen in OA.
- Novel approaches to the detection of BCP crystals in synovial fluid have highlighted their pathogenic potential.
- The treatment of periarticular and intraarticular BCP-associated arthropathies remains largely symptomatic as no treatment currently exists to specifically antagonize the pathogenic effects of BCP crystals.
- The absence of any disease-modifying osteoarthritic drugs has led to a renewed interest in anticrystal agents such as phosphocitrate as a potential medical treatment for OA.

may involve tendons, ligaments, intravertebral discs, joint capsule, synovium, and cartilage. There is an emerging body of evidence that these crystals may also play a key pathogenic role in degenerative osteoarthritis (OA), the most common of human joint disorders.

The purpose of this chapter is to outline the historical perspective and epidemiology of BCP crystal disease, discuss in detail the clinical features of the recognized periarticular and intraarticular syndromes associated with BCP crystal deposition, and to explore the emerging potential pathogenic role of these crystals in OA. Calcification of articular cartilage is a well-recognized feature of OA, with current evidence suggesting that it contributes directly to joint degeneration.[1] However, data on the distribution and frequency of BCP crystals in OA synovial fluid and articular cartilage vary widely, mainly due the lack of simple and reliable methods of detection.[3] Thus, a substantial section of this chapter is directed toward recent published developments regarding improved methods of detection of these BCP crystals and their clinical implications. The treatment of the traditional BCP crystal–associated arthropathies is then discussed in terms of both medical and surgical management. Finally, future avenues of investigation regarding the role of BCP crystals in degenerative joint disease are also addressed, with a particular emphasis on the potential development of effective disease-modifying medical interventions in OA, which are currently unavailable.

Introduction

Basic calcium phosphate (BCP) crystals are a group of ultramicroscopic crystalline particulates that give rise to a number of particular clinical syndromes affecting both periarticular and intraarticular joint structures. BCP collectively describes calcium phosphate crystals, including hydroxyapatite (HA), octacalcium phosphate, tricalcium phosphate, and magnesium whitlockite.[1] The most abundant of these crystal species in BCP crystal–associated clinical syndromes is HA, with smaller amounts of its precursors: octacalcium phosphate and the rarely found tricalcium phosphate.[2] The use of the generic term "BCP" crystal deposition was proposed because all crystals identified were basic (as opposed to acidic) calcium phosphates. BCP crystals frequently deposit in articular tissues but may also be found in arteries, skin, breast, and other tissues.[1] The clinical manifestations of BCP crystal deposition and their pathologic sequelae in the musculoskeletal system

Historical Perspective

Specific clinical syndromes manifesting with both periarticular and intraarticular structural pathology and subsequently found to be associated with BCP crystal deposition have long been recognized in the rheumatology literature.

Calcific Periarthritis

Calcific scapulohumeral periarthritis was first described in 1870 and radiographic demonstration of periarticular shoulder calcifications was accomplished by 1907.[4] Initially these calcifications were thought to have arisen in the subdeltoid bursa but were subsequently demonstrated to occur chiefly in the supraspinatus tendon or the shoulder joint capsule. Years later in 1938, further descriptions of calcific periarthritis of the shoulder heralded a revival of interest in the syndrome and also the recognition of periarticular calcifications at other sites.[5] Another generation later in 1966, it was recognized that the calcific material consisted primarily of HA.[6] This paved the way for the development of the theory that the pathogenic mechanism of calcifying tendonitis is a unique disorder of the musculotendinous junction involving primary tendon necrosis leading to secondary calcification.[7] Subsequently, aggregated clumps of what have become known as BCP crystals and their various crystalline structures, chemical compositions, and physical properties have been further defined using various ultrastructural and microanalytical techniques. These modern tools include standard microscopy with staining, electron microscopy, x-ray diffraction, atomic force microscopy, Raman and Fourier transformation infrared spectroscopy, radioactive assays, and some novel developments involving tetracycline binding and modified paramagnetic beads.[2,8] These developments have enhanced our understanding of the bioactive nature of BCP crystals and have led to a renewed interest in their pathogenic potential.

Intraarticular BCP Crystal Disease

Robert Adams, the famed nineteenth-century Irish surgeon, in what he termed "chronic rheumatic arthritis of the shoulder" in 1857, is credited with the earliest description of the pathologic consequences and anatomic structural damage due to intraarticular BCP crystal deposition.[9] In 1934, Codman reported what he called a "subacromial space hygroma" in a middle-aged woman who presented with recurrent shoulder joint effusions, absent rotator cuff, cartilaginous bodies attached to the synovial tissue, and severe destructive glenohumeral arthritis.[10] These clinical descriptions were made without the benefit of modern radiologic investigations or diagnostic tests and were primarily based on direct visualization during operative surgery or at postmortem examination. This condition has subsequently been known by many different names. In the French literature, the terms *les caries séniles hémorragique de l'épaule* and *l'arthropathie destructrice rapide de l'épaule* have been used,[11] and in the English literature, terms such as "cuff-tear arthropathy" appear.[12] Common to all of these descriptions is the preponderance of elderly female patients with primary involvement of the shoulder joint.[13]

The identification of BCP crystal deposition in articular cartilage (both hyaline and meniscal) and its association with joint disease is a much more recent discovery. Electron microscopic evaluation of synovial fluid led to the first description in 1976 of BCP crystal aggregates in patients with OA,[14] albeit that the presence of solid deposits of BCP crystals in knee menisci had been noted 10 years previously in a report detailing pathologic postmortem findings.[15] This finding that clumps of BCP crystals are present in the synovial fluid of patients with degenerative joint disease was later confirmed by others.[16,17] In a seminal paper, Dan McCarty's group described a large joint destructive arthropathy, most commonly affecting the shoulder joint and mostly seen in elderly women, and called it "Milwaukee shoulder."[18] They noted the presence of large quantities of BCP crystals and collagenase in the synovial fluid, and they hypothesized that the BCP crystals played a major causal role in the associated joint destruction.[18] Subsequently, others noted that many large joints could be involved and terms such as *apatite-associated destructive arthritis* and *idiopathic destructive arthritis of the shoulder* were added to the list of names. BCP crystals were also described in the joint fluids of a few patients with acute synovitis and other forms of arthropathy.[17]

Epidemiology

The true epidemiology of the BCP crystal–associated arthropathies is unknown. To date, few systematic studies of the incidence or prevalence of periarticular deposits of BCP crystals have been carried out. Similarly, the prevalence of intraarticular BCP crystal deposition in the normal population has not been established.

Calcific Periarthritis

Juxtaarticular BCP crystal deposits are often asymptomatic and are most commonly discovered as an incidental finding on plain film radiography. One large scale study of approximately 12,000 shoulder joints of white collar workers published in 1941 reported a prevalence of approximately 3% of calcific shoulder deposits in a predominantly Caucasian population, of which only slightly more than one third were associated with clinical problems.[19] Interestingly, the prevalence was highest (about 20%) in the younger cohort (31 to 40 years of age), with a clear female predominance. No comparable epidemiologic data have been reported subsequently, although a number of smaller pathologic and radiographic studies have documented the relatively high frequency of periarticular calcification. In contrast to intraarticular BCP crystal deposition, calcific periarthritis has been reported in children as young as 3 years old but appears to be relatively uncommon in the elderly. This suggests that many of the calcific deposits seen in young adults must disappear spontaneously. However, there remains a paucity of hard epidemiologic data related to this relatively common phenomenon.

Intraarticular BCP Crystal Deposition

While calcification of articular cartilage (both hyaline and meniscal) is a well-recognized feature of degenerative joint disease, the prevalence and type of calcium crystal deposition in normal joints at different ages are not known. BCP crystals are found in up to 60% of synovial fluid samples from unselected OA patients at knee arthroplasty.[20] Although ample in vitro evidence demonstrates the potent biologic effects of BCP crystals, controversy exists as to whether these crystals play a causal role or are merely reflective of the joint damage seen in OA.[21] This question will be addressed here. The prevalence of the large joint destructive arthropathy of the elderly known as Milwaukee shoulder syndrome and related BCP crystal–associated arthropathies is unknown, with current evidence suggesting that they are uncommon and tend to occur in elderly individuals, with females predominantly more affected than males.

Clinical Features

There are several specific syndromes associated with BCP crystals involving the musculoskeletal system. These arise mainly due to crystal deposition in and around joints but also include a number of secondary forms of BCP deposition that occur in association with certain connective tissue diseases, chronic renal failure, and inherited disorders of phosphate metabolism. These are listed in Table 22-1 and discussed next.

Periarticular BCP Deposition

Juxtaarticular BCP crystal deposition may occur in bursae, tendons, ligaments, joint capsules, and soft tissues. These periarticular crystal deposits are often asymptomatic but are also associated with a number of clinical syndromes. The most well-recognized presentation is that of acute calcific periarthritis. This is an acute inflammatory syndrome mainly affecting the shoulder but it can occur in association with almost any joint. The vast majority of cases present spontaneously with a sudden onset, and if there is a history of trauma, it is usually mild and related to overuse. Presenting features include all the cardinal signs of acute inflammation. Patients complain of sudden onset of severe pain followed by local swelling, heat, and erythema of the overlying skin. The pain is exacerbated by both active and passive movement of the joint, and there is extreme local tenderness. When the shoulder is affected, the pain is usually felt in the subacromial region with radiation distally, and there is marked rotator cuff tenderness. Both glenohumeral and scapulothoracic movements are voluntarily restricted due to pain. As symptoms typically take up to 3 weeks to resolve, the lack of shoulder mobilization may lead to the development of a "frozen shoulder."

Table 22-1 Clinical Features of BCP Crystal Deposition

	Incidental Finding
Periarticular crystal disease	Calcific periarthritis, e.g., rupture of supraspinatus tendon calcific deposit
	Hydroxyapatite pseudopodagra
	Polyarticular disease may mimic seronegative arthritis
Secondary BCP crystal deposition	Tumoral calcinosis, e.g., hyperparathyroidism and renal failure, familial
	Calciphylaxis, e.g., dialysis dependent patients with raised calcium/phosphate product
	Calcinosis associated with scleroderma
	Fascial plane calcification in dermatomyositis
	Iatrogenic, e.g., injection tract calcification
	Myositis ossificans, e.g., post traumatic brain injury
Intraarticular BCP crystal disease	Incidental asymptomatic finding
	Milwaukee shoulder syndrome
	Acute synovitis, e.g., rupture of calcific deposit communicating with joint space
	Chronic monoarthritis, e.g., erosive OA
	Emerging role in the pathogenesis of OA

The syndrome of calcific periarthritis is thought to arise following rupture of a previously quiescent calcific deposit into the adjacent soft tissue or bursa, thus initiating an acute inflammatory reaction.[22] However, it remains unclear why this rupture occurs as most cases arise spontaneously in the absence of any clear precipitant. When the shoulder joint is affected, this rupture of crystalline material (arising most commonly from the supraspinatus tendon) often induces an intense inflammatory reaction involving the subacromial bursa. The dense radiographic appearance of calcium deposits with well-defined borders seen in asymptomatic individuals before an attack is in contrast to often blurred and poorly defined calcification on plain film radiographic imaging during an acute attack (Fig. 22-1). Consequently, patients presenting with suspected calcific periarthritis may require further imaging during an acute episode. Figure 22-2 illustrates the contemporaneous CT images in the sagittal (Fig. 22-2, A) and axial (Fig. 22-2, B) planes of the same shoulder joint depicted in the plain radiograph of Figure 22-1, with a much clearer delineation of the size, location, and extent of the calcific deposit in the supraspinatus tendon. While the shoulder joint is by far the most commonly affected site, other large peripheral joints such as the hip, knee, elbow, wrist, and ankle may also be affected. The smaller peripheral joints of the hands and feet are rarely involved,[23] apart from the first metatarsophalangeal joint of the foot (which may simulate an attack of gout in an otherwise healthy young woman), a condition known as "hydroxyapatite pseudopodagra," which is characterized by amorphous calcium crystal deposition in periarticular tendons, bursae, and ligaments.[24] Acute neck pain attributed to calcifications surrounding the odontoid process has been described and called the "crowned dens" syndrome. These calcifications appear to be composed of apatite or calcium pyrophosphate dihydrate (CPPD), or a combination of both, although analytical data of the exact biochemical nature of these calcified deposits are limited.[25]

Some patients with multifocal deposits develop symptoms simultaneously at several different sites. This can cause significant diagnostic confusion as the presentation mimics an autoimmune seronegative polyarthritis. There are also reports

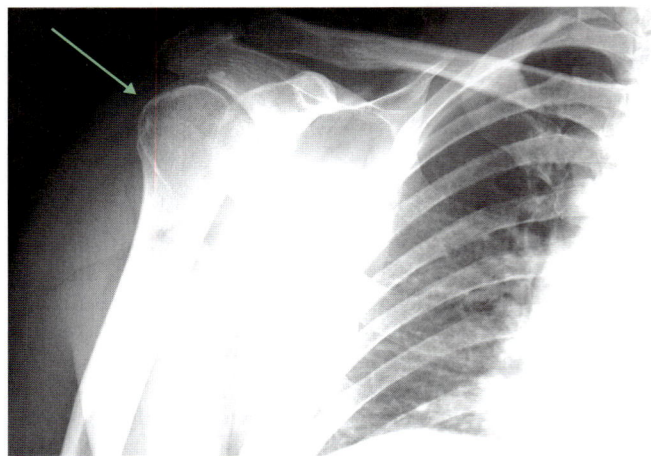

Figure 22-1 Plain film radiograph (AP view) of the right shoulder in a patient with clinical calcific periarthritis. Note the blurred hyperintensity close to the insertion of the supraspinatus tendon (*arrow*), most likely representing a calcific deposit within the supraspinatus tendon.

of calcific periarthritis occurring in families,[26] although no particular inheritance pattern or specific genetic loci have been identified.

Calcific deposits in periarticular tissues may also be associated with chronic pain syndromes. However, as calcific deposits are a common finding in the shoulder area, it is difficult to say what contribution, if any, they make to chronic shoulder pain in the absence of an acute inflammatory reaction. In some patients, recurrent attacks of acute calcific periarthritis result in significant damage to the musculotendinous junctions of the rotator cuff and thus lead to the development of chronic rotator cuff arthropathy.

Secondary BCP Crystal Deposition

Clinically significant periarticular BCP crystal deposition may also occur in association with chronic renal failure and hyperparathyroidism (with or without renal failure) and in the systemic autoimmune diseases of scleroderma and dermatomyositis.[22,27] A number of secondary forms of BCP crystal–associated arthropathies have been described. BCP crystal deposits have been reported in the joints and periarticular tissues of renal failure patients, mostly when undergoing dialysis. Renal failure predisposes to virtually all forms of crystal deposition including monosodium urate (MSU), CPPD, calcium oxalate, and aluminum phosphate, in addition to BCP.[28] Chronic end-stage renal failure requiring dialysis is therefore associated with several different crystal arthropathies, most commonly manifesting as gout (MSU) or pseudogout (CPPD). These conditions are extensively reviewed in Chapter 23 of this book, and the reader is referred here for a more detailed discussion of the increasingly important contribution of end-stage renal failure to joint pathology.

It is only when these conditions and infection have been excluded that BCP crystal deposition is considered in the diagnosis of an acute monoarthritis in a dialysis-dependent patient.

Tumoral calcinosis is a rare condition characterized by the progressive deposition of calcified masses in cutaneous and subcutaneous tissue. It is typically associated with chronic renal failure and either secondary or tertiary hyperparathyroidism. A rare inherited form of familial tumoral calcinosis is characterized by markedly elevated plasma phosphate levels, normal or elevated serum 1,25-dihydroxyvitamin D levels, and severe ectopic calcifications in various different sites. Mutations in both fibroblast growth factor-23 and GALNT3, which encodes a glycosyltransferase responsible for initiating mucin-type O-glycosylation, have been found in this condition.[22] A dreaded and often lethal complication of chronic dialysis that is also associated with elevated phosphate and calcium levels is calciphylaxis.[22] This condition is characterized by nodular subcutaneous and intradermal calcification with painful tissue necrosis often leading to ulceration, secondary infection, and high mortality rates.

BCP deposition is also associated with systemic autoimmune connective tissue disease, in particular scleroderma and dermatomyositis. Following dermatomyositis in childhood, massive sheets of fascial calcification can occur. In scleroderma, the deposits are usually subcutaneous and are associated with the CREST syndrome, although they may also be seen in mixed connective tissue disease. However, in some patients there is extensive subcutaneous calcification known as calcinosis cutis, which may occur in isolation without any other major features of the disease.[22]

A recognized iatrogenic cause of BCP crystal deposition is associated with the intraarticular injection of triamcinolone hexacetonide. This can sometimes lead to the formation of periarticular calcifications along the injection tract, which may become apparent months after the injection and are gradually resorbed over a period of months to years.[22] Finally, major trauma resulting in significant neurologic damage (brain, spinal cord, or peripheral nerve) is sometimes followed by massive heterotopic ossification in periarticular tissues and may drastically limit patients' functional rehabilitation.[29]

Intraarticular BCP Crystal Deposition

Articular cartilage calcification due to BCP crystal deposition (composed mainly of HA) and clumps of BCP crystal aggregates in synovial fluid are associated with specific clinical entities.

Milwaukee Shoulder

A particular type of large joint destructive arthropathy mainly affecting elderly women with a predilection for the shoulder joint and associated with the presence of abundant

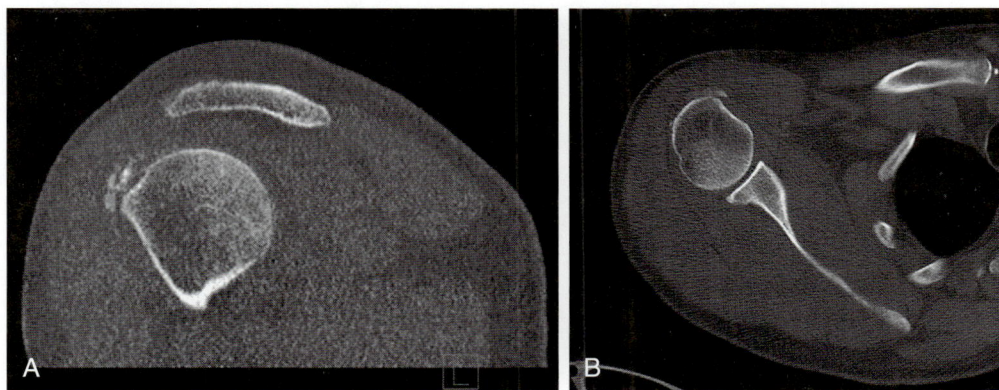

Figure 22-2 A, CT scan (sagittal view) of the same shoulder shown in Figure 22-1 with a much clearer depiction of the ruptured calcific deposit within the supraspinatus tendon anterior to the humeral head. **B,** CT scan (axial view) of the shoulder in Figure 22-1 depicting a large ruptured calcific deposit anterior to the humeral head.

BCP crystalline material, rotator cuff tears, and marked cartilage degeneration was described by Dan McCarty's group.[18] This entity has been termed Milwaukee shoulder syndrome, cuff tear arthropathy, or apatite-associated destructive arthritis.[27] The clinical presentation of this condition typically involves a history of chronic pain, swelling, decreased joint mobility, and gross impairment of function. Patients are nearly always over 70 years old, and approximately 90% are women. The dominant side is most often the presenting problem, although more than half of those affected have objective evidence of bilateral involvement.[30] The pain may be mild but is usually most apparent at night and on joint use. There is often total disruption of the rotator cuff apparatus, manifested by upward migration of the humeral head on plain film radiography (Fig. 22-3). Extensive damage to the periarticular soft tissues as well as to cartilage and subchondral bone on both sides of the joint may also occur (Fig. 22-4). There is reduced active range of motion in all planes, and examination of passive movement usually reveals pronounced joint instability. Crepitation and pain may be noted, especially when the humerus is grated passively against the glenoid. Joint effusion is typically present and may be massive, extending into the subdeltoid region. Aspiration of affected shoulder joints typically yields large volumes (more than 100 ml) of serosanguinous synovial fluid containing relatively low numbers of mononuclear leukocytes.[27] Rupture of the effusion can lead to a massive extravasation of blood and synovial fluid into the surrounding tissues.[31] Although the shoulder predominates, knees, hips, elbows, and other joints may be involved.[32]

The natural history of the condition is unclear, but many cases seem to enter spontaneous stable remission after 1 or 2 years, with a reduction of symptoms, decreased joint effusions, and no further radiographic changes. However, if sufficient damage to articular surfaces and periarticular structures has occurred, particularly if associated with joint instability, functional rehabilitation is severely curtailed and joint replacement surgery is sometimes the only viable therapeutic option (Fig. 22-5).

Acute Synovitis

Episodic attacks of acute monoarthritis associated with intraarticular BCP crystals in relatively young individuals, mainly affecting the knee joint, and resembling gout have been described.[33] These attacks appear to be rare and the diagnosis is difficult to establish, mainly due to the lack of readily available methods of accurately detecting BCP crystals. Occasionally, crystals from a periarticular deposit can rupture into the joint itself, causing acute synovitis. This only occurs where there is a direct connection between the site affected by the calcific rupture and the joint space itself, and it is most commonly seen in elderly individuals when the subacromial bursa also communicates with the glenohumeral joint.[22]

Chronic Monoarthritis

A chronic, sometimes erosive monoarthritis has also been linked with intraarticular BCP crystals. BCP crystals have been particularly implicated in finger joint arthropathies,

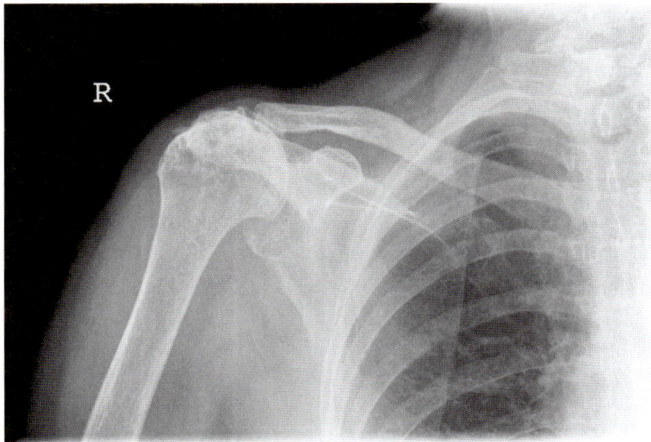

Figure 22-3 Plain film radiograph of the right shoulder in a patient with rotator cuff rupture. Note the upward migration of the humeral head and close approximation to the degenerative acromion process.

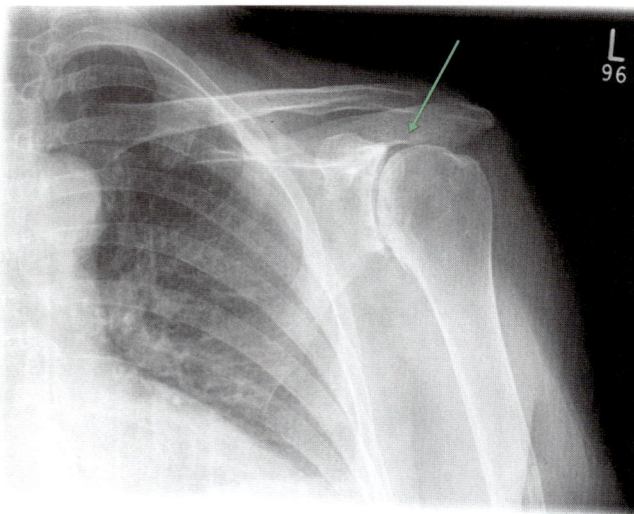

Figure 22-4 Plain film radiograph of the left shoulder in a patient with "Milwaukee shoulder" syndrome. Note the sclerotic changes in the subchondral bone on both sides of the glenohumeral joint (arrow). Also, there is extensive damage to the articular surface of the humeral head.

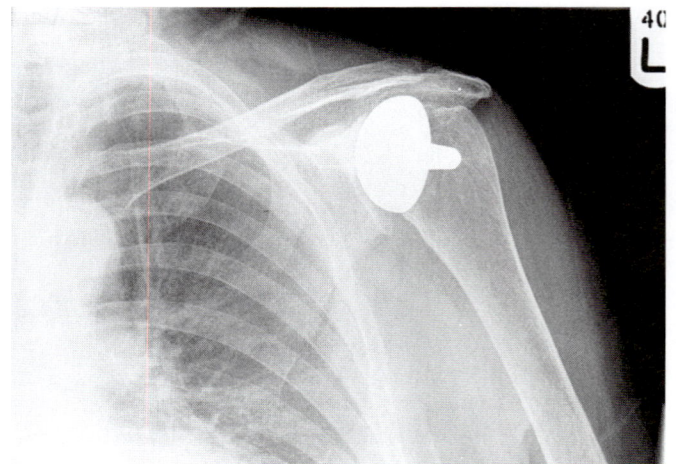

Figure 22-5 Plain film radiograph of the same joint depicted in Figure 22-4, following left shoulder hemiarthroplasty.

including erosive or inflammatory forms of OA.[34] However, this appears to be a very rare phenomenon and the exact contribution of BCP crystals to the pathogenesis of these types of conditions remains unclear.

Osteoarthritis

OA is the leading cause of joint disease in humans. Its complex pathogenesis remains poorly understood but appears multifactorial. OA is slowly progressive and involves all components of the joint, including bone, cartilage, meniscus, and synovium. No specific therapy has been identified to reverse or retard the consequences of OA. Therefore, joint replacement surgery is often ultimately the only therapeutic option.[21]

Calcification of articular cartilage (both hyaline and meniscal) is a well-recognized feature of OA, and current evidence suggests that it contributes directly to joint degeneration.[1] Calcium-containing crystals are found in more than 60% of synovial fluid samples from unselected OA patients at knee arthroplasty.[20] Although ample in vitro evidence demonstrates the potent biologic effects of calcium-containing crystals, controversy exists as to whether these crystals play a causal role or are merely a consequence of the joint damage seen in OA.[1]

CPPD and BCP are the two most common forms of calcium crystals found in articular cartilage.[35] Their presence is associated with a number of clinical manifestations. For example, CPPD crystals cause acute attacks of articular pseudogout,[36] and the presence of intraarticular BCP crystals correlates strongly with the severity of radiographic OA.[37] Both types of crystals are found in OA, but data on the distribution and frequency of BCP crystals vary considerably, mainly due to the lack of simple and reliable methods of detection.[38] Furthermore, the precise source of these crystals is unclear. Recent work by Fuerst et al. clearly demonstrates that BCP is the predominant crystal type in OA hyaline articular cartilage and that chondrocytes derived from OA hyaline cartilage produce BCP crystals in vitro.[38] This suggests that cartilage mineralization with BCP crystals by chondrocytes is part of the disease process in OA.

While meniscal degeneration and calcification are key features of OA knee joints,[39] few studies have investigated the potential role of OA meniscal cells in the pathogenesis of OA. In addressing this neglected area, recent work by Sun et al. offers novel insights into the pathogenesis of meniscal calcification in OA knee joints.[40] Therefore, both meniscal calcification (mediated by meniscal cells)[40] and hyaline calcification (mediated by chondrocytes derived from OA hyaline cartilage)[38] are potentially important contributory factors in the pathogenesis of OA and are discussed in detail later, along with their clinical implications.

Differential Diagnoses of BCP-Related Arthropathy

Due to its clinical presentation of sudden-onset pain, swelling, and erythema of overlying skin, the differential diagnoses of acute calcific periarthritis should include gout, pseudogout, and infection. However, there is often a characteristic distribution and plain film radiographs that demonstrate the calcific deposit(s) are virtually pathognomonic.[22] If there is a clinical concern of a possible septic bursitis, this should always be aspirated and fluid should be sent immediately for Gram stain, bacterial culture, and antibiotic sensitivity.

In cases of chronic tendinitis where calcium crystals are not visualized on radiographic imaging, the main differential diagnoses are mechanical impingement and trauma, and these should be confirmed by appropriate clinical history and functional testing of the affected joint. Dynamic ultrasound of the shoulder is particularly useful in confirming the diagnosis of rotator cuff impingement.

The main differential diagnoses of the large joint destructive arthropathies of the elderly (e.g., Milwaukee shoulder syndrome) include chronic infection, neuropathic or Charcot joints, rheumatoid arthritis (RA), CPPD deposition disease, and OA. Radiographically, the relative paucity of osteophytes and often large joint effusions help distinguish Milwaukee shoulder syndrome from primary OA of the glenohumeral joint.[27] The absence of neurologic findings associated with syringomyelia, diabetes, or chronic alcoholism excludes the diagnosis of neuropathic arthropathy.[41] Aspiration of synovial fluid and appropriate analysis aid the differentiation from pseudogout and infection.

Acute inflammatory arthritis that may mimic gout, pseudogout, or other systemic inflammatory rheumatic disease has been attributed to BCP crystals.[14,33] Erosive arthritis with recurrent episodes of pain and swelling involving the wrists and the finger joints has also been associated with BCP crystal deposition.[34] BCP crystals are often detected in OA joints and appear to promote the degenerative process since their presence is associated with more advanced radiographic change and larger joint effusions than in joints without BCP crystals.[42,43] Specific approaches to the detection of BCP crystals in synovial fluid are discussed later.

Clinical Investigations

The investigations that should be used in the work-up of patients with suspected BCP crystal–related arthropathy involve radiographic imaging, serologic testing, and synovial fluid analysis.

Imaging

Plain radiographs are a simple and cost-effective tool in the detection of periarticular calcific deposition. These deposits are usually visualized in the rotator cuff, typically a few centimeters proximal to the supraspinatus insertion or sometimes within the subacromial bursa. Conventional anteroposterior and lateral films are usually sufficient, but special views, with internal or external rotation of the shoulder, may be necessary to detect retrohumeral deposits. Other imaging modalities such as arthrography may be used to confirm the diagnosis of rotator cuff rupture, and computed tomography (CT) or magnetic resonance imaging (MRI) may be useful in demonstrating small, less radiopaque crystal deposition and other subtle inflammatory changes in the adjacent soft tissues but are rarely necessary in arriving at the diagnosis of calcific periarthritis. Imaging of the contralateral joint should also be carried out, as bilateral calcification is common. Similarly, radiographs of other asymptomatic sites (hips, knees, wrists) will sometimes reveal multiple calcific deposits. It should be remembered that these deposits are often reabsorbed during acute attacks of pericalcific arthritis, only to reappear subsequently.[22]

Heterotopic ossification can sometimes look like periarticular calcification, but these generally contain a trabecular pattern, unlike calcific deposits of BCP crystals. CPPD rarely deposits in periarticular tendons and nearly always manifests as linear deposits of chondrocalcinosis within intraarticular cartilage. This is in contrast to intraarticular BCP crystal deposits, which are rarely visible with any of the aforementioned imaging tools. This is largely due to the fact that individual aggregates of BCP crystals, within cartilage or synovial fluid, are generally tiny and therefore beyond the current limits of detection of conventional radiographic imaging.[2]

Radiographic features of the Milwaukee shoulder syndrome typically involve evidence of rotator cuff rupture (upward migration of the humeral head); degenerative changes of the humeral head, acromioclavicular joint, glenoid, and scapula; and cystic degeneration of the humeral tuberosities, and pseudoarthrosis formation between the humeral head and acromion process is common.[44] MRI is often used to further define these marked anatomic changes.

Serologic Testing

As gout and pseudogout are the main differential diagnoses for BCP-related joint disease, serum urate, renal function, and hematinics are often tested. BCP crystal deposition usually occurs in the absence of any detectable metabolic abnormality, but calcium and phosphate levels should always be checked. Recent evidence indicates that high serum phosphate levels seem more likely to predispose to BCP crystal deposition than abnormalities of calcium alone.[22]

BCP Crystals in Synovial Fluid

Aspiration of bursae involved in acute calcific periarthritis often reveals a creamy mixture of calcific and inflammatory matter that resembles chalky toothpaste.[22] In cases of suspected intraarticular BCP crystal deposition, the synovial fluid findings may vary. Gout (negatively birefringent needle-shaped MSU crystals) and pseudogout (positively birefringent rhomboid-shaped CPPD crystals) are generally excluded using compensated polarized light microscopic analysis of a fresh synovial fluid sample. Infection is ruled out by the absence of any organisms and few, if any, pus cells. Fluid from patients with large joint destructive arthropathy is frequently blood stained with low numbers of white cells (predominantly monocytes) and is usually quite viscous.[27]

In light of the emerging pathogenic role of BCP crystals in OA, the identification of these crystals from the synovial fluid of patients with intraarticular pathology is now of much greater importance. Synovial fluid acts as both a lubricant and a source of biochemical nutrients to the relatively avascular articular surfaces. It is a viscous ultrafiltrate of plasma with a high glycoprotein and hyaluronic acid content, and its complex biologic matrix presents significant analytical challenges.[2] BCP crystals are mainly composed of HA, with smaller amounts of its precursors (octacalcium phosphate and tricalcium phosphate).[1] Individual crystals are typically less than 1 μm (20 to 100 nm), and they aggregate in OA synovial fluid to form clumps (5 to 20 μm), which

appear as amorphous-looking globules that are nonbirefringent in polarized light.[2] Thus, their presence in joints is often unrecognized.

Identification of BCP Crystals

Current approaches employed in detecting BCP crystals are summarized in Table 22-2. These are composed of radiographic imaging, microscopic methods, spectroscopic techniques (including Raman), and other more specialized bioanalytical assays.[45] The following is a brief overview of the available methods in each of these areas. Recent developments in the field are also highlighted, with particular reference to their potential clinical applicability.

Radiologic Imaging

MRI is an excellent tool for detecting inflammatory disease and evaluating soft tissue structure, including periarticular calcific deposits.[46] It has none of the inherent radiation risks of CT but, unlike CT scanning, it poorly resolves bone mineral and has low sensitivity for detecting intraarticular calcifications.[47] However, MRI still has a role in evaluating intraarticular joint structures, especially in OA, due to its ability to generate high-resolution images depicting the morphology and integrity of ligaments and cartilage.[2]

CT scanning is a much more sensitive technique for detecting crystal deposits. In particular, dual energy CT (DECT) has been shown to adequately distinguish between urate and calcium renal stones and has an emerging role in differentiating between both urate and calcium crystal deposition in joints.[48] It also has a role in determining the overall burden of calcification present in particular tissues. However, DECT is unable to identify the subtype of calcium crystal deposition, and although the radiation dose is lower than that of conventional CT, it is significantly high to preclude its use in the routine detection of joint crystal calcification.

As well as depicting many well-recognised features of OA (e.g., joint space narrowing, osteophyte formation) and large joint destructive arthropathy (upward migration of rotator cuff, osteonecrosis, degenerative changes), plain radiographs can also detect periarticular BCP crystal calcification and chondrocalcinosis due to CPPD deposition. Thus, plain radiography remains the first-line imaging method of choice due to its cost-effectiveness, availability, and relatively low radiation exposure.[2] However, none of these imaging methods (radiography, CT, or MRI) can adequately detect intraarticular BCP crystals unless present in extremely large quantities.

Microscopy

While conventional light microscopy is capable of detecting the MSU crystals seen in gouty arthritis, the CPPD crystals of pseudogout, and the calcium oxalate monohydrate (COM) crystals sometimes present in the joint fluid of patients on long-term dialysis, its limit of resolution (1 μm) renders it incapable of resolving BCP crystals unless they have aggregated into large clumps.[2] Compensated polarized light microscopy (CPLM) uses the phenomenon of birefringence (based on a color change with rotation) to more easily identify MSU (negative birefringent needles) and CPPD crystals (weakly

Table 22-2 Methods Used for Detection of BCP Crystals

Method/Tool	Positives	Negatives
RADIOLOGIC IMAGING		
Computed axial tomography (CT)	Good resolution of bone mineral.	High radiation dose precludes routine use.
Magnetic resonance imaging (MRI)	No radiation risks. High resolution of soft tissue structures.	Poorly resolves bone mineral. Low sensitivity for intraarticular calcifications.
Plain film radiography (x-rays)	Inexpensive. Relatively low radiation exposure.	None of x-ray, CT, or MRI can adequately detect intraarticular BCP crystals unless present in very large quantities.
MICROSCOPIC METHODS		
Microscopy	Easy to operate, widely available, and inexpensive.	Limit of detection (> 1μm) insufficient for most BCP crystals unless aggregated in clumps
Microscopy with staining	Improved sensitivity for BCP crystal clumps.	High false-positive rate, non-specific for BCP.
Electron microscopy	Higher magnification and greater resolution than conventional microscopy.	Equipment is expensive, needs specialist training, operator dependent.
Atomic force microscopy	Suitable for very small sample sizes, chemical force microscopy offers potential.	High level specialist training, operator dependent, expensive, difficulties with liquid samples.
SPECTROSCOPIC METHODS		
Infrared	FTIR absorption spectra can distinguish different crystal types, sensitivity and specificity enhanced using a synchrotron light source.	Requires prior sample purification. Not widely available, expensive, highly specialized equipment.
Raman	Unique "Raman shift" spectral patterns for each crystal type (MSU, CPPD, HA/BCP); water causes little interference.	Expensive equipment, specialized training.
Near-infrared fluorescence	NIR fluorescent bisphosphonates are potentially more selective for BCP crystals	Dyes and equipment are expensive.
OTHER METHODS		
Calcium and phosphate analysis	Colorimetric/spectophotometric methods based on sound scientific rationale and are reasonably selective.	Problems with interference from other matter present in synovial fluid.
X-ray diffraction	Highly sensitive and specific when used on an appropriately prepared sample.	Requires complex drying and purification steps prior to analysis.
Radioassay	Enables quantitative estimation of BCP crystals in synovial fluid samples.	Radioactive agents preclude its use in the clinical setting.
NEW DEVELOPMENTS		
Tetracycline staining	Easy to use method. Equipment required is inexpensive and widely available.	High false-positive rate. Needs further refinement.
Extraction by magnetic beads	One-step method for extraction of calcium phosphate crystals. Highly selective. Potential for clinical applicability.	Requires combination with other imaging tools.

positive birefringent rods).[49] However, accuracy of detection is somewhat operator dependent,[50] especially regarding CPPD crystals as they are only weakly birefringent.[51] Due to their lack of birefringence and amorphous appearance, clumps of BCP crystals are often mistaken for artefacts or debris with both conventional light microscopy and CPLM.[2]

Staining of joint fluid samples with dyes is often used to improve the detection of BCP crystal clumps and small CPPD crystals, especially those missed by CPLM.[2] The Alizarin red S stain is recommended by many as a useful complementary test to CPLM for both CPPD and HA/BCP crystal aggregates.[52] Alizarin red does not distinguish between different types of calcium compounds, and therefore CPPD and HA crystals can only be distinguished by morphology when both

are present together.[53] Furthermore, the sensitivity of Alizarin red S staining is closely related to the pH of the sample solution and the concentration of the dye, with considerable overlap in the optimal detection ranges between CPPD and BCP crystal types.[2] Preparation of the sample by centrifugation and resuspension of the synovial fluid sediment has been reported to enhance the specificity of Alizarin red in crystal identification.[54]

Fluorescent dyes have been extensively applied throughout the bioanalytical sciences to suit a variety of different disciplines. Fluo-4 is a calcium-specific fluorescent dye that enhances greater than 100-fold upon binding Ca^{2+} ions.[55] It has recently been applied to selectively stain calcium-containing crystals in synovial fluid. In synovial fluids spiked

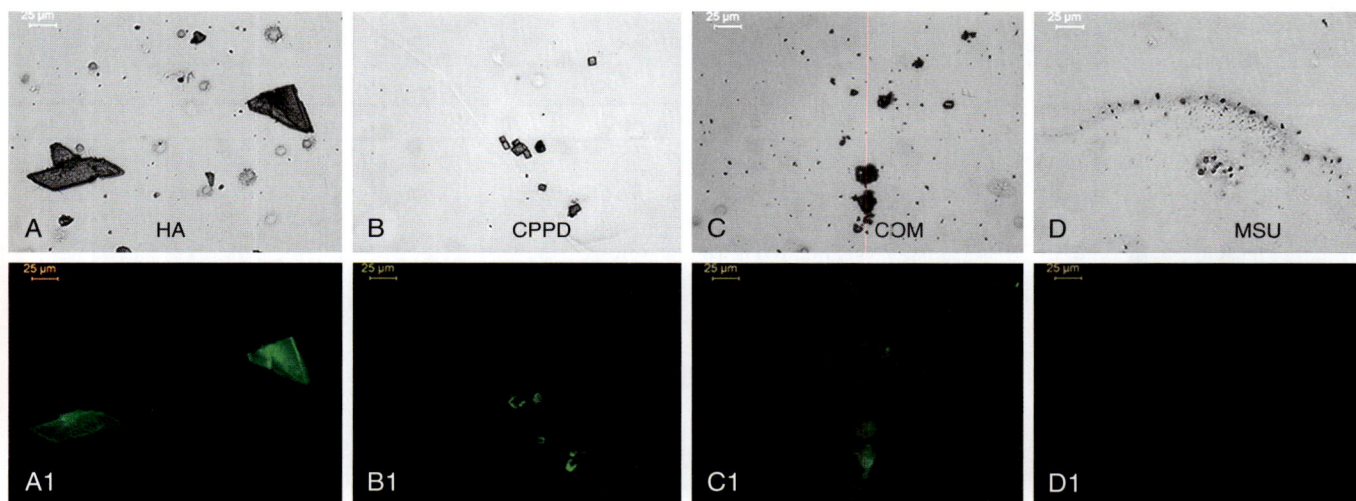

Figure 22-6 Phase contrast images of synovial fluid samples (**A–D**) spiked with HA, CPPD, COM, MSU, respectively, using Fluo-4. The corresponding fluorescence images of HA (**A1**), CPPD (**B1**), COM (**C1**), and MSU (**D1**) show bright green fluorescence for all crystals except MSU.

with HA, CPPD, COM, and MSU crystals, Fluo-4 demonstrated bright green fluorescence for all crystals except MSU (Fig. 22-6) (McMahon et al., unpublished data). However, as Fluo-4 is not specific for calcium phosphate, further analysis is required to differentiate between different crystal subtypes.

Scanning electron microscopy (SEM) generates images by scanning a focused electron beam across the surface of a sample, which then interacts with the sample to produce secondary signals, including electron emission, cathode luminescence, and x-rays.[2] In combination with Alizarin staining, SEM has been frequently used to examine crystal deposits in cartilage and synovial fluid.[56] However, its sensitivity is dependent on the presence of a high concentration of crystals in the sample, and as fluids with CPPD crystals also stain positively with Alizarin red, it is not a definitive method for BCP crystals.[2] Synovial samples also contain significant amounts of other biologic material that can burn and coagulate under the high voltages required for imaging.[2] Methods have been developed to filter such material and enhance crystal identification.[57] Transmission electron microscopy (TEM) is another useful technique as its enhanced resolution also allows visualization of crystal–cell interaction and the granular materials (presumably protein coating) often associated with both CPPD and HA crystals.[58] However, it also displays artefacts (e.g., silicon-containing particles from glassware) that can be mistaken for crystals.[59] Notwithstanding these limitations, recent work demonstrates the superiority of TEM over light microscopy (with Alizarin red staining) in identifying BCP crystals in OA synovial fluid samples.[60]

Another highly specialized and expensive tool is atomic force microscopy (AFM), a variant of scanning probe microscopy used in surface imaging, down to the level of atoms.[2] AFM is a powerful technique for the detection and surface topologic analysis of microcrystals in synovial fluid.[61] Its specificity can be further enhanced by coating the AFM microscope tip with chemical materials that are selective for particular crystal subtypes, so-called chemical force microscopy (CFM).[2]

While SEM, TEM, and AFM all have important roles in OA research, the cost of the required equipment, complexity of the techniques, need for specialized training, and aforementioned difficulties with synovial sampling all present practical barriers to their use in the routine diagnosis of suspected BCP crystal–related joint disease.[45]

Spectroscopic Techniques

Spectroscopy relies on the identification of substances via the spectra emitted or absorbed by them and comparing these with specific emission/absorbance spectra of known compounds.[45] Analysis of the absorbance, reflectance, and transmittance properties of synovial fluid has been widely studied in OA research using a number of different techniques based mainly on Fourier-transform infrared, Raman, and near-infrared spectra.[2]

Fourier-transform infrared spectroscopy (FTIR) has been applied to quantify the various components of several bodily fluids (e.g., blood, plasma, serum, urine, saliva, and synovial fluid).[2] Based on statistical pattern recognition methods, FTIR has been shown to effectively distinguish between synovial fluid samples from patients with OA, RA, and spondyloarthropathy, by their absorption spectra in the infrared region.[62] The FTIR absorption spectrum of HA has been reported[63] and is different than that of CPPD.[64] This could potentially aid the correct diagnoses of crystal-related joint diseases, but its accurate application would likely require prior isolation of the crystals from the biologic matrix of synovial fluid.[2] Furthermore, this spectral pattern recognition approach will also require thorough statistical validation as there is considerable variation between individuals within the various different joint disease populations.[2] Recent work has shown that the sensitivity and specificity of FTIR in identifying small amounts of CPPD and BCP crystals in synovial fluid can be significantly enhanced by using a synchrotron-generated beam as the light source.[65] However, access to this technology is extremely limited and is only available in a small number of specialized centers.

Raman spectroscopy is based on the phenomenon that occurs when molecules are excited by monochromatic light (usually from a laser source) to a higher energy state and subsequently emit light of a different frequency when they "relax," the difference in frequency being the so-called Raman shift.[66] It can probe the molecular composition of a wide range of materials and, as water causes very little interference, it can be readily applied to investigate fresh tissue or an aqueous solution like synovial fluid.[2] Raman spectroscopy has been applied to the identification of CPPD in pathologic samples,[67] and different Raman spectra for HA/BCP, COM, CPPD, and MSU crystals have recently been described[2] and are illustrated in Figure 22-7. Thus, notwithstanding the significant cost of the technology involved and the necessary sample purification required to distinguish between various crystal types, Raman spectroscopy offers considerable future potential as a research tool for the detection of BCP crystals in OA.

As in Raman, near-infrared (NIR) fluorescence (wavelengths of 700 to 900 nm) detection avoids the background fluorescence interference of many natural biomolecules, thus providing sufficient contrast between target substances and background tissue.[2] A particularly relevant application of this technique is the analysis of crystalline mineralization using an NIR fluorescent bisphosphonate (BP) derivative (Pamidronate-IRDye78).[68] This has been shown to bind tightly to HA crystals (both in vitro and in vivo) to give specific peak absorption and emission spectra.[68] It has recently been applied in the investigation of microcalcifications in breast cancer[69] and may well have a future in evaluating BCP crystals in OA.

BCP Detection Methods Based on Physical Chemistry

BCP crystals contain calcium, phosphate, hydroxyl, and carbonate ions. Therefore, it seems reasonable to apply methods that can determine the concentration of these ions in a given sample. Colorimetric/spectrophotometric methods involve the addition of various reagents (e.g., eriochrome blue, Phosphonazo III), which then form a colored complex with the specific element to be detected.[2] However, there are a number of problems with this approach when aiming to detect BCP crystals in synovial fluid: the high turbidity of synovial fluid complicates the direct determination of calcium without additional crystal purification/extraction steps; magnesium may also interfere with calcium detection in a pH-sensitive manner; and these reagents do not work well with crystal-bound calcium.[63]

X-ray diffraction (XRD) is another common method in physical chemistry for the characterization of many minerals, including calcium phosphates.[70] However, it requires a number of drying and purification steps prior to analysis.[2] An x-ray beam is targeted at a preprepared powdered sample, which is then scattered in various directions depending on the crystal structure.[70] While this technique has been successfully applied to the identification of both BCP and CPPD clusters that were missed by light microscopy,[71] the complex preparation and expertise required preclude its routine diagnostic use in the clinical setting.

The application of a specific binding assay for the detection of HA using a radioactive isotope has enabled semiquantitative estimation of HA crystals in synovial fluid samples.[72] Developed by Dan McCarty's group, this assay uses ^{14}C ethane-1-hydroxy-1,1-disphosphonate (EHDP), which tightly binds HA crystals while having much lower affinity for synthetic CPPD. The resultant nuclide binding provides a semiquantitative assessment of the amount of ultramicroscopic BCP material present in a sample.[72] While this assay has certainly provided evidence at a conceptual level for a likely role of BCP crystals in OA, the use of radioactive agents likely precludes its routine use in the clinical setting. Also, subsequent work using (^{14}C) EHDP in OA demonstrated significant nuclide binding to CPPD in some patient samples, a finding that brings into question the specificity of (^{14}C) EHDP for HA/BCP crystals but also underlines the fact that both types of crystals are likely to coexist in severe degenerative arthritis.[2]

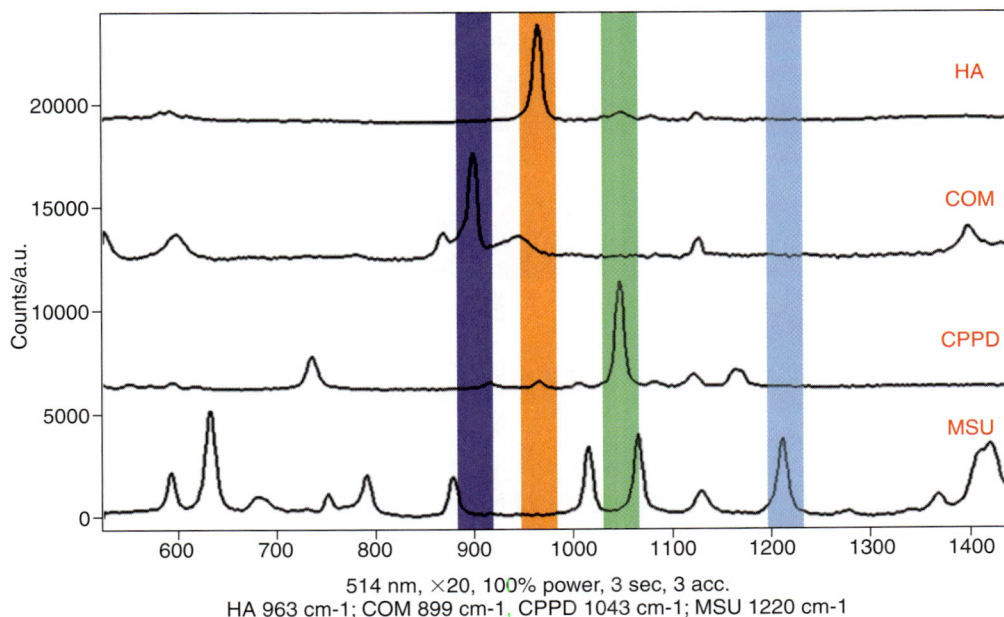

514 nm, ×20, 100% power, 3 sec, 3 acc.
HA 963 cm-1; COM 899 cm-1; CPPD 1043 cm-1; MSU 1220 cm-1

Figure 22-7 Raman reference spectra of synthetic hydroxyapatite (HA), calcium oxalate monohydrate (COM), calcium pyrophosphate dihydrate (CPPD), and monosodium urate (MSU) crystals.

Recent Developments

Two recent developments offer significant potential for the improved detection of BCP crystals in the clinical setting; one is based on a modification of light microscopy with tetracycline staining,[52] and the other involves capture of crystals from synovial samples using BP-modified magnetic beads.[3]

The ability of tetracycline antibiotics to bind HA material and their fluorescence has enabled their use as labels of mineralization in bones and teeth.[73] This property has recently been successfully adapted to the detection of HA/BCP crystals in synovial fluid.[52] The authors used oxytetracycline staining and ultraviolet light microscopy to identify and quantify increasing concentrations of synthetic BCP crystals in spiked porcine synovial fluid samples, as well as native BCP crystal material in human synovial fluid from a patient with Milwaukee shoulder syndrome.[52] When compared to Alizarin red S staining, the oxytetracycline method had significantly fewer (35% versus 58%) false-positive results,[52] although far in excess of what would be required for a reliable clinical test. Nonetheless, with further refinement and subsequent validation in larger numbers of specimens, this simple and inexpensive approach certainly has potential.

Certain methods of calcium phosphate crystal identification (e.g., SEM, AFM) require sample purification and extraction of the crystals prior to analysis, due to the presence of crystalline cholesterol, lipid particles, and other artefacts in human synovial fluid.[2] Indeed, even prior corticosteroid injections, a common intervention in patients with OA, can give a false-positive result for calcium phosphate crystals.[74] Previous attempts at extraction of BCP material have applied deproteination,[56] enzymatic degradation,[72] and multistep extraction procedures

with some success in improving diagnostic yield.[75] However, they are generally cumbersome to carry out, involve significant adulteration of the synovial fluid sample, and are ineffective when the crystals are present in low quantities.[45] The recent development of a simple, one-step crystal extraction procedure using modified paramagnetic beads addresses this problem. This novel approach involves the use of micrometer-sized paramagnetic beads coated with a BP analog. The success of BPs in the treatment of osteoporosis relies on their strong affinity for solid-phase calcium phosphate in bone mineral, but they are also known to avidly bind BCP and CPPD crystals.[76] The use of superparamagnetic beads to capture analytes has been widely exploited in the biomedical sciences.[77] The beads used in this technique are conjugated to a synthetic BP analog (neridronate 4) via an amine group while leaving the BP moiety intact.[3] The BP-coated beads are added to the synovial sample, where they selectively bind any calcium phosphate crystals which may be present. They are then easily removed from the fluid using a simple laboratory magnet.[3] The viability of the technique was first established using synovial fluid spiked with HA, BCP, and CPPD synthetic crystals followed by SEM imaging of the extracted material (Fig. 22-8). The technique was then used to confirm the presence of BCP and CPPD crystals in native synovial fluid samples from patients with OA and peudogout, respectively.[3] This nondestructive extraction method has the potential to be used in the routine clinical setting, while still allowing further diagnostic testing to be carried out on the synovial fluid sample. The combination of this extraordinarily simple approach with other imaging tools could significantly improve the diagnosis and characterization of BCP crystal–related arthropathy and help clarify the pathologic potential of these crystals in OA.

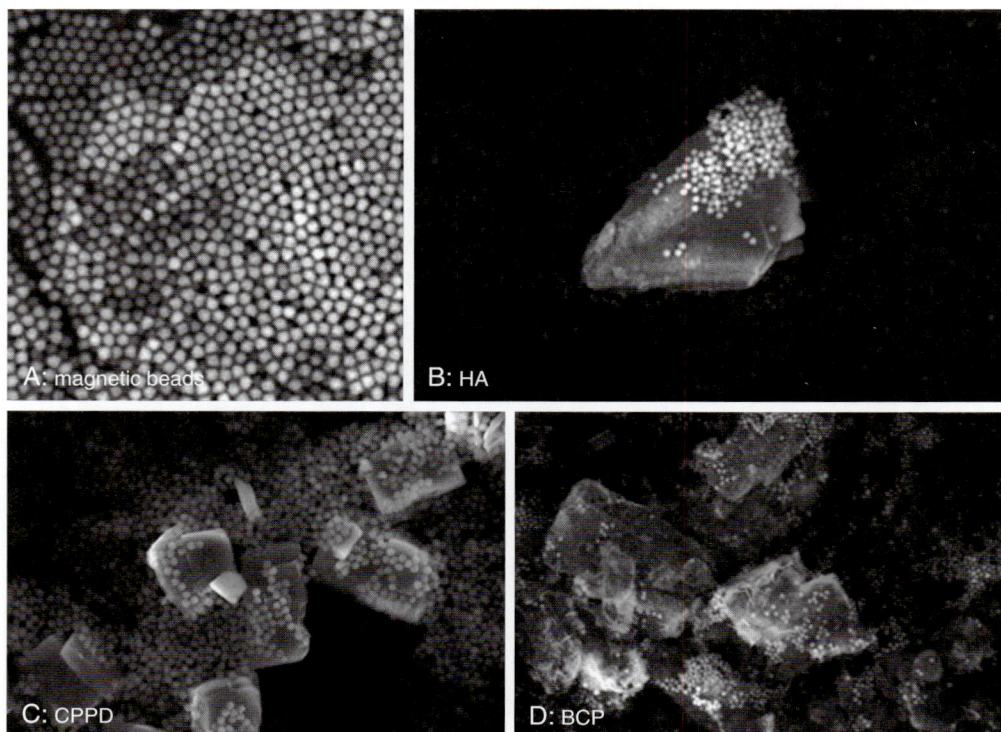

Figure 22-8 **A,** Bisphosphonate-coated magnetic beads. **B, C, and D,** SEM images of extracted synthetic crystals demonstrating capture of HA, CPPD, and BCP crystals, respectively.

Pathogenesis of BCP Crystal Arthropathy

The relatively avascular connective tissue matrices of articular hyaline cartilage, fibrocartilaginous menisci, joint capsule, ligaments, and tendons are particularly susceptible to calcification.[27] There appear to be certain pathologic differences between the etiology of periarticular calcium deposition and intraarticular calcification associated with the large joint destructive arthropathies and degenerative OA. It should also be remembered that physiologic deposition of BCP in the form of HA is essential, as this is the principal mineral phase laid down in growth cartilage and bone.[27]

Calcific Periarthritis

The exact mechanisms involved in periarticular calcification are largely unknown. Intratendinous deposits are thought to occur following injury; however, the classic description of a relationship between repetitive strain injury of the shoulder and the formation of calcific deposits in the rotator cuff has not been firmly established. Certain systemic conditions with a known predisposition to calcific deposits (e.g., diabetes mellitus and hyperparathyroidism) often lead to the involvement of multiple bilateral sites. These same sites (e.g., shoulder, hip, wrist) are also most often involved in cases of sporadic calcific periarthritis with no known metabolic cause. Even in familial clusters of severe periarticular calcium deposition, a relationship with specific HLA alleles or other genetic markers remains to be established.[22]

The commonly accepted pathophysiology of calcific tendonitis is primary tendon degeneration leading to secondary calcification through a dystrophic process.[78] A common clinicopathologic correlation is three distinct phases of the disease process: the precalcific or formative phase, which is usually painless; the calcific phase, which is asymptomatic and may last months to years; and the resorptive or postcalcific phase, during which the acute painful presentation occurs as calcium crystals are resorbed.[79]

In cases that involve the shoulder, localization of the calcific deposits within the supraspinatus has been attributed to chronic impingement against the acromion process leading to local degeneration of the tendon fibers.[80] However, the same area of the supraspinatus tendon (just medial to its humeral attachment) is also involved in patients without impingement. This a watershed area in its blood supply (derived from an anastomotic network of local vessels), which is vulnerable to ischemia during overhead upper limb activities and referred to as the "critical zone."[81]

Some evidence has indicated that calcifying tendinitis is an active, cell-mediated process in which local vascular and mechanical changes result in focal transformation of tendinous tissues into fibrocartilaginous material containing chondrocytes. This is followed by local deposition of hydroxyapatite crystals within extracellular matrix vesicle-like structures derived from these chondrocytes.[82]

Acute calcific periarthritis appears to be induced by rupture of the deposit and the shedding of crystals into more cellular and better vascularized areas. BCP crystals have been shown to be intrinsically proinflammatory. They are phagocytosed in vitro resulting in the release of inflammatory mediators.[83] Similarly, in vivo models of inflammation show a brisk inflammatory reaction to apatite and injection into the tissues of human volunteers results in an inflammatory response.[84] Phagocytosis may be one of the main ways in which the crystals are removed. However, there is currently a lack of good animal or in vitro models to adequately study the formation of periarticular calcific deposits and their subsequent resorption. Aging and degeneration of collagen fibers, with or without a compromised vascularity, do not seem to be a sufficient explanation for the phenomenon.

Intraarticular BCP Crystal Deposition and Joint Degeneration

Calcium deposition due to either BCP or CPPD crystals tends to develop in different zones of articular cartilage and probably in distinct phases of cartilage degeneration.[27] CPPD crystal deposition has a clear predilection for the middle zone of articular cartilage, whereas BCP crystals tend to be concentrated in the pericellular matrix of chondrocytes in the superficial zone.[85] However, both crystal subtypes are often found within the same joint.[21] Evidence suggests that both normal human articular cartilage and diseased osteoarthritic cartilage contain matrix vesicles (MVs) which are capable of progressive mineralization and can generate either BCP or CPPD in vitro [86] (see Chapter 20). While the underlying triggers and regulatory mechanisms are not completely clear, more than one source of formation is likely. For example, the *ANK* gene product, a cell membrane protein (ANKH) that regulates extracellular inorganic pyrophosphate (ePP$_i$), has recently been identified. ePP$_i$ is an important inhibitor of nucleation and growth of BCP. This has led to the theory of ANKH-mediated control of ePP$_i$ levels as a possible mechanism of regulation of tissue calcification.[87] Defective ANKH-mediated PP$_i$ channeling is directly implicated in several forms of familial CPPD leading to the accumulation of excessive ePP$_i$ and precocious OA with chondrocalcinosis.[27] While linkage to the *ANK* gene on chromosome 5 has been established in several studies of familial CPPD deposition,[88-90] a unique mutation was identified in only 1 of 95 subjects with sporadic chondrocalcinosis.[89] Conversely, increased activity of tissue-nonspecific alkaline phosphatase (TNAP) which is the product of the *AKP2* gene, decreases ePP$_i$ levels by hydrolysis, thereby providing a source of extracellular inorganic phosphate (eP$_i$) and subsequent BCP crystal generation.[91,92] Variant genotypes for both ANKH and TNAP were observed more frequently in cases compared with controls in a recent study of patients with cuff-tear arthropathy.[93] In addition, abundant cartilage nitric oxide (NO) production may promote mitochondrial dysfunction, chondrocyte extracellular ATP depletion, and lowering of ePP$_i$, thus favoring HA/BCP over CPPD deposition.[94] However, it should be noted that joint fluid from patients with large joint destructive arthropathy often contains high levels of ePP$_i$,[95] although this may be more reflective of end-stage disease. Thus, dysregulated ePP$_i$/P$_i$ metabolism in the setting of an altered pericellular milieu is a key driver of the type (BCP or CPPD or both) and extent of matrix calcification by chondrocytes in specific disease states, including OA.

The degree of damage that can occur in apatite-associated destructive arthropathies is marked (see Fig. 22-4). The basis of cartilage damage by calcium-containing crystals is still somewhat speculative. Theoretically, crystals in cartilage may directly injure chondrocytes. However, in pathologic specimens crystals are rarely seen in immediate contact with chondrocytes and even less frequently found engulfed by chondrocytes.[22]

It is more likely that cartilage damage ultimately results from effects of the crystals on the synovial membrane and subsequent release of proinflammatory cytokines from fibroblast-like synoviocytes. BCP crystals have been shown to induce mitogenesis in vitro, a theoretical explanation for the synovial proliferation characteristic of both Milwaukee shoulder syndrome and apatite-associated OA.[96,97] Increased cell numbers in the synovial lining enhance the capacity for further secretion of cytokines, which may promote chondrolysis. Furthermore, BCP crystals induce the secretion of proteolytic enzymes leading to degradation of intraarticular collagenous structures, an observation that correlates with the detection of high levels of collagenase and neutral protease in synovial fluid from patients with Milwaukee shoulder syndrome.[98] BCP crystals also enhance the production of collagenase 1, stromelysin, and 92-kDa gelatinase from human fibroblasts and collagenase-1 and -3 from porcine chondrocytes.[97] Last, BCP crystals induce cyclooxygenase-1 and -2 followed by increased prostaglandin E_2 in human fibroblasts.[99,100]

Calcification of articular cartilage (both hyaline and meniscal) is a well-recognized feature of OA and current evidence suggests that it contributes directly to joint degeneration.[1] Calcium-containing crystals are found in more than 60% of synovial fluid samples from unselected OA patients at knee arthroplasty.[20] Although ample in vitro evidence demonstrates the potent biologic effects of calcium-containing crystals, controversy exists as to whether these crystals play a causal role or are merely a consequence of the joint damage seen in OA.[1]

The presence of intraarticular BCP crystals correlates strongly with the severity of radiographic OA,[37] BCP is the predominant crystal type in OA hyaline cartilage, and chondrocytes derived from OA hyaline cartilage produce BCP crystals in vitro.[38] Thus, cartilage mineralization with BCP crystals by chondrocytes is an indissociable part of the disease process in OA. Another likely source of BCP particulates in advanced OA are the bony shards embedded in damaged cartilage and the bony debris resulting from the exposure of subchondral bone due to cartilage erosion.[85,101] It is particularly important to note here that cartilage mineralization is also a physiologic process involving chondrocyte differentiation and hypertrophy at the growth plate, which, along with other factors, promotes HA mineralization of the surrounding matrix and ossification.[102] However, it is unclear how and why crystals form in normally unmineralized articular cartilage. Hypertrophic chondrocytes at the growth plate and in OA cartilage share particular features, including synthesis of type X collagen, upregulated expression of various enzymes, and the release of MVs responsible for the initial formation of HA/BCP or CPPD crystals.[38,103] Articular cartilage MVs are chondrocyte-derived organelles that are the primary source of crystal formation within joints.[103] These MVs have been shown to generate both CPPD and BCP in vitro, with BCP preferentially produced in the absence of ATP.[104] The role of these MVs in pathologic calcification in OA has been confounded by the fact that they are also found in normal cartilage and, while OA cartilage contains a greater concentration of MVs compared to normal cartilage, they do not display a greater mineralization capacity in vitro.[104] This strongly suggests that substances within the extracellular matrix strongly

influence the mineralizing activity of these MVs in vivo. Recent data supporting this concept clearly demonstrate that type 1 collagen (which is greatly increased in OA cartilage) dose-dependently stimulates MV mineralization and that this is inhibited by certain large proteoglycans (which are severely depleted in OA) in a novel in vitro model using porcine articular cartilage.[103] This indicates that extracellular components that are known to be altered in OA regulate the type and extent of crystal formation in articular hyaline cartilage. Release of these crystals (BCP or CPPD or both) into the joint space, due to altered mechanical loading, trauma, or other factors, promotes a vicious cycle of joint degradation mediated by the aforementioned pathogenic effects of these crystals on the synovium with subsequent release of proinflammatory cytokines, proteolytic enzymes, collagenases, prostaglandin E_2 and matrix metalloproteinases (MMPs), which promote further chondrocyte hypertrophy[85] and may lead directly to cartilage degeneration and chondrolysis.[1,35,105] A schematic model of the pathogenic significance of hyaline cartilage calcification in OA, incorporating chondrocyte differentiation, release of MVs, dysregulated ePP_i metabolism, and an altered extracellular environment is represented in Figure 22-9.

Furthermore, meniscal degeneration and calcification are also key features of OA knee joints,[39] and recent work by Sun et al. offers novel insights into the pathogenesis of meniscal calcification in OA knee joints.[40] First, calcium crystal deposition is common in the menisci of end-stage OA patients, and the pattern of calcification seen is different from that of primary chondrocalcinosis. Second, OA meniscal cells, when cultured, induce significantly more calcium deposition than do normal control meniscal cells. Third, the expression of genes known to cause articular calcification (*ANKH* and *ENPP1*) is upregulated in OA meniscal cells.[21] Finally, calcium deposition by OA meniscal cells is inhibited by phosphocitrate, an

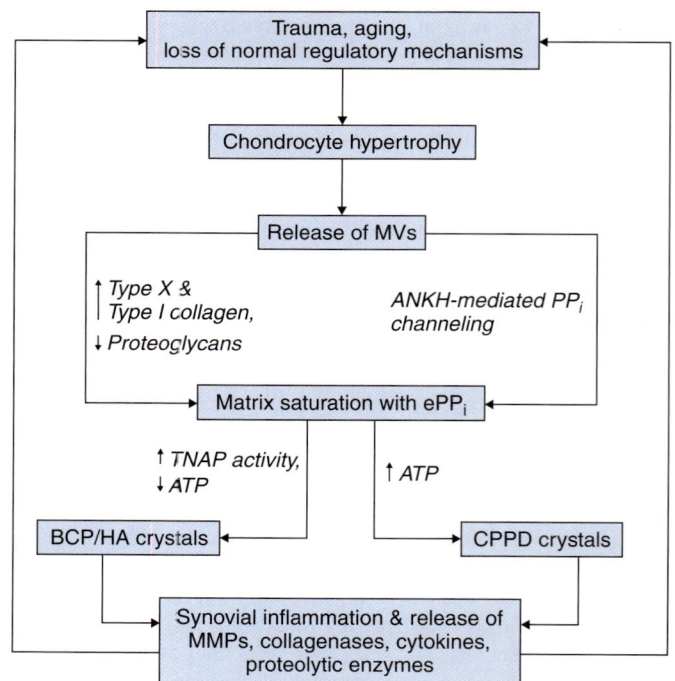

Figure 22-9 Schematic diagram of the contribution of calcium containing crystals to the vicious cycle of articular cartilage degradation in OA.

observation that is also supported by complementary work using an animal model of OA.[105]

The potential impact of the study by Sun et al. is hampered by the fact that the specific type of crystals (CPPD or BCP or both) present in both the clinical samples and the cultured cells was not established.[21] Furthermore, the phenotype of the meniscal cells and their ability to produce type X collagen as a marker of chondrocyte hypertrophy and other potential differences between OA meniscal cells and control cells were not addressed.[21] This is important, as previous work clearly distinguishes specific phenotypes of meniscal cells (with different functional capabilities) in OA menisci compared to normal menisci.[106]

Nonetheless, both meniscal calcification (mediated by meniscal cells)[40] and hyaline calcification (mediated by chondrocytes derived from OA hyaline cartilage)[38] are potentially important contributory factors in the pathogenesis of OA and may represent new modulatory targets in the search for an effective medical intervention in OA. Recent work examining a novel formulation of phosphocitrate (PC) in the Hartley strain guinea pig model (which histologically mimics human OA) led to some important observations.[105] The authors found that the calcium depositis in the menisci of these animals were primarily HA/BCP crystals and that intraperitoneal injections of PC blocked the calcification-induced cartilage degeneration and arrested OA disease progression via inhibition of new calcification of the menisci (thus preventing abnormal joint loading) and via specific inhibition of BCP crystal-induced cellular response.[105] Furthermore, this PC treatment had no therapeutic effect in a rabbit hemi meniscectomy model of OA, in which there is no known crystal involvement. While the authors propose that their observations were most likely due to the recognized inhibitory effect of PC on HA formation[107] and by the influence of PC on the interaction of calcium crystals with biomembranes,[108] they also concede that the therapeutic effect of PC may be due to other, as yet unidentified, mechanisms.[105]

Management
Calcific Periarthritis

Asymptomatic calcific deposits require no treatment. Acute calcific periarthritis can be managed with a variety of nonsteroidal antiinflammatory drugs (NSAIDs) and colchicine.[22] Cases involving the rotator cuff and subacromial bursa are often treated by needle aspiration, irrigation, and steroid injections.[27] However, local corticosteroid injections are controversial as they may increase the likelihood of further attacks but ultrasound-guided techniques may enhance the success of such approaches.[27] For patients with chronic periarticular syndromes, the treatment approach is much the same as whether the deposits were present or not.

Large Joint Destructive Arthropathy

At the time of diagnosis of BCP crystal–associated destructive arthropathies, such as Milwaukee shoulder syndrome, advanced destructive changes are usually present and may even be asymptomatic. A conservative approach, including analgesics and NSAIDs, repeated shoulder aspirations, and decreased joint use, has sometimes controlled symptoms

satisfactorily. In theory, nonselective cyclooxygenase (COX) inhibition should be more effective since BCP crystals induce the upregulation of both COX-1 and COX–2 enzyme pathways.[92,93] Surgical therapy involves arthroscopic lavage and/or debridement, humeral tuberoplasty, arthrodesis, arthroplasty, or hemiarthroplasty and is sometimes successful for the relief of pain and restoration of function but may be difficult because of the extent of joint damage.[10]

Osteoarthritis

No specific therapy has been identified to reverse or retard the consequences of OA. Therefore, joint replacement surgery is often ultimately the only therapeutic option.[21]

Future Directions

The clinical implications of improved detection methods BCP crystals are wide-ranging. Calcification of articular cartilage is now well recognized as an indissociable feature of OA and predominantly involves BCP crystal deposotion.[35] There is strong in vitro evidence that demonstrates that such calcium deposition is inhibited by phosphocitrate[40] and is supported by complementary work using an animal model of OA.[105] To truly test the hypothesis that calcium phosphate crystals play a causative role in OA, animal studies in which BCP crystals are injected intraarticularly are warranted.[1] Should such studies demonstrate the induction or acceleration of joint degeneration that could then be arrested or reversed by an agent such as phosphocitrate, this would provide proof-of-concept evidence for the pathogenicity or otherwise of these crystals in OA. Currently, assessments of therapeutic interventions in OA rely on end-stage radiographic outcome measures (such as joint space narrowing), which often take years to develop and are therefore unsuitable for placebo-controlled trials. This has been a major barrier to developing effective disease-modifying drugs in OA. Thus, improved detection methods for BCP crystals (which are reliable, inexpensive, technically simple, and specific), coupled with the adoption of articular cartilage calcification as a surrogate marker of OA disease, could enable trials of targeted anticrystal therapies with biologic endpoints and a fast turnaround time.[21] This could significantly advance the search for an effective medical intervention in the most common of human joint disorders.

Acknowledgments

The authors would like to acknowledge the assistance of Dr Niamh Long (Specialist Registrar in Radiology) and the Radiology Department of the Mater Misericordiae University Hospital in collating the clinical images for this chapter.

References

1. McCarthy GM, Cheung HS. Point: hydroxyapatite crystal deposition is intimately involved in the pathogenesis and progression of human osteoarthritis. Curr Rheumatol Rep 2009;11(2):141–7.
2. Yavorskyy A, Hernandez-Santana A, McCarthy G, et al. Detection of calcium phosphate crystals in the joint fluid of patients with osteoarthritis: analytical approaches and challenges. Analyst 2008;133(3):302–18.

3. Hernandez-Santana A, Yavorskyy A, Olinyole A, et al. Isolation of calcium phosphate crystals from complex biological fluids using bisphosphonate-modified superparamagnetic beads. Chem Commun (Camb) 2008;21(23):2686–8.

4. Painter CF. Subdeltoid bursitis. Boston Med Surg J 1907;156:345–9.

5. Sandstrom C. Peritendinitis calcarea. A common disease of middle life: its diagnosis, pathology and treatment. Am J Radiol 1938;40:1–21.

6. McCarty DJ, Gatter RA. Recurrent acute inflammation associated with focal apatite crystal deposition. Arthritis Rheum 1966;9:804–19.

7. Uhthoff HK, Sarker K, Maynard JA. Calcifying tendonitis. A new concept of its pathogenesis. Clin Orthop 1976;118:164–8.

8. Rosenthal A, Mandel N. Identification of crystals in synovial fluids and joint tissues. Current Rheumatol Rep 2001;3:11–6.

9. McCarty DJ. Robert Adams' rheumatic arthritis of the shoulder: "Milwaukee shoulder" revisited. J Rheumatol 1989;16:668–70.

10. Jensen K, Williams G, Russell I, et al. Rotator cuff tear arthropathy. J Bone Joint Surg Am 1999;81-A(9):1312–24.

11. Lequesne M, Fallut M, Couloumb R. L'arthropathie destructice rapide de l'epaule. Rev Rheum 1982;49:427–37.

12. Neer CS, Craig EV, Fakuda H. Cuff-tear arthropathy. J Bone Joint Surg 1983;65A:1232–44.

13. Campion GV, McCrae F, Alwan W, et al. Idiopathic destructive arthritis of the shoulder. Semin Arthritis Rheum 1988;17:232–45.

14. Dieppe PA, Huskisson EC, Crocker P, et al. Apatite deposition disease: a new arthropathy. Lancet 1976;1:266–9.

15. McCarty DJ, Hogan JM, Gatter RA, et al. Studies on pathological calcifications in human cartilage. J Bone Joint Surg 1966;48:309–25.

16. Halverson PB, McCarty DJ. Identification of hydroxyapatite crystals in synovial fluid. Arthritis Rheum 1979;22:389–95.

17. Schumacher HR, Cherian PV, Reginato AJ, et al. Intraarticular apatite crystal deposition. Ann Rheum Dis 1983;42(Suppl. 1):54–9.

18. McCarty DJ, Halverson PB, Carrera GF, et al. Milwaukee shoulder:association of microspheroids containing hydroxyapatite crystals, active collagenase, and neutral protease with rotator cuff defects, i:clinical aspects. Arthritis Rheum 1981;24:464–73.

19. Bosworth BM. Calcium deposits in the shoulder and subacromial bursitis. A survey of 12,222 shoulders. JAMA 1941;116:2477–82.

20. Derfus BA, Kurian JB, Butler JJ, et al. The high prevalence of pathologic calcium crystals in pre-operative knees. J Rheumatol 2002 Mar;29(3):570–4.

21. Macmullan PA, McCarthy GM. The meniscus, calcification and osteoarthritis: a pathologic team. Arthritis Res Ther 2010 May 20;12(3):116.

22. McCarthy GM. Basic calcium phosphate crystal deposition disease. Rheumatology, 4th ed. vol. 2. 2010; Section 14, Chapter 187.

23. McCarthy GM, Carrera GF, Ryan LM. Acute calcific periarthritis of the finger joints: a syndrome of women. J Rheumatol 1993;20:1077–80.

24. Fam AG, Rubenstein J. Hydroxyapatite pseudopodagra. A syndrome of young women. Arthritis Rheum 1989;32:741–7.

25. Bouvet J-P, le Parc J-M, Michalski B, et al. Acute neck pain due to calcifications surrounding the odontoid process: the crowned dens syndrome. Arthritis Rheum 1985;28:1417–20.

26. Hajeroussan VJ, Short CL. Familial calcific periarthritis. Ann Rheum Dis 1983;42:469–70.

27. Terkeltaub R. Diseases associated with articular deposition of calcium pyrophosphate dihydrate and basic calcium phosphate crystals. In Textbook of Rheumatology, 8th ed. vol. 2. 2009. p. 1507–24.

28. Halverson PB. Arthropathies associated with basic calcium phosphate crystals. Scann Microsc 1992;6:791–7.

29. Fitzsimmons AS, O'Dell MW, Guiffra LJ, et al. Radial nerve injury associated with traumatic myositis ossificans in a brain injured patient. Arch Phys Med Rehabil 1993;74(7):770–3.

30. Halverson PB, Carrera GF, McCarty DJ. Milwaukee shoulder syndrome: fifteen additional cases and a description of contributing factors. Arch Int Med 1990;150:677–82.

31. McCarty D, Swanson A, Ehrhart R. Hemorrhagic rupture of the shoulder. J Rheumatol 1994;21:1134–7.

32. Dieppe PA, Doherty M, Macfarlane DG, et al. Apatite associated destructive arthritis. Br J Rheumatol 1984;23:84–91.

33. Schumacher HR, Smolyo AP, Tse RL, et al. Arthritis associated with apatite crystals. Ann Intern Med 1977;87:411–6.

34. Schumacher HR, Miller JL, Ludivico C, et al. Erosive arthritis associated with apatite crystal deposition. Arthritis Rheum 1981;24:31–7.

35. Molloy ES, McCarthy GM. Calcium crystal deposition diseases: update on pathogenesis and manifestations. Rheum Dis Clin North Am 2006;32(2):383–400, vii.

36. McCarty DJ. Crystal-induced inflammation of the joints. Annu Rev Med 1970;21:357–66.

37. McCarthy GM. Inspirational calcification: how rheumatology research directs investigation in vascular biology. Curr Opin Rheumatol 2009;21(1):47–9.

38. Fuerst M, Bertrand J, Lammers L, et al. Calcification of articular cartilage in human osteoarthritis. Arthritis Rheum 2009;60(9):2694–703.

39. Bennett LD, Buckland-Wright JC. Meniscal and articular cartilage changes in knee osteoarthritis: a cross-sectional double-contrast macroradiographic study. Rheumatology (Oxford) 2002;41(8):917–23.

40. Sun Y, Mauerhan DR, Honeycutt PR, et al. Calcium deposition in osteoarthritic meniscus and meniscal cell culture. Arthritis Res Ther 2010;12(2):R56.

41. Hatzis N, Kaar TK, Wirth MA, et al. Neuropathic arthropathy of the shoulder. J Bone Joint Surg Am 1998;80(9):1314–9.

42. Halverson PB, McCarty DJ. Patterns of radiographic abnormalities associated with basic calcium phosphate and calcium pyrophosphate crystal deposition in the knee. Ann Rheum Dis 1986;45:603–5.

43. Carroll GJ, Stuart RA, Armstrong JA, et al. Hydroxyapatite crystals are a frequent finding in osteoarthritic synovial fluid, but are not related to increased concentrations of keratan sulfate or interleukin 1b. J Rheumatol 1991;18:861–6.

44. McCarty DJ, Halverson PB, Carrera GF, et al. "Milwaukee shoulder": association of microspheroids containing hydroxyapatite crystals, active collagenase, and neutral protease with rotator cuff defects. I. Clinical aspects. Arthritis Rheum 1981;24(3):464–73.

45. MacMullan PA, McMahon G, McCarthy GM. Detection of basic calcium phosphate crystals in osteoarthritis. Jt Bone Spine 2010:In Press.

46. Kieft GJ, Sartoris DJ, Bloem JL, et al. Magnetic resonance imaging of glenohumeral joint diseases. Skeletal Radiol 1987;16(4):285–90.

47. Reid G, Esdaile JM. Rheumatology: 3. Getting the most out of radiology. CMAJ 2000;162(9):1318–25.

48. Choi HK, Al-Arfaj AM, Eftekhari A, et al. Dual energy computed tomography in tophaceous gout. Ann Rheum Dis 2009;68(10):1609–12.

49. Dieppe P, Swan A. Identification of crystals in synovial fluid. Ann Rheum Dis 1999;58(5):261–3.

50. Ivorra J, Rosas J, Pascual E. Most calcium pyrophosphate crystals appear as non-birefringent. Ann Rheum Dis 1999;58(9):582–4.

51. Pascual E, Jovani V. Synovial fluid analysis. Best Pract Res Clin Rheumatol 2005;19(3):371–86.

52. Rosenthal AK, Fahey M, Gohr C, et al. Feasibility of a tetracycline-binding method for detecting synovial fluid basic calcium phosphate crystals. Arthritis Rheum 2008;58(10):3270–4.

53. Lazcano O, Li CY, Pierre RV, et al. Clinical utility of the alizarin red S stain on permanent preparations to detect calcium-containing compounds in synovial fluid. Am J Clin Pathol 1993;99(1):90–6.

54. Ortiz-Bravo E. [The test of the synovial fluid in microcrystalline joint diseases]. Rev Prat 1994;44(2):174–7.

55. Gee KR, Brown KA, Chen WN, et al. Chemical and physiological characterization of fluo-4 Ca(2+)-indicator dyes. Cell Calcium 2000;27(2):97–106.

56. Cunningham T, Uebelhart D, Very JM, et al. Synovial fluid hydroxyapatite crystals: detection thresholds of two methods. Ann Rheum Dis 1989 Oct;48(10):829–31.

57. Ali SY. Apatite-type crystal deposition in arthritic cartilage. Scan Electron Microsc 1985; (Pt 4):1555–66.

58. Schumacher HR, Cherian PV. Transmission electron microscopic studies on articular calcium crystals and associated protein coatings. Scan Electron Microsc 1984(Pt 2):965–8.

59. Bardin T, Schumacher HR, Lansaman J, et al. Transmission electron microscopic identification of silicon-containing particles in synovial fluid: potential confusion with calcium pyrophosphate dihydrate and apatite crystals. Ann Rheum Dis 1984;43(4):624–7.

60. Nero P, Nogueira I, Vilar R, et al. [Synovial fluid crystal identification by electron microscopy]. Acta Reumatol Port 2006;31(1):75–81.

61. Blair JM, Sorensen LB, Arnsdorf MF, et al. The application of atomic force microscopy for the detection of microcrystals in synovial fluid from patients with recurrent synovitis. Semin Arthritis Rheum 1995;24(5):359–69.

62. Shaw RA, Kotowich S, Eysel HH, et al. Arthritis diagnosis based upon the near-infrared spectrum of synovial fluid. Rheumatol Int 1995;15(4):159–65.

63. Hornez JC, Chai F, Monchau F, et al. Biological and physico-chemical assessment of hydroxyapatite (HA) with different porosity. Biomol Eng 2007;24(5):505–9.

64. Shah JS. Application of physical methods in the investigations of crystal-related arthropathies. Ann Rheum Dis 1983;42(Suppl 1):68–72.

65. Rosenthal AK, Mattson E, Gohr CM, et al. Characterization of articular calcium-containing crystals by synchrotron FTIR. Osteoarthritis Cartilage 2008;16(11):1395–402.
66. Carden A, Morris MD. Application of vibrational spectroscopy to the study of mineralized tissues. J Biomed Opt 2000;5(3):259–68.
67. McGill N, Dieppe PA, Bowden M, et al. Identification of pathological mineral deposits by Raman microscopy. Lancet 1991 Jan 12;337(8733):77–8.
68. Zaheer A, Lenkinski RE, Mahmood A, et al. In vivo near-infrared fluorescence imaging of osteoblastic activity. Nat Biotechnol 2001;19(12):1148–54.
69. De Grand AM, Lomnes SJ, Lee DS, et al. Tissue-like phantoms for near-infrared fluorescence imaging system assessment and the training of surgeons. J Biomed Opt 2006;11(1):014007.
70. Calafiori AR, Di Marco G, Martino G, et al. Preparation and characterization of calcium phosphate biomaterials. J Mater Sci Mater Med 2007;18(12):2331–8.
71. Swan A, Chapman B, Heap P, et al. Submicroscopic crystals in osteoarthritic synovial fluids. Ann Rheum Dis 1994;53(7):467–70.
72. Halverson PB, McCarty DJ. Identification of hydroxyapatite crystals in synovial fluid. Arthritis Rheum 1979;22(4):389–95.
73. Dahners LE, Bos GD. Fluorescent tetracycline labeling as an aid to debridement of necrotic bone in the treatment of chronic osteomyelitis. J Orthop Trauma 2002;16(5):345–6.
74. Brannan SR, Jerrard DA. Synovial fluid analysis. J Emerg Med 2006;30(3):331–9.
75. McCarty D. Crystals, joints, and consternation. Ann Rheum Dis 1983;42(3):243–53.
76. Catterall JB, Cawston TE. Drugs in development: bisphosphonates and metalloproteinase inhibitors. Arthritis Res Ther 2003;5(1):12–24.
77. Haukanes BI, Kvam C. Application of magnetic beads in bioassays. Biotechnology (N Y) 1993;11(1):60–3.
78. Sarkar K, Uhthoff HK. Ultrastructural localization of calcium in calcifying tendinitis. Arch Pathol Lab Med 1978;102(5):266–9.
79. McKendry RJ, Uhthoff HK, Sarkar K, et al. Calcifying tendinitis of the shoulder: prognostic value of clinical, histologic, and radiologic features in 57 surgically treated cases. J Rheumatol 1982;9(1):75–80.
80. Neer 2nd CS. Anterior acromioplasty for the chronic impingement syndrome in the shoulder: a preliminary report. J Bone Joint Surg Am 1972;54(1):41–50.
81. Rathbun JB, Macnab I. The microvascular pattern of the rotator cuff. J Bone Joint Surg Br 1970;52(3):540–53.
82. Sarker K, Uhthoff HK. Ultrastructural localization of calcium in calcifying tendinitis. Arch Pathol Lab Med 1978;102:266–9.
83. Dayer J-M, Evequoz V, Zavadil-Grob C, et al. Effect of synthetic calcium pyrophosphate and hydroxyapatite crystals on the interaction of human blood mononuclear cells with chondrocytes, synovial cells and fibroblasts. Arthritis Rheum 1987;30:1372–81.
84. Dieppe P, Doherty M, Papadimitriou GM. Inflammatory responses to intradermal crystals in healthy volunteers and patients with rheumatic diseases. Rheumatol Int 1982;2:55–8.
85. Terkeltaub RA. What does cartilage calcification tell us about osteoarthritis? J Rheumatol 2002;29(3):411–5.
86. Kranendonk S, Ryan L, Buday M, et al. Human osteoarthritic vesicles generate both monoclinic calcium pyrophosphate dihydrate and apatite crystals in vitro. J Bone Joint Surg 1994;18:502–3.
87. Ho A, Johnson M, Kingsley D. Role of the mouse ank gene in control of tissue calcification and arthritis. Science 2000;289:265–9.
88. Andrew LJ, Brancolini V, de la Pena LS, et al. Refinement of the chromosome 5p locus for familial calcium pyrophosphate dihydrate deposition disease. Am J Hum Genet 1999;64(1):136–45.
89. Pendleton A, Johnson MD, Hughes A, et al. Mutations in ANKH cause chondrocalcinosis. Am J Hum Genet 2002;71(4):933–40.
90. Williams CJ, Zhang Y, Timms A, et al. Autosomal dominant familial calcium pyrophosphate dihydrate deposition disease is caused by mutation in the transmembrane protein ANKH. Am J Hum Genet 2002;71(4):985–91.
91. Johnson K, Hashimoto S, Lotz M, et al. Up-regulated expression of the phosphodiesterase nucleotide pyrophosphatase family member PC-1 is a marker and pathogenic factor for knee meniscal cartilage matrix calcification. Arthritis Rheum 2001;44(5):1071–81.
92. Terkeltaub RA. Inorganic pyrophosphate generation and disposition in pathophysiology. Am J Physiol Cell Physiol 2001;281(1):C1–11.
93. Peach C, Zhang Y, Dunford J, et al. Cuff tear arthropathy: evidence of functional variation in pyrophosphate metabolism genes. Clin Orthop Relat Res 2007;462:67–72.
94. Johnson K, Jung A, Murphy A, et al. Mitochondrial oxidative phosphorylation is a downstream regulator of nitric oxide effects on chondrocyte matrix synthesis and mineralization. Arthritis Rheum 2000;43(7):1560–70.
95. Rachow JW, Ryan LM, McCarty DJ, et al. Synovial fluid inorganic pyrophosphate concentration and nucleotide pyrophosphohydrolase activity in basic calcium phosphate deposition arthropathy and Milwaukee shoulder syndrome. Arthritis Rheum 1988;31(3):408–13.
96. Cheung HS, Story MT, McCarty DJ. Mitogenic effects of hydroxyapatite and calcium pyrophosphate dihydrate crystals on cultured mammalian cells. Arthritis Rheum 1984;27:668–74.
97. McCarthy G, Westfall P, Masuda I, et al. Basic calcium phosphate crystals activate human osteoarthritis synovial fibroblasts and induce matrix metalloproteinase-13 (collagenase-3) in adult porcine articular chondrocytes. Ann Rheum Dis 2001;60:399–406.
98. McCarthy GM, Mitchell PG, Struve JS, et al. Basic calcium phosphate crystals cause co-ordinate induction and secretion of collagenase and stromelysin. J Cell Physiol 1992;153:140–6.
99. Molloy E, Morgan M, Doherty G, et al. Mechanism of basic calcium phosphate crystal-stimulated cyclo-oxygenase-1 up-regulation in osteoarthritic synovial fibroblasts. Rheumatology (Oxford) 2008;47:965–71.
100. Morgan M, Whelan L, Sallis J, et al. Basic calcium phosphate crystal-induced PGE2 production in human fibroblasts: role of cyclo-oxygenase-1 and -2, and interleukin-1b. Arthritis Rheum 2004:In press.
101. Gordon GV, Villanueva T, Schumacher HR, et al. Autopsy study correlating degree of osteoarthritis, synovitis and evidence of articular calcification. J Rheumatol 1984;11(5):681–6.
102. Kronenberg HM. Developmental regulation of the growth plate. Nature 2003;423(6937):332–6.
103. Jubeck B, Gohr C, Fahey M, et al. Promotion of articular cartilage matrix vesicle mineralization by type I collagen. Arthritis Rheum 2008;58(9):2809–17.
104. Derfus BA, Kurtin SM, Camacho NP, et al. Comparison of matrix vesicles derived from normal and osteoarthritic human articular cartilage. Connect Tissue Res 1996;35(1-4):337–42.
105. Cheung HS, Sallis JD, Demadis KD, et al. Phosphocitrate blocks calcification-induced articular joint degeneration in a guinea pig model. Arthritis Rheum 2006;54(8):2452–61.
106. Verdonk PC, Forsyth RG, Wang J, et al. Characterisation of human knee meniscus cell phenotype. Osteoarthritis Cartilage 2005;13(7):548–60.
107. Tew WP, Mahle C, Benavides J, et al. Synthesis and characterization of phosphocitric acid, a potent inhibitor of hydroxylapatite crystal growth. Biochemistry 1980;19(9):1983–8.
108. Dalal P, Zanotti K, Wierzbicki A, et al. Molecular dynamics simulation studies of the effect of phosphocitrate on crystal-induced membranolysis. Biophys J 2005;89(4):2251–7.

Chapter 23

Crystalline Disorders Associated With Renal Disease Including Oxalate Arthropathy

Elisabeth Matson and Anthony M. Reginato

KEY POINTS

- Rheumatic syndromes are a common complication of chronic kidney disease (CKD); regardless of renal disease etiology, musculoskeletal symptoms have been reported in up to 82% of patients receiving hemodialysis.
- The pathogenesis of abnormal mineral metabolism in CKD involves inadequate renal conversion of 25-hydroxyvitamin D to its active forms, 1,25-dihydroxyvitamin D, further exacerbated by concomitant nutritional deficiency of 25-hydroxyvitamin D. Deficiencies in vitamin D axis impair dietary calcium absorption and release the parathyroid glands from feedback inhibition.
- Impaired phosphorous excretion with worsening renal function and decreased expression of calcium sensing receptor in the parathyroid gland also promotes increased parathyroid hormone levels, leading to secondary hyperparathyroidism and refractory hyperparathyroidism.
- CKD–mineral and bone disorders are closely interlinked with deposition of calcium-containing crystals, such as basic calcium phosphate, hydroxyapatite, calcium pyrophosphate dihydrate, calcium oxalate, and, to a lesser extent, monosodium urate.
- Calcium oxalate deposition can lead to arthritis and vascular disease, which often are delayed in diagnosis.

Clinical Disease

Chronic kidney disease (CKD) is a growing public health epidemic that affects up to 13% of the U.S. population. CKD exerts a toxic toll in a variety of tissues and other organ system and tissues beginning early in its course, resulting in numerous complications leading to decrease on the quality of life and premature death in affected patients.[1] Rheumatic syndromes are a common complication of CKD; regardless of renal disease etiology, musculoskeletal symptoms have been reported in up to 82% of patients receiving hemodialysis[2] with increasing incidence during long-term maintenance hemodialysis. These rheumatic disorders have been well described and carefully studied for many years (Table 23-1).[3] This chapter will briefly review CKD–mineral and bone disorders (CKD-MBD) and the clinically relevant crystalline disorders with emphasis on oxalate arthropathy.

Chronic Kidney Diseases

Crystal-induced arthropathies and CKD-MBD, as manifest by several laboratory abnormalities, bone diseases, and vascular calcification,[4] are well-recognized complications that occur in all stages of CKD as well as in hemodialysis. The pathogenesis of disordered mineral metabolism in CKD involves inadequate renal conversion of 25-hydroxyvitamin D to its active forms. 1,25-Dihydroxyvitamin D may be further exacerbated by concomitant nutritional deficiency of 25-hydroxyvitamin D. Deficiencies in vitamin D axis impair dietary calcium absorption and release of parathyroid glands from feedback inhibition. Impaired phosphorous excretion with worsening renal function and decreased expression of calcium-sensing receptor in the parathyroid gland also promotes increased parathyroid hormone (PTH) levels leading to secondary hyperparathyroidism and refractory hyperparathyroidism.[5] Furthermore, decrease in circulating 1,25-dihydroxyvitamin D concentrations in early CKD is mediated by fibroblast growth factor 23 (FGF23) by inhibiting the synthetic 1α-hydroxylase and stimulating the catabolic 24-hydroxylase leading to release of the parathyroids from feedback inhibition and further contributing to secondary hyperparathyroidism. CKD-MBD are closely interlinked with deposition of calcium-containing crystals, such as basic calcium phosphate (BCP), hydroxyapatite (HA), calcium pyrophosphate dihydrate (CPPD), calcium oxalate (CaOX), and, to a lesser extent, monosodium urate (MSU). Deposition of these crystals in and around the joints and soft tissues leads to several clinical presentations, including bursitis, tenosynovitis, synovitis, and arthritis in patients with progressive CKD and hemodialysis. The clinical presentations of crystal-induced arthropathies in CKD and hemodialysis are often similar, requiring diagnostic arthrocentesis, with examination of synovial fluid for crystals undercompensated polarized microscopy and sometimes requires the additional use of special stains for their proper identification. Although the exact molecular mechanisms leading to crystal deposition

Table 23-1 Noncrystalline and Crystalline Manifestations of Chronic Kidney Disease/End-Stage Renal Disease (CKD/ESRD)

NON–CRYSTALLINE-ASSOCIATED DISORDERS

Chronic Kidney Disease–Mineral and Bone Disorders (CKD-MBD)

Secondary hyperparathyroidism (sHPP)

Osteopenia/osteoporosis

Low and high bone turnover

Osteomalacia

Mixed osteodystrophy (hyperparathyroidism and osteomalacia)

Adynamic bone disorder (ABD)

Osteosclerosis

Soft tissue and vascular calcification (VC)

Hemodialysis related

Aluminum toxicity

β_2-Microglobulin amyloidosis

Upper extremities

    Scapulohumeral periarthritis

    Carpal tunnel syndrome (CTS)

    Flexor tenosynovitis

Spine

    Destructive spondyloarthropathy

    Periodontoid pseudotumor

    Extradural amyloid deposits

Bone cysts

    Pathologic fractures

Nephrogenic systemic fibrosis (NSF)

Avascular necrosis (AVN)

Infection

Septic arthritis/bursitis

Discitis

Osteomyelitis

Tendon disorder

Tendon rupture

Tendinitis

Olecranon bursitis

Uremic myopathy

CRYSTALLINE-ASSOCIATED DISORDERS

Arthropathy associated with partially carbonate-substituted apatite crystals

Calcium pyrophosphate dihydrate

Monosodium urate

Calcium oxalate

---

studies have identified many proteins that act as stimulators or inhibitors of crystal formation and could contribute to crystal-induced arthropathies in patients with CKD.

An imbalance between these proteins in uremic and hemodialysis patients may accelerate crystal formation and deposition in the extracellular matrix and may lead to the initiation and propagation of inflammation as these crystals are deposited and released from tissues. In addition, alterations of mineral metabolism in CKD associated with elevated levels of serum calcium (Ca), phosphorus (P), Ca-P product (Ca × P), and PTH are also associated with increased cardiovascular morbidity and mortality.[6,7] Cardiovascular disease is up to 20-fold more frequent in end-stage renal disease (ESRD) patients and accounts for up to 50% of all deaths, with accelerated atherosclerosis being consistently implicated in this process.[8] Among abnormalities of mineral metabolism, one of the most prominent and relevant is hyperphosphatemia,[8] an event already present in the early phases of renal failure.[9] Elevated serum phosphorous has been related to cardiovascular morbidity and mortality in both hemodialysis and predialysis patients. Vascular and coronary artery calcification have been suggested as the link between abnormal mineral metabolism in general and hyperphosphatemia in particular cardiovascular events in this population.[9-11] Hyperphosphatemia has been pointed out as the primary culprit in the process of cardiovascular calcification,[9,11-13] an event that is present in the early phases of CKD.[12,14] A significant association between the progression of coronary artery calcification and serum phosphorous concentration was observed in CKD patients, despite serum phosphorous being in the normal range. Faster vascular calcification progression was found in patients with a high-normal serum phosphorous, which was accompanied by more frequent cardiovascular events.[15] However, despite these various findings, the mechanisms by which serum phosphorous contributes to vascular calcification and cardiovascular disease are not completely understood.

Soft Tissue and Vascular Calcification

Calcium and phosphate ions in biologic fluids exist in concentrations near the point at which mineral salt precipitation can occur. The balance between extracellular inorganic pyrophosphate (ePP_i) and extracellular inorganic phosphate (eP_i) levels in local tissues regulates both normal and pathologic mineralization. The normal ratio of ePP_i/eP_i is tightly regulated and lower values are associated with increased calcification.

Three molecules closely regulate the ePP_i/eP_i levels: tissue nonspecific alkaline phosphatase,[16] enzyme ectonucleotide pyrophosphatase/phosphodiesterase-1 (ENPP1),[17] and the ePP_i transporter ANKH (or *ank*).[18] Inactivation of ENPP1 in humans markedly reduces plasma PP_i levels and results in extensive large artery calcification and variable periarticular calcifications.[19] ENPP1 (ENPP1K121Q) polymorphisms in hemodialysis patients are associated with higher coronary calcification and increased aortic stiffness.[20] PP_i is hydrolyzed by extracellular phosphatases, most notably by tissue nonspecific alkaline phosphatase. In patients with calcific uremic arteriolopathy, increased levels of serum alkaline phosphatase activity are observed.[21] The kidney normally clears pyrophosphate but, in patients with stage 5 CKD, plasma pyrophosphate is very efficiently removed by hemodialysis.[22] This contributes

Table 23-2 Inhibitory Proteins of Soft Tissue and Vascular Calcification (VC) With Potential Roles in Uremia and Chronic Kidney Disease/End-Stage Kidney Disease

Name/Class	Chemistry	Production/ Distribution	Action	Null Mice	Notes
PP$_i$ inorganic	Chain of P linked through oxygen plasma solute	VSMCs, chondrocytes osteoblasts/ubiquitous	Inhibits mineralization, oxalate crystallization		Hydrolyzed by TNAP
MGP GLA protein	Noncollagenous bone protein, 84 amino acids; 14 kDa 5 g-GLA residues	VSMCs, chondrocytes/ calcified tissues (cartilage, vessels)	Inhibits calcification	Arterial calcification, aortic rupture, osteopenia, fractures	Requires vitamin K–dependent g-carboxylation
BMP-7 TGF-β superfamily	Protein, 431 amino acids; 7-cystatin-residue ring	Adult: kidney Embryo: skeleton, kidney, eye, CV/collecting tubules, glomerulus, adventitia	Cell proliferation/ differentiation/ apoptosis; osteoblasts, VSMC differentiation	Uremia	Anti-TGF-β, anti-inflammatory effect (IL-1,-6,8 inhibition)
OPG TNF-R superfamily	Glycoprotein 40 amino acids; 60 kDA M; 120 kDa D	Heart, arteries, veins, bone, marrow, lung, kidney, intestine/ several tissues (bone, vessels); cytokine receptor glomerulus, adventitia	Inhibits osteoclastogenesis, protective for vascular (endothelial cell survival factor)		High turnover, osteoporosis, VC

Ca, Calcium; CV, cardiovascular; D, dimeric; GLA, glutamic acid; IL, interleukin; M, monomeric; P, phosphate. PP, inorganic pyrophosphate; R, receptor; TGF-β, transforming growth factor-β; TNF, tumor necrosis factor.

to an altered ratio of ePP$_i$/eP$_i$, thereby promoting soft tissue, periarticular, and vascular calcification.

As mentioned, the spontaneous formation of Ca^{2+}:PO$_4$$^{-3}$ solid phases in extracellular fluids may be prevented by a number of proteins that inhibit precipitation or sequester ions to reduce their bioavailability. In bone, normal mechanisms inhibiting mineral deposition are blocked in a carefully regulated manner. It is thought that, under normal physiologic states, similar proteins expressed in soft tissues and in blood vessels prevent precipitation of calcium with other minerals. However, this process is believed to be dysregulated in stage 5 CKD. Prominent among these many inhibitors are matrix c-carboxyglutamic acid protein (MGP) in the extracellular matrix and α$_2$-Heremans-Schmid glycoproteins/fetuins in serum (Table 23-2). MGP can directly sequester calcium, acting as a buffering agent, but it also serves as an inhibitory partner of bone morphogenic protein (BMP)-2.[23] BMP-2, a potent morphogen of the transforming growth factor-β superfamily, normally functions during skeletal development, but under unusual circumstances, it can induce ectopic cartilage and bone formation in soft tissues. Interestingly, serum concentrations of BMP-2 in uremic patients are twice those found in normal serum.[24] Local concentrations of MGP seem important in reducing ectopic calcification. In situ hybridization and immunohistochemistry studies of MGP in vascular smooth muscle cells demonstrate downregulation of this molecule in calcific human tissue and in animal models of calcification. MGP knockout mice develop overwhelming vascular calcification of the vascular tree,[25] an effect that appears to be regulated locally in cells in an autonomous manner.[26] Warfarin, which is administered to patients undergoing hemodialysis, inhibits vitamin K–dependent c-carboxylation of MGP[27] and results in reduced MGP function. Finally, MGP polymorphisms are of prognostic significance in predicting progression to stage 5 CKD, cardiovascular mortality, and vascular calcification in patients with CKD.[28] Another systemic factor

that functions as a potent inhibitor of HA crystal formation is α$_2$-Heremans-Schmid glycoprotein-A produced by the liver.[29] Fetuin-A binds calcium and phosphorus in extracellular fluids and helps maintain the solubility of calcium in plasma. Fetuin-A plasma levels are reduced in patients with stage 5 CKD compared with healthy control subjects.[30]

The toxic environment associated with late-stage CKD can induce trans-differentiation of vascular smooth muscle cells into an osteoblastic phenotype with subsequent deposition of BCP and HA into tissues through matrix vesicles.[31] This occurs when genes for regulatory transcription factors, such as Cbfa1/Runx2, Msx2, and Sox9, which are pivotal to determine chondroblastic and osteoblastic differentiation, are induced.[32] A number of key mechanisms, including hyperphosphatemia, BMP-7, and osteoprotegerin (OPG), contribute to the induction of these genes. Elevated phosphate concentrations, such as those in patients with late-stage CKD, may increase intracellular phosphate levels through Pit-1, a type II sodium/phosphate cotransporter that induces Cbfa1 expression and vascular smooth muscle cell trans-differentiation.[33] BMP-7 deficiency in CKD further contributes to the differentiation and transformation of vascular smooth muscle cells into cells with an osteoblastic phenotype.[34] OPG, a soluble protein inhibitor of the RANK/RANKL system, maintains a balance between bone formation and bone breakdown; increased levels of OPG lead to increased bone formation. Deletion of OPG in mice results in osteoporosis and also, surprisingly, to extensive vascular calcification. Concentrations of soluble plasma OPG are significantly higher in patients undergoing hemodialysis compared to age-matched healthy volunteers. OPG is upregulated at sites of tissue calcification,[35] which supports a role for local tissue phenotype-determining factors in promoting aberrant ectopic calcification.

Extracellular phosphate levels are tightly regulated through the activity of multiple secreted signaling peptide hormones. Fibroblast growth factor 23 (FGF23) is a recently identified hormone regulator of mineral and vitamin D metabolism. FGF23 is an osteoclast-derived secreted protein that works in conjunction with PTH to induce phosphaturia; levels of FGF23 are markedly elevated in CKD.[36,37] The principal actions of FGF23 are to inhibit sodium-dependent phosphate reabsorption and to suppress circulating $1,25(OH)_2$-vitamin D levels. Mutations in the gene for FGF23 result in hyperphosphatemic familial tumoral calcinosis.[38] In stages 3 and 4 CKD, FGF23 levels are quite elevated to compensate for persistent phosphate retention, which results in reduced renal production of 1,25-dihydroxyvitamin D and thereby stimulate secretion of PTH, suggesting its critical role in the pathogenesis of altered mineral homeostasis in CKD. Furthermore, it has recently been shown that FGF23 directly acts on parathyroid gland and mediates secretion of PTH.[39] It has been postulated that, as the major phosphaturic hormone, this may be a counterbalancing mechanism to increase the fractional excretion of phosphate by the reduced mass of functioning kidney. To function, FGF23 must bind to an FGF receptor complexed to its cofactor Klotho, which is a 130-kilodalton transmembrane glucuronidase,[40] the expression of which in the kidney is reduced in CKD. Besides its function in the proximal tubule of the kidney, FGF23 signals in the parathyroid glands to reduce PTH gene transcription and translation in rats. This result is paradoxical, because transgenic mice overexpressing FGF23 develop hyperparathyroidism. However, greater understanding of the mechanism by which FGF23 regulates extracellular phosphate levels may allow development of targeted therapies to better control hyperphosphatemia in stages 4 and 5 CKD.[39] Whether FGF23 also has local effects that contribute to calcium-containing crystal formation and deposition has not yet been studied.

Crystal-Induced Inflammation and Chronic Inflammation in CKD

Crystal release from soft tissue and joints induces inflammation through mechanisms that involve innate immunity and interleukin (IL)-1β.[41] Conflicting data have been reported regarding the role of TLRs in crystal-induced inflammation (see Chapter 5), although some of the observed differences may be accounted for by the different animal models from which these disparate data were derived.[42-44] However, the IL-1 receptor (IL-1R), which signals through its TLR adaptor protein myeloid differentiation factor 88 (MyD88), is critical for mediating inflammation induced by MSU, CPPD, and HA crystals.[44-46] These crystals stimulate the activation of mononuclear phagocytes involving the NLRP3 inflammasome (see Chapter 5). The pivotal role of the inflammasome and IL-1 signaling in response to certain crystals has been exploited by successful use of the IL-1R antagonist (anakinra, rilonacept, canakinumab) to treat refractory cases of gout and pseudogout.[47] Similar studies have not been performed in other crystal arthropathies such as CaOX crystal deposition disease, which likely use similar inflammatory mechanism.

Interestingly, an attenuated inflammatory response to MSU crystals has been observed in patients receiving chronic hemodialysis, with decreased monocyte release of IL-1α, IL-6, and tumor necrosis factor as compared with individuals having normal renal function.[48] In addition, it is possible to speculate that the increased P_i concentration seen in CKD may also trigger phosphorylation-driven signaling inflammatory cascade[49] that correlates with chronic inflammatory state seen in patients with CKD as one the pivotal factor contributing to increased cardiovascular risk.[50]

HA and BCP Disease

HA and other forms of BCP (i.e., carbonate-substituted hydroxyapatite, octacalcium phosphate, and tricalcium phosphate) may cause significant extraskeletal calcification in patients with late-stage CKD by depositing in periarticular tissue, viscera, and arteries. HA may deposit in the small joints of the hands, wrists, elbows, hips, and ankles, but the shoulders are the joints most commonly affected. Prospective studies conducted during the years soon after the introduction of hemodialysis found the prevalence of extraskeletal calcification to be 52%, a number that has decreased gradually over time with more aggressive management of hyperphosphatemia and secondary hyperparathyroidism. This reduction in the prevalence of extraskeletal calcification among patients with CKD has resulted from a reduction of the elevated calcium × phosphorus quotient, as well as from changes in the local (tissue) and circulating (serum) levels of calcification-inhibitory and calcification-stimulatory proteins.[51]

CPPD Deposition Disease (Pseudogout)

Acute attacks of pseudogout occur when CPPD crystals are shed from hyaline cartilage and fibrocartilage into joints or periarticular tissues, inducing a sterile inflammatory response.[52] CPPD crystal–induced arthritis affects large or medium-sized joints, including the knees, wrists, hips, and shoulders, although small joints can also be involved. The prevalence of CPPD deposition disease increases with age, both among patients with late-stage CKD and among the remainder of the general population. One study reported a prevalence of CPPD arthropathy as high as 43% among patients receiving chronic dialysis.[53]

Patients with late-stage CKD and CPPD deposition disease may develop secondary osteoarthritis due to crystal-induced activation of MMP-13 mediated by IL-1β.[54] In the setting of CPPD deposition disease, degenerative changes may occur in atypical joints such as the metacarpophalangeal joints. Accelerated spinal osteoarthritis could also occur, the appearance of which may be remarkably similar to that of Charcot-type joint involvement.[55] The frequent occurrence of metabolic abnormalities common to CPPD deposition disease and CKD (e.g., hypercalcemia, hyperphosphatemia, vitamin D deficiency with secondary and tertiary hyperparathyroidism, and iron overload) accounts for the higher prevalence and greater severity of attacks of CPPD-induced arthritis among patients receiving hemodialysis.[56] In contrast, attacks of MSU crystal–induced arthritis are much less frequent and less severe among patients receiving dialysis treatment, compared with those with CKD who have not yet initiated dialysis. Chondrocalcinosis in patients with CKD is not pathognomonic of CPPD deposition disease, as similar calcifications can be seen in radiographs of patients with CKD who have deposition of CaOX or HA crystals.[57] Thus, diagnostic arthrocentesis is critical when evaluating an inflamed joint in a patient with CKD.[58]

MSU Deposition Disease (Gout)

The clinical presentation of gout is similar to that of pseudogout, although small joints such as the first metatarsophalangeal joints are commonly affected. Gout disproportionately affects persons with CKD, because declining GFR reduces urate clearance and results in hyperuricemia. Hyperparathyroidism, a common complication of moderate to severe CKD, can also promote hyperuricemia by enhancing urate absorption.[59] MSU crystal–induced arthritis continues to develop after the onset of uremia; however, symptoms are milder than before its onset.[60] In hemodialysis patients, hyperuricemia is attenuated by urate removal, especially when high-flux hemodialysis membranes are used.[61] Further descriptions of CPPD and MSU in relationship to CKD are described in their respective chapters.

Calcium Oxalate Deposition Disease

Oxalate is a metabolic end product of glycine, serine, other amino acids, and ascorbic acid. Large amounts of oxalate are also present in certain foods, such as spinach and rhubarb. Oxalate is readily absorbed after ingestion, cannot be metabolized in mammals, and is primarily eliminated through renal excretion. Oxalate is freely filtered by the glomerulus and is secreted by the tubules. Hyperoxalemia, hyperoxaluria, oxalate kidney stones, and crystalline tissue deposits may result from several contributing factors that may affect oxalate metabolism. Familial or primary hyperoxaluria (PHs) are rare genetic disorders of glyoxylate metabolism in which specific hepatic enzyme deficiencies result in the overproduction of oxalate by the liver leading to severe hyperoxaluria, recurrent urolithiasis or progressive nephrocalcinosis, ESRD, and tissue deposition. Secondary oxalosis results from either dietary or other exposures to large amounts of oxalate or oxalate precursors or underlying disorders such as ESRD, inflammatory bowel disease, or infections (Table 23-3).

Excess oxalate in the diet or increased absorption in patients with chronic inflammatory bowel disease, small bowel resection, intestinal bypass, external biliary drainage, and intestinal lymphangiectasia can lead to hyperoxalemia.

Table 23-3 Types of Oxalosis

FAMILIAL

Primary hyperoxaluria
Type 1 (HP1): AGT deficiency
Type 2 (HP2): GR deficiency
Type 3 (HP3): mutation in the mitochondrial dihydrodipicolinate synthase-like gene DHDPSL

ACQUIRED

Diet rich in oxalate, e.g., rhubarb
Increased ingestion or administration of oxalate precursors, e.g., ascorbic acid, ethyleneglycol, and xylitol
Increased absorption, e.g., small bowel resection or bypass, inflammatory bowel disease, or external biliary drainage
Increased production, e.g., deficiency in thiamine or pyridoxine, Aspergillus niger infection
Decreased renal excretion: uremia
Dystrophic: retinal damage

AGT, Alanine:glyoxylate aminotransferase; *DHDPSL,* gene encoding 4-hydroxy-2-oxoglutarate aldolase, catalyzing the final step in the metabolic pathway of hydroxyproline; *GR,* glyoxylate reductase/ᴅ-glycerate dehydrogenase.

Bowel abnormalities such as Crohn's disease[62,63] and small bowel resection[64,55] have been reported to result in secondary oxalosis. Patients with cystic fibrosis are at increased risk for hyperoxaluria due to intestinal malabsorption and a lack of intestinal *Oxalobacter formigenes* from frequent antibiotic use. *O. formigenes* absorbs oxalate to create adenosine triphosphate, so decreased bacterial counts contribute to oxalosis.[66] Arthritis is a rare complication of cystic fibrosis classified as either cystic fibrosis–related arthropathy or hypertrophic pulmonary osteoarthropathy, and no evidence of oxalate crystals has been reported as a cause of the arthritis.[67]

Ascorbic acid or vitamin C replacement is often recommended for long-term dialysis patients due to dialysis loss and potential benefit in opposing erythropoietin resistance. However, ascorbate is partially metabolized to oxalate, leading to higher levels of oxalate in dialysis patients.[68] The appropriate level of ascorbic acid repletion to achieve benefits but avoid risk of oxalosis is unknown.[69] Methoxyflurane, ethyleneglycol, and xylitol are all metabolized to oxalate as well. Infections caused by the *Aspergillus* sp., particularly *Aspergillus niger* cause localized oxalate deposition. Oxalate is a fermentation product of the fungus and may participate in the invasive nature of aspergillomas.[70] Aspergillomas have been reported to cause systemic oxalosis with renal failure related to oxalate deposition.[71] HIV-infected patients have been reported to have oxalate deposition in coronary arteries.[72] Oxalate deposition has also been reported in the globe of the eye,[73] eyelid,[74] and a renomedullary interstitial cell tumor[75] in AIDS patients. Thiamine and pyridoxinene deficiencies may inhibit glyoxylate metabolism, thereby increasing oxalate production.

Three rare autosomal recessive disorders of primary oxalosis are associated with oxalate arthropathy (Fig. 23-1). Primary hyperoxaluria type I (HP1) is an autosomal recessive disorder characterized by an accumulation of CaOX in various bodily tissues, especially the kidney, resulting in renal failure. Affected individuals have decreased or absent liver-specific peroxisomal enzyme alanine-glyoxylate aminotransferase (AGXT) activity and a failure to transaminate glyoxylate, which causes the accumulated glyoxylate to be oxidized to oxalate. Almost 100 disease-causing mutations in the *AGXT* gene, located on chromosome 2q36-q37, have been reported thus far. They include mostly point mutations leading to missense, nonsense, and a number of splicing mutations through the 11 exons of the gene. Minor deletions/insertions and a few major deletions spanning several exons account for the remaining third. This overproduction of oxalate results in the accumulation of nonsoluble CaOX in various body tissues, with pathologic sequelae.[76]

Primary hyperoxaluria type 2 (HP2) is caused by mutation in the glyoxylate reductase/hydroxypyruvate reductase gene (*GRHPR*) on chromosome 9.[77] To date, approximately 15 causative mutations in the *GRHPR* gene have been described with the base pair deletion G (c.103delG) in exon 2 the most common in patients of Caucasian descent (40%). As a result of reduced enzyme activity, increased amounts of glyoxylate and hydroxypyruvate are available for conversion by lactate dehydrogenase to both oxalate and ʟ-glyceric acid. Excessive amounts of both metabolites are excreted by the kidney. The hyperoxaluria leads to recurrent nephrolithiasis and, less frequently, nephrocalcinosis. Although the clinical course of HP2 is very similar to that of HP1, HP2 appears to have less

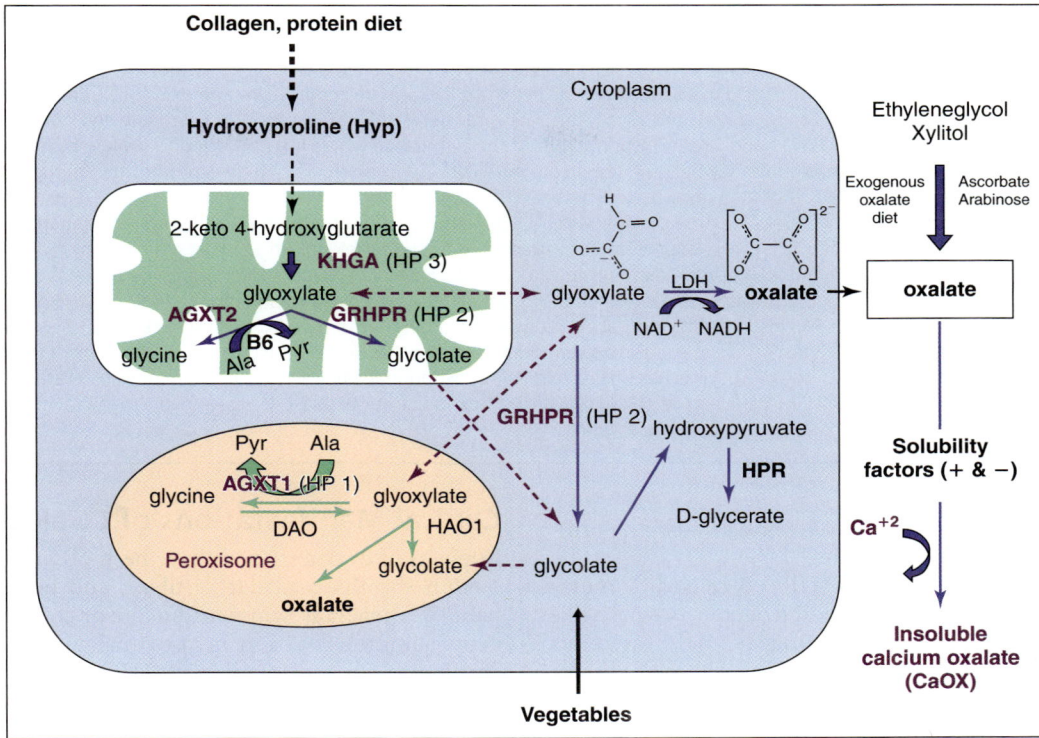

A

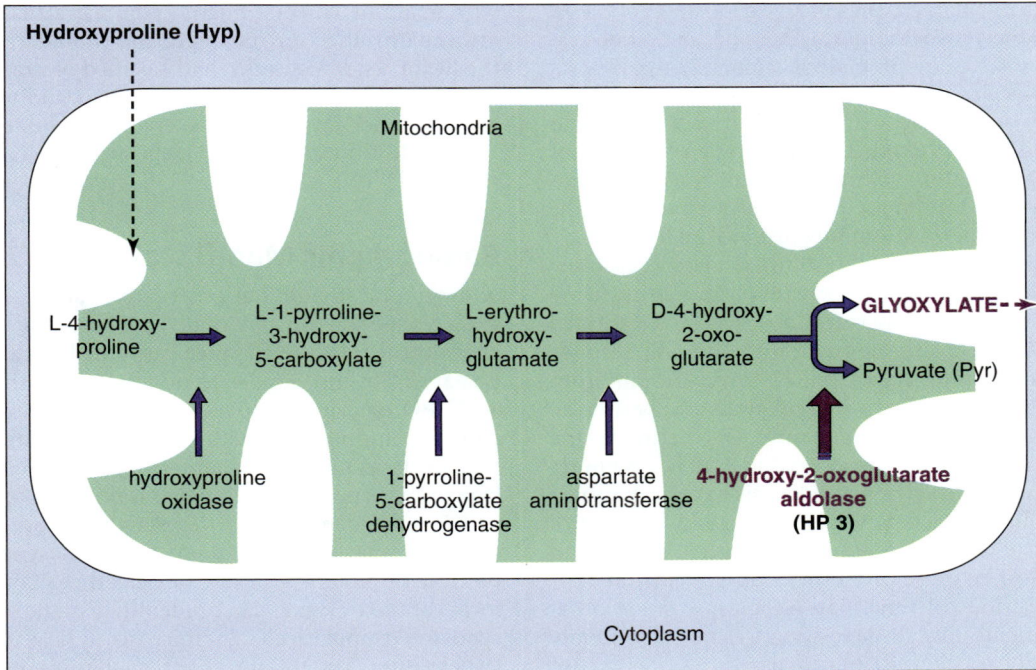

B

Figure 23-1, Cont'd.

Figure 23-1 A, The metabolic pathways to glyoxylate and oxalate production in humans. Both genetic and environmental factors likely contribute to oxalate production. The major sites of production of endogenous glyoxylate are the peroxisomes and the mitochondria. Glycolate is the major precursor of glyoxylate. In the peroxisomes glyoxylate can be derived from glycine through the reaction of D-aminoacid oxidase or, more significantly, from imported glycolate by the reaction with hydroxyacid oxidase 1 (HAO1). Glyoxylate can also be imported into peroxisomes from the cytoplasm. Glyoxylate is removed from transamination with alanine and alanine:glyoxylate aminotransferase (AGXT1), producing pyruvate and glycine. Excess glyoxylate in peroxisomes is converted to oxalate by HAO1 and Or is transported out of the cytoplasm, where it is converted to oxalate by lactate dehydrogenase (LDH). The former reaction plays a minor role but may become significant in AGXT1 deficiences, Glyoxylate is produced in mitochondria through the metabolism of 4-hydroxyproline (Hyp). Mitochondrial glyoxylate is converted to glycolate through the action of glyoxylate reductase/hydroxypyruvate reductase (GRHPR) or to glycine by alanine-glyoxylate aminotransferase (AGXT2). AGXT2 is distinct from AGXT1 with localization in the mitochondria. In the absence of glyoxylate reductase (AGXT2), glyoxylate will be converted to oxalate. **B,** Metabolism of hydroxyproline (hyp) as a significant source of glyoxylate. Hyp is derived from meat and gelatin in the diet and from normal turnover of collagen. Hydroxyproline is metabolized by four distinct mitochondrial enzymes into glyoxylate and pyruvate. Gain-of-function mutations in 4-hydroxy-2-oxoglutarate aldolase (KHGA) are responsible for the primary hyperoxaluria type III (HP 3). Peroxisomal enzymes: alanine:glyoxylate aminotransferase (AGXT1) (deficient in HP1); hydroxyacid oxidase 1 (HAO1), D-amino acid oxidase (DAO). Cytosolic enzymes: glyoxylate reductase/hydroxypyruvate reductase (GRHPR) (deficient in HP2), lactate dehydrogenase (LDH), hydroxypyruvate reductase (HPR). Mitochondrial enzymes: mitochondrial alanine-glyoxylate aminotransferase (AGXT2), glyoxylate reductase/hydroxypyruvate reductase (GRHPR) (deficient in HP2), 4-hydroxy-2-oxoglutarate aldolase (KHGA) (overactivity in HP3) *Ala,* alanine; *Pyr,* pyruvate. *Solid arrows:* enzymatic reactions; *broken arrows:* transport.

severe stone formation, less nephrocalcinosis, and better preservation of renal function over time.

Type III primary hyperoxaluria (HP3) is caused by mutation in the mitochondrial dihydrodipicolinate synthase-like gene (*DHDPSL*) on chromosome 10q24.[78] HP1 accounts for the majority (70% to 80%) of all cases. Although disease severity and resulting phenotype vary widely within affected families, about 90% of all HP1 cases become symptomatic in childhood to adolescence with cardinal features of urolithiasis and/or nephrocalcinosis. In both HP1 and HP2, renal insufficiency is associated with rapid progressive deposition of CaOX crystals in the kidney, myocardium, skin, bone, and blood vessels as GFR decreases below 30 to 40 ml/min/1.73 m².[79]

Oxalate crystals deposition has been described in musculoskeletal tissues such as synovium, tendon sheaths, articular cartilage, and bone,[80] producing multitude of symptoms including an inflammatory arthritis that can resemble rheumatoid arthritis or autoimmune disorders/vasculitis, and the correct diagnosis is not uncommonly overlooked for years.

Chronic renal failure can lead to serum oxalate levels fourfold to eightfold greater than normal levels. Serum levels oxalate levels parallel those of creatinine, becoming saturated when levels of serum creatinine reach 8 to 9 mg/dl. Secondary oxalosis complicating stage 5 CKD, which results from inefficient removal of oxalate by hemodialysis and peritoneal dialysis, has been reported infrequently. Furthermore, the overall incidence of secondary oxalosis due to ESRD is poorly understood. Patients receiving hemodialysis have been shown to have higher plasma oxalate levels compared with control subjects.[81] Oxalate deposition occurs in multiple organs and has been shown to be more pronounced in patients on dialysis for longer periods of time.[82] In an autopsy study of 80 hemodialysis patients, oxalate deposition was most frequently noted in the kidneys, thyroid, and myocardium. It was also noted in spleen, lungs, bone, central nervous system, and vessel walls, suggesting diffuse deposition.[83] Regardless of the etiology of oxalosis, when renal function declines below 30 to 40 ml/min/1.73 m² body surface area, oxalate can no longer be efficiently excreted by the kidneys and achieves supersaturation levels. Normal levels of serum oxalate are 1 to 6 μmol/L and can precipitate out as CaOX crystals at greater than 30 μmol/L, resulting in crystal deposition in multiple tissues including retina, myocardium, blood vessels, skin, bone, and central nervous system.[84]

Clinical Manifestations of Oxalosis

Deposits of oxalate crystals have been observed in synovium, tendon sheaths, articular cartilage, and bone. The arthritis pattern is generally symmetric, acute or chronic arthritis with most common location in proximal interphalangeal joints and metacarpophalangeal joints. However, it can present in other joints including knees, elbows, ankles, and first metatarsophalangeal joints. The associated clinical manifestations are similar to those of CPPD or MSU deposition.[85-88] Clinical features of CaOX deposition include polyarticular pain with acute or chronic microcrystalline arthritis, destructive arthropathy affecting the finger and shoulder, calcification of the flexor tendon sheaths, and calcified olecranon bursitis. In addition to these findings, periarticular and tendon deposits as well as Achilles tendonitis, epiphyseal bone densities, and soft tissue tumoral calcium deposits have been described[89] (Fig. 23-2).

Radiographic Manifestation of Oxalosis

Radiographic manifestations of oxalosis resemble those of CPPD, especially in the hands and feet, and may appear as chondrocalcinosis of the metacarpophalangeal or metatarsophalangeal joints. Similar to other crystal arthropathies such as CPPD or calcium apatite disease, chondrocalcinosis is a common finding along with vascular calcifications. Therefore, diagnostic arthrocentesis and examination of synovial fluid by compensated polarizing light microscopy are required to properly identify CaOX crystals from other crystals that exhibit similar radiographic pattern. The synovial fluid may be clear or cloudy with low nucleated cell count. Two main forms of these crystals can be identified in the synovial fluid or synovium by polarized light microscopy: CaOX monohydrate (whewellite) crystals appear as irregular birefringent squares, chunks, or rods that can be confused with CPPD crystals, and CaOX dihydrate (weddellite) crystals have a typical envelope-like or bipyramidal shape. Positive Alizarin red S staining of CaOX on fresh synovial fluid preparations may facilitate diagnosis (Fig. 23-3).

The most common skeletal findings on plain radiograph in a pediatric population of HP1 were dense and radiolucent metaphyseal bands and vertebral osteocondensations. The bands appeared in areas of growth and are more prominent than those seen in renal osteodystrophy.[90] In adult patients,

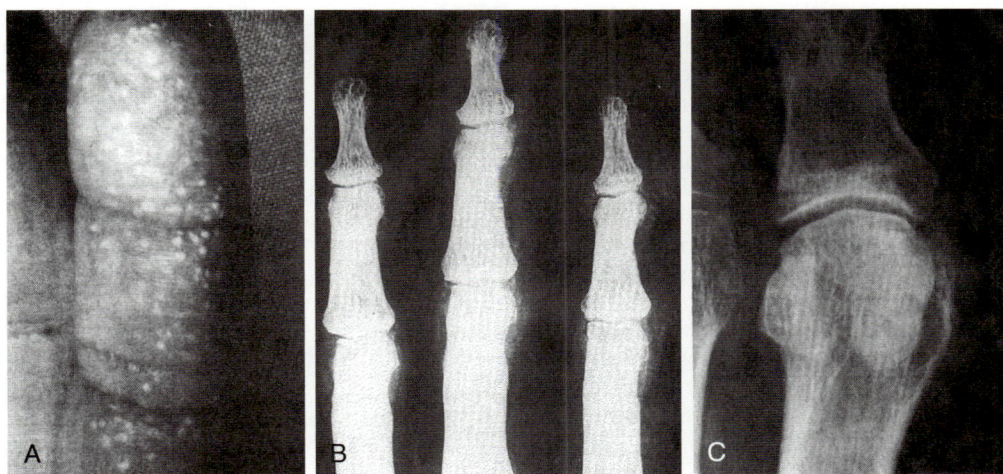

Figure 23-2 Clinical presentation and radiographs of oxalosis. **A,** Miliary skin deposits in a patient with hemodialysis oxalosis. **B,** Radiograph of a patient with hemodialysis oxalosis showing skin, vascular, and periarticular calcification. **C,** First metarsophalangeal joint showing synovial calcification and chondrocalcinosis. *(From Reginato AJ, Kurnik B. Calcium oxalate and other crystals associated with kidney disease and arthritis. Semin Arthritis Rheum 1989;18: 198-224, with permission.)*

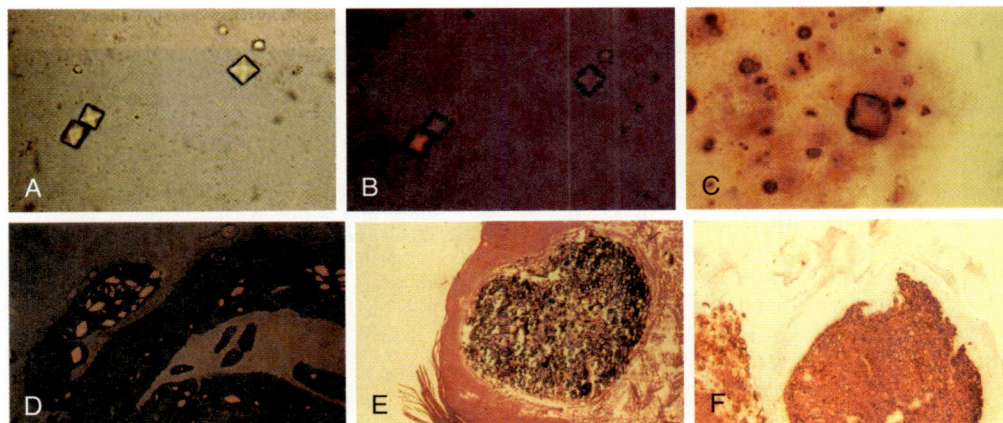

Figure 23-3 Calcium oxalate deposition in synovial fluid and tissues. **A,** Polymorphic calcium oxalate dihydrate crystals "envelope" in synovial fluid from a patient with secondary oxalosis and ESRD on hemodialysis (ordinary light ×400). **B,** Polymorphic calcium oxalate dihydrate crystals under compensated polarized light microscopy with positive birefringence, no birefringence (compensated polarized microscopy ×400). **C,** Calcium oxalate crystals stained with Alizarin red S stain. Abundant polymorphic calcium oxalate crystals (×400). **D,** Calcium oxalate crystals in the synovial membrane of the first metatarsophalangeal joint (hematoxylin and eosin stain, ×180). **E,** Tophaceous deposit of calcium oxalate in the skin. Pizzolato's stain is generally used for the demonstration of calcium oxalate crystals on paraffin. **F,** Tophus-like deposit of calcium oxalate in the skin. Stained with Alizarin red S stain (ordinary light ×300). *(Antonio J. Reginato synovial fluid slide collection.)*

abnormalities due to oxalosis include diffuse osteopenia, osteosclerosis of the peripheral and axial skeleton, subperiosteal resorption, and a coarse trabecular pattern—all of which can be confused with secondary hyperparathyroidism.[91,92] Periarticular erosions surrounding intracancellous deposits of oxalate resembling an erosive arthropathy have been noted in an adult patient presenting late at age 61 with HP1. Fractures and pseudofractures have also been noted.[93] Oxalate osteopathy occurs in patients with primary hyperoxaluria who are on dialysis for ESRD and may present with bone pain. Oxalate crystals are formed within the bone and seen on iliac crest biopsy samples of both HP1 and HP2 patients. Bone resorption is also noted to increase while there is a decrease in bone formation, mimicking secondary hyperparathyroidism.[94-96] In children with primary hyperoxaluria, a higher incidence of spondylolysis was noted and possibly related to pathologic

fracture of the pars interarticularis. Oxalate crystal deposition can also occur in the bone marrow leading to cytopenias.[97] In addition, hyperostosis of the ligamentum flavum was reported to cause central spinal stenosis.[98] Deposition of CaOX can occur in other soft tissues such as skin, vascular beds, cardiac, endocrine, eye, and nervous system. Other imaging modalities such as unenhanced computed tomography evaluation may assist in the evaluation of CaOX deposition as seen in a patient with PH1 with dense kidneys as well as increased attenuation of the myocardium.

Treatment of Oxalosis

It is recommended that fluid intake be increased to 3 to 4 L/day and large quantities of oxalate precursors such as ascorbic acid should be avoided. Foods rich in oxalate such as chocolate, rhubarb, tea, spinach, and starfruit should be avoided. In HP1, pyridoxine (B6), a cofactor of AGT, can be administered on a trial basis but has varied effects due to the gene mutation heterogeneity. HP1 patients with the G170R mutation in the *AGXT* gene are most likely to respond to pyridoxine and can maintain near normal levels of urinary oxalate excretion for many years.[99] Hemodialysis has been most effective in oxalate removal with additional sessions rather than prolonged sessions because the rate of mobilization of CaOX from tissue is at a slow rate.[100] The oral use of intestinal bacteria, *Oxalobacter formigenes*, to break down oxalate in the intestines was shown to decrease urinary oxalate secretion.[101] Ultimately, either a combined liver and kidney transplant or a kidney transplant in HP1 patients and renal transplants in all other HP patients may need to be conducted. There is no standard approach to transplanting patients with primary hyperoxaluria; however, transplant survival has improved significantly since the 1990s. In a cohort of patients who received kidney transplants since 2000 in the International Primary Hyperoxaluria Registry (IPHR), survival rates were similar to those for patients who received transplants for all reasons.[102] With regard to HP1, the European data suggest that the combined liver and kidney transplant carries the best survival for HP1 patients[103]; however, data from the United States suggest kidney transplantation alone to be equally as effective.[104,105] This is likely related to the risk of conducting a complete liver removal and orthotopic transplant, which would require all possible oxalate-producing cells to be removed. Even after removal of the oxalate-producing liver, renal graft oxalosis is possible for many years after transplantation due to overall body stores of oxalate. In patients with primary HP2, kidney transplant alone has been the recommended approach if necessary given the enzymatic defect is found in multiple body tissues. It is unclear what effect treatment of general oxalosis has on the musculoskeletal sequelae. Unfortunately, the synovitis associated with oxalosis tends to follow a chronic course and does not respond to nonsteroidal antiinflammatory drugs, colchicine, intraarticular corticosteroids, or increasing frequency of dialysis. Similarly, the use of IL-1R antagonist (anakinra, rilonacept, canakinumab) as used to treat refractory cases of gout and pseudogout has not been tested or employed in the management of recurrent oxalosis.

Conclusions

CKD exerts a toxic toll in a variety of tissues and other organ system and tissues beginning early in its course, resulting in numerous complications that leading to decrease on the quality of life and premature death in affected patients. Rheumatic syndromes are a common complication of CKD and patients receiving hemodialysis with increasing incidence during long-term maintenance hemodialysis. The relative new term "chronic kidney disease–mineral bone disorder" (CKD-MBD) reflects the growing research of chronic kidney disease into the realm of system physiology, involving renal, skeletal, and vascular tissues and other structures, and points to a variety of biochemical factors that act beneficially or adversely to the development of the various musculoskeletal manifestations in CKD including crystal-induced arthropathies. Patients with chronic and end-stage kidney disease and on chronic hemodialysis develop several crystal-induced arthropathies that can

exhibit similar clinical presentations and require diagnostic arthrocenthesis and examination of the synovial fluid under compensated polarized microscopy and/or the use of specialized staining to properly differentiate MSU, CPPD, HA, or oxalate deposition diseases. These findings emphasize the importance of viewing CKD as a systems approach instead of as a single-organ viewpoint.

References

1. Coresh J, Selvin E, Stevens LA, et al. Prevalence of chronic kidney disease in the United States. JAMA 2007;298:2038–47.
2. Keith DS, Nichols GA, Gullion CM, et al. Longitudinal follow-up and outcomes among a population with chronic kidney disease in a large managed care organization. Arch Intern Med 2004;164:659–63.
3. Sarraf P, Kay J, Reginato AM. Non-crystalline and crystalline rheumatic disorders in chronic kidney disease. Curr Rheumatol Rep 2008;10:235–48.
4. Martin KJ, González EA. Metabolic bone disease in chronic kidney disease. J Am Soc Nephrol 2007;18:875–85.
5. Komaba H, Tanaka M, Fukagawa M. Treatment of chronic kidney disease-mineral and bone disorder (CKD-MBD). Intern Med 2008;47:989–94.
6. Block GA, Klassen PS, Lazarus JM, et al. Mineral metabolism, mortality, and morbidity in maintenance hemodialysis. J Am Soc Nephrol 2004;15:2208–18.
7. Slinin Y, Foley RN, Collins AJ. Calcium, phosphorus, parathyroid hormone, and cardiovascular disease in hemodialysis patients: the USRDS waves 1, 3, and 4 study. J Am Soc Nephrol 2005;16:1788–93.
8. Amann K, Tyralla K, Gross ML, et al. Special characteristics of atherosclerosis in chronic renal failure. Clin Nephrol 2003;60(suppl 1):S13–21.
9. Blacher J, Guerin AP, Pannier B, et al. Arterial calcifications, arterial stiffness, and cardiovascular risk in end-stage renal disease. Hypertension 2001;38:938–42.
10. Raggi P, Boulay A, Chasan-Taber S, et al. Cardiac calcification in adult hemodialysis patients. A link between end-stage renal disease and cardiovascular disease? J Am Coll Cardiol 2002;39:695–701.
11. Goldsmith D, Ritz E, Covic A. Vascular calcification: a stiff challenge for the nephrologist: does preventing bone disease cause arterial disease? Kidney Int 2004;66:1315–33.
12. Tomiyama C, Higa A, Dalboni MA, et al. The impact of traditional and non-traditional risk factors on coronary calcification in pre-dialysis patients. Nephrol Dial Transplant 2006;21:2464–71.
12a. Guérin AP, Pannier B, Métivier F, et al. Assessment and significance of arterial stiffness in patients with chronic kidney disease. Curr Opin Nephrol Hypertens 2008;17:635–41.
13. Tomiyama C, Carvalho AB, Higa A, et al. Coronary calcification is associated with lower bone formation rate in CKD patients not yet in dialysis treatment. J Bone Miner Res 2010;25:499–504.
14. Russo D, Palmiero G, De Blasio AP, et al. Coronary artery calcification in patients with CRF not undergoing dialysis. Am J Kidney Dis 2004;44:1024–30.
15. Russo D, Corrao S, Miranda I, et al. Progression of coronary artery calcification in predialysis patients. Am J Nephrol 2007;27:152–8.
16. Moss DW, Eaton RH, Smith JK, et al. Association of inorganic-pyrophosphatase activity with human alkaline phosphatase preparations. Biochem J 1967;102:53–7.
17. Terkeltaub R, Rosenbach M, Fong F, et al. Causal link between nucleotide pyrophosphohydrolase overactivity and increased intracellular inorganic pyrophosphate generation demonstrated by transfection of cultured fibroblasts and osteoblasts with plasma cell membrane glycoprotein-1. Relevance to calcium pyrophosphate dihydrate deposition disease. Arthritis Rheum 1994;37:934–41.
18. Ho AM, Johnson MD, Kingsley DM. Role of the mouse ank gene in control of tissue calcification and arthritis. Science 2000;289:265–70.
19. Rutsch F, Ruf N, Vaingankar S, et al. Mutations in ENPP1 are associated with 'idiopathic' infantile arterial calcification. Nat Genet 2003;34:379–81.
20. Eller P, Hochegger K, Feuchtner GM, et al. Impact of ENPP1 genotype on arterial calcification in patients with end-stage renal failure. Nephrol Dial Transplant 2008;23:321–7.
21. Mazhar AR, Johnson RJ, Gillen D, et al. Risk factors and mortality associated with calciphylaxis in end-stage renal disease. Kidney Int 2001;60:324–32.
22. Lomashvili KA, Khawandi W, O'Neill WC. Reduced plasma pyrophosphate levels in hemodialysis patients. J Am Soc Nephrol 2005;16:2495–500.

23. Zebboudj AF, Imura M, Bostroânm K. Matrix GLA protein, a regulatory protein for bone morphogenetic protein-2. J Biol Chem 2002;277:4388–94.
24. Chen NX, Duan D, O'Neill KD, et al. The mechanisms of uremic serum-induced expression of bone matrix proteins in bovine vascular smooth muscle cells. Kidney Int 2006;70:1046–53.
25. Luo G, Ducy P, McKee MD, et al. Spontaneous calcification of arteries and cartilage in mice lacking matrix GLA protein. Nature 1997;386:78–81.
26. Murshed M, Schinke T, McKee MD, et al. Extracellular matrix mineralization is regulated locally; different roles of two gla-containing proteins. J Cell Biol 2004;165:625–30.
27. Nishimoto SK, Price PA. The vitamin K-dependent bone protein is accumulated within cultured osteosarcoma cells in the presence of the vitamin K antagonist warfarin. J Biol Chem 1985;260:2832–6.
28. Brancaccio D, Biondi ML, Gallieni M, et al. Matrix GLA protein gene polymorphisms: clinical correlates and cardiovascular mortality in chronic kidney disease patients. Am J Nephrol 2005;25:548–52.
29. Schafer C, Heiss A, Schwarz A, et al. The serum protein alpha 2-Heremans-Schmid glycoprotein/fetuin-A is a systemically acting inhibitor of ectopic calcification. J Clin Invest 2003;112:357–66.
30. Ketteler M, Bongartz P, Westenfeld R, et al. Association of low fetuin-A (AHSG) concentrations in serum with cardiovascular mortality in patients on dialysis: a cross-sectional study. Lancet 2003;361:827–33.
31. Proudfoot D, Skepper JN, Hegyi L, et al. Apoptosis regulates human vascular calcification in vitro: evidence for initiation of vascular calcification by apoptotic bodies. Circ Res 2000;87:1055–62.
32. Reynolds JL, Joannides AJ, Skepper JN, et al. Human vascular smooth muscle cells undergo vesicle-mediated calcification in response to changes in extracellular calcium and phosphate concentrations: a potential mechanism for accelerated vascular calcification in ESRD. J Am Soc Nephrol 2004;15:2857–67.
33. Tyson KL, Reynolds JL, McNair R, et al. Osteo/chondrocytic transcription factors and their target genes exhibit distinct patterns of expression in human arterial calcification. Arterioscler Thromb Vasc Biol 2003;23:489–94.
34. Dorai H, Vukicevic S, Sampath TK. Bone morphogenetic protein-7 (osteogenic protein-1) inhibits smooth muscle cell proliferation and stimulates the expression of markers that are characteristic of SMC phenotype in vitro. J Cell Physiol 2000;184:37–45.
35. Doumouchtsis KK, Kostakis AI, Doumouchtsis SK, et al. sRANKL/osteoprotegerin complex and biochemical markers in a cohort of male and female hemodialysis patients. J Endocrinol Invest 2007;30:762–6.
36. Imanishi Y, Inaba M, Nakatsuka K, et al. FGF-23 in patients with end-stage renal disease on hemodialysis. Kidney Int 2004;65:1943–6.
37. Westerberg PA, Linde T, Wikstroânb B, et al. Regulation of fibroblast growth factor-23 in chronic kidney disease. Nephrol Dial Transplant 2007;22:3202–7.
38. Benet-Pages A, Orlik P, Strom TM, Lorenz-Depiereux B. An FGF23 missense mutation causes familial tumoral calcinosis with hyperphosphatemia. Hum Mol Genet 2005;14:385–90.
39. Nakai K, Komaba H, Fukagawa M. New insights into the role of fibroblast growth factor 23 in chronic kidney disease. J Nephrol 2010;23:619–25.
40. Urakawa I, Yamazaki Y, Shimada T, et al. Klotho converts canonical FGF receptor into a specific receptor for FGF23. Nature 2006;444:770–4.
41. Church LD, Cook GP, McDermott MF. Primer: inflammasomes and interleukin 1beta in inflammatory disorders. Nat Clin Pract Rheumatol 2008;4:34–42.
42. Liu-Bryan R, Pritzker K, Firestein GS, et al. TLR2 signaling in chondrocytes drives calcium pyrophosphate dihydrate and monosodium urate crystal-induced nitric oxide generation. J Immunol 2005;174:5016–23.
43. Liu-Bryan R, Scott P, Sydlaske A, et al. Innate immunity conferred by Toll-like receptors 2 and 4 and myeloid differentiation factor 88 expression is pivotal to monosodium urate monohydrate crystal-induced inflammation. Arthritis Rheum 2005;52:2936–46.
44. Martinon F, Petrilli V, Mayor A, et al. Gout-associated uric acid crystals activate the NALP3 inflammasome. Nature 2006;440:237–41.
45. Chen CJ, Shi Y, Hearn A, et al. MyD88-dependent IL-1 receptor signaling is essential for gouty inflammation stimulated by monosodium urate crystals. J Clin Invest 2006;116:2262–71.
46. Reginato AM, Olsen BR. Genetics and experimental models of crystal-induced arthritis. Lessons learned from mice and men: is it crystal clear? Curr Opin Rheumatol 2007;19:134–45.
47. Burns CM, Wortmann RL. Gout therapeutics: new drugs for an old disease. Lancet 2010 Aug 16.
48. Schreiner O, Wandel E, Himmelsbach F, et al. Reduced secretion of proinflammatory cytokines of monosodium urate crystal-stimulated monocytes in chronic renal failure: an explanation for infrequent gout episodes in chronic renal failure patients? Nephrol Dial Transplant 2000;15:644–9.
49. Viatour P, Merville MP, Bours V, et al. Phosphorylation of NF kappaB and IkappaB proteins: implications in cancer and inflammation. Trends Biochem Sci 2005;30:43–52.
50. Navarro-González JF, Mora-Fernández C, Muros M, et al. Mineral metabolism and inflammation in chronic kidney disease patients: a cross-sectional study. Clin J Am Soc Nephrol 2009;4:1646–54.
51. Schoppet M, Shroff RC, Hofbauer LC, et al. Exploring the biology of vascular calcification in chronic kidney disease: what's circulating? Kidney Int 2008;73:384–90.
52. Ellman MH, Brown NL, Katzenberg CA. Acute pseudogout in chronic renal failure. Arch Intern Med 1979;139:795–6.
53. Menerey K, Braunstein E, Brown M, et al. Musculoskeletal symptoms related to arthropathy in patients receiving dialysis. J Rheumatol 1988;15:1848–54.
54. Johnson K, Terkeltaub R. Upregulated ank expression in osteoarthritis can promote both chondrocyte MMP-13 expression and calcification via chondrocyte extracellular PP_i excess. Osteoarthritis Cartilage 2004;12:321–35.
55. Kuntz D, Naveau B, Bardin T, et al. Destructive spondyloarthropathy in hemodialyzed patients. A new syndrome. Arthritis Rheum 1984;27:369–75.
56. Kart-Koseoglu H, Yucel AE, Niron EA, et al. Osteoarthritis in hemodialysis patients: relationships with bone mineral density and other clinical and laboratory parameters. Rheumatol Int 2005;25:270–5.
57. Braunstein EM, Menerey K, Martel W, et al. Radiologic features of a pyrophosphate-like arthropathy associated with long-term dialysis. Skeletal Radiol 1987;16:437–41.
58. Ferrari AJ, Rothfuss S, Schumacher Jr HR. Dialysis arthropathy: identification and evaluation of a subset of patients with unexplained inflammatory effusions. J Rheumatol 1997;24:1780–6.
59. Newcombe DS. Endocrinopathies and uric acid metabolism. Semin Arthritis Rheum 1972;2:281–300.
60. Buchanan WW, Klinenberg JR, Seegmiller JE. The inflammatory response to injected microcrystalline monosodium urate in normal, hyperuricemic, gouty, and uremic subjects. Arthritis Rheum 1965;8:361–7.
61. Sombolos K, Tsitamidou Z, Kyriazis G, et al. Clinical evaluation of four different high-flux hemodialyzers under conventional conditions in vivo. Am J Nephrol 1997;17:406–12.
62. Buño Soto A, Torres Jiménez R, Olveira A, et al. Lithogenic risk factors for renal stones in patients with Crohn's. Arch Exp Urol 2001;54:282–92.
63. Maldonado I, Prasad V, Reginato AJ. Oxalate crystal deposition disease. Curr Rheum Rep 2002;4:257–64.
64. Chadwick VS, Modha K, Dowling RH. Mechanism for hyperoxaluria in patients with ileal dysfunction. N Engl J Med 1973;289:172–6.
65. Cornelis T, Bammens B, Lerut E, et al. AA amyloidosis due to chronic oxalate arthritis and vasculitis in a patient with secondary oxalosis after jejunoileal bypass surgery. Nephrol Dial Transplant 2008;23:3362–4.
66. Andrieux A, Harambat J, Bui S, et al. Renal impairment in children with cystic fibrosis. J Cyst Fibros 2010;9:263–8.
67. Thornton J, Rangaraj S. Disease modifying anti-rheumatic drugs in people with cystic fibrosis-related arthritis. Cochrane Database Syst Rev 2009(21):CD00733668.
68. Alkhunaizi AM, Chan L. Secondary oxalosis: a cause of delayed recovery of renal function in the setting of acute renal failure. J Am Soc Nephrol 1996;7:2320–6.
69. Canavese C, Petrarulo M, Massarenti P, et al. Long-term, low-dose, intravenous vitamin C leads to plasma calcium oxalate supersaturation in hemodialysis patients. Am J Kidney Dis 2005;45:540–9.
70. Roehrl MH, Croft WJ, Liao Q, et al. Hemorrhagic pulmonary oxalosis secondary to a noninvasive Aspergillus niger fungus ball. Virchows Arch 2005;451:1067–73.
71. Vaideeswar P, Sakhdeo UM. Pulmonary aspergilloma with renal oxalosis: fatal effect at a distance. Mycoses 2009;52:272–5.
72. Fishbein GA, Micheletti RG, Currier JS, et al. Atherosclerotic oxalosis in coronary arteries. Cardiovasc Pathol 2008;17:117–23.
73. Pecorella I, McCartney AC, Lucas S, et al. Histological study of oxalosis in the eye and adnexa of AIDS patients. Histopathology 1995;27:431–8.
74. Pecorella I, Ciardi A, Maedsco A, et al. Histological findings in the eyelids of AIDS patients. Acta Ophthalmol Scand 1999;77:564–7.
75. Pecorella I, Lucas SB, Ciardi A, et al. Calcium oxalate precipitates in a reno-medullary interstitial cell tumor. Pathol Oncol Res 2003;9:47–8.
76. Williams EL, Acquaviva C, Amoroso A, et al. Primary hyperoxaluria type 1: update and additional mutation analysis of the AGXT gene. Hum Mutat 2009;30:910–7.
77. Williams HE, Smith Jr LH. L-glyceric aciduria. A new genetic variant of primary hyperoxaluria. N Engl J Med 1968;278(5):233–8.
78. Belostotsky R, Seboun E, Idelson GH, et al. Mutations in DHDPSL are responsible for primary hyperoxaluria type III. Am J Hum Genet 2010;87:392–9.

79. Hillman RE. Primary hyperoxaluria. In: Scriver CR, editor. The Metabolic Basis of Inherited Diseases. Primary Hyperoxalurias. 6th ed. New York: McGraw-Hill; 1989:933–44.

80. Reginato AJ, Kurnik B. Calcium oxalate and other crystals associated with kidney disease and arthritis. Semin Arthritis Rheum 1989;18:198–224.

81. Balcke P, Schmidt P, Zazgornik J, et al. Secondary oxalosis in chronic renal insufficiency. N Engl J Med 1980;303:944.

82. Salyer WR, Keren D. Oxalosis as a complication of chronic renal failure. Kidney Int 1973;4:61–6.

83. Fayemi AO, Ali M, Braun EV. Oxalosis in hemodialysis patients: a pathologic study of 80 cases. Arch Pathol Lab Med 1979;103:58–62.

84. Hoppe B, Beck B, Milliner D. The primary hyperoxalurias. Kidney Int 2009;75:1264–71.

85. Hoffman GS, Schumacher HR, Paul H, et al. Calcium oxalate microcrystalline-associated arthritis in end-stage renal disease. Ann Intern Med 1982;97:36–42.

86. Reginato AJ, Ferreiro Seoane JL, Barbazan Alvarez C, et al. Arthropathy and cutaneous calcinosis in hemodialysis oxalosis. Arthritis Rheum 1986;29(11):1387–96.

87. Abuelo G, Swartz ST, Reginato AJ. Cutaneous calcinosis after long-term hemodialysis. Arch Int 1992;152:1517–20.

88. Reginato AJ, Falasca GF, Usmani Q. Do we really need to pay attention to the less common crystals? Review about the clinical significance of rare crystals found in synovial fluid in articular tissues. Curr Opin Rheumatol 1999;11:446–52.

89. Reginato AJ. Calcium oxalate and other crystals or particles associated with arthritis. In: Koopman WJ, editor. Arthritis and Allied Conditions. 14th ed. Baltimore: Williams & Wilkins; 2002:2393–414.

90. El Hage S, Ghanem I, Baradhi A, et al. Skeletal features of hyperoxaluria type I, revisited. J Child Orthop 2008;2:205–10.

91. Sadeghi N, De Pauw L, Vienne A, et al. Late diagnosis of oxalosis in an adult patient: findings on bone radiography 1998. AJR Am J Roentgenol 1998;170:1248–50.

92. Canavese C, Salomone M, Massara C, et al. Primary oxalosis mimicking hyperparathyroidism diagnosed after long-term hemodialysis. Am J Nephrol 1990;10:344–9.

93. Kuo LW, Horton K, Fishman E. CT evaluation of multisystem involvement by oxalosis. AJR Am J Roentgenol 2001;177:661–3.

94. Benhamou CL, Bardin T, Tourlière D, et al. [Bone involvement in primary oxalosis: study of 20 cases]. Rev Rhum Mal Osteoartic 1991;58:763–9.

95. Schnitzler CM, Kok JA, Jacobs DW, et al. Skeletal manifestations of primary oxalosis. Pediatr Nephrol 1991;5:193–9.

96. Desmond P, Hennessy O. Skeletal abnormalities in primary oxalosis. Aust Radiol 1993;37:83–5.

97. Marangella M, Vitale C, Petrarulo M, et al. Bony content of oxalate in patients with primary hyperoxaluria or oxalosis-unrelated renal failure. Kidney Int 1995;48:182–7.

98. Knight RQ, Taddonio RF, Smith FB, et al. Oxalosis: cause of degenerative spinal stenosis: a case report and review of the literature. Orthopedics 1998;11:955–8.

99. Monico CG, Rossetti S, Olson JB, et al. Pyridoxine effect in type I primary hyperoxaluria is associated with the most common mutant allele. Kidney Int 2005;67:1704–9.

100. Illies F, Bonzel KE, Wingen AM, et al. Clearance and removal of oxalate in children on intensified dialysis for primary hyperoxaluria type I. Kidney Int 2006;70:1642–8.

101. Hoppe B, Beck B, Gatter N, et al. Oxalobacter formigenes: a potential tool for the treatment of primary hyperoxaluria. Kidney Int 2006;70:1305–11.

102. Bergstralh EJ, Monico CG, Lieske JC, et al. IPHR Investigators. Transplantation outcomes in primary hyperoxaluria. Am J Transplant 2010;10: 2493–501.

103. Jamieson NV. The European Primary Hyperoxaluria Type 1 Transplant Registry report on the results of combined liver/kidney transplantation for primary hyperoxaluria 1984-1994. European PH1 Transplantation Study Group. Nephrol Dial Transplant 1995;10:33–7.

104. Scheinman JI, Alexander M, Campbell ED, et al. Transplantation for primary hyperoxaluria in the USA. Nephrol Dial Transplant 1995;10:42–6.

105. Sarborio P, Scheinman JL. Transplantation for primary hyperoxaluria in the United States. Kidney Int 1999;56:1094–100.

Section IV

Imaging of Gout and Other Crystal Deposition Arthropathies

Chapter 24

Plain Radiography and Advanced Imaging of Gout

Amilcare Gentili

KEY POINTS

- Radiography is the main imaging modality for evaluation of progression of gout, but there is a 5- to 10-year latent period between first clinical symptoms and the appearance of specific radiographic findings.
- The classic radiographic appearance of gout is the presence of well-defined erosions with overhanging edges, normal bone mineralization, and relative sparing of the joint space.
- Tophi appear as soft tissue masses with higher density than surrounding soft tissue and occasionally are calcified.
- Computed tomography is useful in the evaluation of complex areas such as the spine and sacroiliac joints.
- Dual-energy computed tomography (DECT) is specific in detecting urate crystal deposition and in distinguishing tophi from calcific crystal deposits. There is noteworthy utility of DECT in diagnosis of gout, and in following the outcome of therapeutic urate lowering.
- Magnetic resonance imaging is primarily used for evaluation of spinal involvement by gout. Tophus deposits often have low to intermediate signal on all sequences.

Introduction

The gold standard for making the diagnosis of gout is the detection of urate crystals in the symptomatic joint. Imaging is often inconclusive early in the disease, as the only finding is nonspecific soft tissue swelling. In typical cases, there is a latent period of about 5 to 10 years between the first clinical symptom and the appearance of specific plain radiographic signs,[1] such as well-defined erosions and tophi. In more advanced disease, imaging provides documentation of extent and distribution of the disease and allows assessment of response to treatment. High-resolution ultrasound, an increasingly useful modality for detection of early disease in gout, and for differential diagnosis of gout and calcium pyrophosphate dihydrate (CPPD) deposition disease, is reviewed in detail in Chapter 26.

Plain Radiography

Since the initial description of the radiographic appearance of gout by Huber in 1896,[2] radiography has become the main imaging modality to evaluate progression of gout,[3-5] as radiographs are readily available and relatively inexpensive.

General Considerations

Soft Tissue

An early finding of gout is soft tissue swelling around the joint during the acute gouty attach (Fig. 24-1), this soft tissue swelling resolves when the symptoms subside. Later in the disease, with chronic gout there is deposition of urate crystals in the soft tissues with the formation of tophi. On radiographs, tophi appear as masses slightly denser than surrounding soft tissues (Fig. 24-2). Occasionally, tophi may calcify (Fig. 24-3) and rarely ossify. Calcification of tophi suggest the presence of coexisting calcium-containing crystals such as hydroxyapatite or an underlying abnormality of calcium and mineral metabolism such as renal failure or hyperparathyroidism.

Joint Space

Although erosion can be present, the joint space is often well maintained until late in the disease (Fig. 24-4). The presence of a relatively normal joint space in patients with extensive erosions helps in distinguishing gout from other type of arthritis. Obliteration of the joint space and bony ankylosis are rare.

Bone Mineralization

Mild osteopenia is occasionally observed in films taken during an acute gouty attack, but more often the bone mineralization is normal; when osteopenia is present, it may be mediated by effects of urate crystals on osteoblast and osteoclast function, as well as disuse.

Erosions

Bone erosions can be marginal (Fig. 24-5), intraarticular (Fig. 24-6), or away from the joint (Fig. 24-7). Erosions are usually well defined and may have a sclerotic border. A characteristic of gouty erosion is the presence of overhanging edges. These spurlike formations are thought to be related to a combination of the bony resorption beneath the gradually enlarging

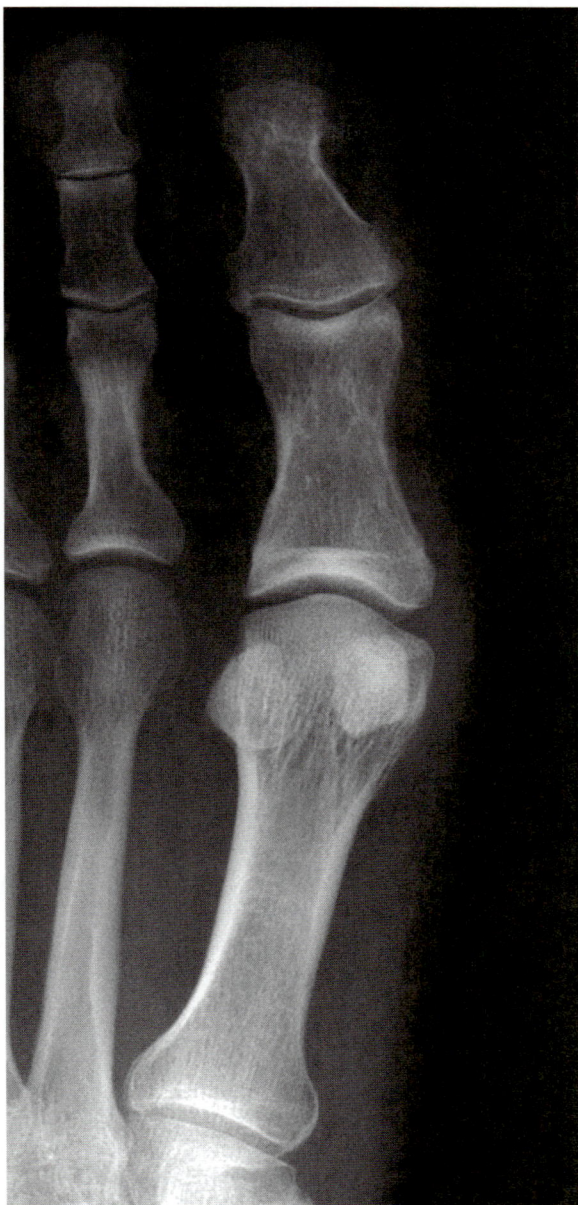

Figure 24-1 Soft tissue swelling. Dorsoplantar radiograph shows mild soft tissue swelling medial to the first metarsophalangeal joint. The joint space is preserved and no erosions are present. Bone mineralization is normal. This radiograph was obtained at the time of the first attack of gouty arthritis.

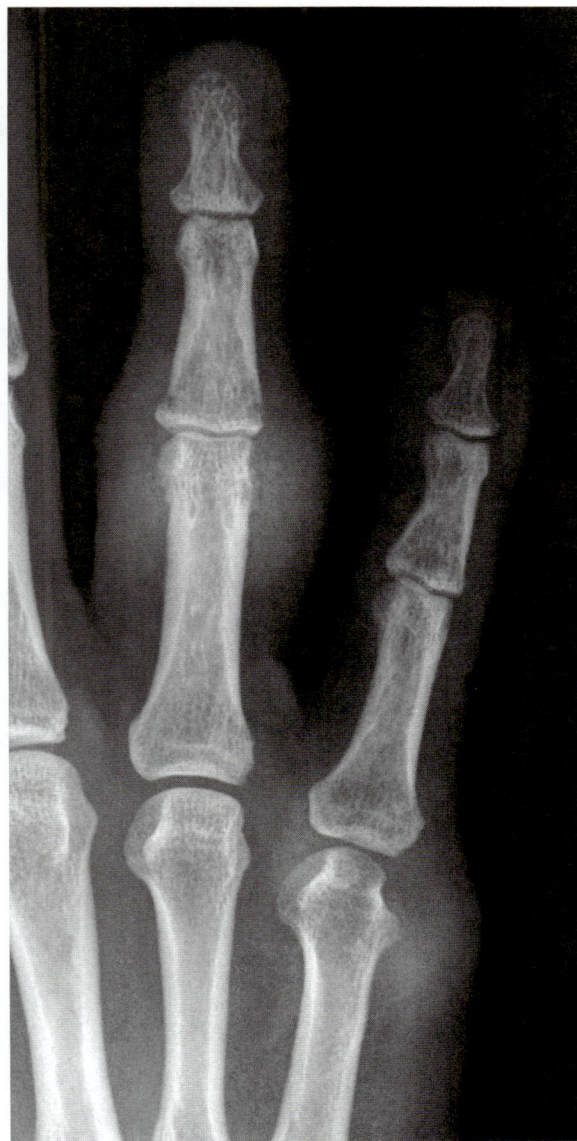

Figure 24-2 Tophus. Dorsopalmar radiograph shows soft tissue masses around the fourth proximal interphalangeal joint and radial to the fifth metacarpophalangeal joint. The joint spaces are normal.

tophus and the concomitant bony thickening at the edge of the involved cortex.

Bone Proliferation

Bone proliferation is an uncommon finding in gout.

Intraosseous Calcifications

Intraosseous calcifications (Fig. 24-8) can be seen especially in the hand and foot and are caused by intraosseous tophi.[6-8] Intraosseous tophi are usually seen in patients with longstanding tophaceous gout with hyperuricemia and chronic renal failure.

Differential Diagnosis

When reviewing radiographs of patients with arthritis, it is important to remember the "ABCDs of arthritis" (**A**lignment, **B**one mineralization and proliferation, **C**artilage, **D**istribution and **S**oft tissues). The alignment of the joints is usually normal with gout, while it is frequently abnormal in rheumatoid arthritis, in spondyloarthritis malalignment is a late manifestation. Bone mineralization is usually normal with gout as in spondyloarthritis; with osteoarthritis, bone density is normal or increased; and with rheumatoid arthritis, osteopenia is common. Bone proliferation is rare in gout, it is absent in rheumatoid arthritis, and it is common with spondyloarthritis

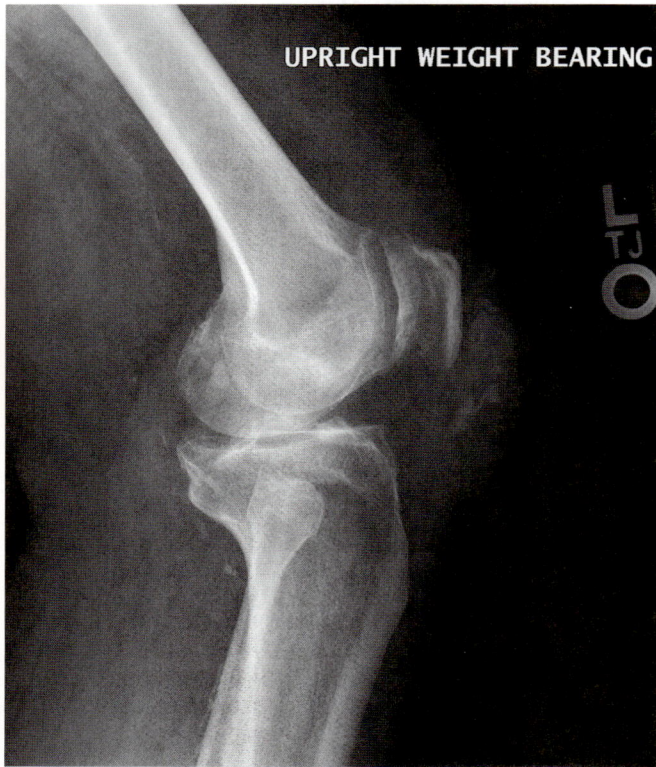

Figure 24-3 Calcified tophus. Lateral radiograph of the knee demonstrates a large prepatellar tophus with calcifications.

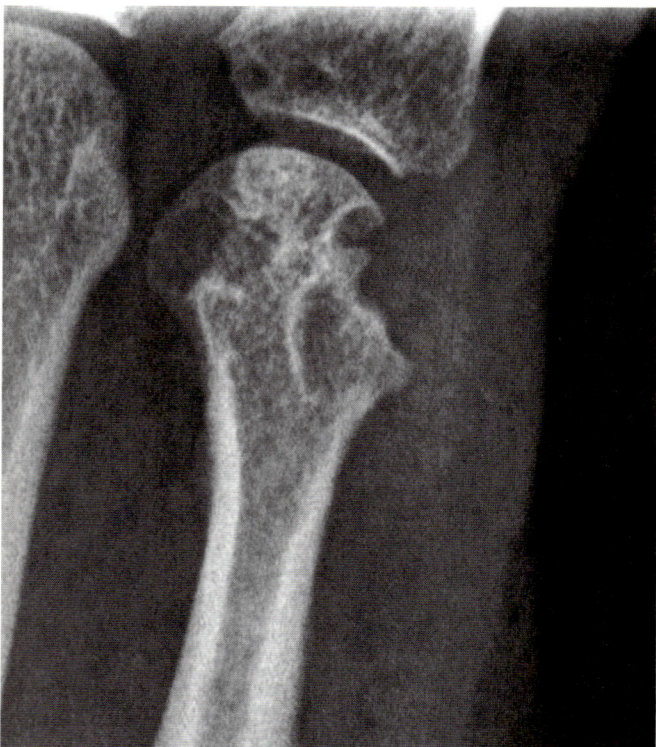

Figure 24-4 Erosions with normal joint space. Dorsopalmar radiograph shows large well defined erosions with sclerotic borders of the fifth metacarpophalangeal joint; the joint space is preserved.

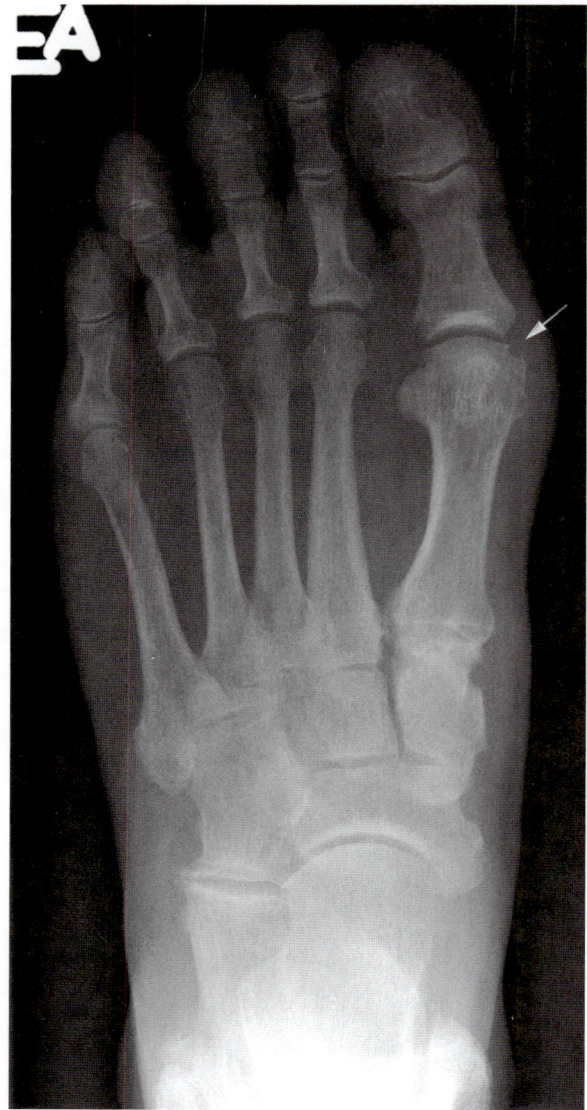

Figure 24-5 Marginal erosion. Dorsoplantar radiograph of the foot shows a well defined erosion of the medial aspect of the first metatarsal head.

and juvenile idiopathic arthritis. The joint space is often normal in gout; joint space narrowing is an early finding in rheumatoid arthritis and osteoarthritis and a late manifestation in spondyloarthritis. Erosions in gout are eccentric, intraarticular or extraarticular, with sclerotic borders and overhanging edges. In rheumatoid arthritis, erosions are marginal or intraarticular and do not have sclerotic borders unless treated. In spondyloarthritis, erosion may be marginal or intraarticular and often associated with periosteal bone proliferation. The distribution of joint involvement is usually asymmetric in gout, while it is symmetric in rheumatoid arthritis. Distribution is variable with spondyloarthritis. Soft tissue swelling is often eccentric in gout and is fusiform in rheumatoid arthritis. In spondyloarthritis, it can be fusiform or involve an entire digit (sausage digit). With osteoarthritis, soft tissue swelling is often absent except in erosive osteoarthritis. Soft tissue calcifications are seen occasionally in gout, but are rare in rheumatoid arthritis and spondyloarthritis. Soft tissue

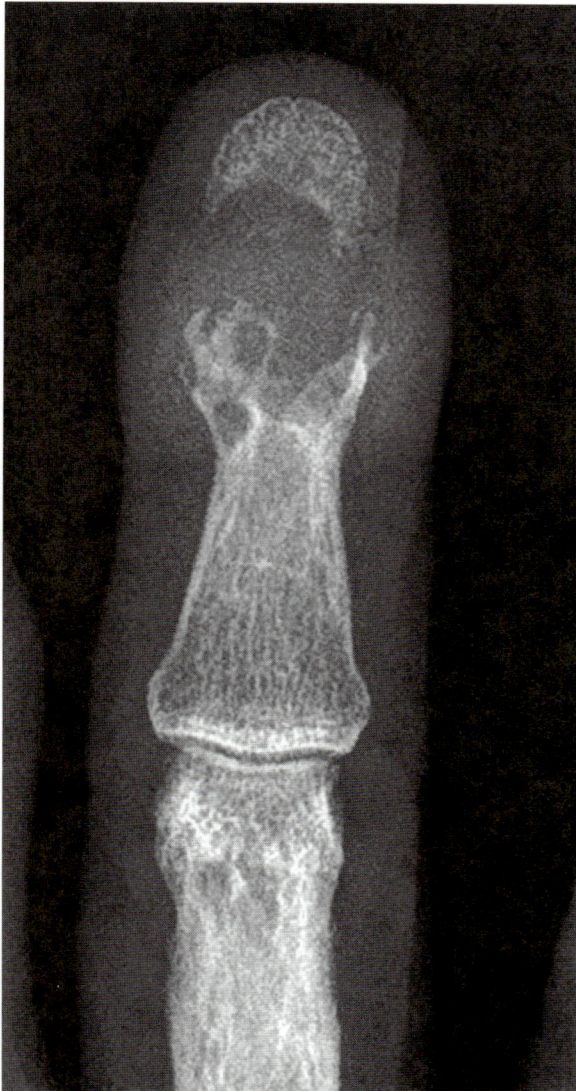

Figure 24-6 Intraarticular erosion. Dorsopalmar radiograph of the ring finger shows large erosions of the head of the middle phalanx and base of the distal phalanx.

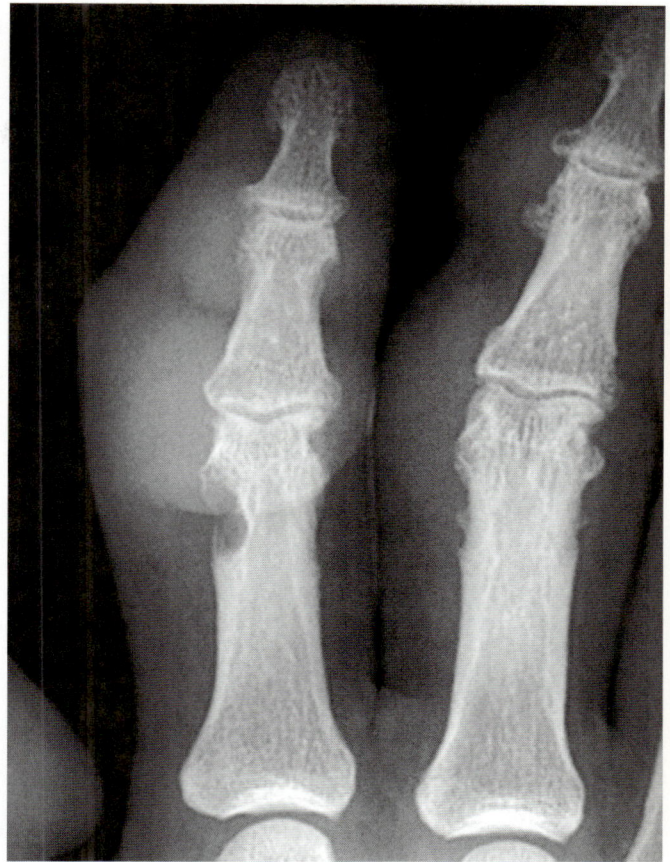

Figure 24-7 Overhanging edges. Dorsopalmar radiograph of the hand shows a large erosion with overhanging edges of the distal diaphysis of the middle phalanx of the index finger. There are large tophi around the proximal and distal interphalangeal joints of the index and middle finger.

calcifications are common in calcium pyrophosphate deposition disease, hydroxyapatite deposition disease, scleroderma, dermatomyositis, and polymyositis (Table 24-1).

Computed Tomography

The differentiation of tissues in computed tomography (CT) is based on their x-ray attenuation as quantified in Hounsfield units and displayed in shades of gray at different window levels in CT scans. Attenuation is caused by absorption and scattering of radiation by the tissues examined. The attenuation of different tissues varies based on the energy of the x-rays. The variation in attenuation with different beam energy is small for low atomic number tissues such as soft tissues and tophi but is larger for high atomic number materials such as calcium. The main advantage of dual-energy CT (DECT) is that the ratio or change in CT values is independent of density or concentration of the tissue. Using DECT it is possible to color coding for dual energy properties of different materials (i.e., uric acid uroliths, urate crystalline tophi, and calcific crystals).

Single-Energy Computed Tomography

Single-energy CT is used in evaluation of the extent of gout in areas that are difficult to visualize on radiographs, such as sacroiliac joints and spine. The density of sodium urate crystals is approximately 170 Hounsfield units (HU) $\pm$ 30 HU (Figs. 24-9 and 24-10), which is very different from muscles (less than 50 HU) or calcium (greater than 400 HU), but differentiation of a calcified tophus from other calcified lesion is difficult on CT.[9,10] CT is more useful in differentiating tophi from other noncalcified soft tissue masses such as xanthomas[11] or rheumatoid nodules.[12]

Dual-Energy Computed Tomography

DECT is useful to evaluate mixed lesion containing both calcium deposits and urate deposits.[13,14] DECT can help in difficult cases including atypical gout and subclinical tophi. DECT can distinguish confidently gout from other inflammatory arthritis and calcific deposits of CPPD deposition disease. (Fig. 24-11)

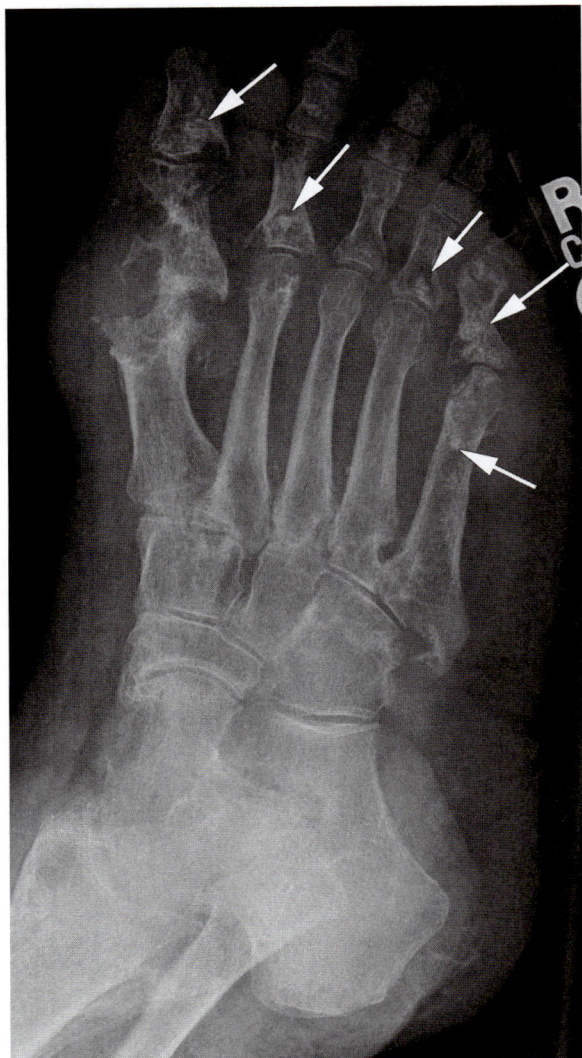

Figure 24-8 Intraosseous tophi. Oblique radiograph of the foot shows multiple calcific densities (*arrows*) within several bones, consistent with intraosseous tophi.

It also provides accurate and reproducible volumetric assessment of the tophi size. The specificity of DECT in detecting tophaceous disease could eliminate the need of arthrocentesis in some cases, unless septic arthritis needs to be ruled out (as a prime example).

Nuclear Medicine

Nuclear medicine is rarely used in the evaluation of patients with gout. Abnormal uptake in patients with gout is often an incidental finding on a nuclear medicine examination performed for other reasons.

Scintigraphy

Skeletal scintigrams are obtained 3 to 4 hours after intravenous injection of ^{99m}Tc methylene diphosphonate; this 3- to 4-hour delay is used to give time for urinary excretion to decrease the amount of radiotracer in the soft tissues. The uptake on these delayed images is proportional to the bone turnover. Increased uptake is present on skeletal scintigraphy in the bones affected by gout due to increased bone turnover, but it is not specific. Similar increased uptake can be seen with other types of arthritis such as rheumatoid arthritis or osteoarthritis. To distinguish osteomyelitis from cellulitis, three-phase bone scans are used, but they do not help in distinguishing acute gouty arthritis from septic arthritis or osteomyelitis (Fig. 24-12). During an acute gouty attack, increased uptake is present on all three phases of a bone scan.[15-18] In the first phase (blood flow phase), increased activity is seen due to hyperemia; in the second phase (blood pool phase), increased activity is seen due to the local inflammation; and in the third phase (delayed images), increased uptake is present due to bone remodeling.

Radionuclide-labeled leukocyte studies are not useful in distinguishing infection from an acute gouty attack. Labeled leukocyte scintigraphy during acute gouty arthritis shows accumulation of labeled leukocytes in the affected joints in a pattern indistinguishable from septic arthritis

Table 24-1 Differential Diagnosis

	Gout	Rheumatoid Arthritis	Seronegative Arthritis
Alignment	Normal	Frequent malalignment	Occasional malalignment
Bone proliferation	Rare	Absent	Common
Bone mineralization	Normal or mild osteopenia	Moderate to severe osteopenia	Normal or mild osteopenia
Cartilage: joint space	Often normal	Early narrowing	Late narrowing
Cartilage: erosions	Eccentric, sclerotic borders, overhanging edges, intraarticular or extraarticular	Marginal, no sclerotic borders, intraarticular, no overhanging edges	Marginal, intraarticular
Distribution	Asymmetric	Symmetric	Asymmetric or symmetric
Soft tissue swelling	Eccentric	Fusiform	Fusiform or sausage-digit
Soft tissue calcifications	Occasional	Rare	Rare

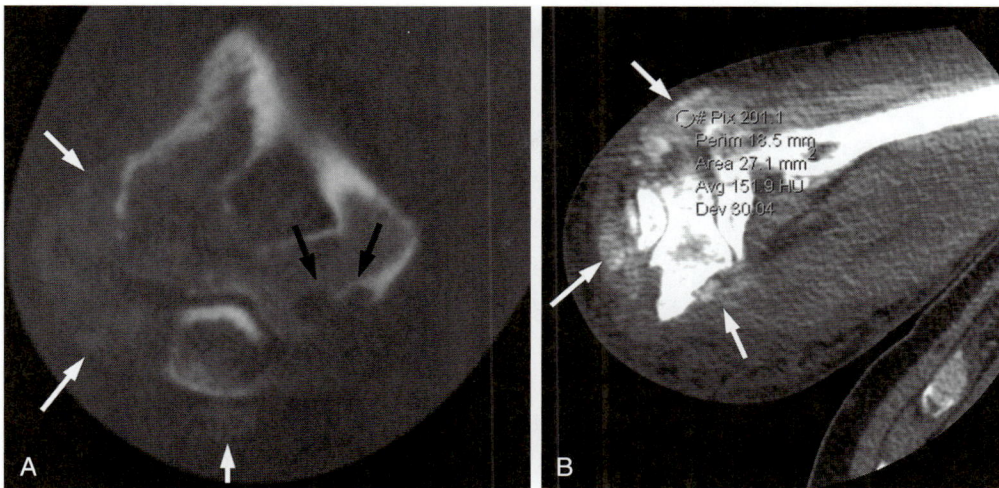

Figure 24-9 Dense tophus of the elbow. **A,** Coronal image of the distal humerus displayed using bone window shows faint densities in the soft tissues (*white arrows*) and erosion of the distal humerus (*black arrows*). **B,** Coronal image of the proximal ulna displayed soft tissue window shows increased density in the soft tissue; the density of this lesion is approximately 150 Hounsfield units, which is in the expected range of urate crystals, but less than calcium.

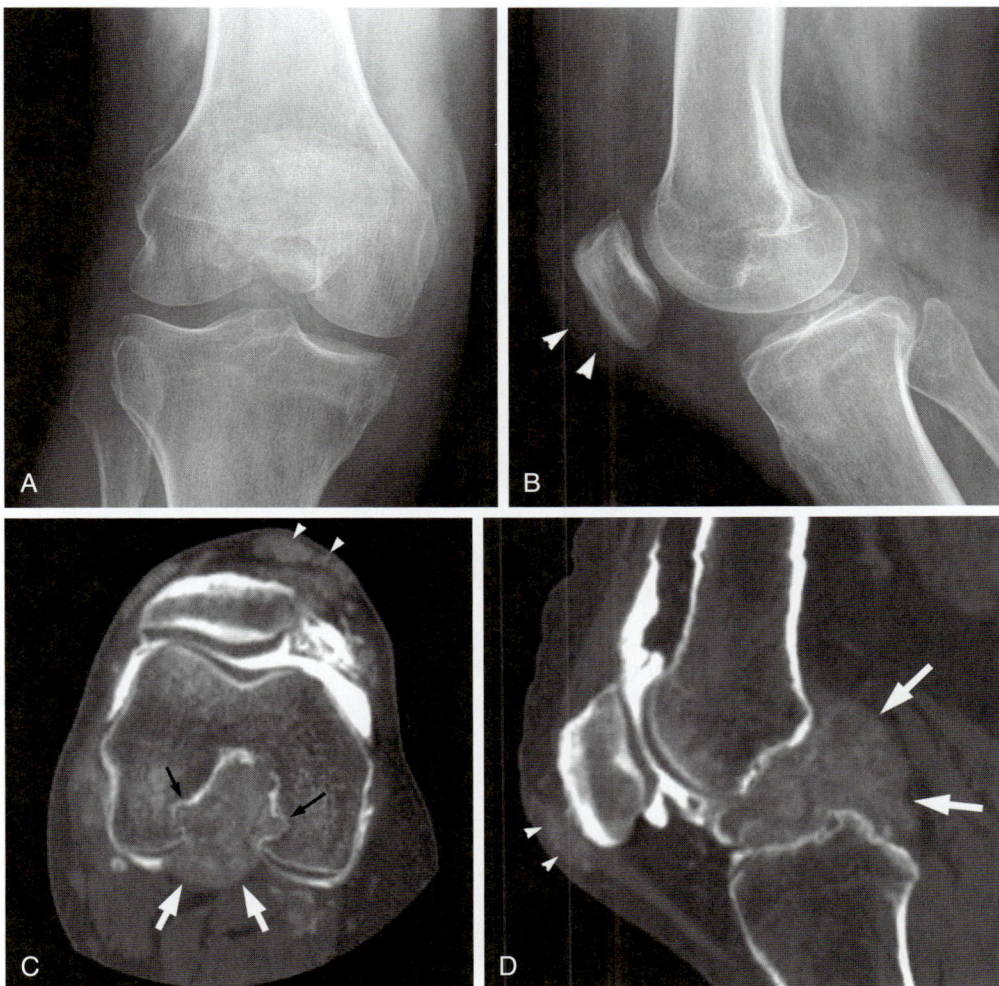

Figure 24-10 Tophi of the knee. **A,** Anteroposterior radiograph shows normal joint space narrowing. **B,** Lateral radiograph shows soft tissue prominence anterior to the patella (*arrowheads*). Axial (**C**) and sagittal (**D**) computed tomography arthrogram demonstrate extensive tophi in the prepatellar soft tissues (*white arrowheads*) and intercondylar notch (*white arrows*) with erosions of the femur (*black arrows*).

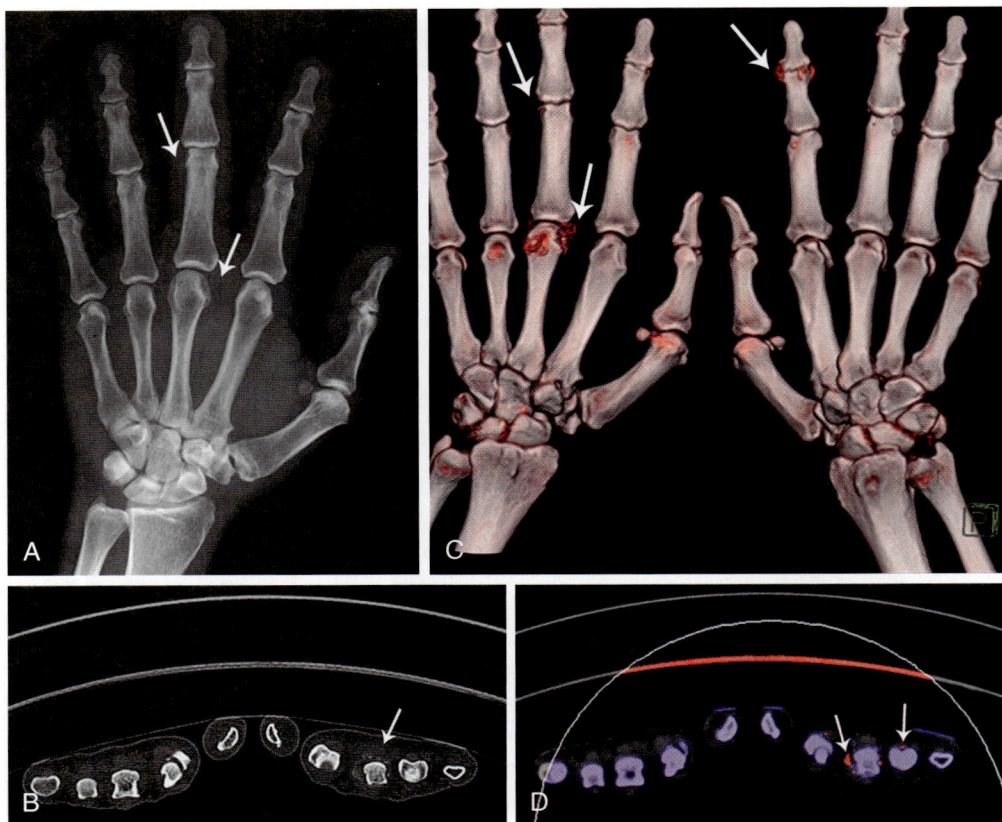

Figure 24-11 A 71-year-old man who presented with painful left hand. **A,** Radiograph shows moderate amount of faint calcification surrounding third metacarpophalangeal joint (*arrows*). **B,** Conventional axial unenhanced computed tomography (CT) image shows areas of nodular thickening with high-attenuating material present along third metacarpophalangeal joint (*arrow*). **C,** Three-dimensional volume-rendered coronal reformatted dual-energy CT (DECT) image confirms that high-attenuating material (*arrows*) represents monosodium urate deposition, in keeping with diagnosis of gout. **D,** Axial color-coded DECT two-material decomposition image confirms presence of monosodium urate deposition (*arrows*). *(From Nicolaou S, Yong-Hing CJ, Galea-Soler S, et al. Dual-energy CT as a potential new diagnostic tool in the management of gout in the acute setting. AJR Am J Roentgenol 2010;194:1072-8.)*

or osteomyelitis (see Fig. 24-12), but after treatment and remission of the acute attack, labeled leukocyte scintigraphy returns to normal.

Positron Emission Tomography Scanning

There are only a few case reports of the appearance of gout on positon emission tomography (PET).[19-21] Gout can present with moderate increased uptake of ^{18}F-fluoro-2-deoxy-D-glucose (FDG), but the standardized uptake value (SUV), which indicates the accumulation semiquantitatively, is less than in malignant lesions and is in the range of that of benign lesions.

Magnetic Resonance Imaging

MRI is used as the primary imaging modality only in the rare cases of gout involving the spine; otherwise, MRI is not used for the diagnosis or management of patients with gout; but MRI may reveal tophaceous gout as an incidental finding. As with conventional radiographs, the typical

radiographic manifestations of marginal and paraarticular erosions of gout may be demonstrated with MRI. The MRI may show cartilage sparing, typical of the disease. Tophi have homogeneous low signal intensity, similar to muscle on T1-weighted images. On T2-weighted images, the signal characteristics of tophi vary from homogeneous high signal intensity to homogeneous low signal intensity (Fig. 24-13). However, signal intensity on the T2-weighted images may be heterogeneous due to urate crystals or calcium deposition, making distinction from neoplasm difficult in a patient without clinically diagnosed gout. The variability in signal intensity on T2-weighted images could be due to differences in urate or calcium concentration within a tophus. Hemosiderin deposition in a tophus has also been reported as a cause of low signal on T2-weighted images.[16] The pattern of enhancement is variable from intense homogeneous, to peripheral and heterogeneous enhancement[15]; near homogeneous enhancement is the most common pattern. The enhancement of the tophus is likely caused by hypervascularity of the affected synovium and the hypervascular granulation tissue surrounding the tophus.[18]

Although the MR appearance of tophi is nonspecific, the diagnosis of gout should be considered when a mass

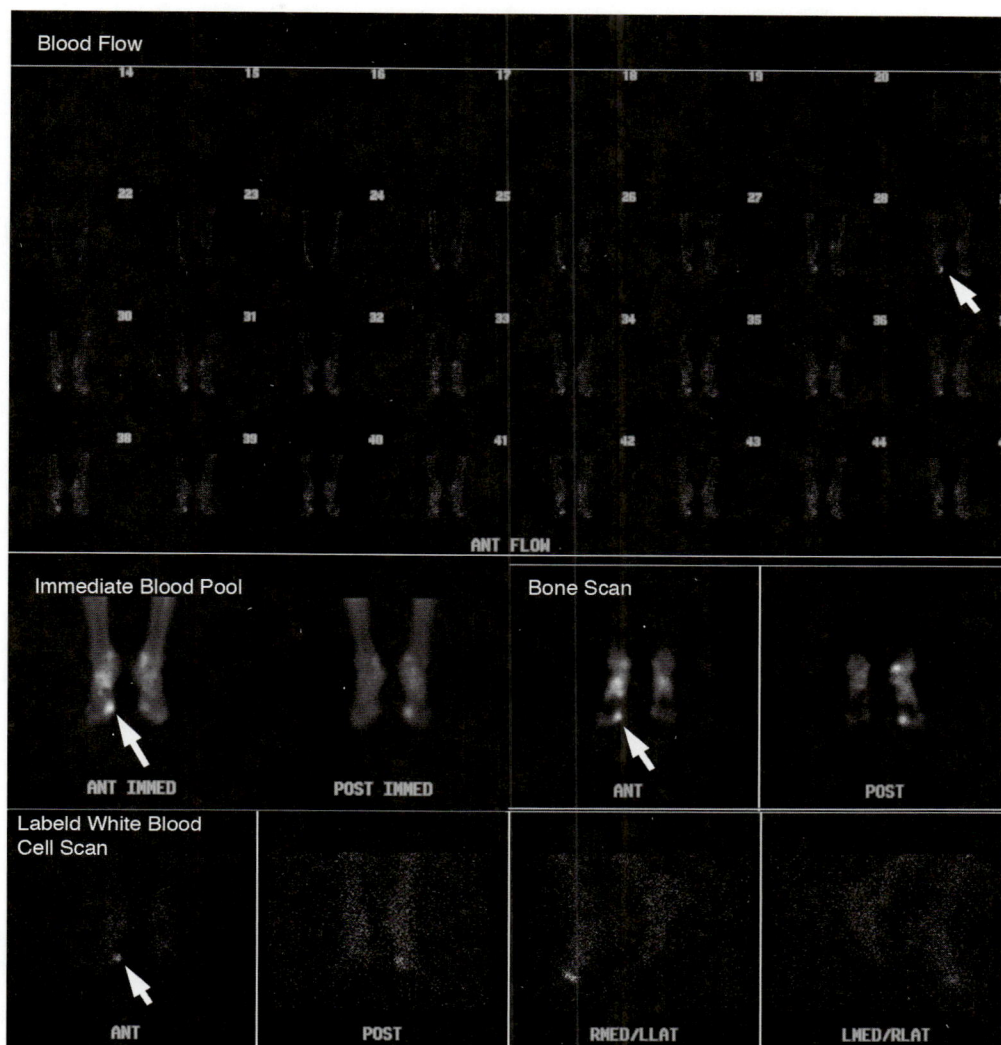

Figure 24-12 Acute gouty arthritis of the first metatarsophalangeal joint. A three-phase bone scan and indium-labeled white blood cell scan shows increased blood flow, increased blood pool, and increased uptake on both bone scan and labeled white blood cell scans. This pattern of increased activity can be seen in acute gouty arthritis but is indistinguishable from septic arthritis/osteomyelitis.

has heterogeneous low to intermediate signal intensity on T2-weighted images, especially if the mass erodes adjacent bones.[18] MRI can demonstrate extraarticular deposition of monosodium urate crystals in bones,[22, 23] tendons,[24] and bursae.[23] MRI is useful in distinguishing ulcerated tophi from nonhealing ulcer due to osteomyelitis (Fig. 24-14). In ulcerated tophi, the tophus and underlying bone have low to intermediate signal intensity on the T2-weighted images, while in nonhealing ulcer due to osteomyelitis, the underlying bone has high signal intensity on T2-weighted images.

Lesions that can have similar signal characteristic on MR are pigmented villonodular synovitis (PVNS) (Fig. 24-15), amyloidosis (Fig. 24-16), and fibromatosis (Fig. 24-17). PVNS usually has areas of lower signal intensity than gout on T2-weighted images due to the presence of hemosiderin deposits. In addition, PVNS involves a single joint while gout often is multiarticular. Amyloidosis is often associated with chronic renal failure and has a different distribution than gout. Amyloidosis has a predilection for spine, hips,

and shoulders, which are rarely affected by gout. Although a plantar fibroma can have similar characteristics as a tophus, the classic involvement of the plantar fascia and the lack of joint involvement help in differentiating plantar fibromas from tophi.[22-29]

Specific Joints: Imaging Gout "From Toe to Head"

Common Joints
Foot and Ankle

The foot is one of the most common areas affected by gout. A classic location is the involvement of the first metatarsophalangeal joint (Fig. 24-18). Often, early erosions are seen in the medial and dorsal aspect of the first metatarsal head and are best seen on oblique views. Less frequently, erosions are present in the base of the first proximal phalanx. The

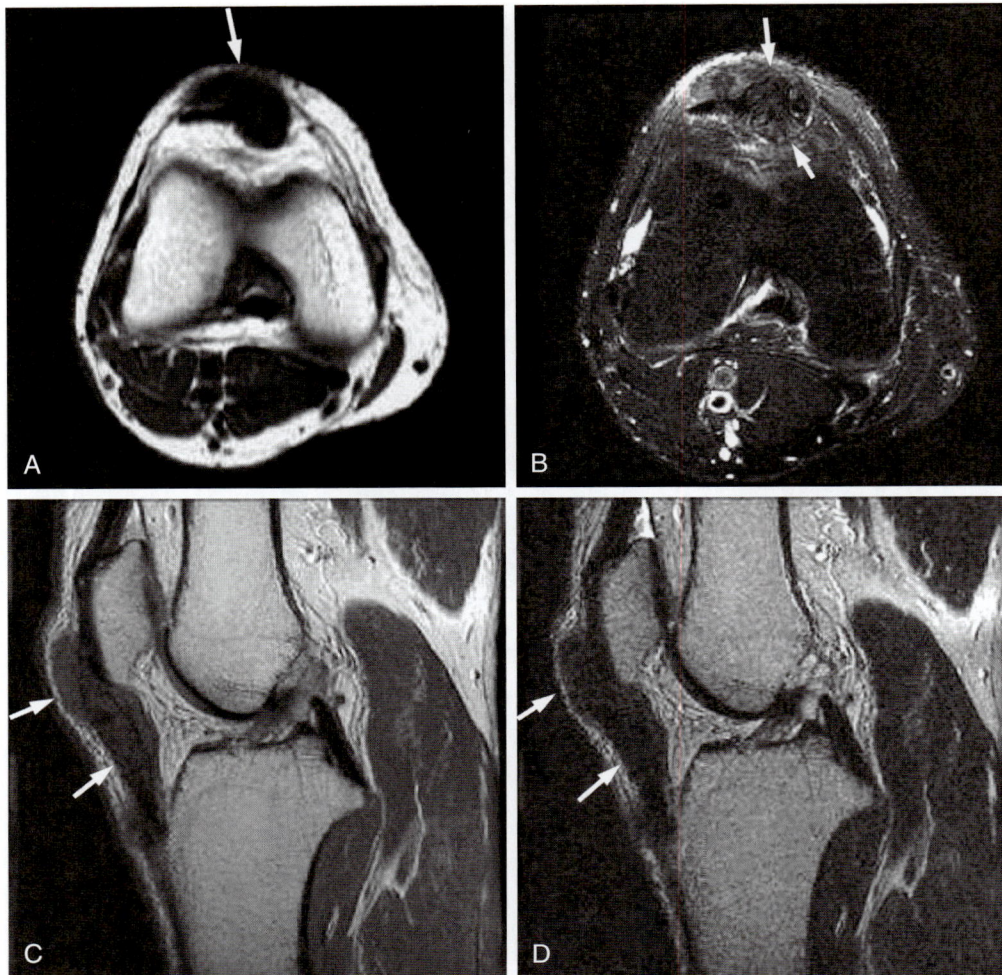

Figure 24-13 Tophus of the patellar tendon. Magnetic resonance imaging of the right knee: axial T1-weighted (**A**), axial fat-saturated T2 (**B**), sagittal proton density (**C**), and sagittal T2-weighted (**D**) images show a mass (*white arrows*) with low to intermediate signal on all sequences involving the medial aspect of the patellar tendon and extending superiorly anterior to the patella. This mass is a large tophus.

fifth metatarsophalangeal joint is also frequently involved. The other joints of the foot—metatarsophalangeal, interphalangeal, tarsometatarsal, and intertarsal joints—are also frequently involved, but usually not in isolation (Fig. 24-19). Involvement of only the ankle joint is rare; when the ankle joint is involved, other joints are also affected. [1, 30-32] Tophi in the Achilles tendon and pre-Achilles and retrocalcaneal bursae can be occasionally detected with CT or MRI. CT allows one to distinguish thickening of the Achilles tendon due to gout from xanthomas.

Radiographs are usually sufficient to evaluate the extent of involvement of the foot; occasionally, MRI is used to evaluate for tendon rupture, nerve entrapment, or infection (Figs. 24-20 and 24-21).

Hand and Wrist

The hand and wrist are also commonly involved, usually with bilateral, but asymmetric articular and soft tissue abnormalities. In the hand, the joints most commonly involved (in decreasing order of frequency) are the distal interphalangeal joints, the proximal interphalangeal joints, and the metacarpophalangeal joints (Fig. 24-22). In the wrist, erosions can be present in the intercarpal and carpometacarpal joints (Fig. 24-23). Tophi can rarely cause carpal tunnel syndrome. MRI is the study of choice to evaluate the presence, location, and complexity of gouty lesions in patients with carpal tunnel syndrome. [24,26,33-35]

Knee

Marginal erosions of the tibia and or femur (Fig. 24-24), with sparing of the joint space, are typical, but isolated lesions of the patella have been reported. [36] Intraosseous lesions in the patella may also predispose to pathologic fractures. [37] Intraosseous lesions in the patella and femur may be confused with neoplasms.

Intraarticular and periarticular tophi limiting knee joint range of motion are a rare but important cause of walking disability in gout patients [38] (see Fig. 24-10). Although most patients do not display visible subcutaneous tophi over the knee on physical examination, the differential diagnosis should consider intraarticular tophi and MRI is valuable in this clinical setting [28,37] as radiographs may not demonstrate

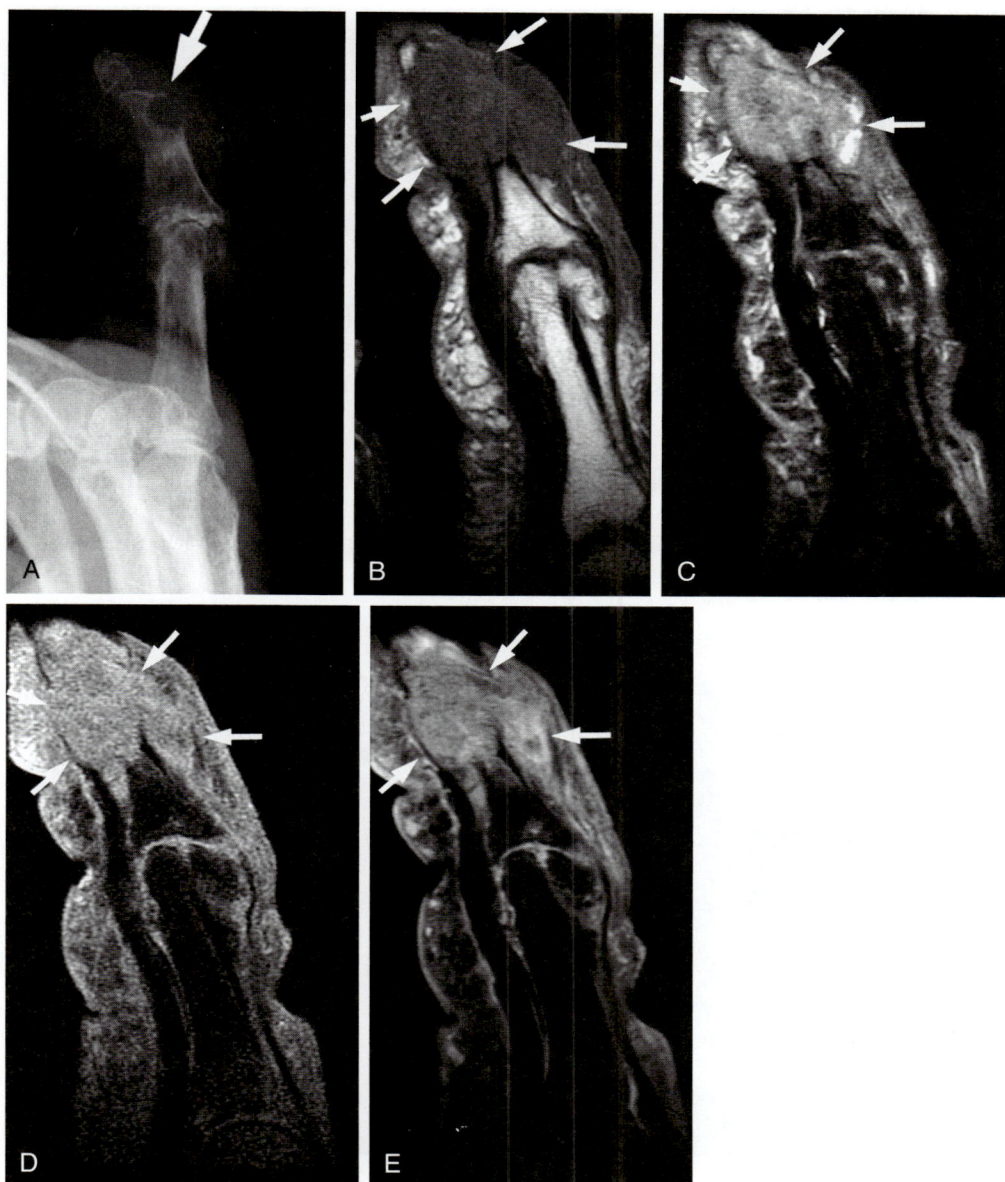

Figure 24-14 Ulcerated tophus. This elderly man presented with soft tissue swelling and drainage from the interphalangeal joint not responding to antibiotics. **A,** Oblique radiograph of the index finger demonstrates destruction of the distal interphalangeal joint and a large erosion with overhanging edges (*arrow*) of the middle phalanx. T1-weighted (**B**), T2-weighted fat-saturated (**C**), and T1-weighted fat-saturated before (**D**) and after (**E**) administration of intravenous contrast show a large tophus destroying the distal interphalangeal joint, with minimal adjacent bone marrow edema and no significant enhancement. The lack of surrounding edema and of enhancement confirms the diagnosis of gout and excludes osteomyelitis. The patient had a rapid improvement after treatment for gout was initiated.

intraarticular tophi. Rarely, gout of the knee can present as a Baker's cyst.[39] Tophi can involve the quadriceps and the patellar tendons and can predispose to rupture of these tendons (see Fig. 24-13).

Elbow

In the elbow, the most common presentation is soft tissue swelling caused by either olecranon bursitis or soft tissue tophi. The increased density (Fig. 24-25; see Fig. 24-9) and occasional calcifications (Fig. 24-26) of the olecranon bursa help in distinguishing olecranon bursitis caused by gout, from olecranon bursitis from other causes such as rheumatoid

arthritis, infection, and trauma. The presence of bony erosion is uncommon in the elbow.[24,40]

Uncommon Joint Involvement in Gout

Spine

Spinal tophi are rare and difficult to diagnose, but the number of reports has increased in the past decade probably due to the wider use of cross-sectional imaging. On radiographs, bony erosions and secondary proliferative osseous changes are the prominent but nonspecific feature of spinal gout. Gout

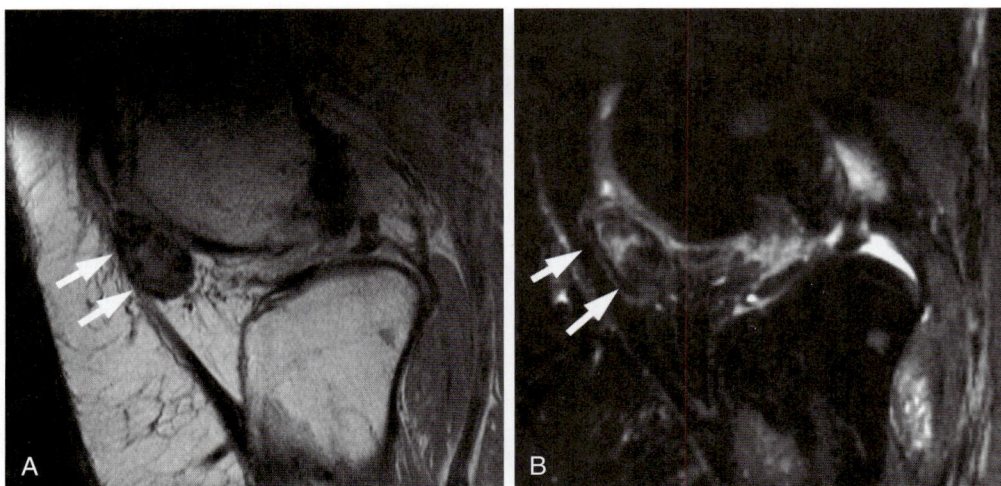

Figure 24-15 Pigmented villonodular synovitis. Proton density (**A**) and T2-weighted (**B**) images of the knee demonstrate a large mass (*arrows*) in the Hoffa fat pad with low to intermediate signal on all sequences. This mass is abutting but not involving the patellar tendon.

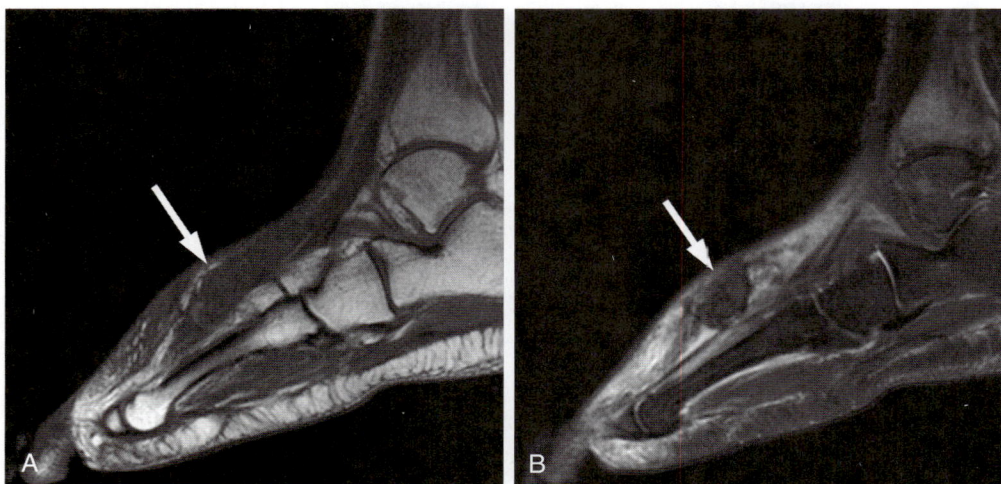

Figure 24-16 Amyloidosis. Sagittal T1-weighted (**A**) and sagittal T2-weighted fat-saturated (**B**) images of the foot demonstrate a large mass (*arrows*) in the dorsum of the foot with low to intermediate signal on all sequences. This patient had a long history of hemodialysis.

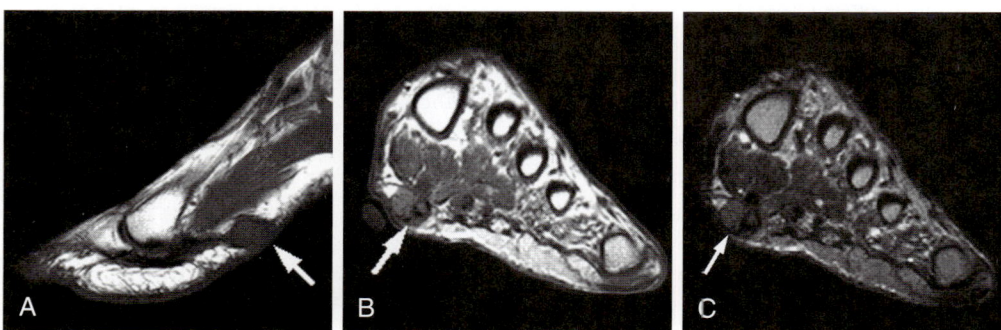

Figure 24-17 Plantar fibromatosis. Sagittal T1-weighted (**A**), short-axis proton density (**B**), and short-axis T2-weighted fat-saturated (**C**) magnetic resonance images of the foot demonstrate a mass (*arrows*) plantar to the first metatarsal with low to intermediate signal on all sequences. This mass invades the plantar fascia and is consistent with plantar fibromatosis.

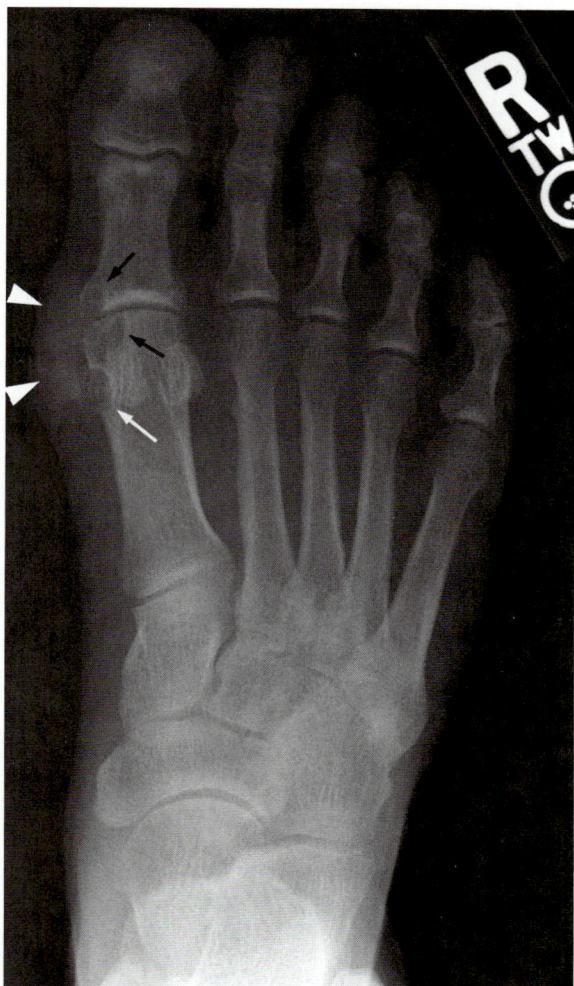

Figure 24-18 Isolated first metatarsophalangeal involvement. Dorso-plantar radiograph of the right foot shows a tophus medial to the first metatarsophalangeal joint (*white arrowhead*) as well as intraarticular erosions (*black arrows*) and a more proximal erosion (*white arrow*) with overhanging edges.

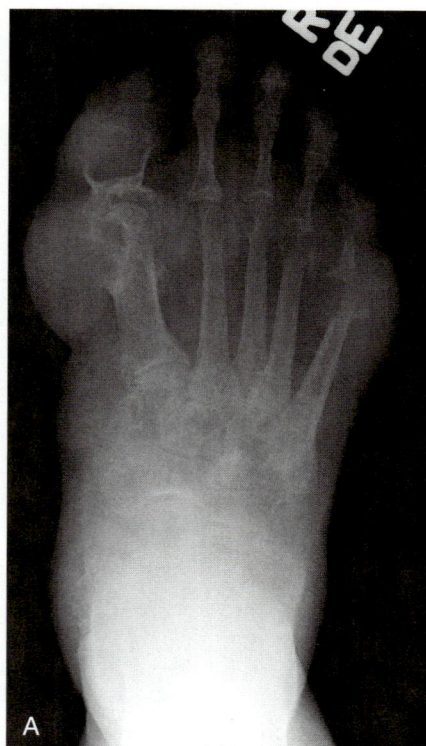

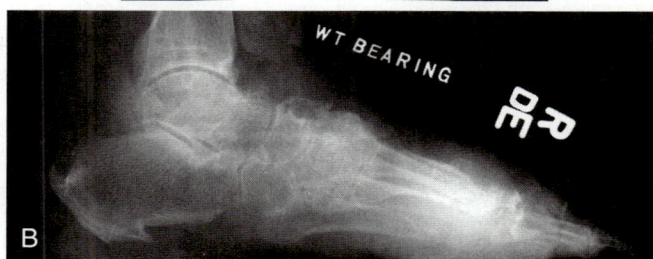

Figure 24-19 Advanced tophaceous gout. Dorsoplantar and lateral radiographs of the right foot show extensive involvement of the soft tissues by multiple tophi. There are erosions of the first interphalangeal joint, the metatarsophalangeal joints, and mid foot. The ankle joint is also affected.

can cause erosions of the facet joints, posterior elements, and vertebral bodies and results in disc space narrowing, and vertebral subluxation. CT and MRI are more useful in these complex areas.[41-49] CT is helpful in delineating bone and soft tissue changes and in showing tophi (Fig. 24-27). MRI is the modality of choice to evaluate the spinal canal. Involvement of the disc space can simulate discitis.[41] Tophi in the spinal canal can be mistaken for an epidural abscess[50,51] or can cause spinal canal stenosis and myelopathy.

Sacroiliac Joints

Sacroiliac joints are an uncommon site of involvement and usually other sites are also affected. Radiographic changes are nonspecific, as with most other arthritis characterized by sclerosis and erosions of the sacroiliac joints. CT (Fig. 24-28) and MRI are more useful as the sacroiliac joints are difficult to visualize on radiographs.[52]

Shoulder

Erosions of the glenohumeral joint (Fig. 24-29) and of the acromioclavicular joint (Fig. 24-30) are rare in gout. Occasionally, tophaceous gout of the rotator cuff can be present, and it can be confused with calcific tendinitis.[53,54]

Hip

Involvement of the hips is rare (Fig. 24-31). If intraosseous tophi are present, they can be confused with avascular necrosis.

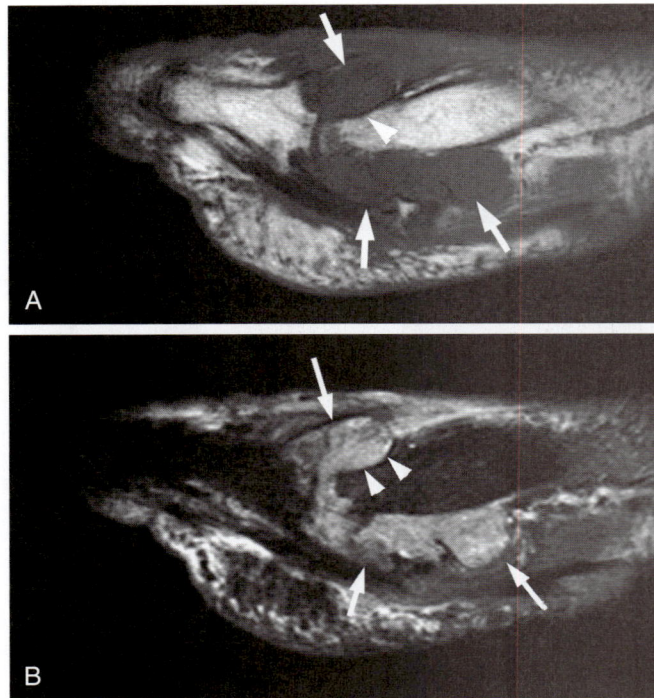

Figure 24-20 Tophaceous gout. Sagittal T1-weighted (**A**) and sagittal T2-weighted fat-saturated (**B**) magnetic resonance images of the first metatarsophalangeal joint show large tophi (*arrows*) with pressure erosion of the first metatarsal head (*arrowheads*). These images were obtained to evaluate for osteomyelitis.

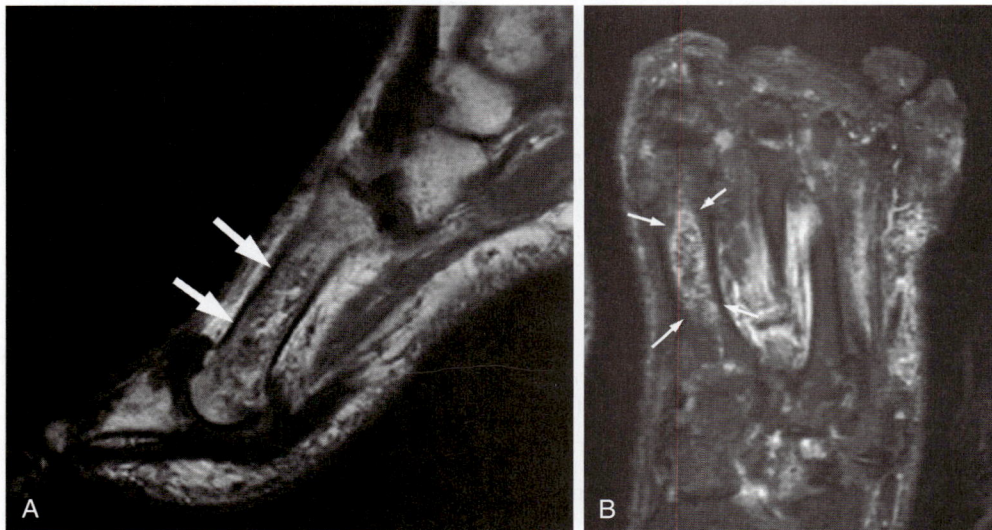

Figure 24-21 Intraosseous tophus. Sagittal T1-weighted (**A**) and long-axis T2-weighted fat-saturated (**B**) magnetic resonance images of the first metatarsal bone show large intraosseous tophus *(arrows)* within the first metatarsal shaft. These images were obtained to evaluate for osteomyelitis.

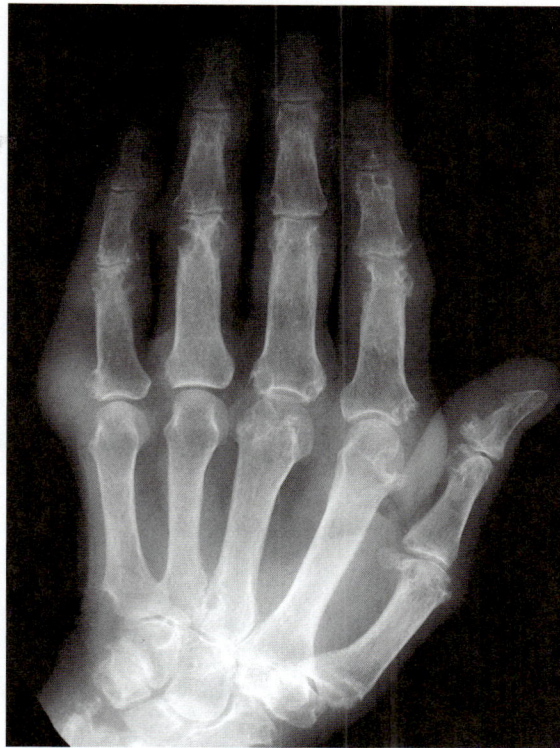

Figure 24-22 Tophaceous gout. Dorsopalmar radiograph of the hand shows multiple soft tissue tophi. There are erosions involving multiple joints, but the joint spaces are preserved.

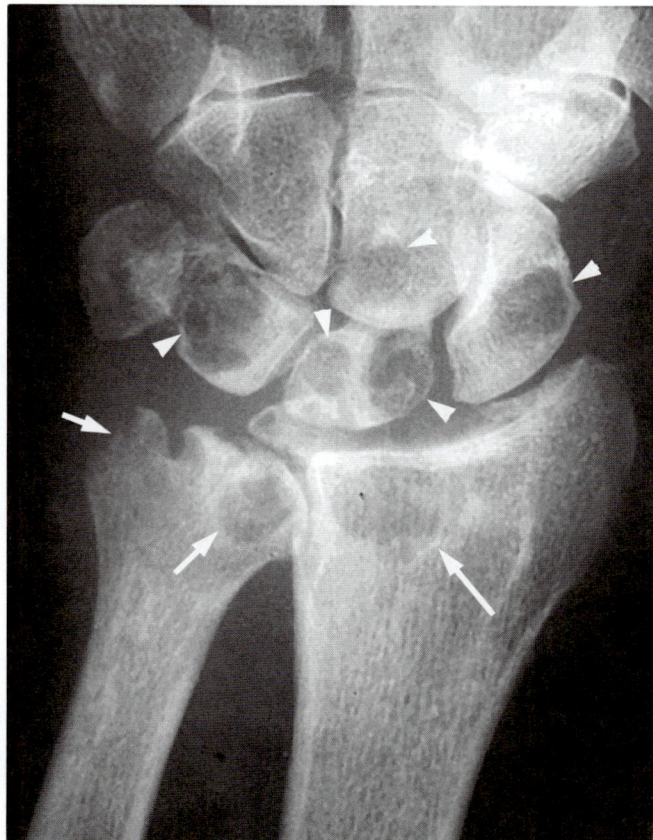

Figure 24-23 Spotty carpal sign. Dorsopalmar radiograph of the wrist shows multiple erosions of the carpal bones (*white arrowheads*) creating the spotty carpal sign. There are also erosions of the distal radius and ulna (*white arrows*).

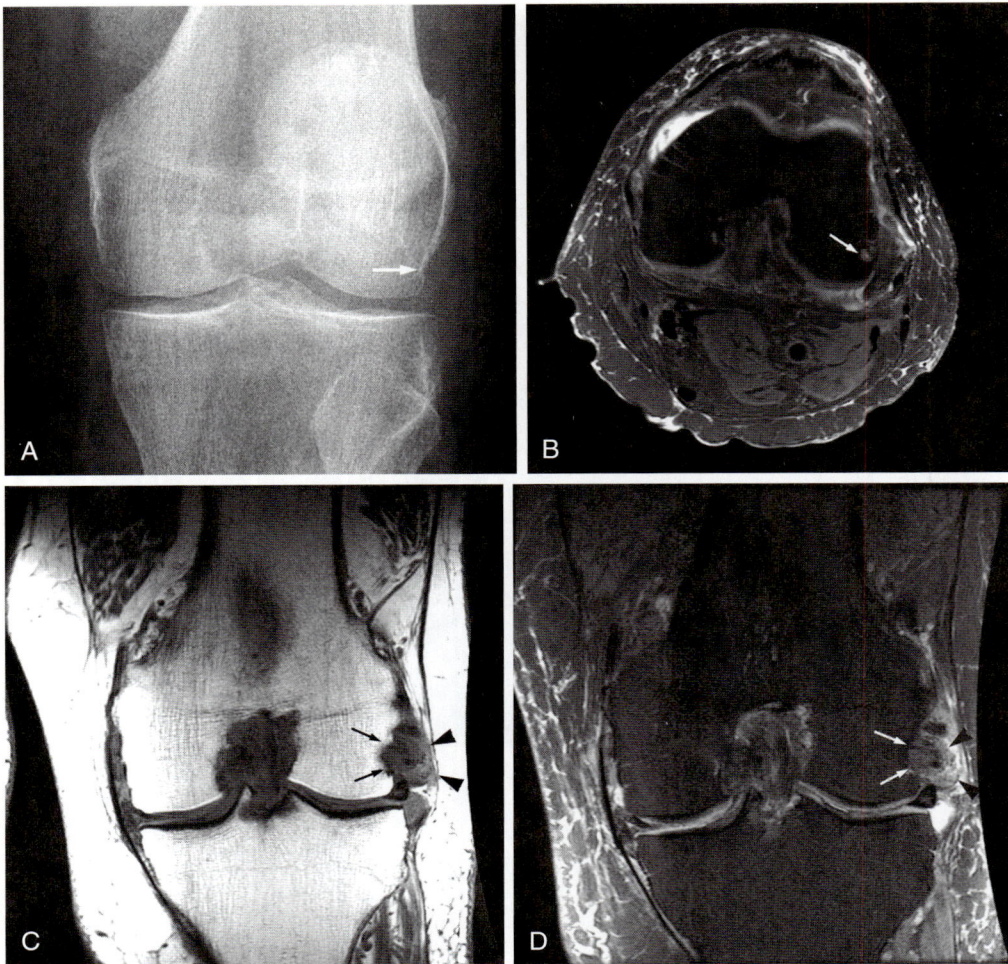

Figure 24-24 Marginal erosion. **A,** Anteroposterior radiograph of the knee shows subtle erosion of the lateral femoral condyle. Proton density fat-saturated axial (**B**), coronal T1-weighted (**C**), and coronal T2-weighted fat-saturated (**D**) magnetic resonance images show a small erosion (*arrows*) of the lateral femoral condyle with adjacent small tophus (*arrowheads*).

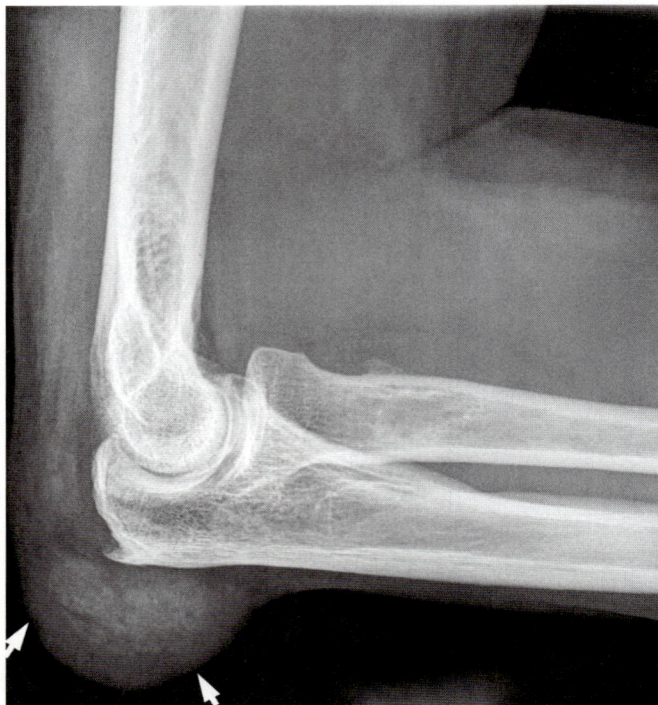

Figure 24-25 Olecranon bursitis (dense bursa). Lateral radiograph of the elbow shows a dense soft tissue mass posterior to the olecranon consistent with olecranon bursitis; as the bursa is denser than normal soft tissues this is consistent with gout.

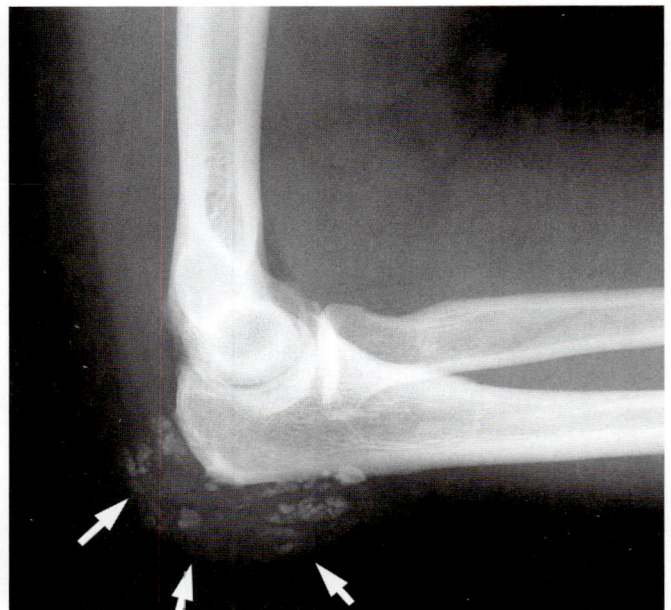

Figure 24-26 Olecranon bursitis (calcified bursa). Lateral radiograph of the elbow shows a dense soft tissue mass containing large calcifications consistent with olecranon bursitis; the presence of calcification is a rare presentation of gout.

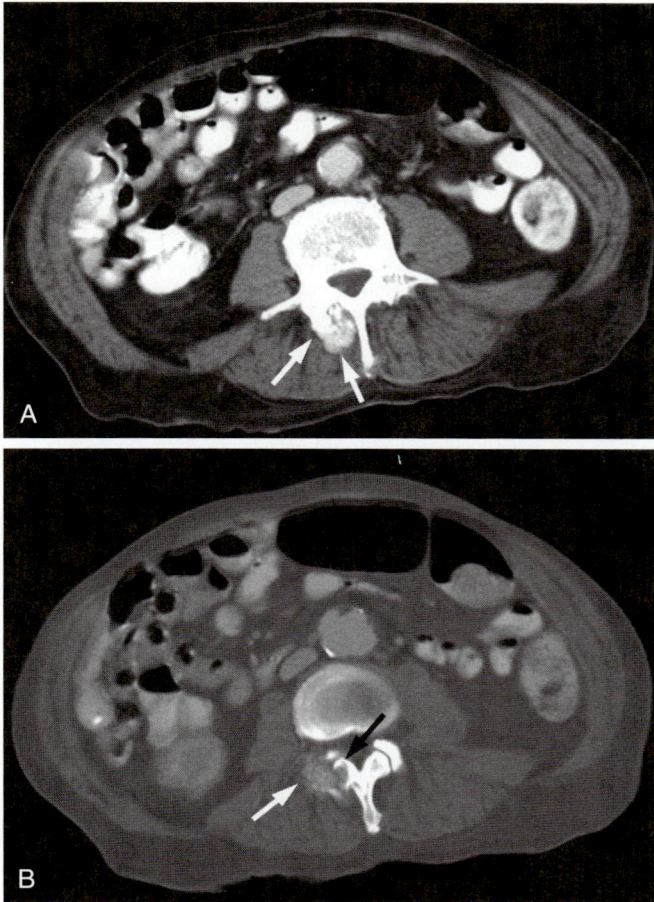

Figure 24-27 Tophaceous gout of the spine. Axial images from a CT of the abdomen displayed with (**A**) soft tissue and (**B**) bone windows show a large tophus (*white arrows*) eroding the right facet joint (*black arrow*).

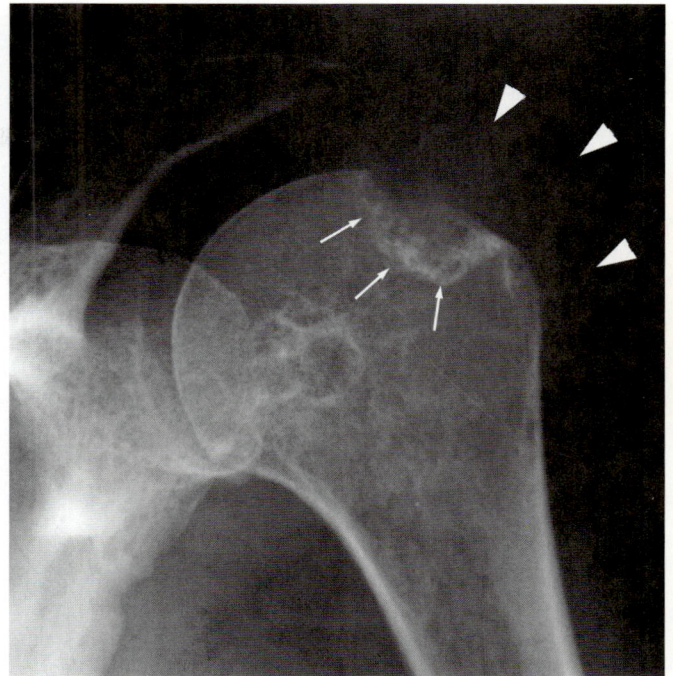

Figure 24-29 Erosions of the humeral head. Anteroposterior radiograph of the shoulder demonstrates large erosions (*white arrows*) of the humeral head with adjacent soft tissue density (*arrowheads*) consistent with a tophus.

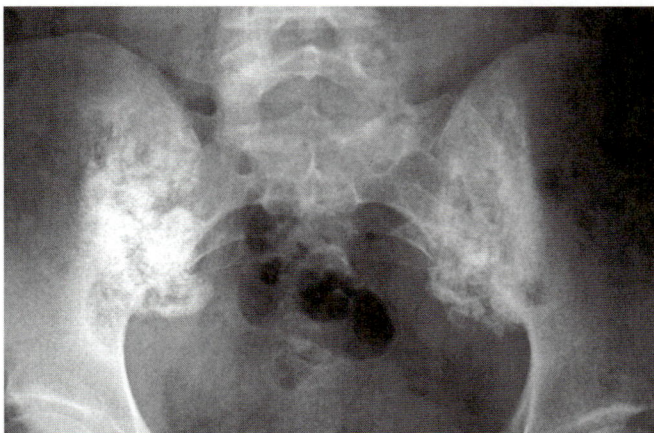

Figure 24-28 Sacroiliitis. Anteroposterior radiograph of the sacroiliac joint shows bilateral sacroiliitis with erosions and sclerosis.

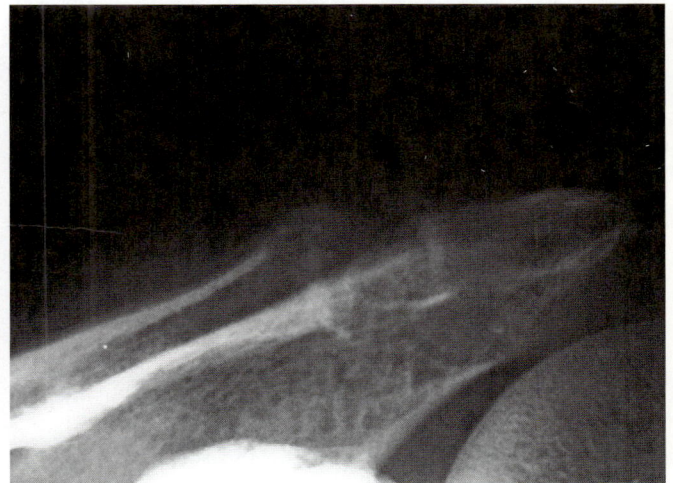

Figure 24-30 Erosion of the acromioclavicular joint. Anteroposterior radiograph of the clavicle shows erosion of the distal clavicle with widening of the acromioclavicular joint.

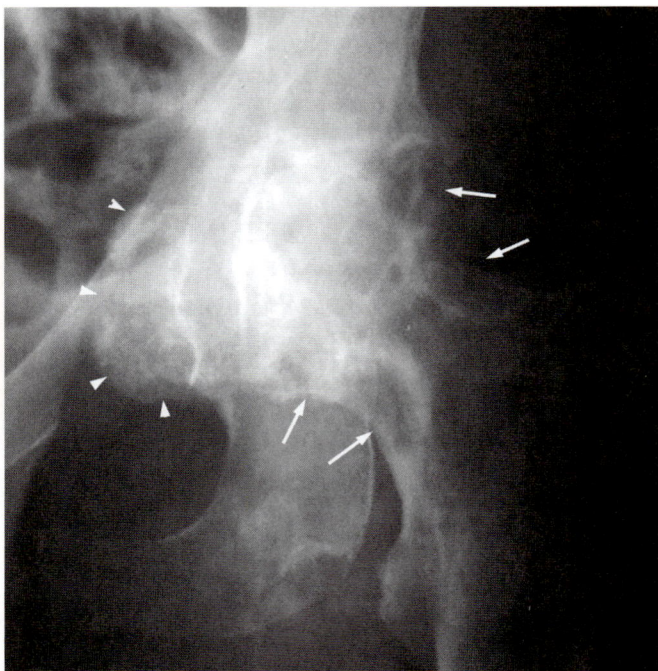

Figure 24-31 Tophaceous gout of the hip. Anteroposterior radiograph of the hip shows multiple erosions of the femoral head and neck (*white arrows*) and a large soft tissue density (*arrowheads*) consistent with a tophus. The joint space is also narrow.

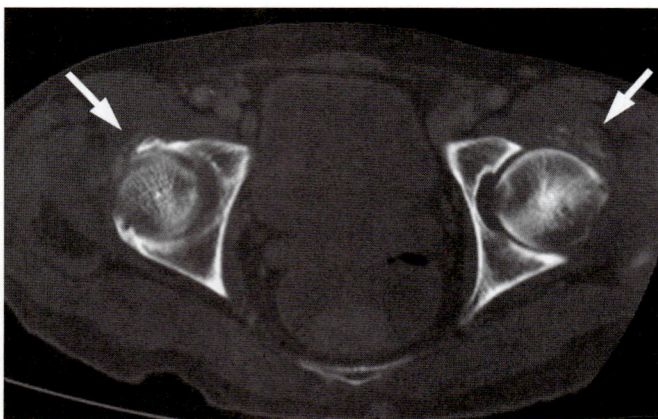

Figure 24-32 Tophaceous gout of the hips. Axial computed tomography image at the level of the femoral heads shows tophi (*white arrows*) anterior to both femoral heads.

References

1. Bloch C, Hermann G, Yu TF. A radiologic reevaluation of gout: a study of 2,000 patients. AJR Am J Roentgenol 1980;134(4):781–7.
2. Huber N, Zur Verwertung der Röntgenstrahlen im Gebiete der inneren Medizin. Deutsche Med Wochnschr 1896;22(12):182–4.
3. Rubenstein J, Pritzker KP. Crystal-associated arthropathies. AJR Am J Roentgenol 1989;152(4):685–95.
4. Rosenberg EF, Arens RA. Gout: clinical, pathologic and roentgenographic observations. Radiology 1947;49(2):169–77.
5. Dalbeth N, Collis J, Gregory K, et al. Tophaceous joint disease strongly predicts hand function in patients with gout. Rheumatology 2007;46(12):1804–7.
6. Resnick D, Broderick TW. Intraosseous calcifications in tophaceous gout. AJR Am J Roentgenol 1981;137(6):1157–61.
7. Liu S-Z, Yeh L, Chou Y-J, et al. Isolated intraosseous gout in hallux sesamoid mimicking a bone tumor in a teenaged patient. Skeletal Radiol 2003;32(11):647–50.
8. Chen YJ, Hsu RW, Hsueh S. Intraosseous tophaceous pseudotumor in the trigonal process of the talus. Clin Orthop Relat Res 1998(346):190–5.
9. Johnson PT, Fayad LM, Fishman EK. CT of the foot: selected inflammatory arthridites. J Comput Assist Tomogr 2007;31(6):961–9.
10. Carotti M, Salaffi F, Ciapetti A. Computed tomography in tophaceous gout. J Rheumatol 2010;37(6):1267–8.
11. Kelman CG, Disler DG, Kremer JM, et al. Xanthomatous infiltration of ankle tendons. Skeletal Radiol 1997;26(4):256–9.
12. Gerster JC, Landry M, Duvoisin B, et al. Computed tomography of the knee joint as an indicator of intraarticular tophi in gout. Arthritis Rheum 1996;39(8):1406–9.
13. Choi HK, Al-Arfaj AM, Eftekhari A, et al. Dual energy computed tomography in tophaceous gout. Ann Rheum Dis 2009;68(10):1609–12.
14. Nicolaou S, Yong-Hing CJ, Galea-Soler S, et al. Dual-energy CT as a potential new diagnostic tool in the management of gout in the acute setting. AJR Am J Roentgenol 2010;194(4):1072–8.
15. Coombs RJ, Pinsky ST, Padanilam TG. Bone scan findings of combined gout and septic arthritis in the same digit. Clin Nucl Med 2001;26(5):442–3.
16. Goshen E, Schwartz A, Zwas ST. Chronic tophaceous gout: scintigraphic findings on bone scan. Clin Nucl Med 2000;25(2):146–7.
17. Herrmann T, Granjon D, Loboguerrero A, et al. Tc-99m HMPAO leukocyte uptake in articular gout. Clin Nucl Med 1991;16(6):457.
18. Kumar ASR, Bui C, Szwarc G, et al. Florid polyarticular gout mimicking septic arthritis. Clin Nucl Med 2004;29(4):262–3.
19. Blumer SL, Scalcione LR, Ring BN, et al. Cutaneous and subcutaneous imaging on FDG-PET: benign and malignant findings. Clin Nucl Med 2009;34(10):675–83.
20. Steiner M, Vijayakumar V. Widespread tophaceous gout demonstrating avid F-18 fluorodeoxyglucose uptake. Clin Nucl Med 2009;34(7):433–4.
21. Sato J, Watanabe H, Shinozaki T, et al. Gouty tophus of the patella evaluated by PET imaging. J Orthop Sci 2001;6(6):604–7.
22. Miller LJ, Pruett SW, Losada R, et al. Clinical image. Tophaceous gout of the lumbar spine: MR findings. J Comput Assist Tomogr 1996;20(6):1004–5.
23. Jbara M, Patnana M, Kazmi F, et al. MR imaging: arthropathies and infectious conditions of the elbow, wrist, and hand. Magn Reson Imaging Clin N Am 2004;12(2):361–79:vii.
24. Jbara M, Patnana M, Kazmi F, et al. MR imaging: arthropathies and infectious conditions of the elbow, wrist, and hand. Radiol Clin North Am 2006;44(4):625–42:ix.
25. Chung C, Dailiana T, Yu JS, et al. MR-imaging of tophaceous gout. Radiology 1995;197:466.
26. Carter JD, Kedar RP, Anderson SR, et al. An analysis of MRI and ultrasound imaging in patients with gout who have normal plain radiographs. Rheumatol (Oxford) 2009;48(11):1442–6.
27. Gentili A, Sorenson S, Masih S. MR imaging of soft-tissue masses of the foot. Semin Musculoskelet Radiol 2002;6(2):141–52.
28. Chen CK, Yeh LR, Pan HB, et al. Intra-articular gouty tophi of the knee: CT and MR imaging in 12 patients. Skeletal Radiol 1999;28(2):75–80.
29. Yu JS, Chung C, Recht M, et al. MR imaging of tophaceous gout. AJR Am J Roentgenol 1997;168(2):523–7.
30. Lee YA, Lee SH, Yang HI, et al. Clinical images: aggressive gouty arthritis with concurrent involvement of the ankle and cervical spine. Arthritis Rheum 2009;60(12):3581.
31. Bancroft L, Peterson J, Kransdorf M. Cysts, geodes, and erosions. Radiol Clin N Am 2004;42(1):73–87.
32. Monu JUV, Pope TL. Gout: a clinical and radiologic review. Radiol Clin N Am 2004;42(1):169.
33. Andracco R, Zampogna G, Parodi M, et al. Dactylitis in gout. Ann Rheum Dis 2010;69(1):316.
34. Chen CK, Chung CB, Yeh L, et al. Carpal tunnel syndrome caused by tophaceous gout: CT and MR imaging features in 20 patients. AJR Am J Roentgenol 2000;175(3):655–9.
35. Rand B, McBride TJ, Dias RG. Combined triggering at the wrist and severe carpal tunnel syndrome caused by gouty infiltration of a flexor tendon. J Hand Surg Eur Vol 2010;35(3):240–2.
36. Recht MP, Seragini F, Kramer J, et al. Isolated or dominant lesions of the patella in gout: a report of 7 patients. Skeletal Radiol 1994;23(2):113–6.
37. Yu KH, Lien LC, Ho HH. Limited knee joint range of motion due to invisible gouty tophi. Rheumatology (Oxford) 2004;43(2):191–4.
38. Chen CKH, Yeh LR, Pan HB, et al. Intra-articular gouty tophi of the knee: CT and MR imaging in 12 patients. Skeletal Radiol 1999;28(2):75–80.
39. Levitin PM, Keats TE. Dissecting synovial cyst of popliteal space in gout. AJR Am J Roentgenol 1975;124(1):32–3.

40. Gerster JC, Landry M, Dufresne L, et al. Imaging of tophaceous gout: computed tomography provides specific images compared with magnetic resonance imaging and ultrasonography. Ann Rheum Dis 2002;61(1):52–4.

41. Duprez TP, Malghem J, Vande Berg BC, et al. Gout in the cervical spine: MR pattern mimicking diskovertebral infection. AJNR Am J Neuroradiol 1996;17(1):151–3.

42. Oaks J, Quarfordt SD, Metcalfe JK. MR features of vertebral tophaceous gout. AJR Am J Roentgenol 2006;187(6):W658–9.

43. Pfister AK, Schlarb CA, O'Neal JF. Vertebral erosion, paraplegia, and spinal gout. AJR Am J Roentgenol 1998;171(5):1430–1.

44. Bonaldi VM, Duong H, Starr MR, et al. Tophaceous gout of the lumbar spine mimicking an epidural abscess: MR features. Am J Neuroradiol 1996;17(10):1949–52.

45. Hsu CY, Shih TT, Huang KM, et al. Tophaceous gout of the spine: MR imaging features. Clin Radiol 2002;57(10):919–25.

46. Yen PS, Lin JF, Chen SY, et al. Tophaceous gout of the lumbar spine mimicking infectious spondylodiscitis and epidural abscess: MR imaging findings. J Clin Neurosci 2005;12(1):44–6.

47. Ko KH, Huang GS, Chang WC. Tophaceous gout of the lumbar spine. J Clin Rheumatol 2010;16(4):200.

48. Ntsiba H, Makosso E, Moyikoua A. Thoracic spinal cord compression by a tophus. Joint Bone Spine 2010;77(2):187–8.

49. Feydy A, Liote F, Carlier R, et al. Cervical spine and crystal-associated diseases: imaging findings. Eur Radiol 2006;16(2):459–68.

50. Barrett K, Miller ML, Wilson JT. Tophaceous gout of the spine mimicking epidural infection: case report and review of the literature. Neurosurgery 2001;48(5):1170–2:discussion 2–3.

51. Gines R, Bates DJ. Tophaceous lumbar gout mimicking an epidural abscess. Am J Emerg Med 1998;16(2):216.

52. Alarcons D, Cetina JA, Diazjoua E. Sacroiliac joints in primary gout: clinical and roentgenographic study of 143 patients. AJR Am J Roentgenol 1973;118(2):438–43.

53. Chang CH, Lu CH, Yu CW, et al. Tophaceous gout of the rotator cuff. A case report. J Bone Joint Surg 2008;90(1):178–82.

54. Olsen KM, Chew FS. Tumoral calcinosis: pearls, polemics, and alternative possibilities. Radiographics 2006;26(3):871–85.

Chapter 25

Plain Radiography and Advanced Imaging of Calcium Pyrophosphate Dihydrate Crystal Deposition Disease and of Arthropathy Associated With Basic Calcium Phosphate Crystal Deposition

Diego F. Lemos and Tudor H. Hughes

KEY POINTS

- Cartilage calcification (chondrocalcinosis) can occur in both fibrocartilage and hyaline cartilage. Fibrocartilaginous calcifications are most common in the menisci of the knee, triangular fibrocartilage of the wrist, symphysis pubis, annulus fibrosus of the intervertebral disc, and acetabular and glenoid labra but also can be seen also within the discs of the sternoclavicular and acromioclavicular joints.

- Fibrocartilaginous deposits appear more thick, shaggy, and irregular when compared to the deposits in hyaline articular cartilage.

- Hyaline cartilage calcifications may be detected by plain radiography in many joints but most commonly in the knee, wrist, hip, elbow, and shoulders. These deposits are typically thin, punctate and linear or curvilinear and are parallel to but separated from the subchondral bone plate.

- Synovial calcification is a relatively common feature of calcium pyrophosphate dihydrate (CPPD) crystal deposition disease. Such synovial deposits are most frequently detected by plain radiography in the knee, wrist, and metacarpophalangeal and metatarsophalangeal joints.

- CPPD crystal arthropathy affecting the joint can have features similar to those seen in osteoarthritis, such as joint space narrowing, sclerosis, and cyst formation;

however, distribution of involved joints (and/or specific joint compartments) can help differentiate this particular arthropathy from primary, degenerative joint disease. Examples are isolated involvement of the patellofemoral compartment of the knee, isolated radiocarpal or trapezioscaphoid joint involvement in the wrist, and isolated talocalcaneonavicular joint involvement.

- Prominent subchondral cyst formation, variable osteophyte formation, and, in some cases, destructive bone changes that are severe and progressive (resembling those seen on neuropathic arthropathy) also help in distinguishing primary CPPD deposition disease from osteoarthritis.

- The characteristic homogeneous cloudlike appearance of basic calcium phosphate (BCP) crystal deposition and a predilection for characteristic sites help distinguish it from other disorders that can be also associated with periarticular calcifications.

- BCP crystal deposition can be confused sometimes with gout due to radiographic and clinical similarities, and the fact that some tophi are faintly calcified, but BCP deposition should not be confused with the more linear, punctate and diffuse CPPD crystal calcifications.

- BCP and CPPD crystal deposition can coexist in the same joint.

Introduction

In this chapter, we review the imaging appearance of calcium pyrophosphate dihydrate (CPPD) crystal deposition disease and of basic calcium phosphate (BCP) crystal deposition related arthropathy (which is here termed hydroxyapatite deposition disease [HADD]). This chapter focuses on plain radiography but also discusses advanced imaging. High-resolution ultrasound is separately reviewed (see Chapter 26) in this book. Importantly, Chapter 24 describes the use of dual-energy computed tomography (DECT) to specifically distinguish tophi from pathologic calcifications, and DECT will not be further discussed here.

Calcium Pyrophosphate Dihydrate Crystal Deposition Disease

A variety of terms have been used to describe different manifestations of CPPD crystal deposition disease. The European League Against Rheumatism (EULAR) has proposed a specific nomenclature.[1] However, in this review, nomenclature will be employed that features use of the terms "chondrocalcinosis" and "pyrophosphate arthropathy." Chondrocalcinosis is a more general term that should be reserved for radiologically or pathologically evident cartilage calcification. Such cartilage deposition can be due to CPPD, dicalcium phosphate dihydrate, or calcium hydroxyapatite crystals, or a combination of the three.

"CPPD crystal deposition disease" is a more specific term for a specific disorder characterized by the exclusive presence of CPPD crystals in or around joints.

The term "pseudogout" is not a radiologic diagnosis; this term should be reserved for the gout-like clinical syndrome produced by CPPD crystal deposition and characterized by intermittent acute attacks of arthritis.

The term "pyrophosphate arthropathy" (discussed later) here refers to a particular pattern of structural joint damage that can develop in patients with CPPD crystal deposition disease.[2-7]

General Imaging Features

ARTICULAR AND PERIARTICULAR CRYSTAL DEPOSITION

Crystalline deposits of CPPD can be located in the cartilage, synovium, capsule, tendons, bursae, ligaments, and soft tissues.

Cartilage calcification (chondrocalcinosis) can occur in both fibrocartilage and hyaline cartilage. Fibrocartilaginous calcifications are most common in the menisci of the knee, triangular fibrocartilage of the wrist, symphysis pubis, annulus fibrosus of the intervertebral disc, and acetabular and glenoid labra. These deposits can be seen also within the discs of the sternoclavicular and acromioclavicular joints. Fibrocartilaginous deposits appear more thick, shaggy, and irregular compared to the deposits in hyaline cartilage. Hyaline cartilage calcifications may occur in many joints but are most common in the knee, wrist, hip, elbow, and shoulders. These deposits are typically thin, punctate and linear or curvilinear and are parallel to but separated from the subchondral bone plate.[2-7]

Synovial calcification is a relatively common feature of CPPD crystal deposition disease. Such synovial deposits are most frequent in the knee, wrist, and metacarpophalangeal and metatarsophalangeal joints. When present, synovial calcifications are usually combined with chondrocalcinosis but in some instances can be the dominant radiographic feature. These synovial deposits may be cloudlike, particularly at the margins of the joint. In addition, detached pieces of calcified synovium can be seen. The overall appearance may resemble idiopathic synovial chondromatosis.[2-7]

Capsular calcification is more frequently seen in the elbow, knee, metacarpophalangeal, and glenohumeral joints. These deposits usually appear as fine or irregular linear calcifications along the capsule spanning the joint.[2-7]

Tendon, bursa, and ligament calcification is another feature that can be seen in patients with CPPD crystal deposition disease. Commonly involved tendons include the Achilles, triceps, quadriceps, gastrocnemius, popliteus, gluteal, and sometimes the tendons of the rotator cuff. Such calcifications along tendons appear thin and linear and may be quite extensive. Common involved ligaments include the intercarpal ligaments of the wrist as well as the cruciate ligaments of the knee.[2-7]

Soft tissue calcification can occasionally be seen in patients with CPPD crystal deposition disease particularly about the elbow, pelvis, and wrist. These calcifications are usually poorly defined and sometimes can be quite prominent and tumor-like, particularly around the digits and the temporomandibular joint, as well as in the retro-odontoid region. Other reported sites include the elbow, hip, wrist, knee, glenohumeral, and acromioclavicular joints. Because of the overall imaging appearance of these lesions, which can be fairly impressive and sometimes aggressive-looking with erosion of the adjacent osseous structures, different designations have been coined on reported cases including terms such as "tophaceous pseudogout," "pseudotumor," "massive CPPD," "tumoral CPPD," and "destructive CPPD arthropathy," among others.[2-8]

PYROPHOSPHATE ARTHROPATHY

The term "pyrophosphate arthropathy" is not a generally adopted nomenclature but it can be used for a specific type of arthropathy related to CPPD crystal deposition disease, with characteristic structural changes depending on the joint involved. The wrist, knee, and metacarpophalangeal joints are the most commonly affected but it may occur in any joint. Although usually bilateral, symmetric changes may not be always present. Features similar to those seen in osteoarthritis, such as joint space narrowing, sclerosis, and cyst formation occur; however, there are several characteristics that differentiate this particular arthropathy from the classic degenerative joint disease. For instance, although pyrophosphate arthropathy can be found in weight-bearing joints (i.e., knee and hip), it can also occur in articulations that are less commonly involved in degenerative joint disease such as the wrist, elbow, and glenohumeral joints. Furthermore, its distribution is unusual in some joints. For instance, isolated patellofemoral compartment of the knee, isolated radiocarpal or trapezioscaphoid joint involvement in the wrist, and isolated talocalcaneonavicular joint involvement in the foot are highly suggestive of pyrophosphate arthropathy. Additional features such as prominent subchondral cyst formation, variable osteophyte formation, and, in some cases, destructive bone changes that are severe and progressive (resembling those seen on neuropathic arthropathy) also help in its distinction.[2-7]

Specific Sites

KNEE

The knee is the most commonly involved joint in CPPD crystal deposition disease. Chondrocalcinosis affecting both the fibrocartilage of the meniscus and the hyaline articular cartilage can be seen as well as synovial and capsular calcifications (Fig. 25-1). Tendinous and ligamentous deposits of CPPD, particularly along the quadriceps, gastrocnemius, and popliteus tendons, as well as along the cruciate and collateral ligaments, can be also seen.[2,9,10] Rarely, large calcified pseudotumoral soft tissue masses can be found about the knee.[11]

Pyrophosphate arthropathy of the knee most commonly involves the medial femorotibial compartment followed by the patellofemoral compartment and, less frequently, the lateral femorotibial compartment. However, isolated or severe patellofemoral compartment changes should suggest this particular diagnosis. Along with these changes, the presence of a distal femoral excavation or erosion along the anterior cortex of the distal femur is highly suggestive of pyrophosphate arthropathy[2,12,13] (Fig. 25-2). Isolated involvement of the lateral femorotibial compartment should also suggest this diagnosis. Stress fractures and collapse of the articular surface in either the medial or lateral compartment resembling the features of spontaneous osteonecrosis of the knee can be seen.[2,14]

WRIST

The wrist is another commonly involved joint in CPPD crystal deposition disease. Chondrocalcinosis can be seen affecting the triangular fibrocartilage as well as the hyaline cartilage of the radiocarpal, midcarpal, and common carpometacarpal joints (Fig. 25-3). Synovial and capsular calcifications can occur as well as ligamentous deposits, particularly along the scapholunate and lunotriquetral intrinsic ligaments, which

may rupture with resultant widening of the interosseous distances and carpal malalignment. Depending on the location of the deposits, areas of significant synovitis, tenosynovitis, and even tendon ruptures can also occur.[2-7,15-19]

Pyrophosphate arthropathy in the wrist has characteristic features including the predilection for the radiocarpal compartment with evidence of joint space narrowing, subchondral sclerosis, and cyst formation. The scaphoid can move proximally close to the radius while the lunate may move distally close to

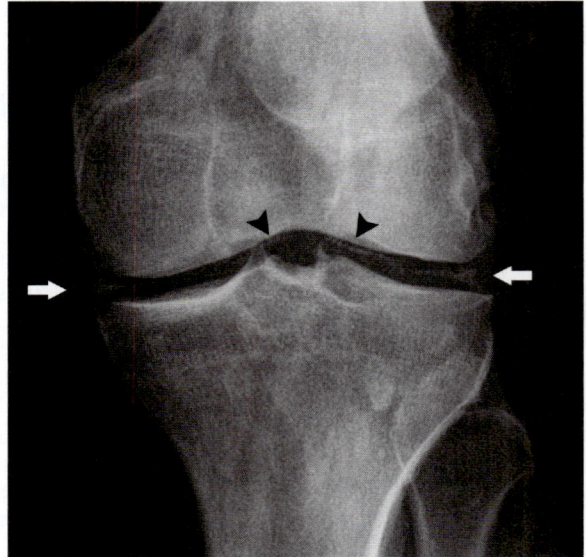

Figure 25-1 Chondrocalcinosis of the knee. Frontal radiograph of the knee demonstrates CPPD deposition in the fibrocartilage of the menisci (*white arrows*) as well as along the hyaline articular cartilage (*black arrowheads*).

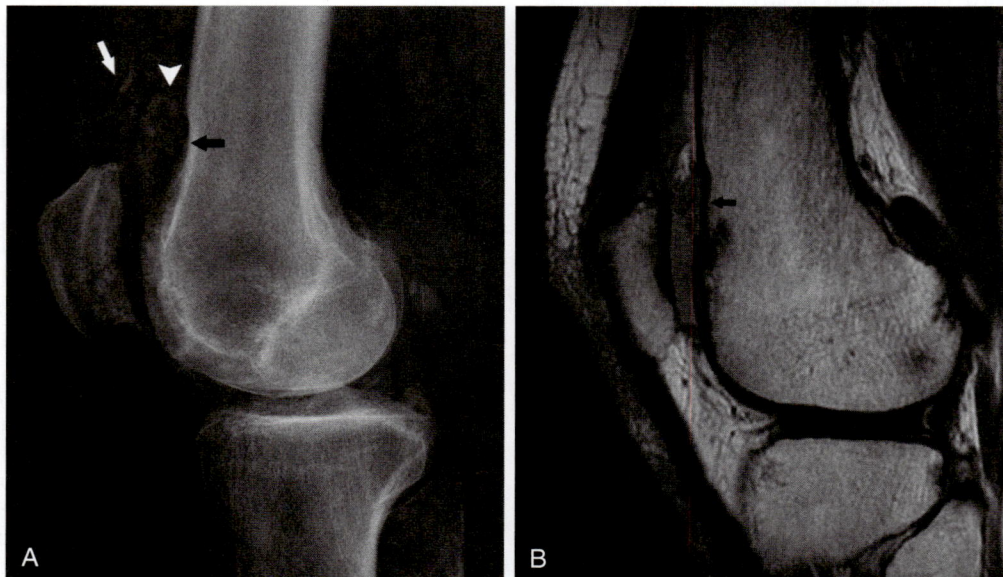

Figure 25-2 Pyrophosphate arthropathy of the knee. **A,** Lateral radiograph of the knee shows CPPD deposition along the synovium and capsule particularly along the suprapatellar recess (*white arrow*) as well as a masslike deposit of crystals in the prefemoral region (*white arrowhead*) with an associated excavation or erosion of the adjacent anterior cortex of the distal femur (*black arrow*). **B,** Sagittal proton density MR image of the knee in a different patient demonstrates also a femoral excavation or erosion in the anterior cortex of the distal femur (*black arrow*). Note the severity of the structural joint changes seen on the patellofemoral compartment including cartilage denudation and reactive bone marrow changes, which were out of proportion with those in the medial and lateral compartments.

the capitate with a resultant "stepladder' appearance, which is characteristic of this arthropathy (Fig. 25-4). The overall appearance is similar to the so-called scapholunate advanced collapse (SLAC) initially described in the setting of a wrist injury. The midcarpal compartment is the second most commonly involved after the radiocarpal compartment. Moreover, isolated changes of the trapezioscaphoid joint are suggestive of the disease.[2-7,15-19] Cases of carpal tunnel syndrome have been reported in the setting of CPPD crystal deposition disease.[20]

METACARPOPHALANGEAL JOINTS

Features of CPPD crystal deposition disease at the level of the metacarpophalangeal joints include calcifications in the cartilage, capsule, and synovium as well as changes of arthropathy including joint space narrowing, subchondral sclerosis, and cyst formation, in addition to collapse of the metacarpal heads. Such structural joint changes show a characteristic predilection for the second and third metacarpophalangeal joints[2-7,21] (Fig. 25-5). Milder changes can be seen occasionally in the interphalangeal joints. The bone collapse is more prominent in this arthropathy than in degenerative joint disease, which, in addition to the predilection of the metacarpophalangeal involvement over the interphalangeal joint, helps in its differentiation from osteoarthritis. The structural changes seen in the second and third metacarpophalangeal joints can also be seen in hemochromatosis; however, in this latter condition, similar changes in the fourth and fifth metacarpophalangeal joints are common. The "drooping" or hooklike osteophytes along the radial aspects of the metacarpal heads that can be seen in patients with CPPD crystal deposition disease are also characteristic of hemochromatosis.[2-7,22]

A different metacarpophalangeal arthropathy related to manual labor, the "Missouri metacarpal syndrome," can have structural changes similar to pyrophosphate arthropathy; however, in patients with this syndrome, there is no evidence of CPPD crystal deposition disease or hemochromatosis.[23]

ELBOW

Chondrocalcinosis, capsular, and synovial calcifications, as well as deposits along the flexor, extensor, distal biceps, and triceps tendons, can occur (Fig. 25-6). Features of

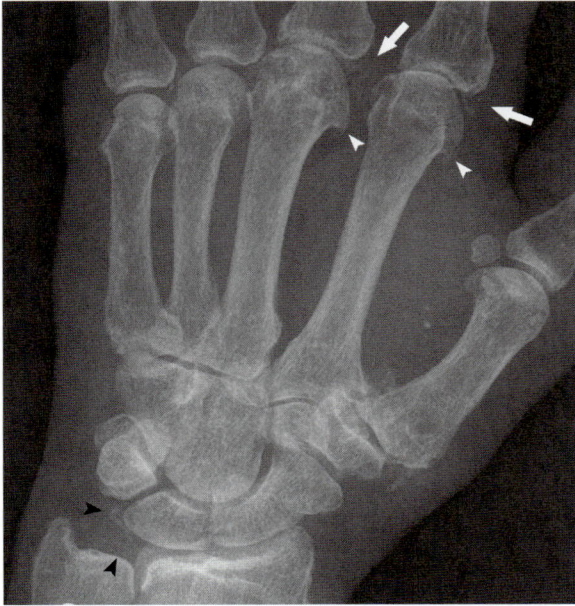

Figure 25-3 CPPD crystal deposition hand and wrist. Oblique radiograph of the hand shows chondrocalcinosis at the level of the triangular fibrocartilage (*black arrowheads*) as well as along the capsule of the metacarpophalangeal joints, particularly the second and third (*white arrows*). Note the "drooping" or "hooklike" osteophytes along the radial aspects of the heads of the second and third metacarpals (*white arrowheads*). Severe structural changes are seen in the first carpometacarpal joint in a background of osteoarthritis.

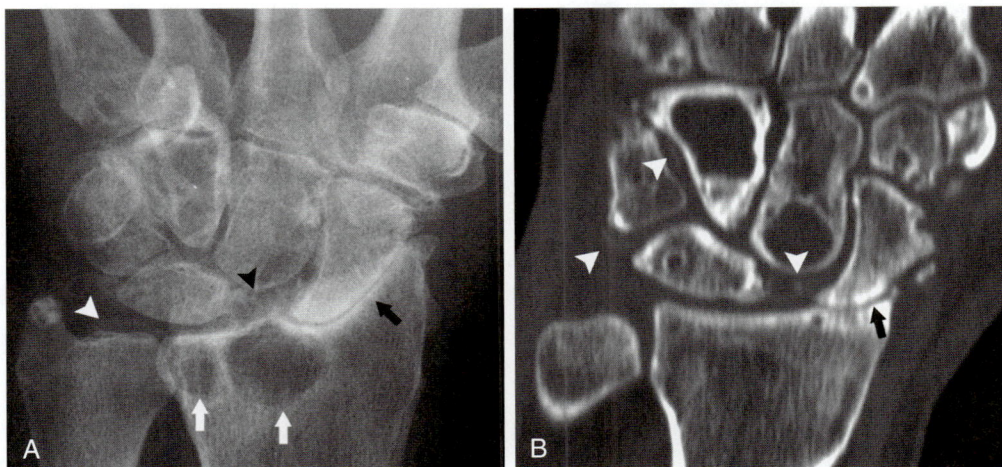

Figure 25-4 Pyrophosphate arthropathy of the wrist. **A,** Posteroanterior radiograph of the wrist demonstrates chondrocalcinosis in the triangular fibrocartilage (*white arrowhead*) as well as within the scapholunate interval, which is markedly widened (*black arrowhead*). In addition, there is severe joint space narrowing in the radiocarpal compartment with subchondral sclerosis and remodeling of the distal radius (*black arrow*). The capitate is proximally migrated. Note the large intraosseous cysts in the distal radius (*white arrows*). Large cysts are also present in some of the carpal bones. **B,** CT coronal reconstruction of the wrist in a different patient shows similar changes of pyrophosphate arthropathy including CPPD deposition in the scapholunate, lunotriquetral, and hamatotriquetral intervals (*white arrowheads*) as well as severe joint space narrowing in the radiocarpal compartment (*black arrow*). The capitate is proximally migrated into a markedly widened scapholunate interval. Note the large intraosseous cysts in the capitate and hamate.

pyrophosphate arthropathy in the elbow include joint space narrowing, subchondral sclerosis, and cyst formation, as well as osseous resorption in the proximal radius and ulna. Surrounding bursae about the elbow, including the olecranon and bicipitoradial (cubital) bursa, can contain CPPD crystals.[2-7,24] Tumoral CPPD or "tophaceous pseudogout" has been reported in the elbow.[25] Depending on the specific location, cases of cubital tunnel syndrome[26] and posterior interosseous nerve entrapment have been described.[27]

HIP

Chondrocalcinosis affecting both the fibrocartilage of the acetabular labrum and the hyaline articular cartilage of the femoroacetabular joint can be seen as well as capsular and synovial calcifications. The fibrocartilaginous deposits can present as small radiodensities along the periphery of the superolateral aspect of the acetabulum (Fig. 25-7). The deposits along the articular hyaline cartilage can present as a radiodense curvilinear line that parallels the femoral head but is separated from the subchondral bone plate.[2-7] Surrounding tendons, including the rectus femoris, hamstrings, and adductor insertion, may also calcify.[2-7,28] CPPD crystals can deposit in the surrounding bursae of the hip including the trochanteric bursa.[29] The initial structural changes in CPPD-related arthropathy of the hip can resemble osteoarthritis, with subchondral sclerosis, lateral osteophyte formation, and joint space narrowing in the superolateral aspect of the joint.

However, concentric joint narrowing with axial migration can also occur, mimicking the appearance of an inflammatory arthropathy such as rheumatoid arthritis.[2-7] A pattern of rapid and extensive destruction of the hip has been described, and although its cause is not entirely clear, some of the cases may be related to CPPD crystal deposition disease[30,31]

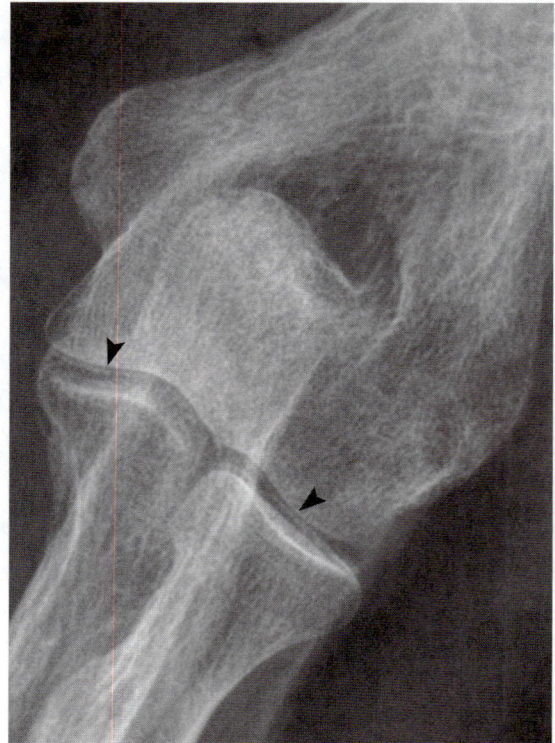

Figure 25-6 CPPD crystal deposition of the elbow. Frontal radiograph of the elbow demonstrates the linear and punctate nature of the crystal deposits of CPPD along the hyaline articular cartilage of the radiocapitellar and ulnotrochlear compartments of the elbow joint (*black arrowheads*).

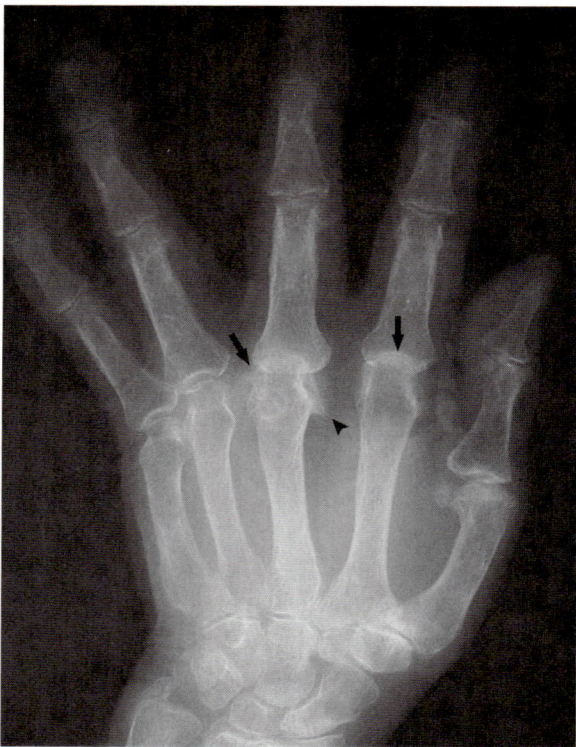

Figure 25-5 Pyrophosphate arthropathy of the hand. Posteroanterior radiograph of the hand shows the predilection of the structural joint changes in this specific arthropathy for the second and third metacarpophalangeal joints manifested mainly by severe joint space narrowing and subchondral sclerosis (*black arrows*). Note the bone proliferation including a hooklike osteophyte on the radial aspect of the head of the third metacarpal (*black arrowhead*). No discernible chondrocalcinosis is seen.

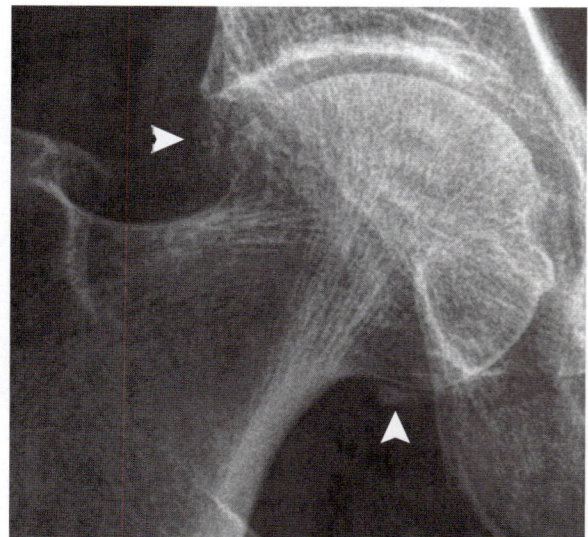

Figure 25-7 CPPD crystal deposition of the hip. Frontal radiograph of the hip shows the deposits of CPPD along the fibrocartilage of the acetabular labrum and along the capsule of the hip joint (*white arrowheads*).

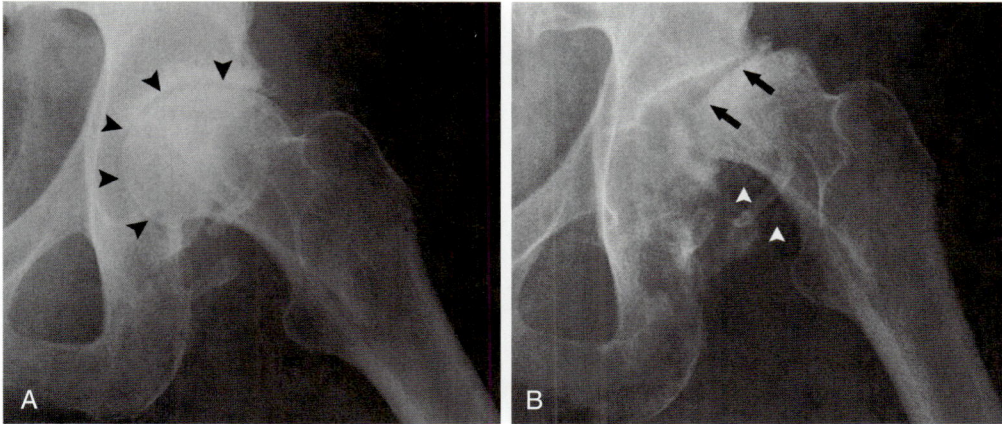

Figure 25-8 Pyrophosphate arthropathy of the hip. **A,** Frog leg lateral view of the hip shows concentric joint space narrowing and subchondral sclerosis (*black arrowheads*). **B,** Frog leg lateral view of the hip on the same patient obtained 3 months after shows the rapid destructive nature of this arthropathy with flattening of the femoral head (*black arrows*) and remodeling of the acetabulum. Multiple faint intracapsular densities (*white arrowheads*) likely correspond to the multiple deposits of CPPD crystals documented after fluid aspiration. There was no evidence of infection or neoplastic cells.

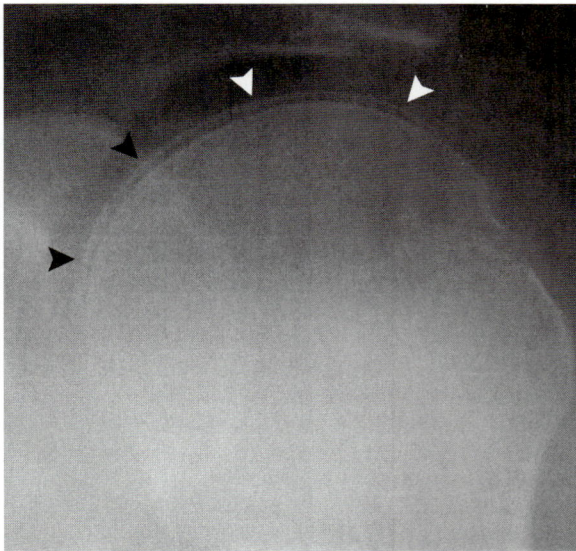

Figure 25-9 CPPD crystal deposition of the shoulder. Frontal radiograph of the shoulder demonstrates the linear nature of the deposits of CPPD along the hyaline cartilage of the glenohumeral joint paralleling the articular surface of the humeral head (*arrowheads*).

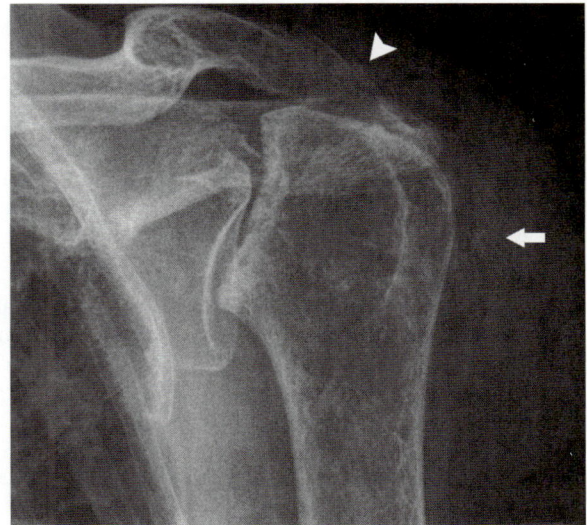

Figure 25-10 Pyrophosphate arthropathy of the shoulder. Radiograph of the shoulder shows the destructive changes with remodeling of the humeral head, which also appears superiorly migrated with respect to the glenoid due to rotator cuff tear. Other changes of rotator cuff arthropathy include the remodeling on the undersurface of the acromion. There are calcifications in the region of the subdeltoid bursa likely corresponding to crystal deposits (*white arrow*). Note the CPPD deposition also at the level of the acromioclavicular joint (*white arrowhead*).

(Fig. 25-8). Cases of tumoral CPPD have also been reported about the hip.[32,33]

SHOULDER

Chondrocalcinosis affecting both the fibrocartilage of the glenoid labrum and the hyaline articular cartilage of the glenohumeral joint can be seen as well as capsular, tendinous, and bursal calcifications. The deposits along the articular hyaline cartilage can present as a radiodense curvilinear line that parallels the humeral head but is separated from the subchondral bone plate (Fig. 25-9). Rotator cuff tears are common in patients with CPPD crystal deposition disease. The structural changes can resemble degenerative joint disease with joint space narrowing, bony eburnation, cysts, and osteophyte formation.[2-7] Similar to the hip, a pattern of advanced destructive changes

may be occasionally apparent[34] (Fig. 25-10). Whether CPPD has a role in the Milwaukee shoulder syndrome (discussed later in this chapter) is controversial and not entirely clear. While CPPD crystals have been found in patients with Milwaukee shoulder, other crystals have also been detected. Some authors believe that the structural joint damage is more related to BCP crystals. Milwaukee shoulder syndrome probably represents a severe example of mixed BCP crystal deposition.[35-38]

In addition to the glenohumeral joint, the acromioclavicular joint can also be affected in patients with CPPD crystal deposition disease about the shoulder. Calcification is most common in the articular disc; however, calcified

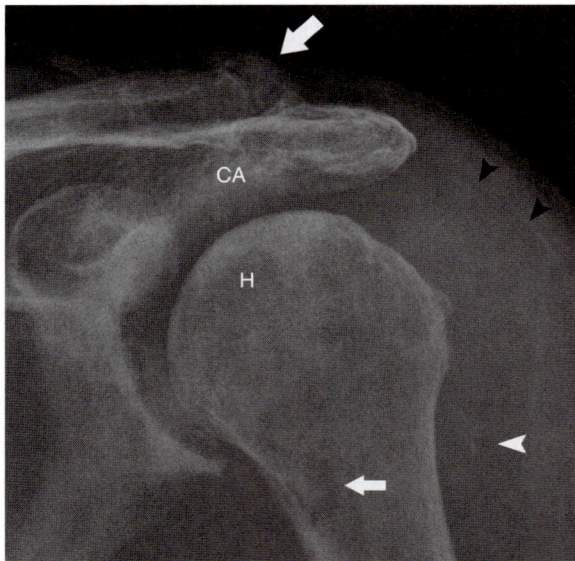

Figure 25-11 CPPD crystal deposition of the acromioclavicular joint. Radiograph of the shoulder demonstrates a calcified masslike deposit of CPPD intimate with the acromioclavicular joint (*white arrow*). Note the changes of rotator cuff arthropathy including femoralization of the humeral head (*H*) and acetabularization of the coracoacromial arch (*CA*) as well as an excavation on the medial cortex of the proximal humerus (*white arrow*) likely due to an erosion-like phenomenon related to the superior migration of the humerus with respect to the glenoid. There is a large effusion that has decompressed into the subacromial-subdeltoid bursa (*black arrowheads*) with punctate calcifications within it (*white arrowhead*) likely corresponding to deposits of crystals.

deposits above the joint can be seen as well as adjacent calcified or cystic masses intimate with the acromioclavicular joint (Fig. 25-11). The joint itself can exhibit arthropathic structural changes and destruction.[39-43]

ANKLE AND FOOT

CPPD crystal deposition disease in the ankle and foot is not that common and pyrophosphate arthropathy in these sites is somewhat unusual. However, the structural joint changes, when present, have a predilection for the talocalcaneonavicular joint[2-7] (Fig. 25-12). Calcifications along the Achilles tendon and plantar fascia can be seen.[44] Capsular calcification may be seen in the forefoot, particularly about the metatarsophalangeal joints. Periarticular calcification and soft tissue swelling medial to the first metatarsophalangeal joint can simulate the changes of gout both radiographically and clinically. However, in some of these cases, the absence of adjacent bone erosion may allow a more accurate differentiation.[2-7,45]

NECK AND SPINE

CPPD crystal deposition disease of the spine is usually asymptomatic; many patients are elderly and have underlying degenerative disease of the spine. However, CPPD crystal deposition by itself can produce severe degenerative disc disease. Moreover, the spine may be the only site affected by CPPD crystal deposition disease. The arthropathy can be so severe and destructive that it can simulate infectious discitis or neuropathic arthropathy.

Calcification of the nucleus pulposus usually appears first in the outer fibers; because of this location, such calcific

deposits may resemble the slender and vertically oriented syndesmophytes of ankylosing spondylitis. Although not that frequent, calcification in the nucleus pulposus can occasionally occur, particularly in patients with a genetic predisposition to this disease. In these patients, the overall appearance of disc calcification can resemble that seen in ochronosis.[2-7] CPPD crystals may deposit in other spinal tissues such as the ligamentum flavum, the posterior longitudinal ligament, the interspinous and supraspinous ligaments, and the interspinous bursae. Furthermore, such deposits lead to myelopathy, cord compression, and spinal stenosis.[2-7,46-49]

CPPD crystal deposition in the spinous tissues, for instance along the ligamentum flavum, can be detected with CT and MR imaging.[50,51] Cross-sectional techniques are also ideal for assessment of patients with calcifications about the odontoid process in the area of the transverse and alar ligaments, the "crowned dens syndrome" (Fig. 25-13). Moreover, depending on the size of the deposits, which can be tumor-like, complications such as spinal cord compression, myelopathy, atlantoaxial subluxation, and spontaneous fractures of the odontoid can occur.[2-7,52-57]

SACROILIAC JOINTS AND SYMPHYSIS PUBIS

Calcification is common in the fibrocartilage of the symphysis pubis (Fig. 25-14). In addition to the chondrocalcinosis, severe erosive changes and fragmentation can occasionally be seen in this joint.[2-7] Structural changes in the sacroiliac joints have been identified in approximately 45% to 50% of the patients with CPPD crystal deposition disease.[58] Such changes include articular calcifications, vacuum phenomena, subchondral erosions, sclerosis, and cyst formation.[2-7] Calcification of the interosseous sacroiliac ligament also has been observed.[46]

TEMPOROMANDIBULAR JOINT

Although uncommon, CPPD crystal deposition disease has been reported in the temporomandibular joints. The crystals can deposit in the fibrocartilage disc. However these calcified deposits can become quite large and tumor-like, and aggressive features such as large erosions and osseous destruction can be seen. Patients can present with preauricular swelling; these tumoral CPPD deposits can mimic external ear canal or parotid tumors on clinical examination[2-7,59-63] (Fig. 25-15).

Differential Diagnosis

CPPD can be sporadic (idiopathic) or associated with other disorders. Differentiation of the nonsporadic cases depends on the presence of features suggestive of the underlying condition associated with CPPD. Some of these conditions include primary hyperparathyroidism, hemochromatosis, hemosiderosis, hypophosphatasia, hypomagnesemia, hypothyroidism, gout, amyloidosis, ochronosis, and Wilson disease, among others.[2-7]

Other conditions that can simulate CPPD crystal deposition disease radiographically include osteoarthritis, neuropathic osteoarthropathy, synovial osteochondromatosis, HADD, septic arthritis, gout, osteonecrosis, and inflammatory arthritides.

Radiographic features that aid in distinguishing CPPD crystal deposition disease from primary osteoarthritis include local calcification and chondrocalcinosis, large subchondral cystlike lucencies, extensive sclerosis, collapse and fragmentation of joint surfaces, variable osteophyte formation, lack of erosion, and osseous debris. Particularly, the involvement of

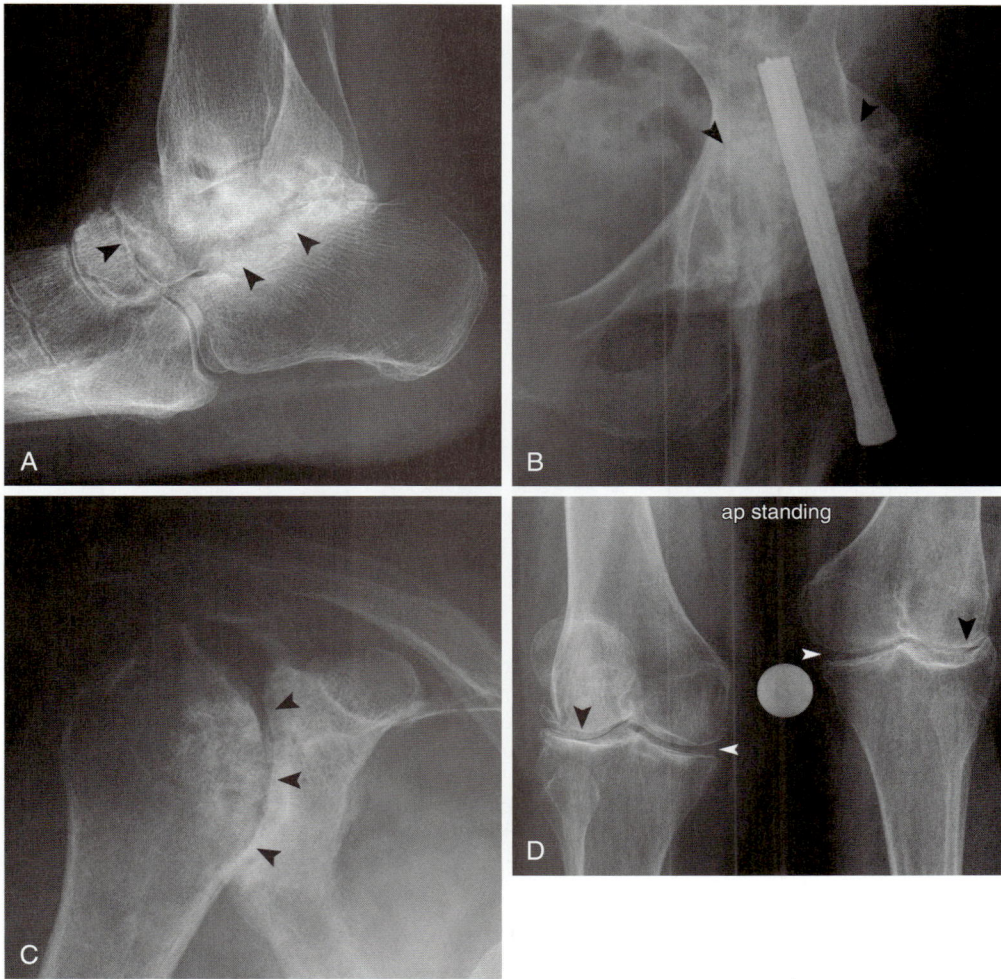

Figure 25-12 A, Pyrophosphate arthropathy of the ankle. Lateral radiograph of the ankle shows severe structural changes along the talocalcaneonavicular joint (*black arrowheads*). **B,** Pyrophosphate arthropathy of the hip. Frontal radiograph of the hip on the same patient demonstrates severe structural changes in the femoroacetabular joint with obliteration of the joint space, destruction and remodeling of the acetabulum and proximal femur (*black arrowheads*) in this patient with attempted fusion of the femoroacetabular joint. **C,** Pyrophosphate arthropathy of the shoulder. Frontal radiograph of the shoulder on the same patient shows severe structural changes in the glenohumeral joint (*black arrowheads*). **D,** Pyrophosphate arthropathy of the knees. Frontal radiograph of both knees shows evidence of chondrocalcinosis (*white arrowheads*) and bilateral structural knee joint changes that were more conspicuous on the patellofemoral (not shown) and lateral femorotibial compartments on both knees (*black arrowheads*).

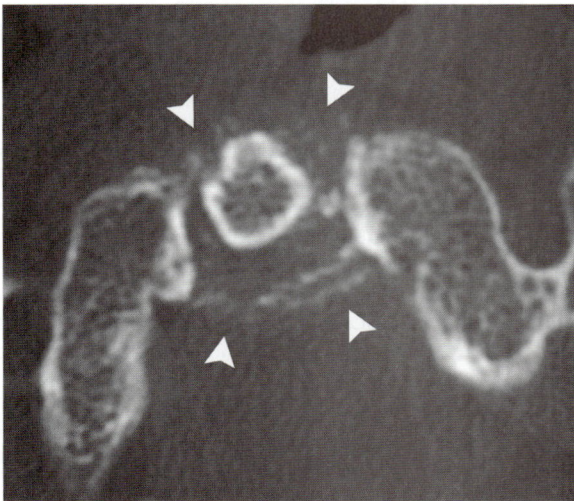

Figure 25-13 CPPD crystal deposition of the atlantoaxial joint. Axial CT image shows multiple deposits of CPPD crystals posterior to the odontoid along the transverse and alar ligaments as well as in the anterior aspect of the C1-C2 interval (*arrowheads*).

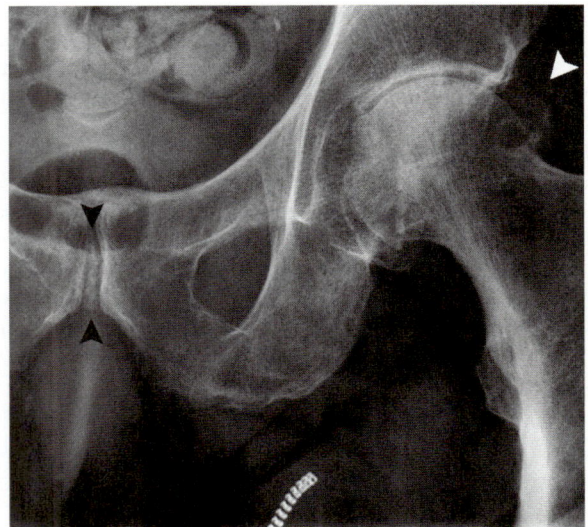

Figure 25-14 CPPD crystal deposition of the symphysis pubis. Frontal radiograph of the pelvis shows crystal deposits along the symphysis pubis (*black arrowheads*) as well on the left hip (*white arrowheads*).

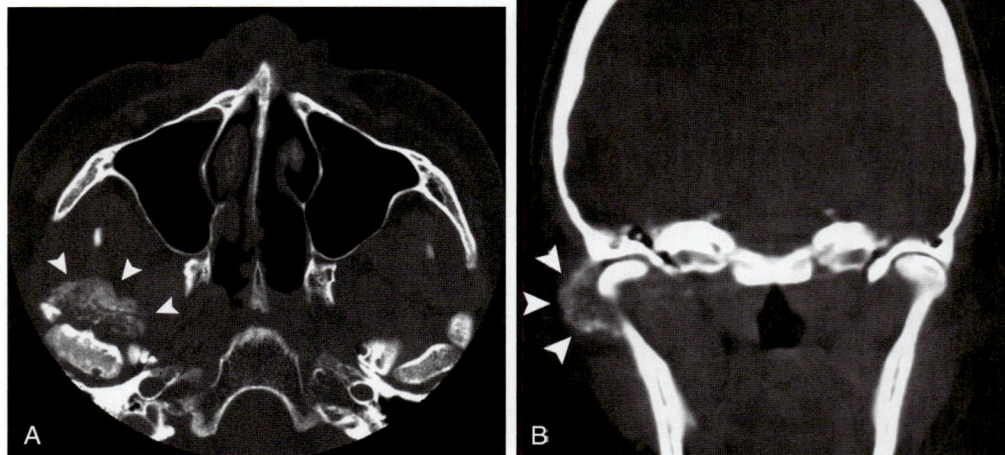

Figure 25-15 CPPD crystal deposition of the temporomandibular joint. **A,** Axial CT image shows large deposit of crystals of CPPD intimate with the right temporomandibular joint (*white arrowheads*). **B,** Coronal CT reconstruction on a different patient also demonstrates deposits of crystals of CPPD intimate with the right temporomandibular joint (*white arrowheads*).

joints or components of joints that are not commonly affected by osteoarthritis is a very useful feature for this distinction.[2-7]

The calcifications in HADD are more homogeneous or cloudlike, and chondrocalcinosis is not nearly as common as seen in CPPD crystal deposition disease.

Regarding pyrophosphate arthropathy, as indicated previously, unusual joint and compartment involvement is key. In the setting of severe structural joint abnormality, osseous density is usually preserved in neuropathic arthropathy, whereas this finding may not be true in CPPD crystal deposition disease.[2-7]

Bone erosion is not a typical feature of CPPD crystal deposition disease; hence, the absence of erosive changes usually helps in differentiating this condition from rheumatoid arthritis and seronegative spondyloarthropathies. However, in chronic cases, joint erosion may be present and quite severe, simulating rheumatoid arthritis.

Because sepsis may coexist with crystal synovitis in 1% or 2% of cases, sampling of the joint fluid for Gram stain and culture should be undertaken if there is any concern for infection, even if CPPD crystals are identified on plain radiographs or in the joint fluid.[2-7]

The differentiation between CPPD crystal deposition disease and gout may be complicated by the occasional coexistence of these two arthropathies in the same joint or person. The presence of the characteristic "punched-out" or juxtaarticular osseous erosion is useful for diagnosing gouty arthropathy. The lack of chondrocalcinosis in association with periarticular calcification may suggest other causes, such as dystrophic calcification, metastatic calcification, or tumoral calcinosis either primary (idiopathic) or secondary.[2-7]

BCP Crystal Deposition (Here Termed Hydroxyapatite Deposition Disease)

HADD is a relatively common condition if simply characterized by the periarticular deposition of crystals of BCP crystals including hydroxyapatite in the soft tissues about a joint, most commonly in tendons near their osseous attachments. However, deposits in bursae, ligaments, and other periarticular soft tissues can also occur. Less commonly, such crystals may also be deposited intraarticularly in a grossly detectable manner, either as a primary phenomenon or secondary to another disease. A variety of terms have been used to describe different manifestations of the disease, including "calcific tendinosis," "calcific tendonitis," "calcific periarthritis," "peritendinitis" or "periarthritis calcarea," "apatite arthropathy," and "hydroxyapatite rheumatism."[64-72]

General Imaging Features

PERIARTICULAR CRYSTAL DEPOSITION

Initially on plain radiographs, the deposits of crystals of hydroxyapatite may appear thin, cloudlike, and poorly defined as they blend into the surrounding soft tissues. With time, they may become more ovoid, denser, homogeneous, and more sharply delineated. HADD is not a static process; on the contrary, the dynamic nature of this disease can result in pitfalls in the diagnosis by imaging. Sequential radiographic examinations in patients with such calcific periarticular deposits may reveal different patterns. In some instances, the deposits may not or minimally change in size, morphology, or location, while in others they may enlarge and change in shape or location. Spontaneous reduction in size and disappearance of the deposits are not infrequent either. Reappearance of the deposits has also been documented. CT, with its excellent signal-to-noise ratio and multiplanar imaging capability, demonstrates the periarticular calcifications to better advantage and can optimally characterize underlying bone erosions, a feature that can be seen in patients with HADD. Magnetic resonance imaging, with its excellent soft tissue resolution, can better evaluate the associated soft tissue swelling, edema, joint effusions, and capsule abnormalities about the affected joint.[64-71]

ARTICULAR CRYSTAL DEPOSITION

Intraarticular deposition of crystals of hydroxyapatite can be divided into calcification and structural joint damage or arthropathy.

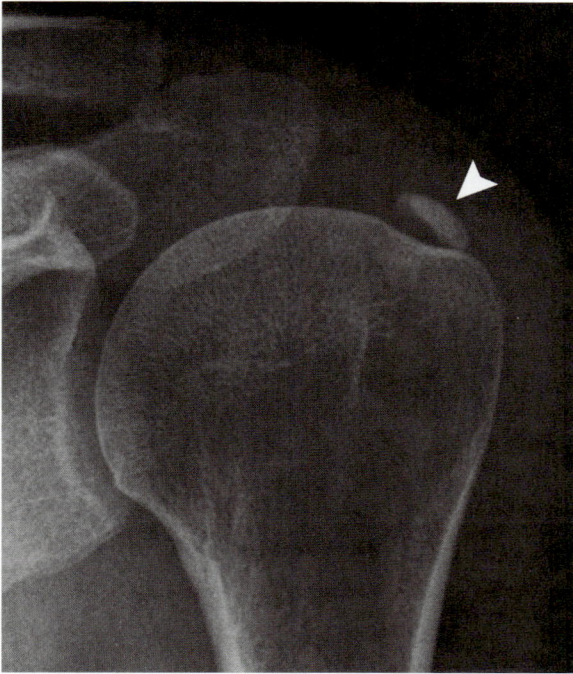

Figure 25-16 Hydroxyapatite deposition of the supraspinatus tendon. Frontal radiograph of the shoulder shows a focus of hydroxyapatite deposition disease in the expected location of the distal aspect of the supraspinatus tendon near its insertion in the horizontal facet of the greater tuberosity (*white arrowhead*).

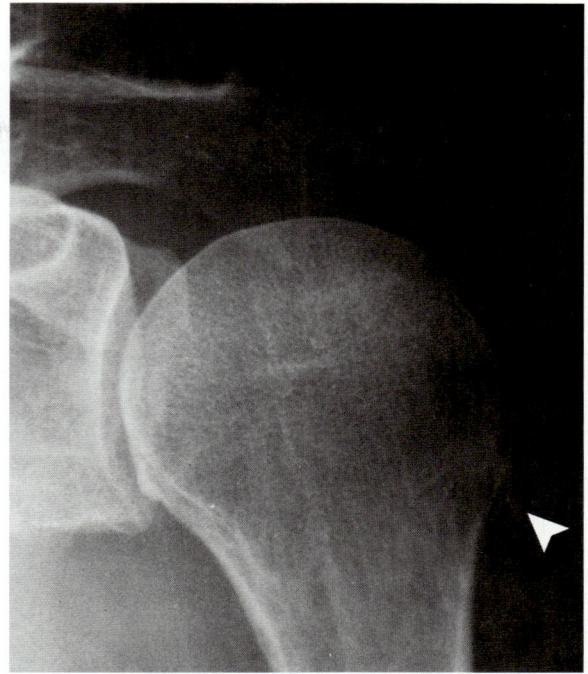

Figure 25-18 Hydroxyapatite deposition of the teres minor tendon. Frontal radiograph of the shoulder shows a focus of HADD in the expected location of the distal aspect of the teres minor tendon near its insertion in the vertical facet of the greater tuberosity (*white arrowhead*).

Gross cartilage calcification has been noted occasionally; however, other patterns of intraarticular calcification are more typical than chondrocalcinosis. For instance, crystal deposition along the synovial membrane or capsule, or both, leading to amorphous or cloudlike radiodensities within a joint, can occur. Of interest, large amounts of crystals of hydroxyapatite can be detected within a joint in the absence of intraarticular calcification.[64,72]

Clinical Milwaukee shoulder syndrome is reviewed in Chapter 22.[35-38] Very similar processes have been described by other investigators including terms such as "cuff tear arthropathy,"[73] "apatite-associated destructive arthritis,"[74] and "apatite-associated arthropathy."[75]

Specific Sites

SHOULDER

The shoulder is the most common site of HADD, accounting for approximately 60% of cases of acute calcific periarthritis. Such periarticular deposits can occur in one or both shoulders in as many as 7.5% of adults.[76] The tendons of the rotator cuff are the most commonly involved and among them the supraspinatus tendon is the most frequent site of hydroxyapatite deposition (Fig. 25-16), followed by the infraspinatus (Fig. 25-17, online only), the teres minor (Fig. 25-18), and the subscapularis (Fig. 25-19, online only). Besides the rotator cuff, calcific deposits can also occur at the origin of the long head of the biceps (Fig. 25-20), origin of the long head of the triceps (Fig. 25-21, online only), the deltoid attachment

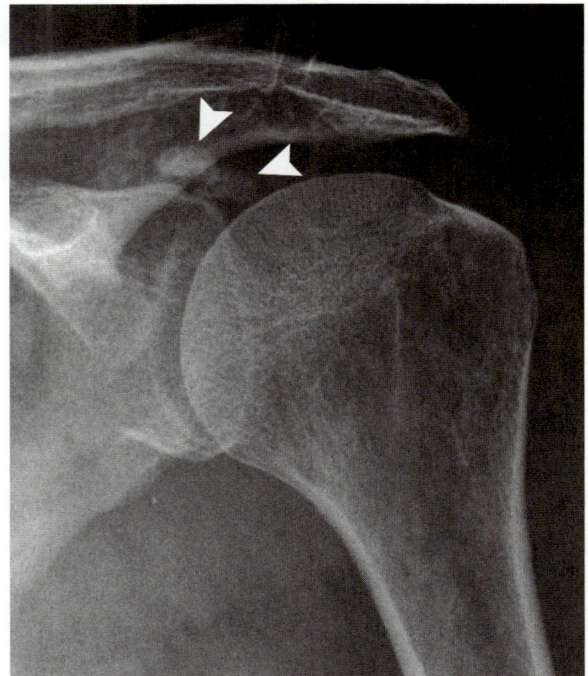

Figure 25-20 Hydroxyapatite deposition of the long head of the biceps tendon. Frontal radiograph of the shoulder shows foci of HADD in the expected location of the proximal aspect of the long head of the biceps tendon near its origin at the level of the supragenoid tubercle (*white arrowheads*).

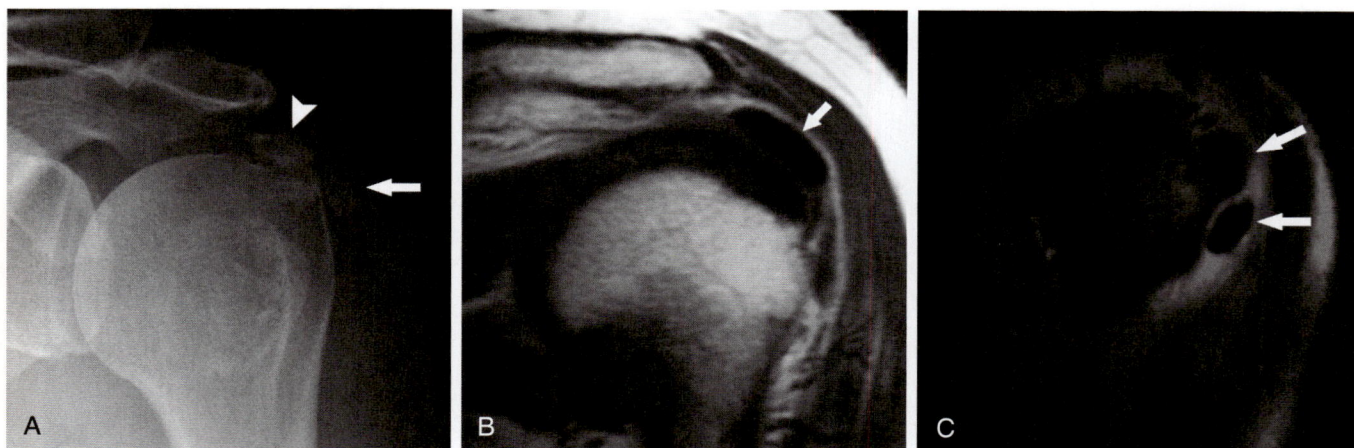

Figure 25-23 Hydroxyapatite deposition of the subacromial-subdeltoid bursa. **A,** Frontal radiograph of the shoulder shows a focus of HADD intimate with the distal aspect of the supraspinatus tendon near or at its footprint in the greater tuberosity (*white arrowhead*). A second focus of HADD appears extruded in the location of the subacromial subdeltoid bursa (*white arrow*). **B,** Coronal intermediate weighted MR image of the shoulder in a different patient shows a focus of HADD outside the rotator cuff tendon in the subacromial-subdeltoid bursal plane (*arrow*). **C,** Sagittal fluid–sensitive MR image of the shoulder in a different patient shows foci of HADD within the subacromial-subdeltoid bursa (*white arrows*).

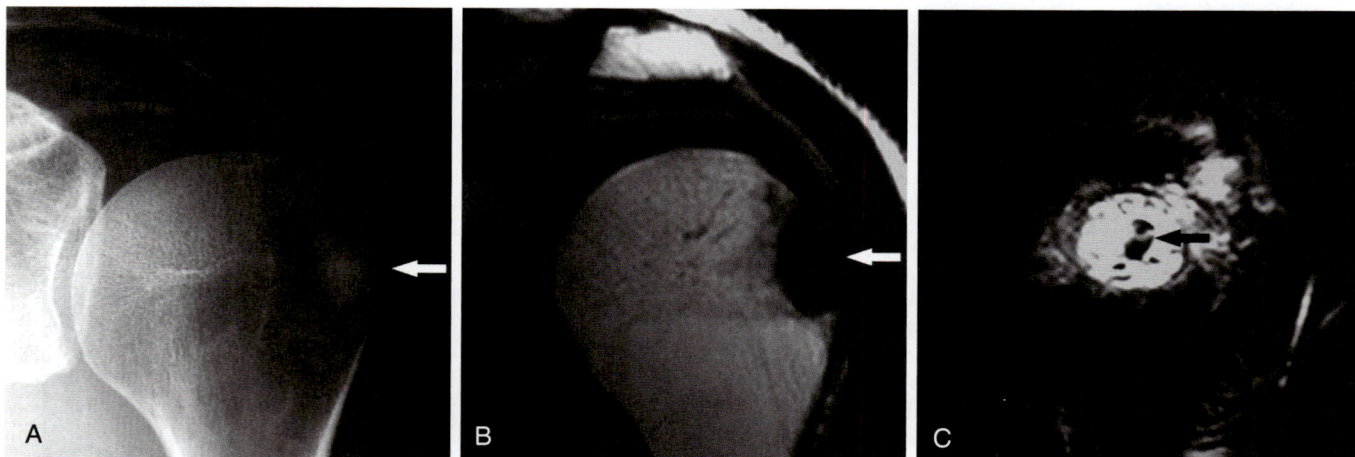

Figure 25-24 Intraosseous focus of hydroxyapatite deposition. **A,** Frontal radiograph of the shoulder shows a focus of HADD projecting on the greater tuberosity of the humeral head (*white arrow*). **B,** Coronal T1W MR image of the shoulder on the same patient confirms the intraosseous loculation of the HADD (*white arrow*). **C,** Sagittal fluid–sensitive MR image of the shoulder on the same patient shows the intraosseous cystic change with the focus of HADD within it (*black arrow*).

to the acromion, insertion of the pectoralis major in the humeral shaft, where associated cortical erosion can be seen (Fig. 25-22, online only).[64-71,77-84]

Moseley has extensively studied the natural history of HADD in the shoulder joint.[85] He reported an initial silent phase in which deposition of hydroxyapatite is completely contained within the involved tendon; this phase is usually asymptomatic. On plain radiographs, this stage corresponds to well-defined, sharply marginated calcifications. During the mechanical phase, there is enlargement of the deposit of hydroxyapatite that may become liquified and can subsequently rupture either into the supraspinatus tendon and collect beneath the subacromial bursa (subbursal rupture) or into the subacromial bursa itself (intrabursal rupture) (Fig. 25-23). This phase is characterized by acute painful attacks. On plain radiographs, this stage corresponds to ill-defined

calcifications. The chronic stage is known as the "adhesive periarthritis phase," in which fibrosis develops in the peritendinous soft tissues. This phase is characterized by chronic pain and restriction of joint motion. Occasionally, extension and loculation of the deposit of hydroxyapatite into the adjacent bone can occur with resultant erosion and cavity formation within the bone including cystic and calcified components of different sizes (Fig. 25-24). Even less commonly, bone marrow edema associated with hydroxyapatite deposition disease may occur even without associated cortical erosion. Such intraosseous loculated deposits of hydroxyapatite can be misinterpreted for an osseous neoplasm if one is not familiar with this appearance or if the imaging chronology is not available. Rarely, a dumbbell deformity of a subacromial bursal deposit of hydroxyapatite can be seen as a result of pressure from the adjacent coracoacromial ligament.[64-71,85-89]

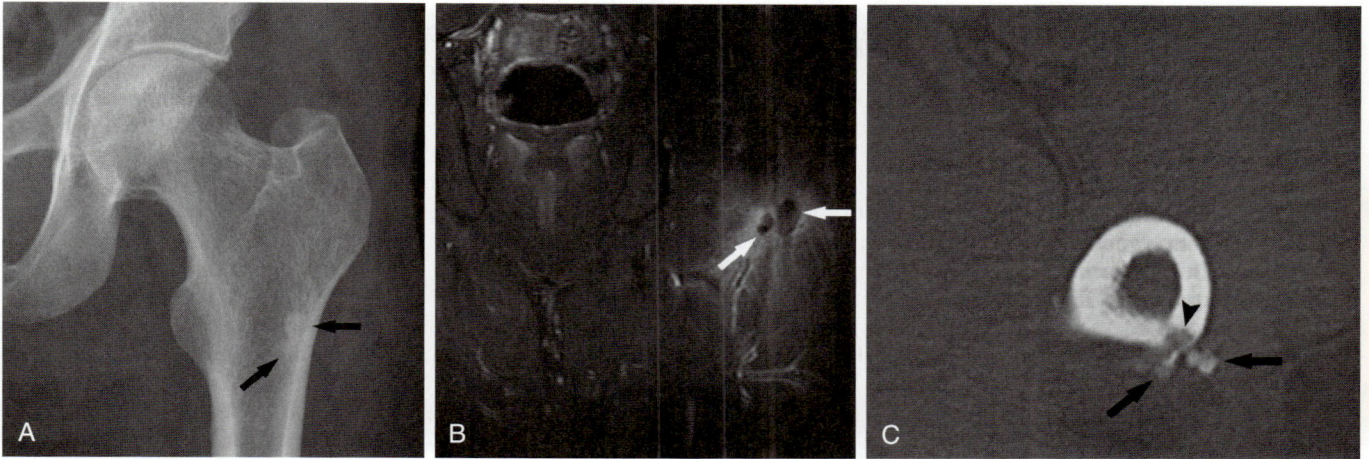

Figure 25-26 Hydroxyapatite deposition of the gluteus maximus tendon. **A,** Frontal radiograph of the hip shows foci of HADD intimate with the distal aspect of the gluteus maximus tendon near its femoral attachment (*black arrows*). **B,** Coronal fluid–sensitive MR image of the hip on the same patient shows the foci of HADD (*white arrows*) and the edema in the surrounding soft tissues. **C,** Axial CT image shows foci of HADD (*black arrows*) intimate with the distal insertion of the gluteus maximus along the posterolateral aspect of the femur with associated cortical irregularity (*black arrowhead*).

HIP

The hip is the second most common site of HADD. The calcific deposits usually occur in the gluteus medius tendon near its insertion in the greater trochanter (Fig. 25-25, online only).[90, 91] More distally, deposits of hydroxyapatite can be seen at the gluteus maximus insertion along the posterolateral aspect of the femoral shaft; erosions at this level are not uncommon (Fig. 25-26).[92,93] Less commonly, nearby deposits of hydroxyapatite can be seen intimate with the vastus lateralis tendon along the femoral shaft.[94] Calcific deposits can also be seen at other sites of tendon attachments in the femur including the iliopsoas tendinous insertion in the lesser trochanter as well as in other sites in the pelvis, such as at the hamstring origins along the ischium (Fig. 25-27, online only), at the attachment of the adductor brevis, and at the origin of the rectus femoris (Fig. 25-28, online only), among others.[95-98] Occasionally, deposits of hydroxyapatite can be seen along the capsule and capsular ligaments such as the iliofemoral ligament[99] as well as in the region of the ligamentum teres.[100] Last, involvement of the bursae about the hip can occur; for example, deposits in the region of the trochanteric bursa can be seen with associated bursitis.

ELBOW

Deposits of hydroxyapatite can be seen intimate with the origin of the flexor and extensor tendons adjacent to the humeral epicondyles (Fig. 25-29) and along the medial and lateral collateral ligaments. Such deposits may also be seen at the brachialis, biceps, and triceps tendon attachments on the ulnar tuberosity, radial tuberosity, and olecranon, respectively (Fig. 25-30, B, online only). Calcifications in the region of the olecranon bursa have also been described.[101-105]

WRIST AND HAND

Calcific deposits of hydroxyapatite are seen in the periarticular structures of the wrist and hand namely along tendons and ligaments. The wrist is more frequently involved than the hand, and the most common site of hydroxyapatite deposition is along the flexor carpi ulnaris tendon near

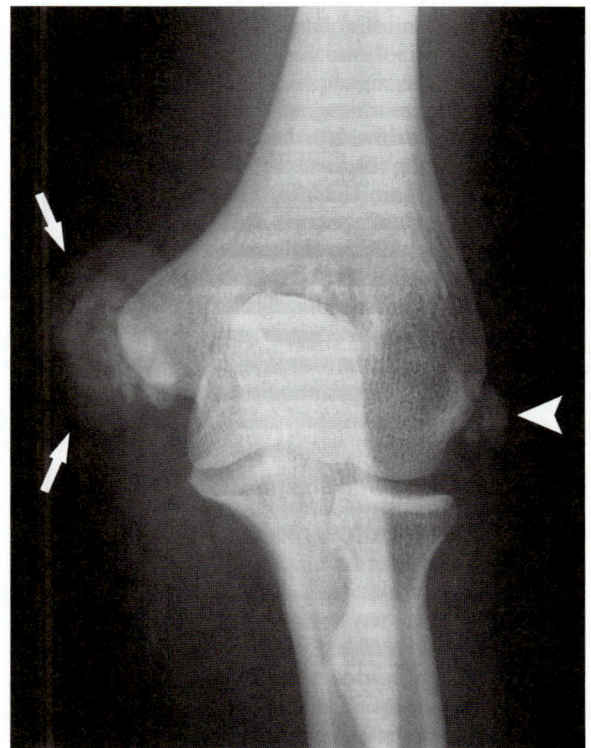

Figure 25-29 Hydroxyapatite deposition of the common flexor and extensor tendon groups. Frontal radiograph of the elbow shows large deposits of hydroxyapatite in the soft tissues intimate with the origin of the common flexor-pronator tendon group on the medial epicondyle (*white arrows*). Smaller deposits of hydroxyapatite are seen in the soft tissues intimate with the origin of the common extensor tendon group on the lateral epicondyle of the humerus (*white arrowhead*).

its attachment to the pisiform (Fig. 25-31).[106-110] Cases of carpal tunnel syndrome associated with HADD have been reported.[111,112] Calcific deposits are also common around the metacarpophalangeal and interphalangeal joints (Fig. 25-32).

KNEE

HADD about the knee has been described with the calcifications being most commonly located adjacent to the femoral condyles, fibular head, and prepatellar region. Calcific deposits intimate with the medial collateral ligament (Fig. 25-33) and lateral collateral ligament (Fig. 25-34) have been reported, as have deposits on the popliteus tendon and quadriceps tendon.[113-119]

ANKLE AND FOOT

Calcific deposits may be occasionally seen about the ankle and foot. HADD has been described in the peroneus longus, flexor hallucis longus, and brevis tendons.[120-123] At the first metatarsophalangeal joint, HADD can cause a clinical picture that can be confused with gout including pain and swelling, the so-called hydroxyapatite pseudopodagra, typically affecting young patients, especially women[124-127] (Fig. 25-35, online only).

NECK AND SPINE

HADD in the neck typically occurs along the longus colli muscle and tendon; tendinosis and peritendinitis in this region may result in acute, severe neck and occipital pain and rigidity, and the symptoms are exacerbated by swallowing and head movement. Radiography and CT can show the calcific deposits to a better extent, while MR imaging can show the degree of edema in the adjacent soft tissues (Fig. 25-36).[128-130]

Calcifications can also occur elsewhere in the spine, including the ligamentum flavum, apophyseal joints, interspinous bursae, infraoccipital region, and around the odontoid process.[64] Actually, in addition to CPPD, HADD is another cause of the so-called "crowned dens syndrome."[131]

Differential Diagnosis

The characteristic homogeneous cloudlike appearance of HADD distinguishes it from other disorders that can be also associated with periarticular calcifications. Moreover, finding calcific deposits in the above-mentioned specific sites favored by HADD also helps to separate this entity from others. HADD can be confused sometimes with gout due to radiographic and clinical similarities. However, gouty tophi are frequently more faintly calcified; in addition, other characteristics of gout such as the typical erosions are not usually present with HADD. HADD should not be confused with the more linear, punctate and diffuse CPPD crystal calcifications. Of note, HADD and CPPD can coexist in the same joint (see later discussion). Periarticular deposits of tumoral calcinosis, either primary (idiopathic) or secondary may mimic HADD, particularly if such deposits are small. Heterotopic

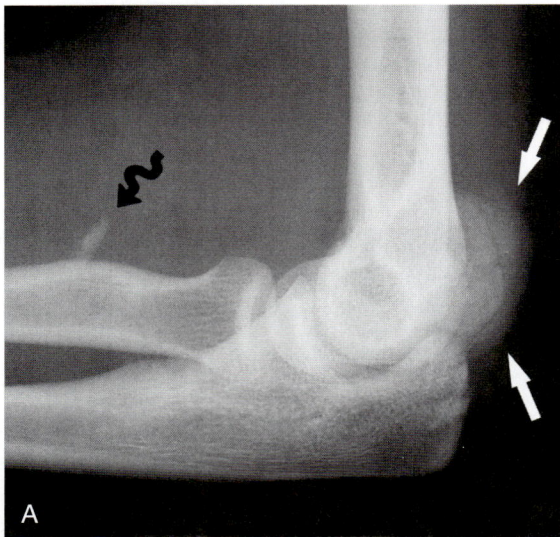

Figure 25-30 **A,** Hydroxyapatite deposition of the distal biceps insertion. Lateral radiograph of the elbow in the same patient on Fig. 25-29 shows a focus of HADD intimate with the distal aspect of the biceps tendon near or at its insertion in the radial tuberosity (*serpentine black arrow*). The larger foci of HADD intimate with the origin of the common flexor-pronator tendon group are redemonstrated (*white arrows*).

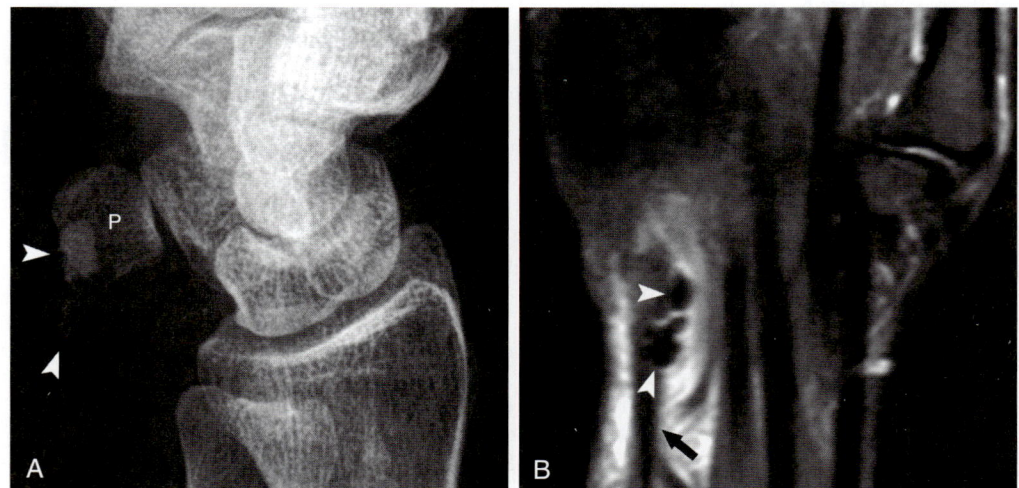

Figure 25-31 Hydroxyapatite deposition of the flexor carpi ulnaris tendon. **A,** Lateral radiograph of the wrist shows foci of HADD (*white arrowheads*) intimate with the distal aspect of the flexor carpi ulnaris tendon near or at its insertion in the pisiform (*P*). **B,** Coronal fluid–sensitive MR image of the wrist on the same patient shows the foci of HADD (*white arrowheads*) intimate with the distal aspect of the flexor carpi ulnaris tendon (*black arrow*). Note the edema in the surrounding soft tissues.

bone and myositis ossificans can be distinguished from HADD due to the trabecular pattern and cortical rim that can be seen in the former two conditions. Collagen vascular diseases such as scleroderma and dermatomyositis can have widespread calcifications in the subcutaneous tissues that help in its differentiation. Periarticular calcifications may also be seen in sarcoidosis, hypoparathyroidism, hyperparathyroidism and renal osteodystrophy, hypervitaminosis D, and milk-alkali syndrome, among others.[64]

Mixed Calcium Crystal Deposition

The coexistence of both HADD and CPPD crystals has been documented in joint tissues (see Chapter 22). The recognition of such mixed crystal deposition can be difficult. Calcification within or outside a joint can be seen in both entities, although subtle differences can be seen in the pattern of calcification, calcific deposits in synovium, capsule, and tendon are common to both diseases. The tendon calcifications in CPPD may appear more diffuse and elongated than those seen with HADD. Another clue is provided by the pattern of chondrocalcinosis, which, when widespread, is much more characteristic of CPPD than HADD. On the other hand, diffuse amorphous calcifications within a joint are more typical of HADD. The presence of both disorders coexisting in the same region should be suspected if plain radiographs demonstrate extensive chondrocalcinosis, indicative of CPPD, and diffuse capsular calcification or dense homogeneous calcific deposits at tendinous attachments, indicative of HADD.[64,132-134] Intraarticular CPPD crystal deposition is common in osteoarthritis, often found together with BCP crystals. Of note, triple crystal disease has been documented (crystals of monosodium urate monohydrate, CPPD, and BCP[135]).

The Milwaukee shoulder syndrome and its manifestations in additional joints probably represent examples of mixed calcium phosphate crystal deposition (Figs. 25-37 and 25-38). In these patients, hydroxyapatite as well as other BCP crystals such as octacalcium phosphate and tricalcium phosphate are identified within the joint, and CPPD crystals are sometimes recovered within the same joint or in other joints. The differential diagnosis for the severe and extensive resultant arthropathy includes other conditions such as neuropathic arthropathy, avascular necrosis, and infection.[35-38]

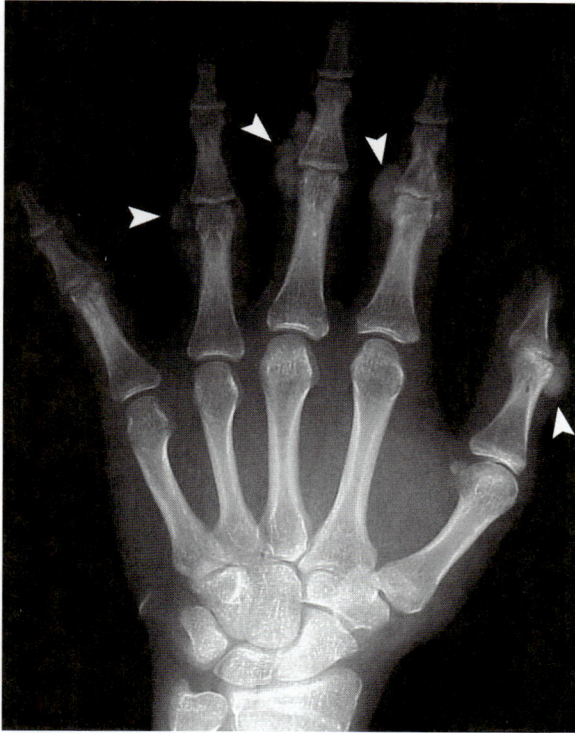

Figure 25-32 Hydroxyapatite deposition in fingers. Posteroanterior radiograph of the hand shows multiple foci of HADD at the level of the second, third, and fourth proximal interphalangeal joints as well as at the level of the interphalangeal joint of the thumb (*white arrowheads*).

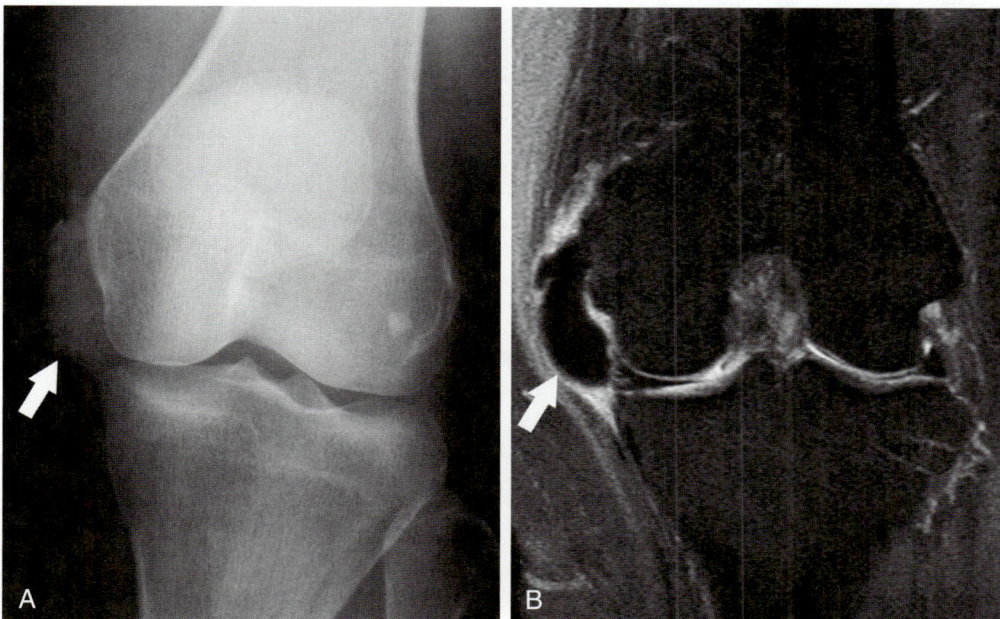

Figure 25-33 Hydroxyapatite deposition of the medial collateral ligament complex. **A,** Frontal radiograph of the knee shows foci of HADD in the soft tissues intimate with the proximal aspect of the medial collateral ligament complex (*white arrow*). **B,** Coronal fluid–sensitive MR image of the knee shows the HADD with some edema in the adjacent soft tissues (*white arrow*).

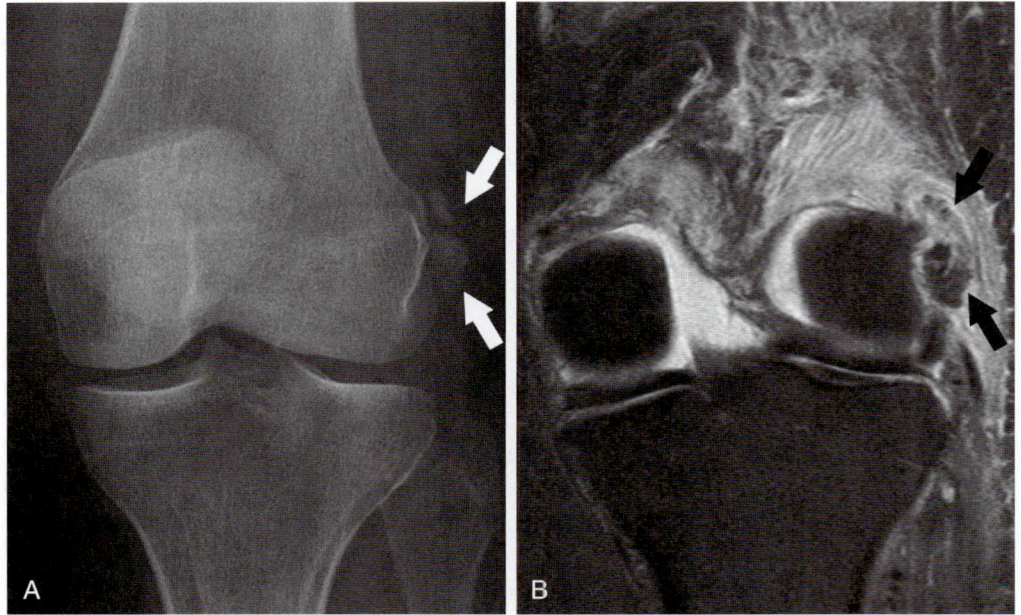

Figure   25-34 Hydroxyapatite deposition of the lateral collateral ligament complex. **A,** Frontal radiograph of the knee shows foci of HADD in the soft tissues intimate with the proximal aspect of the lateral collateral ligament complex (*white arrows*). **B,** Coronal fluid–sensitive MR image of the knee shows the HADD (*black arrows*) with significant amount of edema in the adjacent soft tissues.

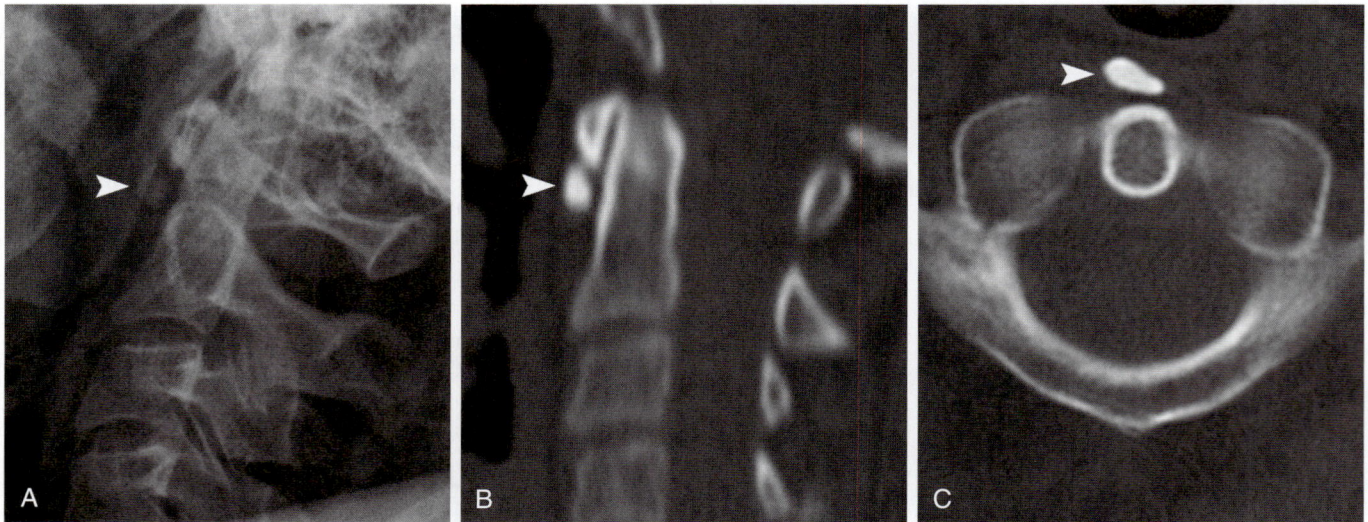

Figure 25-36 Hydroxyapatite deposition of longus colli. **A,** Lateral radiograph of the neck shows a focus of HADD in the preodontoid soft tissues in the expected location of the longus colli muscle (*white arrowhead*). Sagittal (**B**) and axial (**C**) CT images show in a better extent the focus of HADD within the longus colli muscle (*white arrowheads*).

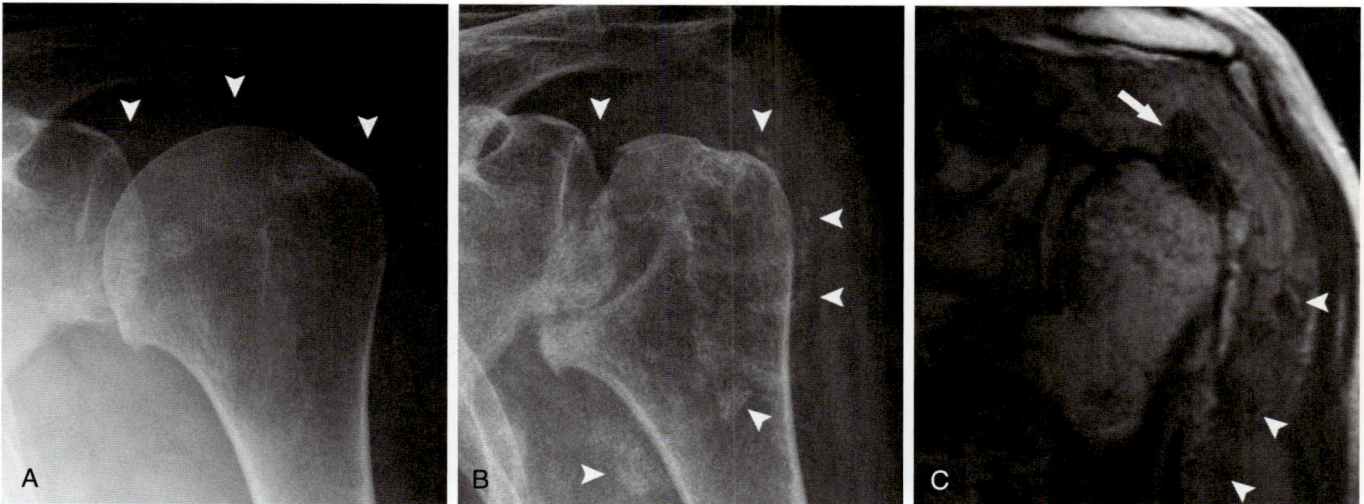

Figure 25-37 Milwaukee shoulder. **A,** Frontal radiograph of the shoulder shows faint calcifications in the soft tissue about the humeral head (*white arrowheads*). There are mild degenerative changes on the glenohumeral joint. Follow-up frontal radiograph of the shoulder on the same patient shows extensive destructive structural changes on the glenohumeral joint with severe remodeling of the humeral head and widespread calcifications (*arrowheads*) corresponding to abundant basic calcium phosphate crystals documented after fluid aspiration. **C,** Coronal intermediate weighted sequence on the same patient shows in a better extent the structural damage of the glenohumeral joint as well as a torn rotator cuff (*white arrow*), large amount of fluid in the subacromial subdeltoid bursa with multiple areas of low signal within it likely corresponding to deposits of basic calcium phosphate crystals (*white arrowheads*).

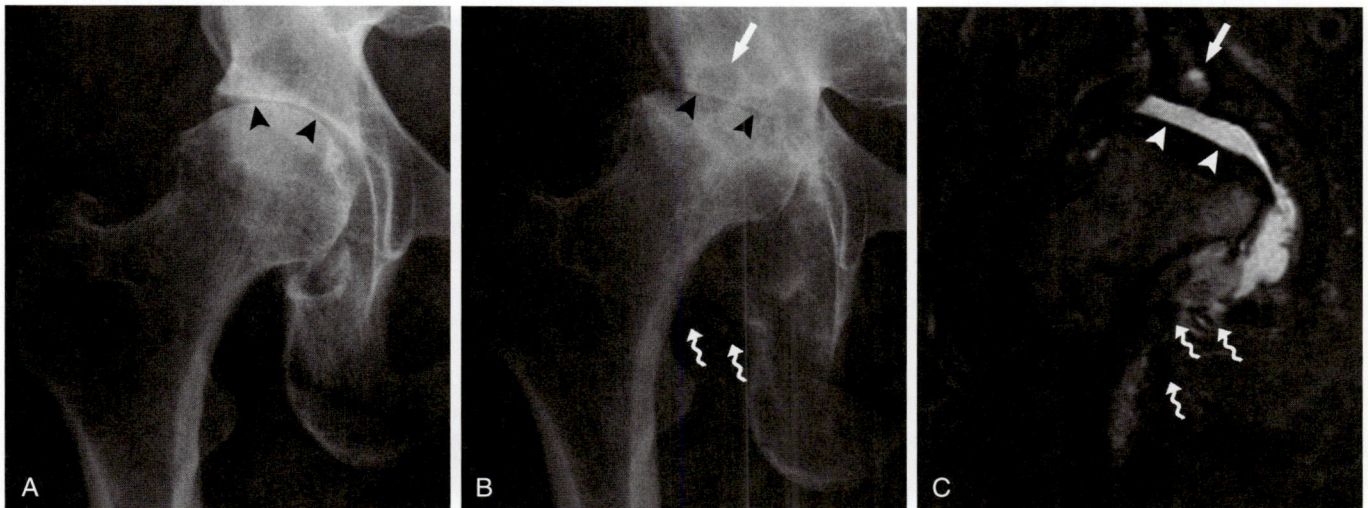

Figure 25-38 Milwaukee hip. **A,** Frontal radiograph of the hip shows joint space narrowing (*black arrowheads*) as well as collar-like proliferative changes and osteophyte formation along the femoral head neck junction. **B,** Follow-up frontal radiograph of the hip on the same patient shows the rapid and extensive nature of the process with flattening and remodeling of the femoral head (*black arrowheads*) and the acetabulum with intraosseous cyst formation (*white arrow*). Calcifications are seen inferomedially likely corresponding to abundant basic calcium phosphate crystals documented after fluid aspiration (*serpentine white arrows*). **C,** Coronal intermediate weighted sequence on the same patient shows in a better extent the structural damage of the femoroacetabular joint including the flattening of the femoral head (*white arrowheads*) and the remodeling of the acetabulum with intraosseous cyst formation (*white arrow*). There is a joint effusion with some areas of low signal inferomedially likely corresponding to deposits of basic calcium phosphate crystals (*serpentine white arrows*).

References

1. Zhang W, Doherty M, Bardin T, et al. European League Against Rheumatism recommendations for calcium pyrophosphate deposition. Part I: terminology and diagnosis. Ann Rheum Dis 2011 Jan 7. [Epub ahead of print].

2. Resnick D. Calcium pyrophosphate dihydrate crystal deposition disease. In: Resnick D, editor. Diagnosis of Bone and Joint Disorders. Vol. 2. 4th ed. Philadelphia: Saunders; 2002:1560–618.

3. Resnick D, Niwayama G, Goergen TG, et al. Clinical, radiographic and pathologic abnormalities in calcium pyrophosphate dihydrate deposition disease (CPPD): pseudogout. Radiology 1977;122(1):1–5.

4. Resnik CS, Resnick D. Crystal deposition disease. Semin Arthritis Rheum 1983;12(4):390–403.

5. Steinbach LS, Resnick D. Calcium pyrophosphate dihydrate crystal deposition disease revisited. Radiology 1996;200(1):1–9.

6. Steinbach LS, Resnick D. Calcium pyrophosphate dihydrate crystal deposition disease: imaging perspectives. Curr Probl Diagn Radiol 2000;29(6):209–29.

7. Steinbach LS. Calcium pyrophosphate dihydrate and calcium hydroxyapatite crystal deposition diseases: imaging perspectives. Radiol Clin North Am 2004;42(1):185–205.

8. Brunot S, Fabre T, Lepreux S, et al. Pseudotumoral presentation of calcium pyrophosphate dihydrate crystal deposition disease. J Rheumatol 2008;35(4):727–9.

9. Yang BY, Sartoris DJ, Resnick D, et al. Calcium pyrophosphate dihydrate crystal deposition disease: frequency of tendon calcification about the knee. J Rheumatol 1996;23(5):883–8.

10. Abreu M, Johnson K, Chung CB, et al. Calcification in calcium pyrophosphate dihydrate (CPPD) crystalline deposits in the knee: anatomic, radiographic, MR imaging, and histologic study in cadavers. Skeletal Radiol 2004;33(7):392–8.

11. Kato H, Nishimoto K, Yoshikawa T, et al. Tophaceous pseudogout in the knee joint mimicking a soft-tissue tumour: a case report. J Orthop Surg (Hong Kong) 2010;18(1):118–21.

12. Handy JR. Pyrophosphate arthropathy in the knees of elderly persons. Arch Intern Med 1996; 25;156(21):2426–32.

13. Lagier R. Femoral cortical erosions and osteoarthrosis of the knee with chondrocalcinosis. An anatomo-radiological study of two cases. ROFO 1974;120(4):460–7.

14. Kwak SM, Resnick D, Haghighi P. Calcium pyrophosphate dihydrate crystal deposition disease of the knee simulating spontaneous osteonecrosis. Clin Rheumatol 1999;18(5):390–3.

15. Resnik CS, Miller BW, Gelberman RH, et al. Hand and wrist involvement in calcium pyrophosphate dihydrate crystal deposition disease. J Hand Surg Am 1983;8(6):856–63.

16. Yang BY, Sartoris DJ, Djukic S, et al. Distribution of calcification in the triangular fibrocartilage region in 181 patients with calcium pyrophosphate dihydrate crystal deposition disease. Radiology 1995;196(2):547–50.

17. Donich AS, Lektrakul N, Liu CC, et al. Calcium pyrophosphate dihydrate crystal deposition disease of the wrist: trapezioscaphoid joint abnormality. J Rheumatol 2000;27(11):2628–34.

18. Chen C, Chandnani VP, Kang HS, et al. Scapholunate advanced collapse: a common wrist abnormality in calcium pyrophosphate dihydrate crystal deposition disease. Radiology 1990;177(2):459–61.

19. Kastan DJ, Ellis BI, Shier CK, et al. Case report 456: Scaphoid-trapezium-trapezoid dissociation in pyrophosphate arthropathy of the wrist. Skeletal Radiol 1987;16(8):685–7.

20. Gerster JC, Lagier R, Boivin G, et al. Carpal tunnel syndrome in chondrocalcinosis of the wrist. Clinical and histologic study. Arthritis Rheum 1980;23(8):926–31.

21. Bourqui M, Vischer TL, Stasse P, et al. Pyrophosphate arthropathy in the carpal and metacarpophalangeal joints. Ann Rheum Dis 1983;42(6):626–30.

22. Adamson 3rd TC, Resnik CS, Guerra Jr J, et al. Hand and wrist arthropathies of hemochromatosis and calcium pyrophosphate deposition disease: distinct radiographic features. Radiology 1983;147(2):377–81.

23. Williams WV, Cope R, Gaunt WD, et al. Metacarpophalangeal arthropathy associated with manual labor (Missouri metacarpal syndrome). Clinical, radiographic, and pathologic characteristics of an unusual degeneration process. Arthritis Rheum 1987;30(12):1362–71.

24. Gerster JC, Lagier R, Boivin G. Olecranon bursitis related to calcium pyrophosphate dihydrate crystal deposition disease. Arthritis Rheum 1982;25(8):989–96.

25. Sander O, Scherer A. Mimicry of a rheumatoid nodule by tophaceous pseudogout at the elbow. J Rheumatol 2008;35(7):1419.

26. Taniguchi Y, Yoshida M, Tamaki T. Cubital tunnel syndrome associated with calcium pyrophosphate dihydrate crystal deposition disease. J Hand Surg Am 1996;21(5):870–4.

27. Taniguchi Y, Yoshida M, Tamaki T. Posterior interosseous nerve syndrome due to pseudogout. J Hand Surg Br 1999;24(1):125–7.

28. Kanterewicz E, Sanmartí R, Pañella D, et al. Tendon calcifications of the hip adductors in chondrocalcinosis: a radiological study of 75 patients. Br J Rheumatol 1993;32(9):790–3.

29. Lagier R, Vasey H. Calcium pyrophosphate dihydrate (CPPD) crystal deposition in the trochanteric bursa of a patient with hip osteoarthritis. J Rheumatol 1986;13(2):473–4.

30. Menkes CJ, Decraemere W, Postel M, et al. Chondrocalcinosis and rapid destruction of the hip. J Rheumatol 1985;12(1):130–3.

31. Rosenberg ZS, Shankman S, Steiner GC, et al. Rapid destructive osteoarthritis: clinical, radiographic, and pathologic features. Radiology 1992;182(1):213–6.

32. Coral A, Hardy G, Harvey A, et al. Case report: tumoral pseudogout of the hip joint. Clin Radiol 1996;51(12):889–91.

33. Sissons HA, Steiner GC, Bonar F, et al. Tumoral calcium pyrophosphate deposition disease. Skeletal Radiol 1989;18(2):79–87.

34. Mizutani H, Ohba S, Mizutani M, et al. Tumoral calcium pyrophosphate dihydrate deposition disease with bone destruction in the shoulder. CT and MR findings in two cases. Acta Radiol 1998;39(3):269–72.

35. McCarty DJ, Halverson PB, Carrera GF, et al. "Milwaukee shoulder"–association of microspheroids containing hydroxyapatite crystals, active collagenase, and neutral protease with rotator cuff defects. I. Clinical aspects. Arthritis Rheum 1981;24(3):464–73.

36. Halverson PB, Cheung HS, McCarty DJ, et al. "Milwaukee shoulder"–association of microspheroids containing hydroxyapatite crystals, active collagenase, and neutral protease with rotator cuff defects. II. Synovial fluid studies. Arthritis Rheum 1981;24(3):474–83.

37. Garancis JC, Cheung HS, Halverson PB, et al. "Milwaukee shoulder"–association of microspheroids containing hydroxyapatite crystals, active collagenase, and neutral protease with rotator cuff defects. III. Morphologic and biochemical studies of an excised synovium showing chondromatosis. Arthritis Rheum 1981;24(3):484–91.

38. Halverson PB, Cheung HS, McCarty DJ. Enzymatic release of microspheroids containing hydroxyapatite crystals from synovium and of calcium pyrophosphate dihydrate crystals from cartilage. Ann Rheum Dis 1982;41(5):527–31.

39. Huang GS, Bachmann D, Taylor JA, et al. Calcium pyrophosphate dihydrate crystal deposition disease and pseudogout of the acromioclavicular joint: radiographic and pathologic features. J Rheumatol 1993;20(12):2077–82.

40. Cooper AM, Hayward C, Williams BD. Calcium pyrophosphate deposition disease–involvement of the acromioclavicular joint with pseudocyst formation. Br J Rheumatol 1993;32(3):248–50.

41. Gerster JC. Cystic distension of the acromioclavicular joint in calcium pyrophosphate dihydrate crystal deposition disease. J Rheumatol 1995;22(2):371–2.

42. Tshering Vogel DW, Steinbach LS, Hertel R, et al. Acromioclavicular joint cyst: nine cases of a pseudotumor of the shoulder. Skeletal Radiol 2005;34(5):260–5.

43. Marcove RC, Wolfe SW, Healey JH, et al. Massive solitary tophus containing calcium pyrophosphate dihydrate crystals at the acromioclavicular joint. Clin Orthop Relat Res 1988;227:305–9.

44. Gerster JC, Baud CA, Lagier R, et al. Tendon calcifications in chondrocalcinosis. A clinical, radiologic, histologic, and crystallographic study. Arthritis Rheum 1977;20(2):717–22.

45. Luisiri P, Blair J, Ellman MH. Calcium pyrophosphate dihydrate deposition disease presenting as tumoral calcinosis (periarticular pseudogout). J Rheumatol 1996;23(9):1647–50.

46. Resnick D, Pineda C. Vertebral involvement in calcium pyrophosphate dihydrate crystal deposition disease. Radiographic-pathological correlation. Radiology 1984;153(1):55–60.

47. Yayama T, Baba H, Furusawa N, et al. Pathogenesis of calcium crystal deposition in the ligamentum flavum correlates with lumbar spinal canal stenosis. Clin Exp Rheumatol 2005;23(5):637–43.

48. Muthukumar N, Karuppaswamy U, Sankarasubbu B. Calcium pyrophosphate dihydrate deposition disease causing thoracic cord compression: case report. Neurosurgery 2000;46(1):222–5.

49. Fidler WK, Dewar CL, Fenton PV. Cervical spine pseudogout with myelopathy and Charcot joints. J Rheumatol 1996;23(8):1445–8.

50. Brown TR, Quinn SF, D'Agostino AN. Deposition of calcium pyrophosphate dihydrate crystals in the ligamentum flavum: evaluation with MR imaging and CT. Radiology 1991;178(3):871–3.

51. Kinoshita T, Maruoka S, Yamazaki T, et al. Tophaceous pseudogout of the cervical spine: MR imaging and bone scintigraphy findings. Eur J Radiol 1998;27(3):271–3.

52. Scutellari PN, Galeotti R, Leprotti S, et al. The crowned dens syndrome. Evaluation with CT imaging. Radiol Med 2007;112(2):195–207.

53. Roverano S, Ortiz AC, Ceccato F, et al. Calcification of the transverse ligament of the atlas in chondrocalcinosis. J Clin Rheumatol 2010;16(1):7–9.

54. Doita M, Shimomura T, Maeno K, et al. Calcium pyrophosphate dihydrate deposition in the transverse ligament of the atlas: an unusual cause of cervical myelopathy. Skeletal Radiol 2007;36(7):699–702.

55. Salaffi F, Carotti M, Guglielmi G, et al. The crowned dens syndrome as a cause of neck pain: clinical and computed tomography study in patients with calcium pyrophosphate dihydrate deposition disease. Clin Exp Rheumatol 2008;26(6):1040–6.

56. Kuzma BB, Goodman JM, Renkens KL. Cervical myelopathy secondary to calcium pyrophosphate crystal deposition in the alar ligament. Surg Neurol 1997;47(5):498–9.

57. Kakitsubata Y, Boutin RD, Theodorou DJ, et al. Calcium pyrophosphate dihydrate crystal deposition in and around the atlantoaxial joint: association with type 2 odontoid fractures in nine patients. Radiology 2000;216(1):213–9.

58. Martel W, McCarter DK, Solsky MA. Further observations on the arthropathy of calcium pyrophosphate crystal deposition disease. Radiology 1981;141(1):1–5.

59. Reynolds JL, Matthew IR, Chalmers A. Tophaceous calcium pyrophosphate dihydrate deposition disease of the temporomandibular joint. J Rheumatol 2008;35(4):717–21.

60. Nicholas BD, Smith 2nd JL, Kellman RM. Calcium pyrophosphate deposition of the temporomandibular joint with massive bony erosion. J Oral Maxillofac Surg 2007;65(10):2086–9.

61. Goudot P, Jaquinet A, Gilles R, et al. A destructive calcium pyrophosphate dihydrate deposition disease of the temporomandibular joint. J Craniofac Surg 1999;10(5):385–8.

62. Olin HB, Pedersen K, Francis D, et al. A very rare benign tumour in the parotid region: calcium pyrophosphate dihydrate crystal deposition disease. J Laryngol Otol 2001;115(6):504–6.

63. Magno WB, Lee SH, Schmidt J. Chondrocalcinosis of the temporomandibular joint: an external ear canal pseudotumor. Oral Surg Oral Med Oral Pathol 1992;73(3):262–5.

64. Resnick D. Calcium hydroxyapatite crystal deposition disease. In: Resnick D, editor. Diagnosis of Bone and Joint Disorders. Vol. 2. 4th ed. Philadelphia: Saunders; 2002:1619–57.

65. Hayes CW, Conway WF. Calcium hydroxyapatite deposition disease. Radiographics 1990;10(6):1031–48.

66. Chung CB, Gentili A, Chew FS. Calcific tendinosis and periarthritis: classic magnetic resonance imaging appearance and associated findings. J Comput Assist Tomogr 2004;28(3):390–6.

67. Farid N, Bruce D, Chung CB. Miscellaneous conditions of the shoulder: anatomical, clinical, and pictorial review emphasizing potential pitfalls in imaging diagnosis. Eur J Radio 2008;68(1):88–105.

68. Siegal DS, Wu JS, Newman JS, et al. Calcific tendinitis: a pictorial review. Can Assoc Radiol J 2009;60(5):263–72.

69. Garcia GM, McCord GC, Kumar R. Hydroxyapatite crystal deposition disease. Semin Musculoskelet Radiol 2003;7(3):187–93.

70. Choi MH, MacKenzie JD, Dalinka MK. Imaging features of crystal-induced arthropathy. Rheum Dis Clin North Am 2006;32(2):427–46, viii.

71. Bonavita JA, Dalinka MK, Schumacher Jr HR. Hydroxyapatite deposition disease. Radiology 1980;134(3):621–5.

72. Schumacher HR, Cherian PV, Reginato AJ, et al. Intra-articular apatite crystal deposition. Ann Rheum Dis 1983;42(Suppl. 1):54–9.

73. Neer 2nd CS, Craig EV, Fukuda H. Cuff-tear arthropathy. J Bone Joint Surg Am 1983;65(9):1232–44.

74. Dieppe PA, Doherty M, Macfarlane DG, et al. Apatite associated destructive arthritis. Br J Rheumatol 1984;23(2):84–91.

75. Fam AG, Pritzker KP, Stein JL, et al. Apatite-associated arthropathy: a clinical study of 14 cases and of 2 patients with calcific bursitis. J Rheumatol 1979;6(4):461–71.

76. Faure G, Daculsi G. Calcified tendinitis: a review. Ann Rheum Dis 1983;42(Suppl. 1):49–53.

77. Arrigoni P, Brady PC, Burkhart SS. Calcific tendonitis of the subscapularis tendon causing subcoracoid stenosis and coracoid impingement. Arthroscopy 2006;22(10):1139.e1-3.

78. Ji JH, Shafi M, Kim WY. Calcific tendinitis of the biceps-labral complex: a rare cause of acute shoulder pain. Acta Orthop Belg 2008;74(3):401–4.

79. Kim KC, Rhee KJ, Shin HD, et al. A SLAP lesion associated with calcific tendinitis of the long head of the biceps brachii at its origin. Knee Surg Sports Traumatol Arthrosc 2007;15(12):1478–81.

80. Goldman AB. Calcific tendinitis of the long head of the biceps brachii distal to the glenohumeral joint: plain film radiographic findings. AJR Am J Roentgenol 1989;153(5):1011–6.

81. Cahir J, Saifuddin A. Calcific tendonitis of pectoralis major: CT and MRI findings. Skeletal Radiol 2005;34(4):234–8.

82. Dürr HR, Lienemann A, Silbernagl H, et al. Acute calcific tendinitis of the pectoralis major insertion associated with cortical bone erosion. Eur Radiol 1997;7(8):1215–7.

83. Kraemer EJ, El-Khoury GY. Atypical calcific tendinitis with cortical erosions. Skeletal Radiol 2000;29(12):690–6.

84. Fritz P, Bardin T, Laredo JD, et al. Paradiaphyseal calcific tendinitis with cortical bone erosion. Arthritis Rheum 1994;37(5):718–23.

85. Moseley HF. Shoulder Lesions. Baltimore: Williams & Wilkins; 1969.

86. Flemming DJ, Murphey MD, Shekitka KM, et al. Osseous involvement in calcific tendinitis: a retrospective review of 50 cases. Am J Roentgenol 2003;181(4):965–72.

87. Hayes CW, Rosenthal DI, Plata MJ, et al. Calcific tendinitis in unusual sites associated with cortical bone erosion. Am J Roentgenol 1987;149:967–70.

88. Chan R, Kim DH, Millett PJ, et al. Calcifying tendinitis of the rotator cuff with cortical bone erosion. Skeletal Radiol 2004;33:596–9.

89. Bui-Mansfield LT, Moak M. Magnetic resonance appearance of bone marrow edema associated with hydroxyapatite deposition disease without cortical erosion. J Comput Assist Tomogr 2005;29(1):103–7.

90. Sakai T, Shimaoka Y, Sugimoto M, et al. Acute calcific tendinitis of the gluteus medius: a case report with serial magnetic resonance imaging findings. J Orthop Sci 2004;9(4):404–7.

91. Yang I, Hayes CW, Biermann JS. Calcific tendinitis of the gluteus medius tendon with bone marrow edema mimicking metastatic disease. Skeletal Radiol 2002;31(6):359–61.

92. Thornton MJ, Harries SR, Hughes PM, et al. Calcific tendinitis of the gluteus maximus tendon with abnormalities of cortical bone. Clin Radiol 1998;53(4):296–301.

93. Mizutani H, Ohba S, Mizutani M, et al. Calcific tendinitis of the gluteus maximus tendon with cortical bone erosion: CT findings. J Comput Assist Tomogr 1994;18(2):310–2.

94. Ramon FA, Degryse HR, De Schepper AM, et al. Calcific tendinitis of the vastus lateralis muscle. A report of three cases. Skeletal Radiol 1991;20(1):21–3.

95. Hodge JC, Schneider R, Freiberger RH, et al. Calcific tendinitis in the proximal thigh. Arthritis Rheum 1993;36(10):1476–82.

96. Tamangani J, Davies AM, James SL, et al. Calcific tendonitis of the adductor brevis insertion. Clin Radiol 2009;64(9):940–3.

97. Chow HY, Recht MP, Schils J, et al. Acute calcific tendinitis of the hip: case report with magnetic resonance imaging findings. Arthritis Rheum 1997;40(5):974–7.

98. Pierannunzii L, Tramontana F, Gallazzi M. Case report: calcific tendinitis of the rectus femoris: a rare cause of snapping hip. Clin Orthop Relat Res 2010;468(10):2814–8.

99. Kuroda H, Wada Y, Nishiguchi K, et al. A case of probable hydroxyapatite deposition disease (HADD) of the hip. Magn Reson Med Sci 2004;3(3):141–4.

100. Arlet JB, André H, Mutschler C, et al. Unusual acute crystal-induced hip arthritis: hydroxyapatite deposition of the round ligament. Clin Rheumatol 2009;28(4):483–4.

101. Schmitt J. Bursitis calcarea am epicondylus externus humeri. Arch Orthop Unfallchir 1921;19:215.

102. Park JY, Gupta A, Park HK. Calcific tendinitis at the radial insertion of the biceps brachii: a case report. J Shoulder Elbow Surg 2008;17(6):e19–21.

103. Hughes ESR. Acute deposition of calcium near the elbow. J Bone Joint Surg Br 1950;32-B(1):30.

104. Yosipovitch G, Yosipovitch Z. Acute calcific periarthritis of the hand and elbows in women. A study and review of the literature. J Rheumatol 1993;20(9):1533–8.

105. Vizkelety T, Aszodi K. Bilateral calcareous bursitis at the elbow. J Bone Joint Surg Br 1968;50(4):644–52.

106. Doumas C, Vazirani RM, Clifford PD, et al. Acute calcific periarthritis of the hand and wrist: a series and review of the literature. Emerg Radiol 2007;14(4):199–203.

107. Moyer RA, Bush DC, Harrington TM. Acute calcific tendinitis of the hand and wrist: a report of 12 cases and a review of the literature. J Rheumatol 1989;16(2):198–202.

108. Dilley DF, Tonkin MA. Acute calcific tendinitis in the hand and wrist. J Hand Surg Br 1991;16(2):215–6.
109. Ryan WG. Calcific tendinitis of flexor carpi ulnaris: an easy misdiagnosis. Arch Emerg Med 1993;10(4):321–3.
110. Gandee RW, Harrison RB, Dee PM. Peritendinitis calcarea of flexor carpi ulnaris. Am J Roentgenol 1979;133(6):1139–41.
111. Duey RE, Beall DP, Ahluwalia JS, et al. Carpal tunnel syndrome resulting from hydroxyapatite deposition. Curr Probl Diagn Radiol 2006;35(6): 261–3.
112. Verfaillie S, De Smet L, Leemans A, et al. Acute carpal tunnel syndrome caused by hydroxyapatite crystals: a case report. J Hand Surg Am 1996;21(3):360–2.
113. Mansfield HL, Trezies A. Calcific tendonitis of the medial collateral ligament. Emerg Med J 2009;26(7):543.
114. Schindler K, O'Keefe P, Bohn T, et al. The case: your diagnosis? Calcific tendonitis of the fibular collateral ligament. Orthopedics 2006;29(4): 373–85:282.
115. Shenoy PM, Kim DH, Wang KH, et al. Calcific tendinitis of popliteus tendon: arthroscopic excision and biopsy. Orthopedics 2009;32(2):127.
116. Tibrewal SB. Acute calcific tendinitis of the popliteus tendon-an unusual site and clinical syndrome. Ann R Coll Surg Engl 2002;84(5):338–41.
117. Macurak RB, Goldman JA, Hirsh E, et al. Acute calcific quadriceps tendinitis. South Med J 1980;73(3):322–5.
118. Varghese B, Radcliffe GS, Groves C. Calcific tendonitis of the quadriceps. Br J Sports Med 2006;40(7):652–4.
119. Rehak DC, Fu FH. Calcification of tendon of the vastus lateralis. A case report. Am J Sports Med 1992;20(2):227–9.
120. Cox D, Paterson FW. Acute calcific tendinitis of peroneus longus. J Bone Joint Surg Br 1991;73(2):342.
121. Roggatz J, Urban A. The calcareous peritendinitis of the long peroneal tendon. Arch Orthop Trauma Surg 1980;96(3):161–4.
122. Weston WJ. Tendinitis calcarea on the dorsum of the foot. Br J Radiol 1959;32:495.
123. Gruneberg R. Calcifying tendinitis in the forefoot. Br J Radiol 1963;36: 378–9.
124. Fam AG, Rubenstein J. Hydroxyapatite pseudopodagra. A syndrome of young women. Arthritis Rheum 1989;32(6):741–7.
125. Goupille P, Soutif D, Fouquet B, et al. Hydroxyapatite pseudopodagra. J Rheumatol 1991;18(5):786–7.
126. Goupille P, Valat JP. Hydroxyapatite pseudopodagra in young men. Am J Roentgenol 1992;159(4):902.
127. Mines D, Abbuhl SB. Hydroxyapatite pseudopodagra in a young man: acute calcific periarthritis of the first metatarsophalangeal joint. Am J Emerg Med 1996;14(2):180–2.
128. Offiah CE, Hall E. Acute calcific tendinitis of the longus colli muscle: spectrum of CT appearances and anatomical correlation. Br J Radiol 2009;82(978):e117–21.
129. Diaw AM, De Maeseneer M, Shahabpour M, et al. Calcium hydroxyapatite deposition disease of the neck: finding in three patients. J Belge Radiol 1998;81(2):73–4.
130. De Maeseneer M, Vreugde S, Laureys S, et al. Calcific tendinitis of the longus colli muscle. Head Neck 1997;19(6):545–8.
131. Malca SA, Roche PH, Pellet W, et al. Crowned dens syndrome: a manifestation of hydroxy-apatite rheumatism. Acta Neurochir (Wien) 1995;135(3-4): 126–30.
132. Halverson PB, Cheung HS, Johnson R, et al. Simultaneous occurrence of calcium pyrophosphate dihydrate and basic calcium phosphate (hydroxyapatite) crystals in a knee. Clin Orthop Relat Res 1990;257:162–5.
133. Doyle DV, Dieppe PA, Crocker PR, et al. Mixed crystal deposition in an osteoarthritic joint. J Pathol 1977;123(1):1–4.
134. Halverson PB, McCarty DJ. Patterns of radiographic abnormalities associated with basic calcium phosphate and calcium pyrophosphate dihydrate crystal deposition in the knee. Ann Rheum Dis 1986;45(7):603–5.
135. Halverson PB, Ryan LM. Triple crystal disease: monosodium urate monohydrate, calcium pyrophosphate dihydrate, and basic calcium phosphate in a single joint. Ann Rheum Dis 1988;47(10):864–5.

Ultrasound in the Diagnosis of Crystal Deposition Disease

Ralf G. Thiele

KEY POINTS

- Assessment of nephrolithiasis, cholecystolithiasis, and ureteral calcified concrements has been the main indication for ultrasound in internal medicine. Ultrasound can detect uric acid–containing kidney stones that would escape detection with conventional radiography.
- As high-frequency ultrasound transducers become available, more superficial structures including joints, tendons, bursae, and subcutaneous tissues can be evaluated for deposits of calcium or urate.
- Calcium-containing deposits and urate crystal deposits have acoustic properties and preferential areas of precipitation that help identify and distinguish them.
- Crystalline deposits and their relationship to surrounding tissues can be appreciated in vivo using gray-scale ultrasound. Doppler ultrasound can help assess and characterize crystal-related tissue hyperemia.
- Changes of crystal deposits over time, in response to treatment, can be observed using serial ultrasound. This includes change in volume of crystal deposition and change in crystal-related inflammatory response.
- Ultrasound can help guide arthrocentesis and removal of crystals.

Introduction

Ultrasound assessment of crystal arthritis has gained traction over the past few years as improved equipment with higher-frequency transducers became available.[1-4] Ultrasound assessment of calcium deposition has been the main indication for the use of ultrasound in internal medicine over the past 50 years.[5] Calcium-containing gall stones, kidney stones, and ureteric concrements strongly reflect sound waves and provide a bright signal and a pronounced posterior acoustic shadow with brightness-modulated (B-mode) ultrasound (Table 26-1).

Given the ubiquity of gout, new diagnostic modalities were often used for the assessment of gout as soon as they became available. Van Leeuwenhoek used one of the first microscopes to assess tophaceous material and found that gouty tophi consist of aggregates of needle-shaped crystals, and not globules of chalk as was believed until then. The first polarized

microscope was developed by Amici in 1844. In his 1859 treatise on "The Nature and Treatment of Gout," Alfred Baring Garrod emphasized the importance of polarizing microscopy to assess monosodium urate (MSU) crystals from specimen obtained of patients with gout: "The phenomenon can be well observed when we examine the specimen with a linear magnifying power of from ×100 to ×200, either by transmitted or reflected light, and still more satisfactorily by the aid of polarized light."[6] Konrad Roentgen took the first radiograph of his wife's hand on December 22, 1895, and began lecturing on the topic in January 1896. In March 1896, the first article on the radiographic features of tophaceous gout appeared in the medical literature, with a description of the punched-out appearance of erosions with thin cortical overhangs, radiolucency of tophi, and joint destruction that was not detectable by clinical examination alone. Combining physical findings with these radiographic finding led to the conclusion that erosions and cysts in gout would be filled with tophaceous material.[7] Ultrasound examinations of superficial, musculoskeletal structures require higher frequency transducers than the ones used for abdominal ultrasound. Once these became available in the 1980s, ultrasound began to be used for the assessment of gouty tophi.[8]

Ultrasound Technique

In diagnostic ultrasound, sound waves are sent from the transducer into the tissues. Some of the sound wave energy is reflected back at interfaces between different tissues, and some of the sound wave energy passes through the tissues, depending on their acoustic properties. The reflected sound waves, or echoes, are being detected by the transducer and transformed into electric impulses. The length of time that it takes for an echo to return to the transducer gives information about the depth of the reflected echogenic structure, and the strength of the echo gives information about the proportion of the sound wave energy that is being reflected by a tissue. A sound wave reflected of a deeper-seated structure travels a longer time from emission to detection and is displayed as pixels farther away from the transducer, or upper margin of the screen. The precise depth of a structure can be read by markers on the side of the screen or can be measured on the screen with calipers. A tissue structure that reflects most or all of the sound wave energy will return a strong echo to the

Table 26-1 Historical Timeline Leading to Adoption of Use of High-Resolution Ultrasound for Assessment of Urate Crystal Deposits in Gout

1679	Microscopy	Van Leeuwenhoek	Van Leeuwenhoek discovers that gouty tophi consist of needle shaped crystals and not globules of chalk
1776	Isolation of uric acid	Carl Wilhelm Scheele	Crystals in gouty tophi identified as monosodium urate
1809	Polarization of light	Malus	Very small fragments of crystals examined under polarizing light
1844	Polarizing microscope	Amici	
1859	Polarizing microscopy of urate crystals	Alfred Garrod	Polarizing microscopy recommended: "I may here remark in conclusion, that in whatever tissue or situation, urate of soda is deposited, it invariably exhibits a crystalline appearance, although sometimes the prisms are exceedingly small, requiring high magnifying powers and the use of polarized light to define them very clearly."
1895	X-rays	Konrad Roentgen	
1896	Use of x-rays for assessment of gouty arthritis	Huber	Description of typical roentgenographic features of gout, including joint destruction and subluxation not detected by clinical examination, radiolucency of tophi, punched-out appearing lesions with thin cortical overhangs. Suggestion of tophaceous, radiolucent material within erosions.
1961	Use of ultrasound for localizing renal calculi	J.U. Schlegel, P. Diggdon, J. Cuellar	
1975	Ultrasound used in rheumatology	C.P. Moore, D.A. Sarti, J.S. Louie	Ultrasonographic demonstration of popliteal cysts in rheumatoid arthritis
1982	Ultrasound used to assess gouty tophi	N. Tiliakos, A.R. Morales, C.H. Wilson Jr.	Use of ultrasound in identifying tophaceous versus rheumatoid nodules

transducer, and this is displayed on the screen as a bright pixel or pixels. Tissues with high water content such as hyaline cartilage or synovial fluid will allow much of the sound wave energy to pass through them and reflect few echoes. Such tissues are described as not echogenic, or "anechoic." They will appear as dark areas on the ultrasound screen. Tissues with moderate water content, and tissues with high cellular content and interstitial fluid, including synovial tissue or muscle tissue, will cause reflection at interfaces such as cell walls or muscle fiber sheaths and will allow through-transmission of sound waves in the fluid containing tissue compartments. Such tissues can have an echogenicity below average, or less than fatty tissue, and will be called "hypoechoic." Hypoechoic tissue will have a gray appearance on the screen. Some tissues have acoustic properties that cause most or all of the sound wave energy to be reflected. Ultrasound cannot pass through densely packed calcified tissues. All of the sound wave energy is being reflected, and calcium-containing tissues give very bright reflexes with ultrasound. Of physiologically occurring tissues, calcium-containing tissues cause the brightest reflections. Metallic prostheses or hypodermic needles give an even brighter reflex, as all sound energy is being reflected in one direction, unlike the scattered reflection on the rough surface of calcified structures including bony cortices. Such bright reflexes are called "hyperechoic." One consequence of the complete reflection and inability of high-frequency sound waves to pass through calcified tissues is the absence of echoes deep to these structures. This provides the characteristic "posterior acoustic shadow," an artefact that can help with the diagnosis of calcifications. When assessing crystal deposits, this sonographic artefact can help distinguish calcific concrements from MSU crystalline deposit macroaggregates in cartilage and in tophi, which usually will not give an intensive posterior acoustic shadow.

Doppler ultrasound assesses blood flow and is helpful for the assessment of inflammation. Sound waves that are reflected from a moving object change their frequency relative to the detector (ears or ultrasound transducer). Sound waves reflected from an object moving toward the detector become "compressed"; the frequency appears increased. As the object passes the detector and moves away, the reflected sound waves become "stretched" or elongated, and the frequency appears lower. This shift in frequency can be color-coded in color Doppler ultrasound, with objects moving toward the ultrasound probe coded in one assigned color and objects moving away from the transducer in another. Any color can be assigned; red and blue are often used. In the human body, moving objects are primarily erythrocytes. Power Doppler ultrasound gives information about the strength, or power, of blood flow. This is often encoded in only one color; shades of red are often used. Doppler ultrasound is a brilliant tool for the detection of blood flow. However, any movement will be detected. Artefacts need to be distinguished from Doppler signals that represent blood flow. Movement of transducer or patient can create motion artefacts. The ultrasound probe needs to be kept steady for an accurate assessment of blood flow. The patient's extremity should be kept steady as well and may rest on an exam table or desk. Abnormal and physiologic tissues can first be identified using gray-scale ultrasound. A Doppler signal can then be matched with the tissue in question, to help distinguish actual flow from artefacts. Pulse synchronicity of the Doppler signal will also be an identifier of blood flow.[9]

Ultrasound transducers use different frequencies. Higher frequencies (10 to 20 MHz) have less tissue penetration but provide the best images at shallower depths. These will be the frequencies of choice for the assessment of crystalline deposits and their effects on surrounding tissues in the musculoskeletal

Table 26-2 Ultrasound Terminology Relevant to Assessment of Crystal Arthritis

Term	Appearance	Example	Explanation
Anechoic	Dark or "black"	Tissues with high water content, e.g. hyaline cartilage and joint fluid with low cellular content	Bright ultrasound signals are caused by reflections at interfaces between tissues, depending on their acoustic properties. Tissues with high water content and few interfaces, or oligocellular joint fluid allow through-transmission of sound waves and little reflection. This appears as a "dark" area on the screen.
Hypoechoic	Gray	Synovial tissue	Tissues with high cellular content and third space fluid content provide more interfaces that reflect sound waves.
Hyperechoic	Bright or "white"	Fibrous joint capsule, bony cortex	Fibrous tissues strongly reflect sound waves but allow some through-transmission. This gives a bright sonographic appearance. Calcium containing bony cortices or calcified concrements strongly reflect sound waves and usually allow no through-transmission of sound waves. This gives a very bright sonographic appearance with posterior acoustic shadow.
Interface reflex	Bright reflection at interface of two tissues, strongest at perpendicular angle of incidence of sound waves	Meniscus shaped bright reflex at superficial margin of hyaline cartilage	Smooth, sharply defined surfaces reflect sound waves similar to reflection of light from glass or water. When curved structures such as metatarsal or metacarpal heads are insonated, the strongest reflex will be seen at a perpendicular angle of incidence, where most sound waves are reflected back to the transducer.
Scattered reflection	Bright reflexion that follows the outline of rough or granular surfaces that provide multiple small surfaces for sound wave reflection	Bony cortex and crystal deposits over hyaline cartilage	Rough or granular surfaces may reflect sound waves in many directions and will be detected by the transducer from many different angles. This provides the image of a bright outline that follows the shape of the structure, e.g., along the surface of hyaline cartilage affected by gout.

system. Transducer frequencies of less than 10 MHz were found to be unsuitable for the assessment of crystal arthritis.[10] Lower frequencies (3 to 7.5 MHz) have deeper tissue penetration and are best suited for deeper-seated structures in abdominal ultrasound and other indications. In general, image resolution increases with higher frequencies, but quality of hardware and software algorithms will also influence image quality. Linear transducers, with a straight footprint, are mostly used in musculoskeletal medicine (Table 26-2).

Technique of Ultrasound Assessment of Crystal Arthritis in Selected Joints

Published guidelines for the use of musculoskeletal ultrasound in rheumatologic indications should be followed to achieve standardization of the examination. A standardized approach will facilitate repeatability and reproducibility.[11]

First Metatarsophalangeal Joints

Tophaceous deposits in first metatarsophalangeal (MTP) joints can be visualized from dorsal, medial, and plantar.[12] From dorsal, the transducer can be placed midline over the metatarsal head and proximal phalanx. The bony contours of distal metatarsal and proximal phalanx will be the landmarks and should be visible as much as possible on the image. As the first toe may deviate laterally, the probe may need to be adjusted for this. The joint line should be near the center of the

image, but the image can be adjusted to include as much anatomy of interest as possible, in particular the proximal recess of the joint capsule. Identifiable anatomical structures include bony cortices, hyaline cartilage, joint cavity, joint capsule, and extensor tendon. Synovial fluid can best be appreciated from a dorsal view. Of note, small visible fluid collections in first and second MTP joints are the norm. Anechoic or hypoechoic synovial fluid can distend the hyperechoic joint capsule by 3 to 4 mm, measured from the hyperechoic anatomical neck of the metatarsal head.[13,14] From medial, metatarsal head and proximal phalanx will be the bony landmarks. The joint line can serve as the center of the image. The medial collateral ligament can be identified. Tophaceous deposits will typically distend the space between metatarsal head and medial collateral ligament. Bony erosions can be seen here as well. From plantar, the metatarsal head with potential MSU deposits can only be appreciated if a midline view in between the sesamoid bones can be achieved. Bony contour of metatarsal head, hyaline cartilage, and flexor tendon will be structures of interest. Sesamoid bones with potential erosive changes can be seen medially and laterally.

Knee Joint

Fluid in the knee joint will largely collect in the suprapatellar recess and can readily be seen using sonography. Suprapatellar long- and short-axis views are used for this. The knee is positioned in a neutral position or can be slightly flexed if the knee is supported with a cushion for patient comfort. Bony contour of femur, prefemoral fat pad, suprapatellar fat pad, proximal patella, and quadriceps tendon are the structures of interest in a suprapatellar long-axis view. Fluid collections, synovial hypertrophy, and potentially tophi can be seen in this view. Crystal deposits in or on femoral hyaline cartilage can be assessed sonographically. In a neutral position, much of the femoral cartilage will be covered by the patella. Patient positioning is required. With maximal flexion of the knee, the patella will move distally, and much of the distal femoral cartilage will be exposed and accessible to ultrasound. Suprapatellar, long- and short-axis views can show bony contour of femoral condyles and overlying hyaline cartilage. For an assessment of crystal deposition in the fibrocartilage of the menisci, medial and lateral long-axis views can be employed. Similar to the exposed olecranon bursa, the prepatellar bursa can be affected by gout. Based on clinical examination alone, acute gout of the prepatellar bursa can be difficult to distinguish from gout involving the knee joint space, and ultrasound examination can be very helpful. In healthy control subjects, the prepatellar bursa contains very little synovial fluid. For a sonographic assessment, transducer pressure needs to be minimized, as any fluid here is easily displaced by pressure. Floating the probe on a layer of gel can decrease transducer pressure.

Calcium Pyrophosphate Dihydrate (CPPD) Crystal Deposition in the Knee

In hyaline articular cartilage, calcium pyrophosphate dihydrate (CPPD) crystals deposit preferentially in lacunes in the middle zone of hyaline cartilage.[15-17] These deposits provide a very characteristic sonographic appearance of hyperechoic stippling or form a hyperechoic band embedded in the center of the surrounding anechoic or hypoechoic hyaline cartilage.[18,19] This location of hyperechoic deposits distinguishes chondrocalcinosis of CPPD deposition from the deposits of MSU crystals, which typically form a hyperechoic band on the surface of hyaline cartilage.[20] Suprapatellar long- and short-axis views in maximal knee flexion are best suited for an ultrasound assessment (Fig. 26-1).

To assess CPPD crystal deposits in the peripheral portion of the fibrocartilaginous menisci of the knee, medial and lateral long-axis views can be used. Distal femur and proximal tibia will be the bony landmarks, with joint line, triangular menisci, and centrally embedded hyperechoic CPPD deposits in the center of the image (Fig. 26-2, *A*).

Wrist

The triangular fibrocartilage complex of the wrist is a locus with factors including exposure to biomechanical forces that foster precipitation of crystals. In particular, calcium-containing crystals, especially CPPD, will deposit in the fibrocartilaginous tissues. The bony borders of the triangular fibrocartilage complex include distal ulna proximally, triquetrum distally, and lunate radially. The insertion of triangular fibrocartilage fibers into the distal radius is often too deep seated to be accessible for ultrasound. The triangular fibrocartilage complex includes the following components: fibrous tissue originating from the fovea of the distal ulna, which continues

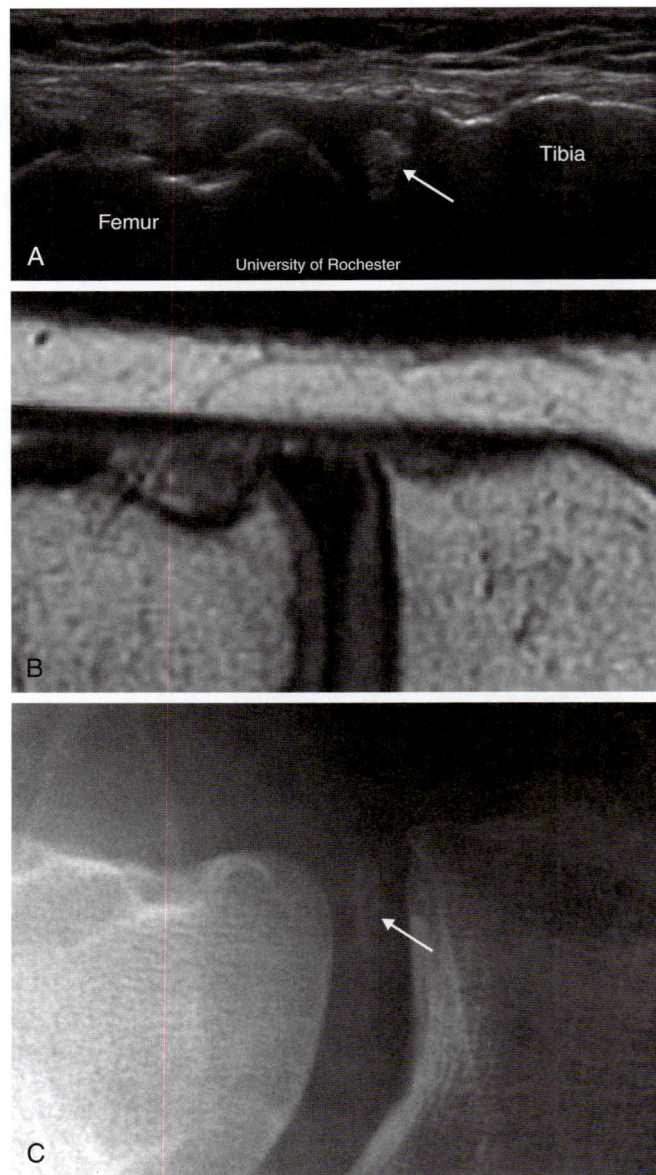

Figure 26-2 Knee **A,** Ultrasound, lateral long-axis view. A hyperechoic, oval-shaped structure of CPPD deposition (*arrow*) is seen between lateral bony outlines of femur and tibia. **B,** Lateral aspect, MRI. Same patient and location as *A.* CPPD deposition cannot be visualized by this MRI. **C,** Radiograph. Same patient and location as in **A** and **B.** Oval-shaped CPPD deposition is seen, similar to ultrasound image.

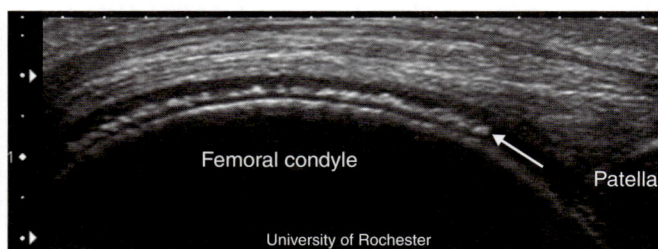

Figure 26-1 Knee, suprapatellar long-axis view in maximal flexion. Convex bony contour of femoral condyle is deepest structure. A bright, hyperechoic, irregular band of CPPD deposition (*arrow*) is seen embedded in the dark, anechoic to hypoechoic hyaline cartilage that covers the femoral condyle. Peripheral fibers of quadriceps tendon are seen on *top* of image.

to become the fibrocartilaginous disc proper that inserts into the radius and separates ulna from lunate; and the triangle-shaped meniscus homologue proximal to the triquetrum. This complex is bordered by fatty tissue deep to the extensor carpi ulnaris tendon on the ulnar aspect. Ulnar (medial) long-axis views are best suited to evaluate crystal deposits here. Dynamic examination with gentle adduction and abduction of the wrist can help express and identify crystal deposits.

Shoulder

Calcium-containing deposits of basic calcium phosphate crystals are a common cause of chronic shoulder pain. Calcium deposits near the insertion of the supraspinatus tendon can be readily assessed sonographically, and surrounding tendon, bursa, and bony structures can be appreciated. In a neutral position, much of the supraspinatus tendon will be located deep to the acromion, and cannot be assessed sonographically. With proper patient positioning, the supraspinatus tendon can be exposed from under the acromion. Maximal internal rotation and adduction of the shoulder are needed for sonographic visualization of the supraspinatus tendon.

CPPD deposition in hyaline cartilage of the humeral head can best be assessed using anterior short-axis views with the shoulder positioned in adduction and internal rotation (i.e., with the ipsilateral hand placed behind the back or at the hip). The anechoic hyaline cartilage will be found superficial to the hyperechoic rounded bony surface of the humeral head and deep to the hyperechoic fibers of the supraspinatus tendon.

To assess CPPD deposits in the fibrocartilage of the glenoid labrum, posterior short-axis views with the ipsilateral hand placed palm up on the contralateral knee or touching the anterior aspect of the contralateral shoulder are used. The probe is placed parallel to the spine of the scapula, with glenoid fossa and humeral head serving as bony landmarks. Fibrous glenoid labrum and overlying joint capsule can also be assessed dynamically with slow internal and external rotation of the shoulder. With this view, joint effusions of shoulder joint (glenohumeral joint) are also best seen,[21] and this may serve as a portal for ultrasound-guided shoulder aspirations.[22, 23]

Hip

Part of the cartilage of the femoral head will be obscured by the acetabulum, but the anterior portion can be assessed sonographically. Similar to menisci of knee and glenoid labrum of the shoulder, the fibrocartilage of the acetabular labrum can be affected by CPPD deposition. Anterior long-axis views will show bony acetabulum, fibrocartilaginous acetabular labrum, femoral hyaline cartilage, bony femoral head, femoral neck, and joint capsule. The probe will be placed over the anterior hip, along the axis of the femoral neck, at an angle of 120 to 130 degrees to the anatomical axis of the femur (caput-collum-diaphyseal angle). CPPD deposition in hyaline cartilage can be seen in this long-axis view and in orthogonal, short-axis views. Crystal deposition in the acetabular labrum is best seen in long-axis views.

Elbow

Chondrocalcinosis of hyaline cartilage covering capitulum and trochlea of distal humerus can be seen in long-axis views centered over humeroradial or humeroulnar joint from anterior in a neutral (extended) position of the elbow. Transverse, short-axis views centered over distal humerus show hyaline cartilage of both trochlea and capitulum in one view.

Ultrasound of Gout

High-frequency diagnostic ultrasound penetrates body tissues to a depth of a few centimeters. Crystalline deposits in joints, tendons, and soft tissues, as well as bony erosions and inflamed tissues adjacent to crystal deposits, can readily be accessed at these depths. Ultrasound waves cannot penetrate the bony cortex—strictly intraosseous tophi cannot be appreciated. The packing of monosodium urate (MSU) crystals in gouty tophi allows for a large proportion of ultrasound waves to pass through between the thin needles. This permits a detailed assessment of the tophus itself and tissues that surround it or permeate it. Where MSU crystals reflect a sound wave, they provide a small, strong echo. This gives tophi a hypoechoic to hyperechoic, inhomogeneous appearance (where crystals give small, bright reflexes and the intervening space provides no strong reflex and appears darker). Tophi can have a sonographic appearance of "wet clumps of sugar."[20] The crystalline core of the tophus is surrounded by a corona of cells including macrophages, plasma cells, and mast cells[24] (see Chapter 5). A large number of the cells of this corona express cytokines, particularly interleukin (IL)-1β.[25] The corona is a few cell layers thick. Sonographically, it appears as a thin anechoic (dark) rim that surrounds the much brighter tophus. Occasionally, blood flow is seen in this corona using sensitive Doppler ultrasound (Fig. 26-3, *A*). Tophi and their surrounding cellular corona are embedded in a fibrovascular matrix.[24] Fibrous tissue is more hyperechoic than the cellular corona and will have a brighter appearance. This fibrous tissue is vascularized. Individual vessels can be seen in the fibrovascular matrix with sensitive Doppler equipment. Pulse synchronicity of the Doppler signals will confirm vascular flow, as opposed to artefact.[9] Flow surrounding tophi can be seen in asymptomatic joints and soft tissues (Fig. 26-4, *A*). Such flow is not seen in asymptomatic controls. It would be a matter of definition, if the presence of unphysiologic, hyperemic tissue in asymptomatic joints can be regarded as subclinical inflammation. As almost all joint destruction in tophaceous gout occurs during an asymptomatic or pauci-symptomatic stage, and chronic subclinical inflammation can drive the increased cardiovascular mortality of gout, subclinical inflammation would be an important feature of gout.[26,27]

Tophi

Aggregates of MSU crystals may be found sonographically in intraarticular or extraarticular locations. Tophus size can be directly measured using ultrasound calipers. Diameters can range from less than 1 mm (microtophi) to centimeters. Changes in tophus volume over time may be of interest. This may help to objectively assess a treatment response. Once measurements are taken, the volume can be calculated for spherical or ellipsoid shaped tophi. Volume functions of the ultrasound machine may be used. Ultrasound probes with three-dimensional capabilities may be used for an operator-independent measurement of volume.

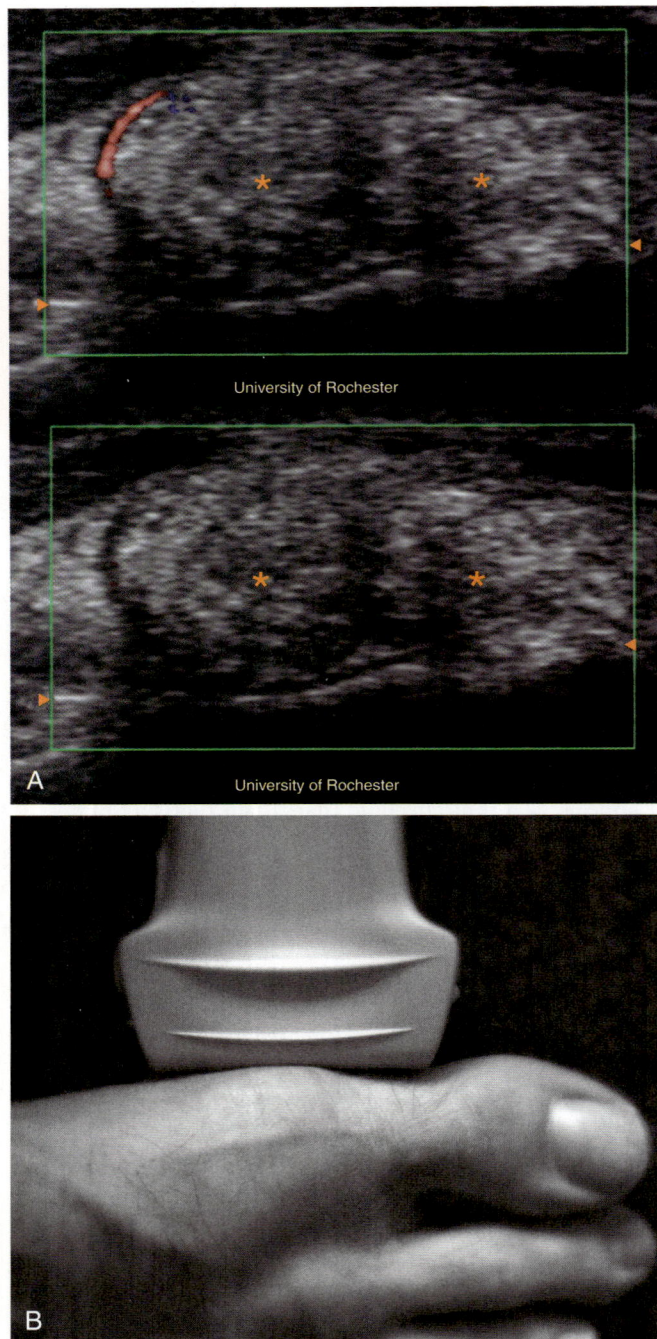

Figure 26-3 **A,** First metatarsophalangeal joint (MTP1), medial long-axis view. Two large tophi (*asterisks*) distend space between bone (in between *arrowheads*), medial collateral ligament and skin (*top* of images). *Green rectangle* denotes Doppler box. *Top* image taken during systole, *bottom* image taken during diastole. Blood flow is seen surrounding tophus on *left* during systole. **B,** Orientation of probe.

Tophi may be formed, or shaped, and assume a fairly regular shape with defined margins. Sonographically, this margin may be accentuated by the anechoic rim formed by the cellular corona. Oval or spherical structures may be found. Irregular shapes may be found just as often, and seemingly shaped tophi may merge with other tophi (Fig. 26-5, *A*).[28] Amorphous tophaceous material may fill out available spaces,

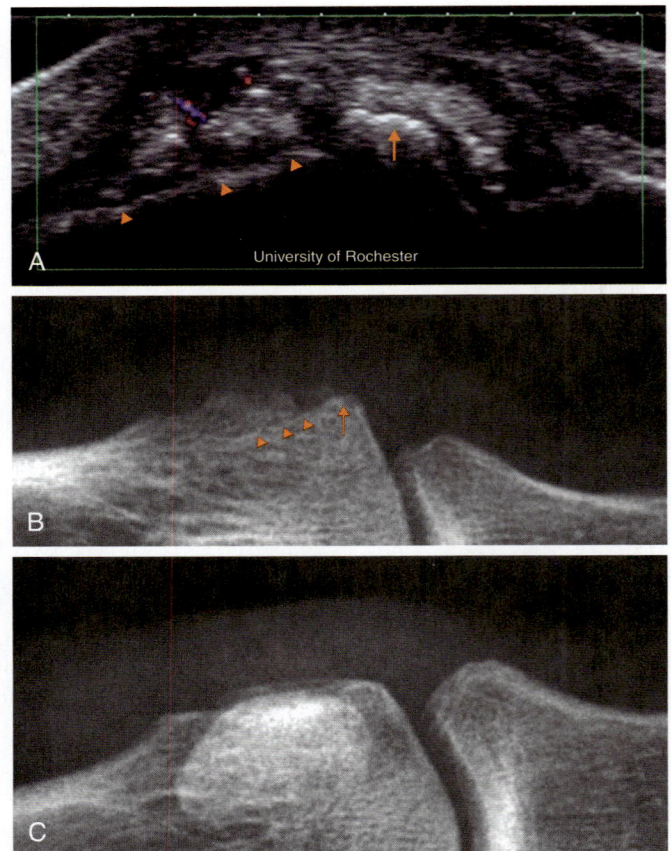

Figure 26-4 First metatarsophalangeal joint (MTP1). **A,** Medial long-axis view. Asymptomatic patient. Hyperechoic tophi are seen adjacent to metatarsal head, distending the space between bone and medial collateral ligament. *A arrowheads* indicate medial contour of metatarsal head. *Arrow* indicates bone spur at medial distal corner of metatarsal head. Hyperechoic, tophaceous material is seen curving around bone spur and pointing into joint space. Note that tophi are not in immediate contact with bone. Rectangular box denotes area of Doppler capture. Doppler signal is seen adjacent to tophi left and center. **B,** Radiograph, oblique view. Same patient as ultrasound image in **A** taken on same day. *Open arrowheads* indicate medial contour of metatarsal head, and *arrow* indicates bone spur, analog to image **A.** Rotation of oblique view projects a second bony contour beyond strictly medial contour of metatarsal head. **C,** MTP1, radiograph, anteroposterior view. Same patient as images in **A** and **B.** Tophaceous material and hyperemia are not seen on radiograph.

which may correspond to the phenomenon of "urate milk" on joint aspiration.

As MSU crystal aggregates tend to be surrounded by a corona of cells, they are rarely found to be in direct contact with adjacent tissues. Hyperechoic tophi or amorphous urate milk will be separated from the hyperechoic fibrous joint capsule or hyperechoic bone by an anechoic rim (Fig. 26-6). This is an important feature; it allows distinction of tophaceous material from proliferative synovial tissue that would be contingent with the fibrous, hyperechoic joint capsule, or would be in close contact with subchondral bone in the case of pannus invasion of an erosion.

Microtophi may be defined as hyperechoic concrements of less than 1 mm in diameter. These may be found embedded in or adjacent to synovial lining tissue. In contrast to larger tophi, they cannot be readily distinguished sonographically

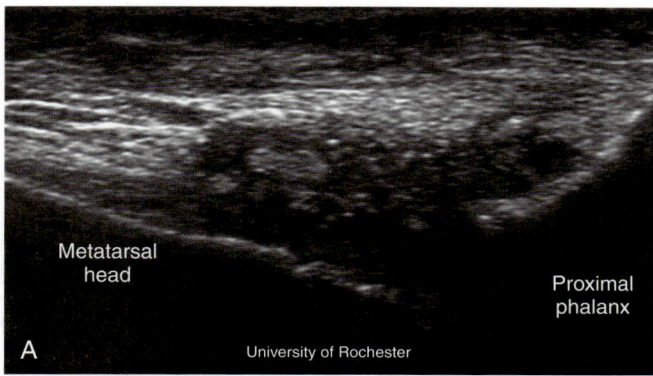

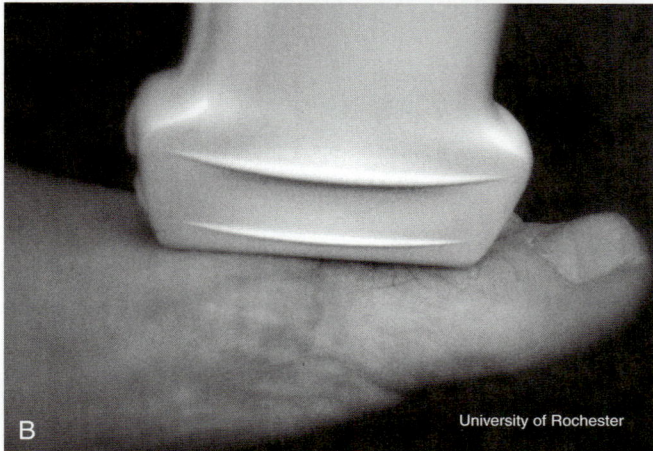

Figure 26-5 A, First metatarsophalangeal joint (MTP1), dorsal long-axis view. Multiple grouped hyperechoic tophi are seen in dorsal compartment of joint space. Punctate, submillimeter, hyperechoic microtophi are seen as well, dispersed throughout joint space. **B,** Orientation of probe for Figures 26-5, *A,* 26-6, and 26-7.

Figure 26-6 First metatarsophalangeal joint (MTP1), dorsal long-axis view. Layered, hyperechoic, tophaceous material is seen in proximal dorsal recess of joint space. Hyperechoic, tophaceous material is separated from adjacent tissue by anechoic corona (*arrowheads*). A deeper layer also shows an anechoic corona. Hyperechoic dots in center represent gas bubbles trapped in viscous anechoic synovial fluid.

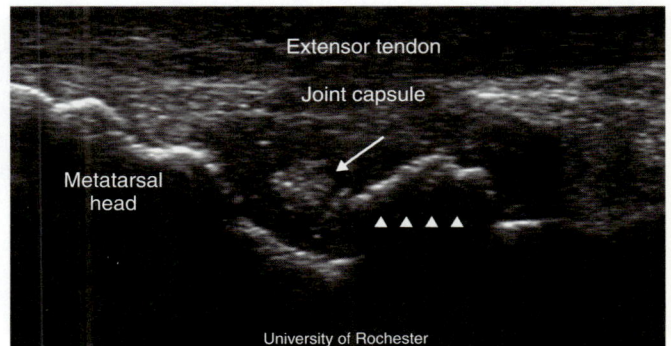

Figure 26-7 First metatarsophalangeal joint (MTP1), dorsal long-axis view. Hyperechoic to hypoechoic formed tophus is seen within dorsal compartment of joint space (*arrow*). This tophus had a characteristic inhomogeneous appearance consisting of brighter echoes and darker areas in intervening spaces. There is no attenuation appreciated of sound waves deep to this tophus. Calcified material is seen with brighter, hyperechoic irregular surface and posterior acoustic shadow (*arrowheads*).

from calcium-containing microtophi, as small concrements may not have a posterior acoustic shadow.

Larger tophi may be not be oval or egg-shaped structures but can be permeated by the fibrovascular matrix. With sensitive Doppler equipment and high-frequency probes, tissue and vessels can be seen invading the crystalline tophus.

MSU tophi will usually not give a profound posterior acoustic shadow. That means ultrasound waves reach structures deep to the tophus, and tophi can be appreciated in their environment. Occasionally, large tophi or very broad tophi can attenuate the sound waves and decrease the echogenicity of deeper tissues. Calcification may occasionally occur in long-standing tophaceous gout, and such calcified tophi will have a posterior acoustic shadow as other calcium concrements will have (Fig. 26-7). If conventional radiography is available for comparison, calcified concrements will be visible radiographically, whereas MSU tophi are typically radiolucent.

Double Contour Sign

MSU in hypersaturated solution precipitates around seed nuclei, or on available surfaces, in particular if these surfaces have properties that foster crystallization.[29] Intraarticularly, hyaline cartilage provides a surface for crystallization.[30,31] Pathologic reviews of joints affected by gout find the hyaline cartilage the locus of MSU precipitation "par excellence."[32,33] MSU crystal deposits

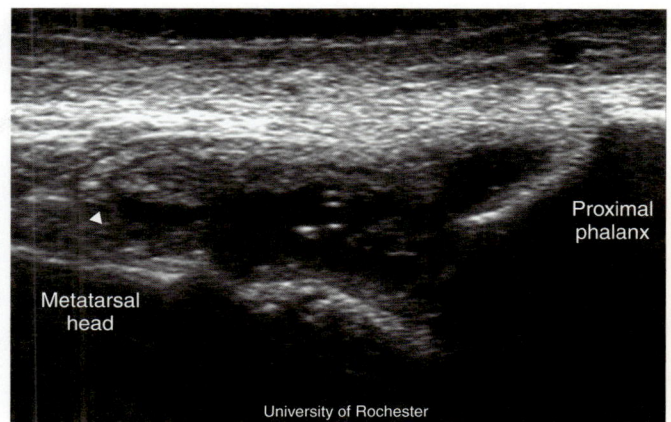

do not penetrate the surface of hyaline cartilage very deeply, but enough to "anchor" the crystal deposits on the joint surface. This phenomenon can be observed in vivo with arthroscopy, or sonographically.[34] Using ultrasound, the contour of bone will appear hyperechoic and bright, the overlying water containing hyaline cartilage anechoic or hypoechoic and dark, and the overlying crystal deposits again bright. As both anechoic hyaline cartilage and overlying crystal deposits follow the contour of the bone surface, the image of a "double contour" is created. Using ultrasound, arthroscopy, or autopsy specimen, the MSU deposits have an appearance of "urate icing" or "urate frosting" on the cartilage (Fig. 26-8, *A*).*

---

*Validation of the specificity of the double contour sign, with urate crystal identification from joint fluids and cartilage samples, would benefit from more development. For example, it is true that prior studies in gout of the double contour sign were done on patients without previous corticosteroid injections. However, one suspects that intraarticular steroids could produce a double contour sign on high-resolution ultrasound, and such a study should be prospectively done.

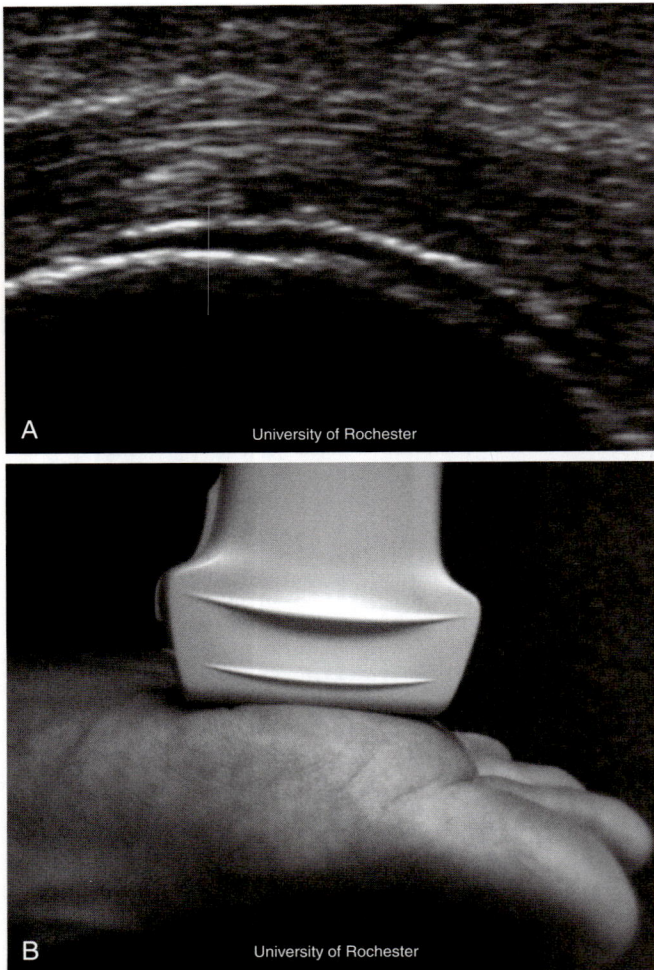

Figure 26-8 A, Metatarsal head, plantar long-axis view. The hyperechoic bony contour of the metatarsal head is the deepest structure, covered by anechoic, dark-appearing hyaline cartilage. A hyperechoic, bright-appearing irregular-shaped band of MSU crystal deposition is seen covering part of the hyaline cartilage. Flexor tendon fibers are seen more superficially. **B,** Orientation of probe.

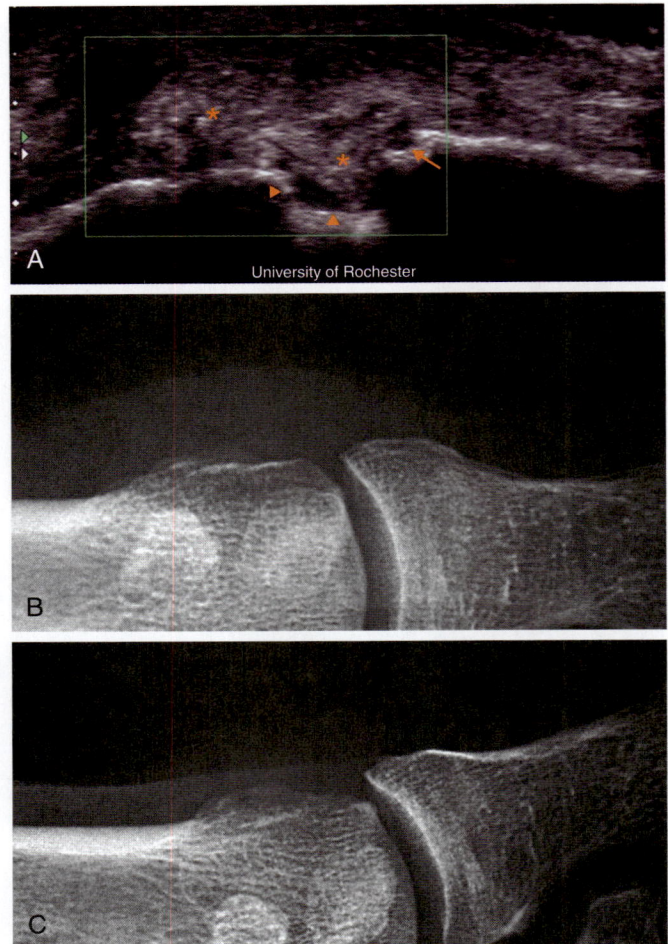

Figure 26-9 First metatarsophalangeal joint (MTP1). **A,** Medial long-axis view. Hyperechoic, tophaceous material is seen adjacent to metatarsal head and proximal phalanx. An erosion is seen at distal medial aspect of metatarsal head (*arrowheads*). A small, punched-out appearing erosion is seen at proximal medial aspect of proximal phalanx (*arrow*). **B** and **C,** Conventional radiograph of same joint and patient. Anteroposterior and oblique views. Radiographs were taken on the same day as the ultrasound image. Erosions and tophi cannot be detected on radiographs.

Erosions

For a long time, conventional radiography was the only imaging modality to assess erosions in vivo. However, due to the physics of radiography where all bony tissues are superimposed on each other on a two-dimensional film, few bony erosions are actually detected using conventional radiography. Bony erosions can only be verified as a break in the bony contour if they are seen in profile. To achieve this, different radiographic views are obtained of a given joint area. In feet, anteroposterior, lateral, and often oblique radiographs are obtained.[35] Nevertheless, adding a third, oblique view improves the yield of radiography only marginally.[36,37] Cross-sectional imaging including ultrasound, MRI, and CT scanning detects more erosions in erosive arthropathies than conventional radiography (Fig. 26-9).[38-40] Sonographically, bony erosions are defined as breaks in the hyperechoic cortical contour seen in two perpendicular planes.[41] Erosions of gout may be filled by hyperechoic tophi and their surrounding anechoic rim.[20] Crystalline material is not regularly seen in direct contact with bone (Fig. 26-10, Table 26-3).

Ultrasound of Calcium Crystalline Arthritides

Detection of calcium deposits has been the main indication for the use of ultrasound in internal medicine for the last decades. Calcified concrements are impermeable to sound waves and produce bright, hyperechoic reflections. The rough surface of calcium concrements reflects incident sound waves in many different directions. This produces a scattered reflection, and calcium-containing concrements can readily be seen from different angles of insonation. As no sound waves pass through densely packed calcific concrements, they will produce pronounced posterior acoustic shadows. This makes such deposits stand out prominently from the surrounding soft tissues.

Small, loosely packed calcifications allow passage of sound waves in between them, and tissues deep to areas of small, loosely packed calcifications can still be assessed sonographically. An example for this is chondrocalcinosis of hyaline cartilage, with multiple small crystal deposits in central lacunes.

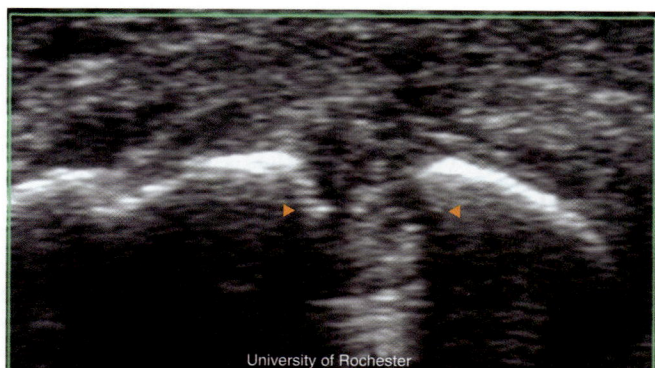

Figure 26-10 Bony erosion. Break in cortex (between *arrowheads*) is filled with typical hyperechoic, inhomogeneous tophaceous material. The intralesional tophus is separated from bony tissue by a fine anechoic margin.

Table 26-3 Ultrasound Features of Tophi

Echogenicity Features	%
Hyperechoic	26.1
Hyperechoic heterogeneous	37.6
Hyperechoic heterogeneous with calcification	32.6
Hypoechoic	0.7
Hypoechoic heterogeneous	2.2
Hypoechoic heterogeneous with calcification	0.7
Contour	**%**
Well-defined	16.7
Poorly defined	83.3
Hypoechoic halo	**%**
Present	55.8%
Absent	44.2
Number of tophi	**%**
Individual	36.2
Multiple isolated	2.2
Multiple grouped	61.6

From de Ávila Fernandes E, Kubota ES, Sandim GB, et al. Ultrasound features of tophi in chronic tophaceous gout. Skeletal Radiol 2010 Jul 31.

Hydroxyapatite (Basic Calcium Phosphate) Crystal Deposition Disease

Deposition of hydroxyapatite and other basic calcium phosphate (BCP) crystals is a common cause of shoulder pain and occasionally pain in other joint areas. Calcific tendinitis of the rotator cuff is a frequent manifestation. The most frequent site is the supraspinatus tendon. Deposits are often found in the "critical zone," a poorly vascularized area of the supraspinatus tendon located 0.5 to 1 cm proximal to its insertion.[42]

An extensive body of literature exists on ultrasonography of calcific tendinitis and bursitis, and ultrasound may be considered the gold standard of localizing BCP crystal deposits in tendons, particularly in the shoulder.

Calcium Pyrophosphate Dihydrate Crystal Deposition Disease

Calcium pyrophosphate dihydrate (CPPD) crystals can deposit in fibrocartilage and hyaline cartilage. Periarticular deposition can occur, although less frequently. CPPD has a predilection for central areas of fibrocartilaginous menisci, including knee, triangular fibrocartilage of the wrist, symphysis pubis, and others. In the menisci of the knees, CPPD deposits in the peripheral third of medial or lateral meniscus, which is accessible to ultrasound examination (see Fig. 26-2, A). In the wrist, the fibrocartilage of the meniscus homologue proximal to the triquetrum is superficial enough for ready ultrasound access, but the fibrocartilage of the disc proper of the triangular fibrocartilage is deeper seated and can require dynamic positioning for visualization of calcium deposits. As with MSU and BCP crystals, many affected patients remain asymptomatic for long periods of time. In a given joint, both hyaline cartilage covering bones and adjacent fibrocartilage may be affected by CPPD deposition, and both can be assessed sonographically.

Osteoarthritis and Crystal Deposition

True osteoarthritis is not a disease characterized by a consistent level of synovitis. Even in "erosive osteoarthritis," invading pannus tissue is essentially never observed sonographically, unlike findings in rheumatoid arthritis. Swollen joints in osteoarthritis are not characterized by proliferative, hyperemic synovial tissue by sonographic criteria, but rather by bone spur formation with local irritation of the joint capsule.[43] The term "inflammatory osteoarthritis" remains therefore a concept in search of a tissue diagnosis. Nevertheless, osteoarthritis and CPPD deposition often coexist. Furthermore, a large percentage of patients with CPPD crystal deposition disease present with an arthritis that simulates osteoarthritis. An occasional acute inflammatory component is seen in 35% to 60% of such patients (Fig. 26-11).[44] Possibly, some of the descriptions of synovitis found sonographically in osteoarthritis refer to such a crystal-induced arthritis or to synovitis related to BCP crystal deposition (Table 26-4).

Use of Ultrasound in the Treatment of Crystal Arthritis

Ultrasound Guidance of Aspirations and Injections

Arthrocentesis in crystal arthritis can be diagnostic and therapeutic. Aspiration of crystalline material and subsequent microscopy, the diagnostic gold standard,[45] requires identification of a potential target area and retrieval of synovial fluid or extraarticular material. However, the location of crystal deposits cannot always be found based on clinical examination and radiography alone. Dry aspiration can be a frustrating experience for caregiver and patient. Ultrasonography can help localize crystal deposits and fluid collections, and sonographic visualization of the needle can improve accuracy and safety of the procedure. In particular, small joints

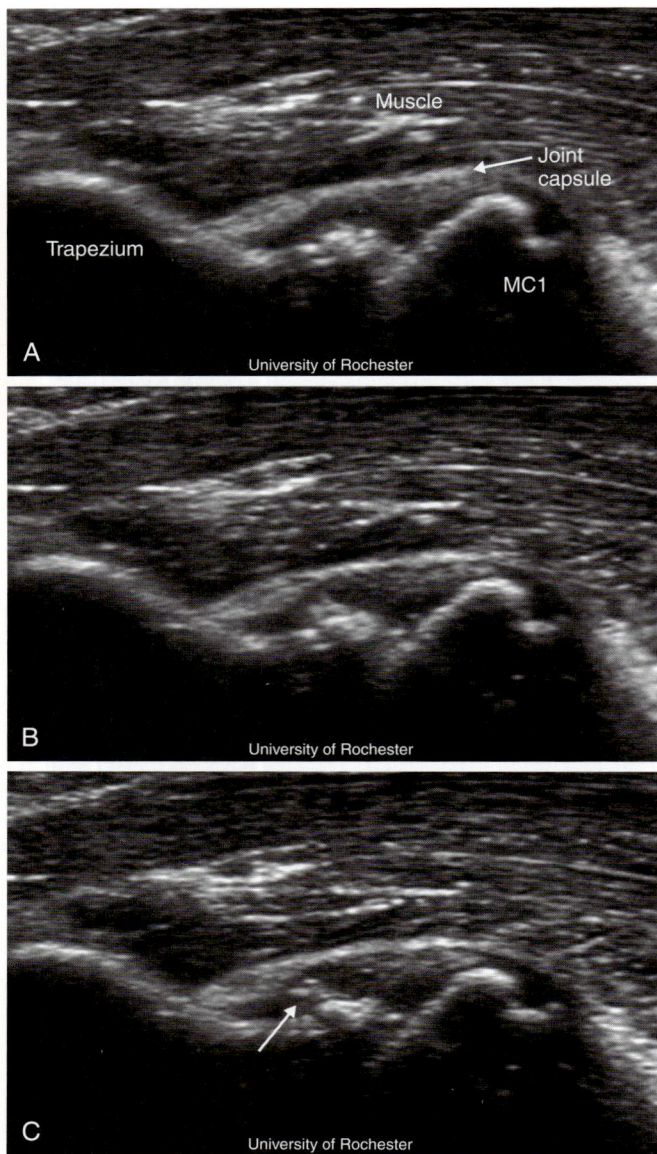

Figure 26-11 First Carpometacarpal joint (CMC1), volar long-axis view. Osteoarthritis. Dynamic examination. Ulnar adduction (**A**); neutral position (**B**) and radial abduction (**C**). Bony prominence is seen at base of metacarpal bone 1 (abbreviated MC1); and bony irregularity with calcification is seen at distal trapezium. Joint capsule changes shape from straight to more convex and distended in radial abduction. Hyperechoic, calcific material is expressed into joint recess with abduction (*arrow* in **C**).

of feet can be difficult to aspirate or inject with needle guidance based on clinical examination alone, even for experienced clinicians. Image guidance including fluoroscopy and sonography was found to drastically increase the yield of such aspirations.[46]

Treatment of Hydroxyapatite Crystal Deposition Disease

Removal of calcific concrements in the shoulder can decrease pain and improve activities of daily living. Ultrasound guided needle aspiration can help decrease the crystal burden. Once

concrements are localized, an approach can be planned. After local anesthesia, a needle attached to a syringe with normal saline can be inserted into the calcification, and a small amount of saline injected into the tophus. The increased intratophaceous pressure will lead to reflux of saline and hydroxyapatite (HA) crystals into the syringe. Active pull on the plunger should be avoided, as this will clog the lumen of the needle. Saline injection and passive reflux can be repeated several times, until a collapse of the HA deposit can be seen sonographically (Fig. 26-12).[47]

Ultrasound Assessment of Treatment Response in Gout

An objective measure of treatment response in gout is desirable. A decrease of the frequency or intensity of acute gout attacks is a working measure, but this provides no information about total body tophus burden, erosion formation with joint destruction and subclinical chronic inflammatory response with associated cardiovascular risk. Similarly, periodic measurement of serum urate is an indirect indicator of treatment response. Urate-lowering therapy (ULT) is intended to decrease the urate burden by lowering the serum urate level below the solubility threshold and facilitate resolution of tophi. This can be assessed objectively by applying external calipers if superficial tophi can be palpated, by performing serial MRI measurements of MSU deposits—if sufficient sensitivity can be achieved—or by serial ultrasonography.[48-50]

Ultrasound assessment of joints affected by gout can be performed at the point of care, in the provider's office, during a patient visit. This makes serial ultrasound assessment of a possible treatment response particularly practicable. Changes in tophus size can be measured and documented using sonographic calipers. Maintaining the same probe orientation is essential for comparison of measurements over time. MSU deposition on hyaline articular cartilage will disappear once normouricemia (serum urate less than 6 mg/dl) is achieved and maintained. Sonographically, disappearance of the double-contour sign of gout can be seen after maintaining serum urate levels of less than 6 mg/dl for 6 months or more.[50] Of interest for the patient will be a reduction of gout-associated acute or chronic inflammation. Gout-associated hyperemia can be assessed and scored using color Doppler or power Doppler ultrasound, and changes over time can be documented.[26]

Ultrasound of Crystal Arthritis in Perspective

Newer technologies need to be evaluated against the current gold standard. Documentation of intracellular crystals is diagnostic of crystal arthritis. However, synovial fluid aspiration and polarizing microscopy analysis of synovial fluid are infrequently performed, and treatment decisions are often based on an assumed diagnosis.[51] Joint aspiration requires technical skill and can be an operator-dependent procedure. In small joints of feet, even experienced operators place their needle correctly in less than 50% of joints if this is guided by clinical examination alone.[46,52] If fluid is obtained, how operator dependent is crystal identification

Table 26-4

	Echogenicity	Posterior Acoustic Shadow of Microtophi <1 mm	Posterior Acoustic Shadow of Larger Aggregates	Anechoic Halo	Preferential Deposition in Hyaline Cartilage	Radiographic Appearance
MSU	Hypoechoic to hyperechoic	No posterior acoustic shadow	Pronounced posterior acoustic shadow infrequent unless calcified	Common	Surface of hyaline cartilage	Radiolucent or poorly visible
CPPD	Hyperechoic	No posterior acoustic shadow	Posterior acoustic shadow of larger concrements	Uncommon	Central lacunes of hyaline cartilage	Visible
Apatite and other BCP crystals	Hyperechoic	No posterior acoustic shadow	Pronounced posterior acoustic shadow	Uncommon	No preference for hyaline cartilage	Visible

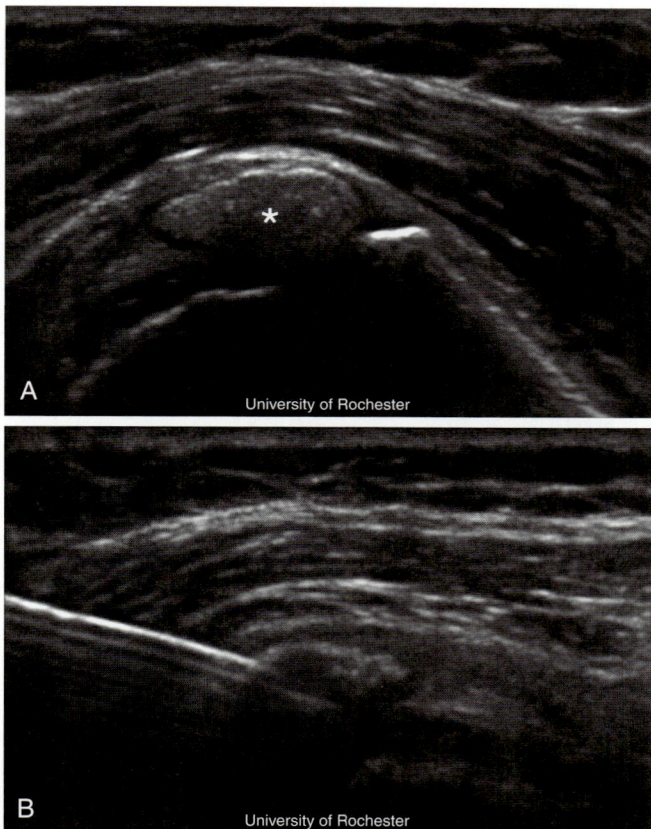

Figure 26-12 Shoulder. **A,** Hydroxyapatite crystal deposition disease. A large HA crystal macroaggregate is seen riding on the greater tubercle and dissecting the supraspinatus tendon. **B,** Same patient as in **A.** A hyperechoic needle is seen entering from left of image and perforating the tophus. Metallic reverberation artefacts are seen deep to needle.

in the laboratory? This is reviewed in Chapter 3, but this author's perspective is that correct identification of MSU crystals is achieved in 43% to 79% in the lab.[53-55] Sensitivities were found to range from 62.5% to 69%.[53,56] False-positive results were found in 24%[57] in some studies. Measurement of serum urate can be helpful, but some patients with acute gout may have normal levels of serum urate[58] (see Chapter 9).

In comparison, concordance between ultrasound readers determining the presence of MSU deposition in knee and toe joints was found to be very high, with agreements of 95% to 100% and kappa values of agreement of 0.942 to 1.000%.[20,59]

Ultrasound was found to be more sensitive in detecting MSU deposits than MRI and conventional radiography if high-frequency equipment was used and less sensitive than conventional radiography if frequencies of less than 10 MHz were used.[10,60]

Ultrasound detects CPPD crystal deposition in hyaline cartilage more readily than conventional radiography and MRI in those with CPPD deposition arthropathy.[61]

Similar to rheumatoid arthritis, ultrasound detects more erosions in feet affected by gout than conventional radiography, regardless if two or three radiographic views are used.[36,62]

Based on the available data, ultrasound assessment of crystal arthritis is less operator dependent than joint aspiration and microscopy and compares favorably to MRI and conventional radiography.

Editor's Note

Since this chapter went into production, a controlled ultrasonographic study of asymptomatic hyperuricemia (>7 mg/dl) versus normouricemia by Pineda et al[63] has been published, analyzing 50 consecutive patients (mean age ~55 years, predominantly male) recruited from rheumatology, nephrology, and cardiology clinics, with the control group being 52 subjects from healthy, normouricemic hospital staff and relatives (mean age ~47 years, predominantly male). Ultrasound findings were changes suggestive of articular gout (double contour sign in ~25%, articular tophi in ~15%, as well as soft tissue changes in the patellar tendon and Achilles tendon suggestive of gout) in the first metatarsophalangeal and knee joints and selected soft tissues of the leg, which were significantly more common than in the normouricemic control group. This controlled study warrants further and deeper corroboration and validation of the crystal deposition, but it does suggest the value of high-resolution ultrasound in discovering early subclinical gout. In this sense, the study points to the possibility of a novel and simple ultrasound approach to potential redefinition and reclassification of gout as a disease.

Author's Note

It is currently unknown whether corticosteroids, injected into a joint, would attach to hyaline cartilage and form an echogenic layer that could be mistaken for MSU deposition. Sonographically, injected crystalline suspensions of corticosteroids show buoyancy relative to synovial fluid and collect away from cartilaginous surfaces. Cartilage degeneration, such as in osteoarthritis, will not resemble a double contour sign, as the radial, or perpendicular, orientation of cartilage fissures will not create a hyperechoic layer over the surface of cartilage, as does MSU deposition. After flares of pseudogout, CPPD may conceivably escape into the synovial fluid and adhere to the surface of cartilage. Other sonographic evidence for CPPD, including deposition in central lacunes, can be helpful in this situation, along with radiographic demonstration of CPPD (MSU deposits would generally remain radiolucent). In the available sonographic studies of gout, aspiration had confirmed the presence of MSU crystals in patients with a double contour sign, and no CPPD was found.

References

1. Dalbeth N, McQueen FM. Use of imaging to evaluate gout and other crystal deposition disorders. Curr Opin Rheumatol 2009;21(2):124–31.
2. Perez-Ruiz F, Dalbeth N, Urresola A, et al. Imaging of gout: findings and utility. Arthritis Res Ther 2009;11(3):232.
3. Grassi W, Gutierrez M, Filippucci E. Crystal-associated synovitis. In: Wakefield RJ, D'Agostino MA, editors. Essential Applications of Musculoskeletal Ultrasound in Rheumatology. Philadelphia: Saunders Elsevier; 2010:187–97.
4. Thiele RG. Role of ultrasound and other advanced imaging in the diagnosis and management of gout. Curr Rheumatol Rep 2011.
5. Schlegel JU, Diggdon P, Cuellar J. The use of ultrasound for localizing renal calculi. J Urol 1961;86:367–9.
6. Garrod AB. The Nature and Treatment of Gout and Rheumatic Gout. London: Walton and Maberly; 1859.
7. Huber N. Zur Verwerthung der Röntgen-Strahlen im Gebiete der inneren Medicin. Dtsch Med Wochenschr 1896;22(12):182–4.
8. Tiliakos N, Morales AR, Wilson Jr CH. Use of ultrasound in identifying tophaceous versus rheumatoid nodules. Arthritis Rheum 1982;25(4):478–9.
9. Thiele R. Doppler ultrasonography in rheumatology: adding color to the picture. J Rheumatol 2008;35(1):8–10.
10. Carter JD, Kedar RP, Anderson SR, et al. An analysis of MRI and ultrasound imaging in patients with gout who have normal plain radiographs. Rheumatology (Oxford) 2009;48(11):1442–6.
11. Backhaus M, Burmester GR, Gerber T, et al. Guidelines for musculoskeletal ultrasound in rheumatology. Ann Rheum Dis 2001;60(7):641–9.
12. Wright SA, Filippucci E, McVeigh C, et al. High-resolution ultrasonography of the first metatarsal phalangeal joint in gout: a controlled study. Ann Rheum Dis 2007;66(7):859–64.
13. Koski JM. Ultrasonography of the metatarsophalangeal and talocrural joints. Clin Exp Rheumatol 1990;8(4):347–51.
14. Schmidt WA, Schmidt H, Schicke B, et al. Standard reference values for musculoskeletal ultrasonography. Ann Rheum Dis 2004;63(8):988–94.
15. Bjelle AO. Morphological study of articular cartilage in pyrophosphate arthropathy. (Chondrocalcinosis articularis or calcium pyrophosphate dihydrate crystal deposition diseases.) Ann Rheum Dis 1972;31(6):449–56.
16. Schumacher Jr HR. Pathology of crystal deposition diseases. Rheum Dis Clin North Am 1988;14(2):269–88.
17. Reginato AJ, Schumacher HR, Martinez VA. The articular cartilage in familial chondrocalcinosis. Light and electron microscopic study. Arthritis Rheum 1974;17(6):977–92.
18. Grassi W, Lamanna G, Farina A, et al. Sonographic imaging of normal and osteoarthritic cartilage. Semin Arthritis Rheum 1999;28(6):398–403.
19. Filippucci E, Riveros MG, Georgescu D, et al. Hyaline cartilage involvement in patients with gout and calcium pyrophosphate deposition disease. An ultrasound study. Osteoarthritis Cartilage 2009;17(2):178–81.
20. Thiele RG, Schlesinger N. Diagnosis of gout by ultrasound. Rheumatology (Oxford) 2007;46(7):1116–21.
21. Schmidt WA, Schicke B, Krause A. [Which ultrasound scan is the best to detect glenohumeral joint effusions?] Ultraschall Med 2008;29(Suppl. 5):250–5.
22. Thiele RG. Musculoskeletal joint interventions. In: Dogra VS, Saad WEA, editors. Ultrasound-Guided Procedures. New York: Thieme; 2010:229–43.
23. Bruyn GA, Naredo E, Moller I, et al. Reliability of ultrasonography in detecting shoulder disease in patients with rheumatoid arthritis. Ann Rheum Dis 2009;68(3):357–61.
24. Palmer DG, Hogg N, Denholm I, et al. Comparison of phenotype expression by mononuclear phagocytes within subcutaneous gouty tophi and rheumatoid nodules. Rheumatol Int 1987;7(5):187–93.
25. Dalbeth N, Pool B, Gamble GD, et al. Cellular characterization of the gouty tophus: a quantitative analysis. Arthritis Rheum 2010;62(5):1549–56.
26. Schlesinger N, Thiele RG. The pathogenesis of bone erosions in gouty arthritis. Ann Rheum Dis 2010;69(11):1907–12.
27. Thiele RG, Schlesinger N. Ultrasonography shows active inflammation in clinically unaffected joints in chronic tophaceous gout. Arthritis Rheum 2009;60(Suppl. 10) S1512.
28. De Avila Fernandes E, Kubota ES, et al. Ultrasound features of tophi in chronic tophaceous gout. Skeletal Radiol 2011;40(3):309–15.
29. McGill NW, Dieppe PA. The role of serum and synovial fluid components in the promotion of urate crystal formation. J Rheumatol 1991;18(7):1042–5.
30. Burt HM, Dutt YC. Growth of monosodium urate monohydrate crystals: effect of cartilage and synovial fluid components on in vitro growth rates. Ann Rheum Dis 1986;45(10):858–64.
31. Katz WA, Schubert M. The interaction of monosodium urate with connective tissue components. J Clin Invest 1970;49(10):1783–9.
32. Sokoloff L. The pathology of gout. Metabolism 1957;6(3):230–43.
33. Sokoloff L. Pathology of gout. Arthritis Rheum 1965;8(5):707–13.
34. Yu KH. Intraarticular tophi in a joint without a previous gouty attack. J Rheumatol 2003;30(8):1868–70.
35. Berquist TH. Foot, ankle and calf. In: Berquist TH, editor. Musculoskeletal Imaging Companion. 2nd ed. Philadelphia: Lippincott, Williams & Wilkins; 2007:308–437.
36. Schueller-Weidekamm C, Schueller G, Aringer M, et al. Impact of sonography in gouty arthritis: comparison with conventional radiography, clinical examination, and laboratory findings. Eur J Radiol 2007;62(3):437–43.
37. Thiele RG, Schlesinger N. Ultrasound detects more erosions in gout than conventional radiography. Arthritis Rheum 2010;62(Suppl 10):S368–9.
38. Wakefield RJ, Gibbon WW, Conaghan PG, et al. The value of sonography in the detection of bone erosions in patients with rheumatoid arthritis: a comparison with conventional radiography. Arthritis Rheum 2000;43(12):2762–70.
39. Weidekamm C, Koller M, Weber M, et al. Diagnostic value of high-resolution B-mode and doppler sonography for imaging of hand and finger joints in rheumatoid arthritis. Arthritis Rheum 2003;48(2):325–33.
40. Wakefield RJ, Kong KO, Conaghan PG, et al. The role of ultrasonography and magnetic resonance imaging in early rheumatoid arthritis. Clin Exp Rheumatol 2003;21(5 Suppl. 31):S42–9.
41. Wakefield RJ, Balint PV, Szkudlarek M, et al. Musculoskeletal ultrasound including definitions for ultrasonographic pathology. J Rheumatol 2005;32(12):2485–7.
42. Ptasznik R. Sonography of the shoulder. In: Van Holbeeck MT, Introcaso JH, editors. Musculoskeletal Ultrasound. 2nd ed. St. Louis: Mosby; 2001:463–516.
43. Thiele RG, Paxton LA, Marston BA, et al. Erosive osteoarthritis is not associated with invading synovial tissue: an ultrasound study. Arthritis Rheum 2010;62(10):S674.
44. Steinbach LS, Resnick D. Imaging of calcium pyrophosphate dihydrate (CPPD) crystal deposition disease. In: Smyth CJ, Holers VM, editors. Gout, Hyperuricemia, and Other Crystal-Associated Arthropathies. New York: Marcel Dekker, Inc; 1999:299–331.
45. McCarty DJ, Hollander JL. Identification of urate crystals in gouty synovial fluid. Ann Intern Med 1961;54:452–60.
46. Khosla S, Thiele R. Baumhauer JF. Ultrasound guidance for intra-articular injections of the foot and ankle. Foot Ankle Int 2009;30(9):886–90.
47. Jacobson JA. Fundamentals of Musculoskeletal Ultrasound. Philadelphia: Saunders Elsevier; 2007.
48. Schumacher Jr HR, Becker MA, Palo WA, et al. Tophaceous gout: quantitative evaluation by direct physical measurement. J Rheumatol 2005;32(12):2368–72.
49. Schumacher Jr HR, Becker MA, Edwards NL, et al. Magnetic resonance imaging in the quantitative assessment of gouty tophi. Int J Clin Pract 2006;60(4):408–14.
50. Thiele RG, Schlesinger N. Ultrasonography shows disappearance of monosodium urate crystal deposition on hyaline cartilage after sustained normouricemia is achieved. Rheumatol Int 2010;30(4):495–503.

51. Chen LX, Schumacher HR. Gout: can we create an evidence-based systematic approach to diagnosis and management? Best Pract Res Clin Rheumatol 2006;20(4):673–84.
52. Khosla S, Thiele RG, Baumhauer JF. Injection of foot and ankle joints: comparison of guidance by palpation, ultrasonography and fluoroscopy with anatomic dissection as gold standard. Arthritis Rheum 2008;58 (Suppl. 9):S408.
53. Schumacher Jr HR, Sieck MS, Rothfuss S, et al. Reproducibility of synovial fluid analyses. A study among four laboratories. Arthritis Rheum 1986;29(6):770–4.
54. Hasselbacher P. Variation in synovial fluid analysis by hospital laboratories. Arthritis Rheum 1987;30(6):637–42.
55. McGill NW, York HF. Reproducibility of synovial fluid examination for crystals. Aust N Z J Med 1991;21(5):710–3.
56. Gordon C, Swan A, Dieppe P. Detection of crystals in synovial fluids by light microscopy: sensitivity and reliability. Ann Rheum Dis 1989;48(9):737–42.
57. Von Essen R, Holtta AM. Quality control of the laboratory diagnosis of gout by synovial fluid microscopy. Scand J Rheumatol 1990;19(3):232–4.
58. Logan JA, Morrison E, McGill PE. Serum uric acid in acute gout. Ann Rheum Dis 1997;56(11):696–7.
59. Howard RG, Pillinger MH, Gyftopoulos S, et al. Reproducibility of musculoskeletal ultrasound for determining monosodium urate deposition: concordance between readers. Arthritis Care Res 2011 [Epub ahead of print].
60. Thiele RG, Anandarajah AP, Tabechian D, et al. Comparing ultrasonography, MRI, high-resolution CT and 3D rendering in patients with crystal proven gout. Ann Rheum Dis 2008;67(Suppl. II):248.
61. Thiele RG, Schlesinger N. Ultrasound detects calcium pyrophosphate dihydrate crystal deposition in hyaline cartilage more readily than conventional radiography and MRI in pyrophosphate arthropathy. Arthritis Rheum 2007;56(Suppl. 9):S1618.
62. Thiele RG, Schlesinger N. Ultrasound detects more erosions in gout than conventional radiography. Ann Rheum Dis 2010;69(Suppl. 3):612.
63. Pineda C, Amezcua-Guerra LM, Solano C, et al. Joint and tendon subclinical involvement suggestive of gouty arthritis in asymptomatic hyperuricemia: an ultrasound controlled study. Arthritis Res Ther 2011;13(1):R4:[Epub ahead of print.]

Epilogue: Creating a Better Future of Diagnosis and Treatment of Gout and Other Crystal Arthropathies

Robert Terkeltaub

Introduction

This textbook has thoroughly covered the current status of gout clinical practice, a subject whose nuances, with respect to evidence-based medicine, have been succinctly addressed in some major, recent reviews.[1,2] This chapter focuses on the future of the diagnosis and treatment of gout.

It is often said, in many different ways, both that predictions are difficult, and that the best way to predict the future is to take an active part in creating it. As such, it is with trepidation, in early 2011, that I present my own brief treatise, thereby concluding this textbook with both prognostication and a call to arms.

Creating a Better Future of Gout Treatment

Better Use of Imaging, Biomarkers, and Quality of Life (QOL) Instruments

Further Development and Application of Imaging Modalities in Gout

Table 27-1 summarizes a proposed action plan for the field of gout, based on the foundation of clinical and translational knowledge put forward in this textbook. We are poised to redefine gout as a disease by earlier diagnosis, including in asymptomatic hyperuricemia, using inexpensive, and increasingly available, high-resolution ultrasound, and well as the dual-energy computed tomography (DECT) approach. These imaging tools also will help in better monitoring outcomes (as opposed to tracking serum urate and gouty arthritis) by visualizing tophus shrinkage and resolution. Further, these imaging approaches, especially refinement of the highly specific DECT application, could ultimately lead to better understanding of

Supported by the VA Research Service.

the range of tissues affected by subclinical tophi at different stages of the disease. For example, we may learn that gouty nephropathy is far more common in this era than currently appreciated. DECT and perhaps other advanced imaging approaches could unlock some of the mysteries that surround the linkage of hyperuricemia and cardiovascular disease.

Monosodium Urate Crystal Macroaggregates at the Articular Surface in Diagnosis and Clinical Decision Making

At several junctures in this book (see Chapters 1, 5, and 26) there has been discussion of the likely importance in gout, including both in diagnosis and attacks of arthritis, of changes in monosodium urate (MSU) crystal deposition at the articular cartilage surface. This clinical-pathological aspect of gout has been under-recognized in recent years. How the sentinel high resolution ultrasound finding in gout of the cartilage surface MSU crystal deposition "double contour sign" impacts on clinical decision making will be critical. Major questions will include whether how often the ultrasound can replace arthrocentesis and synovial fluid crystal analysis for diagnosis in the setting of acute gout. In addition, it is not clear whether the macroaggregates of MSU crystals in cartilage detected by ultrasound have the same implications for initiating pharmacologic urate-lowering therapy as the absolute indication of the finding of bursal, articular, and subcutaneous tophi, as well as tophi detected by erosion on plain radiography. The same questions will hold for DECT.

Biomarkers

Better monitoring of outcomes in gout, and achievement of improved outcomes, should benefit by wider application of advanced quality of life instruments, as reviewed in Chapter 18. Furthermore, better biomarkers in gout than serum urate—C-reactive protein and possibly markers of urate oxidation

Table 27-1 **Keys to Better Future Treatment of Gout**
• Better use of imaging, biomarkers, quality of life (QOL) instruments • Identify and validate new drug targets • Exploit drug combinations • Develop treatment guidelines (beyond EULAR) • Define cost-effectiveness, ideal treatment targets • Better educate patients, physicians for improved adherence and quality of care • Better personalize treatment, possibly including use of gene chip technology targeted for therapy of gout • *Prospectively* decode cardiovascular and renal disease connections of gout and hyperuricemia

Table 27-2 **Examples of New Targets in Gout**
ANTIINFLAMMATORY THERAPY
• Process of tophus deposition • Chemokines such as IL-8 and monocyte chemoattractant chemokines • C5b-9 • TLR2, free fatty acids • Caspase-1 • Mast cell and neutrophil proteases that stimulate endoproteolytic conversion of pro-IL-1β to an active, mature form
URATE-LOWERING THERAPY (ULT)
• Molecularly designed, selective inhibitors of renal urate transporters • Purine nucleoside phosphorylase (PNP) inhibition

Table 27-3 **Potential New Gout Treatments Currently in Clinical Trials**
>100 Ongoing or Completed Clinical Trials in Gout, partially listed on clinicaltrials.gov Phase I to phase III examples: • IL-1 inhibition (prophylaxis and flare therapy): rilonacept, canakinumab • Apremilast (phosphodiesterase PDE4: TNFα, IL-8 are among targets) • Celecoxib • Uricosuric: RDEA594 and others (alone, but more often combined with xanthine oxidase inhibition [XOI]) • PNP inhibition: BCX-4208 (combined with XOI) • Recombinant uricase: pegsitacase

Table 27-4 **Uricosurics and Xanthine Oxidase Inhibitors (XOIs)**

A Fundamental Synergy in Urate-Lowering Therapy (ULT)
XOIs Lower Absolute Amount of Urinary Uric Acid Excretion:
    Decreased risk of uricosuric-induced urolithiasis
    Narrowed route for decreasing body urate stores
    Add-on uricosuric improves ULT if:
Renal function adequate for uricosuric to work
Uricosuric does not markedly increase XOI drug excretion in urine
Uricosuria balanced with XOI lessens risk of urolithiasis (especially in uric acid overproducers)

such as a allantoin, for example—should allow for improved estimation of body urate load and ongoing inflammation specific to gout. A simple test to accurately estimate total body urate stores would be particularly helpful. To date, the isotope-based techniques developed to estimate total body urate burden have not proven applicable on a wide scale for clinical practice.

Identify and Validate New Targets, and Exploit Drug Combinations

Table 27-2 summarizes some novel treatment targets for gouty inflammation and hyperuricemia, and Table 27-3 lists some of the recent and current Food and Drug Administration (FDA)–registered clinical trials in gout. Many of these targets and clinical trials programs have been discussed in detail in this book, including in Chapters 3 through 5, 10, 12, 15, and 16. A prime example is the promising approach of IL-1β inhibition for gouty inflammation.

Other potential targets for advanced therapeutics to improve management of gouty arthritis include the process of tophus deposition itself, which likely involve both inflammation and urate transport, and may involve regulation by adaptive immunity (see Chapter 5). Novel targets for gout arthritis prophylaxis and treatment, also reviewed in Chapter 5, could emerge from knowledge of the effects in experimental MSU crystal inflammation of chemokines such as interleukin (IL)-8 and MCP-1. Other targets include mast cell activation (including release of chymase), and other mechanisms (such as neutrophil elastase and proteinase 3 [PR3] release) that provide alternatives and complementation to caspase-1 for endoproteolytic conversion of pro-IL-1β to an active, mature form. Activation of C5 and assembly of the C5b-9 membrane attack complex of complement, and specific innate immune effects of TLR2 activation via free fatty acids also could be exploited in future therapies.

Combined Xanthine Oxidase Inhibitor and Uricosuric Therapy

An attractive, fundamentally synergistic (Table 27-4), and increasingly applied approach to combination therapy of hyperuricemia is to use combined xanthine oxidase inhibitor (XOI) and uricosuric therapy. The rationale is robust, since XOI therapy reduces urinary uric acid excretion, and thereby limits the major, natural pathway for reduction of total body urate stores. This neglected strategy, actually dating back decades ago for severe, tophaceous gout, is receiving particularly active clinical investigation after and even used in milder cases of tophaceous gout in the 1960s and early 1970s, being "rediscovered" via preliminary, supportive findings employing submaximal probenecid with submaximal allopurinol.[3] Such an approach can significantly increase the proportion of subjects with gout achieving a serum urate target of less than 6 mg/dl, relative to XOI treatment alone. One limitation of the approach is that probenecid increases oxypurinol clearance, and this sort of drug–drug interaction, although surmountable, needs to be considered and addressed.

There is strong impetus now, based on the remarkable, accelerated tophus resolution seen in responders to pegloticase (see Chapter 14) to bring the serum rate down to the 1 to 3 mg/dl range in subjects with severe, chronic tophaceous gouty arthritis, until tophi are resolved. With pegloticase responders, this combined, sustained serum urate-lowering and tophus resolution outcome typically occurs in months to a year. It is hoped that combined XOI and uricosuric therapy could also achieve such dramatic responses of gout to therapy, analogous to the desired American College of Rheumatology 70 (ACR70) outcome score in biologic therapy in rheumatoid arthritis. We still do need to understand if there are unrecognized short- and long-term safty consequences (e.g., neurologic) of profound serum urate lowering to the 0 to 2mg/dL.

Preliminary studies with the uricosuric RDEA594 and febuxostat indicated the capacity to bring the serum down to about 3 mg/dl, without use of potentially dose maximal regimens. Cost, convenience, and potentially safety advantages of such combined oral medication regimens, relative to recombinant uricase regimens, will be offset in patient subsets by delays in response or inadequate response, the latter particularly the case with significant renal impairment. However, combined XOI and uricosuric therapy will not obviate the utility of recombinant uricase therapy for refractory gout. In this light, the clinical development of less immunogenic formulations of uricase should increase management options in gout.

Targeting of PNP for Hyperuricemia in Gout Patients

PNP inhibition is at the proof of concept stage, using BXC4208, which is being evaluated as a combination therapy with XOI for urate-lowering therapy (ULT) in refractory disease. As reviewed in Chapter 3, PNP catalyzes conversion of guanosine to guanine, and of inosine to hypoxanthine. Inherited PNP deficiency is associated with marked hypouricemia, but also associated with severe immunodeficiency mediated by cytotoxic effects on T cells (and likely other lymphocyte subsets) of certain accumulated deoxypurine nucleotides. Hence, the challenge of developing PNP inhibitor therapy of hyperuricemia for gout will be to discover and exploit drug combinations of PNP inhibitors and XOI inhibitors that are additive and potentially synergistic, and also safe for clinical use.

Gout Diagnosis and Treatment Guidelines, Effectiveness of Care

EULAR has published helpful diagnostic and treatment guidelines for gout,[3,4] but other methodologies will be useful to employ, and such guidelines need updating following recent FDA approvals (e.g., low-dose colchicine for early acute gout in 2009, febuxostat in 2009, pegloticase in 2010). Drs. John Fitzgerald, Dinesh, and Puja Khanna and myself as Principal Investigators, with an international panel of multidisciplinary experts, are currently working on the process involved in crafting of the first American College of Rheumatology Treatment Guidelines for Gout. Treatment targets will be one of the major subjects reviewed in this process.

Cost-effectiveness of therapy in gout is an enormous issue,[5,6] and wedded into any consideration of quality of care (see Chapter 17). In most countries, a huge dilemma is the cost difference between allopurinol and febuxostat, weighed against the risks of severe forms of allopurinol hypersensitivity (see Chapter 13). This issue is just beginning to be

Personalized medicine: Concept of "gout section" of DNA chips

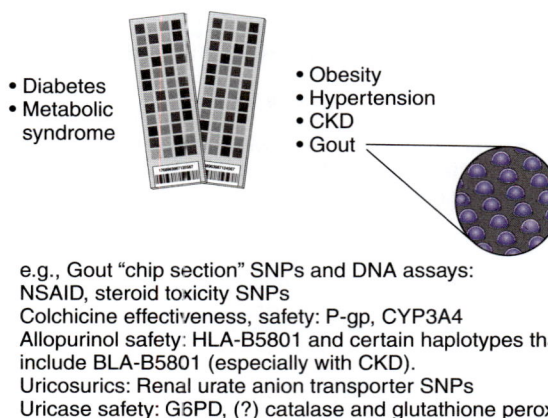

- Diabetes
- Metabolic syndrome

- Obesity
- Hypertension
- CKD
- Gout

e.g., Gout "chip section" SNPs and DNA assays:
NSAID, steroid toxicity SNPs
Colchicine effectiveness, safety: P-gp, CYP3A4
Allopurinol safety: HLA-B5801 and certain haplotypes that include BLA-B5801 (especially with CKD).
Uricosurics: Renal urate anion transporter SNPs
Uricase safety: G6PD, (?) catalase and glutathione peroxidase

Figure 27-1 Futuristic concept for personalization of care in gout: paradigm for a "gout gene chip" section in a "neighborhood" within chips designed for treatment of various metabolic and vascular diseases. In this model, relevant information to help screen for mechanisms of hyperuricemia (renal urate anion transporter single nucleotide polymorphisms [SNPs]), risks of specific drug toxicities (e.g., allopurinol hypersensitivity, hemolysis with uricases), and likelihood of drug efficacy with individual agents would be arrayed on the chips.

addressed on a cost-effectiveness level.[6] With the arrival of relatively costly biologic therapies for gout (IL-1 inhibitors and uricases), there will be much additional work to do. Quality of life in gout, and what metrics that best assess this (see Chapter 18), will also require substantial further consideration, since the disease subsets and stages that merit advanced biologic therapies in gout are just beginning to be defined. Advances in personalization of treatment in gout would help to sort out these questions. Figure 27-1 presents a paradigm for how a "gout section" on "gene chip" sets for specific single nucleotide polymorphisms (SNPs) and other pertinent genetic information for gout, and metabolic and vascular diseases, could help to prevent drug toxicity and assist in choosing appropriate therapy.

Critical Role of Patient Adherence

Ultimately, it is the patient that ensures success of treatment in gout via adherence with optimal medical recommendations. Gout patients are far less adherent than those with many other medical conditions, and this is especially so for younger patients with fewer office visits.[8-10] This huge issue is indicative of systematic failure of both patient education and physician education.[11] There are enormous myths and misunderstandings about gout that are clung to by many patients with the condition.[8] Patients need better understanding of the causes of gout, and of rationale in different diet and lifestyle modifications and therapies that have been discussed extensively in this book. Patients need to get on board, and stay on board, with the diagnostic and therapeutic measures, since better outcomes are linked with better management of expectations (including gout attacks in early ULT) and understanding long-term treatment objectives. Emerging strategies for improved communication between physician and patient are part of the solution.[11,12]

Prospectively Decoding the Cardiovascular and Renal Disease Connections of Gout and Hyperuricemia

Chapter 19 reviewed some of the antioxidant effects of uric acid, but also how uric acid promotes decrease of the vasodilator nitric oxide. We also increasingly recognize that urate can increase oxidative stress and damage, including within intracellular and extracellular compartments, and it can inhibit the function of enzymes sensitive to oxidative stress.[13] The peroxide-dependent oxidation (independent of uricase) by myeloperoxidase (MPO) of uric acid to 5-hydroxyisourate[13] may be a missing link in the association of hyperuricemia with vascular diseases such as hypertension and atherosclerosis, and possibly of release of uric acid by necrotic cells with immune and inflammatory consequences reviewed in Chapter 5. MPO is abundant in neutrophils, catalyzes production of hypochlorous acid from hydrogen peroxide and chloride, and is a peroxidase, and MPO attaches to the endothelium (reviewed by Meotti et al.[13]). Involvement of MPO in consuming nitric oxide, and promoting endothelial dysfunction and promoting foam cell formation while impairing reverse cholesterol transport and atherosclerotic plaque stability, can be coupled with circulating MPO as a risk factor for coronary artery disease (CAD) (and mortality from CAD) into an attractive paradigm for further investigation of vascular effects linked to asymptomatic hyperuricemia.[13] Given that uricases generate 5-hydroxyisourate (and hydrogen peroxide) (see Chapter 14), and that 5-hydroxyisourate itself, within hepatocytes, can exert effects on liver biology and carcinogenesis,[6] further attention to potential pro-oxidative consequences of uricase therapy also is warranted. However, under most circumstances, the antioxidant capacity of whole blood has been suggested to be sufficient to buffer out oxidant effects of uricase, which is delivered in plasma in therapy,[14] as opposed to uricase residing in hepatic peroxisomes in lower species.

Toward Advances in Diseases of Basic Calcium Phosphate (BCP) Crystal Deposition and in Calcium Pyrophosphate Dihydrate (CPPD) Crystal Deposition Disease

Resolution of the role BCP crystals could play in progression of OA is the major need going forward for this form of pathologic calcification. Standardization of detection methods, in the clinic, for articular BCP crystal deposition not visible by plain radiographs, will be valuable. Recent EULAR guidelines endorse high resolution ultrasound as a sensitive diagnostic approach for CPPD crystal deposition disease.[15] Therapy of arthritis of CPPD deposition disease remains largely empiric, and borrows heavily from management of gout, in particular. There is a pressing need for focused clinical trials of therapeutics for different phenotypes of CPPD arthropathies. The future will likely see IL-1 inhibition therapy merit a place in management, as one example. As evident from the reviews of Chapters 19 and 20, therapy of arthritis in CPPD crystal deposition lacks the proven equivalent of urate lowering drug therapy that can decrease tissue PP_i levels and inhibit CPPD crystal deposition. Sources of such treatments to address disordered chondrocyte PP_i metabolism may come not only from molecular drug designs attuned to PP_i generation, degradation, and transport, but also from chondrocyte signaling and differentiation-targeted therapies, perhaps borrowed in part from osteoarthritis chondroprotective agents.

Editor's Note

As cited in the Editor's Note at the end of Chapter 26, since this chapter went into production a controlled ultrasonographic study of lower extremity tissues in asymptomatic hyperuricemia (>7 mg/dl) versus normouricemia by Pineda et al[16] has been published that revealed ultrasound changes in a large proportion of those with asymptomatic hyperuricemia (including the double contour sign in ~25% and articular tophi in ~15%), hence, the potential value of high-resolution ultrasound in identifying early subclinical gout. This may provide the most accessible methodology for impetus to redefinition and reclassification of gout as a disease.

Editor's Note

As reviewed in Chapter 13, the increasingly recognized value of pharmacogenomics has further emerged in publications since this book went into productionY-19. The identification of HLA-B5801 and specific haplotypes that include HLA-B5801 as being highly associated with severe allopurinol hypersensitivity has the potential to be productively applied a priori in high-risk populations (such as stage 3-5 CKD and in Asians) to help prevent clinically devastating drug reactions to allopurinol. The cost of such pharmacogenomic screening, 20 in the Editor's opinion, will likely be proven to be inexpensive relative to the cost-effectiveness of limiting the incidence of severe forms of toxicity to allopurinol.

References

1. Neogi T. Gout. N Engl J Med 2011;364(5):443–52.
2. Terkeltaub R. Update on gout: new therapeutic strategies and options. Nat Rev Rheumatol 2010;6(1):30–8.
3. Reinders MK, van Roon EN, Houtman PM, et al. Biochemical effectiveness of allopurinol and allopurinol-probenecid in previously benzbromarone-treated gout patients. Clin Rheumatol 2007;26(9):1459–65.
4. Zhang W, Doherty M, Bardin T, et al. EULAR Standing Committee for International Clinical Studies Including Therapeutics. EULAR evidence based recommendations for gout. Part II: Management. Report of a task force of the EULAR Standing Committee for International Clinical Studies Including Therapeutics (ESCISIT). Ann Rheum Dis 2006;65(10):1312–24.
5. Zhang W, Doherty M, Pascual E, et al. EULAR Standing Committee for International Clinical Studies Including Therapeutics. EULAR evidence based recommendations for gout. Part I: Diagnosis. Report of a task force of the Standing Committee for International Clinical Studies Including Therapeutics (ESCISIT). Ann Rheum Dis 2006;65(10):1301–11.
6. Stevenson M, Pandor A. Febuxostat for the management of hyperuricaemia in patients with gout: a NICE single technology appraisal. Pharmacoeconomics 2010 Dec 14. doi: 10.2165/11535770-0. [Epub ahead of print]
7. Cattermole GN, Man CY, Cheng CH, et al. Oral prednisolone is more cost-effective than oral indomethacin for treating patients with acute gout-like arthritis. Eur J Emerg Med 2009;16(5):261–6.
8. Harrold LR, Mazor KM, Velten S, et al. Patients and providers view gout differently: a qualitative study. Chronic Illn 2010;6(4):263–71.
9. Wall GC, Koenigsfeld CF, Hegge KA, et al. Adherence to treatment guidelines in two primary care populations with gout. Rheumatol Int 2010;30(6):749–53.
10. Harrold LR, Andrade SE, Briesacher BA, et al. Adherence with urate-lowering therapies for the treatment of gout. Arthritis Res Ther 2009;11(2):R46.

11. Singh JA, Hodges JS, Asch SM. Opportunities for improving medication use and monitoring in gout. Ann Rheum Dis 2009;68(8):1265–70.

12. Doghramji PP, Edwards NL, McTigue J. Managing gout in the primary care setting: what you and your patients need to know. Am J Med 2010;123(8):S2.

13. Meotti FC, Jameson GN, Turner R, et al. Urate as a physiological substrate for myeloperoxidase: implications for hyperuricemia and inflammation. J Biol Chem 2011 Jan 25. [Epub ahead of print]

14. Hershfield MS, Roberts 2nd LJ, Ganson NJ, et al. Treating gout with pegloticase, a PEGylated urate oxidase, provides insight into the importance of uric acid as an antioxidant in vivo. Proc Natl Acad Sci U S A 2010 Aug 10;107(32):14351–6.

15. Zhang W, Doherty M, Bardin T, et al. European League Against Rheumatism recommendations for calcium pyrophosphate deposition. Part I: terminology and diagnosis. Ann Rheum Dis 2011 Jan 7. [Epub ahead of print]

16. Pineda C, Amezcua-Guerra LM, Solano C, et al. Joint and tendon subclinical involvement suggestive of gouty arthritis in asymptomatic hyperuricemia: an ultrasound controlled study. Arthritis Res Ther 2011;13(1):R4. [Epub ahead of print]

17. Cristallo AF, Schroeder J, Citterio A, et al. A study of HLA class I and class II 4-digit allele level in Stevens-Johnson syndrome and toxic epidermal necrolysis. Int J Immunogenet 2011 May 4. doi: 10.1111/j.1744-313x.2011.01011.x. (Epub ahead of print.).

18. Kostenko L, Kjer-Nielsen L, Nicholson I, et al. Rapid screening for the detection of HLA-B57 and HLA-858 in prevention of drug hypersensitivity. Tissue Antigens 2011;78(1):11-20:doi:10.1111/j.1399-0039.2011.01649.x. (Epub 2011 Apr 19.).

19. Jung JW, Song WJ, Kim YS, et al. HLA-B58 can help the clinical decision on starting allopurinol.

Index

Page numbers followed by *t* and *f* indicate tables and figures respectively.